Mosby's
Comprehensive review of
CRITICAL CARE

Mosby's
Comprehensive review of
CRITICAL CARE

Edited by

DONNA A. ZSCHOCHE, R.N., M.A.

Education Director,
National Critical Care Institute of Education,
Orange, California

SECOND EDITION

with 334 illustrations

The C. V. Mosby Company

ST. LOUIS • TORONTO • LONDON   1981

SECOND EDITION

Copyright © 1981 by The C. V. Mosby Company

Previous edition copyrighted 1976

Printed in the United States of America

The C. V. Mosby Company
11830 Westline Industrial Drive, St. Louis, Missouri 63141

Library of Congress Cataloging in Publication Data

Main entry under title:

Mosby's comprehensive review of critical care.

    Includes bibliographies and index.
    1. Critical care medicine. I. Zschoche, Donna A.
II. Title: Comprehensive review of critical care.
[DNLM: 1. Critical care. 2. Emergency medical ser-
vices. 3. Intensive care units. WX218 M894]
RC86.7.M66 1980   616'.028   80-16790
ISBN 0-8016-5697-4

GW/CB/B 9 8 7 6 5 4 3 2 1   03/C/318

Contributors

BRUCE M. ACHAUER, M.D.

Assistant Professor, Division of Plastic Surgery,
University of California Irvine Medical Center,
Orange, California

PATRICIA ALLYN, R.N.

Head Nurse, Burn Center, University of
California Irvine Medical Center,
Orange, California

BERNHARD G. ANDERSON, M.D.

Assistant Professor of Medicine,
Boston University Medical Center,
University Hospital, Boston, Massachusetts

ROBERT BARTLETT, M.D.

Professor of Surgery,
University of California Irvine Medical Center,
Orange, California

THEODORE B. BERNDT, M.D.

Consultant in Cardiology, Washoe County
Medical Center, Reno, Nevada

GEORGE L. BLACKBURN, M.D., Ph.D.

Associate Professor of Surgery,
Harvard Medical School;
Director, Nutrition Support Service,
New England Deaconess Hospital,
Boston, Massachusetts

DAVID R. BOYD, M.D.

Director, Emergency Medical Services,
Department of Health and Human Services,
Washington, D.C.

REBECCA SCHMEECKLE BROWN, M.S.

Coordinator, Infant Follow-Up Project,
Division of Developmental Disabilities
and Clinical Genetics, UAP;
Department of Pediatrics, University
of California Irvine Medical Center,
Orange, California

MARGARET CALDWELL, R.N., M.S.

Director of Nursing,
Tahoe Forest Hospital,
Truckee, California

JACK COPELAND, M.D.

Associate Professor and Chief,
Section Cardiothoracic Surgery,
University of Arizona Health Sciences Center,
Tucson, Arizona

EARLE DAVIS, Ph.D.

Professor, Basic Science Department,
Southern California College of Optometry,
Fullerton, California;
Lecturer, Department of Anatomy,
University of California, Irvine,
California College of Medicine,
Irvine, California

BERTRAM F. FELSHER, M.D.

Chief of Hepatology, Veteran's Administration
Hospital, Long Beach, California;
Associate Professor of Medicine,
University of California, Irvine,
California College of Medicine,
Irvine, California

THOMAS J. FOGARTY, M.D.

Cardiovascular Surgery, Sequoia Hospital
District, Redwood City, California

KAREN LEE FONTAINE, R.N., M.S.N.

Level Chairperson, Evangelical
School of Nursing, Oak Lawn, Illinois;
Private Practice, Sexual Dysfunction Therapy,
Chicago, Illinois

RAYMOND A. FONTAINE, M.Div., M.A.

Pastor, Golgotha Lutheran Church,
Chicago, Illinois; Private Practice, Sexual
Dysfunction Therapy, Chicago, Illinois

HARRY FRIEDMAN, M.D.

Private Practice, Neurosurgeon;
Instructor, Division of Neurosurgery,
University of Tennessee Health Sciences Center,
Memphis, Tennessee

DAVID W. FURNAS, M.D.

Chief, Plastic Surgery, Professor of Surgery,
Division of Plastic Surgery,
University of California Irvine Medical Center,
Orange, California

VIRGINIA L. GAMBLE, R.N., B.S.N.

Health Facilitator, Healthworks, Inc.,
South Laguna, California;
Nursing Instructor, Golden West College,
Huntington Beach, California

D. E. GENTILE, M.D.

Clinical Professor of Medicine,
University of California, Irvine,
California College of Medicine, Irvine, California;
St. Joseph Hospital Renal Center,
Orange, California

FREDERICK L. GLAUSER, M.D.

Chief, Pulmonary Division,
Medical College of Virginia,
Virginia Commonwealth University,
Richmond, Virginia

DONALD C. HARRISON, M.D.

William G. Irvin Professor and Chief of
Cardiology, Cardiology Division,
Stanford University School of Medicine,
Stanford, California

JOYCE R. HOSTETLER, R.N., M.S.N.

Kidney Transplant Coordinator,
Department of Surgery/Division of Urology,
University of California Irvine Medical Center,
Orange, California

ROBERT F. HUXTABLE, M.D.

Professor of Pediatrics, Director of
Pediatric Perinatal Medicine,
University of California, Irvine,
California College of Medicine,
Irvine, California

ROBERT E. INGHAM, M.D.

Assistant Clinical Professor,
Internal Medicine, University
of California, Davis;
Chairman, Department of Cardiology,
Non-Invasive Division,
John Muir Memorial Hospital,
Walnut Creek, California

MELODY JACOBSON, M.S.

Lecturer-Coordinator, High Risk
Infant Follow-Up Program,
Division of Pediatric Perinatal Medicine,
Department of Pediatrics,
University of California, Irvine,
California College of Medicine,
Irvine, California

STANLEY M. KEGEL, M.D.

Assistant Clinical Professor of
Pediatrics (Cardiology),
University of California,
Los Angeles, California;
Chairman, Department of Cardiology,
Children's Hospital of Orange County,
Orange, California

†WILLIAM F. KIELY, M.D.

Professor of Clinical Psychiatry and
Clinical Medicine, Department of Psychiatry,
University of Southern California
School of Medicine,
Los Angeles, California

RICHARD C. LILLEHEI, M.D., Ph.D.

Professor, Department of Surgery,
University of Minnesota Hospitals,
Minneapolis, Minnesota

G. MADANI, M.D.

Neonatology Fellow, University of
California Irvine Medical Center,
Orange, California

PROFESSOR DR. CHESTER B. MARTIN

Department of Obstetrics and Gynecology,
St. Radborrd Hospital;
Catholic University, Nijmegen,
The Netherlands

DONALD C. MARTIN, M.D.

Chief, Urology, Professor of Surgery,
University of California Irvine Medical Center,
Orange, California; Consultant,
Veteran's Administration Hospital,
Long Beach, California

IRENE MATOUSEK, R.N., M.S.

Assistant Professor, School of Nursing,
University of Minnesota,
Minneapolis, Minnesota

DENNIS L. MING, Pharm.D.

Assistant Director of Pharmaceutical Services,
Department of Pharmaceutical Services,
University of California Irvine Medical Center,
Orange, California; Assistant Clinical Professor,
Division of Clinical Pharmacy,
School of Pharmacy, University of California,
San Francisco, California

†Deceased.

K. S. MIRAHMADI, M.D.

Acting Chief of Nephrology Section,
Veteran's Administration Hospital,
Long Beach, California

ORHAN MUREN, M.D.

Professor of Medicine, Coordinator,
Respiratory Therapy Department,
Medical College of Virginia,
Virginia Commonwealth University,
Richmond, Virginia

ARLENE La BAW NICCOLI, R.N., B.S.

Senior Instructor, Department of
Physical Medicine and Rehabilitation;
Clinical Director, Rehabilitation
Research and Training Center,
Department of Medicine, University
of Colorado Health Sciences Center,
Denver, Colorado

MARY C. PEDUZI, R.N., M.S.N.

Assistant Clinical Professor,
Division of Pediatric Perinatal Medicine;
Coordinator, Nurse Education,
Department of Pediatrics,
University of California, Irvine,
California College of Medicine,
Irvine, California

THOMAS A. PRESTON, M.D.

Associate Professor of Medicine,
University of Washington School of Medicine;
Co-Director, Cardiology Service,
U.S. Public Health Service Hospital,
Seattle, Washington

ALLAN PRIBBLE, M.D.

Chief, Department of Cardiology,
Kaiser Foundation Hospital; Associate
Professor of Medicine, University of Hawaii,
Honolulu, Hawaii

WARREN R. PROCCI, M.D.

Assistant Professor of Psychiatry,
Department of Psychiatry, University of
Southern California School of Medicine,
Los Angeles, California

LORA B. ROACH, R.N., M.S.N.

Associate Professor, University
of Texas at Arlington, School of Nursing,
Arlington, Texas

MARY ANNE ROBINSON, R.N.

Head Nurse, Hemodialysis Unit,
University of California Irvine Medical Center,
Orange, California

TERESA L. ROMANO, R.N.

Director, Medical Systems Development,
Chicago, Illinois

ELLEN BEAM RUDY, R.N., Ph.D.

Associate Professor, School of Nursing,
Kent State University, Kent, Ohio

ARTHUR H. SALIBIAN, M.D.

Assistant Professor, Division of Plastic Surgery,
University of California Irvine Medical Center,
Orange, California

LOUIS SCHWARTZ, R.N., M.N.

Assistant Professor, Department of Nursing,
California State University,
Long Beach, California

STEPHEN R. SEVERANCE, M.D.

Department of Gastroenterology, Long Beach
Memorial Hospital, Long Beach, California

CLAYTON H. SHATNEY, M.D.

Chief, Surgery and Traumatology, Maryland
Institute for Emergency Medical Services;
Assistant Professor of Surgery, Department of
Surgery, University of Maryland Hospital,
Baltimore, Maryland

PERRY M. SHOOR, M.D.

Cardiovascular Surgery,
Sequoia Hospital District,
Redwood City, California

MELVILLE I. SINGER, M.D.

Associate Clinical Professor of Pediatrics
(Cardiology), University of California,
Los Angeles, California;
Cardiologist, Children's Hospital
of Orange County,
Orange, California

WILLIAM RICHARD SMITH, M.D.

Cardiologist, Doctors Hospital,
Modesto, California;
Clinical Associate Professor of Medicine,
University of California, Irvine,
California College of Medicine,
Irvine, California

PAUL E. STANLEY, Ph.D.

Professor Emeritus, Engineering,
Purdue University,
West Lafayette, Indiana

**ROBERT A. STEEDMAN, M.D.,
F.A.C.S.**

Associate Clinical Professor of Surgery,
University of California, Irvine,
California College of Medicine,
Irvine, California;
Chairman, Thoracic and Cardiovascular Surgery,
Santa Ana–Tustin Community Hospital,
Santa Ana, California

JAMES R. STEWART

Chief Diving Officer, Scripps
Institute of Oceanography,
La Jolla, California

PAUL A. THORNTON, Ph.D.

Professor and Department Head,
Department of Clinical Nutrition,
University of Kentucky Medical School,
Lexington, Kentucky

MARY JO TIERNEY, R.N., M.S.

Clinical Specialist, Sequoia Hospital District,
Redwood City, California

JAMES F. TOOLE, M.D.

Chairman, Department of Neurology,
Bowman Gray School of Medicine,
Wake Forest University,
Winston-Salem, North Carolina

N. D. VAZIRI, M.D., F.A.C.P.

Associate Professor of Medicine;
Chief, Division of Nephrology,
University of California Irvine Medical Center,
Orange, California

BERNHARD A. VOTTERI, M.D.

Director of Critical Care,
Sequoia Hospital District,
Redwood City, California;
Assistant Clinical Professor of Medicine,
University of California,
San Francisco, California

JACQUELINE F. WADE, R.N.

Research Associate, Nurse Instructor,
Sequoia Hospital District,
Redwood City, California

LAURA WALL, R.N., CNRN

Nurse Specialist, Department of Neurology,
Bowman Gray School of Medicine,
Wake Forest University,
Winston-Salem, North Carolina

CARMEN GERMAINE WARNER, R.N., Ph.N.

Consultant, Emergency Medicine,
Community Health Systems and
Social and Domestic Violence;
Faculty, San Diego State University,
College of Extended Studies,
San Diego, California

DONALD E. WATSON, M.D.

Medical Director, Santa Ana Psychiatric
Hospital; Assistant Clinical Professor
of Psychiatry, University of California,
Irvine, California College of Medicine,
Irvine, California

KARIN ZENK, Pharm.D.

Senior Pharmacist, University of
California Irvine Medical Center, Orange,
California; Assistant Clinical Professor,
Division of Clinical Pharmacy, School
of Pharmacy, University of California,
San Francisco; Assistant Clinical Professor,
Department of Pediatrics, University of California,
Irvine, California College of Medicine,
Irvine, California

DONNA A. ZSCHOCHE, R.N., M.A.

Education Director, National
Critical Care Institute of Education,
Orange, California

Consultants

MARY JO ASPINALL, R.N., M.S.N.

Cardiovascular Nurse Specialist,
Veteran's Administration Hospital,
Long Beach, California

SUE BULL, R.N.

Clinical Nursing Supervisor,
Swedish Hospital Medical Center,
Seattle, Washington

DIANA R. FIELD, R.N., M.S.

Project Director, Critical Care
Clinical Specialist Program,
California State University, Long Beach,
Long Beach, California

PHILLIS GOODRICH, R.N., M.S.N., CCRN

Education Coordinator; Instructor,
Critical Care Nursing Program,
Sequoia District Hospital,
Redwood City, California

JAN GREEN, R.N., M.A.

Instructor, Psychiatric Technology;
Assistant Director, Psychiatric
Technology Program,
San Bernardino Valley College,
San Bernardino, California

PENELOPE MARTIN, R.N.

Supervisor Coronary Care Unit,
Santa Ana–Tustin Community Hospital,
Santa Ana, California

SANDRA PFLAUM, R.N., M.S.N., N.P., CCRN

Specialist, Critical Care Education;
Faculty, National Critical Care Institute
of Education,
Newport Beach, California

DEBORAH PUGH, M.S.N., CCRN

Critical Care Instructor, St. Joseph Hospital,
Orange, California

SHARON L. ROBERTS, R.N., M.S.

Associate Professor of Nursing,
California State University, Long Beach,
Long Beach, California

ELLEN BEAM RUDY, R.N., Ph.D.

Associate Professor, School of Nursing,
Kent State University,
Kent, Ohio

JUDY SITZMAN, R.N., D.N.S.

Professor of Nursing, School of Nursing,
Boston University,
Boston, Massachusetts

To

The critically ill

Foreword to second edition

As the stresses of our society continue, as the life span lengthens, and as people continue to suffer life-threatening problems, well-prepared health care personnel will continue to be needed. This second edition of a most important volume is designed to help the critical care professional maintain the knowledge necessary for safe and effective practice, thus significantly contributing toward the goal of providing high-quality critical care.

In the first edition (a compilation of the writings of experts in the subspecialties that comprise critical care—a major subdivision of health care delivery) as in this text, Ms. Zschoche appropriately points out that no one individual member of the critical care team can claim exclusive knowledge or skill or provide total care. Critical care specialists, perhaps more than any other group of health specialists, have long accepted the concept that all members of the team must share a common base of knowledge and skill, that each member of the team brings very special expertise to the problem-solving endeavor, and that continuing education to upgrade knowledge and skill is essential. This second edition of *Mosby's Comprehensive Review of Critical Care* implements this concept. As a reference volume for all critical care professionals, it continues to provide the best and most up-to-date information based on advances in the health sciences. It also provides the practitioner with an ever-present resource that will ultimately help the seriously ill patient toward recovery.

Rheba de Tornyay, Ed.D., F.A.A.N.

Dean, School of Nursing,
University of Washington,
Seattle, Washington

Foreword to first edition

The need for care of the critically ill will always exist even though the ability to prevent disease improves as the years pass.

The prevention of disease should be the goal of every citizen, nurse, physician, and health worker. Unfortunately, the prevention of all disease is not yet possible for the following reasons: (1) Even though a certain illness may be preventable, the individual citizen may not cooperate in the effort of prevention. For example, everyone does not take the injections for tetanus immunization. (2) The knowledge that might enable prevention of a certain disease may be incomplete. For example, the prevention of coronary atherosclerosis cannot be promised to every person who eliminates all of the "risk factors." Since the preventive measures are difficult to implement and since they are not universally successful, it is difficult to "sell" the preventive concept to everyone (although I personally subscribe to it). (3) There is no satisfactory prevention for many conditions, such as a gunshot wound in the abdomen of a suburban housewife who is carrying her groceries to her car and is attacked by an unknown assailant.

The point is that acute, serious illnesses will always exist. We must not succumb to the trend of being in favor of preventive medicine *or* emergency medicine. The problem we face cannot be reduced to a simple either-or formula. The fact is that we must all support the work in preventive medicine *and* the efforts to improve emergency care for patients who are seriously and critically ill.

The medical advances of the last few years have produced intensive/critical care units of many types, a new profession of emergency and critical care for physicians, nurses, and other allied health professionals, and new educational programs for the care of the critically ill. Every physician knows that it is not possible to care for seriously ill patients without the help of informed and skilled nurses and technicians who have responded to the modern needs in many exciting ways—not the least of which is their intense interest in continuing education.

Mosby's Comprehensive Review of Critical Care was written by experts in many fields and will be read and reread by nurses, physicians, and technicians alike, but we must thank a nurse for conceiving and stimulating its creation.

J. Willis Hurst, M.D.

Professor and Chairman,
Department of Medicine,
Emory University School of Medicine,
Atlanta, Georgia

Preface

Critical care, as presented in the first edition of this book, has now become an established mode of treatment and practice throughout the world. The concept of the one-body system or multiple-organ approach to critical care continues to encompass critical care, critical care clinicians, and the critical care environment.

Mosby's Comprehensive Review of Critical Care is a book about and for the critically ill patient/client and critical care practitioner, albeit physician, nurse, or allied critical care professional.

As with the first edition, this text is not intended to be a primer for the beginning critical care practitioner, but rather it is designed to assist the practicing critical care clinician in maintaining currency of knowledge with subsequent currency in practice. That is not to say, however, that the novice entering the critical care arena for the first time would not reap great benefits from perusing its contents.

Mosby's Comprehensive Review of Critical Care is designed to serve as a resource and reference for anyone—physicians, nurses, and other critical care professionals—seeking expert opinion or instruction on a particular question or an entire subject. The format is a simple one, structured to pinpoint questions and answers, with emphasis on the flow and continuity of information.

The critical care practitioner who utilizes the whole-body system and multiple-organ approach in practice will benefit from the chapter devoted to anatomy, physiology, and pathophysiology as they relate to the altered regulatory mechanisms present in the seriously ill patient. Other chapters focus on specific diagnoses and clinical care related to disease and trauma entities.

Since professionals prepared to function at the entry level both in mobile intensive care and hospital critical care units, including the emergency department and operating and recovery rooms, continue to be a scarce commodity, it often becomes the hospital's responsibility to provide basic critical care education for new employees. Thus one chapter is devoted to critical care education and a course content that individual educators in community, state college, and university systems, as well as hospital in-service programs, may utilize in developing a personalized curriculum.

Throughout the text an attempt has been made to avoid pronouns that express bias. However, this has not always been possible, since to do so in some cases makes for awkward construction. In these cases pronouns have been used for better readability.

We hope that this literary contribution will be of value to the readers and of long-term benefit to patients.

Donna A. Zschoche

Acknowledgments

Few books are the product of a single mind, and this one is no exception. It is with the deepest respect and gratitude that I acknowledge and thank the contributing authors who have made the preparation of this text possible. Their generous contributions of time, expertise, and knowledge have appreciated the value of this book far above that which words may describe.

I am grateful for the thoughtful foreword prepared by Dr. Rheba de Tornyay, Dean of the School of Nursing at the University of Washington, and I also wish to acknowledge the helpfulness of my many critical care nurse colleagues, with whom I exchanged ideas and who so willingly and graciously offered numerous suggestions and much information during the early stages of this book's development.

My sincere thanks to the National Critical Care Institute of Education staff, Barbara Arnold and Pat Johnson, who have typed this manuscript more than once and dedicated many long hours to its completion. To all—thank you.

Contents

Mosby's
Comprehensive review of
CRITICAL CARE

CHAPTER 1

Critical care education

Donna A. Zschoche

Traditionally, the care of critically ill people has been divided arbitrarily according to biologic age groups. In the past, it has generally been accepted that the critically ill person who is 7 years old will respond altogether differently than the critically ill person who is 70 years old. This assumption has come under close scrutiny during recent years with the result that members of the critical care team are looking for more logical approaches to the concept of critical care.

Although a human being may be large or small, old or young, at the time he suffers a critical illness, it becomes more and more apparent that we must heed the wisdom of expert physiologists who urge us to remember that the living organism functions according to absolute biologic laws and that the balance between physiologic parameters permits extremely narrow deviation whether we consider large or small people, old or young people. Thus the biologic age of a critically ill person can affect the *amount* of a given drug he receives but not the *reason* for receiving it. The *size* of the patient can affect the size of the equipment used in his care but not the *reason* for its use.

For example, hypoxemia occurs when the buffering systems of the patient are no longer able to compensate for respiratory or metabolic deficiencies. Blood gas levels must be maintained at precise levels—levels identical for the infant or the adult—if the patient is to survive. Ventilatory assistance, drug therapy, and fluid and electrolyte corrections differ only in quantities for the infant and the adult—their influence on the patient's condition is based on physiologic needs common to both.

Physiologists further urge us to consider critical care at the micro level as well as the macro level, at the cell level as well as the organ level. For an organ to survive, its *cells* must be maintained in an internal and external homeostatic environment. Although an infant's cells exist in different stages of maturation, they require the *same* environmental balance as adult cells if they are to survive and fully mature. It is this exquisite balance based on absolute biologic laws that must become the primary focus in the care of the critically ill.

It is none too soon in the evolution of critical care for us to recognize that the similarities in infant and adult physiology are far greater than the differences. Experts now recognize that if one enters the field of critical care, one must come prepared to meet the needs of critically ill people, regardless of their size or age. Therefore *Mosby's Comprehensive Review of Critical Care* provides its readers with information that will assist critical care team members to meet this advanced concept.

It is now well recognized that critical care practice encompasses definitive care for the seriously ill and injured adult or child at the scene of an emergency, during transport, or at any place in the hospital where the application of critical care knowledge and techniques is required. The critical care practitioner should have expertise in cardiopulmonary resuscitation and treatment of the seriously ill or injured as well as a theoretical and practical understanding of the common disease states and injuries that result in life-threatening conditions. Care may be extended independently or as a part of a team effort; the team may be composed of any combination of the following persons: physician, registered professional nurse, vocational/practical nurse, pharmacist, respiratory therapist, critical care technician, paramedic/emergency medical technician, or social worker.

Any one individual member of the critical care team may be required to render or supervise technologic treatment involving physiologic measurements as well as to administer to the patient's psychologic, social, and environmental needs . . . total care! *Such areas are not the exclusive concern of one profession or discipline!*

Because critical care may be needed anywhere and should be available anywhere, each member of the critical care team should be able to demonstrate skills in emergency life support until more comprehensive restorative care is available. Therefore any critical care team member may at any time be required to resuscitate and/or maintain life-support systems until professional help arrives, and it is recommended that educational preparation reflect a minimum level of performance.

This preparation commences with the study of the major organ systems, that is, the respiratory, cardiovascular, renal, central nervous, and endocrine systems, with a foundation of anatomy and physiology *as they relate to the altered regulatory mechanisms affecting the critically ill.* These sciences provide the theoretical base required to knowledgeably incorporate technology into practice.

Critical care specialists now accept the concept and need for a basic "core" of instruction—a preparatory base for entry into the critical care arena. The concept of the core or basic critical care preparation views the patient en toto; it focuses on the patient as a whole and is as basic as the concept of the critical care center and system itself. All subspecialties, which can include respiratory, coronary, burn, neonatal, pediatric, hemodialysis, and emergency/trauma medicine, revolve around this whole-body concept. A well-prepared clinician will think physiologically, correlating all body systems in both healthy and dis-

ease states and comprehending the many parameters that are or that should be monitored through gross observation or utilization of advanced biomedical instrumentation. The goal is expertise and management of the definitive therapy required in life support.

Basic critical care preparation may be derived from the core curriculum, which may be modified for various levels of practice. Optimum preparation for the critical care clinician should be supplemented by internship (or bedside clinical experience) in the care of both adult and pediatric patients suffering shock, respiratory distress, myocardial infarction, a major burn or renal failure, or undergoing pre- and postoperative heart catheterization, surgery, or pacemaker implantation, as well as the care of certain other specifically selected critically ill patients. Inasmuch as the emergency department and mobile intensive care unit are staffed by front-line critical care professionals, internship in those areas should be scheduled if possible.

Through isolating the commonalities and precepts in all critical care subspecialties, the basic course content, or core curriculum, becomes a dynamic tool to serve the entry-level practitioner. The progress and development of critical care preparation is reinforced when the practitioner has a central base of knowledge. For example, it has long been recognized and acknowledged that arrhythmia identification and interpretative skills are equally as important in caring for the open-heart surgery patient (or the respiratory care, burn, or hemodialysis patient) as they were in the first coronary care unit. We know, too, that alveolar ventilation shares priority with data relative to cardiac output, central venous pressure, and arterial and pulmonary wedge pressures. Temperature control is seen to be as vitally important in the care of the neonate, the critically burned patient, or the neurosurgical patient as is renal function and fluid and electrolyte management.

Consideration should also be given to the critical care environment—the esoteric devices that sustain and measure, the plan of care that will serve to avoid sensory overload, dream deprivation, and time and space disorientation.

In our perception of the patient in the whole-body system, the core curriculum encompasses consideration for eventual recovery and rehabilitation. Thus such entities as these constitute the core or basic preparation for practice.

With didactics drawn from a basic core of knowledge, clinical internship, and return demonstration, the prepared clinician has the ability to apply the skills learned in any of the subspecialties with a minimum of additional knowledge. This core of knowledge is a tremendous asset to hospitals where economics implicitly require full utilization of staff. The well-prepared individual is consequently in a position to provide backup support for colleagues in other critical care units. Efficiency, effectiveness, and economy are also served when this practitioner/clinician serves in the preceptor role without requiring additional extensive specialized education or training.

The core curriculum has already been recognized in the in-service departments of acute care hospitals' continuing education programs and adopted by many community colleges and state universities. It is a product of a new era in medicine. As we see medicine moving toward new standards and with medical science still developing and hospital design changing, the commonalities between disciplines become clear. The multidisciplinary critical care team approach to patient care continues to evolve and is stabilizing. As role changes emerge, it is important to establish guidelines and standards that will provide a measure of security for both the provider and the consumer.

Signaling the congruent roles of the physicians, nurses, and allied health professionals, studies are presently being conducted in some areas of the country that may provide for the more efficient and economic utilization of each team member. The recognized collaborative role of the team was born out of knowledge, skills, and acceptance. There has been a gradual transfer of specific functions, including accountability and responsibility for decision making, from physicians to other critical care professionals and technicians. Such role changes could not occur without reliance on the knowledge and skills found in the core curriculum. The core approach to education provides the foundation on which

critical care can be practiced efficiently, effectively, and dynamically.

Explosive changes are occurring in medical practice and health care itself, and we can be certain of an increased acceleration of change in this decade. Toffler[1] describes the "transient age" in *Future Shock,* which is of marked relevance to health care practitioners. Preparation for these expectations will lessen the trauma, and a "standard" base of knowledge lends a certain degree of security to both the practitioner and the consumer of critical care.

The core course content outlined on the following pages is recommended for entry-level critical care team members as well as those currently in practice. *The educator is cautioned that this course content will not include the minute aspects of care, since it is assumed that the practitioners have a body of basic knowledge in their initial preparation, certification, or professional licensure.* For example, if individuals require a review in basic anatomy and physiology, this should be pursued through *independent study* and not be a part of the critical care curriculum; however, anatomy and physiology *as they relate to the altered regulatory mechanisms seen in the critically ill* should be included. The same is true of basic bedside techniques and approaches for care. Superfluous courses increase program costs and ultimately are reflected in increased hospitalization per diem charges.

The educator or hospital in-service department instructor is encouraged to use the recommended course content as a base, altering or adding specific content and laboratory experience or internship for specializations without sacrificing the whole-body approach.

The recommended course content may be utilized in the development of individualized curriculum and/or written plans for instruction. The course outline that follows clearly provides the reader with information related to what constitutes:

1. Beginning critical care practice
2. **Advanced critical care practice**
3. *The "nice to know" areas, but not required for clinical competence*

Examples of how the recommended course content can be used in the development of critical care continuing education and graduate school (master's in critical care nursing) programs commences on p. 14.

RECOMMENDED COURSE CONTENT FOR USE IN CRITICAL CARE CURRICULA DEVELOPMENT*

I. Review of anatomy and physiology *as they relate to the altered regulatory mechanisms in the critically ill.* See Chapter 2 for a review of the integrative levels at which the body functions in states of health, disease, and/or injury.

II. Cardiovascular system
   A. The heart
      1. Conduction system
         a. Sinoatrial (SA) node
         b. *Atrial preferential pathways*
         c. *Anterior internodal tract*
         d. *Middle internodal tract*
         e. *Posterior internodal tract*
         f. Atrioventricular (AV) node
         g. Bundle of His
         h. **Left bundle branch**
            (1) **Anterior superior fascicle**
            (2) **Posterior inferior fascicle**
         i. **Right bundle branch**
         j. Purkinje fibers
      2. Electrophysiology
         a. **Resting membrane potential**
         b. **Depolarization**
         c. **Repolarization**
         d. **Action potential**
         e. **Integrity and maintenance of the membrane potential**
         f. **Refractory periods**
            (1) Absolute
            (2) Relative (effective)
            (3) Supernormal (vulnerable)
         g. **Membrane responsiveness**
         h. **Vectors**
         i. **Electrical axis**
   B. Muscle mechanics (Chapter 2)
      1. Electrical activation and electromechanics
         a. *Ionic exchange or sodium pump*
         b. *Electrical potential*
         c. **Electromechanical coupling**
         d. *Contractile process*
         e. Muscle function principles
            (1) All-or-none principle

---

*The reader is also referred to the bibliography, which includes a number of excellent references related to the recommended critical care course content.

            (2) Frank-Starling law
   C. Variables related to cardiac contractility
      1. Pharmaceuticals
         a. Inotropic drugs
            (1) Calcium
            (2) Isoproterenol (Isuprel)
            (3) Digitalis
            (4) Catecholamines
            (5) Nitroprusside
         b. Negative inotropic drugs
            (1) Lidocaine (generally no inotropic effect, does suppress the heart but no real negative effect)
            (2) Propranolol
            (3) **Alcohol**
            (4) Barbiturates
            (5) Quinidine
            (6) Procainamide (Pronestyl)
            (7) **Bretylol**
            (8) Dopamine
      2. Other properties related to contractility
         a. Available oxygen
         b. Condition of cardiac muscle
         c. **Preload**
         d. **Afterload status**
         e. Nervous control
         f. Electrical activation
         g. Irritability
         h. Automaticity
         i. Conductivity
   D. Cardiac evaluation
      1. Physical examination and assessment
         a. Inspection
         b. **Palpation**
         c. **Percussion**
         d. **Auscultation**
      2. Cardiac catheterization
         a. Patient preparation
         b. Care before and after catheterization
         c. Diagnostic purpose
         d. **Technique**
         e. Complications
         f. **Diagnostic data obtained**
      3. **Coronary angiography**
      4. *Cine- and coronary arteriography*
      5. *Echocardiography*
      6. *Phonocardiography*
      7. *Tracings of bundle of His*
      8. **Vectorcardiography**
   E. Physiologic measurements
      1. Arterial pressure
      2. Pulmonary artery and capillary (wedge) pressure
      3. Central venous pressure

4. **Cardiac output and cardiac index**
5. **LAP—some institutions still measure direct LAP**
F. Electrocardiography
  1. Rhythm strip
  2. **12- and 13-lead ECG**
  3. **Esophageal leads**
  4. Lewis leads
  5. **Intra-atrial lead**
  6. **ECG leads**
    a. Bipolar (extremities)
    b. Unipolar (augmented)
    c. Unipolar (precordial)
  7. **Electrical axis**
    a. Einthoven's triangle
    b. Axis calculation
  8. **Vectorcardiography (future ECG's)**
G. Arrhythmias (Chapter 12)
  1. Cardiac monitoring
  2. Arrhythmia recognition and interpretation
  3. Pacemaker
    a. Temporary
    b. Demand
    c. Fixed
    d. Atrial pacing vs ventricular pacing
H. Cardiac and/or respiratory arrest (see ACLS standards as designed by American Heart Association)
  1. Cardiovascular collapse and electromechanical dissociation
  2. Ventricular tachycardia
  3. Ventricular fibrillation
  4. Ventricular asystole
    a. Cardiopulmonary resuscitation (adult, pediatric, and neonatal patient)
      (1) Ventilation
      (2) External cardiac compression
      (3) **Internal cardiac massage**
    b. Definitive therapy
      (1) Drugs
      (2) Airway adjuncts
      (3) Counter shock
      (4) Intravenous fluids
      (5) Monitoring and control of dysrhythmia
      (6) Care after resuscitation (stabilization and transport)
I. Heart sounds
  1. **Sound characteristics**
    a. Duration
    b. Pitch
    c. Frequency
    d. Timbre
    e. Intensity

  2. Heart sound origin
    a. Blood flow
    b. Muscle vibration
    c. Muscle contraction
    d. Valves
  3. Cardiac auscultation techniques
    a. *Phonocardiography*
    b. **Stethoscopy**
  4. **Normal heart sounds**
    a. First (S_1)
    b. Second (S_2)
    c. Third (S_3)
    d. Fourth (S_4)
    e. Heart sound variants (splitting)
  5. Abnormal heart sounds
    a. **Gallop rhythms**
      (1) Ventricular diastole (S_3)
      (2) Atrial contraction (S_4)
      (3) Summation gallop (both atrial and ventricular)
    b. Murmur classification
      (1) **Systolic**
        (a) Tricuspid insufficiency
        (b) Aortic stenosis
        (c) Mitral valve insufficiency
        (d) Pulmonic stenosis
        (e) Coarctation of aorta
        (f) Intraventricular septal defect (maladie de Roger)
        (g) Foramen ovale
      (2) **Diastolic**
        (a) Aortic insufficiency
        (b) Pulmonic insufficiency
        (c) Mitral stenosis
        (d) Tricuspid stenosis
      (3) **Continuous**
        (a) "Machinery" murmur (begins in systole and continues through diastole)
        (b) Types
          (i) Aortopulmonary connections
          (ii) Arteriovenous connections
          (iii) Disturbance in flow patterns in arteries
          (iv) Disturbance in flow patterns in veins
    c. **Murmur characteristics**
      (1) Loudness
      (2) Quality
      (3) Intensity
      (4) Time
      (5) Pitch

(6) Transmission

(7) Location

6. *Heart sound variations caused by dysrhythmias*

    a. Atrial fibrillation

    b. Premature extrasystole

    c. Bundle branch block

    d. Complete heart block

7. Extracardiac sounds

    a. **Mediastinal "crunch"**

    b. **Pericardial "friction rub"**

    c. **Ejection sounds**

        (1) Pulmonary

        (2) Aortic

    d. *Systolic click*

    e. *Systolic whoop or honk*

    f. *Opening snaps*

        (1) Mitral valve

        (2) Tricuspid valve

    g. *Pericardial knock*

    h. **Artificial valves**

J. Clinical management of medical emergencies (Chapter 13)

1. Review of pathophysiology, etiology, precipitating factors, clinical manifestations, and physical signs

    a. Myocardial infarction

    b. Congestive heart failure

    c. Hypertensive crisis

    d. **Thyroid storm**

    e. Cardiac tamponade

    f. Pulmonary edema

    g. Cardiogenic shock

    h. Ventricular rupture

    i. Cor pulmonale

    j. **Disseminated intravascular coagulation**

    k. Adult respiratory distress syndrome

    l. Cardiopulmonary arrest

K. Shock (Chapter 41)

1. Definition and diagnosis

2. Pathophysiology

3. Types

4. Clinical management

L. **Pericarditis**

1. Diagnosis

2. Clinical management

M. **Subacute bacterial endocarditis**

1. Diagnosis

2. Clinical management

N. Cardiovascular surgery (Chapters 17-20)

1. Pre- and postoperative clinical management (not acute)

2. **Acute postoperative clinical management**

3. **Cardiopulmonary bypass**

    a. Procedure complications (arrhythmias, conduction defects, shock, tamponade, and so forth)

    b. Extracorporeal oxygenation

    c. Intra-aortic balloon pump

4. **Surgical procedures**

    a. Aneurysm

        (1) Classification

            (a) Location

            (b) Type

        (2) Repair

            (a) Surgical resection

            (b) Grafting

    b. Occlusive lesions

        (1) Surgical resection and grafting

        (2) Revascularization (bypass grafting)

        (3) Thromboendarterectomy

        (4) Embolectomy

        (5) Angioplasty (patch graft)

    c. Pericardiectomy

    d. Valve replacements

    e. Ventriculectomy

    f. Commissurotomy

    g. Myocardial revascularization

        (1) Vein and artery grafts

        (2) Internal mammary artery to coronary artery bypass

        (3) Gas endarterectomy

        (4) Congenital cardiac lesion repairs

        (5) Aneurysmectomy

    h. Venous surgical intervention

        (1) Embolism (embolectomy) or vena cava ligation, and so forth

        (2) Thrombosis (thrombectomy)

III. Pulmonary system

NOTE: Topics for classroom discussion should include the following conditions:

Acute respiratory distress syndrome (ARDS)

Disseminated intravascular coagulation

Coccidioidomycosis

Fat emboli

Oxygen toxicity

Chronic obstructive pulmonary disease

Status asthmaticus

Pulmonary edema

Cor pulmonale

Tracheal or bronchial lacerations

Esophageal rupture

Pulmonary emboli

Embolectomy

Vena caval ligation

Vena cava umbrella

Carbon monoxide poisoning

Acute idiopathic polyneuritis (Guillain-Barré
 syndrome)
Tetanus (lockjaw)
Myasthenia gravis
Poliomyelitis
Tracheal esophageal fistula
Pneumonoconiosis
Pneumothorax
Cholothorax
Hemothorax
A. Respiration
  1. External respiration
  2. Internal respiration
  3. Gas diffusion
    a. **Partial pressures**
    b. **Pressure gradients**
    c. **Inspired and expired gases**
    d. **Mixed venous levels**
  4. Oxygen and carbon dioxide transport
    a. Oxygen measurements
    b. **Oxyhemoglobin and myoglobin dissociation curves**
    c. Dissolved carbon dioxide measurements
    d. **Carbon dioxide transport and elimination**
      (1) Hydrogen ions, acids, and bases
      (2) Buffers
      (3) Acidosis and alkalosis (acid-base balance)
        (a) Respiratory
        (b) Metabolic
        (c) Compensated
        (d) Partially compensated
  5. Blood gases
    a. Sampling
      (1) Arterial catheter
      (2) **Arterial puncture**
      (3) **Analysis and assessment (P_{O_2}, P_{CO_2}, pH, O_2 saturation, base excess, bicarbonate, constant exhaled CO_2 monitoring)**
B. Ventilation
  1. **Ventilation and perfusion rates**
    a. Shunting
    b. Diffusion barriers
C. Respiratory care terminology
  1. Large capital letters
    a. V—gas volume
    b. F—fractional concentration of a gas
    c. Q—volume of blood
    d. **S—percent saturation Hb with O_2**
    e. **P—partial pressure of a gas or its tension**

  2. Small capital letters
    a. I—inspired
    b. E—expired
    c. A—alveolar
    d. D—dead space gas
    e. B—barometric
    f. L—lung
    g. T—tidal volume
  3. Lowercase letters
    a. a—arterial blood
    b. v—venous blood
    c. f—frequency
    d. c—capillary blood
  4. Breathing patterns
    a. Eupnea
    b. Tachypnea
    c. Bradypnea
    d. Cheyne-Stokes
    e. Apneusis
    f. Cluster
    g. Kussmaul's
  5. *Nomograms used in pulmonary care*
    a. Hastings-Singer
    b. Henderson-Hasselbalch equation
    c. Radford
    d. Sigaard-Anderson
D. Physical examination of the chest
  1. Inspection
  2. **Palpation**
  3. *Percussion*
  4. **Auscultation**
E. Lung sounds
  1. **Sound characteristics**
    a. Pitch
    b. Duration
    c. Inspiration vs expiration
  2. **Auscultation and normal lung sounds**
    a. Vesicular
    b. Bronchovesicular
    c. Bronchial or tubular
    d. Tracheal
  3. **Abnormal lung sounds**
    a. Absent
    b. Cogwheel
    c. Bronchial
    d. Asthmatic
    e. Metamorphic
  4. **Adventitious sounds**
    a. Crackles
      (1) Fine, medium rales
      (2) Moist rales or rhonchus
    b. Wheezes
F. Disease states leading to respiratory failure
  1. Obstructive and restrictive conditions

    a. Impaired ventilation
    b. Restricted defects
    c. Limited thorax expansion
    d. Decreased diaphragmatic movement
    e. Pulmonary embolism
G. General respiratory insufficiency
    1. Bronchopulmonary disease
    2. Common parenchymal disease
    3. Neoplastic disease
    4. Cardiopulmonary disease
    5. Neuromuscular disease
H. Traumatic respiratory insufficiency
    1. Cerebral dysfunction
    2. Cardiovascular dysfunction
    3. Biochemical dysfunction
    4. Thoracic trauma
I. Postoperative respiratory insufficiency
    1. Atelectasis
    2. Pneumonia
    3. Aspiration pneumonitis
    4. Pneumothorax
    5. Hemothorax
J. **Pediatric insufficiency**
    1. Congenital anomalies
    2. Infant (acute) respiratory distress syndrome
       a. Incidence
       b. Pathology
       c. Management
    3. Cystic fibrosis
    4. Croup syndrome (laryngotracheobronchitis)
K. Acute respiratory failure
    1. Definition
    2. Diagnosis
    3. Symptoms
       a. Hypoxia
       b. Hypoxemia
       c. Hypercapnia
    4. Clinical management
       a. Assurance of patent airway
       b. Ventilatory support (ventilator management)
       c. **Chest physiotherapy**
       d. Control of secretions and bronchospasms—initiation or discontinuance of drug therapy
       e. Infection control
       f. **Maintenance of physiologic blood gases**
       g. Patient support
         (1) Reassurance
         (2) Alleviation of fears and apprehension

         (3) Relief of anxiety
            (a) Comfort measures
            (b) Drug therapy
L. Airway management
    1. Equipment
    2. Procedure
    3. Endotracheal pathway
    4. Nasopharyngeal pathway
    5. **Esophageal pathway (Chapter 15)**
    6. Tracheostomy
       a. Indications
       b. Procedure
       c. Complications
       d. Clinical bedside care
    7. Suctioning
       a. Equipment
       b. Procedure
         (1) For intubated patients
         (2) For nonintubated patients
       c. Tracheostomy and tracheostomy tube management
       d. Potential complications of suctioning
         (1) Arrhythmias, cardiovascular collapse, and cardiac arrest
         (2) Hypoxemia and atelectasis
         (3) Airway trauma
    8. Ultrasonic nebulization, therapeutic humidity, and aerosol treatment
M. Mechanical ventilators
    1. Indications for use
    2. Side-effects and complications of use
    3. Classification of ventilators
       a. Cycling
         (1) Volume
         (2) Pressure
         (3) Time
       b. How cycle initiated
         (1) Assisted
         (2) Controlled
         (3) Combination
       c. Power source
    4. Positive pressure ventilators
       a. Bird Mark VII and VIII
       b. Puritan Bennett—PR II
    5. Volume ventilators
       a. Emerson
       b. Bennett MA-1
       c. Ohio 560
       d. Monaghan
       e. Bourns
    6. **Gravity rocking bed**
    7. *Negative pressure—iron lung*
    8. *Cuirass ventilation*
N. **Phrenic pacing**

O. Special techniques
1. Indications for weaning and complications
2. **Procedures and methods used**
3. **Positive end-expiratory pressure (PEEP)**
4. **Continuous positive air pressure (CPAP and EPAP)**
5. **Intermittent mandatory ventilation (IMV)**

P. **Postural drainage**
1. Indications
2. Methods
3. Clinical support

Q. Chest physiotherapy
1. Percussion
   a. Mechanical
   b. Manual
2. Vibration
3. Breathing exercises—incentive spirometers

R. Clinical bedside management of artery lines
1. Intravenous
2. Arterial
3. **Pulmonary**

S. Pharmaceuticals used in respiratory management
1. Indications
2. Actions
3. Contraindications
4. Untoward reactions
5. Dosages and administration
6. Types
   a. Bronchodilators
   b. Mucolytics
   c. Steroids

IV. Renal system
A. Pathophysiology of renal failure (Chapter 24)
1. Definition
   a. Acute
   b. Chronic
2. Laboratory studies
   a. Urinalysis
   b. Specific urine gravity
   c. **Osmolality of serum and urine**
   d. Urinary pH
   e. Urinary sodium
   f. Glucose determination
   g. Protein evaluation
   h. **Microscopic examination**
   i. Serum creatinine level
   j. Creatinine clearance
   k. Blood urea nitrogen concentration
   l. **Renal biopsy**
      (1) Precautions
      (2) Complications

3. Normal mechanisms of control
   a. Fluid, electrolytes, and acid-base balance
   b. Bedside physical assessment
      (1) Central nervous system status
      (2) Respiratory status
      (3) Cardiovascular system status
      (4) Renal system status
      (5) Psychosocial status

B. Causes of renal failure
1. Prerenal failure
   a. Precipitating factors
      (1) Fluid and electrolyte imbalance
      (2) Decreased renal blood flow
         (a) Shock
         (b) Plasma or blood loss
         (c) Decreased blood pressure
      (3) Decreased glomerular filtration rate
      (4) Tubular ischemia
      (5) Accumulated metabolic waste products in blood (decreased secretion of solutes)

2. **Intrarenal failure**
   a. Acute vasomotor nephropathy
   b. Acute cortical necrosis
   c. Acute and chronic glomerulonephritis
   d. Nephrosis
   e. Kidney trauma
   f. Transfusion reaction

3. Postrenal failure
   a. Obstruction
   b. Structural abnormalities
   c. Vascular occlusion
   d. Calculi
   e. Blood clots
   f. Uric acid crystals

4. Uremia
   a. Anemia (normocytic/normochromic)
   b. Hypertension
   c. Pericarditis
   d. Gastrointestinal manifestations
   e. Neurologic manifestations
   f. Uremic pneumonitis
   g. Dermatologic manifestations
   h. Role of diet

C. **Management and treatment of renal failure (Chapters 24-26)**
1. Medical and bedside management of renal failure
2. Diagnosis and treatment of underlying cause
3. Special nutrition and total parenteral nutrition

4. Protein catabolism (to be minimized)
   a. Hyperkalemia management
   b. Calcium and phosphorus control
5. Fluid and electrolyte balance
6. Blood transfusion reactions
7. Hemodialysis (Chapters 27-29)
   a. Acute
   b. Chronic
   c. Care of shunt and fistulas
8. Peritoneal dialysis (Chapters 30 and 31)
   a. Acute
   b. Chronic
   c. Peritoneal machines
      (1) Pump
      (2) Cycler
9. Kidney transplant
D. Pharmaceuticals as they relate to the renal failure patient
   1. Narcotics and barbiturates
   2. Salicylates
   3. Diuretics
   4. Carbonic anhydrase inhibitors
   5. Immunosuppressive agents
      a. Azathioprine (Imuran)
      b. Steroids
   6. Antibiotics
   7. Antacids
   8. Vitamin and mineral supplements
E. Prevention of renal failure
F. Kidney transplant (Chapters 25 and 26)
   1. Indication
   2. Patient preparation
      a. Tissue typing
         (1) Antigens
         (2) Antibodies
      b. Donors
         (1) Live related
         (2) Cadaver
      c. Organ harvesting
   3. Recovery period
   4. Potential complications and their management
   5. Organ rejection
G. Drug metabolism and renal failure
V. The nervous system (Chapters 35 and 36)
   A. Neurologic evaluation
      1. **Physical examination**
      2. Assessment and diagnosis
         a. Neurologic check
            (1) Level of consciousness
            (2) **Corneal reflexes**
            (3) Pupil reaction
               (a) Constriction to light
               (b) Consensual

(c) Accommodation
(d) Unusual
   (i) Ciliospinal
   (ii) Argyll Robertson
(4) Gag reflex
(5) Motor and sensory responses
   (a) Decorticate
   (b) Decerebrate
   (c) Normal or weakened movement
(6) **Doll's eyes**
(7) **Calorics**
(8) Babinski
(9) Meningeal irritation
   (a) Nuchal rigidity
   (b) Kernig's
   (c) Brudzinski's
3. **Continuous intracranial monitoring**
4. Psychologic and sociologic factors
5. Human evoked responses (pain, tactile, and so forth)
B. Neurologic emergencies
   1. Trauma
      a. Spinal cord injuries
         (1) Paralysis
         (2) Loss of sensation
         (3) Loss of reflexes
         (4) Hyperreflexia
      b. Head and neck injuries
         (1) Contusion
         (2) Concussion
         (3) CVA
   2. **Vascular disorder**
      a. Epidural hematoma
      b. Ruptured aneurysm
      c. Subarachnoid hemorrhage
      d. Subdural hematoma
      e. Arterial-venous malformation
   3. Supratentorial herniation
   4. **Tumors and brain abscesses**
      a. Pituitary
      b. Hypothalamus
   5. **Microbial invasion**
      a. Guillain-Barré syndrome
         (1) Etiology
         (2) Pathology
         (3) Clinical evaluation
         (4) Diagnosis
         (5) Management modalities
      b. **Myelitis**
         (1) Etiology
         (2) Pathology
         (3) Clinical evaluation and assessment
         (4) Diagnosis

(5) Management and modalities
  c. **Meningitis**
    (1) Etiology
    (2) Pathology
    (3) Clinical evaluation and assessment
    (4) Diagnosis
    (5) Management and modalities
  6. Electrochemical disorders
    a. Seizure disorders, status epilepticus
    b. **Myasthenia gravis**
    c. **Parkinson's disease**
C. Treatments
  1. Neurosurgery
    a. Craniotomy
    b. Burr holes
    c. **Transphenoidal hypophysectomy**
    d. **Ventriculostomy**
    e. **Bone flaps**
  2. Pre- and postoperative care
  3. Complications
    a. **Increased intracranial pressure (Scott cannula)**
    b. Spinal shock hypotension
    c. Pneumonia (respiratory insufficiency)
    d. Urinary tract infection
    e. Malnutrition
    f. Decubiti
    g. Spasms
    h. Chronic pain
    i. **Chronic depression**
    j. Temporary and permanent motor and sensory losses (aphasia, paraplegia, hemiplegia, quadriplegia)
    k. Thermal imbalance
    l. Hemorrhage
    m. Fluid and electrolyte imbalance
  4. **Radiation therapy**
  5. **Hormone replacement**
  6. Drug therapy
VI. Endocrine and metabolic disorders (Chapter 23)
  A. **Adrenal disorders**
    1. Adrenocortical insufficiency
      a. Addison's disease
      b. Acute adrenal crisis
    2. Cushing's disease
    3. Pheochromocytoma
  B. **Thyroid disorders**
    1. Thyrotoxic storm (hyperthyroidism)
    2. Myxedema coma (hypothyroidism)
  C. **Parathyroid disorders**
    1. Hypercalcemia
    2. Hypocalcemia
  D. Diabetes mellitus
    1. Pathophysiology

2. Primary disorders
  a. Diabetic ketoacidosis
  b. Hyperglycemic hyperosmolar nonketotic coma
3. **Secondary disorders**
  a. Stress-induced hyperglycemia
  b. Hypoglycemia
4. **Lactic acidosis**
E. **Pituitary disorders**
  1. Diabetes insipidus
  2. Inappropriate ADH syndrome
  3. Cushing's syndrome
VII. Psychosocial aspects of critical care (Chapters 3-5)
  NOTE: The critical care practitioner, whether physician, nurse, respiratory therapist, or other allied critical care team member, is prompted to recognize his or her personal impact on each situation or individual encountered in practice. Self-awareness along with in-depth perceptual skills relative to the dynamics of human behavior, communication, and environmental effects are vital therapeutic components of care. Consideration of the psychosocial aspects of care is an integral part of any critical care education program. It is therefore recommended that the aspects of care listed here be included in the case presentation portion of any critical care curriculum or course of instruction.
  A. Interpersonal relationships (psychosocial dynamics)
    1. Patient
    2. Behavioral adaptation to pathophysiologic changes
    3. Family
    4. Health team
  B. **Transcultural nursing**
  C. **Crisis intervention**
  D. Effects of critical care environment
    1. Patient
    2. Sensory and/or dream deprivation
    3. Sensory overload
    4. Stress
    5. Loneliness
    6. Dependencies and/or independencies
    7. Space and/or time orientation
    8. **Staff (personnel)**
    9. Families
  E. The dying patient
    1. Patient
    2. Family
    3. Health team
  F. **Progressive care and rehabilitation**
VIII. Bioelectronic instrumentation (Chapter 45)

2. Precautionary measures to be employed when providing direct patient care in the hospital setting

H. **Disaster planning**

XI. Pharmacology (Chapter 6)
A. Analgesics
B. Anesthetics
C. Antiarrhythmics
D. Antibiotics
E. Anticoagulants
F. Anticonvulsants
G. Antispasmodics
H. Cardiotonics
I. Diuretics
J. Drugs used in cardiac arrest
K. Drugs used in controlled ventilation procedures
L. Drugs used in electrolyte replacement
M. Drugs used in respiratory therapy
N. Nitrates
O. Vasodilators
P. Vasopressors
Q. Steroids

XII. Recommended clinical practice and return demonstration (based on hospital nursing policies)
A. Skills and techniques
1. Laboratory data interpretation
2. Venous and arterial catheters
3. Central venous pressure and arterial pressure monitoring
4. Pulmonary wedge pressure monitoring (PAP monitoring)
5. **Cardiac output determinations**
6. Cardiopulmonary resuscitation (adult and infant)
7. Defibrillation
8. Arrhythmia identification and interpretation
9. **Electrocardiogram (ECG) monitoring (12-lead)**
10. **Esophageal lead**
11. **EEG monitoring**
12. Pacemakers and pacing
a. Internal and external
b. Intrathoracic pacing
13. Synchronized cardioversion
14. Care of chest tubes
15. Determination of alveolar ventilation
a. Tidal volume
b. Minute volume
c. Dead space
d. Minute alveolar ventilation
16. Spirometry
17. *Use of nomograms*

18. **Blood gas sampling and analysis**
19. **Arterial puncture**
20. **Intubation**
a. Endotracheal procedure
b. Esophageal airway
c. Cricothyrotomy
(1) Needle thyrotomy
(2) Other procedures
21. Heimlich maneuver
22. **Breath sounds (auscultation and percussion)**
23. **Heart sounds**
24. Chest physiotherapy
a. Vibration
b. Percussion
c. Tracheostomy care
d. Suctioning and secretion management
e. Sepsis control
f. **Postural drainage**
25. Use of mechanical ventilators
a. Assisted and controlled ventilation
(1) Volume control
(2) Pressure limitation
(3) Accessories and modifications
(4) Intermittent positive pressure breathing (IPPB)
(5) Continuous positive airway pressure (CPAP)
(6) Positive end-expiratory pressure (PEEP)
(7) Intermittent mandatory ventilation (IMV)
26. Use of manual ventilatory devices
27. **Peritoneal dialysis**
28. **Hemodialysis**
a. Atrioventricular shunt care
b. **Atriovenous fistula**
(1) Side-to-side
(2) End-to-end
29. Patient/family teaching

XIII. Recommended clinical experience
A. In-hospital patient care experience
1. Shock
a. Cardiogenic
b. Septic
2. Heart catheterization (pre- and postcatheterization)
3. **Open-heart surgery (pre- and postoperative)**
4. Pacemaker
5. Myocardial infarction
6. Respiratory distress (adult and child)
7. **Acute renal failure**

8. Neuromedical and neurosurgical care
9. **Severe burns**
10. Acute pulmonary edema
11. **Major trauma**
12. Patient and family teaching
B. Nursing process and intervention
    1. Patient data base (history)
    2. **Physical examination**
    3. **Nursing diagnosis**
    4. **Plan of care**
    5. Observation
    6. Interpersonal relationships (development of trust between nurse and patient)
C. **Prehospital patient care experience (mobile intensive care/field experience) is highly recommended. This should include experience in the following:**
    Patient data base (history)
    Physical examination
    Observations in the field
    Diagnosis
    Intervention
    Transportation

Examples: Critical care nursing continuing education course

A NONPROFIT CORPORATION LEARNING CENTER PROGRAM*
Critical care nursing: a pathophysiologic approach

The critical care nursing continuing education course is a five-tract program presenting principles of normal and altered physiology leading to clinical disease. Each 2-day tract will focus on a major body system and the disorders and nursing care relevant to that system. Each tract may be taken as a separate course.

On completion of the five critical care nursing tracts of instruction, the well-motivated learner will have acquired an excellent base of knowledge that will encourage future search of new information as it becomes available and will enable the individual to function more knowledgeably as a critical care bedside practitioner.

---

*Critical care nursing course presented at the National Critical Care Institute of Education Learning Center in Orange, California. Instructor and course author: Sandra Pflaum, R.N., M.S.N., N.P., CCRN; Specialist, Critical Care Education.

This preparation will provide specific information that may be useful in successful completion of a number of written examinations that may become a nationwide employment requirement in the future for nurses functioning in the critical care arena.

Tract I: Cardiovascular System

Tract I is a 2-day course designed for the critical care nurse and allied professional responsible for the care of patients with disease of the cardiovascular system. The instruction includes a review of anatomy and physiology, assessment techniques, hemodynamic principles, and selected clinical disorders. Emphasis is placed on the increasing responsibility of the nurse in the assessment and care of the critically ill. The course content includes:

Review of cardiovascular anatomy and physiology
Hemodynamic principles and circulatory pressure gradients
Introduction to hematology
Cardiovascular assessment including chest auscultation
Myocardial infarction
Cardiogenic shock
Hypovolemic shock
Pericarditis and cardiac tamponade

Learner objectives. On completion of this course the well-motivated learner will be able to:
Sketch circulation through the heart and pulmonary system, labeling all chambers, valves, and normal pressures
List and discuss the hemodynamic principles of blood flow and pressures
List each heart sound including its underlying physiology; list four abnormal sounds including the pathophysiology
Correctly interpret a CBC report
Compare right and left heart failure
Discuss the pathophysiology of cardiogenic shock including etiologies, clinical presentation, assessment techniques, and therapy
List and discuss two examples of hypovolemic shock citing differences and similarities
Describe the clinical sequence of cardiac tamponade and the nursing responsibilities

Tract II: Respiratory System

Tract II is a 2-day course designed for the critical care nurse and allied professional who care for patients with respiratory dysfunction. Instruction includes a review of anatomy and pulmonary physiology with emphasis on gas diffusion and transportation. The role of the respiratory system in acid-base maintenance, blood gas interpretations, and ventilator principles will be stressed. Selected clinical disorders are discussed to assist the learner in understanding assessment techniques and principles of therapeutics. The course content includes:

Pulmonary and cellular respiration

O_2 and CO_2 transport

Types and causes of hypoxia

Principles and practice of arterial blood gas studies

Calculation of Po_2 and FIO_2

Principles of O_2 and ventilator therapies

Respiratory assessment including chest auscultation

Acute respiratory failure

Chronic obstructive airway disease

Pulmonary embolus

Adult respiratory distress syndrome

Learner objectives. On completion of this course the well-motivated learner will be able to:

Describe how O_2 is carried to the cell and how CO_2 is carried from the cell

State the role of the respiratory system in maintaining acid-base balance

State the normal range for arterial blood Po_2, Pco_2, pH, and HCO_3^-

Correctly interpret 20 arterial blood gas reports and suggest a clinical condition compatible with each

Calculate a predicted alveolar Po_2 when given a respiratory minute volume and O_2 liter flow

Compare volume ventilators with pressure cycled ventilators

List the four types of hypoxia; give an example of each and an appropriate intervention

Demonstrate on selected patients the physical findings (1) rales, (2) rhonchi, (3) egophony, and (4) bronchophony

List and discuss the three types of chronic obstructive airway disease

List three signs of a pulmonary embolus

Discuss the clinical characteristics of adult respiratory distress syndrome

Tract III: Renal System

Tract III is a 2-day course designed for the critical care nurse and allied professional responsible for caring for patients with altered renal function. Instruction includes renal anatomy and physiology with emphasis on the excretory, regulatory, and secretory roles of the renal system. Acute and chronic renal failure are viewed as clinical states with implications for all body systems. Principles of dialysis and equipment discussion provide insight for the practitioner. The course content includes:

Functional renal physiology

The roles of ADH, renin, angiotensin, and aldosterone

Renal regulation of electrolytes

The renal role in acid-base balance

Acute renal failure

Etiologies of chronic renal failure

The nephrotic syndrome

Systemic effects of renal failure

Nursing assessment in renal failure patients

Principles of dialysis filtration, osmosis, and diffusion

Blood access for hemodialysis

Psychosocial aspects of acute and chronic renal failure

Learner objectives. On completion of this course, the well-motivated learner will be able to:

Draw and label a nephron including tubular and vascular components

State the functional categories of renal function and give two examples of each

List three ways the kidney influences acid-base balance

List two conditions that alter glomerular filtration; tubular reabsorption

Diagram the origin and actions of renin, angiotensin, and aldosterone

List two nursing measures that can be performed on urine to aid in renal assessment

Discuss six systemic complications of chronic renal failure

Diagram the pathophysiology of nephrotic syndrome

List and discuss the three principles of hemodialysis

Tract IV: Endocrine System

Tract IV is a 2-day course designed for the critical care nurse and allied professional involved
in the care of patients with metabolic dysfunction. Instruction includes a review of all endocrine glands and hormones, including actions
and control mechanisms. The interrelatedness of
this system and its effects on the total body are
examined in depth. Selected clinical disease
states and related nursing responsibilities are
presented. The course content includes:
Endocrine gland anatomy
Hormones: actions and controls
Hormonal regulation of glucose, water, and
electrolytes
Hypothalamic and autonomic nervous system
functions
Diabetes mellitus
Diabetes insipidus
Addison's disease—adrenal crisis
Cushing's disease and syndrome myxedema
Grave's disease—hyperthyroidism
Learner objectives. On completion of this course
the well-motivated learner will be able to:
Name the hormone(s) that help control blood
sugar, serum calcium, serum sodium, and
serum potassium
Diagram the mechanisms of control for each
of the above
Name the hormone(s) that help regulate
growth and repair, secondary sex characteristics, fluid balance, and adrenal cortical activity
List possible endocrinologic and clinical manifestations of a hypothalamic tumor
Discuss why a patient with adrenal cortical disease might have fluid and electrolyte disturbances
Discuss the systemic effects of diabetes mellitus
List nursing care objectives for a patient with
myxedema; Grave's disease

Tract V: The Nervous System

Tract V is a 2-day course designed for the critical care nurse and allied professional involved
in the care of patients with neurologic dysfunction. Instruction includes a review of neuroanatomy and physiology, neurologic assessment techniques, and selected clinical disorders. This
course enables the practitioner to base her neurologic nursing practice on a sound base of understanding to complement her clinical skills. The
course includes:
Anatomy and physiology of the central, peripheral, and autonomic nervous systems
Neurologic assessment principles and techniques
Neurologic diagnostic studies
Seizure disorders
Spinal cord injuries
Meningitis and encephalitis
Myasthenia gravis
Guillain-Barré syndrome
Care of the postcraniotomy patient
Learner objectives. On completion of this course
the well-motivated learner will be able to:
Diagram the cerebral vascular supply labeling
major vessels
List the cranial nerves and give one function
for each
Perform a neurologic assessment including ori-
entation and mood, memory and reasoning,
cranial nerve integrity, and motor and sen-
sory function
List three diagnostic studies performed for
neurologic assessment; give a reason why
each might be done
List four factors to observe during a seizure
List two immediate complications of spinal
cord injury; two long-term complications
Discuss nursing care objectives for a patient
with meningitis; encephalitis
Compare myasthenia gravis with Guillain-
Barré syndrome including etiology, clinical
presentation, treatment principles, prognosis, and patient education
Write a nursing care plan for the postcraniotomy patient

A HOSPITAL IN-SERVICE EDUCATION PROGRAM*

Since 1970, Sequoia Hospital District has provided a formal in-service education program de-

*Sequoia Hospital District; Redwood City, California; Phyllis
Goodrich, R.N., M.S.N., CCRN, Education Coordinator.

signed to train professional nursing personnel, with varied educational preparation, to care for patients in an intensive care setting. For the majority of over 200 orientees who have completed the program this was their initial experience working as registered nurses in a special care area. The purpose of this section is to present an overview of the programs and methods of implementation that have pragmatically been proven to facilitate the orientees' adjustment to critical care nursing practice.

Environmental setting

A staff of approximately 90 registered nurses is required to care for the patients assigned to the 37-bed special care unit (SCU): transitional care, 17; intensive care, 13; cardiac care, 7. Nurses assigned to these units are required to successfully complete the planned orientation program and critical care nursing courses that are implemented by the Education Coordinator, Cardiovascular Nurse Specialist, and Medical-Surgical Clinical Nurse Specialist for 3 to 11 and 11 to 7 shifts.

Prerequisite criteria for assignment to SCU

Eligible personnel must be registered nurses who have completed:
A minimum of 6 months work experience in an acute hospital setting
A basic CPR certification program
An intravenous and intracannula training program
An introductory ECG interpretation course (10 hours)
An interview with the SCU coordinator/administrator

Orientation program

The orientation program is adapted to meet the individual nurse's learning needs in the area of critical care nursing. The length of the program has varied from 2 to 8 weeks depending more on the work experience of the orientees rather than their educational preparation.

Status	Orientation time
Inexperienced R.N., new graduate (special 320 hour program)	2 months

Status	Orientation time
Experienced R.N. (minimum 6 to 12 months general nursing)	3 to 5 weeks
Experienced R.N., ICU (minimum 12 months plus 6 to 12 months ICU-CCU experience)	2 to 3 weeks
Experienced R.N., "float" to SCU prn (minimum 6 to 12 months general nursing)	3 to 4 days

Types of critical care nursing courses

Three types of critical care nursing courses were designed and utilized at Sequoia Hospital for training the following groups of inexperienced orientees.

Special training program

A special training program was designed to prepare recent R.N. graduates to effectively care for critically ill patients by providing an intensified orientation program (320 hours) that integrated basic theory (134 hours) with supervised patient care in the transitional (TCU), cardiac (CCU), and intensive care (ICU) units. Twenty nurses completed the program, which was conducted once in 1974 and once in 1975 with 10 orientees in each group. The program was discontinued in 1976 as the emergency need for staff members no longer existed. Furthermore, the graduates of the program had recommended that prior to assignment to the SCU, new graduates needed an opportunity for testing their nursing practice abilities in a less stressful and complex patient care environment. Nursing personnel who had assisted with the implementation of the program wholeheartedly supported this recommendation. Ultimately, the existing SCU prerequisite criterion that nurses acquire a minimum of 6 months experience working in an acute hospital area was established.

Mini–critical care nursing course

A mini–critical care nursing course was designed to train the staff nurses in a "float" position to assist in the care of selected patients when requested to work in the ICU. This "crash" program was implemented when a sudden increase in cardiovascular surgery patients resulted in a temporary shortage of experienced ICU nurses.

Although the "float" nurse worked under the direction of an experienced ICU nurse and was not assigned to care for immediate postoperative patients, the insecurity experienced and expressed by these nurses was justifiable. The 21 hour (3 days) course was conducted three times in 1979 for a total group of 21 "float" nurses. The basic clinical knowledge and skills necessary for these nurses to assess and report pertinent observations to their charge nurses were emphasized. The purposes of the special cardiac and pulmonary monitoring equipment were presented briefly and observations of equipment in bedside use were included. All the program participants expressed an increase in self-confidence concerning their patient assignments and were less reluctant to work in the intensive care units.

Basic critical care nursing course

A basic critical care nursing course is a progressive phase of the ongoing in-service education program for all nurses assigned to the SCU with the exception of the two categories of nurses previously mentioned. The 70 hour course is conducted over a 2-week time period (Monday thru Friday) for a scheduled group of from five to nine nurses. The head nurses and staffing director arrange release time for the eligible nurses to attend class. Most often nurses are scheduled to attend 5 to 8 months after completing their orientation program, rather than attending the course during their orientation period. Active participation in course activities has been overtly enhanced when the nurses have had an opportunity to deal firsthand with a variety of complex patient care problem situations. An indepth description of the program curriculum follows.

Description of course

The program provides the learner with a practical review of core critical care nursing theory as applied to the clinical management of patients with major problems such as craniocerebral trauma, cardiac arrhythmias and cardiopulmonary arrest, acute respiratory failure, and fluid-electrolyte and acid-base imbalances. The holistic approach to patient care is emphasized along with the nurses' role in assuming responsibility for assessing and monitoring the patient's status and implementing appropriate interventions.

Central objective

The primary purpose of the course is that the nurse participants develop their working knowledge, skills, and ability to assess, make decisions, and cope effectively with the complex clinical problems encountered in caring for critically ill patients and their families.

Behavioral objectives

During the course the emphasis for learning is that the nurse increase his/her ability to:
1. Identify the scientific knowledge underlying physiologic processes involved in maintaining homeostasis of major systems
2. Conduct a systematic physical assessment of the patient's status utilizing the techniques of inspection, palpation, percussion, and auscultation to:
   a. Assess the neurologic patient's level of consciousness, pupillary status, motor function, respirations
   b. Locate areas for cardiac auscultation and identify normal and abnormal heart sounds
   c. Identify normal and adventitious breath sounds
   d. Identify signs of fluid-electrolyte imbalances
3. Demonstrate technical and operational knowledge of special monitoring equipment used in the daily care of patients
   a. Hemodynamic monitoring: arterial-venous lines (CVP, Swan Ganz); cardiac output
   b. Pulmonary ventilators; MA-1, IPPB
   c. Electrocardiogram monitors: lead cardioscope placement; telemetry
4. Identify major stress factors and related coping mechanisms encountered by patients, families, and staff in an intensive care setting
5. Develop theoretical knowledge of the types of leadership roles, assertive behavior, and the decision-making process for application to management of patient care problem situations

Specific behavioral objectives are compiled for

each major content area presented. For an example of the neurologic seminar and workshop objectives see the box below.

Description of content

An example of the specific content presented is illustrated in the sample 2-week class schedule on pp. 20 and 21. The order of presentation and amount of time spent in discussing a particular content area vary among class groups as the schedule is adapted to meet the expressed theoretical and clinical learning needs of the participants.

Instructors and teaching methods

The education coordinator is the primary instructor responsible for planning, coordinating, and implementing the program. A multidisciplinary faculty consisting of physicians (director of critical care units, cardiologist, cardiovascular surgeon, neurosurgeon, and so forth), clinical nurse specialists, unit head nurses, and allied health personnel such as pulmonary therapists discuss the prescribed material with a small group of from five to eight participants in an informal classroom setting. The class is located

Example: Basic critical care nursing program

NEUROLOGIC NURSING OBJECTIVES

SEMINAR

I. Craniocerebral trauma: assessment and management of the comatose patient

Objectives

At the conclusion of this session, the participant should be able to:
Describe the anatomic structures concerned with consciousness
State the major functions for the lobes of the brain
Trace the flow of cerebrospinal fluid
Describe the steps in the pathogenesis of increased intracranial pressure (ICP)
List the Harvard criteria for determining brain death
Describe four types of head injury
Describe the clinical signs of increased ICP from a space-occupying lesion herniated downward and compressing the brain stem

Nursing observations
Level of consciousness
Pupillary status
Motor function
Respiratory
Cardiovascular status

WORKSHOP

II. The neurologic examination: assessment and interpretation of deficits

Objectives

At the conclusion of this workshop, the participant should be able to:
Perform a neurologic examination covering the following areas:
Consciousness-mentation
Cranial nerves
Motor function
Cerebellar function
Sensory
Reflexes
Apply assessment information to selected patient care situations

Sequoia Hospital District Staff

Primary instructor

Phyllis Goodrich, R.N., M.S.N., CCRN
Educational Coordinator
Special Care Units

Guest speakers

George Koenig, M.D.
Neurosurgeon

Michael Finerty, M.D.
Neurologist

TOTAL TIME: 10 hours

SEQUOIA HOSPITAL IN-SERVICE EDUCATION

Week 1 class schedule: November 6-10, 1978

Time	Monday	Tuesday	Wednesday	Thursday	Friday
8:00	*Overview of course* Assessment of learning needs	*Cardiovascular workshop* Cardiac auscultation heart sounds	*Pulmonary system* Anatomy/physiology AV slide/tape program: "Anatomical Landmarks of the Chest"	*Bedside assessment* Clinical rounds DR. VOTTERI	*Cardiovascular surgery* A/P coronary arteries Types of open heart surgery Pre/postop teaching Nursing care (TCU)
8:30					
9:00			Clinical rounds DR. VOTTERI		SUE JOHNSON, R.N.
9:30				*Acid/base problems*	
10:00	*Seminar* Critical care nursing role				
10:30			Anatomy/physiology AV slide/tape program: "Anatomical Landmarks of the Chest"		
11:00	*Assessment of patient needs* (Maslow's hierarchy)			*ABG*	
11:30		LUNCH			
12:00	LUNCH		LUNCH	LUNCH	LUNCH
12:30			*Common medications ICU/CCU* K. ROESCH, R.N.		
1:00	*Update review* Pretest Cardiovascular system anatomy/physiology	*Hemodynamic monitoring workshop* SUE HENNINGSEN, R.N.		*Pulmonary workshop* G. GUNNARSON, CTRT	*Seminar: leadership roles* MARY JO TIERNEY, R.N.
1:30					
2:00			*Pulmonary workshop* Auscultation chest breath sounds		
2:30					
3:00					
3:30				OFF	OFF
4:00	OFF				
4:30	Home study assignment	OFF	OFF		Have a nice weekend!
5:00					

Primary instructor: Phyllis Goodrich, R.N., M.S.N., CCRN.
Others specified: Sue Johnson, R.N., B.S.N., C-V Surgery Coordinator; Sue Henningsen, R.N., M.S.N., Clinical Specialist, CVS; Mary Jo Tierney, R.N., M.S.N., Clinical Specialist, M/H/Psych; Kari Roesch, R.N., ACLS, CPR Instructor; Carol Manchester, R.N., M.S.N., Clinical Specialist, Endocrinology.

SEQUOIA HOSPITAL IN-SERVICE EDUCATION

Week 2 class schedule: November 13-17, 1978

Time	Monday	Tuesday	Wednesday	Thursday	Friday
8:00	*Nervous system* Pretest Practical neuro- anatomy phys- iology	*Nervous system workshop* The neurologic ex- amination	*Endocrine* Management of the acute diabetic patient	*Renal system* Anatomy/physiology DR. SCHIFFNER	*Cardiac cath* A. RIDER, M.D.
8:30					
9:00			C. MANCHESTER, R.N.		*Elective review and post course test- ing*
9:30					
10:00			*Clinical rounds and observation ICU*	*Renal workshop* Fluid electrolyte problems	
10:30					
11:00			*Nurses' role ICU/ stress*	*Management of patient* Pulmonary surgery	
11:30		LUNCH	M. MONJHAN, R.N., H.N.	D. ROWLES, M.D.	
12:00	LUNCH		LUNCH		LUNCH
12:30				LUNCH	
1:00	*Assessment co- matose patient*	*Workshop* ECG update			*Summarization- evaluation of learning*
1:30			Film: "Renal Trans- plants"	*Patient care and role in TCU*	
2:00			*Fluid/electrolyte problems*	LYNDA ALEXANDER, R.N.	
2:30				*Seminar: Decision making in ICU*	
3:00				DR. VOTTERI	
3:30	OFF		OFF		OFF
4:00		OFF		OFF	
4:30			*PMC meeting* Massive transfusions		
5:00			8:00-9:00 PM (optional)		

California State University, Long Beach
Department of Nursing
Graduate Program*

CRITICAL CARE CLINICAL SPECIALIST

The terminal objectives for the critical care program include the following:
1. Operationalize the nursing process to function as an *advanced clinician* by demonstrating the ability to:
   a. Synthesize relevant knowledge from nursing, medical science, psychology, and social science in planning care, written assignments, oral assignments, and examinations
   b. Prepare in writing patient teaching models including objectives, content, methods, and evaluation criteria
   c. Plan in writing staff development programs including objectives, content, methods and evaluation
   d. Identify and discuss for selected clinical conditions, in writing and on examinations, pathophysiology, clinical presentation, assessment, complications, and management
   e. Show through satisfactory evaluation by the clinical instructor the ability to assess and manage critical care problems
   f. Communicate findings, problems, and management clearly through oral and written reports and assignments
2. Foster a *research climate* in the practice of nursing and expand nursing theory by demonstrating the ability to:
   a. Analyze and integrate relevant research and literature as it applies to assessment, diagnosis, management, and evaluation of problems encountered in clinical practice
   b. Analyze and integrate relevant research in discussion of roles and functions of the clinical specialist
3. Identify and implement a *professional leadership role* by demonstrating the ability to:
   a. Maintain individual competence in nursing practice (as evaluated by clinical evaluations and oral and written presentations and examinations), initiate actions, demonstrate judgments, and be accountable for decisions
   b. Initiate assessment of own knowledge, abilities, and performances in terms of strengths and areas that need improvement in the clinical area
   c. Implement a plan to strengthen those areas identified as needing improvement by self or clinical instructors
   d. Show through satisfactory evaluation the ability to work interdependently with other members of the health care team
   e. Demonstrate through satisfactory clinical evaluation the functions of change agent and role model
   f. Teach patient and staff members using appropriate teaching strategies as evidenced by clinical evaluation

*The program is funded in part by the United States Department of Health, Education and Welfare, Public Health service, Division of Advanced Nurse Training, Grant number 1D23 NU 000 87, California State University Long Beach, Department of Nursing, Critical Care Clinical Specialist Program, 1331 Palo Verde Ave., Long Beach, Ca. 90840.

within the special care area so that the group can readily move to the intensive care unit to accompany the physician on bedside rounds, observe procedures, and utilize special monitoring equipment for workshop practice sessions. In addition to participating in clinical patient rounds and workshops, other teaching methods have included lectures, demonstrations, patient-nurse interviews, psychodrama, viewing audiovisual materials, pre- and posttesting, group projects, and home study assignments. Daily seminars are popular for sharing information and exchanging ideas about problem solving selected patient care situations (case histories reviewed).

Critical care clinical specialist program curriculum

The masters degree curriculum includes (1) prerequisite requirements, (2) nursing process sequence, (3) clinical sequence, and (4) research sequence. Each element is discussed in the following:

Prerequisite requirements

Prerequisite requirements for entry into the critical care specialist program include a baccalaureate degree in nursing. Courses in pathophysiology and physical assessment will be taken prior to entry into the program. These courses provide a background for the clinical sequence that builds on basic pathophysiology and requires continuous assessment skills. Statistics will also be required as a prerequisite to the research content of the program. Recently, baccalaureate programs have incorporated all three prerequisite content areas into the basic curriculum, but many students seeking to enter the program will have to take these as separate prerequisite courses. Physical assessment and pathophysiology are available in the Extension Division of the Department of Nursing to facilitate completion by potential candidates.

Nursing process sequence

The nursing process sequence is composed of three subject areas. The first is a course designed to acquaint the student with theory in areas of communication, counseling, teaching, learning, cultural implications, and change theory (660A). The second course is an in-depth course of the psychophysiologic and psychosocial needs of the critically ill patient and family of the patient and defines various roles and functions of the clinical specialist (660B).

Clinical series

The graduate clinical series is designed to prepare an advanced critical care nurse who can assess and appropriately intervene in any critical care area. It stresses advanced pathophysiology and management skills and includes substantial medical content. The first two semesters (N680A and N680B) will utilize a systems approach to content including pulmonary, cardiovascular, central nervous, renal, and metabolic systems. The trauma patient will be included at the end of this segment. The final course will be utilized as a speciality preparation course with the students selecting their area of special interest for concentrated study (N680C). In each of the three semesters N680L is the coordinated laboratory practice setting for the N680 content material.

Research sequence

The research sequence includes two courses, N696—Research Methodology, which will build on the prerequisite statistics course and N698—Thesis. This sequence is designed to assist students to develop investigative skills, critically read research literature, test hypotheses related to clinical practice, and participate in the research team.

NOTE: To receive general information on the University Graduate Program, send a request to the University Forty-niner Bookstore for a Graduate Bulletin. Enclose a check for $1.75.

Methods of evaluation

An advantage of the small group method of teaching is the opportunity the instructor has to interact continually with the participants concerning their learning needs and progress. Daily assessments are made of the activities experienced in classroom and clinical areas. Pre- and post- written tests are utilized to assess theoretical learning on the major content areas discussed. Participants submit a written evaluation rating the content in relation to their own learning progress at the conclusion of each week.

Postcourse follow-up evaluations in the clinical areas are considered the most important test of

Master of Science degree critical care specialist curriculum

Sequence	Summary of content					
	Semester I		Semester II		Semester III	
	Course	Units	Course	Units	Course	Units
Research sequence	N696—Research Methods in Nursing	3	N696—Thesis	1	N698—Thesis	3
Nursing process sequence	N660A—Theoretical Base for Advanced Nursing Practice	3	N6603—Theoretical Base for Advanced Nursing Practice	3		
Clinical studies sequence	N680A—Extended Nursing Roles	3	N680B—Extended Nursing Roles	3	N680C—Extended Nursing Roles	3
	N680L—Clinical Practicum (hospital setting)	3	N680L—Clinical Practicum (hospital setting)	3	N680L—Clinical Practicum (hospital setting)	3
Electives			Elective	2	Elective	3
UNIT TOTALS		12		12		12

Prerequisites: B.S. nursing; pathophysiology; statistics; physical assessment; 1 to 2 years critical care experience preferred.

learning that had been acquired during the course. This achievement is demonstrated when, in the performance of patient care, the nurse evidences an increased ability to identify and apply appropriate facts and principles as rationale for setting priorities and making decisions in determining nursing actions. This change in behavior is often observed by staff members, instructors, and the nurse him/herself.

Nurses are awarded a "certificate of attendance" for successfully completing the course and earn 70 continuing education contact hours toward their California Board of Registered Nursing relicensure requirements (30 hours in 2 years mandatory).

Conclusion

The critical care nursing program content and methods of implementation are continually being evaluated and revised to help nurses develop and maintain clinical expertise in their performance of patient care. A measure of the effectiveness of in-service personnel and staff members in achieving this central goal will be reflected in the degree to which patients on the special care units consistently receive high-quality nursing care.

REFERENCE

1. Toffler, A.: Future shock, New York, 1970, Random House, Inc.

BIBLIOGRAPHY

Abdellah, F. G., and Levine, E.: Better patient care through nursing intervention, Riverside, 1979, Macmillan, Inc.

Abels, L. F.: Mosby's manual of critical care: practices and procedures, St. Louis, 1979, The C. V. Mosby Co.

Abram, H. S.: Adaptation to open heart surgery: a psychiatric study of response to the threat of death, Am. J. Psychiatry **122:**659, 1965.

Abram, H. S.: Psychological aspects of the intensive care unit, Hosp. Med. **2:**22, 1969.

Adams, C. W.: Recognition and evaluation of cardiogenic shock, Heart Lung **2:**893, 1972.

Albanese, J. A.: Nurse's drug reference, New York, 1979, McGraw-Hill Book Co.

Altman, J.: Ecological aspects of interpersonal functioning, In Esser, A. H., editor: Behavior and environment, New York, 1971, Plenum Publishing Corp.

Altshuler, A.: Complete transposition of the great arteries, Am. J. Nurs. **71:**96, 1971.

Amacher, N. J.: Touch is a way of caring, Am. J. Nurs. **73:**852, 1973.

American Academy of Orthopaedic Surgeons: Emergency care and transportation of the sick and injured, 1979, P.O. Box 7195, Chicago, Ill. 60680.

American College of Cardiology: Advanced cardiac nursing, Philadelphia, 1970, The Charles Press, Publishers.

Andreoli, K., Hunn, V. K., Zipes, D. P., and Wallace, A. G.: Comprehensive cardiac care, a text for nurses and other health professionals, ed. 3, St. Louis, 1979, The C. V. Mosby Co.

Artiss, K. L., and Levine, A. S.: Doctor-patient relations in severe illness, N. Engl. J. Med. **288:**1210, 1973.

Artz, C., Moncrief, J., and Pruitt, B.: The treatment of burns, Philadelphia, 1979, W. B. Saunders Co.

Aspinall, M. J.: Nursing the open heart surgery patient, New York, 1973, McGraw-Hill Book Co.

Ayres, S. M., and Giannelli, S., Jr.: Care of the critically ill, ed. 2, New York, 1974, Appleton-Century-Crofts, Inc., p. 246.

Ayres, S. M., and Laguson, J.: Pulmonary physiology at the bedside; O_2 and CO_2 abnormalities, Cardiovasc. Nurs. **9:**1, 1973.

Ayres, S. M., and Mueller, H.: The overall approach to the patient with hypotension, Heart Lung, **3:**463, 1974.

Baden, C. A.: Teaching the coronary patient and his family, Nurs. Clin. North Am. **7:**563, 1972.

Baek, A. M., Makabali, G., Bryan-Brown, C. W., Kusek, J., and Shoemaker, W. C.: The influence of parenteral nutrition on the course of acute renal failure, Surg. Gynecol. Obstet. **141:**405, 1975.

Barber, J. M.: Handbook of emergency pharmacology, St. Louis, 1978, The C. V. Mosby Co.

Barber, J. M., and Budassi, S. A.: Mosby's manual of emergency care: practices and procedures, St. Louis, 1979, The C. V. Mosby Co.

Bartlett, R. H., and Gazzaniga, A. B.: Extracorporeal circulation for cardiopulmonary failure, Curr. Probl. Surg. **40:**1, 1978.

Bartlett, R. H., Gazzaniga, A. B., Fong, S. W., and Burns, N. E.: Prolonged extracorporeal cardiopulmonary support in man, J. Thorac. Cardiovasc. Surg. **68:**918, 1974.

Bartlett, R. H., Gazzaniga, A. B., Wilson, A. F., Geraghty, T., and Wetmore, N.: Mortality prediction in adult respiratory insufficiency, Chest **67:**680, 1975.

Bates, B.: A guide to physical examination, ed. 2, Philadelphia, 1979, J. B. Lippincott Co.

Baxter, S.: Psychological problems of intensive care, Nurs. Times **71:**63, 1975.

Beall, C., Braun, H., and Cheney, F., Jr.: Physiologic bases for respiratory care, Missoula, Mont., 1974, Mountain Press Publishing Co.

Beland, I.: Clinical nursing: pathophysiological and psychosocial aspects, New York, 1971, Macmillan Inc.

Bendixen, H. H., et al.: Respiratory care, St. Louis, 1965, The C. V. Mosby Co.

Bendixen, H. H.: Rational ventilator modes for respiratory failure, Crit. Care Med. **2:**225, 1974.

Benotti, P. N., et al.: Safe cannulation of the internal jugular vein for long-term hyperalimentation, Surg. Gynecol. Obstet. **144:**574, 1977.

Berger, E.: The physiology of adequate perfusion, St. Louis, 1979, The C. V. Mosby Co.

Bergersen, B. S.: Pharmacology in nursing, ed. 14, St. Louis, 1979, The C. V. Mosby Co.

Bernard, H., and Huickers, W.: Dynamics of personal adjustment, Boston, 1971, Holbrook Press, Inc.

Beyers, M., Dickelmann, N., and Thompson, M.: Developing a modular curriculum, Nurs. Outlook **20:**643, 1972.

Bilodeau, C. B.: The nurse and her reactions to critical care nursing, Heart Lung **2:**358, 1973.

Blackburn, G. L., and Bistrian, B. R.: Curative nutrition: protein-calorie malnutrition. In Schneider, H. A., Andersen, C. E., and Coursin, D. B.: Nutritional support of medical practice, Hagerstown, Md., 1977, Harper & Row, Publishers, p. 80.

Blackburn, G. L., Maini, B. S., and Pierce, E. C.: Nutrition in the critically ill patient, Anesthesiology **47:**181, 1977.

Blackburn, G. L., et al.: Nutritional and metabolic assessment of the hospitalized patient, Parenteral Enteral Nutrition **1:** 11, 1977.

Blake, P. J., and Perez, R. C.: Applied immunological concepts, New York, 1978, Appleton-Century-Crofts.

Bolin, R. H.: Sensory deprivation: an overview. Nurs. Forum **13:**240, 1974.

Bolognini, V.: The Swan-Ganz pulmonary artery catheter: implications for nursing, Heart Lung **3:**976, 1974.

Branthwaite, M. A.: Detection of neurological abnormality following open-heart surgery, Thorax **28:**464, 1973.

Brault, G. L., and Pflaum, S. S.: Planning and development of a masters degree program in critical care, Heart Lung 8(5):933, 1979.

Broughton, J. O.: Chest physical diagnosis for nurses and respiratory therapists, Heart Lung **1:**200, 1972.

Brunner, L. S., and Suddarth, D. S.: The Lippincott manual of nursing practice, Philadelphia, 1979, J. B. Lippincott Co.

Bruno, F.: Psychology: a life-centered approach, Santa Barbara, Ca., 1974, Hamilton Publishing Co.

Bryan-Brown, C. W., Savitz, M. H., Elwyn, D. H., and Shoemaker, W. C.: Cerebral edema unresponsive to conventional therapy in neurosurgical patients with unsuspected nutritional failure, Crit. Care Med. **1:**125, 1973.

Bryk, D.: Infrapulmonary effusion, Radiology **120:**33, 1976.

Burch, G. E.: Myocardial infarction: is a CCU really so important? Med. Times **104:**79, 1976.

Burke, S.: Composition and function of body fluids, St. Louis, 1972, The C. V. Mosby Co.

Burrell, L. O., and Burrell, Z. L., Jr.: Critical care, ed. 3, St. Louis, 1977, The C. V. Mosby Co.

Bushnell, S. S.: Respiratory intensive care nursing, Boston, 1973, Little, Brown & Co.

Carlson, C. E.: Behavioral concepts and nursing intervention, Philadelphia, 1970, J. B. Lippincott Co.

Cassem, N. H., and Hackett, T. P.: Psychiatric consultation in a coronary care unit, Ann. Intern. Med. **75:**9, 1971.

Cassem, N. H., and Hackett, T. P.: Psychological rehabilitation of myocardial infarction patients in the acute phase, Heart Lung **2:**382, 1973.

Cassem, N. H., Hackett, T. P., Bascom, C., and Wishnie, H. A.: Reactions of coronary patients to the CCU nurse, Am. J. Nurs. **70:**319, 1970.

Chernick, R. M., et al.: Respiration in health and disease, ed. 2, Philadelphia, 1972, W. B. Saunders Co.

Children's Hospital Medical Center, Boston: Manual of pediatric therapeutics, Boston, 1974, Little, Brown & Co.

Chusid, J. G.: Correlative neuroanatomy and functional neurology, ed. 17, Los Altos, Ca., 1979, Lange Medical Publications.

Clark, N. F.: Pump failure, Nurs. Clin. North Am. **7:**529, 1972.

Clowes, G. H. A., Jr., O'Donnell, T. F., Jr., Ryan, N. T., and Blackburn, G. L.: Energy metabolism in sepsis: treatment based on different patterns in shock and high output stage, Ann. Surg. **179:**684, 1974.

Cogen, R. G.: Cardiac catheterization: preparing the adult, Am. J. Nurs. **73:**77, 1973.

Cohen, R. G.: Providing emotional support, R.N. Magazine **37:** 62, 1974.

Cole, J. S., and McIntosh, H. D.: Electroshock hazards in the coronary care unit, Heart Lung **1:**481, 1972.

Colley, R., and Phillip, K.: Helping with hyperalimentation, Nursing '73 **3:**6, 1973.

Colling, A., Dellipiani, A. W., and McCormack, P.: Coronary care units, Am. Heart J. **91:**537, 1976.

Comroe, J. H.: The lung, Chicago, 1962, Year Book Medical Publishers, Inc.

Comroe, J. H.: Physiology of respiration, ed. 2, Chicago, 1974, Year Book Medical Publishers, Inc.

Conn, H. L., et al.: Cardiac and vascular diseases, vols. I-II, Philadelphia, 1971, Lea & Febiger.

Conover, M. H.: Cardiac arrhythmias: exercises in pattern interpretation, ed. 2, St. Louis, 1978, The C. V. Mosby Co.

Conover, M. H., and Zalis, E. G.: Understanding electrocardiography—physiological and interpretive concepts, ed. 2, St. Louis, 1976, The C. V. Mosby Co.

Conway, B. L.: Carini and Owens' neurological and neurosurgical nursing, ed. 7, St. Louis, 1978, The C. V. Mosby Co.

Copeland, E. M., MacFayden, B. V., McGowan, C., and Dudrick, S. J.: The use of hyperalimentation in patients with potential sepsis, Surg. Gynecol. Obstet. **138:**377, 1974.

Cox, J. M. R.: Prolonged pediatric ventilatory assistance and related problems, Crit. Care Med. **1:**158, 1973.

Craven, R.: The effects of illness on family function, Nurs. Forum **11:**191, 1972.

Craven, R.: Anaphylactic shock, Am. J. Nurs. **72:**718, 1972.

Crawford, W. O., Jr.: Pulmonary injuries in thoracic and nonthoracic trauma, Radiol. Clin. North Am. **11:**527, 1973.

Cullen, D. J., Civetta, J. M., Briggs, B. A., and Ferrara, L. C.: Therapeutic intervention scoring system: a method for quantitative comparison of patient care, Crit. Care Med. **2:**57, 1974.

Daly, C. R., and Kelly, E. A.: Prevention of pulmonary embolism: intracaval devices, Am. J. Nurs. **72:**2004, 1972.

Davis, M. Z.: Socioemotional component of coronary care, Am. J. Nurs. **75:**132, 1975.

Delman, A. J., and Stein, E.: Dynamic cardiac auscultation and phonocardiography, Philadelphia, 1979, W. B. Saunders Co.

DeVillier, B.: Preoperative teaching of the cardiovascular patient, Heart Lung **2:**522, 1973.

Dlin, B. M.: Risk factors, life style, and the emotions in coronary disease, Psychosomatics **18:**28, 1977.

Downes, J. J., and Raphaely, R. C.: Pediatric intensive care, Anesthesiology **43:**238, 1975.

Drain, C. B., and Shipley, S. B.: The recovery room, Philadelphia, 1979, W. B. Saunders Co.

Dublin, D.: Rapid interpretation of ECG's, ed. 2, Tampa, Fla., 1977, Cover Publishing Co.

Dudrick, S. J., MacFayden, B. V., Van Buren, C. T., Ruberg, R. L., and Maynard, A. T.: Parenteral hyperalimentation, metabolic problems and solutions, Ann. Surg. **176:**259, 1972.

Ebel, R.: Essentials of education measurement, Englewood Cliffs, N.J., 1972, Prentice-Hall, Inc.

Egan, D. F.: Fundamentals of respiratory therapy, ed. 3, St. Louis, 1977, The C. V. Mosby Co.

Eliott, R., and Miles, R.: What to tell the cardiac patient about sexual intercourse, Consultant **13:**23, 1973.

Escher, D. J.: Medical aspects of artificial pacing of the heart, Cardiovasc. Nurs. **8:**1, 1972.

Evans, G. W.: Personal space, Psychol. Bull. **80:**334, 1973.

Fisher, J. E., editor: Total parenteral nutrition, Boston, 1976, Little, Brown & Co.

Flint, T., and Cain, H. D.: Emergency treatment and management, Philadelphia, 1970, W. B. Saunders Co.

Foster, S. B.: Pump failure, Am. J. Nurs. **74:**1830, 1974.

Frankenhauser, M.: Experimental approaches to the study of human behavior as related to neuroendocrine functions. In Levi, L., editor: Society, stress and disease, London, 1971, Oxford University Press.

Friedman, M., and Rosenman, R. H.: In Greenwich, C. T., editor: Type A behavior and your heart, New York, 1974, Fawcett Publications, Inc.

Friedman, W.: Patent ductus arteriosus in premature infants, J. Pediatr. **90:**338, 1977.

Friedman, W., Hirschklau, M., Pritz, P., Pitlick, P., and Kirkpatrick, S.: Pharmacologic closure of patent ductus arteriosus in the premature infants, N. Engl. J. Med. **295:**526, 1976.

Garfield, C. A.: Stress and survival: the emotional realities of life-threatening illness, St. Louis, 1979, The C. V. Mosby Co.

Gentry, W. D., Foster, S. B., and Freeling, S.: Psychologic response to situational stress in intensive and nonintensive nursing, Heart Lung **1:**793, 1972.

Germain, C. P.: Helping your patient with an implanted pacemaker, R.N. Magazine **37:**3, 1974.

Gernert, C. F., and Schwartz, S.: Pulmonary artery catheterization, Am. J. Nurs. **73:**1182, 1973.

Goldberger, A. L.: Myocardial infarction: electrocardiographic differential diagnosis, St. Louis, 1979, The C. V. Mosby Co.

Goldman, M. J.: Principles of clinical electrocardiography, ed. 10, Los Altos, Ca., 1979, Lange Medical Publications.

Gould, E. P.: The emotional effects of surgical illness, Heart Lung **2:**368, 1973.

Govoni, L. E., and Hayes, J. E.: Drugs and nursing implications, New York, 1978, Appleton-Century-Crofts.

Green, A.: Sexual activity and the post-myocardial infarction patient, Am. Heart J. **89:**246, 1975.

Greyton, A.: Textbook in medical physiology, ed. 4, Philadelphia, 1971, W. B. Saunders Co.

Griffith, G.: Sexuality and the cardiac patient, Heart Lung **2:** 70, 1973.

Gutch, C. F., and Stoner, M. H.: Review of hemodialysis for nurses and dialysis personnel, ed. 3, St. Louis, 1979, The C. V. Mosby Co.

Guyton, A.: Textbook of medical physiology, ed. 2, Philadelphia, 1976, W. B. Saunders Co.

Guyton, A.: Basic human physiology: normal function and mechanisms of disease, ed. 2, Philadelphia, 1977, W. B. Saunders Co.

Hackett, T., and Cassem, N.: Psychological adaptation in myocardial infarction patients. In Naughton, J., and Hellerstein, H., editors: Exercise testing and exercise training in coronary heart disease, New York, 1973, Academic Press, Inc.

Hall, E. T.: The hidden dimension, Garden City, N.Y., 1966, Doubleday & Co., Inc.

Hamilton, W. P., and Lavin, M. A.: Decision making in the coronary care unit—a manual and workbook for nurses, ed. 2, St. Louis, 1976, The C. V. Mosby Co.

Hampe, S. D.: Needs of the grieving spouse in a hospital setting, Nurs. Res. **24:**113, 1975.

Harrington, J., and Brener, E.: Patient care in renal failure, Philadelphia, 1973, W. B. Saunders Co.

Harris, C. C.: A primer of cardiac arrhythmias: a self-instructional program, St. Louis, 1979, The C. V. Mosby Co.

Hay, D., and Oken, D.: The psychological stress of intensive care unit nursing, Psychosom. Med. **34:**109, 1972.

Hedley-Whyte, J., Burgess, G. E., III, Feeley, T. W., and Miller, M. G.: Applied physiology of respiratory care, Boston, 1976, Little, Brown & Co.

Hilberman, M., et al.: An analysis of potential physiological predictors of respiratory adequacy following cardiac surgery, J. Thorac. Cardiovasc. Surg. **71:**711, 1976.

Hilt, N. E., and Cogburn, S. B.: Manual of orthopedics, St. Louis, 1979, The C. V. Mosby Co.

Himathongkam, T., et al.: Acute adrenal insufficiency, J.A.M.A. **230:**1317, 1974.

Hodgkin, J. E., Bowser, M. A., and Burton, G. G.: Respiratory weaning, Crit. Care Med. **2:**96, 1974.

Horney, K.: The neurotic personality of our time, New York, 1964, W. W. Norton & Co.

Hudak, et al.: Critical care nursing, Philadelphia, 1977, J. B. Lippincott Co.

Hudak, et al.: Work manual for critical care nursing, ed. 2., Philadelphia, 1977, J. B. Lippincott Co.

Hurst, J. W., and Logue, R. B.: The heart, New York, 1978, McGraw-Hill Book Co.

Hurwitz, L. J.: Helping the aphasic to communicate again, Geriatrics **28:**102, 1973.

Hymovich, D.: Incorporating the family into care, J. N.Y. Nurs. Assoc. **5:**9, 1974.

Isler, C.: Blood, the age of components, R.N. Magazine **36:**31, 1973.

Isler, C.: I.V. therapy, R.N. Magazine **36:**23, 1973.

Jackle, M., Ceronsky, C., and Petersen, J.: Nursing student's experience in critical care: implications for staff development, Heart Lung **6:**689, 1977.

Jackson, B. S.: Chronic peripheral arterial disease, Am. J. Nurs. **72:**928, 1972.

Jacox, A. K., editor: Pain: a source book for nurses and other health professionals, Boston, 1979, Little, Brown & Co.

Jarrard, M. M., and Freeman, J. B.: The effects of antibiotic ointments and antiseptics on the skin flora beneath subclavian catheter dressings during intravenous hyperalimentation, J. Surg. Res. **22:**521, 1977.

Jenkins, C. D.: Psychologic and social precursors of coronary disease, N. Engl. J. Med. **284:**244, 307, 1971.

Jenkins, C. D.: The coronary-prone personality. In Gentry, W. D., and Williams, R. B.: Psychological aspects of myocardial infarction and coronary care, ed. 2, St. Louis, 1979, The C. V. Mosby Co., p. 5.

Jenkins, C. D., Rosenman, R. H., and Zyzanski, S. J.: Prediction of clinical coronary heart disease by a test for the coronary prone behavior pattern, N. Engl. J. Med. **290:**1271, 1974.

Johns, M. P.: Case studies in drug therapy, Riverside, 1979, Macmillan Inc.

Johns, M. P.: Drug therapy and nursing care, New York, 1979, Macmillan Inc.

Johnson, B., Cantwell, J., and Fletcher, G.: Eight steps to inpatient cardiac rehabilitation: the team effort- methodology and preliminary results, Heart Lung **5:**97, 1976.

Kahn, A.: Stranger in the world of ICU, Am. J. Nurs. **75:**2022, 1975.

Kannel, W. B., McGee, D., and Gordon, T.: A general cardiovascular risk profile: the Framingham study, Am. J. Cardiol. **38:**46, 1976.

Kee, J. L., and Gregory, A. P.: The ABC's and mEq's of fluid imbalance in children, Nursing '74 **4:**28, 1974.

Kenigsberg, D., et al.: The coronary-prone behavior pattern in hospitalized patients with and without coronary heart disease, Psychosom. Med. **36:**344, 1974.

Kersten, L.: Chest tube drainage system—indications and principles of operation, Heart Lung **3:**97, 1974.

Khosla, T., Newcombe, R. G., and Campbell, H.: Who is at risk of a coronary? Br. Med. J. **1:**341, 1977.

Kiely, W. F.: Critical care psychiatric syndromes, Heart Lung **2:**54, 1973.

Kinney, J. M.: Energy requirements for parenteral nutrition. In Fischer, J. E., editor: Total parenteral nutrition, Boston, 1976, Little, Brown & Co.

Kintzel, K. C., et al.: Advanced concepts in clinical nursing, Philadelphia, 1972, J. B. Lippincott Co.

Klaus, M., and Fanaroff, A.: Care of the high risk neonate, Philadelphia, 1979, W. B. Saunders Co.

Knapp, M. L.: Nonverbal communication in human interaction, New York, 1978, Holt, Rinehart & Winston, Inc.

Kochar, M., et al.: Hypertension control for nurses and other health professionals, St. Louis, 1978, The C. V. Mosby Co.

Kolobow, T., Stool, E. W., Sacks, K. L., and Vurek, G. G.: Acute respiratory failure-survival following ten days' support with a membrane lung, J. Thorac. Cardiovasc. Surg. **69:**947, 1975.

Kolodny, R. C., Masters, W. H., Johnson, V. E., and Biggs, M. A.: Textbook of human sexuality for nurses, Boston, 1979, Little, Brown & Co.

Kornfeld, D. S., Simberg, S., and Malm, J. R.: Psychiatric complications of open-heart surgery, N. Engl. J. Med. **273:**287, 1965.

Korones, S. B.: High-risk newborn infants—the basis for intensive nursing care, ed. 2, St. Louis, 1976, The C. V. Mosby Co.

Kostis, J.: Patent ductus arteriosus, N. Engl. J. Med. **296:**106, 1977.

Kubler-Ross, E.: On death and dying, New York, 1976, Macmillan Inc.

Lee, M. M.: Emotional reactions to trauma, Nurs. Clin. North Am. **5:**33, 1970.

Lehman, J.: Auscultation of heart sounds, Am. J. Nurs. **72:**1242, 1972.

Levine, R. R.: Pharmacology: drug actions and reactions, Boston, 1973, Little, Brown & Co.

Light, I. J., Atherton, H. D., and Sutherland, J. M.: Decreased colonization of newborn infants with *Staphylococcus aureus* 80/81: Cincinnati General Hospital, 1960-1972, J. Infec. Dis. **131:**281, 1975.

Lillehei, R. C., et al.: The pharmacologic approach to shock, I. Defining traumatic, septic and cardiogenic shock, Geriatrics **27:**73, 1972.

Lillehei, R. C., et al.: The pharmacologic approach to shock, II.

Diagnosis of shock and the plan of treatment, Geriatrics **27:** 81, 1972.

Lindbalm, J., et al.: Coronary care units, Am. Heart J. **91:**673, 1976.

Littman, D.: Stethoscopes and auscultation, Am. J. Nurs. **72:** 1238, 1972.

Long, M. L., Scheuling, M. A., and Christian, J. L.: Cardiopulmonary bypass, Am. J. Nurs. **74:**860, 1974.

Lumb, P. D., Dalton, B., Bryan-Brown, C. W., and Donnelly, C.: An approach to intravenous feeding for the critically ill patient, Heart Lung **7:**71, 1978.

Maini, B., et al.: Cyclic hyperalimentation: an optimal technique for preservation of visceral protein, J. Surg. Res. **20:** 515, 1976.

Marchiondo, K.: CVP: the whys and hows of central venous pressure monitoring, Nurs. '74 **4:**21, 1974.

Marlow, D.: Textbook of pediatric nursing, ed. 5, Philadelphia, 1977, W. B. Saunders, Co.

Maslow, A. H.: Personality development and the self. In Hamachek, E. E., editor: The self in growth, teaching and learning, Englewood Cliffs, N.J., 1965, Prentice-Hall, Inc.

Maslow, A. H.: Toward a psychology of being, New York, 1968, Van Nostrand Reinhold Co.

Masters, W., and Johnson, V.: Human sexual response, Boston, 1966, Little, Brown & Co.

Mather, H. F., et al.: Myocardial infarction: a comparison between home and hospital care for patients, Br. Med. J. **1:** 925, 1976.

McGrath, R.: Patent ductus arteriosus, N. Engl. J. Med. **296:** 106, 1977.

Mehrabian, A.: Public places and private spaces, New York, 1976, Basic Books, Inc., Publishers.

Melia, K. M.: The intensive care unit: a stress situation? Nurs. Times **73:**17, 1977.

Meltzer, L. E., et al.: Textbook of coronary care, Philadelphia, 1973, The Charles Press, Publishers.

Merrill, S. A.: A nursing contribution to cardiac rehabilitation programs, Milit. Med. **142:**129, 1977.

Metheny, N. M., and Snively, W. D., Jr.: Nurses handbook of fluid balance, ed. 2, Philadephia, 1979, J. B. Lippincott Co.

Moore, V. B.: I.V. fluids, Nursing '73 **3:**32, 1973.

Mosby's Current Practice and Perspectives in Nursing Series: Current practice in critical care, Vol. I, St. Louis, 1979, The C. V. Mosby Co.

Mountcastle, V. B., editor: Medical physiology, vols. I-II, ed. 14, St. Louis, 1980, The C. V. Mosby Co.

Munn, H. E.: Developing and improving your communication skills, Hosp. Top. **53:**40, 1975.

Nadas, A.: Patent ductus arteriosus revisited, N. Engl. J. Med. **295:**563, 1976.

National Critical Care Institute of Education: Psychiatric liaison services, vol. 4, No. 3, Critical Care Update!, March, 1977.

National Critical Care Institute of Education: Cranial trauma; Library series, 1978, Orange, Ca.

National Critical Care Institute of Education: Blood gas and fluid-electrolyte notebook; Library series, 1979, Orange, Ca.

National Critical Care Institute of Education: Intra-aortic balloon pump; Library series, 1979, Orange Ca.

National Critical Care Institute of Education: Parenteral medication compatibility guide; Library series, 1979, Orange, Ca.

National Critical Care Institute of Education: Radiological accidents, Critical Care Update!, Orange, Ca., 1979.

National Critical Care Institute of Education: The Swan-Ganz flow directed catheter; Library series, 1979, Orange, Ca.

Naughton, J.: Accelerated restoration of cardiac patients, Cardiol. Dig. **12:**14, 1977.

Nursing '79: Nurse's guide to drugs, Hicksville, New York, 1979, Skillbook Co.

O'Brien, M. T., and Pallett, P. J.: Total care of the stroke patient, Boston, 1979, Little, Brown & Co.

O'Neill, N., and O'Neill, G.: Shifting gears, New York, 1975, Avon Books.

Pace, N. L.: Positive end-expiratory pressure (PEEP) in treating salt water near-drowning, West. J. Med. **122:**165, 1975.

Petty, T. L.: Intensive and rehabilitative respiratory care, ed. 2, Philadelphia, 1974, Lea & Febiger, p. 59.

Phibbs, B.: The cardiac arrhythmias, ed. 3, St. Louis, 1978, The C. V. Mosby Co.

Philips, K. J.: Nursing care in parenteral nutrition. In Fischer, J. E., editor: Total parenteral nutrition, Boston, 1976, Little, Brown & Co.

Phipps, W. J., Long, B. C., and Woods, N. F.: Shafer's medical-surgical nursing, ed. 7, St. Louis, 1980, The C. V. Mosby Co.

Physician's desk reference: Oradell, N.J., 1976, Medical Economics, Inc.

Picklesiner, L.: The nurse-challenging syndrome DIC, R.N. Magazine **37:**46, 1974.

Pinneo, R.: Symposium concepts in cardiac nursing, Nurs. Clin. North Am. **7:**411, 1972.

Placek, M. Y.: Territoriality and the patient's life space, Va. Nurse **45:**17, 1977.

Plum, F., and Posner, J. B.: Diagnosis of stupor or coma, Philadelphia, 1972, F. A. Davis Co.

Pyle, R. B., et al.: Clinical use of membrane oxygenator, Arch. Surg. **110:**966, 1975.

Rahe, R. H.: Epidemiological studies of life change and illness, Int. J. Psychiatry Med. **6:**133, 1975.

Rahe, R. H., and Paasikivi, J.: Psychosocial factors and myocardial infarction, J. Psychosom. Res. **15:**33, 1971.

Rahe, R. H., et al.: Subjects' recent life changes and coronary heart disease in Finland, Am. J. Psychiatry **130:**1222, 1973.

Rahe, R. H., et al.: Recent life changes, myocardial infarction, and abrupt coronary death, Arch. Intern. Med. **133:**221, 1974.

Reichle, M. J.: Psychological stress in the intensive care unit, Nurs. Digest **3:**12, 1975.

Respiratory diseases: Task Force Report, United States Department of Health, Education and Welfare, National Institutes of Health, March, 1977.

Rhodes, M. J., et al.: Alexander's care of the patient in surgery, ed. 6, St. Louis, 1978, The C. V. Mosby Co.

Ridley, M., Barrie, D., Lynn, R., and Stead, K. C.: Antibiotic-resistant *Staphylococcus aureus* and hospital antibiotic policies, Lancet **1:**230, 1970.

Roberts, F. B.: The child with heart disease, Am. J. Nurs. **72:** 20, 1972.

Roberts, S. L.: Behavioral concepts and the critically ill patient, Englewood Cliffs, N.J., 1976, Prentice-Hall, Inc.

Robinson, J. R.: Fundamentals of acid-base regulation, ed. 3, Philadelphia, 1967, F. A. Davis Co.

Rodman, M. J., and Smith, D. W.: Pharmacology and drug therapy in nursing, Philadelphia, 1979, J. B. Lippincott Co.

Rodman, T., Myerson, R. M., Lawrence, L. T., Gallagher, A. P., and Kaspar, A. J.: The physiologic and pharmacologic basis of coronary care nursing, St. Louis, 1971, The C. V. Mosby Co.

Russel, R. O., and Rackley, C. E.: Hemodynamic monitoring in a coronary intensive-care unit, New York, 1974, Futura Publishing Co., Inc.

Ryan, J. A., Jr.: Complications of total parenteral nutrition, In Fischer, J. E., editor: Total parenteral nutrition, Boston, 1976, Little, Brown & Co.

Ryschkewitsch, W. K.: How to walk in someone's shoes, some ideas toward better communication, Am. J. Med. Technol. **43**:451, 1977.

Sarason, I. G.: Abnormal psychology: the problem of maladjustive behavior, New York, 1972, Appleton-Century-Crofts.

Scalzi, C. C.: Nursing management of behavior responses following an acute myocardial infarction, Heart Lung **2**:62, 1973.

Schumer, W.: Steroids in the treatment of clinical septic shock, Ann. Surg. **184**:333, 1976.

Schumer, W., and Erve, P. R.: Cellular metabolism in shock, Circulatory Shock **2**:109, 1976.

Shapiro, B. A., Harrison, R. A., and Trout, C. A.: Clinical application of respiratory care, Chicago, 1975, Year Book Medical Publishers, Inc.

Shapiro, H. M.: Intracranial hypertension: therapeutic and anesthetic considerations, Anesthesiology **43**:445, 1975.

Sharp, M. A., et al.: Nursing in the coronary care unit, Philadelphia, 1970, J. B. Lippincott Co.

Silver, H. K., Kempe, C. H., and Bruyn, H. B.: Handbook of pediatrics, ed. 12, Los Altos, Ca., 1977, Lange Medical Publications.

Smith, C. M.: Identifying blocks to communication in health care settings and a workshop plan, J. Continuing Educ. Nurs. **8**:26, 1977.

Sorensen, K. C., and Luckmann, J.: Basic nursing: a psychophysiologic approach, Philadelphia, 1979, W. B. Saunders Co.

Spencer, R. T.: Patient care in endocrine problems, Philadelphia, 1978, W. B. Saunders Co.

Sproul, C. W., and Mullanney, P. J., editors: Emergency care: assessment and intervention, St. Louis, 1974, The C. V. Mosby Co.

Stein, R. F., et al.: A multimedia independent approach for improving the teacher-learning process in nursing, Nurs. Res. **21**:436, 1972.

Stephenson, H. E., Jr., editor: Immediate care of the acutely ill and injured, St. Louis, ed. 2, 1978, The C. V. Mosby Co.

Stross, J. K., et al.: Effectiveness of coronary care units in small community hospitals, Ann. Intern. Med. **85**:709, 1976.

Stuart, G. W., and Sundeen, S. J.: Principles and practice of psychiatric nursing, St. Louis, 1979, The C. V. Mosby Co.

Stude, C.: Cardiogenic shock, Am. J. Nurs. **74**:1636, 1974.

Sweetwood, H.: Nursing in the intensive respiratory care unit, New York, ed. 2, 1979, Springer Publishing Co., Inc.

Swift, N., and Mabel, R.: Manual of neurological nursing, Boston, 1979, Little, Brown & Co.

Sykes, M. K., McNicol, M. W., and Campbell, E. J. M.: Respiratory failure, ed. 2, Oxford, 1976, Blackwell Scientific Publications.

Taylor, J. P.: Manual of respiratory therapy, ed. 2, St. Louis, 1978, The C. V. Mosby Co.

Teres, D., Schweers, P., Bushnell, L. S., Hedley-Whyte, J., and Feingold, D. S.: Sources of *Pseudomonas aeruginosa* infection in a respiratory/surgical intensive therapy unit, Lancet **1**:415, 1973.

Tesler, M., and Hardgrove, C.: Cardiac catheterization: preparing the child, Am. J. Nurs. **73**:80, 1973.

Thiel, H. G., Parker, D., and Bruce, T. A.: Stress factors and the risk of myocardial infarction, J. Psychosom. Res. **17**:43, 1973.

Thompson, M.: Learning: a comparison of traditional and autotutorial methods, Nurs. Res. **21**:457, 1972.

Tilkian, A. G., and Conover, M. B.: Understanding heart sounds and murmurs, Philadelphia, 1979, W. B. Saunders Co.

Tilkian, S. N., Conover, M. H., and Tilkian, A. G.: Clinical implications of laboratory tests, St. Louis, 1979, The C. V. Mosby Co.

Torrex, M. R.: Educational needs of the coronary care nurse, Heart Lung, **1**:254, 1972.

Tyzenhouse, P. S.: Myocardial infarction: its effect on the family, Am. J. Nurs. **73**:1012, 1973.

Vinsant, M. O., Spence, M. I., and Chapell, D. E.: A common-sense approach to coronary care—a program, ed. 2, St. Louis, 1975, The C. V. Mosby Co.

Volicer, B. J.: Perceived stress levels of events associated with the experience of hospitalization: development and testing a measurement tool, Nurs. Res. **22**:491, 1973.

Wade, J. F.: Respiratory nursing care—physiology and technique, ed. 2, St. Louis, 1977, The C. V. Mosby Co.

Walts, L. F.: The use of muscle relaxants to facilitate crisis care. In Weil, M. H., and Shubin, H., editors: Critical care medicine handbook, New York, 1974, John N. Kolen, Inc., p. 21.

Warner, C. G.: Emergency care: assessment and intervention, St. Louis, 1978, The C. V. Mosby Co.

Watson, J. E.: Medical/surgical nursing and related physiology, Philadelphia, 1979, W. B. Saunders Co.

Weldy, N. J.: Body fluids and electrolytes—a programmed presentation, ed. 2, St. Louis, 1976, The C. V. Mosby Co.

West, N. D.: Stresses associated with I.C.U.'s affect patients, families and staff, Hospitals **49**:62, 1975.

Widmann, F. K., editor: Clinical interpretation of laboratory tests, Philadelphia, 1979, F. A. Davis Co.

Wilson, L. M.: Intensive care delirium—the effects of outside deprivation in a windowless unit, Arch. Intern. Med. **130**:225, 1972.

Woods, N. F.: Human sexuality in health and illness, St. Louis, 1979, The C. V. Mosby Co.

Woods, N. F., and Falk, S. A.: Noise stimuli in the acute care area, Nurs. Res. **23**:144, 1974.

Woods, S. L., and Mansfield, L. W.: Effect of position upon pulmonary artery and pulmonary capillary wedge pressures in noncritically ill patients, Heart Lung **5**:83, 1976.

Wu, R.: Behavior and illness, Englewood Cliffs, N.J., 1973, Prentice-Hall, Inc.

Ziegel, E. E., and Cranley, M. S.: Obstetric nursing, ed. 7, New York, 1978, Macmillian Inc.

CHAPTER 2

Anatomy, physiology, and altered regulatory mechanisms

Earle Davis

Characteristic interrelationships coexist at different stages in the normal maturation of the body and during the existence of pathologic conditions in any individual's life cycle. Since the integration of these interrelationships involves physiologic anatomy at the cellular through body system levels, potentially involving the entire field of medicine, the degree of comprehension sought in understanding these processes will determine the extent to which the individual reader will search the references beyond the minimum coverage summarized at the end of this chapter. The relative weighting of the material in this chapter is based on the premise that, although all of the body systems are important to proper integration, treatment of the critically ill patient will commonly be more involved with a limited number of these systems.

■ What are the integrative levels at which the body functions?

The cell theory states that the body is made up of *cells* (Fig. 2-1) and cell products. Although the definition of the cell as "the unit of structure, function, and heredity of which the body is composed" has the problems inherent in defining basic words, it nonetheless provides on a gross level a substantial basis for initiating discussion.

The living substance of the cell is known as *protoplasm*. It consists of a nucleus and cytoplasm and is surrounded by a plasma membrane. The nucleus exerts control over the cellular metabolic processes and transmits the genetic information. Cytoplasm constitutes that portion of the protoplasm other than the nucleus.

Tissues are collections of similar cells and cell products that are organized for the performance of a given function. The classic categories are epithelial, connective (general and special, for example, blood), muscle, and nerve.

Organs are collections of tissues organized for the performance of a given function. Examples are the stomach, for storing food, and the brain, for integrating the actions of the nervous system.

Systems are collections of organs organized for the performance of a given function. The classic categories are integumentary, musculoskeletal, circulatory, respiratory, digestive, urogenital, endocrine, and nervous.

The total energy expenditures within the body are referred to as *metabolism*. In this constant interchange of energy, there is a building up of some substances (anabolic processes) and a tearing down of others (catabolic processes).

■ What is the histologic nature of the cytoplasm and what are its functions?

Although a considerable portion of the volume of most cells consists of substances (the solutes) dissolved in water (the solvent), many undissolved substances are held in suspension. The passage of these substances through selectively permeable membranes by diffusion is known as *osmosis*.

30

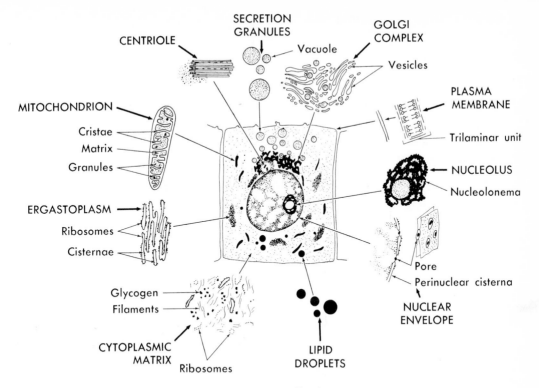

Fig. 2-1. Cell.

Some of the cytoplasmic substances are submicroscopic, that is, at the molecular level; others, known as *organelles* and *inclusions,* produce the characteristic features of specific cells as seen under the light microscope. It is significant that the submicroscopic and microscopic features of a cell and its chemical composition and pH vary according to the function(s) of the cell, for example, in the serous vs the mucous cells of a single submaxillary acinus or, more grossly, in muscle vs adipose tissue.

■ What are some examples of cytoplasmic organelles and what are their functions?

An *endoplasmic reticulum,* consisting of an irregular network of branching and anastomosing tubules and often associated with saccular structures called *cisternae,* attracts ribonucleoproteins called *ribosomes.* The ribosomes, some of which are also free in the cytoplasmic matrix, are the sites of protein synthesis.

Organelles known as *mitochondria* generate a supply of *adenosine triphosphate* (ATP), which in turn acts as an energy source for many cellular chemical transformations.

The role of the *Golgi apparatus* is to add carbohydrate to proteins brought to the organelle from the endoplasmic reticulum. The glycoprotein formed is released into the cytoplasm (as enzymes or enzymatic precursors) in membranous vesicles known as zymogen granules and lysosomes. Ultimately the *zymogen granules* are released through the cell surface to carry on their enzymatic processes extracellularly, while the *lysosomes* remain within the cell, digesting substances brought in by phagocytosis or pinocytosis.

■ What is the structural and functional nature of the nucleus?

The nucleus contains *deoxyribonucleic acid* (DNA), or genetic material that determines the specific morphologic and biochemical characteristics of each cell type and controls each cell type's metabolic activities, including the cell division phenomena of mitosis and meiosis. Although aberrations at the level of the gene and/or chromosome become manifest as both anatomic and physiologic pathologies, in general these are not of the type involved with producing the critical illnesses discussed in this book.

■ **How does the structure of the cell membrane (or plasmalemma) adapt itself for its functions?**

Cytoplasmic membranes consist, theoretically, of bimolecular layers of lipids that orient themselves with their polar groups projecting into the polar solvent (water) on either side of the membrane and their nonpolar portions buried in the membrane interior. This results in a trilaminar structure. The membrane formed by these glyco- and phospholipids contains numerous motile proteins and glycoproteins embedded in it that act as enzymes or function as pumps, moving material into and out of the cell. It is the diversity of the protein activity that gives each particular membrane its characteristic distinctions. Although the basic principles of Donnan equilibrium underlie the cell's ultimate ionic balance, the processes of dialysis, ultrafiltration, and secretion each play a part in metabolism. The ease with which solutes pass through the plasmalemma is determined by such factors as polarity (nonpolar molecules pass through readily), temperature, lipid solubility (lipid-soluble compounds pass through readily), and size. The speed with which molecules diffuse across cell membranes implies that pores with an average diameter of about 8 Å occupy less than 1% of the total plasmalemma surface area.

All nutrients must enter the cell by crossing the membrane, and all substances synthesized by the cell as useful or waste products must leave the cell through the membranes.

■ **What are pinocytosis and phagocytosis?**

The additional methods by which substances may be moved through the plasma membrane are comparable to those used by protozoa in feeding. In these phenomena a portion of the cell membrane invaginates and then detaches itself from the surface, forming an intracellular vesicle. To what extent pinocytosis may occur with smaller particles in the lining of the digestive and respiratory systems or the endothelium of capillaries is currently unknown.

The phagocytic activity of leukocytes and macrophages of the reticuloendothelial system on bacteria has long been recognized. The production of acid hydrolases contained in lysosomes is implicit to the normal functioning of phagocytic cells and may, at cell death, be considered the self-destructive "suicide sac" of many cell series.

BASIC CATEGORIES OF TISSUES

Tissues have been defined as specialized groups of cells organized for the performance of a given function. The four basic types of tissues are epithelial, connective, muscle, and nervous. The latter two will be discussed in association with their respective body systems.

Epithelial tissues
■ **What is the histologic nature of the basic types of epithelium and what are the functions of these basic types?**

Epithelial tissues (Fig. 2-2) are classified (1) according to the shape of the individual cells, that is, squamosal, cuboidal, columnar, and transitional, and (2) as to whether they constitute a single cell layer, that is, nonstratified, or multiple cell layers, that is, stratified. The term "pseudostratified" applies to modified types of nonstratified epithelium.

Cytologic metamorphosis is seen in the follicle cells of the thyroid gland. When the follicle is distended with thyroglobulin, the cells assume a squamosal shape. As the follicle shrinks because of metabolic changes, the cells successively pass through stages in which they are cuboidal, then columnar. The process of modification in the internal epithelial lining of the ureters and bladder to accommodate size changes differs somewhat from that of the thyroid gland, involving the presence of *transitional cells.*

Cilia sometimes extend from the epithelial surfaces into adjacent lumina, providing a basis for using the terms "ciliated" and "nonciliated" epithelial tissues.

Squamosal cells lining body cavities form *mesothelia,* which are more commonly called *pleura* (in the chest) and *peritoneum* (in the abdomino-

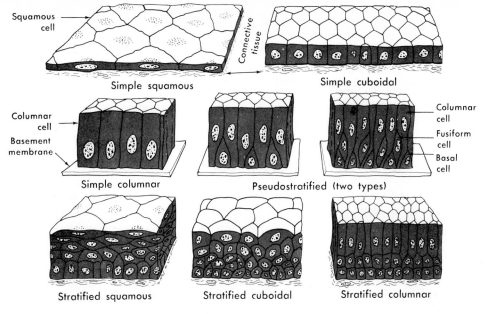

CLASSIFIED TYPES OF EPITHELIUM

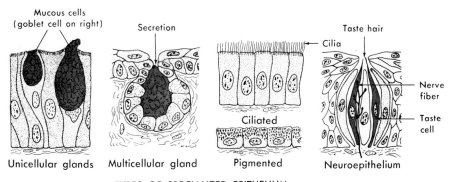

TYPES OF SPECIALIZED EPITHELIUM

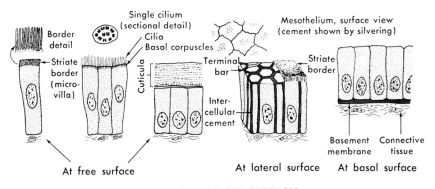

DIFFERENTIATIONS AT CELL SURFACES

Fig. 2-2. Epithelial tissue. (From Arey, L. B.: Human histology, ed. 4, Philadelphia, 1974, W. B. Saunders Co.)

pelvic cavity). As the lining of a blood vessel, squamous cells form an *endothelium*.

Epithelial tissues exposed to the external environment, that is, those at the surface of the integument, lose their moisture content and replace it with the horny substance characteristic of *keratinized epithelium*. The presence of the cornified layer diminishes the dehydration of deeper cell strata. Where epithelial cells line the body's lumina, they remain moist (nonkeratinized) and can thus participate vigorously in the process of osmosis. By comparison, the inward penetration of substances from ointments is relatively slow into keratinized surface structures.

Connective tissues

The body is composed of three materials: cells, intercellular substances, and fluids. Intercellular substances are the prime constituents of connective tissue, being largely responsible for structural strength.

The relationship between various intercellular substances can be represented schematically.

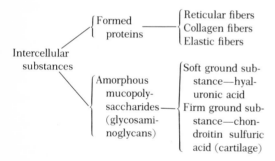

■ **What is the histologic nature of the formed intercellular substances and what are their functions?**

Both reticular and collagen fibers are formed by the crystallization of tropocollagen molecules, many of which unite to form fibrils that in turn join to form fibers. This takes place in the ground substance surrounding formative cells called *fibroblasts*, the number and arrangement of component fibrils and the relation of the fibrils to the intercellular cement being different in each particular type of connective tissue. The reticular fibers tend to form delicate networks, as in areolar tissue, and the collagen fibers form stronger

structures, such as tendons, fasciae, and aponeuroses. Whereas collagen is relatively unyielding, elastin (of which elastic fibers are composed) can be stretched to 150% of its original length.

The design of the body is such that the relative amounts of collagen and elastin in a given structure relate directly to the function of that tissue. If tissues composing the origins and insertions of muscle contained much elastin, when the muscle belly contracted, stretching of the tendon would result rather than skeletal movement. Although a moderate amount of bone separation during flexion, extension, and so forth is normal, an excessive stretching and separation of the joint would result under strain if the articular capsule of joints was composed primarily of elastin. This would result in ineffective muscle movement; therefore collagen predominates. On the contrary side, it is an advantage to have the skin loosely attached (by elastin) to the underlying epimysium in some places, for example, on the forearm, and firmly attached at others, as on the fingers.

Cicatrix is formed by a combination of the intercellular substances in which the white collagen fibers predominate. *Keloid* formation constitutes a familiar collagen disorder.

■ **What is the histologic nature of the amorphous intercellular cement and what is its function?**

The amorphous intercellular cement substances *chondroitin sulfuric acid* and *hyaluronic acid* act as adhesives to bind together cells and/or formed intercellular substances. Although chondroitin sulfuric acid is widely distributed throughout the body, it is proportionately in far greater abundance in cartilage. Since the amount of cartilaginous tissue in the body is relatively small, hyaluronic acid assumes the dominant role as the intercellular cement. Synovial fluid may be considered an example of hyaluronic acid admixed with an unusually high proportion of water. Since hyaluronidase (Wydase) decomposes the intercellular cement, it is used in injecting anesthetic drugs as an adjunct to speed up the drugs' diffusion to and through the epineurium. However, it also is equally able to break down the normal barrier of the blood vessel wall. Accordingly, rather than just producing local anesthesia, injections that include hyaluronidase may result in dramatic, sudden—and disconcertingly unexpected—total anesthesia if injected too near a vessel.

As in the case with other body tissues, intercellular substances are constantly being replaced and modified in type and composition as an adaptation to the environment. From the time of birth the process of aging consists of a gradual shift in tissue composition, with formed intercellular substances substituting more and more for amorphous substances, as is well evidenced in the wrinkling of the skin. This process is subject to considerable modification during pathologic processes, sometimes speeding up, sometimes slowing down, sometimes favoring the formation of one type of formed or amorphous intercellular substance, and sometimes sustaining another.

■ **What is the histologic nature of loose connective tissue and what are the functions of its components?**

The use of the terms "loose" and "dense" to describe connective tissue connotes the relative compactness of the formed intercellular substances collagen and elastin. The loose type is characterized by an admixture of fixed fibrous components (with their associated fibrocytes and adipose cells) and wandering cells, such as macrophages, plasma cells, mast cells, and white blood cells, that is, lymphocytes and eosinophils. Areolar tissue is the classic example. *Macrophages* (or *histiocytes*) are the equivalent of the phagocytic polymorphonuclear cells of the blood. Interstitial monocytes can develop into macrophages.

Plasma cells produce antibodies that in turn collect on mast cells. *Mast cells* produce histamine (and presumably inconsequential amounts of heparin). The combination of an antigen with an antibody causes histamine release, the subsequent contraction of smooth muscle, and the dilatation and increased permeability of capillaries that are associated with the anaphylactic phenomenon known as *allergy*. Considerable research is being done on the role of lymphocytes in rejecting tissue and organ transplants by activating destructive pyroninophilic cells.[1] Eosino-

phils phagocytize antigen-antibody complexes; basophils are also involved in allergic responses, containing about half of the histamine present in the blood.

It is generally believed that in adult tissues of mesodermal origin there typically remain a scattering of undifferentiated *mesenchymal* cells. Depending on the nature of the stimulus received, on occasion some of these cells may differentiate into tissue similar to that of the immediate area, for example, loose connective tissue. However, on receiving a different stimulus they may develop into another type of tissue of mesodermal origin, for example, bone. In addition to connective tissue and bone, mesoderm also gives rise to cartilage and muscle and, accordingly, they have the same propensities.

Normally one type of adult tissue does not form another type of adult tissue; for example, muscle does not become bone. However, under pathologic conditions such changes do occur and are referred to as *metaplasia*, a classic example being the replacement of pseudostratified ciliated columnar (respiratory) epithelium by stratified squamous epithelium.

■ **What is the histologic nature of dense connective tissue and what are the functions of its components?**
Tendons and aponeuroses

In the form of tendons and aponeuroses dense connective tissue consists primarily of collagen with an admixture of collagen and elastin. Where more stretch is desired, proportionately more elastin is present. Where more nonyielding strength is desired, proportionately more collagen is present. The cornea is basically pure collagen; the nuchal ligament is basically pure elastin. In all of these tissues the intercellular cement is hyaluronic acid. Fibroblasts secrete both the hyaluronic acid and tropocollagen, the precursor of collagen. Although the origin of elastin is uncertain, it is believed to come sometimes from fibroblasts and at other times from myofibers.

Cartilage

Cartilage is simply dense connective tissue in which chondroitin sulfuric acid has substituted for hyaluronic acid, giving greater strength and rigidity to the tissue. *Hyaline cartilage* differs from fibrocartilage basically in that in hyaline cartilage the optic index of refraction of the intercellular cement is the same as that of the fibers, but the two optic indices are different in *fibrocartilage*. In *elastic cartilage* the elastic fibers and matrix also have different optical indices. Hyaline cartilage is located at the ends of long and short bones; elastic cartilage is found in the epiglottis and ear; fibrocartilage occurs in the symphysis pubis and intervertebral discs.

Bone

Bone has achieved considerable strength, durability, and supporting power through the supplementation of the fibroelastin and cement complex with calcium phosphate salts. Since a review of the nature of both intramembranous and endochondral bone formation is essential to understanding the repair of fractures, bone transplants, malignancies, and so forth, the reader is encouraged to pursue appropriate details in a standard histology book.

THE INTEGUMENTARY SYSTEM

The integumentary system consists of the skin (Fig. 2-3) and its modifications, which in man includes hair (variously modified to include the eyelashes and eyebrows) and the nails of the fingers and toes. Skin is stratified into a more superficial epidermis and a deeper dermis. The dermis is contiguous with the underlying hypodermis which, when rich with adipose tissue, is referred to as the superficial fascia. Depending on the area of the body considered, the hypodermis rests on the epimysium or aponeurosis of muscle, periosteum, or perichondrium.

■ What is the histologic nature of the epidermis?

The *epidermis* is unique in that its major purposes are achieved by producing dead cells. In the orderly accomplishment of this objective a stratification of cell layers results, in which new cells, constantly formed in the basal layer (in the stratum germinativum) are pushed to the surface, from which they are eventually sloughed off. Since the epidermis contains no blood vessels but is dependent on diffusion from the dermis for maintenance, the osmotic gradient established produces a gradual change in the shape and chemical composition of these cells. These cytologic stratifications are identifiable centripetocentrifugally as basal stratum germinativum (for cell replication), stratum spinosum, stratum granulosum, stratum lucidum, and stratum corneum, the latter being composed of anuclear keratinized cells.

■ What is the histologic nature of the dermis?

The *dermis* is composed of a more superficial papillary layer and a deeper reticular layer, the former possessing papillae that correspond to the epidermal ridges recognized, for example, as fingerprint lines. Sensory corpuscles for touch, pressure, and temperature plus capillaries are found in the papillae. Fibers for pain reception extend into the stratum granulosum. The basic tissue of the *papillary layer* is a closely interwoven mesh composed of thin collagen and elastic fibers, plus some reticular fibers.

The *reticular layer* is a densely interlacing fibroelastic layer varying from less than 0.5 mm (in the eyelid) to 4.0 mm or more (on the back). The roots of hair, sebaceous glands, and sweat glands originate in this layer.

■ What is the histologic nature of the subcutaneous layer, the hypodermis?

In adipose individuals considerable fat is stored in the *hypodermis*, or *superficial fascia*, and the layer may attain considerable thickness. With lesser amounts of fat the layer is thin and consists of a greater abundance of fibroelastic tissue.

■ What is the importance of the keratinized layer?

The horny nature of the stratum corneum acts as a physical barrier to the entrance of chemicals and foreign objects, such as splinters and disease-producing organisms (whole bodies or parts thereof). It also acts as a physical barrier to water, making it possible to bathe either in salt water, without losing water, or in fresh water, without the body becoming swollen. On the other hand, the use of dermal ointments indicates that the fact that a certain degree of absorption takes place through the skin is of therapeutic advantage.

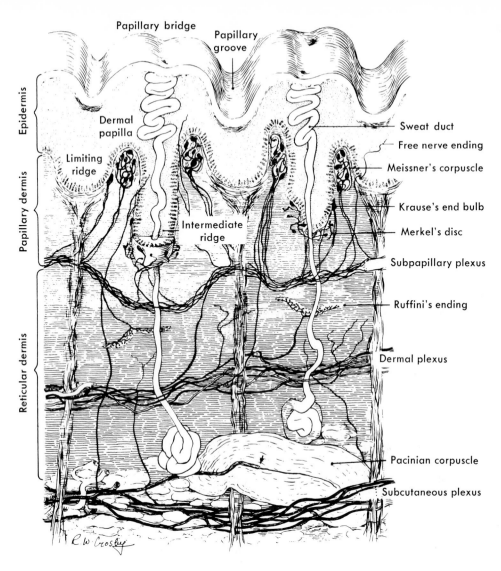

Fig. 2-3. Skin. (From Mountcastle, V. B.: Medical physiology, ed. 14, vol. I, St. Louis, 1980, The C. V. Mosby Co.)

■ **Of what diagnostic value is the skin in medicine?**

Many allergies and infectious diseases are identifiable by the skin rashes they produce. In certain vitamin deficiencies and hormonal imbalances the texture of the skin assumes characteristic features. The color of the skin may indicate jaundice, cyanosis, infection, hormonal imbalance, or malignancy. Skin temperature and/or the relative amounts of moisture are of diagnostic value also. In the event that the patient is unable to communicate or in the case of a cadaver, the character of the skin is often of value in determining the sites of mechanical trauma, burns, and frostbite.

■ How do skin wounds heal?[2]

In a V-shaped wound extending into the hypodermis some fibrin forms near the bottom, and the epidermis soon starts to grow down into the groove. About a week later the epidermis has extended well down the sides of the slit, attaching to the adjacent healthy tissue. Meanwhile, at the junction between the dermis and hypodermis a ridge of new tissue forms from fibroblasts and capillaries derived from the subcutaneous tissues. By the end of the second week the epidermal downgrowths on the two sides meet in the center, only to be pushed outward (toward the surface) during the next 2 weeks by the proliferating ridge until the area is flattened out.

■ What are the general categories of skin grafts?

Regardless of the type of tissue transplanted, transplants are classified as autologous grafts, homografts, or heterografts. In *autologous* grafts the tissue, usually skin, is moved from one part of the body to another site on the same individual. In *homografts* (or *allografts*) the tissue is transplanted from another individual of the same species. In *heterografts* the tissue is transplanted from another species. Homografts and heterografts, like skin and bone, do not "take" but are sometimes used as temporary filling until the patient can regenerate the tissue. Heart, lung, and kidney transplants are (hopefully) permanent.

■ What are the two general methods used in autologous grafting?

One method is to move skin from one part of the body to another without the transplant tissue ever being completely separated from its blood supply. There are two versions of this procedure. One is by "walking" the graft tissue from its original to its intended site by a series of retransplantations with a pedicle at one end of the graft being left connected to its original blood supply until the other portion has established new vascular connections. Then the earlier pedicle is transected, a new one is created, and the patch is relocated again with the newly created pedicle. A

modification of this method is to bring one part of the body close to another, freeing up the graft from the donor site, except for its pedicle, and suturing the graft to its recipient site. The transplant tissue is permitted to establish new anastomoses with the subjacent tissue of the recipient site before the pedicle is detached.

A second method is to use free skin grafts.

■ How are skin grafts performed and what is the rationale?

There are two general types of autologous skin grafts: split grafts and full-thickness grafts. In *split grafts* the skin to be transplanted may be cut at a level about halfway down the dermis and placed on the denuded area. Temporarily the transplanted tissue will derive its nourishment by diffusion from the raw surface to which it is transposed. In about a week capillaries in the graft bed will connect with capillaries of the transplant.

Concurrent with the take of the graft, the denuded area from which the new graft was taken will be recovered with new epidermis that grows from the germinal cells of the external sheath of hair follicles and the ducts of sweat glands.[1]

In *full-thickness grafts* both dermis and epidermis are transplanted.

■ How is recovery of burned areas accomplished histologically?

In moderate burns the dermis may not be destroyed. Repair in these cases is comparable to that experienced in areas from which split grafts are removed, that is, as long as viable hair follicles and/or bases of the sweat glands remain, reepithelialization will take place. In more severe burns if grafting is not done, cicatrix will form, the fibroelastic plug being derived from fibroblasts located in the subcutaneous tissue and/or brought in on the surface of local capillaries.

CARDIOVASCULAR SYSTEM

The cardiovascular system is committed to expediting the exchange of gases and of food and waste products involved in metabolism. This is achieved with the aid of a pump (the heart), a system of tubes (the blood vessels), and the blood itself. The food (energy) supply is made potentially available by being brought into the digestive tract and acted on by various enzymes. From

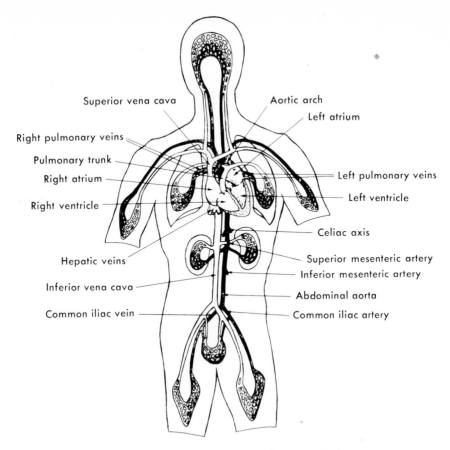

Fig. 2-4. Schematic of systemic and pulmonary circulation.

there on, for further appropriate distribution, the body depends on the cardiovascular system. Less than 2% of the metabolic waste products are finally returned (by the bloodstream) to the digestive tract for elimination. Other by-products are eliminated via the lungs, the kidneys, and the skin, all of which are in turn dependent on the cardiovascular system for normal functioning (Fig. 2-4). Depending on the degree of finite knowledge of vessel distribution sought, the reader should select appropriate references.

■ What is the nature of plasma and what are its roles?

Blood consists of *cellular elements* and a liquid, *plasma*, in which the cellular elements are suspended. After an anticoagulant is added, if blood is permitted to stand or is centrifuged, the cells settle to the bottom 45% of the tube, constituting the *hematocrit reading*. The supernatant, 55%, is the plasma, which is 90% water by volume. When the fibrinogen is removed from plasma, the remaining fluid is known as *serum*.

A normal sedimentation (sed) rate does not exclude the possibility of disease, but further study is indicated if the rate is increased. Among the conditions associated with a rapid sed rate are: extensive inflammation, pregnancy, tuberculosis, active rheumatic fever, and all types of shock. A slow sed rate is usually found in the newborn, polycythemia, congestive heart failure, and allergic conditions.

As the principal solvent in the blood, naturally most of plasma's functions relate to acting as a transport mechanism for respiratory gases, food, wastes, antibodies, hormones, electrolytes, and proteins. In addition, it acts as a suspensory agent for the blood's cellular elements and provides for fluid balance and temperature regulation, the latter being closely tied to the phenomenon of perspiring.

Plasma proteins are classified as albumins and globulins, and they are synthesized by the liver, except for the immunologically related gamma globulins, which are formed in the lymph nodes and spleen. Proteins used in cell synthesis are usually manufactured locally rather than drawn from the plasma proteins. Although proteins are the most abundant solute by weight, *osmolarity* depends on the number of particles. Accordingly sodium (144 mM/L) and secondly chloride (100 mM/L) are the most important determinants of plasma osmolarity, proteins falling in line with calcium (at 2.5 mM/L) after bicarbonate (4.4 mM/L) and potassium (4.4 mM/L).

The heart

■ What is the basic course of the blood through the heart?

It is convenient clinically to speak of the heart as being composed of right and left halves, the blood vessels of the right half consisting of the venae cavae. After passing into the first chamber, the right atrium, blood passes through the right atrioventricular (tricuspid) valves to the right ventricle, and from there to the pulmonary trunk, backflow from which is prevented by semilunar valves. The trunk splits into right and left pulmonary arteries, which conduct the blood to the right and left lungs for an exchange of gases. Purified blood returns via the pulmonary veins to the left atrium. The right ventricle, pulmonary vessels, lungs, and left atrium constitute the *pulmonary system* of circulation. From the left atrium, blood passes through the left atrioventricular (bicuspid or mitral) valves into the left ventricle. In both the right and left halves of the heart the atrioventricular valves function to prevent regurgitation from the ventricles into the respective atria. From the left ventricle, blood flows out the aorta to be distributed to the nonpulmonary portions of the body, backflow being prevented by semilunar valves. The left ventricle, the aorta and its subdivisions, the associated venous network (including capillaries) returning blood to the heart, and the right atrium constitute the *systemic system*. Depending on the degree of finite knowledge of vessel distribution sought, the reader should select appropriate references on the systemic and/or pulmonary system(s).

■ On what does the heart depend for its mechanical effectiveness?

To derive its force as a pump the heart depends on the effective contraction of the cardiac muscle and the proper functioning of its valvular system. Effective contraction involves (1) proper stimulation of the cardiac myofibers, (2) the normal sequence of events associated with contraction of myofibers, and (3) an efficient transmission of the contractive force to propel the blood.

■ What is the nature of the contractile force of cardiac muscle?

The physiologic chemistry of cardiac myofiber contraction is basically similar to that of striated muscle, where the phenomenon has been worked out in greatest detail. Depolarization of the myofiber's T-tubal system results in the critical release of calcium ions among the actinomycin filaments, activating adenosine triphosphatase (ATPase). The ultimate splitting of ATP and the associated release of energy cause the change in the shape of the myosin cross-bridges, which results in fiber contraction. Although the mechanism whereby the electric charge causes calcium ion to be released is unknown, clinically a proper balance of available ionic calcium is extremely important.

■ How is the rate of the heartbeat controlled?

In in vitro experiments dissociated heart cells each beat with their own independent rhythm. When two of them are joined, they assume the speed of the faster one. This intrinsic phenomenon is known as *autorhythmicity*. However, in the normal heart integration is achieved via the sinoatrial (SA) and atrioventricular (AV) nodes, the former located where the superior vena cava joins the right atrium and the latter situated on the posterior junction of the right atrium and ventricle near the interatrial septum.

The SA node is the normal pacemaker for the entire heart. Special conduction fibers travel from the SA node throughout the right and left atria and also from SA node to the AV node. Atrial systole lasts approximately 0.1 seconds. There is a 0.1-second delay before the AV node is activated by atrial excitation, permitting the atria to contract before the ventricles do.

The AV node impulse travels down the interventricular bundle of His and spreads out in the Purkinje fibers. The impulse spreads over the right and left ventricles, resulting in ventricular systole, which lasts approximately four times as long as atrial systole—about 0.38 seconds.

■ What are the etiologies of some of the anomalous heartbeats?

Atrial fibrillation is associated with the development of ectopic atrial foci. *Ventricular fibrillation* is associated with unusual conduction routes, so that the main impulse constantly meets an area that is no longer refractory. For example, in electrocution the normal pathways conducting impulses of 60 beats/min are overwhelmed by 60 Hz.

In *partial cardiac blocks* only a fraction of the impulses reach the ventricles. As a consequence, there may be a rhythm of 85 beats/min in the atria, but only 65 beats/min in the ventricles, resulting in faulty filling. In *complete cardiac block* the atria may maintain a rhythm of 75 beats/min and the ventricles 25 to 40 beats/min, the two rhythms being completely independent.

Cardiac blackouts are associated with recurrent complete blocks, resulting in decreased flow to the brain and fainting.

■ What does the term "PQR-ST complex" mean?

The electromagnetic fields created by the beating of the heart are recorded as the electrocardiogram (ECG). In it P equals atrial depolarization; QRS, ventricular depolarization; and T, ventricular repolarization. Because it is masked by the QRS complex, atrial repolarization is not seen. Discussion of the PQR-ST waves receives appropriate detailed analysis in standard textbooks of physiology and/or cardiology.

■ What phenomena are associated with diastole and systole?

Typically when the terms "systole" and "diastole" are used without an adjective, for example, "during systole," reference is made to ventricular rather than atrial systole or diastole.

In *late diastole* the AV valves open, and 80% of ventricular filling takes place before atrial systole. This is of considerable physiologic importance during periods of rapid heartbeat as it allows the major portion of ventricular filling to occur despite the overall reduction of beat time. The amount of blood in the ventricles just prior to systole is known as *end-diastolic volume*. During *systole* most of the blood is ejected rapidly, followed by a tapering off. The amount of blood remaining after contraction is the *end-systolic volume*. *Early systole* is the rapid ventricular filling taking place after the AV valves open.

■ What are the common heart sounds and their causes?

In the normal heartbeat, *lub-dub,* the lub is caused by closure of the AV valves and coincides with the later part of the QRS wave. The dub is caused by closure of the semilunar valves and coincides with the T wave at the onset of diastole.

Murmurs are heard when the normal, smooth flow becomes turbulent. A *systolic murmur* results from a narrowed pulmonary or aortic valve or a hole in the interventricular septum. *Diastolic murmurs* are caused by faulty valve closure. *Atrial murmurs,* heard laterally, are produced by a patent foramen ovale.

■ How much is the normal cardiac output?

Cardiac output is determined by stroke volume and rate. The normal volume is about 60 ml/stroke, and the normal rate about 70 beats/min, thus totaling well over 4000 ml/min. Since the average person has about 5 L of blood—the weight of the blood equals about 7% of the body weight—this means that, at rest, all of the blood presumably passes through the heart once each minute, allowing that flow is sluggish in some areas and rapid in others and that the rate of flow in a given area varies with variations in physiologic conditions. The concept of "a gallon a minute" is more meaningful to those on the English measuring system.

■ What mechanisms are involved in modifying the cardiac output?

Among the factors modifying the cardiac activity are: a series of sensors, the autonomic nervous system, restricting blood flow to certain organs according to the type of activity, and response according to Starling's law of the heart (see below). *Baroreceptors* found in the carotid sinus and aortic arch respond reflexly to changes in arterial pressure, activating the sympathetic nerves to speed up the heart (if pressure is inadequate) or the parasympathetic nerves to reduce the speed (and the pressure). Reaching the heart by the vagus nerve, the parasympathetic nerves cause the SA and AV nodes to reach their thresholds more slowly. The sympathetic nerves, via the cardiac plexus, cause the pacemakers to reach their thresholds more rapidly. If both sympathetic and parasympathetic nerves are cut, the heartbeat goes to about 100 beats/min, illustrating the dominance of the parasympathetic system here.

According to *Starling's law of the heart*, there is a direct proportion between the diastolic volume and the contractile force of the following systole. With increased end volume there is increased stroke volume and vice versa. However, overstretching will produce a decreased contractile force and a reduction in stroke volume.

In exercise, because of increased heart rate and stroke volume, the flow of blood to skeletal muscle is increased. Additional compensation consists of decreasing the flow to the kidneys and decreasing the total peripheral resistance.

Arteries

■ **How does the structure of arteries adapt them for their functions?**

Arteries and veins share the structural pattern of being composed of an outer tunica adventitia, an interposed tunica media, and an inner tunica intima.

In arteries the *tunica adventitia* is a relatively thin fibroelastic layer.

The *tunica media* varies with the size of the artery. In large arteries it is characterized by many layers of elastic membranes (to absorb the shock of the systolic pressure and begin the establishment of a smooth, steady blood flow to the capillaries). In smaller ("muscular") arteries, the tunica media consists of many layers of smooth muscle cells. There are gradual admixtures of elastic fibers and muscle cells in the tunica media of intermediate-sized vessels. The tunica media aids

further in absorbing the pulsatile nature of the blood flow. Its musculature is under the control of the sympathetic nervous system.

The *tunica intima* is lined with a single layer of *squamosal endothelium* and may possess some subendothelial tissue.

■ **How is the structure of arterioles adapted to their functions?**

As compared with arteries, the major modification of the three basic tunicae in arterioles is the prominence of the purely muscular tunica media. Relative to the lumen, the vessel wall is thicker than in any other blood vessel.

Although the elastic and muscular arteries do much toward removing the pulsatile nature of the blood flow, the sympathetic nerves, reacting to baro- and chemoreceptors, ultimately regulate peripheral resistance to meet local needs by setting the diameter of the arterioles (via the muscles of the tunica media). If less blood is needed, the medullary cardiovascular center increases sympathetic activity, and less blood passes through the narrowed arterioles; if more blood is needed, the sympathetic nerves are deactivated, and more blood passes through the dilated arterioles. There are probably also local effects produced by carbon dioxide (CO_2), lactic acid, epinephrine, angiotensin, and vasopressin.

In *surgical shock* there is a dilatation of the arteriolar bed, possibly from histamine released from injured tissues. The associated decrease in blood pressure causes a weak, rapid pulse and increased respiration.

Medically vasoconstriction may be brought about by the use of epinephrine and other sympathomimetic drugs. The vasodilatation sought for *pectoral angina* is induced with the aid of amyl nitrite.

■ **What factors control the arterioles?**

An obvious response to exercise is the increased blood supply to the muscles known as *hyperemia,* the increase in blood flow being directly proportional to increased activity. Unknown chemical factors probably underlie the cause of the phenomenon. Sympathetic fibers maintain a characteristic tone in the arterioles of all organs, usually releasing epinephrine as the neurohumor. (The amount of epinephrine released from the adrenal medulla is normally of no physiologic consequence.) Increased sympathetic activity causes increased vasoconstriction; decreased sympathetic activity results in dilatation. However, at the arterioles of skeletal muscles sympathetic fibers release acetylcholine (ACh), which causes vasodilatation and increased flow.

At the moment of an injury mast cells located peripheral to the tunica adventitia of the vessels release histamine. This causes vasodilatation, possibly as an evolutionary effort to assure an immediate blood plethora that might be associated with rapidly revitalizing the traumatized area.

■ How do the structure and distribution of capillaries adapt them to their functions?

The thin-walled structure, ubiquitous distribution, and total surface area provided by the capillaries are direct reflections of their functions in providing sites for the exchange of metabolites. Although the capillary lumen is only wide enough to pass the red blood cells (RBC's) in single file and although the tubule itself averages only 1 mm long, since no cell is more than 0.005 inch from a capillary, normally an adequate exchange of metabolites occurs. However, the ubiquitous network results in a total storage capacity of 7 L, considerably more than the 5 L constituting the total blood volume. An explanation as to why one "does not bleed to death into the capillaries" relates to the fact that most persons have a dual capillary system: arteriovenous shunts and true capillaries. The shunts connect arterioles and venules directly. The true capillaries are like branches of the shunts, each possessing a sphincter at its origin that opens and closes intermittently. At any one time most of the capillaries are closed, containing little, if any, blood. Although the total cross-sectional area of the capillary system is 800 times that of the aorta, the capillary flow rate is only 0.4 mm/sec, compared with 320 mm/sec in the aorta. The single layer of endothelial cells constituting the wall provides a minimum osmotic barrier consistent with retaining the circulating formed elements (RBC's, WBC's,

and platelets) and preventing an infinite loss of fluids to the tissue spaces. It is not clear to what extent the diffusion of solutes is carried out from endothelial cell to subjacent cell as opposed to diffusion through the interstices between adjacent endothelial cells.

■ Why is there an exchange between the capillaries and the tissue fluid?

In arteries and arterioles and in veins and venules the thickness of the walls prevents significant osmotic exchange between the blood and adjacent extravascular cells. For capillaries the potentials for exchange that exist depend on the reciprocal interaction of blood pressure and osmotic strength. In the proximal end of the capillary there is typically found a relatively high blood pressure and a high concentration of crystalloids, plus the normal concentration of proteins. The capillary wall acts much like a highly porous filter, and a process of *ultrafiltration* takes place in which much of the plasma fluid and crystalloids leave the capillary, but the protein molecules remain because of their relatively large size. By the time the blood has reached the midpoint of the capillary the continued pressure of the capillary wall and the loss of fluid have further reduced the blood pressure and considerably elevated the concentration of the proteins, producing an equilibrium state. In the area of the distal capillary the difference in plasma protein and interstitial concentration produces an osmotic flow greater than the effect of the remaining capillary hydrostatic pressure, resulting in a return of crystalloids and water to the capillary and a reestablishment of a plasma concentration resembling the arteriolar state. Allowed for in the latter is the interposed exchange of metabolites of total equivalent isosmotic strength.

Any physiologic state, normal or pathologic, that increases the blood pressure causes the ultrafiltration to predominate, and edema results, as in exercise. Decreased blood pressure results in a movement of fluids from the tissues into the bloodstream. When protein synthesis decreases, as in liver disease, the resultant drop in plasma protein concentration causes an increased fluid accumulation in the tissues, edema. Edema may also result from changes in capillary permeability (as in trauma) or from obstruction of the lymphatics associated with node infection. Increased filtration from the capillaries as a result of elevated venous or capillary pressure may be the chief feature of ventricular failure.

Normally the interstitial fluid volume is three to four times the plasma volume.

Veins

Systemic blood pressure drops steadily on its return to the heart; the values are arteries, 120/80 mm Hg; arterioles, 35 to 40 mm Hg; capillaries and venules, 15 mm Hg; veins, 10 mm Hg; and right atrium, 0 to 5 mm Hg.

■ What is the structural nature of veins?

Although veins are composed of the same basic layers that characterize arteries, the wall is proportionately thinner and the lumen correspondingly larger, the pressure being only one tenth that in the aorta. Compared with arteries, the tunica adventitia is proportionately much thicker; the tunica media is proportionately small and accordingly possesses less muscle. Unlike arteries, many veins possess valves to prevent the reflux of blood.

■ What part do veins play in regulating blood pressure?

The return of blood to the heart is constantly favored by the movements of the thorax and abdomen during respiration. During exercise veins are compressed by the adjacent musculature and, aided by the presence of valves, propel the venous blood toward the heart. Stimulation of the medullary cardiovascular center activates the venous as well as the arterial side of the circulatory system, raising the pressure within the veins. Consistent with the view that there is a direct relation between the diastolic volume of the heart and the force of contraction of the following systole—Starling's law of the heart—the rate of venous return directly relates to determining the stroke volume and in turn to determining atrial pressure. However, concurrently the increased sympathetic activity also causes a more rapid and stronger ventricular contraction, resulting in a more complete ventricular ejection—lower end-diastolic volume. Accordingly, during exercise,

although the blood pressure goes up, the normal heart usually does not distend.

Lymphatic system
■ How are the structure and distribution of the lymphatic vessels related to their functions?

Histologically the lymphatic vessels begin peripherally as blind tubules, resembling capillaries in that they consist only of an endothelium. Their continuations toward the heart also resemble their venous counterparts in the relative increase in size of the tubules and associated tunicae (intima, media, and adventitia). As in the case of veins, these vessels are classified as superficial and deep and generally form chains that accompany the arteriovenous bundles. While they are also similar to veins in that they possess valves as an augmentation to lymph flow, they have in addition a series of nodes dispersed along their courses.

The lymphatic vessels from all of the lower half of the body and from the left upper half of the body drain into the junction of the left subclavian and left internal jugular veins. Lymphatic vessels from the right upper half of the body drain into the junction of the right subclavian and right internal jugular veins.

Over most of the body the lymphatic vessels act as adjuncts to the veins in returning tissue fluid to the heart. Once the tissue fluid enters the lymphatic vessels, it is called *lymph*. Compared with venous plasma, lymph is relatively rich in lipids and proteins, the protein molecules being of small size unless intercellular disruption of endothelium occurs, as in inflammation.

The nodes interspersed along the lymphatic chain act as filtering areas and add lymphocytes to the lymph. Lymphatic vessels that originate in the villi of the small intestine are called *lacteals*. Although they return a small amount of the local tissue fluid, their principal function is to transport lipids into the circulatory system in the form of *chyle*. They return collectively to nodes known as the *cisterna chyli*, which join the *thoracic duct* in returning their contents to the junction of the left subclavian and left internal jugular veins.

IMMUNE SYSTEM

■ Of what is the body's immune system composed?

The body's defense system may be in the nature of response at the level of the whole individual, for example, flight or fight, or at the level of the cell. At the cellular level the defense may be by way of forming acids, for example, HCl of the stomach, by phagocytosis, or by the development of an immune system, the latter often preparing the invader for consumption by phagocytosis.

During embryonic development the body comes to recognize its various organic components as being parts of itself, that is, to recognize its own particular species of carbohydrates, fats, and proteins, as well as recognizing food and other substances transmitted by the placenta. After birth many of the new substances encountered are similar enough to components of the prenatal environment and fetus to be recognized as being compatible. In fact some organic and inorganic substances, even though foreign, for example, stainless steel, plastic prostheses, and suture thread, may be universally tolerated and may not induce immune reactions. In other cases there may be universal immune responses, for example, against the toxins of food poison. Then there are situations in which a certain portion of the population will display an immune reaction to the presence of a given foreign substance—the *responders*—while other segments of the population will not react—the *nonresponders*.

Antigens (Ag's) are substances capable of producing an immune response. They may be in the nature of particular matter, for example, bacteria or RBC's of the wrong (blood) type, or of solutions, for example, toxins from bacteria, mushrooms, or venoms. *Antibodies (Ab's)*, the gamma globulins of the serum, are secreted by lymphocytes and (principally) by plasma cells to counteract the antigens and are, therefore, called *immunoglobulins*, or *Ig's*.

There are two types of lymphocytes, T lymphocytes (or T cells) and B lymphocytes (or B cells), named according to their origins. T lymphocyte is the term applied to thymocytes once they leave the thymus. B lymphocytes are formed in bone marrow, lymph nodes, gut-associated lymphatic tissue (GALT), and the spleen. About 95% of the lymphocytes of the peripheral blood are recirculating cells, with only 5% being derived as fresh components when the lymph is returned from lymphoid tissue. In the peripheral blood about 75% of the lymphocytes are T cells and 25% are B cells, with the majority being small—vs medium and large—lymphocytes representing what are referred to as memory cells. While the genetic mechanisms are still unresolved,[3] it is currently thought that each virgin T and B cell has secreted onto the outer surface of its plasmalemma an antibody that is genetically programmed to react with a specific antigen. Theoretically each of the body's T and B cells is capable of defending the body against some specific antigen. (Some authorities would argue that the substance on the surface of T cells is an antibody-like substance rather than a real immunoglobulin.) Prior to encountering their appropriate antigen, the T and B cells are referred to as *virgin cells*. When the T or B cell encounters its appropriate antigen, it is stimulated to undergo cloning, in what is known as a *primary response*. From the clones two populations of cells are produced: effector cells and memory cells. *Effector cells* produce an immediate immune response and, as short-lived lymphocytes, survive an average of several weeks to months. For T cells this consists of producing killer cells and helper cells (see Immune System Chart A,3). For B cells it involves the formation of clones producing either IgM or IgG (see Immune System Chart B,3 and the section on the types of immunoglobulins). Actually the clones that produce IgM are B lymphoblasts. About a week after the B lymphoblasts have been producing cells (and IgM), some of the cells metamorphose into plasmablasts and begin producing IgG. The plasmablasts, of course, mature into adult cells, mitoses occurring every 6 hours at the height of an infection. Plasma cells have a life span of about 1 to 2 weeks. The relative quantities of IgM produced by such cloning B cells peak in about 2 weeks and essentially terminate in 3 weeks (Fig. 2-5). The production of IgG peaks in about 3 weeks, then rapidly declines. Considering the average longevity of mankind, typically the individual produces enough antibody to overcome the first at-

IMMUNE SYSTEM CHART

A. T lymphocytes
  1. Formed in thymus and go to lymph nodes and spleen
  2. There are genetically determined, specific antibody-producing T and B cells for every possible antigen. They develop a coating of specific antibody before encountering the antigen.

  3. After encounter with antigen, T cells form blasts $\xrightarrow[\text{form nodules}]{\text{proliferate and}}$

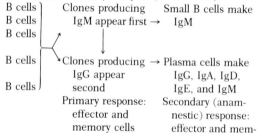

  4. T cell killer cells $\xrightarrow[\text{antigen}]{\text{contact}}$ Lymphokines → For example MIF, MAF, neutrophilic chemotactic factor, interferon, and lymphocytotoxins
  5. T cell helper cells (see B,3 below)
B. B lymphocytes
  1. Formed in bone marrow, lymph nodes, Peyer's patches, GALT, spleen, and so forth
  2. Genetically programmed; has coating of specific antibody before encountering antigen
  3. Activated by T helper cell humors directly or by antigen-antibody complex (substance X)
    a. Noncomplexed antigen floats to   B cells ⎫ Clones producing   Small B cells make
    b. T helper cell humor floats to   B cells ⎪   IgM appear first →   IgM
    c. Noncomplexed antigen transferred by   B cells ⎪
       macrophage to   ⎬
    d. Substance X floats from or transferred   B cells ⎪ Clones producing → Plasma cells make
       physically by T helper cell to   ⎪   IgG appear   IgG, IgA, IgD,
    e. Substance X floats from or transferred   B cells ⎭   second   IgE, and IgM
       physically by T helper cell to macro-   Primary response: Secondary (anam-
       phage, then transferred to   effector and   nestic) response:
                                                           memory cells   effector and mem-
                                                           formed   ory cells formed

tack and recover, although the "battle time" is longer in the primary response than in subsequent encounters with the same antigen. This is true whether the foreign substance be in the nature of bacteria or a skin graft.

Coincident with and subsequent to the first encounter many of the T and B cells become inactive *memory cells,* remaining distributed in lymphoid tissue throughout the body, seemingly just waiting for the next encounter with the appropriate antigen—waiting to produce a secondary response.

The reaction to a second encounter, the *sec-ondary response,* is different in T vs B cells. For T cells the reaction by *memory cells* consists of simply producing more clones of killer and/or helper cells appropriate to the recurring antigen. However (as seen in Fig. 2-5 and B,3 on the Immune System Chart), for B cells the amount, pattern, and nature of antibody produced as a result of memory cell activity is significantly different from the primary response. Therefore the secondary response for B cells is referred to as an *anamnestic response.* In this case the onset of IgM and IgG production is more rapid, with IgM reaching a slightly higher titer than in the pri-

IMMUNE SYSTEM CHART—CONT'D

C. Immune reactions
  1. Cell mediated
    a. By lymphokines (as in A, 4)
    b. By phagocytosis
      (1) By macrophages, including reticuloendothelial cells
      (2) By WBC's
        (a) Neutrophils—most active WBC in first phase of inflammatory response
        (b) Monocytes—become macrophages outside of the blood vessels; as macrophages they dominate the inflamatory response after about 12 hours
        (c) Eosinophils—important in certain parasitic infections and in destroying antigen-antibody complexes
        (d) Basophils—moderately phagocytic
  2. Humoral (as in B,3)
    a. By T cell helpers that bind Ig's that may be transferred directly to B cells or indirectly via macrophages (T cells = 75% of peripheral lymphocytes; B cells = 25% lymphocytes)
    b. By B cells via primary and secondary responses
D. Courses of action of immunoglobulins
  1. Neutralize specific toxins (precipitins) by combining with them
  2. Complexing of Ig's and virus renders virus unable to attach to plasmalemma and virus dies
  3. Specific ⟶ Mast cells $\xrightarrow{\text{arrival of antigen}}$ Merocrine ⟶ Anaphylaxis $\begin{cases}\nearrow \text{Smooth m. contraction} \\ \searrow \text{Capillary dilatation}\end{cases}$
     IgE's ⟶ Basophils   Histamine release
  4. Assist in preparing foreign substances for phagocytosis
    a. Opsonization: Ig's rough up bacterial surface, making it sticky
    b. Complement: when added to antigen-antibody complex causes cytolysis
    c. Agglutination serum Ab's (agglutinins) cause various particulate antigens (agglutinogens, for example, bacteria and foreign RBC's) to clump
  5. Phagocytosis: prepares antigens for consumption (phagocytosis) by WBC's and macrophages, including reticuloendothelial cells

mary response and declining in about 10 days to 2 weeks. However IgG production, while also occurring earlier than in the primary response, becomes several thousandfold greater than in the primary response and lasts much longer.

■ How do T lymphocytes function?

As indicated in the preceding, T cells produce effector cells and memory cells, the effector cells being of two types: killer cells and helper cells (see Immune System Chart A,3). When a *T lymphocyte killer cell* has been stimulated by an appropriate antigen, it forms a clone of cells that produce *lymphokines* that physically act over short distances. Among the dozen activities attributed to lymphokines are producing (1) a macrophage migration inhibiting factor (MIF) for keeping macrophages at the site of infection, (2) chemotatic factors to attract basophils, (3) interferon, and (4) lymphotoxins. Interferon, which is produced by macrophages as well as T killer cells, protects susceptible host cells from translating viral-coded messages and is host-species specific; that is, human interferon protects human cells, not mouse cells, and vice versa. Lymphotoxins are generalized cytotoxins released onto the appropriate antigen when it is encountered. Killer cell lymphokines are also involved in graft rejection and in the destruction of cancer cells, since the targets involved are recognized as being foreign bodies. Once the breakdown or neutralization of antigen is instituted by the immune system, macrophages and granulocytic WBC's assume the responsibility of "cleaning up."

IMMUNOGLOBULINS

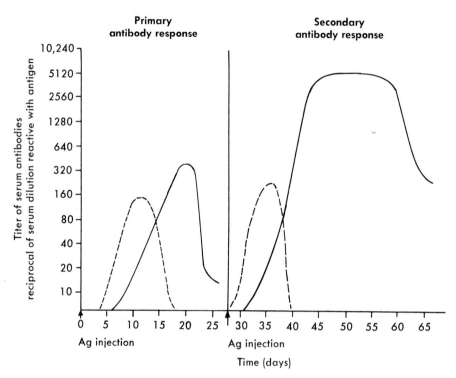

Fig. 2-5. Hypothetical primary and secondary antibody responses. (Modified and reproduced with permission from Bigley, N. J.: Immunologic fundamentals. Copyright © 1975 by Year Book Medical Publishers, Inc., Chicago.)

The majority of antigens do not have the ability to directly stimulate B cells to form antibody without the participation of T cells. However, if an antigen reacts with an appropriately programmed *T lymphocyte helper cell,* microhumoral substances might be released (see Immune System Chart B,3,b), and/or antigen-antibody complexes may be formed as a result of the interaction between antigen and antibody. For purposes of discussion an *antigen-antibody complex* may be referred to as *substance X.* Among the fates of substance X, two are listed on the Immune System Chart under B,3, specifically as d and e. Substance X may detach from the helper cell and simply float to an appropriately programmed B cell, or it may be transferred physically. However substance X more commonly passes from the

T cell helper to a macrophage, only to be relayed to an appropriate B cell. Or the T cell helper may, by physical contact, directly relay substance X to an appropriate B cell. Any of the mechanisms in B,3,a to B,3,e on the Immune System Chart can result in the B cell forming a clone of IgM- and/or IgG-producing blastic cells in the form of a primary response. As indicated previously, when the antigen is contacted again, blastic B lymph memory cells produce a secondary (anamnestic) response, in which B cells produce IgM and plasma cells make IgG, IgM, IgA, IgD, and IgE.

■ How do lymphocytes function?

While the preceding discussion of T cells per force included coverage of most of the B cell activities, there is still one more modus operandi to cover. As indicated on the Immune System Chart under B,3,a, only certain antigens may float unassisted by T cells or macrophages in the plasma or interstitial fluid to an appropriate, acceptable B cell, form antigen-antibody complexes, and stimulate the B cell by a primary response to form IgM- and IgG-producing effector cells. While IgM is the first immunoglobulin produced in an immune response, it is more effective in agglutination and opsonization than in inducing lysis of foreign cells.

■ What are the various types of immunoglobulins?

IgG's constitute the bulk of normal human blood immunoglobulins, provide the major antimicrobial immunity, and are the only Ig's in humans that combine directly with the macrophage surface. They are the only protection of the newborn, having been transported by the placenta. While the IgG's last longer than the other immunoglobulins, their half-life is only 20 to 25 days. Therefore the infant must quickly come to produce its own *IgM* as a protection against the many gram-negative enteric bacteria encountered early on. IgM is more efficient in agglutination and opsonization than in inducing lysis of foreign cells. Since these functions are carried out primarily against bacteria within the bloodstream, IgM's are said to "function primarily in bacteremias." *IgA's* are produced in maternal colostrum and in postnatal saliva, tears, and nasal and tracheobronchial mucosas. By combining with potentially harmful ingested and inhaled antigens before they can be absorbed through the mucous membrane, IgA's prevent the antigens from inducing sensitization. It is speculated that *IgD* may have a significant role as a fetal immunoglobulin and that *IgE* may be involved with immunity in the cranial sinuses and the pulmonary tract. IgE's, as indicated under D,3 of the Immune System Chart, cause mast cells and basophils to release histamine. This results in a secondary, anamnestic response, inducing a condition known as *anaphylaxis* in which there is smooth muscle contraction (associated with bronchial asthma) and capillary dilatation (associated with lacrimal tearing and hypersecretion of the nasal mucosa), plus skin wheal formation

and itching. Since IgE-mediated histamine release is inhibited by increased levels of intracellular cyclic adenosine monophosphate (cAMP), drugs such as isoproterenol may be used to enhance cAMP concentration in mast cells, or theophylline may be given to prevent cAMP degradation. The acute symptoms of serum sickness are attributed to IgE-mediated responses to foreign serum proteins encountered in prophylactic shots.

■ How may the activities of immunoglobulins be summarized?

Five of the *mechanisms of immunoglobulin action* follow: (1) They *may be instrumental in the production of more Ig's* in the sense that the antibody initially present on the virgin B cell became part of the complex that stimulated clone production and, ultimately, the production of more IgG and IgM blasts. This in turn led to the production of Ig secretion by plasma cells and small lymphocytes. (2) Ig's *neutralize toxins by combining with them.* Soluble proteins identified as toxins are referred to as *precipitins.* The liver contributes by its detoxification processes, and the kidneys assist through the process of filtration. (3) By combining with viruses Ig's *render the virus unable to attach to the potential host's plasmalemma.* The viruses then die. (4) Ig's may assist in *preparing a foreign substance for phagocytosis* by opsonization, working with complement, or causing precipitation: (a) In the process of *opsonization* Ig's rough up the surface of the antigens, for example, bacteria, making them sticky and more palatable. (b) *Complement* consists of 11 related plasma proteins of obscure origin that may be activated by IgM or IgG antigen-antibody complexes or by aggregated Ig's. Once the complement reaction sequence ("cascade") is initiated by the binding of the first component—called C1—to the Ig region of the antigen-antibody complex, several sequential phenomena associated with the inflammatory response occur. These include opsonization, anaphylactic activity, chemotatic influences on phagocytic monocytes and polycytes, and alternation of the membrane of the foreign substance, for example, bacteria or RBC's, resulting in death and/or lysis. (c) Particulate antigens, called *ag-*

glutinins, for example, bacteria, RBC's, and WBC's, may cause agglutination, which, as in the admixing of incompatible blood types, may result in clogging of the capillaries and asphyxiation. If the reaction is less severe, the agglutinins are removed by phagocytosis. (5) Some antibodies *may adhere to the surfaces of mast cells,* others *to the surfaces of basophils.* When the appropriate *antigen complexes with them,* histamine is released from the mast cells and basophils by merocrine secretion, *producing an anaphylactic response.*

■ **How are immune reactions classified didactically?**

Didactically immune reactions are classically referred to as being of two types: cell mediated and humoral. Customarily the former alludes to the lymphokinin activity mediated through T killer cells, while the latter relates to the immunoglobulins being transported by the serum—the humor, or liquid. Such a classification fails to carry the process to completion by neglecting the phagocytic actions of macrophages, reticuloendothelial cells, and leukocytes (see Immune System Chart C,1 and 2).

■ **What are the clinical bases for classifying immunities?**

The activities of the various antibodies are collectively known as *immunologic reactions.* Immunity may be natural or acquired. *Natural immunity* is regulated by the individual's genetics. Examples would be the antibodies found in the plasma against incompatible blood types or the large number of species-specific bacterial diseases, that is, diseases that will grow in one species of animal but not another. *Acquired immunity* may be active or passive. The host may attain *active acquired immunity* (1) as a result of having had a disease, (2) by injection with a vaccine consisting of bacteria or viruses that have been highly attenuated by special treatment, for example, influenza or typhoid fever, or (3) by injection with two spaced shots of modified toxins, known as toxoid, that stimulate the production of the related antitoxin, for example, diphtheria and tetanus. *Passive acquired immunity* is attained by injecting toxin into an animal, permitting antibodies to form, then collecting the antibodies

for subsequent injection into the patient. This method has been used against measles, hepatitis A, scarlet fever, botulism, and the venoms of spiders and snakes. Many artificial active immunizations (by vaccines and toxoids) last a lifetime, but some are of short duration. Passive immunizations by antisera and antitoxins typically provide protection of shorter duration. Happily numerous antibiotics may now be used as supplemental armamentaria against bacterial antigens.

■ **How are immune problems treated clinically?**

Alteration of the immune system may be attempted by several methods, including immunization, bone marrow transplants, and correcting dietary deficiencies. In addition to the methods of immunization against bacteria in the preceding question (What are the clinical bases for classifying immunities?), attention should also be brought in treating cancers to the use of the vaccine BCG (bacillus Calmette-Guerin), which stimulates T cells in general, to the use of the animal-worming drug levamisole, and to the increasingly popular use of "transfer factor."

Immunotherapy research received considerable impetus with modern efforts to transplant kidneys and other organs. Initially surgeons used cytotoxic agents to suppress the immune system. Realizing that this left the patient without resistance to bacterial and viral infections, efforts then concentrated on using drug doses and combinations that would suppress the immune system just enough to prevent organ rejection without weakening it to the point of allowing lethal infections. Examples of currently used immunosuppressing drugs include nitrogen mustard, azathioprine (Imuran), and corticosteroids. Greater emphasis came to be placed on better matching of organs and recipients.

From the realization that transplant patients who had been subjected to immunosuppression therapy were more prone to cancer, the concept developed that normal body cells are always becoming malignant in small numbers and that one function of the immune system is to identify and destroy them. However, as with fighting microorganisms and viruses, the body can be overwhelmed by cancer cells. Then it is best to resort to irradiation, surgery, chemotherapy, and/or anticancer drugs. Thereafter, if all goes well, the immune system can once more dominate the scene.

Problems relating to the immune system may be characterized as belonging to the classic categories of preventive medicine and curative medicine. The immune system is sometimes depressed and/or defective, especially in the very young and the aged. This may relate to heredity or to the effects of drugs, burns, or overwhelming infections. Recurrent infections and cancer are classic symptoms of immune deficiency. A diagnosis of leukopenia implies an inability to phagocytize antigens, while lymphopenia indicates an inability to produce antigen.

Immune diseases of the newborn include (1) DiGeorge's syndrome, in which there is no thymus present and therefore no T cells and no Ig response, (2) Bruton type agammaglobulinemia, in which there are no B cells, and (3) Swiss type agammaglobulinemia, in which there are neither T nor B cells. Children with DiGeorge's syndrome can attain normal immunologic vigor subsequent to transplantation of human fetal thymus tissue. Bone marrow transplants, when carefully matched, can reconstitute B–cell deficient systems.

Unfortunately with age the production of disease-fighting antibodies declines while the level of autoantibodies, those directed against the body's own tissues, increases. In line with that, some current research—successful in mice—involves freezing T and B cells during youth and injecting the frozen supply—after thawing, of course—in old age.

RESPIRATORY SYSTEM

It is convenient to discuss the exchange of gases occurring in metabolism as *external respiration,* relating to the exchange of gases in the lungs and pulmonary circulation, and *internal respiration,* relating to events occurring in the systemic circulation between the blood and nonpulmonary tissues.

■ What is the course of air when traveling into the lungs?

From the nasal cavity, air travels through the nasopharynx to the oropharynx, where it is admixed with air drawn in through the mouth. It then passes through the larynx and into the tra-

chea, which bifurcates within the chest into right and left bronchi, each of which enters its respective lung. The bronchi initiate a series of bifurcating branches that become progressively smaller and less complex in structure. The hierarchy of tubules thus established includes successively bronchi, bronchioles, respiratory bronchioles, alveolar ducts, atria, alveolar sacs, and alveoli.

■ What are the anatomic characteristics of the lungs?

The right lung is divided into three lobes, the left into two lobes. Lobes are composed of lobules, consisting of a bronchiole and its anatomic hierarchial subunits. The surface of the lung is covered by a mesothelium called the visceral pleura. (The inner lining of the chest wall is covered with a comparable parietal pleura.)

■ How does the microscopic structure of the alveoli adapt them for their physiologic functions?

The stroma of an alveolus consists of elastic fibers, phagocytes, and occasional cuboidal septal cells of a type secreting surfactant, a substance that, by lowering surface tension, reduces the work of breathing. The parenchyma consists of capillaries adherent to a squamosal type of septal cell, a basement membrane being interposed between the two. Accordingly, as interpreted with the aid of electron microscopy, air would have to pass through the epithelial cell, the basement membrane, and the capillary endothelium in admixing with the blood.

■ How is the flow of air created between the atmosphere and the alveoli?

The movement of air into the lungs is known as *inspiration;* the outward movement is *expiration.* The flow of air involved is created by the combined action of the diaphragm, the rib muscles, and surface tension.

The thoracic cavity is a closed compartment whose floor is formed by the diaphragm and sidewalls by the rib cage. During expiration the lungs are deflated, the rib cage decreases in volume, and the diaphragm assumes a dome shape. In inhalation the size (volume) of the thoracic cavity increases because the diaphragm contracts (flattens out), and the intercostal muscles cause the ribs to move upward and rotate outward. A negative internal pressure results. Surface tension created between visceral and parietal pleurae causes the two layers to adhere, much as two sheets of glass would stick together if they were adjoined by a thin layer of water. Air rushes into the lungs until the internal and external pressures are equal.

When the diaphragmatic and intercostal muscles cease to contract, passive relaxation initiates exhalation, the elastic tissues surrounding the hierarchial subdivisions (from respiratory bronchiole to alveolus) supplementing the outflow by what is referred to as "elastic recoil."

Perforating the chest wall equalizes the intra- and extrathoracic pressures and causes lung collapse, a condition known as *pneumothorax*.

Removal of a lung segment results in classic symptoms: upward movement of the diaphragm, shifting of the mediastinum (heart) toward the side of the surgery, depression of the chest wall on the side of extirpation, and expansion of the adjacent lung segments.

■ What are the respiratory volumes?

Tidal volume is the amount of air moved into and out of the lungs with each breath and usually averages about 500 cc. Of the 500 cc, about 150 cc remains in the "anatomic dead space" of the trachea, bronchi, and bronchioles, resulting in only 350 cc of fresh air being exchanged within the alveoli. Increased depth of breathing is far more effective in elevating alveolar ventilation than an equivalent increase in breathing rate.

Pulmonary ventilation is computed by multiplying the tidal volume by the respiratory rate and averages about 5000 cc/min. Since the atmosphere is about 20% oxygen, about 1000 cc of oxygen is breathed per minute. However, only 200 cc is utilized, and the remaining 800 cc is returned to the atmosphere.

In respiratory therapy it frequently becomes necessary to know more of the patient's breathing capacity than just the normal rate of ventilation. Accordingly, a series of categories have been devised indicating the amount of air exchanged with varying depths of respiration.

The *inspiratory reserve volume* is the amount that can be forcibly inspired after the tidal volume has been taken in; this volume amounts to about 2500 cc. *Expiratory reserve volume* is the amount that can be forcibly expired after the tidal volume has been exhaled; it averages 1000 cc. *Vital capacity* is the cumulative volume of inspiratory and expiratory reserve plus tidal volume. *Residual volume* is the amount left in the lungs after the maximum forcible expiration and is estimated at 1000 cc. Thus the *total lung capacity* of the average individual is about 5000 cc.

■ What clinical terms are applied to variations in the rate of ventilation?

Eupnea is normal, quiet breathing and averages 15 to 18 times/min in the adult, varying with age and position. *Hyperpnea* is increased ventilation; *dyspnea* implies labored breathing; and *apnea* is the cessation of breathing.

■ What is the significance of the respiratory quotient?

The *respiratory quotient* (RQ) is the ratio of CO_2 produced compared with the amount of oxygen (O_2) used in a unit of time; or:

$$\frac{CO_2}{O_2} = RQ$$

Here CO_2 and O_2 are measured in cubic centimeters. The RQ varies with the type of food utilized, being 1.0 for carbohydrates and 0.7 for fats and proteins. Whereas the brain has an RQ of 1.0, indicating that it uses only carbohydrates in respiration, the average for the body is 0.8.

■ What is meant by the partial pressure of gases?

The total of all gases in the dry atmosphere at 0° C creates a pressure of 760 mm Hg at sea level. Such a gas pressure measurement—dry atmosphere, 0° C, and at sea level—is said to be taken under "standard conditions," and appropriate corrections in calculations must be made for variations from the standard. Each gas exerts its own pressure independently of the others; the amount of pressure created by any one gas is referred to as its *partial pressure* (PP), for example, P_{O_2}, represents the PP of O_2. Since the air consists of about 79% nitrogen (N_2), the pressure exerted by N_2 is 79 × 760, or 600 mm (written $P_{N_2} = 600$). The P_{N_2} remains relatively unchanged during respiration. Therefore it is common to speak of O_2 and

Table 2-1. Presence of oxygen and carbon dioxide in selected body components

Component	O_2		CO_2	
	Vol%	Tension (mm Hg)	Vol%	Tension (mm Hg)
Arterial blood	20	100	50	40
Venous blood	15	40	58	46
Tissues		30		50

Table 2-2. Calculation of partial pressure for major respiratory gases

Alveolar air	% by volume	PP (mm Hg)
O_2	14.0	$14/100 \times 713 = 99.8$
CO_2	5.5	$5.5/100 \times 713 = 39.2$
N_2	80.0	$80/100 \times 713 = 570.4$

CO_2 as though they were the only respiratory gases. At standard conditions the Po_2 is about 159 mm Hg, and the Pco_2 is about 0.3 mm Hg.

However, at sea level and 0° C the vapor pressure within the alveoli and/or blood equals 47 mm, or approximately 6% of the total 760 mm. Therefore 47 is subtracted from 760, giving a figure of 713, in deriving the basis for calculating PP's within the body (Tables 2-1 and 2-2).

■ **What is meant by volumes percent of gases dissolved in water or blood?**

Within the alveoli 0.46 cc of O_2 and 3 cc of CO_2 can be dissolved in water. The physiologist would express this as 0.46 volume percent (vol%) of O_2 and 3 vol% of CO_2. This much higher solubility of CO_2 compared with O_2 permits it to diffuse through tissue about 20 times more rapidly than O_2 and bears a number of physiologic implications. A linear relationship exists between the amount of O_2 and CO_2 dissolved in pure water and the O_2 and CO_2 tensions.

■ **How do the principles of gas diffusion apply in respiration?**

Substances diffuse from areas of higher concentration to areas of lower concentration, and if a selectively permeable membrane is interposed between the two areas, the phenomenon is known

as osmosis. Since O_2 is utilized and CO_2 produced in the process of metabolism, there is an ongoing inward movement of O_2 in accordance with the different Po_2 gradients found in the atmosphere, the alveoli, the blood, and the tissues. The Pco_2 gradient is established in the opposite direction, being greatest in the tissues, then successively less in the blood, the alveoli, and the atmosphere.

Atmospheric air contains 21% O_2 (at a PP of 159 mm Hg) and 0.04% CO_2 (at a PP of 0.3 mm Hg), whereas expired air contains 16% O_2 (at 120 mm Hg) and 4% CO_2 (at 32 mm Hg).

■ **What are some of the factors affecting the rate of gas diffusion?**

Any factors that affect the rate of diffusion (osmosis) of gases through the tissue would affect the rate of lung ventilation, lowering or raising it according to whether or not it hinders or abets the rate of diffusion. *Fick's law* states that the amount of gas that moves across a sheet of tissue is proportional to the area of the sheet but inversely proportional to its thickness. A decreased ambient O_2 (to 12% or less) or an increased environmental CO_2 (to 2% or more) stimulates respiration. With impaired diffusion there is an increased respiratory effort and chronic respiratory alkalosis as seen in emphysema, pulmonary edema, and beryllium poisoning (which causes a thickening of the alveolar walls). Depending on the extent of stress, the total number of functional alveoli—total alveolar surface—and the total number of functional capillaries—total blood flow—will vary, increasing threefold if necessary. Finally, a number of chemical reactions involving the plasma and RBC's interrelate.

■ **How is O_2 transported in the blood?**

As stated previously, only 0.46 cc of O_2 can be dissolved physically in water or in the blood, which is 90% water. The rest of the O_2 in the blood is in chemical combination with hemoglobin, which can combine (at the 100 mm Po_2 of arteriolar blood) at the ratio of 1.34 cc of O_2/g of hemoglobin. Since 100 cc of blood contains 13 to 15 g of hemoglobin, this provides a total of about 20 vol% of O_2 in arterial blood at a Po_2 of 100 mm Hg (see Table 2-1). In venous blood there are only 15 vol% of O_2, but the Po_2 is only

40 mm Hg. Oxygen tension—100 mm—and CO_2 tension—40 mm—are due to dissolved O_2 and CO_2, not that held by hemoglobin or bicarbonate.

■ What is the significance of the O_2 dissociation curve?

Hemoglobin (Hb) is slightly acid. Combined with O_2, it forms oxyhemoglobin (HbO_2). The reaction is reversible and is regulated by the Po_2, Pco_2, temperature, and acidity, being more readily dissociated at higher temperatures and greater acidity. The potential advantage can be seen in exercise, where the muscle is increasing in temperature and forming more CO_2.

If samples of blood are placed in a barometric (compression) chamber with air containing O_2 at various PP's, O_2 will continue to be absorbed until the Po_2 reaches 150 mm Hg. At this point the blood hemoglobin is said to be 100% saturated. In contrast, at a Po_2 of 0 mm Hg there would be no O_2 absorbed by the blood, and its percentage of saturation would be 0. However, a plot of the amount of O_2 in the blood against the PP's is not linear but is sigmoid, or S shaped (Fig. 2-6). At the alveolar Po_2 the blood is 97% saturated. The reader should consider the physiologic advantages of having only 10% loss in available O_2 with a drop of environmental tension from 100 to 60 mm Hg, but a 50% dissociation between the blood and tissues as the Po_2 drops from 60 to 20 mm Hg. (Tissue tension is 20 to 30 mm Hg.)

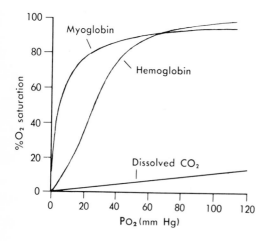

Fig. 2-6. Oxygen dissociation curve.

■ How is CO_2 transported in the blood?

About 5% to 8% of the CO_2 is dissolved in plasma and RBC's as CO_2. Usually about 20% to 25% of the CO_2 combines with hemoglobin, forming carbaminohemoglobin ($HbCO_2$). The remaining 70% is carried in plasma as (sodium) bicarbonate.

■ In the lungs in external respiration, how do the physiochemical factors involved result in an exchange of gases?

For didactic purposes it is convenient to discuss respiration in two phases: external respiration (the exchange of gases taking place within the lungs) and internal respiration (the exchange of gases taking place within tissues other than the lungs).

As stated on p. 53, the relative pressure gradients in the alveoli and pulmonary capillaries result in an exchange of O_2 and CO_2. Additionally, the diffusion of CO_2 from the lung capillaries favors the combination of O_2 and hemoglobin, while concurrently oxygenation of the blood renders hemoglobin more acid and speeds up the release of CO_2. Within the RBC's the enzyme carbonic anhydrase expedites the intermediate, reciprocal exchange of H_2CO_3 with CO_2 and H_2O, speeding up the reaction approximately 5000 times. There is also a slow-acting local control in which an increase of CO_2 causes the bronchioles to expand, permitting more O_2 to enter; increased O_2, in turn, causes the arterioles to dilate. Decreases of CO_2 and O_2 have the opposite effect.

■ In the tissues in internal respiration, how do the physiochemical factors involved result in an exchange of gases?

As stated on p. 53, the relative pressure gradients in the tissue capillaries and systemic tissues results in an exchange of CO_2 and O_2. The loading of CO_2 in the capillaries and the unloading of O_2 are mutually helpful processes. An increase of capillary blood Pco_2 with its attendant decrease of pH facilitates the unloading of O_2 (*Bohr effect*). At the same time the unloading of O_2 facilitates the loading of CO_2 (*Haldane effect*). As in external respiration, within the RBC the intermediate, reciprocal exchanges between H_2O, O_2, and H_2CO_3 are expedited 5000-fold by the enzyme carbonic anhydrase.

■ How does the chloride shift work?

The CO_2 formed in cellular metabolism diffuses progressively from the cell to intercellular fluid, to plasma, and into the RBC, where carbonic anhydrase speeds up the conversion of CO_2 and H_2O into H_2CO_3. In the immediate dissociation into hydrogen and bicarbonate ions, the H^+ joins Hb^- in the RBC to form reduced hemoglobin (HHb); the HCO_3^- joins potassium ions in the RBC to form $KHCO_3$. With the potassium concentration in the RBC coming to exceed that in the plasma, a "chloride shift" takes place in which plasma Cl^- exchanges places with the HCO_3^- of the RBC.

When the HHb reaches the alveolar capillaries and becomes oxygenated, forming $HHbO_2$, the latter reacts with bicarbonate salts to form carbonic acid ($HHbCO_2 + KHCO_3 \rightleftharpoons H_2CO_3 + KHbO_2$). Because of the increased CO_2 formed, as carbonic anhydrase rapidly decomposes the H_2CO_3, a second chloride shift occurs. As a result, both Cl^- and CO_2 leave the RBC and return to the plasma, while the K^+ reacts with the HCO_3 to form $KHCO_3$ again. Ultimately, the CO_2 within the pulmonary capillaries equilibrates with the alveolar air. In fulfilling its role Hb becomes quantitatively the most important blood buffer.

■ What neurologic controls are involved in ventilation?

During eupneic inhalation lung inflation receptors, acting through the *Hering-Breuer reflex,* carry afferent impulses from the stretching lungs through the vagus nerve to the respiratory center in the medulla, ultimately resulting in the cessation of inhalation. The neuronal relays that follow result in efferent impulses through the intercostal (T1-12) and phrenic (C3-5) nerves, producing contraction of the intercostal muscles and the diaphragm. In hyperpnea the pneumotaxic centers of the pons modify the rhythms of the medullary centers. For further details any standard physiology textbook may be consulted.

■ What factors modify the action of the respiratory centers?

One mechanism affecting the respiratory center is a system of O_2 sensors found in the carotid body and aortic bodies that monitor dissolved O_2. It is unfortunate that they do not monitor the O_2 associated with hemoglobin because in carbon monoxide (CO) poisoning the CO is combining with the hemoglobin, not with the dissolved O_2 being sensed. Another mechanism is sensitive to hydrogen ion, which increases as CO_2 increases. Actually the respiratory response in CO_2 accumulation is associated with an increase in pH and not with the CO_2 per se, as can be demonstrated experimentally.

Overventilating results in blowing off the CO_2 and a corresponding lack of respiratory stimulation.

■ What are some additional clinical entities relating to the respiratory system?

In *asthma* the allergic response produces both an edematous response and spasms of the bronchioles, doubly complicating the clinical picture. In *bronchitis* primarily the bronchi are inflamed.

Emphysema is characterized by a breakdown of alveolar walls and a corresponding reduction in the total surface area available for gaseous exchange. In contrast, tuberculosis, pneumonia, and lung cancer reduce the area for respiratory exchange by occlusion of the potential space with fibrosis, cellular hypertrophy, or fluid. Children born with a deficiency of surfactant develop *hyaline membrane disease,* in which the lack of a surface tension reducing agent produces respiratory distress because of unequal and incomplete expansion of the alveoli.

Cheyne-Stokes breathing is characterized by periods in which respirations increase in force and frequency alternating with gradual reversals to short periods of apnea. In addition to being associated with heart and kidney diseases, it may be caused by any damage to the brain stem from narcotics, anesthesia, or increase in intracranial pressure. Various *drugs* affect the respiratory pattern, the positive effects providing therapeutic adjuncts, but the secondary effects often being detrimental.

Decompression sickness, or *bends,* is experienced in deep underwater diving when the diver ascends too rapidly, forcing an abnormal amount of N_2 into the blood. Breathing pure O_2 during decompression assists in eliminating the N_2.

Several terms used in respiratory therapy relate to the relative abundance of CO_2. The term *"acapnia"* indicates a lack of CO_2; the term *"hypocap-*

nia," or *hypocarbia,* designates a low patient CO_2 content; and the term *"hypercapnia"* implies a high patient CO_2, resulting in an overactive respiratory system.

URINARY SYSTEM

It is the function of the urinary system to regulate the levels of various substances within the body and to eliminate certain wastes. This is accomplished by the kidneys and their associated organs: the calyces, renal pelves, ureters, bladder, and urethra.

■ **What is the general disposition and structure of the kidney and its proximal drainage system?**

The kidneys are bilaterally disposed, bean-shaped organs about 4 to 5 inches long lying to the sides of the vertebral column in the lumbar region, with the right kidney disposed slightly lower than the left. The expanded, upper portion of the ureter, the *pelvis,* originates from the concave indentation on the medial border of the kidney known as the *hilus.* The hilus opens into a cavelike structure, the *renal sinus,* that houses the renal artery and vein and the calyces.

The interior of the kidney is almost wholly parenchyma and is divisible macroscopically into a peripheral *cortex* and a central *medulla.* The medulla consists of 10 to 15 pyramids whose apices point into the sinus. Some of the pyramids fuse, but whether or not this is the case, the single or fused apices are referred to as *papillae.*

In relation to each papilla is an infolded, double-walled cup, the *minor calyx,* whose inner wall fits over the papilla. Seven to 12 minor calyces are definable. Several adjacent minor calyces unite to form a total of two or three *major calyces.* Urine formed within the parenchyma drains by a system of tubules to the pyramidal papillae and into the lumina of the minor, and, in turn, the major calyces. The major calyces unite to form the ureteric pelvis. Each renal pelvis drains into a *ureter* that, in turn, drains into the bladder.

■ **What is the anatomic functional unit of the kidney and what are its subdivisions?**

The *nephron* constitutes both the anatomic and the functional unit of the kidney. There are ap-

proximately 1 million of these per kidney. Sequentially, the parts of a nepron include the renal (or malpighian) corpuscle, proximal convoluted tubule, descending tubule, Henle's loop, ascending tubule, and distal convoluted tubule. The distal convoluted tubules join collecting tubules that, much like branches of a tree uniting with the trunk, join the papillary ducts that open on the pyramidal apices. Each portion of the nephron has distinctive histologic features that are adaptive to its particular functions. The only one requiring further elucidation here is the corpuscle. For additional details concerning the other portions, any standard histology textbook may be consulted.

The renal (or malpighian) corpuscle consists of a tuft of capillaries called the glomerulus and its associated covering, named Bowman's capsule. Bowman's capsule is like a partially inflated balloon into which a fist has been shoved. The indented surface of the balloon may be visualized as wrapping around the fingers, just as the inner, visceral layer of Bowman's capsule wraps around the capillaries or glomerulus. The outer layer of the balloon would then be comparable to the peripheral parietal layer of Bowman's capsule, with the air space of the balloon being comparable to the lumen of Bowman's capsule, which is known as Bowman's space. The open end (or stump) of the balloon with its lumen would be continuous with the proximal convoluted tubule and its lumen.

■ **What vascular patterns characterize the kidney?**

After arising from the aorta the renal artery branches on entering the hilus. The branches pass between the pyramids and course to the plane separating the cortex and medulla, spreading out in this region as the arcuate artery and its branches. Since renal corpuscles (plus the proximal and distal convoluted tubules) are located in the cortex, about 95% of the arteries are directed peripherally into the glomeruli. Henle's loops and portions of the descending and ascending loops are found in the medulla, along with the collecting tubules and 5% of the total renal blood flow.

Blood is brought to the proximal part of a glomerular capillary by an afferent arteriole and leaves the distal end by way of an efferent arteriole, rather than a venule as would be expected. As the efferent arteriole leaves the capsule, it spreads out around the other components of the nephron, providing rich capillary networks to them. The venous return consists of arcuate veins and branches of the renal vein, which unite to form the main vein before returning to the inferior vena cava.

■ What happens in the renal corpuscle?

Of the three processes taking place in the kidney (glomerular ultrafiltration, tubular secretion, and tubular resorption), the first is characteristic of the malpighian corpuscle. The glomerulus acts as a type of filter, permitting approximately one fifth of the plasma to escape into Bowman's space, but retaining four fifths of the plasma, the cellular components, the proteins, and the large colloids. Although there is a glomerular capillary pressure of 50 mm Hg, there is a capsular hydrostatic pressure of 10 mm Hg resisting further filtration and an opposing osmotic gradient equivalent to 30 mm Hg caused by the high concentration of protein. (All the crystalloids have essentially identical concentrations in the plasma and in Bowman's space.) The net result is an outward force of about 10 mm Hg. Appropriate tests can be made for the *glomerular filtration rate* (GFR), which varies daily and with the state of health. Although the systemic blood pressure may vary, within limits the pressures in the glomerulus (and the GFR) are kept homeostatic by alterations in the size of the lumen of the efferent, as compared with the afferent, arteriole. Thus increased blood pressure results in narrowing of the afferent arteriole and expansion of the efferent arteriole, producing a reduced pressure to entering the glomerulus, less hydrostatic pressure, and less resistance to exiting via the efferent arteriole. A decreased blood pressure (BP) would be at least partially compensated for by opening the afferent arterioles and narrowing the efferent ones (but this would also result in an overall lower GFR if the pressure drop were significant).

During strenuous exercise and/or subsequent to hemorrhage, blood is shunted from some parts of the body to others as a compensatory mechanism. In such situations the blood supply to the kidneys—and to the gut—may be reduced to half the normal.

■ Of what significance is passive tubular reabsorption?

On leaving Bowman's capsule the efferent arteriole distributes itself among the distal components of the nephron, forming extramural capillaries in relation to each of these structures. At the proximal convoluted tubule there is considerable (passive) osmosis of water and crystalloids, passing from the tubules into the capillaries in reestablishing the normal blood composition that has been temporarily imbalanced by the relatively high protein concentration left in the blood of the efferent arterioles. About 80% of the water and dissolved substances that are reabsorbed are regulated in this way. In this process urea reabsorption is directly proportional to water reabsorption. Ultimately, of the 180 L of filtrate formed daily, about 178 L is reabsorbed.

■ Of what significance is active reabsorption?

In an effort to retain certain substances once they are secured, the body will expend energy to reabsorb them against a concentration gradient—a phenomenon known as *active reabsorption*. A system of enzymes ("carriers") in the tubule wall with energy provided by ATP will actively transport these substances, such as sodium, bicarbonate, glucose, and amino acids, from the glomerular filtrate back into the capillary bloodstream. However, each material has a characteristic threshold or tubular maximum, and once this plasma saturation point has been reached, if additional amounts appear in the filtrate, they are permitted to pass on to become part of the urine—to "spill over." In *diabetes* the lack of insulin and consequent inability to utilize carbohydrates results in extremely high plasma glucose levels. The glucose in excess of the threshold spills over—glucosuria. In glucosuria there is *nothing wrong* with the tubular glucose transport mechanism. Since the threshold mechanism results in the release of the excess sugars, the diabetic occasionally experiences the compromising situation in which the injected insulin does not stop the reduction of blood sugar at its normal level.

Weakness and prostration may result. In such cases it is necessary to administer glucose-containing substances and/or insulin. Under normal circumstances all of the glucose in the filtrate is reabsorbed, and no glucose is found in the urine.

■ What is the countercurrent mechanism?

Depending on the body's relative need to lose or conserve water, the loop of Henle is important in effecting the proper dilution or concentration of the glomerular filtrate. In the ascending limb of the loop sodium is actively reabsorbed by the metabolic pump, and chlorine follows to help maintain an electrolyte balance. The movement of electrolytes, however, results in a filtrate of lower and lower osmolarity, since the water is unable to enter the ascending limb unless the permeability of its cells is changed by a hormone known as antidiuretic hormone (ADH). The total result is that, as sodium chloride increases in the interstitial fluid, it diffuses back into the neighboring descending tubules, increasing the osmolarity of the filtrate moving toward the loop and creating a countercurrent.

■ What part do the kidneys play in acid-base balance?

Although some small amount of acid hydrogen ion (H^+) may be consumed as such in food, on a daily average the total net gain of H^+ comes primarily from protein degradation, for example, the formation of sulfuric acid on a high protein diet. (During the catabolism of carbohydrates and lipids H^+ may exist temporarily, but there is little, if any, net gain in H^+.) In normal respiration the H^+ temporarily released from carbonic acid is completely reincorporated into H_2O molecules, and there is no real gain or loss of hydrogen. When CO_2 levels increase, there is an elevation in the ventilation rates, and more CO_2 is exhaled. However, in any lung disease causing inadequate elimination of CO_2, respiratory acidosis develops—excess H^+ does accumulate.

Even in normal metabolism the body initially neutralizes the temporary excess of H^+ with its buffers (bicarbonate, proteins, phosphates, and hemoglobin) but must ultimately secrete the H^+ through the renal tubules to maintain homeostasis. Much of the significance of eliminating this excess H^+ relates to the fact that enzymes require optimal pH's in which to work, and without proper enzyme functioning the body would soon develop overwhelming complications. Since the actual elimination of H^+ from the body is normally performed only by the kidneys, it is imperative to understand the significant role played by the kidneys in this regard.

One process by which H^+ is secreted relates to the reciprocity between lungs and kidneys in eliminating CO_2, in which both organs utilize carbonic anhydrase to convert CO_2 and H_2O to H_2CO_3. In the walls of the distal and collecting tubules the carbonic acid is dissociated into H^+ and bicarbonate ions (HCO_3^-). The H^+ is then secreted into the filtrate in exchange for sodium ions (Na^+). Once in the tubal cell the Na^+ and the HCO_3^- diffuse into the capillary plasma.

Second, in the process of ultrafiltration, by which Na^+ and HCO_3^- enter the renal tubules, Na^+ is again exchanged for the secreted H^+. The H^+ combines with the filtrate's HCO_3^-, then dissociates into CO_2 and H_2O. Depending on the state of hydration, the water may diffuse back into the tubule. (About 10% to 15% of the filtrate H_2O may be reabsorbed in the distal and collecting tubules.) If the H_2O is voided, two H^+ have been eliminated. Since the CO_2 referred to in the preceding paragraph returned to the plasma with the Na^+ as HCO_3^-, the CO_2 alluded to in this paragraph may diffuse into the tubule as a substitute.

Third, when excess HCO_3^- is formed, as in respiratory and/or metabolic alkalosis, the HCO_3^- is flushed through the glomeruli, but, lacking sufficient H^+ to join it, the excess is voided and produces an alkaline urine. In the contrasting case of excess H^+, phosphates (produced by the dissolution of bone salts and in the catabolism of phospholipids) can act as buffers. The dissociation of sodium phosphate releases two Na^+ and one phosphate ion. A secreted H^+ can exchange for one Na^+. The blood pH is raised because of the gain in sodium.

A fourth process for the elimination of H^+ relates to the fact that ammonia (NH_3) can diffuse through the tubule wall, but ammonium ion (NH_4^+) cannot. NH_3 is formed within the tubular cells primarily by the deamination of the amino acid glutamine. It then diffuses into the lumen, from which it may be excreted as NH_3. However, the H^+ secreted into the filtrate may convert NH_3 to NH_4^+, and the latter, in turn, may join with chloride ion (Cl^-). In states of metabolic acidosis NH_3 may be eliminated as ammonium salts. However, it is usually excreted as urea, the principal end product of protein metabolism, normally comprising 80% to 90% of the total urinary nitrogen. While urea is the major urinary solute under ordinary conditions, its concentration varies with changes in urinary volume, 80% to 90% being reabsorbed if urine flow is low but only 30% to 50% being reabsorbed when urine flow is high. Its excretion is elevated whenever protein catabolism is increased, for example, with diabetes, fever, or excess adrenocortical activity.

■ How is hormonal control involved in renal function?

The hormonal influence is provided mainly by aldosterone and ADH. When the sodium concentration decreases, it stimulates certain renal cells to produce renin. Renin, in turn, is responsible for the formation of angiotensin. Angiotensin is a very potent vasoconstrictor, thereby causing increased blood pressure, and also causes the adrenal cortex to release aldosterone. Aldosterone, in some unknown way, causes an increased absorption of sodium and a secretion of potassium.

ADH (or vasopressin) is produced by the hypothalamus and stored in the posterior lobe of the pituitary gland until released into the blood. It increases the size of the pores of the distal tubules and collecting ducts, permitting reabsorption of water from the filtrate and preventing diuresis. Absence of ADH results in diuresis and a lowering of the plasma level. Its release is determined conjointly by baro- and osmoreceptors located in the hypothalamus. The baroreceptors, being sensitive to changes in blood pressure, cause an increased release of ADH if the arterial and venous pressures are decreased, as would be the case in low plasma volume. If the plasma volume were low, the resultant stimulation of the hypothalamic osmoreceptors would also produce the release of ADH.

Caffeine causes diuresis by initiating a dilatation of the afferent glomerular arteriole and a proportionate increase of glomerular filtrate volume.

While assuring that the blood calcium level is high enough through regulating the movement of calcium into and out of bones and from the intestinal tract, parathormone (PTH) also increases the renal tubular reabsorption of calcium and reduces the tubular reabsorption of PO_4^-.

■ How does congestive heart failure relate to renal function?

In congestive heart failure the patient's low cardiac output results in a decreased GFR. There is also an unexplained increase of aldosterone, which results in increased sodium retention. The decreased GFR and increased sodium retention result in edema. A major factor in treating these patients consists of administering diuretics.

■ How do diuretics work?

Diuretics increase the output of urine by promoting the excretion of excess water and sodium chloride from the body. Among the mechanisms involved are the following: (1) They may *block the reabsorption of Cl^-* from the renal tubular epithelium. Thiazide diuretics, mercurials, ethacrynic acid, and furosemide (Lasix) are common examples. (2) They may *inhibit carbonic anhydrase* from decomposing H_2CO_3 into H^+ and HCO_3^-, thereby preventing Na^+ and H^+ exchange. The classic medication in this group is acetazolamide (Diamox). (3) They may *antagonize the reabsorption of Na^+ and excretion of K^+ by aldosterone*. Since less than 1% of the Na^+ is reabsorbed by this mechanism, such drugs are used primarily in combination with other drugs because of their potassium-sparing action.

■ What is the purpose of renal dialysis and how is it accomplished?

Typically substances found in the plasma exist in "normal" concentrations. However, in renal failure toxic substances and nitrogenous wastes that would ordinarily be excreted accumulate. To correct this, the patient's blood is passed through a hemodialysis machine, usually connected to the radial artery and the basilic or median vein. Blood from the artery flows into a device consisting of two plastic sheets surrounded by dialyzing fluid, whose consistency is determined in accordance with the findings of a prior blood analysis. The composition of the solution is adjusted so that hyperosmotic plasma substances will diffuse out of and substances in hyposmotic plasma concentration will diffuse into the blood through the cellophane. The pore size of the cellophane must permit diffusion without allowing plasma proteins and other desirable colloids to escape.

In the older peritoneal dialysis technique the abdominopelvic cavity substitutes for the machine, and a proper solution of osmotically balanced substances is introduced into the cavity for a period of 30 minutes, then withdrawn and discarded.

■ How does the anatomy of the ureters and bladder adapt them for the performance of their functions?

The bladder is shaped somewhat like a balloon shoved into the anteroinferior half of the pelvis, then partially deflated with the palm of the hand from above and behind, creating relatively triangular walls. The superior surface rises and falls according to the amount of urine contained and is slightly higher in the male than in the female because of the presence in the male of the prostate gland below the bladder. In the female it is circumscribed posteriorly by part of the vaginal wall and the uterus. The ureters and vesicular, or bladder, blood vessels travel from the pelvic wall to the lateral superior corners of the bladder in ligaments that help to hold the bladder (and prostate gland or uterus) in position. Urine drains from the bottom of the bladder into the proximal part of the urethra. On the internal aspect the triangular area on the posterior wall between the ureters and the origin of the urethra is recognized clinically as the *trigone*. While the histologic nature of the ureters and bladder is essentially similar to that of other abdominal and pelvic viscera, there are, of course, some modifications. Both ureters and bladder are lined internally with the type of transitional epithelium referred to on p. 32. This type of epithelium is an adaptation to the constantly changing size of the organs. The tunica muscularis of the bladder, called the *detrussor muscle,* is especially thick and is characterized by an intersecting of the smooth muscle cells of the basic laminae. It is

modified at its junction with the urethra to form the internal urinary sphincter.

■ How does the anatomy of the urethra adapt itself for its functions?

The male urethra is divided into three parts. The prostatic portion is contained within the prostate gland. The membranous portion perforates the urogenital diaphragm, which, from its adjacent fibers, forms an external urinary sphincter around this portion of the urethra. Passing through the corpus spongiosum of the penis is the distal cavernous portion. For details of the structure and physiology of erection of the penis standard histology and general anatomy and physiology textbooks may be consulted.

The female urethra is comparatively short, since there is no prostate gland, and the portion distal to the urogenital diaphragm is only 3 to 5 cm long, lying immediately anterior to the vagina. It is because of this anatomic disposition that it is more susceptible to irritation and infection. However, the passage of catheters and cystoscopes is a much easier process.

As the bladder fills, it goes through a series of stages of stretching to accommodate the influx of urine. Both internal and external sphincters remain closed. When about 200 to 400 ml of urine have accumulated, the pressure receptors initiate a reflex in which the sphincters relax, and the detrussor muscle contracts (through innervation from the parasympathetics). The reflex is sustained until the voiding is complete. Abrupt, voluntary closure of the external sphincter helps to terminate the micturition.

WATER, ELECTROLYTE, AND ACID-BASE BALANCE
■ What are the typical variations in body water content?

The total body water makes up 50% to 60% of the total body weight—or approximately 70% of the body weight of a fat-free individual—and is affected by such variables as age, sex, amount of activity, state of health, and diet. Other than in temporary states of over- and underhydration, the variations are related principally to fat content, sex, and age. Since fat contains only 5% to 10% water and since fat can vary from 10% to 40% of a person's body weight, an obese person will have relatively less water than a thin person. Variations in body weight are as follows:

Category	Percentage of body weight
Infant less than 1 year old	65
Children 1 to 10 years old	60
Men below 40 years old	60
Men 40 to 60 years old	50
Women below 40 years old	50
Women 40 to 60 years old	45

In a normal state of health generally the water intake from drink, food, and metabolism equals the water loss from urine, respiration, perspiration, and stools. While typically there are self-compensating balances within the various subcategories, in ill health daily checks must be made for changes in skin tone, weight, and urine output.

Factors related to dehydration

1. Sensible perspiration
   a. Increases with fever (10% to 12% for each degree centigrade of fever), muscular work, and increased ambient temperature and humidity
2. Insensible perspiration
   a. Breathing: 400 ml/day; increases with hyperventilation and high altitude
   b. Sweating: 15 ml/kg/day in adults; 30 ml/kg/day in newborns; averages 400 ml/day
3. Diuresis (from renal dysfunction, cardiac and/or pulmonary failure, drugs, and so forth)
4. Diarrhea
5. For every 1000 calories of intake 40 ml of water is lost in stools

Factors related to overhydration

1. About 400 ml of free water is contained in 1000 calories of food
2. About 120 ml of water is produced metabolically from each 1000 calories of food
3. Edema (from renal dysfunction, cardiac and/or pulmonary failure, drugs, and so forth)

■ How is the body's water distributed?

Total body water is divided into three compartments: *intracellular, intravascular (plasma),* and *interstitial,* with the latter two often combined under the term *"extracellular."* Whole blood constitutes about one third of the total extracellular fluid. About 93% of the plasma is wa-

ter. The main difference between plasma and interstitial fluid is that plasma contains about 70 g of protein per liter, while interstitial fluid contains relatively little. Urine, sweat, gastrointestinal secretions, and various other exudates and transudates are usually categorized as special portions of the extracellular water. Two excellent examples of the constant movement of water from one compartment to another are the temporal formation of glomerular filtrate from the blood— of the 180 L formed daily, 178 L are reabsorbed— and the daily internal release of approximately 3 L of intestinal secretion, of which approximately 90% is reabsorbed.

Water compartments	Percentage of body weight	Volume in liters (70 kg man)
Plasma water	4	2.8
Interstitial water	16	11.2
TOTAL extracellular water	20	14.0
Intracellular water	40	28
TOTAL average body water in a man	60	42
TOTAL average body water in a 70 kg woman	50	35

Typically the patient who appears to be dehydrated has lost about 5% of his total body water; however, in extreme cases this may amount to 10%. Of these losses about half come from the intracellular and half from the extracellular fluid compartments.

■ What are electrolytes and what is their physiologic significance?

While some substances are in suspension in the body fluid, for example, fat, most are dissolved. Some dissolved substances, such as acids, bases, and salts, dissociate to form charged particles, or ions—the negatively charged ones being anions and the positively charged ones being cations. Such charged particles, capable of conducting electricity, are referred to as *electrolytes.* Other dissolved substances, such as glucose and urea, do not develop electrical charges in solution and are called *nonelectrolytes.*

The concentration of electrolytes is expressed in equivalent weights (Eq Wt). *Equivalent weight* equals the molecular weight of the substance expressed in grams—which is called the *gram molecular weight*—divided by its chemical valence. As an example, in NaCl sodium has a molecular weight of 23.0 and chlorine equals 35.5, totaling 58.5. If a salt is composed of univalent ions, as in NaCl, the equivalent weight is the same as the gram molecular weight, since it is divided by a valence of 1. However, in a salt containing a divalent ion, for example, magnesium chloride ($MgCl_2$), the equivalent weight is half the molecular weight, since the gram molecular weight is divided by 2. To make a solution with a concentration of one *equivalent* per liter, one equivalent weight of that substance, for example, NaCl is put in solution. Since one equivalent is equal to 1000 milliequivalents (mEq), a univalent salt such as NaCl would contain 1000 mEq of NaCl and/or 1000 mEq of Na^+ and 1000 mEq of Cl^- per liter.

The concentrations of electrolytes in body fluids are usually so low that they are expressed in milliequivalents/liter (mEq/L). Each liter of plasma contains a *total* of 153 mEq of electrolytes, the significant *cations* (in mEq) being as follows: Na^+ (142), Ca^{++} (5), K^+ (4), and Mg^{++} (2); the most significant *anions* are Cl^- (104), HCO_3^- (27), protein$^-$ (13 or more), organic acids$^-$ (6), HPO_4^- (2), and sulfate$^-$ (1). Remember, when discussing mEq/L, reference is made basically to the electrolyte combining power—the number of electrical charges—not to the number of particles in solution.

■ **What is osmolarity and what is its physiologic significance?**

Osmosis is the diffusion of particles through a selectively permeable membrane. Osmotic force, or osmotic activity, referred to as *osmolarity,* is the measure of the relative ability to equalize the concentration of the solute(s) and solvent(s) on opposite sides of a selectively permeable membrane. As compared with electrolytic strength, where the force relates to the number of electrical charges, osmolar strength depends on the number of particles dissolved in the solution and bears no relation to the molecular weight or the valence of the particles. For substances that do not dissociate in solution, for example, glucose and urea, a gram molecular weight of the substance dis-

solved in 1 L of water creates an *osmotic strength* (effect) of 1 *mole/liter* (*M/L*). In cell physiology this is referred to as 1 osmole/liter (Osm/L). When one gram molecular weight of a salt that dissociates into two univalent ions, for example, NaCl, is dissolved in 1 L of water, it creates an osmotic effect of 2 moles (or osmoles), since there are twice as many particles. One gram molecular weight of a salt such as $CaFl_2$, which dissociates into three particles, would have a strength of 3 moles/liter (or osmoles/liter). Furthermore, just as there were 1000 milliequivalents to one equivalent, so there are 1000 millimoles to 1 mole (or 1000 milliosmoles to 1 osmole). The osmolarity of the body is usually expressed clinically in mOsm/L in view of the relatively low concentrations of dissolved particles. This is the same in all body compartments and in man is equal to 285 mOsm/L. In discussing toxins, vitamins, and so forth the nanimole (naniosmole) may be used. One millimole (milliosmole) contains 1000 nanimoles (naniosmoles).

The principal electrolytes responsible for maintaining the osmolarity of *extracellular fluid* are Na^+ and Cl^-. In the majority of practical cases the osmolarity of the body can be adequately estimated from a single plasma sodium determination. The composition of *intracellular fluid*, on the other hand, is quite different, with K^+ replacing Na^+ as the principal cation and HPO_4^- replacing Cl^- as the principal anion. From the standpoint of maintaining cellular homeostasis, it is important that there is normally about four times as much protein anion intracellularly as in the plasma.

Since the plasma protein cannot pass the capillary endothelium and since, except for a lesser amount of exocytosis, intracellular proteins are made within the cells where they are found, interstitial fluid may correctly be expected to lack much protein. As was mentioned earlier, the main difference between plasma and interstitial fluid is that plasma contains about 70 g of protein per liter, the interstitial fluid relatively little. Since interstitial fluid lacks the 17 mmoles/L of protein ions present in the plasma, anions other than proteins must make up this (17 mmol/L) deficit by being 1.05 more concentrated than they are in the plasma. Just as the anions of the plasma and interstitial fluid are in balance but different in species concentration in the two media, so the cations of the plasma and interstitial fluid are in balance but different in species concentration in plasma vs interstitial fluid.

According to the law of *iso-osmolarity*, the osmolarity is the same in the various compartments between which water is exchanged, that is, plasma, interstitial fluid, and intracellular fluid. If the laws of electrolytic neutrality and iso-osmolarity interfere with each other, as occurs when semipermeable membranes separate two compartments, the water moves freely but the ions toward which the membrane is selectively permeable are more or less impeded in their transport. Furthermore, metabolic pumps may even become involved in maintaining local asymmetric ionic concentrations by expending energy derived from ATP. The result of such phenomena is the coincident development of voltage gradients such as are seen in nerve and muscle tissue and the secretion of aniosmotic solutions, for example, secretion of hyperosmotic stomach HCl.

■ What are normal solutions and what are their clinical uses?

It is sometimes desirable to compare in the laboratory the relative acidity or alkalinity of solutions, for example, determine the acidity of a gastric sample. This may be accomplished by preparing a *standard,* or *normal, solution* of a base and then comparing it with the acid solution in question or by comparing a standard, or normal, acid solution with the base in question. The standard acid solution—1N, or 1 normal—is prepared such that it contains 1 gram atomic weight—1.0078 g—of replaceable hydrogen per liter. Thus a 1N solution of HCl, a monobasic acid, would contain $1 + 35$, or 36 g HCl/L. With dibasic acids, 1 L of the normal solution will contain only half of the gram molecular weight of the acid. For example, since H_2SO_4 (whose molecular weight of $2 + 23 + 64 = 89$) is dibasic, a 1N solution of H_2SO_4 would contain 44.5 g of the compound. A normal solution of a base is one that contains 17.0078 g $(1.0078 + 16)$ of the radical OH^- per liter. Thus a 1N solution of any acid will neutralize 1 molecular weight of any monoacid base. In the laboratory one-tenth normal (N/10 or

0.1N) solutions are frequently used. Applied clinically, if 10 ml of 0.1N NaOH (molecular weight, 40) neutralized a 1000 ml gastric sample—admittedly, more probably some fraction thereof—collected by a Rehfuss tube from a patient, the sample would contain a 0.001N solution of HCl.

■ How is water balance maintained normally and clinically?

The main route by which water loss is balanced is urination, which is under the control of antidiuretic hormone (ADH). Pituitary dysfunction may involve hypo- or hypersecretion of ADH. In hyposecretion, for example, the plasma fluid content decreases via an increased urine formation—water loss—thereby increasing the osmolarity of the residual plasma solution. In turn, ultimately water throughout the body moves from the cells into the interstices, causing intracellular dehydration. By contrast, in hypersecretion of ADH, more interstitial fluid is retained, which in turn causes cellular edema. Obviously the departure from the normal state of homeostasis in either case will result in cell dysfunction and lead in turn to further imbalance on the part of cells dependent on the faulty product of the edematous cells.

Clinically the dehydrated patient—see "Factors Related to Dehydration" on p. 61—has usually lost more fluid than salt—has a greater water deficit. Therefore, although administering water alone—without salt—will result in a quick loss of much of the replacement fluid, isotonic salt solution need not be used as the sole supplement but may be used alternately with a glucose solution, the glucose being metabolized to carbon dioxide and water.

A 0.9% NaCl solution is isotonic with the 153 mEq/L of the total plasma electrolytes, containing 154 mEq/L of sodium ions and an equal amount of chlorine ions but being deficient with reference to all the other plasma anions and cations. Furthermore, it is actually hyperosmotic for the Na^+ and Cl^-, especially for the chlorine. Accordingly, for each liter of 0.9% NaCl administered, the patient will suffer a base deficit of 3 to 4 mM/L. In an attempt to simulate nature newer solutions substitute acetate to obtain ionic balance, and since the acetate metabolizes to bicarbonate, no acid-base change should result.

In overhydration—see "Factors Related to Overhydration" on p. 61—corrective therapy is directed primarily at instituting diuresis, whether this entails (1) the use of osmotic substances, for example, mannitol and glucose; (2) carbonic anhydrase inhibitors, for example, acetazolamide and thiazides; or (3) aldosterone antagonists, for example, spironolactone. Unfortunately, the prolonged use of diuretics may itself cause excessive, unbalanced loss of electrolytes.

■ What is pH and what is its physiologic significance?

The concentration of hydrogen ions is referred to as *pH,* defined as the negative logarithm of the hydrogen ion concentration. At 25° C pure water has an equal number of hydrogen and hydroxyl ions per liter and, therefore, this is referred to as its neutral point. It contains 0.0000001 g, or 10^{-7} g, of H^+/L. In the laboratory this is expressed as pH 7. At body temperature (38° C) the neutral point is pH 6.8. Therefore the blood is actually more alkaline (at pH 7.4) than it initially seems.

Solutions containing more than 10^{-7} g of H^+/L are said to be *acid*; they have a decreased pH, the pH is lower—it is closer to pH 0. Solutions containing fewer hydrogen ions are said to be *alkaline;* they have an increased pH, the pH is higher—it is closer to pH 14. Unfortunately, acid-base terminologies used by clinicians are not always the same as those used by chemists. Currently chemists define an acid as any compound capable of donating a hydrogen ion or a proton to a base. Thus not only are there conventional acids, such as HCl and H_2CO_3 acid, but ammonium ion (NH_4^+) is also an acid, since it can donate an H^+ to a base. The clinicians tend to stay with the older terminology, classifying Cl^-, SO_4^{--}, and PO_4^{---} as acids and the cations Na^+, K^+, Ca^{++}, and Mg^{++} as bases. The clinicians have two exceptions: the cation H^+ is classified as an acid and the anion OH^- is classified as a base. (OH^- is the strongest base in the body.) According to the newer terminology Na^+, K^+, Ca^{++}, and so forth are neither acids nor bases as they will not accept or donate H ions or protons.

When an acid goes into solution, it dissociates into H^+ and a base. The base of a given acid is called the *conjugate base* of that acid; for example, HCO_3^- is the conjugate base of carbonic acid, and Cl^- is the conjugate base of hydrochloric acid. There is a reciprocity between the strength of an acid and its attachment to its conjugate base; that is, a strong acid is one that is very weakly attached to its conjugate base, yielding a larger number of hydrogen ions, for example, HCl. A weak acid contains proportionately more undissociated molecules—fewer H^+—per liter, for example, H_2CO_3.

Whether directly or indirectly (by way of the Krebs cycle), the major end product of the metabolism of carbohydrates, fats, and proteins is the production of carbon dioxide, which in turn reacts with water to form carbonic acid.

$$CO_2 + H_2O \rightleftharpoons H_2CO_3 \rightleftharpoons H^+ + HCO_3^-$$

The formation of H_2CO_3 from CO_2 and H_2O is referred to as the *hydration* of CO_2, and the reverse action is called *dehydration.* Normally the concentration of CO_2 dissolved in water is about 1000 times greater than the H_2CO_3 concentration, and the preceding equation is pushed to the left by added acids as long as any HCO_3^- remains in the body's reservoir. At least 15,000 mEq of CO_2 escape by the lungs and 50 mEq by the kidneys each day. During the breakdown of protein various nonvolatile acids are formed, such as phosphoric, uric, and sulphuric acids.

■ How is the pH maintained at normal?

Being such an acid-producing machine, the body has developed several mechanisms to regulate its pH between 7.38 and 7.42 in an average state of health. Of the *four main buffer systems* in the body for maintaining pH homeostasis the *bicarbonate–carbonic acid buffer system* is quantitatively the largest and is the principal buffer system in the extracellular fluid. The *phosphate buffer system* is important in the RBC's and in the kidney tubules, where it helps with the excretion of hydrogen ions. The *protein buffer system* operates primarily inside of the tissue cells, there being about four times as much protein anion intracellularly as in the plasma. The *hemoglobin buffer system* works only in the RBC's. However, because the red blood cell also contains carbonic anhydrase (discussed later in the section on respiration), it is the principal source of the bicarbonate involved in both the extracellular water and the RBC's bicarbonate–carbonic acid buffer systems.

Normally the concentration of bicarbonate in the extracellular water is 27 mEq/L (27 mM/L), and the concentration of carbonic acid is 1.35 mEq/L (1.35 mM/L), which can be calculated to equal a ratio of 20:1 at pH 7.4. It is this *ratio* of the two components of the buffer system rather than the absolute amounts that determines the pH.

Although most of the acids formed and encountered (from food and so forth) within the body are stronger than carbonic acid, for example, acetic, citric, glutaric, and hydrochloric acids, they are, nonetheless, buffered by $NaHCO_3$ and similarly converted in part to H_2CO_3. Likewise, any base that enters the body can be immediately converted into bicarbonate and quickly eliminated through the respiratory system. If a strong acid is buffered in the blood, about 7% is buffered by plasma HCO_3^-, 11% by blood proteins, 25% by interstitial HCO_3^-, and 57% by tissue cell water and bone. The clinician follows primarily the percentage reduction in plasma HCO_3^- rather than what goes on in each of these individual entities, as changes in plasma HCO_3^- reflect the approximate amount of change in the total buffer stores.

When analyzing acid-base and electrolyte balance, reference may be made clinically to the *"buffer base"* (BB), the HCO_3^-, and protein content. These are bases according to the newer definition since they are hydrogen ion acceptors. Buffer base amounts to 41 (or 42) mEq/L and is a better index of the acid-base balance than bicarbonate alone, since the HCO_3^- concentration is so much influenced by the Pco_2 level. Likewise, since the slope of the buffer line depends in part on the protein content of the blood, the slope will vary with the Hb concentration in whole blood, that is, it will vary with hematocrit changes.

■ What are the primary acid-base disturbances?

In varying from normal the pH of the body fluids may shift to the acid side, producing an acidotic condition known as *acidosis*, or it may

swing toward the base side, producing an alkaline condition known as *alkalosis*. Any time the concentration of either bicarbonate or carbonic acid is shifted, the normal 20:1 ratio of the buffer components changes and characteristic patient symptoms appear. Based on relationships within the bicarbonate–carbonic acid buffer system, acid-base balance disorders are classified clinically in four large categories: (1) respiratory acidosis, (2) respiratory alkalosis, (3) metabolic acidosis, and (4) metabolic alkalosis.

Respiratory acidosis occurs when the lungs are unable to eliminate CO_2 efficiently and, for this reason, occurs most often in patients with chronic lung diseases, such as emphysema. It is synonymous with hypercapnia, that is, high patient CO_2 levels and an associated overactive respiratory system. As a compensatory mechanism, the kidneys break down more H_2CO_3, thereby both eliminating the acid-forming H^+ and gaining additional HCO_3^- as buffer.

In *respiratory alkalosis* the alveolar Pco_2 has been decreased by hyperventilation, resulting in a lowering of plasma levels of carbonic acid and dissolved CO_2 and a rise in blood pH. This is referred to clinically as hypocapnia, or hypocarbia. Plasma bicarbonate is lowered by increasing renal excretion of bicarbonate. The continued excessive "blowing off of CO_2" in hyperventilation results from excessive stimulation of the respiratory center brought on by drugs, disease, or anxiety.

Metabolic acidosis occurs when the concentration of bicarbonate falls because it has been consumed in neutralizing excess acid, whether (1) volatile CO_2 or volatile nonbicarbonate or (2) nonvolatile acid (such as sulphuric, uric, or phosphoric acid from protein metabolism). The order of the frequency with which the precipitating factors are seen clinically is (1) *uremia*, caused by various types of kidney disease; (2) *ketosis*, where fat is the primary source of energy or associated with diabetic ketone body production; and (3) *lactic acidosis*, where there is an inadequate oxygen supply, as in heart failure or shock. In compensation the acidosis stimulates the respiratory center to increase the depth and rate of respiration, and the kidneys produce more HCO_3^- and excrete more H^+.

In *metabolic alkalosis* there is an increase in the concentration of plasma HCO_3^- relative to the concentration of H_2CO_3, whether from a gain in fixed base or a loss in fixed acid. Major causes of metabolic alkalosis include (1) the loss of chlorine from vomiting, diarrhea, or the use of some diuretics; (2) an excess of aldosterone, which leads successively to K^+ loss, ultimately increased H^+ excretion, and ultimately increased bicarbonate levels; and (3) ingestion of excessive amounts of $NaHCO_3$ or other antacids. Treatment of metabolic alkalosis is complicated and inefficient, relating in part to the correction of potassium deficiency.

■ **How may acid-base disturbances be expressed graphically?**

Since the determination of intracellular electrolyte concentrations requires special techniques, the physician must rely on changes in extracellular electrolytes, particularly in plasma or serum, in treating patients. In doing this, determinations of the concentrations of the blood bicarbonate, the blood pH, and (sometimes) the level of carbonic acid in the plasma are used as indices of the patient's acid-base balance. Once any two of

these three concentrations has been determined in the laboratory, the third concentration may be determined by the use of the Henderson-Hasselbalch equation, which is:

$$pH = 7.62 - \log \frac{P_{CO_2}}{(HCO_3^-)p}$$

Having ascertained the aforesaid concentrations, the patient's data may be matched to a graph similar to that presented in Fig. 2-7 in an effort to determine his/her particular degree and type of metabolic disturbance. On this graph, for convenience, the numbers across the abscissa are given as both pH and in nanomoles of H^+/L. Isobars for P_{CO_2} (in mm Hg) are numbered across the top and to the right. The P_{CO_2} 40 isobar is considered to be the mean. The mM/L of HCO_3^- is given on the ordinate (Fig. 2-7). An introductory concept of how the graph works may be gained if one imagines that the P_{CO_2} is fixed at isobar 40 and a strong, nonvolatile acid is added to a bicarbonate solution. With the addition of H^+ the concentration of bicarbonate would then decrease down the P_{CO_2} 40 isobar and to the left, indicating the decrease in pH and bicarbonate. Contrariwise, if base were added, the reading

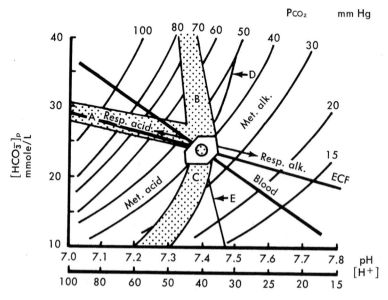

Fig. 2-7. Acid-base diagram. (From Jung, R. C.: Crit. Care Update **3:**5, 1976.)

would move upward and to the right along the P_{CO_2} isobar. The buffering power of the extracellular fluid is represented by the line labeled *ECF* and that of the blood by the line at a slight angle to it. The patient's progress and compensatory mechanisms can be followed as successive tests are made and plotted and analyzed. For further discussion, any standard text on respiratory physiology should be consulted.

NERVOUS SYSTEM

The nervous and endocrine systems are specialized for integrating the body's activities. They accomplish this by providing secretions that stimulate the other organs and even other portions of their own systems. In the case of the endocrine system, the secretion (or stimulus), called a hormone, is released into the bloodstream, and the reaction produced is a relatively slow one. The secretion produced by nerves (or neurotransmitter) is released in the immediate proximity of the structure it will activate, producing almost instantaneous reaction in the structure "innervated," for example, the muscle innervated. The activation, or "excitation," of the nerve cell (called a *neuron*) to release its secretion is characterized by the propagation, or transmission, of an electrical impulse from one of its extremities to the other. Structures innervated by neurons include other neurons, myofibers, and gland cells. When one neuron innervates another, they are said to *synapse* with one another. Synaptic chains are formed when the first neuron in the chain, called a first-order neuron, stimulates a second, second-order neuron, which stimulates a third, third-order neuron, and so forth. Neurons interposed between the first and final order of neurons are referred to as internuncial, or intermediate, neurons. Of the 14 billion neurons in the body, 97% are internuncials.

■ **What is a convenient system for classifying the component parts of the nervous system?**

For didactic purposes it is convenient to divide the nervous system into the following categories:

CENTRAL NERVOUS SYSTEM (CNS)
  Brain
  Spinal cord

PERIPHERAL NERVOUS SYSTEM (PNS)
  Cranial nerves
  Spinal nerves
AUTONOMIC NERVOUS SYSTEM (ANS)

■ **What is the histologic nature of the neuron?**

As shown in Fig. 2-8, in man the nucleus of a neuron is surrounded by a mass of cytoplasm, forming a *cell body* (synonyms are *soma* and *perikaryon*) from which project two or more processes, or *fibers*, called *axon(s)* and *dendrite(s)*. Embedded in the cytoplasm are microtubules, neurofibrils, mitochondria, and Nissl bodies. The plasmalemma is known as the axolemma. The portion of the soma from which the axon originates is known as the *axon hillock,* or *initial segment*. Although some cells, called *bipolar cells,* possess only one dendrite and one axon, the majority of them, called *multipolar cells,* have many dendrites. The relative and absolute lengths of the axons and dendrites will vary depending on the part of the body in which they are located. Initially physiologists used the term "dendrite" to describe the process that transmits an impulse from the synapse toward the cell body and the term "axon" to identify the process carrying the impulse from the cell body to the terminal branches. Unfortunately, it has become a common practice to designate as an axon any neuronal process that is covered with a myelin sheath (see p. 68). Since both the afferent and efferent processes of peripheral neurons may be covered in part with myelin, reference to afferent "axons" can be quite disconcerting to the uninitiated.

■ **How do modifications of the peripheral ends of the dendrites adapt them to their functions?**

The distal ends of dendrites and axons are called *end-organs* and are named, respectively, *receptors* and *telodendria*. While some receptors have free, naked endings, for example, pain receptors, in others there may be a fibrous capsule, variously shaped, surrounding the nerve tip. During the 1950's neurophysiologists espoused Müller's law of specific nerve energies, which maintained that any one neuron carried only one type of stimulus, for example, touch or tempera-

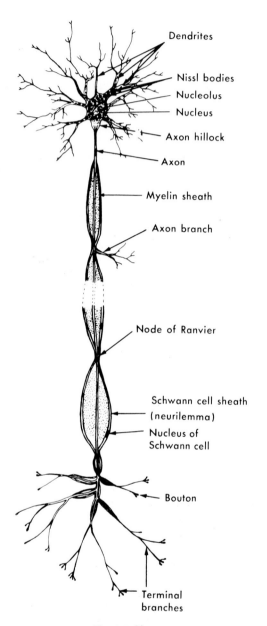

Dendrites

Nissl bodies

Nucleolus

Nucleus

Axon hillock

Axon

Myelin sheath

Axon branch

Node of Ranvier

Schwann cell sheath
(neurilemma)

Nucleus of
Schwann cell

Bouton

Terminal
branches

Fig. 2-8. Neuron.

ture. This is no longer held to be true. For further details, standard texts of neurophysiology may be consulted.

■ **How does the structure of axons adapt them for the performance of their functions?**

The normal current flow of a neuronal impulse starts in a dendritic receptor, passes to and through the soma, and is distributed out the arborizations of the axon to the telodendria. While the branches of dendrites make angular junctions with one another, the branches of axons, called *collaterals*, leave the main trunk at right angles. Depending on their location, the total ("cable") length of the main axon and its collaterals may be less than, equal to, or greater than the total (cable) length of the dendrites. Each collateral branch is potentially capable of innervating some structure(s), that is, cell or cells. For example, the arborization of a neuron going to the biceps muscle of the thigh may have as many as 100 to 150 branches, each going to a separate myofiber, which it can activate. Furthermore, the myofibers innervated by any one neuron do not constitute a localized group but may have a considerable distribution throughout the muscle. Consequently, contraction is general throughout the muscle rather than local.

The exact structural nature of the telodendria and the structural relationship between a telodendron and the cell(s) it innervates take several forms. Some telodendria end by forming spirals around their effector cells. At myoneural junctions the telodendria form *motor end-plates*. Regarding synaptic chain connections, the telodendria of first-order neurons may form bulbous boutons that come into proximity either with the distal ends or the sides of the second neuron's dendrites or with the soma of the second-order neurons.

■ **What are the sheath of Schwann (neurilemma or neurolemma) and myelin and what are their functions?**

Embryologically, as the axons and dendrites of the PNS grow toward the periphery, they are accompanied by *Schwann cells,* or *neurilemmae,* each of which is 0.1 to 0.5 mm long, which invest themselves as a single-cell layer like a tunnel around the neuronal plasma membrane (or axolemma), somewhat like a capillary whose lumen is filled with a nerve fiber. The neurilemma is interrupted at regular intervals by *nodes of Ranvier*, the spaces between successive nodes being referred to as internodes. The nodes mark the areas of discontinuity between successive Schwann cells laid end-to-end along the length of the fiber.

Although all nerves of both the CNS and PNS possess a neurilemma, some neurons, as they mature, remain gray whereas others become white. This depends on whether or not a myelin sheath develops. Electron microscopy (EM) has demonstrated that the *myelin* is actually part of the Schwann cell wrapped in a jelly roll fashion around the neural plasma membrane so as to produce alternating layers of mixed lipids and proteins. The myelin sheath seems to act as an electrical insulator, enhancing the rate of impulse flow in neurons thus shielded. The speed of conduction of a neuronal impulse is also dependent on the diameter—the larger the diameter, the faster the conduction—and the length—the longer the neuron, the longer the conduction time.

Individual peripheral neurons, with or without myelin, are encompassed with reticular and fine collagen fibers; individual CNS fibers are similarly invested by *glial cells*. In each instance the surrounding structure is referred to as an *endoneurium*. A number of nerves going to or coming from a specific area is usually grouped together as a bundle called a *fasciculus*. Each fasciculus also has a (collagen or glial) sheath around it, termed a *perineurium*. The classic "nerve" named in anatomy books, for example, the sciatic nerve, is composed of a number of fasciculi, the entire nerve being surrounded by a sheath known as an *epineurium*.

■ What processes are occurring in a patient who has traumatized a nerve?

If the peripheral portion of a nerve is devitalized by trauma, the portion of the nerve and neurilemma distal to the site of injury, referred to as the distal segment as compared with the proximal segment, will soon degenerate in a process known as *wallerian degeneration*. In this process

the myelin and nerve fiber degenerate, then are consumed by macrophages, leaving a hollow tunnel within the endoneurium. Soon neurilemmal cells at the proximal and distal ends of the degenerate apex proliferate and grow toward one another, filling in the gap. Then the neuron sprouts into the slitlike spaces between the proliferating Schwann cells, toward the distal stump, and the Schwann cells spiral around the fiber, forming myelin. In the extremities proximal regeneration, for example, in the brachium, occurs at a rate of about 1 to 4 mm/week; more distal regrowth, for example, in the fingers, is slower. If a large nerve trunk is crushed, as the neurons regenerate they may grow back into the wrong endo- or even perineurium, for example, in the sciatic nerve, possibly to an entirely different group of muscles; accordingly, this requires that the patient be reeducated on the mental control over the muscle. Cicatrix may form at the site of injury, preventing reinnervation, and possibly even being associated with the growth of a neuroma. Even under the most favorable conditions, there will be anesthesia of the skin and some degree of paresis of the muscles normally innervated until the processes of wallerian degeneration and fiber regrowth have occurred.

In *nerve transplants* a sensory nerve, for example, the sural nerve, may be sacrificed and sewn into the position initially occupied by the motor nerve that has been destroyed. Surgically attention is directed to suturing the epineurium of the substitute to the epineurium of the remaining stumps in end-to-end anastomoses. Wallerian degeneration occurs in the neurons of the nerve transplant and the distal end of the injured nerve. Then the slow process of neural regeneration previously described takes place, with the same inherent problems that accompany normal regrowth.

■ How are nerve fibers classified?

As in the classification of many gross and microscopic anatomic structures and physiologic processes, there are numerous ways of categorizing the material, depending on the purpose(s). To indicate whether an impulse is going into or out of a structure, the neuron may be described as afferent (incoming) or efferent (outgoing). The terms *"presynaptic"* and *"postsynaptic"* are commonly used. Fibers carrying impulses toward a ganglion (see below) are *preganglionic;* those moving away from it are *postganglionic*. The impulse may be sensory or motor, depending on the nature of its stimulus. Impulses moving toward the brain are said to be *ascending;* those moving away from it are *descending.* Neurons surrounded by a myelin sheath are described as *myelinated;* those lacking the sheath are *non-myelinated.* If the axon is long, as in peripheral neurons, the cell is referred to as a *Golgi type I neuron;* if it is short, as those within the gray matter of the cord, it is designated as a *Golgi type II neuron.*

The thicker the nerve, the faster impulses travel in it. Also, generally the thicker the nerve, the thicker is the myelin sheath. Combining these two characteristics, neurons may be classified as A, B, or C fibers, although they vary from one animal group to another with the criteria selected, among other factors, and, accordingly, provide a basis for the different statistics appearing in different books. Fibers of the A group[6] are heavily myelinated, 11 to 20 μ in diameter, and conduct at speeds of 5 to 120 m/sec. Included are somatic motor and proprioceptive fibers. Fibers of the B group are moderately myelinated, 5 to 10 μ in diameter, and conduct at speeds of 3 to 15 m/sec. In addition to fibers for touch and pressure, they include the preganglionic ANS fibers. C fibers are unmyelinated, 0.5 to 4 μ in diameter, and conduct at speeds of 0.5 to 4 m/sec. In addition to fibers for pain, temperature, taste, and touch, the C fiber group includes postganglionic ANS fibers.

■ **What are some of the terms the neurologist uses in discussing anatomic and physiologic nerve groups?**

In some regions of the body the nerves intertwine to form a complex network known as a plexus, for example, the brachial plexus.

The term *"ganglion"* is usually used in reference to a group of cell bodies lying outside the CNS, for example, dorsal root ganglion, autonomic ganglion, or ganglion of a cranial nerve. However, it has been used in reference to components of the CNS, for example, basal ganglion.

Orthopedists also use the term in reference to fluid-filled cystic structures that are usually associated with fibrous tissue. The term *"nucleus"* is the typical counterpart of the term "ganglion" when the aggregate of cell bodies is found within the brain. Each pair of cranial nerves possesses two nuclei—more specifically, the right member of each pair possesses a nucleus and the left member of each pair possesses a nucleus.

Spinal cord and spinal nerves
■ **What are the gross characteristics of the spinal cord and the spinal nerves?**

The spinal cord, lying in the vertebral canal of the spinal column, is continuous through the foramen magnum with the medulla; it extends downward to the level of the second lumbar vertebra, where it ends as the medullary cone. At each vertebral level and attached to the sides of the cord are a pair (right and left) of spinal nerves that communicate with the periphery via openings between vertebrae known as *intervertebral foramina.** The spinal nerves are named in relation to the associated vertebral level of their origins. The first pair of spinal nerves, indicated as C1, leave the canal between the base of the skull and the first cervical vertebra. The C2 pair emerges below the first cervical vertebra between the first and second; the C8 pair appears below the seventh cervical vertebra. T1 is found below the first thoracic vertebra, and so forth. In summary, there are eight pairs of cervical spinal nerves; 12 pairs of thoracic nerves, five pairs of lumbar nerves, five pairs of sacral nerves, and one pair of coccygeal nerves, totaling 31 pairs.

Each spinal nerve is divided into a dorsal (sensory or afferent) root and a ventral (motor or efferent) root near its attachment to the cord. In its dorsal root ganglion the sensory root possesses the cell bodies of the afferent neurons, the dendrites being derived distally and the axons continuing proximally. The ventral root consists of the axons of motor neurons.

There is a cervical enlargement of the cord from the level of the fourth cervical vertebra to

---

*Bony or ligamentous irregularities in the openings can apply pressure to the nerve, producing moderate to severe neurologic symptoms.

the second thoracic vertebra and a lumbosacral enlargement between the levels of the fourth lumbar and third sacral vertebrae because of the concentration of nerves passing to the arms and legs in these areas.

Since the cord ends at the level of the second lumbar vertebra, but its nerves are distributed as far as the coccyx, the nerves in the lower end of the cord become obliquely disposed as components of the *cauda equina* around a central nonsensory terminal filament lying in the midline.

Superficially the cord is divided longitudinally into right and left halves by a dorsal sulcus and a ventral fissure. In cross section a centrally disposed butterfly (or H-shaped) area of *gray matter* is seen to be surrounded by an area of *white matter*. The limbs of the H form the dorsal and ventral horns. In the regions of T1 to L2 and S2 to S4, intermediate gray columns house the cell bodies of autonomic neurons. A central canal that lies in the center of the gray matter runs through the spinal cord, being continuous rostrally with the fourth ventricle of the medulla.

■ How does the anatomy of the spinal gray and white matter adapt them for their functions?

The gray matter consists primarily of cell bodies and, most commonly, the proximal portions of their associated axons and dendrites. Since cell bodies are unmyelinated, the area is gray. The myelin surrounding the axons and dendrites comprising the white matter is produced by oligodendrocytes, the counterparts of the Schwann cells of the PNS. Within the white matter the fibers are grouped into sensory or motor fasciculi that form ascending and descending "tracts," going to or coming from certain parts of the brain and/or ascending or descending to various vertebral levels to make synapses within the cord. Fasciculi are also grouped into dorsal, ventral, and lateral *funiculi*. For example, fibers of the dorsal funiculi are chiefly ascending (sensory), and their dysfunction, as in syphilis, results in tabes dorsalis, or locomotor ataxia, in which disturbances of joint and muscle sensation produce problems with walking. The virus producing infantile paralysis, or poliomyelitis, at-

tacks the anterior horn cells, resulting in motor paralysis of the associated muscles.

As the (sensory) fibers from the periphery join the spinal cord, fibers from the lower part of the body lie most medially. Those entering at progressively higher levels are found progressively more laterally, the cord itself thickening in a caudocephalad direction as a result of this accretion. Conversely, part of the cephalocaudad reduction in diameter is because of the concurrent attrition in the cord's content of motor fibers.

■ What are the anatomic and functional characteristics of a reflex arc?

If the finger is burned, the arm is rapidly withdrawn. The impulse activated by the painful stimulus travels along the dendrites of the involved spinal nerve to the cell bodies located in the dorsal root ganglion and in turn via their axons into the spinal cord. For any one neuron, on reaching the cord, several collateral branches may be given off, including one going into the dorsal (gray) horn of the spinal level of entrance, as well as branches that may descend one or more vertebral levels or ascend one or more vertebral levels before entering the dorsal horn. After entering the dorsal horn, the collateral synapses with a second-order neuron, called an internuncial or intermediate neuron, whose axon, in turn, may do any of the following:

1. Synapse with a third-order neuron whose cell body lies in the ipsilateral ventral (gray) horn
2. Cross over to the contralateral ventral horn to synapse with a third-order neuron
3. Split, one of its collaterals synapsing on the ipsilateral side and one on the contralateral side

In a reflex arc the axon of the third-order neuron leaves the cord by the ventral root (also designated as the motor root because the nerve is carrying out a motor function), as contrasted with the dorsal sensory root, whose nerves perform sensory functions. The dorsal and ventral roots are also labeled as afferent and efferent because of the direction of impulse flow through them. Components of the ventral root join the main nerve to pass distally to an area containing muscles that would be involved in retracting the arm.

Any one neuron would be distributed to 100 or so myofibers of some specific muscle, for example, the brachialis muscle, to participate in the reflex withdrawal.

The brain

In studying any of the body systems some knowledge of anatomy is necessary to develop a meaningful concept of the physiology of that system. This principle is especially applicable to the nervous system in view of its relative complexity. Whether a fundamental or advanced knowledge of the nervous system is sought, some appreciation of neurologic embryogenesis is inherent in making any sense of the maze of pathways and interrelationships.

Early in its development the forerunner of the brain and spinal cord is a hollow neural tube that enlarges at one (the cephalic) end. This swelling develops two transverse strictures, producing three bulbous structures identified serially, rostrocaudally, as the *prosencephalon, mesencephalon,* and *rhombencephalon.* The pros- and rhombencephalon in turn also develop transverse strictures, dividing the prosencephalon into a *telencephalon* and a *diencephalon* and the rhombencephalon into a *metencephalon* and a *myelencephalon.* The *neuroblasts* (formative cells) in the five initial blastema develop in different anatomic patterns and at different speeds, resulting in the formation of (1) swollen and constricted areas; (2) discrete aggregates of cell bodies, which will form the thalamus, cranial nuclei, and so forth vs more homogeneous areas; and (3) rostral modifications of the original central canal into four ventricles that remain in continuity with the initial canal as it persists (in a proportionately narrower state) in the spinal cord.

Much as the digestive tube attains greater length and surface area by coiling and developing inpouchings and outpouchings, the embryonic brain develops flexures and folds. Just as certain parts of the digestive tract are modified to perform special functions and yet are interdependent, so the brain has developed a number of specialized, interrelated subdivisions. The five major subdivisions of the brain may be used as points of reference in describing the various specialized regions and their interrelationships.

For didactic purposes the brain is generally divided into three regions: *cerebrum* (or cerebral hemispheres), *brain stem,* and *cerebellum* (or cerebellar hemispheres). The brain stem consists of medulla, pons, mesencephalon, and diencephalon.

■ What anatomic features of the cerebrum explain its functions?

For the purposes of this discussion the telencephalon will be considered to be composed of cerebral hemispheres, the basal ganglia, and cranial nerves I and II as outgrowths of the brain.

The cerebrum consists of two cerebral hemispheres incompletely separated by a deep, medial longitudinal fissure, at the base of which is the corpus callosum composed of axons interconnecting the two hemispheres anatomically and functionally. The surface of the hemisphere possesses shallow grooves called *sulci* and deep grooves called *fissures.* Of the two major grooves on the lateral surface, the ones beginning near the top and running almost vertically form the *central sulcus of Rolando.* The area anterior to this fissure is called the *frontal lobe;* the area immediately posterior to it is called the *parietal lobe.* The horizontal lateral groove is called the *lateral (sylvian) fissure;* it separates the frontal and parietal lobes above from the *temporal lobe* below. A parieto-occipital fissure, aligned with the lambdoid suture of the skull, separates the posteriorly located *occipital lobe* from the anterior lobes.

The cerebral hemispheres consist of a peripheral *cortex* and a deeper *medulla.* The cortical portion is gray because it consists primarily of cell bodies; the medulla is white because its principal components are myelinated fibers passing to and from the cortex.

Different areas of the cortical gray matter are specialized for the performance of specific functions, for example, the speech area or motor eye field, and are designated as various *Brodmann's areas* by Arabic numerals accorded them by a turn of the century neurologist. For general purposes areas anterior to the central fissure are of a motor nature; those posterior to it are of a sensory nature. For example, sensory fields associated with various parts of the body, such as the foot, knee, chest, or head, can be represented on a "sensory homunculus" projected in relation to the postcentral gyrus (Brodmann's area 3). The part of the cortical gray matter representing the foot is near the corpus callosum; the part representing the head is near the inferior border of the temporal lobe. A comparable "motor homunculus" is represented in the precentral gyrus (area 4).

Three major pathways exist in the cerebral white matter. *Transverse,* or *commisural, fibers* connect one hemisphere to the other, for example, the corpus callosum. In contrast, *association tracts* of various lengths and degrees of complexity connect different Brodmann's areas of the same hemisphere. *Projection tracts* pass to and from the brain stem, becoming part of the corona radiata that is continuous with the internal capsule.

For discussions of the coordinating centers known as the basal ganglia, of the olfactory brain, and of cranial nerves I and II, any standard neurology text may be consulted.

The telencephalon contains the first and second ventricles (see p. 78).

■ What are the anatomic and physiologic characteristics of the cranial nerves?

For ease of didactic discussion scientists have identified the 12 pairs of cranial nerves associated with the brain with both Roman numerals, I to XII, rostrocaudally, and with names. Cranial nerves (CN's) I and II, the olfactory and optic nerves, respectively, are actually outgrowths of the brain associated with smell and vision. Some of the CN's, that is, V, VII, VIII, IX, and X, possess extracephalic (outside of the brain) nuclei, which are analogous with the dorsal root ganglia of the spinal nerves. Within the brain, all of the CN's, except I, II, and VIII, possess motor nuclei formed of neuronal cell bodies that are analogous with the cell bodies of spinal cord ventral horn neurons that give rise to the axons forming the ventral (motor) roots of the spinal nerves.

For a detailed discussion of the location of the nuclei and of the anatomic distribution and the function of the CN's, textbooks of anatomy and/or physiology should be consulted to the depths desired.

■ What anatomic features of the diencephalon explain its functions?

For purposes of simplifying this discussion, the diencephalon will be considered to be composed of the thalamus, hypothalamus, pituitary stalk and associated posterior lobe, and parts of the visual apparatus lying outside of the principal portion of the brain. For further discussion of the pituitary gland, texts of anatomy and/or physiology may be consulted. The study of the visual system is out of the realm of discussion of this text.

With the exception of the olfactory nerves, every sensory impulse must synapse in the thalamus before being relayed to the cerebral cortex. Axons leaving the thalamus on their way to the cortex initially become part of the internal capsule, then perforate the corpus callosum and fan out as the corona radiata to become part of the various projection tracts going to specific cerebral sensory areas.

Inferior to the thalamus is the hypothalamus, which is an "emotional center" containing the origin of some of the sympathetic and parasympathetic fibers.

The third ventricle is located in the diencephalon (see p. 78).

■ What anatomic features of the mesencephalon explain its functions?

For the purposes of this discussion the mesencephalon, or midbrain, will be considered to consist of the corpora quadragemina and the cerebral peduncles, or crus cerebri.

The term *"corpus quadrigeminum,"* or *tectum,* applies to the four bodies distributed as anterior and posterior pairs on the dorsum of the midbrain. The anterior pair, called *superior colliculi,* or *optic tectum,* is a relay station for receiving impulses derived earlier in the synaptic chain from the retina. This pair subsequently synapses with neurons involved in moving the eyes and head and also helps to regulate the diameter of the pupil. The posterior pair, called the *inferior colliculi,* or *auditory tectum,* forms a relay station for receiving impulses derived earlier in the synaptic chain from the organ of Corti (for hearing).

The ventral aspect of the mesencephalon contains the nuclei of CN's III and IV, several descending pathways, and several ascending pathways.

The third ventricle passes through the mesencephalon and is continuous with the *aqueduct of Sylvius* (see p. 78).

■ **What anatomic features of the metencephalon explain its functions?**

For the purposes of this discussion the metencephalon will be considered to consist of the pons, cerebellar peduncles, and cerebellum.

The *pons* is divided into a more dorsal *tegmentum* and the more ventral *cerebral crura*. It contains the nuclei of CN's V to VIII. Pathways found in the ventral part are similar to those encountered rostrally in the midbrain. The existence of a pontine reflex respiratory center was mentioned in the section on the respiratory system.

Three bilateral pairs of *cerebellar peduncles* are prominent bundles of fibers connecting the cerebellum with the brain stem. The *inferior peduncles*, also called the *restiform bodies*, carry fibers from the spinal cord to the cerebellum. Fibers of the *middle peduncle*, or *brachium pontis*, arise from pontine nuclei and extend to the cerebellum. The *superior peduncle*, or *brachium conjunctivum*, constitutes the main efferent connection of the cerebellum, containing fibers for the thalamus, reticular formation, and red nucleus, the latter being a synaptic relay nucleus for fibers whose destination is the spinal cord.

Although the *cerebellum* receives many afferent fibers for proprioception and stereognosis, it is not involved in conscious perception. Rather it is a coordinator of muscle group actions, timing their contractions to perform smoothly and accurately. Although voluntary movements can proceed without it, such movements are usually clumsy and disorganized. *Cerebellar ataxia,* or *asynergy*, produced by cerebellar dysfunction, results in a lack of motor skills. To a considerable extent, if sufficient time elapses, other brain mechanisms compensate for cerebellar defects.

Unlike the cerebrum, where the right half of the brain has motor control over the left side of the body and vice versa, the coordination of muscle movements on the right side of the body is associated with the right half of the cerebellum.

Both the met- and myelencephalon contribute to the formation of the fourth ventricle (see p. 78).

■ **What anatomic features of the myelencephalon explain its functions?**

The term "myelencephalon" is synonymous with the term "*medulla.*" CN's VIII to XII are associated with the medulla.

Since the medulla is directly continuous with the spinal cord, many of the descending fibers arising above the medulla continue caudally into the cord, and many of the ascending fiber tracts associated with the cord are represented in the medulla. For example, on the dorsal surface axons of the cord tracts called the *fasciculus gracilis* and *fasciculus cuneatus* synapse in the medullary centers called, respectively, the *clava* and *cuneate tubercle*.

The ventral aspect is characterized by the prominent groups of corticospinal motor fibers forming the pyramids, which cross over in the lower half of the medulla in the *decussation of the pyramids*. As a result, as mentioned previously, the right half of the brain controls the motor functions of the left side of the body.

On the lateral aspect of the medulla, swellings known as the *inferior olivary nuclei* bulge out between the origins of CN's XI and XII. Axons from the perikaryons located here travel via the restiform body to the cerebellum.

The central canal is modified in relation to the met- and myelencephalon to form the fourth ventricle (see p. 78).

■ **What are some of the major fiber tracts?**
Pyramidal system

It was indicated in discussing the anatomic features of the cerebrum (p. 72) that various Brodmann's areas are responsible for the voluntary selection of muscle movements but that area 4 is responsible for their execution, with the entire body being represented by a motor homunculus here. Actions evolving from willed impulses initiated by area 4 are said to be part of the pyramidal system, as compared with those initiated in premotor area 6, considered to be part of the extrapyramidal system.*

As the axons of the pyramidal system descend to striated muscles, two orders of neurons are involved:

UPPER MOTOR NEURONS (PYRAMIDAL FIBERS)
To CN nuclei of III to VII and IX to XII — As corticomesencephalic and corticobulbar tracts
To ventral horn cells — As corticospinal tracts

*Simultaneous discharges from all parts of the motor cortex produce the movements seen in *epileptic attack*, as compared with a small focus of irritation near one part of the motor area that may precipitate *jacksonian seizures*.

LOWER MOTOR NEURONS (PERIPHERAL FIBERS)

From CN nuclei   As CN's
From ventral horn cells   As 31 pairs of spinal
                            nerves

As in the case of most other nerve tracts, compound names are given to the bundles in which these axons travel, the first name being the site of origin, the second the destination, for example, corticospinal. On leaving the cortex all of the upper motor neurons first interdigitate with the ascending sensory fibers and pass alongside of them in the *internal capsule,* which is the area between the thalamus (medially) and the basal ganglia, or corpus striatum (laterally).

Corticomesencephalic tract fibers descend to the levels of the nuclei of CN's associated with the extraocular muscles, that is, III, IV, and VI. Unlike the other upper motor neurons that start from area 4, these neurons have their origins in area 8. During surgery with part of the calvarium removed, stimulation of the right area 8 causes both eyes to turn to the left.

Corticobulbar tract fibers (and those of the corticospinal tract as well) start from area 4 but continue (with the corticospinal tract) through the mesencephalic peduncles to the pons and medulla, where the bulbar fibers synapse with the nuclear cells of CN's V to VII, and IX to XII. Since CN VIII has no motor output, there is no need for corticobulbar fibers to go to its nucleus.

Corticospinal tract fibers constitute what are classically referred to as the *pyramidal (tract) fibers.* While most of them decussate in the medullary pyramids, as indicated previously, some of them remain uncrossed, but in any event, whether they descend in the anterior or lateral funiculus of the cord, they finally synapse with anterior horn cells. The anterior horn cells provide the axons of the ventral (motor) roots of the spinal nerves.

Extrapyramidal system

The term "extrapyramidal system" usually does not allude to "any descending fibers other than those in the pyramidal system," as might well be assumed, for this would include the descending components of the vestibular and cerebellar systems. Rather, clinically the extrapyramidal system refers to the right and left corpora striata and their associated reticulospinal tracts. Each

corpus striatum consists of a caudate nucleus and a lentiform nucleus, the latter in turn being composed of the putamen and the globus pallidus, or pallidum. (By way of relationships, it should be remembered that the internal capsule passes between the thalamus and the corpus striatum.) Ignoring the details of the internal circuits, the outflow of impulses from the corpus striatum probably emerges entirely from the pallidum. Those fibers that extend from the pallidum to the subthalamic nuclei split up, some continuing to the red nucleus and some to the *reticular activating system* (RAS), also called the *reticular activating formation* (RAF).

The RAS controls the state of arousal or sleep and focuses attention. While arousal is a nonspecific phenomenon affected by all sensory inputs, it is characterized by both ascending and descending divisions. The ascending division influences the excitability of the cerebral cortex, cerebellum, and hypothalamus, disinhibiting them and arousing them. The descending division, via the *reticulospinal tract,* makes synapses in the anterior horn, thus influencing the muscle reflexes; it also affects the autonomic nerves.

■ What are the functional relationships of the ANS?

The ANS is composed of two subdivisions, the sympathetic and the parasympathetic systems, each of which is characterized by a two-neuron complex composed of preganglionic (first-order) and postganglionic (second-order) neurons. In both sympathetic and parasympathetic systems the preganglionic fibers are myelinated and the postganglionic fibers are nonmyelinated.

Since ANS responses are widespread, functionally significant, and relate to phenomena commonly recognized by both laymen and medical personnel, some review of the anatomic bases for the potential responses is in order.

Sympathetic system

The sympathetic preganglionic (first-order) neuron has its cell body located in the lateral horn of the gray matter (intermedolateral column) found from spinal nerve levels T1 through L2. For this reason the sympathetic portion is referred to as the thoracolumbar part of the ANS. As a preganglionic sympathetic axon from some ver-

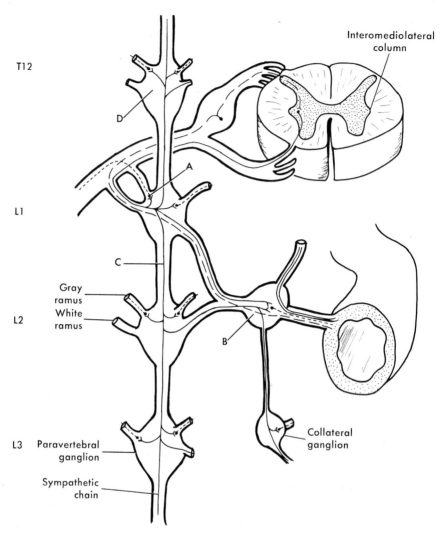

Fig. 2-9. Sympathetic portion of autonomic nervous system. (Redrawn from Netter, F. H.: The Ciba collection of medical illustrations, nervous system, vol. 1, Summit, N.J., 1957, Ciba Pharmaceuticals.)

tebral level between T1 and L2 leaves the cord, it travels as a component of the ventral root and passes to its local level paravertebral sympathetic ganglion (Fig. 2-9). There one of four potential branchings, which will be indicated as types *A, B, C,* and *D,* may occur:

TYPE A: One of the collaterals may synapse in the local *paravertebral ganglion*. The postganglionic fiber,

second-order neurons in the case of L1, would possibly join the first lumbar nerve initially, then shortly join the corresponding artery.

TYPE B: A collateral could leave the paravertebral ganglion without synapsing locally and synapse instead in a nearby *collateral ganglion,* for example, the *celiac ganglion*. In such a case, the postganglionic fiber, as a splanchnic nerve, might go to the tunica muscularis of the gut, causing an inhibition of gastric motility, and/or it might go to a mesenteric artery, potentially causing vasoconstriction.

TYPE C: Another collateral could proceed down to the next several paravertebral ganglia, potentially synapsing at each of these, then act as in A or B branching.

TYPE D: After entering the local paravertebral ganglion, for example, at L1, a collateral could turn rostrally to the next several higher paravertebral ganglia, then act as in A or B branching.

As a result of the presence of the ascending and descending fibers from one paravertebral ganglion to another, a *sympathetic chain* is created on both sides of the spinal column.

In summary, the sympathetic nerves may produce the following phenomena: vasoconstriction, whether the vessel be in smooth muscle or gland; speeding up of the heartbeat; bronchiospasm; uterine contraction; inhibition of gastric motility; and pupillary dilatation.

The neurosecretion at synapses between pre- and postganglionic fibers is ACh; that at the end of the postganglionic fiber is norepinephrine. This provides the basis for referring to the sympathetic nerves as *adrenergic fibers.*

Parasympathetic system

The parasympathetic system is referred to as the *craniosacral* portion of the ANS because it arises in part in association with CN's and in part in the derivatives of spinal nerves S2-4. The sites of origin of the cranial preganglionic (first-order) fibers are nuclei located near the nucleus of the CN with which the preganglionic fiber travels for part of its course. At some point along the course of the nerve the main components of the CN separate from the parasympathetic components, and the latter join an autonomic ganglion in order to synapse with the postganglionic component. Ganglia associated with parasympathetic fibers that are temporarily components of, or travelling with, CN's are: the *ciliary ganglion* (for the ciliary body muscles and sphincter pupillae of the eye), associated with CN III; the *submaxillary ganglion* (for the sublingual and submaxillary glands), associated with CN VII; the *sphenopalatine ganglion* (for secretions of the lacrimal gland, nose, and paranasal sinuses), associated with CN VIII; the *otic ganglion* (for the parotid gland), associated with CN IX; and Meissner's

and Auerbach's plexuses and cardiac nodes (to promote peristalsis of the gut and to slow down the heart), associated with CN X.*

Preganglionic (first-order) fibers of the sacral portion of the parasympathetics, like the sympathetic fibers, arise from cell bodies located in the lateral horn—intermedolateral column—of the spinal cord, but at the level of origin of nerves S2-4. The preganglionic fibers, again similar to the sympathetic fibers, leave the cord with the ventral root of the spinal nerve. However, they do not go to the sympathetic paravertebral ganglia. Rather, they leave the sacral nerves shortly and join one another to form the *pelvic splanchnic nerves.* These pass to the distal ends of the gastrointestinal tract, where they synapse in Meissner's and Auerbach's plexuses within the gut wall and enhance peristalsis when activated.

The parasympathetic fibers secrete ACh at the end of the pre- and postganglionic fibers. This provides the basis for referring to them as *cholinergic fibers.*

■ What are the meninges?

The *meninges* are membranous coverings disposed in three layers around the brain and spinal cord. The most peripheral layer, the *dura mater,* consists of tough, fibrous connective tissue. However, it differs in the cranial cavity and the vertebral canal, being a double layer in the former and a single layer in the latter. In the skull the outer layer constitutes an internal periosteum and stays with the skull when the brain is removed, whereas the inner layer covers the brain. In addition to the numerous branches of the meningeal arteries and veins invested in the dura mater, there are large venous channels known as *venous dural sinuses* that relate in part to the circulation of the cerebrospinal fluid. In the spinal cord an *epidural space* filled with connective tissue exists between the bone and the dura mater. The periosteum of the vertebra forms the outer boundary of the epidural space.

The *pia mater* is adherent to the brain, dipping down between the convolutions as a fine layer of areolar tissue. It is thicker and less vascular in

---

*The vagus nerve is composed primarily of sensory fibers (two-thirds).

relation to the cord than it is in relation to the brain.

The *arachnoid* is a delicate, fibrous tissue forming a cobweblike network of trabeculae between the dura mater and pia mater. The open spaces between the trabeculae constitute the *subarachnoid space,* which contains blood vessels and cerebrospinal fluid.

■ What is cerebrospinal fluid; how does it form and circulate?

Cerebrospinal fluid (CSF) is a clear, slightly viscous solution of inorganic salts with traces of dextrose, protein, urea, and other organic substances. Although it normally contains 0 to 6 WBC's/mm³ (counts over 10 WBC's/mm³ are considered as indicating cerebrospinal infection), the presence of RBC's is considered abnormal.

As was indicated in the sections on the telencephalon through myelencephalon, the brain contains four fluid-filled, communicating ventricles, one of which is located in each cerebral hemisphere (the first and second ventricles), one in the diencephalon (the third), and one on the dorsum of the pons and medulla (the fourth). The third and fourth ventricles are connected by the cerebral aqueduct of Sylvius. CSF is formed by secretion from capillary-like *choroidal plexuses* on the ventricular walls at a rate sufficient to replace its 120 to 135 ml volume about three times daily. To prevent a buildup of pressure above the normal (130 to 150 ml water), it circulates in a definite pattern and then is rejoined with the blood. CSF formed in ventricles I and II flows successively through ventricles III and IV, acquiring additional fluid and draining via foramina into the subarachnoid space. It circulates down and around the spinal cord and through the subarachnoid space around the brain, ultimately passing into and through a number of villi that protrude into the venous dural sinuses. The venous sinuses ultimately join the internal jugular vein.

Obstruction to the normal flow causes increased intracranial pressure, which causes papilledema (swelling at the optic disc), persistent headache, and vomiting. If the condition is present from birth, hydrocephalus results with its typical postnatal enlargement of the head.

While the termination of the cord is at the level of L2, the subarachnoid space extends to the level of about S2. In removing samples of CSF the needle is usually introduced into the subarachnoid space between the third and fourth lumbar vertebrae. Where general anesthesia might not be desirable, caudal blocks may be done, taking advantage of the fact that (relatively large) doses of epidural injections will diffuse into the subarachnoid space when injected into the region of the sacral hiatus.

■ What are the nutritive needs of the nervous system?

It was mentioned earlier that the respiratory quotient (RQ) of the brain is 1.0, indicating that its energy requirements are satisfied completely by carbohydrates. Since neurons do not reproduce after birth, the amount of nucleoprotein and similar substances required for growth from childhood to adulthood is relatively negligible. The need for O_2 is indicated by the speed with which unconsciousness results when the carotid arteries are occluded. Additionally serious brain damage results if the lack of O_2 continues for more than 6 to 8 minutes. Surgical experience has shown that the 4-minute interval quoted in earlier years is not commonly of serious consequence. Whereas in the adult about 20% of the total O_2 utilized by the body is consumed by the nervous system, the amount is even greater in the child, where the brain is proportionately larger.

■ How extensive is the blood supply to the brain?

Since the rate of O_2 utilization by the nervous system is 10 times that of the rest of the body tissues, it requires a rich blood supply. The epineurium of the spinal nerves contains vessels essential for the nerve's vitality. Accordingly, in nerve grafts it is important to preserve the integrity of the nerve sheaths.

An anterior and two posterior spinal arteries run the length of the spinal cord, lying in close proximity to it and nourishing it. The brain has an especially rich blood supply, receiving the internal carotid arteries plus the vertebral arteries as major sources, the latter uniting to form the basilar artery within the skull. The basilar artery unites with the internal carotid arteries to form the circle of Willis, whose functional integrity may provide important collateral in the event of loss of one of its components.

NEUROPHYSIOLOGY

■ **What is meant by membrane potential and how is it maintained?**

Although the positive sodium and potassium ions are found both inside and outside the neuronal membrane, externally the Na^+ concentration is high and the potassium ion (K^+) concentration is low; inside the cell the situation is reversed. The equilibrium potentials of sodium and potassium are such that during the resting or inactive state the inside of the membrane has a negative charge of 90 mV compared with the outside. (For detailed discussion of these equilibrium potentials any standard physiology text may be consulted.) The neuron is said to exhibit a *membrane potential* of −70 mV. The Na^+ and K^+, respectively, constantly leak into and out of the cell. Efforts to compensate for this are at least partially accounted for by an active "Na^+-K^+ pump," in which Na^+ is (1) picked up by an enzyme from the inside of the cell, (2) transferred to the outside of the cell, (3) dumped and exchanged for K^+, which is (4) transferred to the inside of the cell and dumped in exchange for more Na^+, and so forth. Energy to accomplish this active pumping is derived by the breakdown of ATP to ADP.

■ **What is meant by action potential and generator potential?**

The *nerve impulse,* or *action potential,* is a transient reversal of the resting potential, usually from −70 mV (internally) to +30 mV, a total amplitude of about 100 mV, in which the nerve is said to be *depolarized*. The stimulus for depolarization may be initiated (1) by dendritic receptors, for example, those for touch or pressure; (2) by synapses with other neurons, that is, by release of substances such as acetylcholine (ACh); or (3) spontaneously, for example, intrinsic cardiac beat and brain waves of the alpha type, although this is not the transmitter at most synapses. Much research on depolarization has centered on

ACh activity. Therefore the second option is usually chosen as the basis for discussing depolarization.

For an action potential to occur the membrane potential must be reduced to a critical level, called the *threshold potential*. The minimum stimulus capable of producing the threshold potential—and in turn an action potential—is called the *threshold stimulus*. Stimuli of greater capacity are referred to as suprathreshold stimuli. The threshold potential for most neurons is usually only 5 to 15 mV less than the resting membrane potential. Achievement of this 5 to 15 mV depolarization is *generated* by several means and is therefore known as a *generator potential*.

The accumulative depolarization, or generator potential, evolves at the axon hillock, or initial segment, where the axon is beginning but does not yet have a myelin sheath. It is affected by (1) strength, (2) duration, and (3) polarity of the stimulus, among other factors. Although thousands of synaptic knobs may end on a single neuron—a phenomenon referred to as *final common pathway*—potentiating its more rapid firing, no one knob, as a rule, can cause an action potential.* Different dendrites of the same neuron, as well as different neurons themselves, have different thresholds, the result being that as stimulus strength is increased, more and more nerves are "fired," or activated, to stimulate multiple final pathways. The result may be both temporal and spatial summation, which ultimately lowers the recipient neuron's generator potential to threshold. (For further discussion a standard textbook of physiology may be consulted.) Actually some neurons release neurohumors, for example, adenosine 3′,5′-cyclic monophosphate (cyclic AMP) and γ-aminobutyric acid (GABA), that increase the polarity rather than reverse it, that is, make the inside of the cell even more negative. Such *inhibitory neurons* cause increased permeability to K^+ and Cl^- and are said to produce a state of *hyperpolarization* rather than depolarization. ACh and norepinephrine can act as inhibitory or excitatory agents, depending on the nature of the postsynaptic membrane.

---

*This statement applies primarily to an internuncial neuron having multiple synaptic areas, as compared, for instance, with a myofiber that might be activated by a single nerve ending.

■ **What is meant by the "all-or-none" law?**

Regardless of the nature of the stimulus, once sufficient generator potential has been developed to attain the threshold level, an action potential is induced; its shape, magnitude, and duration are the same every time, thus the "all-or-none" law. Within a nerve each neuron is firing independently of the others, according to its individual threshold level. However, once fired the action potential of each neuron in the nerve is basically the same. The response per se gives no indication as to whether the generator potential reached the threshold on the basis of the strength of the stimulus, the frequency of the stimulus, or some other factor.

■ **What histochemical events occur when the threshold is reached?**

When the generator potential reaches threshold, within a fraction of a millisecond the membrane undergoes a change in its permeability to sodium, ions of the latter streaming to the inside at the axon hillock. (The exact relation between reaching threshold and Na^+ permeability is not understood.) The ascending phase of the spike potential represents the Na^+ inflow. Equally suddenly Na^+ reaches its new equilibrium, and the entry of additional ions is shut off, thus this is the apex of the spike. After a brief lag K^+ streams out of the cell, returning the membrane voltage to normal. When the spike has returned to 0, the net effect is that the fiber has exchanged equal amounts of Na^+ for K^+, most of the temporary residual imbalances soon being redressed by the Na^+-K^+ pump. However, the increased permeability to K^+ can continue for some time, causing a hyperpolarization, or positive afterpotential.

■ **How is the impulse propagated along the axon?**

Conduction within the axon is frequently compared with the flow of electrons in a wire. In both the wire and the neuron it is possible for an impulse to produce local changes in potential as ions move short distances internally across the surface of the wire or the membrane and externally produce local currents. In the case of the nerve, when sufficient current flow has been induced, the membrane permeability to Na^+ is changed, and the development of a typical action potential is initiated.

Since the strength of the current decreases exponentially as a function of the distance, in non-myelinated nerves the time required for inducing the depolarization from one area to its adjacent area becomes comparatively significant. Propagation of the impulse here involves sequential depolarization along the entire length of the neuron. In contrast, in myelinated nerves, because of the interrupted electrical insulation created by the myelin, conduction jumps along the axon from node to node—a phenomenon called *saltatory conduction*—and is much more rapid. (See discussion of conduction rates of A, B, and C fibers on p. 70.) When anesthetics are applied to the myelin of the internode, they are relatively ineffective at blocking transmission; when applied at the nodes, they are very effective.

■ **What is involved in the formation, release, response to, and deactivation of ACh?**

Since ACh and some of the catecholamines have been studied most, an introductory review of the activities of ACh will provide a working model of basic neurosecretory activities. The enzyme *choline acetyltransferase*, or *choline acetylase*, is synthesized in the neuronal soma and migrates out the axon to the terminals where ACh is formed and subsequently stored in vesicles as the concentrated ion. On the arrival of an action potential at the terminals, ACh is released from the vesicles and in turn from the neuronal membrane into the synaptic cleft. The process will not occur unless the proper amount of calcium ions (Ca^{++}) is present and even then can be inhibited by the presence of magnesium ions (Mg^{++}). The freed transmitter is attracted to the receptor, where its acceptance results in an almost instantaneous change in membrane permeability. Sequential to the membrane change is the development of an action potential in the postsynaptic structure if the synapse is interneuronal, a muscle contraction if the postsynaptic structure is a myofiber, or the release of a secretion if the postsynaptic structure is a gland cell. Within 1 to 2 msec after its release, ACh is removed from the synaptic cleft. This is the result of the following:

1. Destruction of the neurohormone by interaction at the receptor site
2. Decomposition of some ACh by AChE
3. Reabsorption of some ACh back into the presynaptic terminals for restorage in the vesicles
4. Diffusion of some ACh away from the area

For a similar review of the activities of the catecholamines, refer to the question on monoamines on p. 84.

Related pharmacology
■ **How are the receptor sites and associated drugs classified pharmacologically?**

It has become customary to refer to all neurons secreting catecholamines (CA's) as *adrenergic* and to all ACh-secreting neurons as *cholinergic*. In brief, adrenergic secretory tissues are as follows:

Neurons of the CNS secreting CA's

Postganglionic sympathetic neurons

Adrenal medulla plus similar "chromaffin tissue" scattered throughout the body.

By comparison, the following are classified as cholinergic neurons:

Neurons of the CNS secreting ACh

Peripheral (skeletal) motor nerves (The majority of peripheral sensory nerves are not cholinergic.)

Both sympathetic and parasympathetic preganglionic neurons

Postganglionic parasympathetic neurons

Sympathetic postganglionic neurons to sweat glands

Generally speaking, drugs that simulate the activities of the sympathetic nervous system are referred to as *sympathomimetic*, or *adrenergic*, *drugs* or *agents*, and their receptors are referred to as *adrenergic receptors*. Drugs that simulate the activities of the parasympathetic system are referred to as *parasympathomimetic*, or *cholinergic*, *drugs* or *agents*, and their receptors are referred to as *cholinergic receptors;* both of these types of receptors are shown in Fig. 2-10. Contrariwise, pharmaceutical agents that interfere with the synthesis or release of the body's adrenergic compounds or destroy them, as well as those that block their receptors, are called *antiadrenergic drugs*. Pharmaceuticals having similar relations to the body's cholinergic compounds are referred to as *anticholinergic drugs*.

Nicotine (and certain other drugs) may replace ACh at both sympathetic and parasympathetic autonomic ganglia and at skeletal myoneural junctions. Such postsynaptic tissues are therefore said to possess *nicotinic receptors*. Muscarine (and certain other drugs) may replace ACh at the synapse between the postganglionic

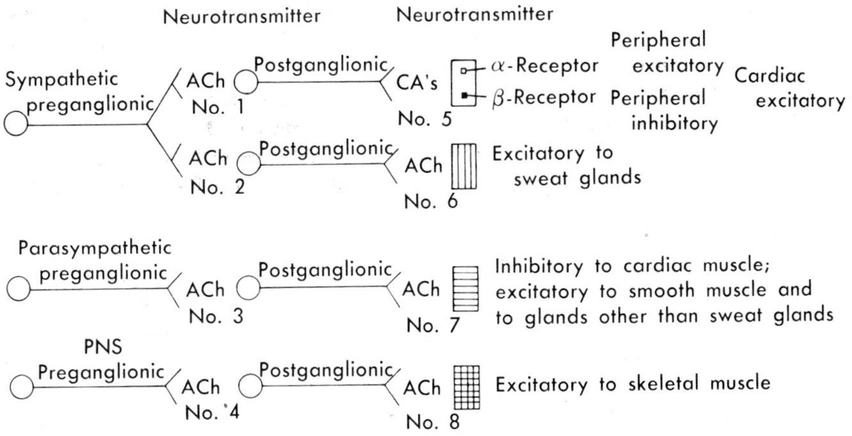

Fig. 2-10. Adrenergic and cholinergic receptors.

parasympathetic neurons and the tissue with which it, in turn, synapses. The reactor sites for such tissues are referred to as *muscarinic receptors.*

■ **What basic pharmacologic principles are needed to understand what is happening at synapses?**

Some compounds act only on smooth muscle, ANS ganglia, or skeletal myoneural junctions, whereas ACh acts on all of these. Presumably ACh has a simple structure, enabling it to react with numerous, basically similar receptors without necessarily being equally effective with all of them. It can easily be anticipated that, in view of the vagaries of drug actions, the rational therapeutic use of cholinergic and adrenergic drugs requires some basic knowledge of drug interactions. The review of the basics presented here will incorporate only a few selected examples of some of the commonly used cholinergic and adrenergic drugs. The reader is encouraged to seek additional specific information from comprehensive books on pharmacology.[7-9]

Drugs produce many reactions within the body, for example, blocking enzyme reactions within various body systems or within invasive, disease-producing micro-organisms or blocking osmotic effects, as in the kidneys or in using enemas. However, in this portion of the chapter, the terms "drugs" and "pharmaceutical agents" will be used in the context of neuropharmacologic reactions. Although topographically applied drugs admittedly have effects on peripheral nerves, didactic discussions of neuropharmacology are usually oriented in relation to synaptic phenomenon, wherein the termination of the presynaptic fiber, the synaptic cleft, and the postsynaptic sites are treated sequentially.

At axonal terminations drugs may facilitate or impede the synthesis, storage, release, and reabsorption of the neurohumor. In the synaptic cleft antiacetylcholinesterase (anti-AChE) agents are clinically effective. However, anticatechol-O-methyltransferase (anti-COMT) agents find no striking medical application.

Because of their inherent complex nature, a more lengthy description of receptor reactions is in order.

The receptor is generally conceived of as being

responsible only for combination with the drug and not for the subsequent type of response of the postsynaptic tissue. For example, after ACh has combined with the receptor the response in one instance might be contraction of gastrointestinal muscle but in another inhibition of cardiac muscle. However, it is also necessary to rationalize this concept with the realization that at different times two drugs can occupy the same receptor, with drug A having one effect and drug B another. A common interpretation is that the two drugs produced different conformational changes in the receptor.[10] An alternative, partially satisfactory interpretation is that the membrane "pores" of the receptor were blocked by one compound but permitted a postsynaptic reaction with the alternate drug, the postsynaptic response itself being subject to variations depending on various factors, for example, the prior physiologic state of the cell.

If two drugs are essentially equally attractive to the receptor, the law of mass action will prevail, and the agent present in the greatest concentration will "compete" most successfully for the majority of the reactive sites. When this competition exists at a cholinergic receptor, the cholinomimetic effects produced by the second drug may be (1) completely or only partially similar to those produced by the ACh, or (2) the second drug may completely block the reactive site, resulting in no postsynaptic reaction. *If the second agent is more powerfully attracted chemically to the cholinergic receptor,* again, either reaction, (1) or (2) above, could result. Comparable situations exist for pharmaceuticals interacting on adrenergic receptors.

In the event that the drug is introduced intravenously the degree of its success in competing with ACh, or any other drug, will depend on the following: its initial blood serum concentration, the efficiency of diffusion into and away from the receptor site, the relative chemical attractiveness to the receptor, the rapidity with which it is metabolized both within the bloodstream and at the receptor site, whether it is a short- or long-acting drug, and other interactions relating to the prior and present state of the reactive area. Obviously despite the ubiquitous nature of ACh, neither it nor any other drug will be acceptable at all receptors.

■ **What are some drugs whose therapeutic use relates to the synthesis, storage, and release of ACh at nicotinic synapses?**

Hemicholinium (HC-3) interferes with the mechanism for transporting choline from the soma to the nerve terminals, effectively inhibiting the production of ACh. Furthermore, it also inhibits choline acetyltransferase. Carbachol (carbamylcholine) was used for treating urinary retention and gastrointestinal spasm until more effective agents were developed. Its current use is primarily as a pupillary miotic, relating to its presumed release of ACh at parasympathetic ganglia. Botulinus toxin, the causative agent of certain types of food poisoning, prevents the release of ACh and thus causes respiratory failure. Once the toxin is firmly bound to the receptor, it can no longer be neutralized by antitoxins.

■ **How are the actions of the AChE's modified and what effects do these have?**

Drugs inhibiting the action of AChE's allow the buildup of ACh and its associated increased amount and duration of ACh action, for example, increased activity of organs and tissues receiving parasympathetic innervation, increased skeletal muscle activity, and CNS effects. Such *anti-AChE's* can be divided into two groups: *reversible and irreversible.* Reversible agents include the shorter acting (1 to 2 hr) edrophonium (Tensilon) and the longer acting (2 to 8 hr) plant derivative physostigmine and synthetic neostigmine. Because of their toxicity, the nonreversible anti-AChE's find little clinical usage, being limited primarily to the treatment of glaucomas, as with the drug isoflurophate (Floropryl). The nonreversible anti-AChE's find widespread commercial use as insecticides and have considerable potential for use as chemical warfare agents. Patient treatment consists of removing the toxic agent and administering atropine and pralidoxime (2-PAM).

■ **How are ganglionic blocking agents categorized?**

Based on their mode of action, ganglionic blocking drugs are categorized into two classes. In one, the *nondepolarizing agents,* the competing drug occupies the postsynaptic receptor in place of the ACh but has no stimulating effect, a classic example being *hexamethonium.* These drugs act on areas arbitrarily numbered 1 and 2 on Fig. 2-10. The second class, known as *depolarizing agents,* act first to stimulate, then to block the ganglion by causing persistent depolarization. The classic example is *nicotine.* Initially, in light and moderate doses, nicotine is cholinomimetic for gastric mobility, resulting in diarrhea and secretory activity in certain glands (salivary, bronchial, and perhaps gastric), but these effects are followed by depressed activity. In large doses the initial stimulation is very quickly followed by a blockage of transmission. Areas 1, 2, 3, and 8 of Fig. 2-10 are acted on by these depolarizing agents.

■ **What drug interactions take place at the myoneural junction?**

Similar to the ganglionic blocking drugs, pharmaceuticals acting at myoneural junctions may be classified as nondepolarizing and depolarizing. Since the myoneural junction was listed earlier as a nicotinic receptor, it should be noted that, although nicotine produces a depolarizing effect here similar to that at autonomic ganglia, it is much more active on ganglia than on myoneural junctions. Therapeutically the depolarizing compound most frequently used as a surgical adjunct is *succinylcholine chloride* (Anectine). The nonpolarizing drugs *curare* and *gallamine* (Flaxedil) also find clinical usage. Because of their histaminic-releasing action, the nondepolarizing blockers, especially *d-tubocurarine,* are not recommended for use in patients with asthma or other diseases producing histamine-like effects.

■ **What happens at cholinergic muscarinic receptors?**

As indicated at the beginning of this discussion (p. 81) muscarine, the *Amanita* mushroom toxin, and muscarine-like compounds compete with ACh at the synapse between the postganglionic parasympathetic neuron and its postsynaptic cell. Both atropine and scopolamine are derived from the African plant belladonna. When the excessive release of ACh by the vagus and pelvic splanchnic (parasympathetic) nerves produces intestinal spasm, when hyperacidity of the gastrointestinal tract is evidenced, in bronchial spasm, and in spasticity of the ureters and bile ducts, *atropine* provides valuable treatment. The atropine derivative *homatropine* is used by ophthalmologists in eye refraction to produce mydriasis.

Because of its depressant effects on the CNS, *scopolamine* is used mainly as a sedative, although it is also used to relieve motion sickness. Both atropine and scopolamine are used to prevent salivation during surgery. They are also used by the neurologist to reduce the tremors and rigidity of parkinsonism. Their pharmacologic effects sometimes persist from 3 to 10 days or more, unless reversed by some means.

Pilocarpine, a South American shrub alkaloid, has a potent muscarinic action but also has some slight nicotinic effects, explaining the slight hypertension observed after its administration. Its use in chronic, simple glaucoma is based on its ability to cause constriction of the iridial and ciliary muscles. It is used subsequent to ophthalmic examination to counteract the effects of atropine.

Bethanechol chloride (Urecholine) is a long-acting muscarinic drug used to treat urinary retention and constipation, especially that caused by autonomic-blocking, antihypertensive agents.

■ **Which of the body's monoamines are important as neurotransmitters, and how may their cycle be described briefly?**

The monoamines considered to be neurohumors are an indoleamine, 5-hydroxytryptamine (5-HT or serotonin), and a group of three catecholamines (CA's): epinephrine, norepinephrine, and dopamine. The formation of CA's is sequentially related. Technically phenylalanine can be converted to *tyrosine* to start the anabolic process. However, there is so much tyrosine normally available that this step is not ordinarily deemed important within the body. In the soma of the postganglionic sympathetic neuron tyrosine is converted by the enzyme tyrosine hydroxylase to dopa, and dopa is subsequently converted (by another enzyme) to *dopamine* (DA). DA migrates down the axon and enters the storage vesicles where it is changed into *norepinephrine* (NE). In the adrenal gland, first NE is manufactured in the medullary cells and stored in vesicles. It then leaves the granules, is methylated to *epinephrine* (E) in the cytoplasm, then is taken into a different group of vesicles within the cytoplasm where it is stored until released.

As with cholinergic nerves, the arrival of an action potential in a postganglionic sympathetic neuron terminal results in the release of the neurotransmitter, provided the proper amount of Ca^{++} is present and Mg^{++} does not cause inhibition.

Having been released into the synaptic space, the transmitter is potentially picked up by and activates receptor sites of two types: alpha (α) sites, which are excitatory, and beta (β) sites, which are inhibitory and cardiac excitatory (see Fig. 2-10). The postsynaptic cell—smooth muscle or gland cell—may have α- or β-receptors, or both, although there is usually a preponderance of one type.

The fate of the CA neurohumor is somewhat similar to the fate of ACh. Part of it is utilized in producing the postsynaptic reaction; part of it diffuses away. Most of it is taken back into the synaptic vesicles for storage, with the cytoplasmic surplus being decomposed by an enzyme stored in the mitochondria, *monoamine oxidase* (MAO). The transfer into the terminals is brought about by an "amine pump." Comparable to the AChE of cholinergic synapses is the compound *catechol-O-methyltransferase* (COMT). The catabolic phenomenon is remembered with the mnemonic "COMT cleans up the synapse; MAO mops up the intraneuronal surplus CA." However, it is generally held that the process of active reuptake by the pump is of itself adequate to account for removal of NE at the synapse.

A feedback, self-limiting control of NE production has been proposed in which the overproduction of NE inhibits the enzyme tyrosine hydroxylase from converting tyrosine to dopa.

In the medulla of the adrenal gland about 80% of the CA stored in the vesicles is E and about 20% NE. An action potential brought to the medullary cells by a preganglionic sympathetic neuron results in the release of E and/or NE into the bloodstream and the subsequent distribution of these CA's to various receptor sites throughout the body.

■ **What are some drugs whose actions affect the synthesis, storage, release, reuptake, and destruction of CA's at the synapse?**

It was mentioned previously that the rate-limiting enzyme in the formation of CA's was tyrosine hydroxylase, involved in transforming tyrosine to dopa as a presumed, natural feedback mechanism. Pharmacologically administration of α-methyl-p-tyrosine provides a similar blocking action, thereby ultimately depleting the supply of NE.

Sometimes the normal neurohumor is not stored in the vesicles. This may be accomplished by introducing substrates that are analogues of those normally involved in producing the neurosecretion, producing what are referred to as *"false transmitters,"* with lesser excitatory effects at the receptor than the NE they displace. Examples are α-methylmetatyrosine and α-methyldopa (Aldomet). In the brain the former of these two drugs reduces brain NE without affecting 5-HT and produces sedation.

The mechanism for active reuptake of CA's into the vesicles after firing is sufficiently nonselective to permit the acceptance as substitutes of sympathomimetics such as *cocaine, imipramine,* and *chlorpromazine.* As a result, NE collects at extracellular sites and/or acts at the receptors. It is by such means that the tricyclic preparations produce their antidepressant, therapeutic effects. In a more indirect manner some drugs, for example, *ephedrine, amphetamine,* and *tyramine,* act by displacing NE from the neuronal cytoplasm, thereby resulting in the NE sustaining transmitter effects on the receptor cells. The rebound phenomenon following amphetamine administration may be the result of a temporary NE depletion. While ephedrine, amphetamine, and tyramine produce brief effects quickly, *guanethidine* is slow to produce more prolonged effects.

Storage of CA's is also blocked by the use of *reserpine,* a product of the plant rauwolfia, lowering the blood pressure and pulse and acting as a tranquilizer, because the NE is destroyed by the mitochondrial MAO's. The reserpine does not block the formation of CA's, just the ability of the vesicle to concentrate and bind the CA's. It acts the same way in relation to 5-HT, again producing sedation, reduced smooth muscle activity, and parasympathetic effects. It is interesting that peripherally reserpine can produce complete adrenergic blockage, whereas in the CNS adrenergic effects can still be elicited following the administration of reserpine.

By inhibiting MAO's, *iproniazid* (Marsilid), the antituberculosis drug, which is the most thoroughly studied MAO inhibitor, causes the supply of NE to increase, thereby acting as an antidepressant.

■ **What drugs act at adrenergic synapses and receptor sites?**

COMT is inhibited by *pyrogallol.* Therefore when the latter is administered, it prolongs the effects of injected CA's, delaying their disappearance from the body.

Phenylephrine can combine at both α- and/or β-receptors to produce sympathomimetic effects.

The most potent normal activator of α-receptors is E, being up to 10 times more active than NE and more than 100 times as potent as the synthetic isoproterenol. *Isoproterenol* is the most potent β-activator, being up to 10 times more active than E and more than 100 times as potent as NE.

■ **What is the neuropharmacologic significance of 5-HT?**

Another indoleamine of questionable potential for acting as neurotransmitter in the CNS is 5-HT. Whereas DA and NE cannot pass the blood-brain barrier, 5-HT can. The question concerning to what extent the 5-HT found within the brain is formed there vs the amount transported there from extracranial sites is currently under investigation. As a monamine, 5-HT is also deaminated by MAO's. Being an indoleamine rather than a CA, it is not acted on by COMT. Considerable literature has evolved relative to the possible relation of 5-HT to behavior,[11] for example, schizophrenia. *LSD* is recognized as a 5-HT opponent.

■ **How do anesthetics work?**

Although drugs are used in treating all of the body systems, in this section attention is directed of course to drugs affecting the nervous system. The scope of such drugs would include such major categories as anesthetics, drugs acting as CNS depressants sedatives, drugs affecting behavior, anticonvulsive drugs, and drugs acting on the ANS and musculoskeletal system.

Anesthesia may be of a permanent or a temporary nature, whether induced intentionally or accidentally or generally or locally. Permanent palliative treatment for pain may be achieved surgically, or where opportune, locally by injection of alcohol, and so forth. General anesthesia probably works on the reticular activating formation rather than the spinothalamic tracts, affecting both the ascending and descending components.[12] The effect on the descending components is probably responsible for the muscle relaxation seen in deep surgical planes.

While the disadvantages inherent in general anesthesia include the necessity for ongoing attendance by an anesthesiologist, additional equipment, postsurgical recuperative phase requiring an attendant, the risk to cardiac patients, and so forth, compensatory advantages include the absence of multiple problems associated with patient apprehensiveness and the availability of a wide range of volatile, gaseous, and intravenous agents.

It can be demonstrated in the PNS that anesthesia progressively lowers the height of the action potential, slows the rate of its rise, elevates the firing threshold, slows the speed of impulse conduction, and lengthens the refractory period until the threshold of the nerve is no longer reached; the nerve is blocked, since depolarization no longer occurs. The ability to raise the Na^+ permeability and generate an action potential is interfered with.[13]

Good local anesthesia practice demands that the injection be placed near the nerve but not in it. The connective tissue sheaths, the perineurium and, if present, the epineurium, represent the most significant barrier to penetration. Therefore since the roots of the spinal nerves are devoid of perineurium, they provide an excellent site for injection. Once the drug reaches the neurilemma, (high) fat solubility and (low) molecular weight seem to be important attributes in determining penetration rate. Since the nerves are frequently components of neurovascular bundles, when using local anesthetics the drug, in addition to blocking the nerve, usually enters the bloodstream, either by diffusion, especially if a substance such as hyaluronidase (Wydase) is added as an expediter, or by inadvertent intravenous injection.

If local anesthetics do enter the bloodstream, at high levels they act as convulsants; at low levels they exert anticonvulsant effects.

Subsequent to local injection into an extremity, it will be observed clinically that anesthesia progresses gradually proximodistally and that the spatial (temporal) pattern is reversed as the pool of drug injected is gradually diffused away, diluted with tissue fluid, and metabolized. The pattern relates anatomically to the fact that, generally speaking, fibers near the surface of a nerve innervate the proximal portion of the region supplied by the nerve, whereas the deeper fibers innervate the distal portion. The physiologic correlates are that, as the anesthetic diffuses from the surface to the center of the nerve, it will attain threshold doses first centrifugally and later centripetally.

■ How do pain mechanisms work?

Realizing that not only articles but entire books continue to appear in the literature regarding the nature and control of pain, obviously it would be futile to pretend to attempt an adequate coverage of either aspect of the subject in this discussion.

In both human and animal experiments, work with a conscious individual is complicated by the "prior experience of pain" factor, indicating the potential value of EEG studies on patients in the nonwakeful state. Although the idea of a pain "center" has long since been abandoned, the sensation and its general relation to the RAS, the cerebral cortex, and the hypothalamus remain recognized.

Although pain is commonly produced by stimuli that at weaker intensities evoke other somatic sensations such as warmth or cold on mechanical contact, nonetheless, it seems to be a separate sensation with its own first-order neurons. One type of pain, the "fast" type, is transmitted by the slower components of the delta group of A fibers and is associated with the pricking form of cutaneous pain.

The second, "slow" type of pain is transmitted by some of the peripheral, unmyelinated C fibers and is associated with long-lasting burning sensations, an unbearable quality of suffering, and prolonged after-image following removal of the stimulus. Local drug injection may reduce conduction in the peripheral nerves by only 20% in producing typical anesthesia. However, it is not known what effect the local anesthetic may have on C fibers.

From the periphery, nociceptive stimuli arrive at portions of the spinal cord known as Lissauer's tract and the gelatinous substance and cross over to the contralateral side to ascend in the spinothalamic tract of the ventral half of the lateral funiculi. While some argue as to possible control of pain at this level, the *double-gate theory* of pain control,[14] others seriously debate the point. Palliative control of intractable pain and complete elimination of this form of stress are addressed by the use of drugs, surgery, hypnosis, acupuncture, psychic control, and manipulation; it sometimes remains difficult to make objective evaluations of the relative successes and merits of these various modalities.

Whereas the mode selected for treatment will vary with the practitioner's education and background of experience, such factors as the possible association of the pain with pathologic lesions, the severity and duration of noxious periods, and the patient's age are always of prime importance. When the use of other modalities fails, transection of the anterolateral column of the cord may be indicated to induce hemianesthesia (for pain and temperature control) of the contralateral side. Stereotactic electrodes may be used to destroy selected regions of the brain with minimum damage to adjacent structures. Last resort procedures involve lesioning part of the thalamus or transecting the fibers linking it to areas 9 to 12 of the frontal lobe.

An excellent summary of clinical manifestations founded in neurologic origins is presented by Clark.[15]

REFERENCES

1. Ham, A. W., and Cormack, D. H.: Histology, ed. 8, Philadelphia, 1979, J. B. Lippincott Co.
2. Lindsay, N. K., and Birch, J. R.: Thin skin healing, Can. J. Surg. **7:**297, 1964.
3. Mark, J. L.: Antibodies (II): another look at the diversity problem, Science **202:**412, 1978.
4. Bigley, N. J.: Immunological fundamentals, Chicago, 1975, Year Book Medical Publishers, Inc.
5. Jung, R. C.: Analysis and interpretation of acid-base balance, Crit. Care Update **3:**5, 1976.
6. Carpenter, M. B.: Human neuroanatomy, ed. 7, Baltimore, 1976, The Williams & Wilkins Co.
7. DiPalma, J. R., editor: Drill's pharmacology in medicine, ed. 6, New York, 1976, McGraw-Hill Book Co.
8. Goodman, L. S., and Gilman, A.: The pharmaceutical basis of therapeutics, ed. 5, New York, 1975, Macmillan Inc.
9. Carrier, O., Jr.: Pharmacology of the peripheral autonomic nervous system, Chicago, 1972, Year Book Medical Publishers, Inc.
10. Gero, A.: Intimate study of drug action. III. Mechanisms of molecular drug action. In DiPalma, J. R., editor: Drill's pharmacology in medicine, ed. 6, New York, 1976, McGraw-Hill Book Co.
11. Barchas, J., and Usdin, E.: Serotonin and behavior, New York, 1973, Academic Press, Inc.
12. Vandam, L. D.: Uptake and transport of anesthetics and stages of anesthesia. In DiPalma, J. R., editor: Drill's pharmacology in medicine, ed. 6, New York, 1976, McGraw-Hill Book Co.
13. deJong, R. H.: Physiology and pharmacology of local anesthesia, Springfield, Ill., 1970, Charles C Thomas, Publisher.
14. Melzack, R., and Wall, P. D.: Pain mechanisms: a new theory, Science **150:**971, 1965.
15. Clark, R. G.: Essentials of clinical neuroanatomy and neurophysiology, ed. 5, Philadelphia, 1975, F. A. Davis Co.

BIBLIOGRAPHY

Adams, R. D., and Victor, M.: Principles of neurology, New York, 1977, McGraw-Hill Book Co.
Barr, M. L.: Human nervous system, ed. 3, Hagerstown, Md., 1979, Harper & Row, Publishers, Inc.
Crowley, L. V.: Introductory concepts in anatomy and physiology, Chicago, 1976, Year Book Medical Publishers, Inc.
Deutsch, S., and Vandam, L. D.: General anesthesia. I. Volatile agents. In DiPalma, J. R., editor: Drill's pharmacology in medicine, ed. 4, New York, 1971, McGraw-Hill Book Co.
Globus, A., et al.: Effects of differential experience on dendrite spine counts in rat cerebral cortex, J. Comp. Physiol. Psychol. **82:**175, 1973.
Goodman, L. C., and Gilman, A.: The pharmaceutical basis of therapeutics, ed. 5, New York, 1975, MacMillan Inc.
House, E. L., Pansky, B., and Siegel, A.: A systematic approach to neuroscience, ed. 3, New York, 1979, McGraw-Hill Book Co.
Iggo, A.: New specific sensory structures in hairy skin, Acta Neuroveg. **24:**175, 1963.
Mountcastle, V. B.: Medical physiology, ed. 14, vols. I-II, St. Louis, 1980, The C. V. Mosby Co.
Slonim, N. B., and Hamilton, L. H.: Respiratory physiology, ed. 3, St. Louis, 1976, The C. V. Mosby Co.
Vander, A. J., Sherman, J. H., and Luciano, D. S.: Human physiology: the mechanisms of body function, New York, 1970, McGraw-Hill Book Co.

CHAPTER 3

Analysis of the critical care unit as a dynamic system

Donald E. Watson

The behavioral sciences have much to offer organizations seeking to optimize their productivity, stability, efficiency, effectiveness, profitability, and goal achievement. Industrial and occupational psychology and psychiatry have had an integral place in the planning and operation of organizations large and small. Through the practical application of knowledge gained from the systematic study of systems of people, these disciplines have become basic to the principles of modern management.

It is surprising, then, to realize that hospitals, as complex goal-oriented organizations, still suffer from archaic management principles that are in collision with modern expectations of employees and patients alike. If hospitals are to escape the suffocating influence of government control, the costs incurred by mismanagement must be controlled. *Costs expressed as money begin with costs suffered by people, many of which are emotional costs.* This chapter assesses some of those costs and suggests interventions to reduce them.

The typical health professional seeks through his or her career a mechanism for mastering individual fears; for example, the typical nurse is terrified of her own dependency needs. Yet, she chooses a profession in which other people become exquisitely dependent on her. Similarly, physicians as a group demonstrate a terror of personal illness or death, which they seek to overcome by conquering illness and death in others. Others in the health professions and ancillary

fields, ranging from hospital administrators to dietary workers to maintenance personnel, are fascinated by and attracted to the hospital as a hoped-for sanctuary against morbidity and mortality. The individual psychodynamics of all these people, mixed together in the hospital setting, becomes the large and complex social system known as hospital-based health care.

The critical care unit (CCU) is a small subsystem within the hospital. Substantial literature relating to the psychologic issues of both patients and staff of CCU's has accumulated in the past few years. Some of the literature has focused on the psychologic reactions of patients to the 24-hour-a-day maelstrom of activity of the unit (for example, see Chapter 4), while others have emphasized the reactions of the staff.[1,2,3]

GENERAL SYSTEMS THEORY AND THERMODYNAMICS

The complexity of the CCU can be analyzed according to the principles of general systems theory. There are two main virtues in choosing that conceptual framework: (1) to better understand complex systems, and (2) to be able to predict effects. This chapter is structured in a sequence that permits a logical analysis of a CCU and then provides predictions based on those generalized observations.

The reader need not be intimidated by the language of general systems theory. The theory is simply a formalization of the commonsense notion that any system is the sum of all of its parts and that each of those parts is a system itself interacting with each of its neighbors. Accordingly, it is stated as a principle in the science of ecology that one can never change one element of a system without affecting every other element and the system as a whole.

In discussing sets of systems that are interrelated by flows of matter, energy, and information among their boundaries, it is also useful to consider the concepts provided by *thermodynamics*. These include the relationships of flows in and out of the system and the internal energy of the system. The concept of *entropy* is particularly valuable because it is a measure of the cost incurred by a system when it is in negative balance, that is, "running down."

In its simplest form thermodynamics states that (1) the total energy in the universe is constant, and (2) in performing work a system always loses some energy in the form of heat, which represents a loss of "free energy" and a gain in entropy.

It is useful to think of "psychic energy" as analogous to the free energy of thermodynamics. Experience has shown that human beings cannot be indefinitely drained mentally without suffering severe disorganization or collapse. In other words, people suffer a gain in entropy as they do psychic work. Accordingly, a *principle of conservation of psychic energy* can be postulated that states that the energy of the mind/brain is conserved; that is, it is neither created nor destroyed. It can, however, be transformed into intellectual activity, physical activity, "worry," acquisition of possessions, and so forth.

According to the conservation principle, a person whose emotional economy is in negative balance relative to the flow of input and output across his boundary suffers a cost in internal organization; that is, his entropy increases. In psychologic terms a person whose needs are chronically unmet is steadily accumulating a propensity toward emotional disorganization or illness. Similarly, the individual's suprasystem will exhibit increased entropy if its net economy is negative.

The language in this chapter is not rigorous; it is hybridized to help bridge the gaps among theory, clinical practice, and management principles. Several definitions are useful at this point for the purpose of the analysis:

level In a hierarchy of systems the degree of aggregation or complexity is called a level; for example, five levels of organization are: (1) cells, (2) an organ, (3) a person, (4) a CCU, and (5) a hospital.

subsystem Any component or element that belongs to a system that has a level lower than that of the system itself; for example, an organelle is a subsystem of a cell.

suprasystem The system that has a level just higher than a given system; for example, an organ is the suprasystem of a cell.

closed system A system that is encapsulated in such a way that neither matter, energy, nor information leaves or enters the system; this is a theoretical concept only, inasmuch as all systems are open but vary in their degrees of openness.

open system A system in which matter, energy, and information exchange across its boundary; a living organism is a highly open system, whereas an inert metal is relatively closed. A complex system such as a CCU is "open" in more ways than is generally acknowledged within the system or its suprasystem, the hospital. Specifically, the area of emotional interaction among the individuals in the system is often ignored, which leads to disruptive (although usually not deliberate) interactions among the individuals involved.

information The "organizer" of systems—in this chapter "information" is used to indicate the interactional exchange among individuals, including money, formalized goal orientation, written procedures and policy, and spoken or unspoken evidence of emotional support, warmth, rage, or fear.

structure The physical or symbolic arrangement of the elements of a system—in the CCU structure refers to the formalized hierarchy or responsibilities and roles of the individuals therein and can also refer to the geographic distribution of inanimate elements at any given time.

process Functioning—together with structure, process characterizes the entire posture of a functioning dynamic system. Process is to structure as physiology is to anatomy.

equilibrium A state of balance that would characterize a "closed" system; that is, no energy, matter, or information is required to maintain the balance.

steady state A balance that is achieved in an "open" system at the cost of energy, matter, or information that is taken in or released by the system. A complex social system such as a CCU achieves stability as a whole only if steady state relationships exist among all the elements of the system. In the short run Peter can be robbed to pay Paul and stability will be achieved, but in the long run stability will be lost unless Peter's reserves are replenished.

entropy A measure of the degree of disorganization or randomness in a system. High entropy indicates great disorganization and low entropy indicates orderliness. For example, a healthy living organism is in a state of low entropy, whereas entropy increases as illness and death set in. A low entropy system in steady state requires energy, matter, and information from external sources.

economy A mechanism of managing and accounting for resources within a given system; for example, an organism's food intake, digestion, assimilation, metabolism, and excretion are parts of the physical economy of the organism. Similarly, human beings exhibit well-developed and powerfully influential psychologic economies.

program A functional organizer within a system, such as a computer or the human mind, that directs the processing of information. This program is itself organized by information of a different kind; this *programming information* is of two important types in the human mind: (1) genetic and (2) acquired from external sources. Programs that are genetically determined can be called "instinctual" and programs that are acquired can be called "learned."

SUBSYSTEMS OF THE CCU

Each person in a CCU is a subsystem of that unit. The person, in turn, consists of his own subsystems, which include both physical and mental components. The structure and processes of the mental subsystems are the objects of the science of psychiatry, broadly defined. Disciplines of psychiatry include the neurosciences, psychology,

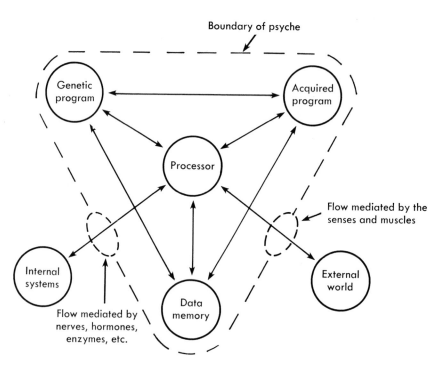

Fig. 3-1. Diagram of human psychic structure with communication paths to other systems both internal and external. Neurotic conflicts occur when genetic and acquired programs give conflicting instructions for processing information. Memory holds data and both programs. *Genetic program, acquired program,* and *processor* correspond to *id, superego,* and *ego,* respectively, of Freud's psychoanalytic theory.

sociology, and economics. The body of knowledge of psychiatry is acquired by formal laboratory methods and clinical observation. Freud based his theory of character organization (called *psychoanalytic theory*) on a systematic study of mental processes observed by both himself and his subjects, the latter observations being called *insights*. Fig. 3-1 is a diagram summarizing the human mental (or psychic) structure and processes. This complex system is one level lower than that of the person and two lower than that of the CCU.

It is not within the scope of this chapter to describe the CCU system in comprehensive detail. Instead, the focus is on analyzing the major problem areas. Toward that end, it is useful to describe the system from the perspective of several of its component parts, keeping in mind that the "real" world can only be described as it is perceived to be by each observer. Accordingly, not one, but four CCU's are described below: (1) the patient's CCU, (2) the nurse's CCU, (3) the physician's CCU, and (4) the administrator's CCU (in this case, the nursing director represents administration). Clearly, this list of descriptions could be extended to include the politician's, the insurance executive's, the clergyman's, the next-of-kin's, and so forth. The emphasis is on the four principals, though, because the bulk of the information exchange is carried on among those people.

The patient's CCU

The hypothetical patient in this case is a 46-year-old man who had never been sick a day in his life and had taken great pride in being a good provider for his wife and three children. He has been striken by a massive myocardial infarction and he is alive at this moment only because the ambulance crew arrived at his side in time to convert a ventricular fibrillation. When he was stricken, he was both surprised and emotionally numb; his conscious mind would not permit him to acknowledge how near death he was. During the excitement of his cardiac arrest and subsequent defibrillation, he became aware for the first time that his life would end; at some time in the future he would cease to exist.

While being transported by the ambulance to the hospital, the patient began to develop a deep

sense of affection for the attendants who were caring for him. Even though their demeanor was to remain detached from him as a person and was even at times frivolous, the patient felt a deep sense of trust for them that could only be explained by his state of enforced dependency. Although he was not consciously aware of it, the affection he felt for the attendants was the same feeling he had felt toward his mother when, as an infant, he had enjoyed her total attention, protection, and nurturance.

By the time the patient arrived at the hospital and was wheeled by gurney into the CCU, other feelings began to emerge: While he could still perceive the hospital as a sanctuary that was filled with fantasied mother figures who would take care of him, he also felt a terror that was only partially softened by the effects of the morphine he received. The terror he felt came from deeply buried memories from his childhhood when he was first struggling to become independent. Unable to verbalize his fear, he was flooded by uncertainty; "What if they don't really love me?" "What if they mutilate me while I am helpless?" "Can they be trusted to know what they are doing?" "What will they do with me while they have me in their control in my helpless, dependent state?" "Will I ever be able to depend on my own body again?"

By this time, the patient has already established in his mind a set of responses and behaviors that he expects from the nursing staff. These expectations are highly individual, based on his own early life experiences and brought to the foreground by the regressive experience of acute illness. It is important to be aware that he expects both positive and negative reactions on the part of the nurse; above all, he expects that he will be totally within the power of these angels/devils that will be ministering to him.

Within the first few hours after being admitted to the CCU, the patient goes through many substantial emotional ordeals. Facing the fact of his mortality for the first time is devastating. The imminent threat of losing everything precious to him is almost overwhelming. Within the span of a few minutes, the patient becomes aware of what is truly important to him in his life. He discovers that even though most of his energies until his illness struck had been spent with his career, the predominant preoccupation of loss is not with his work at all. Instead, it is the fact that he might not be able to see his children grow to adulthood, and that he might not be able to grow old and enjoy his retirement with his wife. Suddently, his entire set of priorities is turned around. He condemns himself for putting off pleasures and he regrets not having made opportunities to be closer to his family. If he appears to be uncooperative to the nurse who is trying to start an IV or attach electrodes to him, it is because his agenda of priorities is considerably different from hers at that moment.

Later, as the patient proceeds with grieving for his lost delusion of immortality, he may express his rage at the CCU—his immediate environment. He may become bitterly intolerant of the constantly lighted room or of the incessantly noisy equipment. Or, in an attempt to regain his sense of mastery and control, he may become obsessively preoccupied with the complex array of devices surrounding him. Above all, he will be anxious constantly because of his totally novel experience with illness and the exotica of the CCU. Unlike the nurse and the physician, he cannot regard the CCU as commonplace.

The nurse's CCU

The hypothetical nurse, 28 years of age, has been part of the elite critical care team for a little over a year. She had decided to become a critical care nurse soon after her first exposure to the CCU while in nursing school. She had been excited by the potential for developing a special competence in a highly technical area of nursing in which her own expertise would sometimes exceed that of the physicians who hospitalize their patients in the unit. She had paid her dues to reach the position she was in now; she had worked nights and evenings all over the hospital and had even "floated" for several months.

Prior to entering nursing school the nurse had worked as a waitress for 2 years to support her husband while he tried out college. The divorce happened about 6 months after the baby was born and about a year after her husband dropped out of college to "find himself." Even though she knew it would be difficult, she entered nurses training

with a sense of determination and strength. She knew she could be a good nurse because she had always taken care of people. She had decided on a career in nursing when she was 13 years old. As the oldest of six children, she functioned as a mother to her younger siblings while her own mother worked long hours to support the family.

She was an ideal critical care nurse: She was bright, dedicated, idealistic, and quietly reliable. She had earned the confidence of her supervisors by frequently working 9- and 10-hour shifts in order to assure that all the work got done. She was proud of the fact that her errors had always been small and had never led to major complications for her patients. She was also proud of the fact that her superiors and her peers alike often turned to her for support during times of crisis.

Despite the high degree of achievement in her career, though, the nurse was also vaguely dissatisfied. She was tired. She was also feeling guilty for neglecting her son. Her routine recently had been to pick him up from the day-care center after her shift, prepare a meal for both of them, get him ready for bed, and retire herself soon after he did. It seemed that in the last few months she had to sleep longer and longer in order to have the energy to return to work the next morning. Secretly, she yearned for an "ideal" man; one she could depend on and who would take care of her. She despaired of ever finding such a man, though, because she knew she would never be able to relinquish her cherished independence. Still, she displayed a bumper sticker that told the world to "Love a Nurse prn."

On this particular day, the nurse was more "tired" than usual. She had developed a special fondness for one of her patients, a man in his late 50's, who was recovering nicely from a myocardial infarct. Over the weeks he had been her patient, they came to know each other fairly well. Developing a relationship with the patient was unusual for her but in this case she permitted herself to make an exception. Perhaps it was because she was vulnerable in her loneliness and perhaps it was because he vaguely reminded her of her father. He was different from her father though in one important respect: He did not abandon her. Also, unlike most of her patients, he seemed to be nurturing and interested in her as a person and was therefore able to provide her with a sense of acceptance and personal worth she had not experienced before. But on this day, 4 days prior to his expected discharge, he suddenly died. She had blindly and instinctively called a code and had personally led the resuscitation team. Completely able to deny her loss at the time, she functioned like a precision-tuned machine. It was to no avail; the hopelessly scarred heart would not start again. So this man, too, left her.

The nurse's peers and even her head nurse tried to give her support. They said they knew how she must feel. They asked if there was anything they could do. They even touched her and stroked her back as she sat holding her head in her hands after the nursing ritual of death had been completed. But she could accept no support from them because she was too isolated in her grief. The nurse fleetingly wondered if she was experiencing depression but quickly dismissed it from her mind; depression was for the weak and the self-pitying. She would have no part of it. Still, she was grateful that only 1 hour was left on her shift and she was left with only one patient to care for next to the empty bed recently occupied by her special patient. It was at that time that the gurney rolled in with a new patient: A 46-year-old, well-respected businessman who had had a massive infarct.

The nurse felt heat at the back of her neck and almost simultaneously a weakness in her legs and arms. Unconsciously, she was enraged at the intrusion of this stranger who was going to be demanding her care but at the same time she became "paralyzed" because her conscience admonished her that rage is forbidden. So, much to the amazement of her colleagues and supervisor, she efficiently and quickly picked up the rhythm of attending to the new admission. It was as if she had no feelings whatsoever.

As she approached the man to start connecting him to the various monitoring devices of the unit, he flailed at her as if he were taking a swing at her. This had happened many times to her before, but she had always shrugged it off as an unexplained phenomenon. This time, though, she took it personally. She shouted at the man to hold

his goddamned arms still or he would pull out the IV's.

Instantly, she felt totally contemptuous of him in his helpless and dependent state. He didn't seem to be affected by her outburst though; he only looked at her in passing as if her presence made only the tiniest impression on the periphery of his consciousness. She quickly regained her composure and silently thanked the morphine, giving it credit for keeping the patient's attention away from her transient loss of control. It did not occur to her that the man's preoccupation with things more important to him than her behavior had accounted for his casual dismissal of her actions.

This rare instance of an outward expression of stress did not go unnoticed by the nurse's conscience. Unconscious mechanisms came into play that would serve to keep her in line thereafter; her rigid, critical, and tyrannical conscience (acquired program) would make sure this new patient would receive the best care she could possibly deliver. She became overly zealous in monitoring the man's vital signs and even went out of her way to ask him if he were comfortable. Even though she had been aware of a sense of guilt after her outburst, she did not consciously connect the guilt with the fact that she stayed 2 hours overtime that day, ostensibly to make sure the PM nurse was adequately informed about taking over the care of the new patient.

By the time she got home that evening, she was snapping at her son and even briefly permitted herself to wish that she did not have him as a dependent. She went to bed exhausted that night but sleep did not come for many hours. Troubling thoughts tumbled through her head but always too quickly for her to be able to grasp them or to understand where they came from. She didn't even think about the death of her special patient. Perhaps she had "forgotten."

The physician's CCU

The physician, 46 years of age, had had a relatively easy day. He had started his hospital rounds at 7:30 in the morning and even had time to wolf down a sandwich at 1:00 before returning to his office to see patients. He had been on call that day for emergency admissions, but the emergency room physician had not called him all day. He was relaxed, bantering back and forth with a long-time patient who was grateful to him for having diagnosed her mysterious illness and for treating it. When the call came from the emergency room physician, there was no doubt about the diagnosis or the course of treatment for the man who just came through the door at the hospital. The clinical signs were unmistakable and the patient had been sent directly to the CCU. The physician hastily excused himself from his waiting patients as he rushed through his waiting room by waving and explaining "Emergency!"

He knew he did not have to run and that other physicians in the community would let the CCU nurses manage the case with only telephone consultations. But he had his own internal ideals that drove him. He rushed to the hospital and went straight to the patient's bedside. He could see at a glance, but did not consciously note it, that the patient was about his size and build and was about the same age. Checking the monitors quickly, his practiced eye flagged the danger signs immediately. All he could say was "Damn!" It was safer to look at the nurse. He was pleased to find that it was his favorite nurse and he knew she would relieve him of a considerable burden because of her competence and dedication. He took the time to notice that she looked different this time. Her face lacked the mobility he was accustomed to, her eyes looked a little sad, and she seemed pale. He thought she could take care of herself, though, so he dismissed it and headed for the patient's chart to write orders.

As he glanced over the cursory workup recorded by the emergency room physician, the physician wondered if he had heard the patient's name before. He seemed to recall being introduced to a man with that name at the handball court a few weeks previously. However, he dismissed that, because there was no way of connecting the energetic, robust, and healthy man at the handball court with the pitiful, helpless mass of tissues he had just seen.

When he saw that the patient's age was the same as his own, the physician could only feel anger at the unfairness of the specter of death attending a man so young. A memory flitted across his mind about the dizzy spells he had suffered

on occasion within the last year. He pushed that out of his mind, though, with a simple denial. Then he chuckled wryly to himself when he became aware of his reliance on his superstition: "I'm a physician, and physicians don't get sick."

Introspection made him nervous, so the physician quickly finished his chart work and returned to the nurse at his patient's bedside. For a moment, he saw her as different from a nurse, almost as a human being. His practiced clinical eye told him that she was in distress and he wished that he could do something to help her. Unfortunately, he needed her to be a nurse at this time. Therefore he only told her that he was really grateful that she was on duty with his patient and that she was the best nurse he had ever known. Hoping that his words would be enough to relieve whatever distress she had, he turned quickly to return to his office and to the patients who were waiting for him.

The administrator's (nursing director's) CCU

The nursing director commanded the respect (or fear) of everyone at the hospital. The only exception to this was the nursing director herself. In 55 years she had come to acquire a great deal of power and was able to either coerce, persuade, or manipulate practically anyone at the hospital into doing her will.

It had not always been so. Before she was 2 years old, the nursing director had experienced more chaos and upheaval in her life than most people do in a lifetime. Her father, whom she does not remember, was the cause of all that. As a child, she had tried to imagine what her father had been like, but since her mother never mentioned him, she had little information to go on. She knew that she had had at least 14 different homes during that 24-month period, including one relatively long stay of 3 months with an aunt. Whether or not her father uprooted his family and moved them so frenetically was because of restlessness, eluding capture, avoiding persecution (either real or imagined), or just mental instability was never known to her. Nevertheless, the experience left her with a deep-felt belief that she would never find security.

Despite her deep-seated sense of insecurity, the

nursing director frequently and vigorously denied feeling insecure, proclaiming to all who would hear that she was able to master any challenge. Thus she compensated for her sense of inadequacy by grandiosity; what others saw as rigidity and strength was actually her defense against fragility. Unconsciously, she was riding a vicious circle: Because she felt insecure and powerless, she garnered all the power and control she could. Rather than relieving her sense of weakness, though, the added responsibility only made her feel more inadequate. To cope with that, she reached for more power, and so on.

The nursing director was herself aware of subtle changes that had taken place in her attitude about herself in the past decade. After having tried and rejected marriage while she was still in her 20's, she had embarked on a career that would combine her professional skills with her dependency instincts. She headed without hesitation toward administration and after an early series of triumphs that were rewarded with promotions and accolades, she developed a satisfying sense of invincibility about her capacity for mastering the world in general. While in her 30's, she stepped from position to position in several hospitals, each representing a major advancement over the previous ones. She decided that she was capable of spending her entire working career moving thus from challenge to challenge, expecting frequent and intense exhilaration from practicing her skills. Something had happened to her somewhere along the line, though, but she did not know what it was. She did know that she had been in her present position for 12 years and she no longer had the inner resources to welcome new challenges.

The only person the nursing director answered to in the entire hospital was the administrator. Fortunately for her, both she and the administrator knew that she was her own boss. The administrator knew that unlike the old generation, the young nurses considered that they owned their own lives and were not chattel of the hospital. Accordingly, he knew that he could not dictate policy without permission from the nursing director. She in turn added to the power she held within the hospital by extending her influence to other hospitals in the area and to the major nursing organizations as well. Although the nurses who feared her wrath considered her to be a tyrant, her own self-perception was that she, in her wisdom, would make more "right" decisions than her subordinate nurses would if they exercised any autonomy.

The nursing director rarely ventured into the clinical areas of the hospital. When she did, it was to assess for herself the accuracy of the reports given her by her immediate subordinates, the supervisors. Some of the physicians in the hospital were faintly bemused by the nursing director's posture: It was ironic that despite her reign of terror in which she held absolute control, her internal feeling of insecurity manifested itself by paranoia. They speculated sometimes among themselves about why the hospital kept her, a relic from the sweat shop days of hospital management. But despite her flaws, there was one thing no one could deny: The nursing director ran a tight, quiet ship and the administrator appreciated that.

On this day, the nursing director visited the CCU at about the same time the patient was wheeled in. She strode briskly over to the desk to check his admission sheet. Noting quickly the upper middle-class neighborhood where the patient lived, the excellent insurance coverage, and the apparent adequacy of documentation of his hospitalization so far, she quickly computed the expected revenue if the patient survived 3 weeks, and felt satisfied that the risk of malpractice litigation would be low.

Then she turned her attention to the nursing personnel on the unit and quickly assessed each of them according to her highly personalized agenda. The head nurse was giving her full attention to the nursing director, disregarding all of the activity on the unit. The nursing director nodded an acknowledgment to the head nurse while reassuring herself that the head nurse was obsequious enough and would cause her no trouble. After glancing over and quickly discounting the significance of the other members of the nursing staff, her eyes fell on the nurse attending the new patient. While she was reflecting that she didn't like the nurse because she was well respected by the doctors and most of the rest of the nursing staff, she was suddenly surprised to witness an emotional outburst by the nurse at the bedside. Smugly, the nursing director concluded that documentation of shouting at a patient in that nurse's personnel file would quench any threatening ambitions she might have, at least for the time being.

The nursing director turned and swept back to her office, already rehearsing the report she would give the administrator: that all was well in the hospital under her direction and the only problem she had observed would be dealt with appropriately.

PSYCHODYNAMICS OF THE FOUR PEOPLE (SUBSYSTEMS) OF THE CCU

The vignettes of the individuals related in the preceding are of hypothetical individuals; in fact, they are composites of real individuals and as such they are "real" people. In the average CCU three of these four people are statistically represented fairly accurately; the majority of physicians and nurses and many nursing directors have personalities very similar to these composites. Patients, of course, have no such uniformity of character. They are placed at the scene for reasons far more diverse than those of career choice. As a result, the analysis following is illustrative of only one set of interactions, in which one variable (the patient) is subject to considerable uncertainty. Nevertheless, the analysis is valid for this particular set of variables at this particular point in time. Indeed, the nature of any dynamic system is the same. For that reason, the methodology must be applied continuously; today's solutions for today's problems will probably not be appropriate for tomorrow's problems.

The style of the preceding presentation is deliberately dramatic. It emphasizes the fact that the emotional activity in the CCU is intense and information about that emotional activity ("affect") is freely exchanged even though it is rarely acknowledged consciously. The impact on the four individuals involved in the exchanges of emotional information is largely destructive. The analysis below of the four parallel subsystems within the CCU is intended to help clarify the processes of those destructive interactions, to assess their impact, and to suggest remedies.

The four human subsystems of the CCU, to-

gether with their own internal organization of emotional information, each comprise a separate but interdependent economy. The CCU is designed to provide a highly sophisticated system of support for the patient's physical economy. The body's healing processes are carefully and continuously monitored so that interventions in the form of input of matter, energy, and information, properly timed, across the patient's system boundaries can reduce the amount of the system's disorganization (illness). In other words, in order to reduce the entropy of the system, the economy of the patient's body requires that external management temporarily supplant his normal internal control mechanisms.

The patient's psychodynamics

As illustrated in the case vignette, the patient's physiologic and anatomic processes are not the only ones affected by his illness. His psychologic steady state has also been severely disrupted. During the same minutes and hours that the CCU team is concentrating on the reorganization of his body, the patient is desperately trying to reconstitute a steady state emotional position. While his long-standing psychologic mechanisms have been abruptly disorganized, the input of organizing information from an external monitor and support systems for his psyche would be helpful. The device best suited for this task is another human being, but that person's own economy must permit the outflow of information without seriously upsetting his or her own steady state. In the preceding vignettes it is obvious that the nurse was unable to provide the external organizing information required by the patient because she was herself in a state of high emotional entropy.

The nurse's psychodynamics

The nurse in the preceding instance offers an example of a long-term process of increasing emotional entropy. Because of her genetic programming, her emotional economy requires contact with human beings. Her natural requirements are for a sense of security, and intimacy with a mate. Unfortunately for her, though, she has been programmed by life experiences to resist having those needs met; that is, she has "learned" that it is not safe to come to depend on someone. As a result, her emotional economy at the moment is in negative balance—she is "giving" more than she is "receiving" emotionally useful information.

Because of her unstable economy, the nurse instinctively "knew" that her survival was at stake. That, in turn, caused her to experience rage when one more demand was made on her in the form of a new patient. In addition, she suffered negative feelings on the death of her special patient because that event triggered a grieving response that was unable to become operative. The grieving process in human beings is a normal healing process triggered by a loss. Grieving permits a reorganization of psychologic variables in order to reduce the entropy gain caused by the loss. In her case, she had never completed the process of reorganizing her psyche after she had been abandoned by her father. Therefore she had entered a state of "pathologic grieving," which left her permanently disorganized and therefore unable to (1) comfortably form dependent attachments to others and (2) satisfactorily complete the process of grieving for this most recent loss. A human system cannot forever remain in a state of negative balance emotionally. Eventually, the system will collapse; the nurse will most likely suffer a state of severe depression eventually.

The physician's psychodynamics

The physician in the vignette demonstrates an economy similar to that of the nurse's. It is in negative balance by virtue of a strong drive to be helpful to others. Organizing information early in his life experience had the result of programming him to respond to the world *as if* his needs for emotional sustenance could be met only if he "earned" it by being useful to others. Accordingly, his fear of becoming dependent on someone was based on the "belief" that to do so would mean annihilation. Even so, his genetically determined psychic organization, like that of the nurse, requires that he receive emotional nourishment in order to maintain a steady state ("happiness").

The primary psychologic mechanism of the physician for dealing with the conflict between his innate and "learned" organization is *denial*. Despite his education and experience he refused to acknowledge the possibility that he too could become ill. The evidence that his body had its limits came from the dizzy spells; the evidence that his emotional economy had limits was that he retreated from giving the nurse the kind of emotional support she needed.

The nursing director's psychodynamics

The nursing director in the vignette reveals still another style of trying to maintain a steady state emotional economy. In her case, information obtained through early life experiences had programmed her to respond to the world *as if* she would never be permitted the security of settling down in a continuous comfortable environment. Still, her genetic programming made such a dependable, structured existence necessary for her to maintain a stable state. Early in her career, she had tried to accommodate her belief that stability was impossible and was successful for a time in the discovery that not only could she deliberately move around a lot but that she could master and thereby enjoy the challenges of moving as well. While doing that, she also developed a mechanism of drawing emotional energy from others by coercion; she became obsessed with gaining power over others and thereby "learned" the illusion that parasitic behavior is a satisfactory substitute for obtaining emotional support that is freely given by others.

As the nursing director aged, the effects of her earlier coping mechanisms came back to haunt her. She had made many enemies and was aware that there were those who wanted her annihilated. Accordingly she became extremely suspicious of others and she continually escalated her reign of terror. She had never been a "giving" person like the majority of her nurse colleagues, but by now her insensitivity to the needs of others—patients, physicians, and subordinates alike—had reached its maximum levels. She was nongiving as a matter of principle; she needed all the security, wealth, and power she could acquire in order to try to satiate the need for tranquility that had been unmet since she was born.

EMOTIONAL ECONOMIES OF THE FOUR PEOPLE

There are no units by which to measure the variables of emotional transactions between people. Instead, quantification is best achieved by using units of time. Consider the analogy of a battery; the economy of a battery can be assessed in terms of the total or amount of charge stored (coulombs) minus the discharge rate (coulombs per second or amperes) plus the recharging rate (coulombs per second) over a given period of time. Such an assessment would require constant monitoring of inflow and outflow and would be awkward for most applications. Instead, it is simpler to rate the battery according to how long it would take to drain (units of time) at a given discharge rate. Similarly, the quantification of a person's "emotional balance" can be made by determining how long a person can give to others before collapsing, depleted. Obviously, the rate at which the person receives the replenishment will contribute to the results.

The individual emotional economies of each of the principals can now be examined in detail. The four individuals with their economies are combined in a later section to assess the overall economy of the CCU.

The patient's economy

Clearly the emotional and physical needs of the patient will vary considerably within the period of time he will be confined to the CCU. During the first hours, he is faced with the psychologic task of reorganizing his own conscious assessment of his mortality and of his priorities in life. In the initial minutes after his heart attack, he is concerned primarily with the physical pain and the effects of the generalized stress reaction. He is facing death at that moment but is not entirely aware of it consciously. Instead, he is fighting the threat of death at very primitive physiologic and biochemical levels. Later, he will face the task of organizing his psychologic structure to cope with the fact of his mortality. He will also need to sort out his wishes and priorities for the future and he will have prominent concerns about his ability to function again in his career. For some of this psychologic reorganization work he needs privacy; for other parts he will need a human being to listen to him as he thinks aloud; and for still other parts he will need active reassurance and accurate information about his physical condition so that he can once more begin to take control of his life and relinquish the dependent, sick role.

The patient's chances for having his need for privacy gratified early in his illness are practically nil; his vital signs and other bodily functions will be monitored with unceasing scrutiny by machines and people. Later, as long as he is in the CCU, the chances for gratifying his need to verbalize his feelings is equally small considering the observation that CCU nurses spend only about 1% of their time talking with their patients.

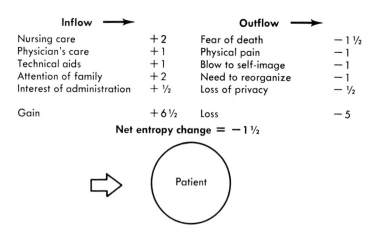

Inflow ⟶		Outflow ⟶	
Nursing care	+2	Fear of death	−1½
Physician's care	+1	Physical pain	−1
Technical aids	+1	Blow to self-image	−1
Attention of family	+2	Need to reorganize	−1
Interest of administration	+½	Loss of privacy	−½
Gain	+6½	Loss	−5

Net entropy change = −1½

Patient

Fig. 3-2. Summary of economy of patient during current interactions. Units of flow are arbitrary and are normalized to values of entropy.

Similarly, it is unlikely that he will obtain the full disclosure of information about his condition that he would like, because his physician is too busy to spend time educating him and the nurse is acting under implicit orders not to give any "medical information" to the patient.

If the patient is fortunate enough to share a close bond of affection and mutual interdependence with his wife, he may find that she is a resource to him emotionally. If, on the other hand, his years of heavy devotion to his career has served to distance him from his wife and family, his wife might meet his new need to talk with her with bewilderment and indifference.

Processes of psychologic reorganization following a severe traumatic event such as the patient has suffered usually take weeks and months to accomplish. By then, the patient will be out of the CCU environment and will have the opportunity to seek emotional support, guidance, and perhaps rehabilitation counseling through friends, a cardiac rehabilitation program, or a relationship with a psychotherapist. Of the four individuals described in this chapter, the patient has the best chance of achieving an emotionally healthy outcome from this encounter. Fig. 3-2 summarizes the patient's economy.

The nurse's economy

The nurse has two major areas in her life that drain her: her job and her child. The income she receives from her job is virtually the only source of replenishment for her, but her life is organized in such a way that she receives very little emotional gratification from the money. A secondary, and largely symbolic, source of support she has is through the dependent relationship she has on the hospital. That relationship is definitely bittersweet. On the one hand, she achieves a vague sense of security by identifying with the larger institution as if it were a nurturing family. Also, the hospital is helping her by providing insurance benefits and a retirement plan, and she has the satisfaction of knowing that her job is secure as long as she does not cross the nursing director. On the other hand, she gives up a lot of autonomy because of her relationship with the hospital: She knows that she could be ordered to float to any floor where the administra-

tion needs "a body" to fill "a slot," she could be pressed into working a double shift at any time because of her susceptibility to manipulation by invoking her guilt feelings, and her chances of career advancement beyond her present salary scale are slim because she knows she could always be replaced by a "cheaper" nurse if she pressed her demands.

A third source of gratification for the nurse's dependency needs is through fantasy. By the mechanism of fantasizing the "ideal" husband, the nurse can pretend to gratify her need to have love and security in her life. That mechanism is not satisfying, however, because there is no real replenishment.

The fourth source of nurturing for the nurse is through the process of identifying with her patients. By that means, she can vicariously enjoy the gratification of their dependency needs by taking care of them herself. Needless to say, that device, like fantasy, only serves as a stopgap measure and will not retard the inexorable pathway to psychologic disorganization and collapse.

The nurse receives very little nurturing from her son; instead, he depends on her and makes his demands known more insistently than all of her patients put together. In return, he offers her little for herself except the occasional time when she permits herself to regress and play with him.

As indicated in the vignette about the physician, the nurse receives very little emotional support from him. Although he accurately identified her distress of the moment and was compassionately drawn to offer her something, the exigencies of his own life at the time required that she be a nurse, not a person. As a result, the well-meant compliment to her professional skills served only to intensify her sense of need for warm human contact.

The nurse receives little more than money from the hospital administration. Her head nurse, insecure in her own job, is motivated to keep the nurse in her present position—quietly efficient, uncomplaining, and generally enhancing the image of the head nurse. The nursing director is more overtly hostile and is interested primarily in devaluing the nurse rather than building her up.

Compared with the other three individuals in

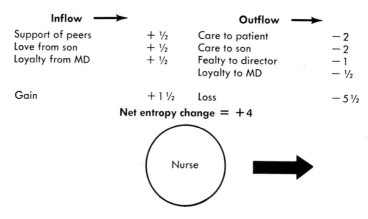

Fig. 3-3. Summary of economy of nurse during current interactions.

this system, the nurse has the poorest outlook for achieving mental health without intensive psychotherapy. Because of the strongly negative balance of her emotional economy (Fig. 3-3), she is a prime candidate for severe depression within the next few months or years. As an alternative to psychotherapy and its attending reorganization of her internal mechanisms (reprogramming), the nurse might change external factors instead, which could lead to an improved economy. For example, she could quit nursing altogether as so many nurses do, she could ally herself with an organization that sympathizes with her feelings such as a union or employees' association, or she could enter administration, thereby hoping to enhance her emotional economy by acquiring power.

The physician's economy

The physician is better able than the nurse to maintain an emotional steady state economy. His output is as great or greater than the nurse's, but he has more sources of replenishment than she does. The respect he holds in the community is much greater than that of the nurse and his patients are much more demonstrative than hers of their feelings of appreciation. Even the nursing director provides support for him; overbearing to her subordinates, nevertheless she is obsequious to those whom she perceives as her superiors. Even at home, the doctor receives a degree of nurture. He and his wife and children are not a

close family emotionally, but his wife appreciates her standard of living and frequently shows her appreciation to the physician.

Unlike the nurse, the physician also uses fantasy to fulfill his emotional needs for dependency. His fantasies tend to be sexual in which his dependency needs are met by passive, responsive women. In that way, he can maintain a position of control while having his needs "serviced." In other areas, fantasy represents a threat to the physician. Because of his acquired programming, the physician feels he is extremely fragile and therefore vulnerable to any change in the status quo. He is programmed to believe that if he has dependency needs, he is weak, and if he is weak, he will not be able to control his emotions and his life, and if he is unable to control those, he will be useless and unnecessary. Predictably then, he recoils from introspection—both psychologic and physical. He refuses to deal with the dizzy spells because he refuses to acknowledge the fact that he might be forced into a state of dependency. Similarly, he refuses to seek emotional help, instead scoffing at psychiatry and calling it "witchcraft."

The emotional prognosis for the physician depends largely at this point on his physical health. Although he is very near an emotional steady state now (Fig. 3-4), if he is stricken by any of the serious illnesses heralded by dizzy spells, his true fragility will be revealed. His programmed internal organization that is designed to maintain

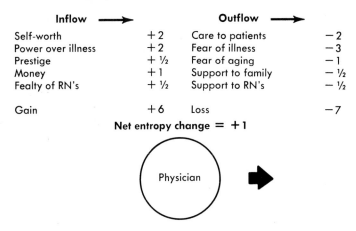

Inflow ➔		Outflow ➔	
Self-worth	+2	Care to patients	−2
Power over illness	+2	Fear of illness	−3
Prestige	+½	Fear of aging	−1
Money	+1	Support to family	−½
Fealty of RN's	+½	Support to RN's	−½
Gain	+6	Loss	−7

Net entropy change = +1

Physician

Fig. 3-4. Summary of economy of physician during current interactions.

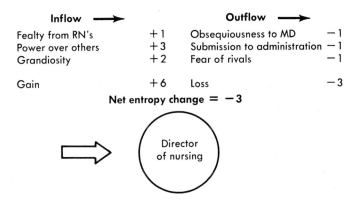

Inflow ➔		Outflow ➔	
Fealty from RN's	+1	Obsequiousness to MD	−1
Power over others	+3	Submission to administration	−1
Grandiosity	+2	Fear of rivals	−1
Gain	+6	Loss	−3

Net entropy change = −3

Director of nursing

Fig. 3-5. Summary of economy of nursing director during current interactions.

his sense of self-esteem will be thrown into a state of chaos as a result of having his primary prop knocked out from under him—his work.

The nursing director's economy

Because of her acquired programming, the nursing director perceives herself as a "closed" system; in her own self-referencing way, she believes she is completely self-contained and needs no one. In fact, she does need others and her uninterrupted obsession with acquiring power over others has kept her in positions by which she cannibalizes her subordinates as if she were an infant sucking at her mother's breast.

The nursing director's programming (character structure) is typical of that of many people who scratch and claw their way to the top. So much energy was involved in organizing her psyche to survive her first 2 years, she has never given up the grandiose, infantile (narcissistic) world view. Incapable of empathy, intimacy, or loyalty to others, she is socially isolated and is able to suck sustenance from others only because she holds power over them. Her emotional economy is satisfactory as long as she holds power. In that way, she is as content and stable as the infant with a slave/mother and a plentiful supply of food, clothing, and shelter (Fig. 3-5.)

Because of her highly self-referenced world view, the nursing director resembles infants in another important way: She uses the same primitive mechanisms of dealing with unpleasant emotional experiences such as hatred and aggression. She simply attributes those feelings to others in a paranoid style, thereby viewing any other important person as a threat to her security. Not surprisingly, many of these projected feelings are accurate; she *is* widely hated and many people wish her dead. In other words, her belief that she is hated and persecuted is accurate, but her way of acquiring that belief was invalid. (The criterion for defining paranoia is not whether a person's beliefs are true, but rather whether his mechanism for acquiring those beliefs is logical within the context of his environment.)

The life crisis that is expected to throw the nursing director's emotional economy into disorganization is suggested in the preceding. If she loses power over people, she will lose her main source of sustenance. Accordingly, as her physical and intellectual energies diminish with age thereby leaving her without the means for satiating her voracious appetite for power, she can be expected to withdraw into a paranoid state equivalent to depression in others.

THE ECONOMY OF THE CCU

The foregoing illustrates that each subsystem within the CCU is itself an incredibly complex system. Examination of the whole CCU system, then, involves examination of the interactive processes among them. In bringing the subsystems together an *organization* is formed.

An organization is a system comprising individual human beings. Organizations can be considered either formal or informal; an example of a formal organization is the CCU, whereas an example of an informal organization is a group of people who come together more or less regularly to drink beer and relax at the end of the work day. Formal organizations are generally established to meet a particular goal. In the case of the CCU, the organizational goal is to provide critical care support for the acutely and severely ill.

The formal goal orientation, however, is not the only orientation to be found in the unit. As seen in the foregoing sections, each subsystem, or individual, within the unit has its own set of goals. Some of these goals are complementary and others are contradictory. For example, the nurse and the physician share the goal of helping others even though each has come to this goal through his or her own experience and programming. The nurse and physician also have contradictory goals: The nurse is longing for personal support and validation of her individual needs, whereas at the same time, the physician's goal is to provide a nurse for his patient. Similarly, the nurse and nursing director have complementary goals: They both want the patient to survive although their reasons for that goal are very different. A contradiction in goals is represented by the nurse's need to be super competent, which conflicts with the nursing director's wish that the nurse will make mistakes and lose her status.

A combination of the complex flows of energy among the four human subsystems of the CCU is represented in Fig. 3-6. Simplification of the diagram is accomplished by considering only the *net* flows of energy for each individual and arranging the subsystems in linear order according to their rates of entropy change (Fig. 3-7). Arrangement of the subsystems in that form is analogous to cascades of batteries connected in series. The potential energy for each level is diminishing and the entropy is increasing with the current drain. Also, by analogy, the flow diagram represents at the top, a "source" of energy and at the bottom a "sink."

Inspection of the flow diagram of the CCU system shows at a glance that the system is not in equilibrium. Further, it is in steady state only if the rate of flow into the system equals the rate of flow out of it. Referring to the individual economies of the source individual (the nurse) and the sink (the nursing director), it is clear that the system is not in steady state. Presumably, the overall gain in entropy of the CCU system must be accounted for outside the CCU.

The principle of conservation of psychic energy dictates that prevention of an increase in the entropy of the CCU must be "paid for" by its suprasystem or set of suprasystems. Qualitatively, payment of this debt can be demonstrated by several factors common to hospital economics: (1) a high rate of turnover of nursing staff,[5] (2) a high inci-

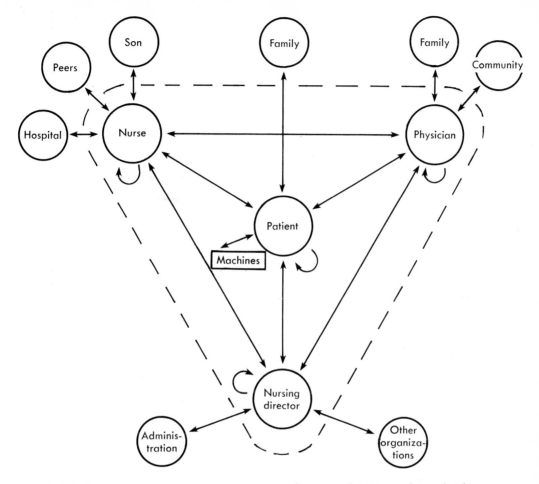

Fig. 3-6. Summary diagram of interactions among subsystems of CCU, together with relations to some of their non-CCU systems. Dashed line represents CCU boundary. Inward-turning arrows represent intrapsychic events: fantasy, grandiose delusions, reorganization by growth, and so on.

dence of absenteeism due to "illness," (3) unconscious sabotage of patients leading to malpractice lawsuits, (4) increases in worker's compensation insurance rates as a result of on-the-job casualties, both physical and emotional, and (5) increased reliance on expensive registry nurses. Low staff cohesiveness and low morale are both measures of high entropy states.

These costs are ultimately measurable financially. The largest single budget item of any hospital is the payroll. Insurance rates, orientation costs, and sick leave compensation contribute significantly. The impact of the cost factors just listed is to raise the cost of hospital care without improving services. These costs, of course, are paid for by the consumer, whether directly, through insurance premiums, or by taxes. It is my assertion that the increase in hospital costs in the past two decades is contributed to significantly by the systematic disregard of the emotional economies of hospital employees.

These emotional forces are potent. To ignore them is to permit no control over their effects, whereas to acknowledge them is to enable constructive channeling of information and energy. Examples of destructive processes within critical

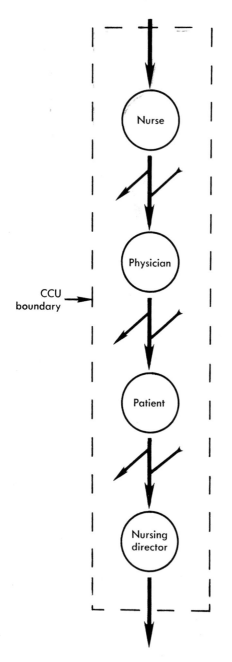

Fig. 3-7. Diagram of net flows of energy and information between the four people in the CCU, arranged in order of their rates of entropy gain (highest at top.) Divergent and convergent arrows represent other sources and sinks.

care units along with the correction of those processes are provided in a study I have made.[3] The principles of liaison psychiatry are not discussed in this chapter except in this general sense: If people in an organization can be helped to understand the emotional undercurrents in the processes of the system, relief can be obtained from disruptive "symptoms" and internal sabotage. Modern management techniques incorporate that principle.

PREDICTIONS BASED ON THE ECONOMIC MODEL

Assessment of the economies of the CCU system and its suprasystem, the hospital, permits several general predictions of effects.

First, because of the intrinsic resistance to change exhibited by hospital management in general, it is easy to predict that things will get worse before they get better; costs will continue to rise as productivity declines.

Second, because the hospital industry has little understanding of the mechanisms of the emotional costs in hospital systems, it has little control over the rapid decrease in cost-effectiveness of hospital care. Predictably, based on the cherished concept of nurse/chattel, administrators will try to squeeze more "giving" out of nurses, but the nurses will resist more.

Third, as a result of the attempts to get more from nurses, nurses will continue to leave their careers early after only brief exposure times. The staff turnover rates will get even higher as job dissatisfaction grows and will be highest at the poorest managed hospitals.

Fourth, in attempts to find more personal autonomy, more nurses will leave hospital staffs and begin working for registries. By this mechanism, nurses have already acquired much more power than hospitals are willing to acknowledge and deal with directly. Instead, they are attempting to form cartels through their own registries.

Fifth, as the adversary lines are drawn more boldly between labor and management, the registries will be supplanted by nurses' unions that will focus on improved working conditions, more nurse representation in hospital decision making, better patient care, and portable pension plans.

As these effects become national in scope,

there will be increased pressure from congress to control hospital costs and thereby to control the quality of medical care. Bureaucratization could supplant professionalism entirely. Professional ideals are internal to professional people and tend to drive them toward flawless performance, which is not possible. Still, the results of externalized application of ideals are well known: Bureaucratic ("socialized") medicine in the United States has proven disastrous. State mental hospitals, county hospitals, Veteran's hospitals, Medicare- and Medicaid-controlled programs offer low-quality, rationed care at exorbitant costs.

Finally, the economic systems analysis suggests solutions to the problems: By sharing the control of patient care institutions with professionals who are motivated to provide that care, the hospital industry can promote establishment of healthy steady-state hospital systems. This would require elimination of exploitative practices and of cannibalistic administrators.

SUMMARY AND CONCLUSION

An organization can obtain steady-state stability only by adhering to, rather than trying to fight, the laws of nature. Modern business management takes into account not only the traditional social science of economics but the science of psychology as well. One reason the hospital industry is saddled with archaic management techniques is the reluctance of people in the allied health professions to emerge from the dark ages and to acknowledge that human beings are systems comprising both physical *and* psychologic subsystems.

One lesson to be learned from the national sociopolitical-economic perturbations of the last 40 years is that while the *economy* can be manipulated, *economics* cannot be. Similarly, the laws of psychology cannot be manipulated. Most members of the health professions are aware that the legislative schemes proposed by some politicians to achieve cost reduction, consumer satisfaction, and quality medical care are spectacles as absurd as trying to repeal the law of gravity. Nevertheless, some of these same people deny the significance of psychologic processes in themselves and in others.

To be cost-effective and stable, a system must conform to certain principles of reality. Specifically, no system is "closed," and no individual or system economy can survive indefinitely in negative balance. Accordingly, it is important to acknowledge that all human systems are "affect-open," which means that the flow of *emotional information* is free and significant. ("Affect" means both the internal experience of feeling and its external expression, as by facial expression, for example.) Therefore an "affect-closed" system does not exist. Nevertheless, hospitals are replete with policies and procedures that are based on the assumption that patients, nurses, physicians, and administrators are each well-encapsulated, highly controlled, and always predictable automatons. In that never-never land, hospital employees can be assumed to have no needs other than those of physical subsistence. Those hospitals operate on the same assumptions of hospitals of a generation ago by which nurses and other employees were the chattel of the hospital and could be deployed as needed without regard to their individual needs and agendas. This is an assumption that contradicts the fact that within our culture, considerations of a worker's needs and wishes are "rights" that were won by bloodshed but are now taken for granted.

There are prominent signs in our current health care crisis that point to serious states of costly disorganization ("disease"): Nurses are extremely ambivalent about their profession and tend to blame "the administration" for most of their problems[4]; nurses from registries are replacing permanent hospital staffs, pushing up the costs of nursing service; administrators are frustrated and angry about being squeezed by the demands of government, physicians, patients, and nurses; nurses are increasingly demanding recognition as "true professionals" on the one hand but seem unwilling to tolerate the demands of 24-hour-a-day professionalism on the other; some members of the public are calling for "free" medical care at the same time that physicians are demanding that they not be asked to "give" so much; and politicians are pushing to take over medical care despite their proven inability to provide quality care. It is obvious that the health professions need to achieve a stable steady state.

To accomplish that, the psychologic needs of all people involved must be considered. Therefore the medical leadership and hospital management must recognize and deal with the emotional needs of the *helping people* as well as those of the helped.

Strategic planning to modernize hospital management can begin immediately, Short-range recommendations include: (1) Hospitals should provide adequate insurance coverage for employees that covers psychotherapy by psychiatrists, psychologists, and psychiatric social workers; (2) hospitals should provide continuous liaison services by mental health professionals to those units with the highest stress levels; and (3) hospitals should develop and formalize measures to promote staff/management interactions and to facilitate feedback from the staff in development of hospital policies.

Longer range recommendations include: (1) Hospital administrators should educate themselves with management consultants to take advantage of knowledge and methods already available; (2) the Joint Commission for the Accreditation of Hospitals (JCAH) should develop criteria for assuring that only well-managed hospitals are accredited; (3) schools should emphasize more the psychology of hospital employees in their curricula for hospital administrators; and (4) researchers in the field of hospital management can assess administrative practices by relying more on the evaluations of supervisors by their subordinates.

ACKNOWLEDGMENTS

I gratefully acknowledge many stimulating and thought-provoking conversations with George A. Michael of the Lawrence Livermore Laboratory as well as the staff and administration of Santa Ana Psychiatric Hospital, but I accept full responsibility for the opinions herein. This work was supported by Donald E. Watson, M.D., Inc., a California professional corporation.

REFERENCES

1. Hay, D., and Oken, D.: The psychological stresses of intensive care unit nursing, *Psychosom. Med.* **34**:109, 1972.
2. Koumans, A. J. R.: Psychiatric consultation in an intensive care unit, J.A.M.A. **194**:163, 1965.
3. Watson, D. E.: Psychiatric liaison services to the critical care nursing staff, Critical care update! **4**:5, 1977.
4. Godfrey, M. A. and Nursing 78: Job satisfaction—or should that be dissatisfaction? Nursing 78 89, 105, 1978.
5. Seybolt, J. W., Pavett, C., and Walker, D. D.: Turnover among nurses: it can be managed, J. Nurs. Admin. **8**:4, 1978.

BIBLIOGRAPHY

Miller, J. G.: General systems theory. In Freedman, A. M., Kaplan, H. I. and Sadock, B. J., editors: Comprehensive textbook of psychiatry/II, Baltimore, 1975, The Williams & Wilkins Co. p. 75.

Porter, L. W., Lawler, E. E., III, and Hackman, J. R.: Behavior in organizations, New York, 1975, McGraw-Hill Book Co.

Kramer, M.: Reality shock: why nurses leave nursing, St. Louis, 1974, The C. V. Mosby Co.

Porter, L. W., and Steers, R. M.: Organizational work and personal factors in employee turnover and absenteeism, Psychol. Bull. **80**:151, 1973.

Tirney, T. R., and Wright, N.: Minimizing the turnover problem: a behavioral approach, Supervisor Nurse **4**:47, 1973.

Brief, P. P.: Turnover among hospital nurses: a suggested model, J. Nurs. Admin. **6**:55, 1976.

CHAPTER 4

Psychiatric aspects of critical care

William F. Kiely and Warren R. Procci

The widespread development of special hospital units for the care of the critically ill and injured during the past decade has brought life-saving benefits for thousands of patients. Multiple organ support systems; monitors of cardiovascular, ventilatory, and renal excretory functions; and techniques for the noninvasive measurement of a variety of circulatory, respiratory, and hemodynamic parameters have been of tremendous value in the care of the dangerously ill patient. A benefit to such patients less heralded but of very great importance has been the sharpened focus brought to bear on altered states of consciousness, emotional responsiveness, and behavioral reaction in the critically ill. Responsibility for the lives of such patients has given the staffs of intensive care facilities increased respect for the integrative action of the CNS, on whose reliable function much of the coordinated action of other body systems depends. Skill in the appraisal and evaluation of the cerebrocortical functions of attention, perception, conception, orientation, and memory as well as of attitudes, feelings, and behavioral responses of the person who is ill are becoming part of the comprehensive care approach of the staffs of critical care units. Practitioners have come to the recognition that anxiety on the one hand or apathetic depression on the other is a danger signal interacting with a precarious balance of forces in the severely ill patient.[1]

Physicians, nurses, and other critical care professionals are becoming increasingly aware of the importance of the patient's previous life experience, coping style, and particular strengths or vulnerabilities in the face of stress and are planning treatment strategies to take account of such factors. It becomes increasingly evident that, although the treatment of disease may be highly impersonal and technologized to a very great extent, the care of a patient must be highly personal. The mind-body relationship, or psychosomatic unity, is nowhere more evident than as exhibited by patients in the grip and under the stress of critical illness.

■ What is stress?

Stress, which originally was a concept of the physical sciences, has come into the parlance of the life sciences to denote a state in which vital functioning of the organism is threatened either from an internal or an external source. Stress involves a sufficiently potent danger to physical or psychologic well-being as to require extraordinary measures for the maintenance of organized, adaptive function. These failing, stress may lead to disorganized emotional reaction, cognitive function, physical behavior, and physiologic or biochemical response patterns.

■ How do physical and psychologic stress differ?

The terms "physical stress," "emotional stress," and "social stress," among similar notions, are often used to denote different sources of threat to organized function. Although all have in common the potential for interfering with integrated organismic function by overtaxing adaptive capacities, they derive from different sources of challenge. In critical care medicine and surgery the stressors are most often multiple, deriving from illness or injury to vital organs or systems, from psychologically threatening challenge to the patient's repertoire of adaptive capacities, and from interruptions of social role functions and the imposition of new role functions involving dependency on and trust in the reliability of total strangers.

■ **What are the most important determinants of psychologic stress and of behavioral reaction among the critically ill?**

There is generally a subtle interweaving of a variety of determinants from several sources, including (1) features reflective of the patient's previous life experience and expressive of personal coping style, (2) factors related to the particular variety of illness or injury being experienced, (3) elements reflective of the critical care unit's distinctive environmental impact on the patient, and (4) patterns reactive to aspects of the treatment program imposed on the patient.

■ **What specifically are such person-related factors?**

The manner in which persons experience and cope with the threat posed by illness or injury and how they accept hospitalization and the imposed sick role will to an important degree reflect their previous life experience in dealing with crisis. If the patient has successfully mastered similar hazards in the past, there is less likelihood that the experience will be overwhelming, because the patient knows what to expect and how to deal with such challenges. Under such circumstances the psychologic threat is likely to be manageable and not spill over into disorganized arousal patterns of emotional, cognitive, behavioral, or psychophysiologic reaction. Coping style with the present challenge will generally reflect personality characteristics typical of that individual's previous manner of functioning, but often in an accented form; for example, the individual may be taciturn, cranky, self-willed, emotionally labile, or depressive. The patient brings to this crisis situation habitual attitudes toward and modes of dealing with novelty and the unfamiliar, dependency, authority figures, and passivity—the hallmarks of the sick role in critical care facilities.

The effect of such adaptive psychologic problems on the patient's current nexus of family relationships—with spouse, parents, and children—and in turn the reactive influence of such family members—particularly their own capacity to cope adaptively—have effects on the patient, and sometimes on the intensive care staff, that may bear importantly on the success or failure of treatment.[2] Previously unrecognized or compensated chronic cerebral insufficiency—related to age, cerebral vascular disease, or previous brain damage—is often thrown into acute decompensation by a sudden change in customary surroundings, particularly if there are deficits in function of the important orienting senses of vision and hearing.[3] Delusional misinterpretation of time, place, and person as well as hallucinatory excitement is sometimes induced in the elderly patient by such minimum degrees of sensory deprivation. In sum, the patient's age, level of cerebral competence, characteristic personality style, emotional state, and nexus of interpersonal relationships all may contribute to the illness experience and determine the reaction to it.[4]

■ **What are some of the disease-related factors?**

The frequency of occurrence of critical care psychiatric syndromes varies considerably with the type of illness and differs in prevalence in the several types of intensive care facilities. The concept of a critical care unit psychiatric syndrome developed originally out of reports of a high incidence of delirium (40% to 70%) following open-heart surgery.[5] Some observers believed that this syndrome, developing typically between the third and fifth postoperative day, reflected the influence of the intensive care unit's environmental impact on the patient. A combination of sleep deprivation, sensory monotony, and loss of a sense of time passage and of a day-night cycle were felt to be major contributing factors to the loss of reality sense.[6] Postcardiotomy delirium has subsequently been found to be highly correlated with neurologic deficit and organically determined cognitive dysfunction[7] perhaps related to the duration of exposure to cardiopulmonary bypass, microemboli originating in the heart, duration of hypothermia, and depth and duration of anesthesia. Significant differences in the incidence of psychiatric disturbances following lung surgery are noted in comparison to open-heart surgery. It would appear that the incidence of such syndromes in well-organized coronary care units is considerably less than that noted in postcardiotomy recovery rooms.[8] Intensive care units treating a wide spectrum of critically ill and injured patients, including the seriously burned, will number among their patients a majority who may suffer from renal, cardiac, or pulmonary failure, serious septic or hypovolemic shock, considerable anemia, fever, and toxemia. Such disease-related elements very probably account for the significantly different incidence of delirium and other psychiatric disorders among such patients as compared to the generally much more physically intact acute coronary patient or even many post-cardiotomy patients.

■ How may the critical care unit's environment affect the patient's coping with illness?

The introduction of critical care facilities has served, among other consequences, to focus attention on the psychobiologic effects of the kinds, variety, and quantity of sensory input that such environments bring to bear on persons who are ill. Reference has already been made to the effect, especially on the elderly, that transfer to such an unfamiliar environment may have. The usual design of critical care units results in windowless, austere, multi-bed rooms with a variety of monitors, respirators, and other bedside equipment whose meaning and purpose to a marginally rational and critically ill patient may be ambiguous at best. Too often the patient lies prone, movement impeded by intubation of some or all of the body orifices, experiencing the persistent stress of pain or discomfort, and with perceptual faculties dulled or impaired by sedatives, tranquilizers, and/or hypnotic analgesics. The compounding influences of azotemia, anoxemia, hypercapnia, and hypovolemic or septic shock may further complicate the task for the patient of making meaningful and purposeful sense of this entire spectrum of input.

In some measure and to variable degrees in the course of treatment of such critical illness there are likely to be elements of (1) sensory underload or deprivation, (2) some periods of sensory overload, (3) much sensory monotony, (4) erratic and interrupted sleep patterns, (5) social isolation, (6) unfamiliarity with the human and situational environment, and (7) prolonged immobilization. Each of these factors has been shown experimentally to be capable of contributing to clouding of consciousness, perceptual distortion, behavioral confusion, and sometimes to frankly delusional and hallucinatory experiences.[9] A number of observers have pointed to the role of reduced or destructured sensory input in the production of delirium such as occurs after eye surgery,[10] with the use of tank-type respirators,[11] and with placement in intensive care units.[12] The passivity and immobilization may reduce very considerably the level of kinesthetic and proprioceptive feedback from muscles and joints on which the midbrain reticular formation and hypothalamus depend to sustain adaptive alertness and orientation in the overlying cerebral cortex.[13] Under such conditions vital subcortical reciprocal balance between arousal and withdrawal systems may break down, resulting in the delivery to the interpretative neocortex of a depatterned, meaningless volley of signals to which cognitive sense is difficult for the patient to assign.[14]

■ What are the neurobiologic bases for the wide spectrum of emotional, behavioral, and psychophysiologic reaction patterns encountered in crisis care of the ill or injured?

Hess,[15] as early as 1925, pointed out that an animal's reaction to environmental challenge is importantly reflective of the influence of subcortical centers that coordinate autonomic, somatic, and psychic functions. He suggested that these centers were organized through reciprocally balanced systems, which he termed *ergotropic* and *trophotropic*. Highly integrated neural functions of the type underlying the cognitive process, generally considered reflective of cortical activity, are under the modulating influence of these primitive, tonically active subcortical systems. All perceptual stimuli, whether of exteroceptive or interoceptive source, as well as memory and logical thought sequences reveal the shaping influence of these balanced systems. Their anatomic basis, physiologic interconnections, and neurochemical transmitters are distinguishable and separable.[16] Their influence is identifiable across the entire continuum of consciousness from sleep to the heights of ecstasy physiologically[13] and from stupor to catatonic excitement psychopathologically.[14]

The ergotropic system integrates functions that prepare the individual for positive action. It is characterized by alerting, arousal, excitement, increased skeletal muscle tone and sympathetic nervous activity, and the release of catabolic hormones. The trophotropic system, on the other hand, integrates systems that promote withdrawal and conservation of energy: raising the stimulus barrier to perceptual input, decreasing skeletal muscle tone, increasing parasympathetic nervous function, and circulating anabolic hormones. A developing body of data indicates that the biogenic amines norepinephrine and dopamine are neurotransmitters for the ergotropic system, whereas 5-hydroxytryptamine (serotonin) and acetylcholine play similar roles for the trophotropic system.[17]

■ **Are there relatively consistent physiologic principles that underlie the operation of these reciprocally opposed systems?**

Yes, a few basic principles play a primary role in the operation of this quite complex psychobiologic process and underlie the resultant patterns of behavior. First, the two systems stand in mutually reciprocal relationship and share tonic, enduring, and balanced physiologic activity. With increasing degrees of activation of the ergotropic "go" (approach) system there is a corresponding degree of inhibition of the trophotropic "no go" (avoidance) system; the converse is also true.

Second, when either system is stimulated, the reactivity of both systems is altered, affecting their state of readiness, set, or tuning,[18] so to speak. In moderate states of activation, or tuning, the reactivity of the various anatomic and physiologic components of the affecting system is heightened, whereas that of the reciprocal system is correspondingly reduced. Thus in situations of moderate, but not extreme, challenge or threat the "go" system expresses itself cortically through alerting, or vigilance; autonomically in a sym-

pathetic stimulation; and behaviorally in a state of muscular readiness. At the same time the reactivity of the several components of the "no go" system is correspondingly suppressed.

Third, at maximum stimulation reciprocal balance between systems breaks down and both discharge simultaneously. A clinical example is the state of anxiety wherein a variety of psychic, skeletal muscular, and visceral disturbances reflect such simultaneous discharge of opposing systems. Flooding of the cerebral cortex by afferents from both systems may be experienced as dread; weak knees may coexist with tremulous hands; and sweating, tachycardia, and hypertension may coexist with nausea, vomiting, and bowel or bladder hyperactivity.

■ **What are the most common varieties of psychiatric syndromes encountered in critical care units?**

The most common syndromes encountered in critical care units are schematically characterized in Table 4-1. They may range from the occasionally encountered overwhelming fear reaction, accompanied by a paralyzing sense of helplessness in which the behavioral-avoidance grip of the "no go" system is evident, through more adaptive but sometimes physiologically stressful states of restless tension. In these polar opposite states of tuning, or adaptation, reciprocal suppression of the opposing system is maintained. At higher degrees of CNS arousal maladaptive, sustained anxiety is encountered with simultaneous discharge to varying degrees of both "go" and "no go" systems as noted psychically, viscerally, and in skeletal muscle groups.

At still higher degrees of stimulation, anxious or agitated depression reactive to the stress of crisis may be encountered. One sometimes sees examples of acute schizophreniform psychotic disintegration with thought disorder, delusions, or hallucinations maintained in the context of clear consciousness and without loss of orientation or memory function. Especially where elements of cardiac, pulmonary, renal failure, or circulatory shock complicate the clinical course of the illness, and particularly in the middle-aged or elderly, one frequently encounters delirium, that is, a state of cerebral insufficiency with im-

Table 4-1. Neurobiology of psychiatric syndromes

State of tuning	Clinical example	Pharmacologic intervention	Site of action
Trophotropic dominance	Acute fear	Benzodiazepine agent (Librium, Valium, Serax, Tranxene)	Limbic forebrain and midbrain serotonergic suppressor sites
Ergotropic dominance	Sustained tension	Benzodiazepine agent (Librium, Valium, Serax, Tranxene)	Limbic forebrain and midbrain serotonergic suppressor sites
Simultaneous "T" and "E" discharge	Anxiety	Benzodiazepine agent (Librium, Valium, Serax, Tranxene)	Limbic forebrain and midbrain serotonergic suppressor sites
	Agitated depression	Benzodiazepine agent (Librium, Valium, Serax, Tranxene)	Limbic forebrain and midbrain serotonergic suppressor sites
	Acute schizophreniform stress reaction	Butyrophenone (Haldol)	Neostriatal and mesolimbic dopamine receptor sites
	Acute delirium	Butyrophenone (Haldol)	Neostriatal and mesolimbic dopamine receptor sites
		Benzodiazepine agent (Librium, Valium, Serax, Tranxene)	Limbic forebrain and midbrain serotonergic suppressor sites

pairment of some or all of such cognitive functions as attention, perception, conception, logical sequence, orientation, and memory. Some degree of clouding of consciousness, not uncommonly punctuated by lucid intervals, is characteristic of this state. The affect of the delirious patient may vary from apathy to irritable restlessness, and the autonomically modulated visceral concomitants may follow a corresponding spectrum.

■ **What principles ought to be followed in the choice of psychoactive drugs for treatment of this spectrum of psychiatric disorders?**

Based on the neurobiologic principle of balance, the disturbance of which is accompanied by psychopathology and often by very undesirable psychophysiologic visceral and behavioral concomitants in critically ill patients, the goal in the use of psychoactive drugs should be the restoration of physiologic reciprocity between opposing ergotropic and trophotropic systems, a situation wherein clarity of cognitive function, smoothness of visceral autonomic activity, and overall behavioral control may be recovered.

Table 4-2 summarizes a fairly reliable approach to the use of a modest number of drugs whose dosage range, site of principal CNS action, and expectable effects are fairly clear. Efficacy is claimed for literally scores of psychoactive drugs produced under a wide variety of trade names, too numerous for the average clinician to develop personal experience with. A wise course, particularly for the physician treating acute, life-threatening illnesses of limited duration, is to master the use of a small group of drugs of antianxiety, antipsychotic, and antidepressant classes and to know their actions and interactions, their modes of administration, dosage ranges, and potential side effects.

■ **What antianxiety drugs are most useful for critical care patients?**

As antianxiety agents, the benzodiazepines are preferable to the meprobamate group, being available in both oral and parenteral form, which the latter are not; likewise the benzodiazepines are preferable to the barbiturates in not significantly depressing cerebrocortical functions in dosage ranges wherein tranquilizing is achievable. The four available benzodiazepines, chlordiazepoxide (Librium), diazepam (Valium), oxazepam (Serax), and clorazepate (Tranxene), are essentially

Table 4-2. Psychoactive drugs for the critically ill and effective dosage ranges

Drug class	Generic name	Trade name	Daily adult dose range (mg)*	
			High	Moderate
Benzodiazepines	Chlordiazepoxide	Librium	150-300	75-150
	Diazepam	Valium	30-60	15-30
	Oxazepam	Serax	75-120	45-75
	Clorazepate	Tranxene	45-90	25-45
Butyrophenone	Haloperidol	Haldol	15-60	6-15

*Reduce by one-half for IM use.

identical except for dose and duration of action, chlordiazepoxide being the longest acting and oxazepam the shortest acting of the group. All rank with the moderate- or long-acting barbiturates, such as phenobarbital, in duration of action. Although oxazepam is an active metabolite of diazepam, poorer bowel absorption necessitates a larger dose. There is pharmacologic evidence to suggest that the antianxiety effects of the benzodiazepines are the result of action in limbic forebrain and limbic midbrain areas rather than on the reticular formation, an important site of barbiturate and nonbarbiturate sedative-hypnotic action. The interruption of serotonergic neurotransmission in limbic suppressor sites appears to block the avoidance (trophotropic) side of approach-avoidance conflict and so reduces fear and tension, permitting more physiologic balance between opposing "go" and "no go" systems.[19]

■ **How may depression be managed among the critically ill?**

The kinds of depressive syndromes encountered in critically ill patients are generally reactive to or concomitants of the overwhelming illness being treated and more often than not are associated with considerable reactive anxiety or agitation. Since the clearest indication for the use of tricyclic antidepressants is in retarded, endogenous, or psychotic depressions, and since an average of 2 to 3 weeks is generally required for clear-cut efficacy to become apparent from the use of these drugs, they are best avoided in critically ill patients. One of the benzodiazepine group of antianxiety agents is often of some use in depressed patients with prominent symptoms of tension, anxiety, or somatic complaints. Controlled trials indicate that antianxiety drugs may be useful in these types of depression.[20] Because of the danger of inhibition of monoamine oxidase (MAO) in critically ill patients, many of whom might require vasopressor circulatory support or sympathomimetic bronchodilator inhalation aerosols, the use of MAO inhibitors is best avoided in the care of the critically ill.

■ **What are the most desirable antipsychotic drugs for the seriously ill or injured patient?**

At present the most widely used antipsychotic agents are of the phenothiazine class, with chlorpromazine (Thorazine) the most thoroughly studied member of the class. In comparison to trifluoperazine (Stelazine) or fluphenazine (Prolixin, Permitil), it is of lower potency and has greater sedative effect. The potential of phenothiazines, particularly chlorpromazine, to block α-adrenergic vasopressor receptor sites and to intensify the vasodilating and other β-adrenergic effects of epinephrine together with other autonomic side effects makes this class of drug less desirable for use in the seriously ill patient than the newer butyrophenone compound haloperidol (Haldol). This agent is rapidly and completely absorbed from the gastrointestinal tract and is available in injectable form as well. It causes little autonomic nervous system receptor blockage and has no adverse interactions with digitalis, diuretics, or other cardiovascular drugs. For the elderly, for those with cardiovascular disease, and for the deliriously excited patient it may be the drug of choice where psychotic behavior and confusion require drug treatment.[21]

■ **What elements in the critical care treatment program itself bear scrutiny with respect to their psychologic effects on the patient?**

Considerations such as those outlined in this chapter should call attention once more, amid a medical technology revolution, to man as the proper measure of relevance for invention. And meaning is the measure by which a man unifies and integrates the world as individually perceived. This refers to the personal significance of the information input for the receiver. How the individual interprets the somatic and visceral sensory input together with the environmental surroundings is of crucial importance for emotional, psychophysiologic, and behavioral response patterns. Where sensory input is dulled by drugs or disease consequences (anoxemia, azotemia, and so forth), or made monotonous by immobilization, fixed lighting, and acoustic input, the additive influence of CNS habituation further isolates and deprives the interpretive cortex of variety and novelty. The net result is diminished meaningfulness of perceptual input, detachment, disengagement from the environmental surroundings, and hypnagogic or dreamlike uprooting from time and place, leading toward outright delusional and hallucinatory experience. Such isolation from the environment deprives the patient of the meaningful information ordinarily depended on to make sensible interpretation of an experience. If the patient cannot organize the input in meaningful terms in relation to past experience, the situation may become chaotic psychologically, the visceral concomitants of this disorganization may sometimes be dangerous (cardiac rate, rhythm, blood pressure, and so forth), and the reactive behavior may call for restraints or further sedation, sometimes with additional consequences in terms of sensory deprivation.

■ **How might supportive treatment be provided in critical care units to best take into account the psychosocial needs of the patient?**

Certain practical therapeutic measures suggest themselves as having both preventive and corrective value for such psychiatric syndromes:

1. Of prime importance preventively, as well as practically, in the presence of beginning mental decompensation is the fact and utilization of the potential of a trusting, confident, caring practitioner-patient relationship.[22] The sense of isolation and helplessness in a potentially hostile environment and the overwhelming feeling of powerlessness accompanying this situation can be devastating for many patients. A number of persons who have been interviewed in depth following harrowing periods of critical care unit experience have testified to the power of trust and hope in tiding them through the experience. The degree of trust and magical power attributed to their physicians appeared proportional to the length of and overall quality of the relationship antedating the critical illness.

2. As a corollary of the point just mentioned, although it is not the rule to anticipate the admission to critical care units for those acutely medically ill, it is possible to anticipate or plan such care for elective surgical patients, as in the case of cardiac, pulmonary, or other major surgical problems. Time spent familiarizing the patient with the broad plan of postoperative care, a visit to the intensive care unit with some explanation of the purpose and the life-supportive power of much of the technologic equipment, and a personal meeting with some of the key nursing and medical staff who will be responsible for the patient's welfare can increase the patient's understanding of and trust in the place and persons in whose care his or her life is to be placed.

3. During the course of critical care periodic physical examination for signs of deteriorating function and mental examination in terms of level of attention, concentration, and time orientation will allow early application of corrective therapy.

4. Overdependency on monitoring and telemetric equipment at the expense of regular, reassuring, and supportive personal contact with the patient by critical care personnel should be avoided.

5. All procedures should be explained to the patient in simple, clear terms. Movement should be as unrestrained as is consistent with the disease under treatment; the patient should be engaged, as much as possible, in the actions of grooming, eating, drinking, and toileting.

6. Where possible, the patient should be surrounded by personally familiar bedside objects,

such as a clock, radio, or family photos, and should be allowed brief visits by the family.

7. Oversedation and excessive use of narcotic analgesics should be avoided, with alertness for the paradoxical responses to such medications that are occasionally seen, especially in the young or the elderly. The benzodiazepines or butyrophenone, which depress cortical functions much less than subcortical ones, are in general preferable to narcotics or barbiturates and can be utilized to lower the required dosages of the latter where indicated.

SUMMARY

Our overall view is that many, if not most, patients meet the challenge of acute, severe illness or injury with admirable equanimity and fortitude. The physical setting of the critical care unit itself, forbidding as it appears to the uninitiated even among medical and nursing staff assigned to duty elsewhere in the hospital, need not be unduly stressful to the patient if the human concern, interest, and caring attitude of the critical care staff in whose hands his or her life and welfare have been placed can be sensed. The humanizing element of person-to-person contact is capable of rapidly desensitizing the patient to the alarm, fear, or bewilderment that strikes the visitor to such intensive care units. An understanding of basic neurobiologic and psychologic principles in constructing a medical and nursing care program for the critically ill is fundamental to improving the quality of the experience for the patient and may well contribute significantly to lowered mortality risk for certain types of illness or injury.

REFERENCES

1. Kiely, W. F.: Psychiatric aspects of critical care, Crit. Care Med. **2**:139, 1974.
2. Kiely, W. F.: Coping with severe illness, Adv. Psychosom. Med. **8**:105, 1972.
3. Engel, G. L., and Romano, J.: Delirium, a syndrome of cerebral insufficiency, J. Chronic Dis. **9**:260, 1959.
4. Lipowski, Z. J.: Physical illness, the individual, and the coping processes, Psychiatry Med. **1**:91, 1970.
5. Blachly, P. H., and Starr, A.: Post-cardiotomy delirium, Am. J. Psychiatry **121**:371, 1964.
6. Kornfeld, D. S., Zimberg, S., and Malm, J.: Psychiatric complications of open-heart surgery, N. Engl. J. Med. **273**:282, 1965.
7. Gilman, S.: Cerebral disorders after open-heart operations, N. Engl. J. Med. **272**:489, 1965.
8. Hackett, T. P., Cassem, N. H., and Wishnie, H. A.: Coronary-care unit: appraisal of its psychologic hazards, N. Engl. J. Med. **279**:1365, 1968.
9. Freedman, S. J., Grunebaum, H. V., and Greenblatt, M.: Perceptual and cognitive changes in sensory deprivation. In Solomon, P., et al., editors: Sensory deprivation, Cambridge, Mass., 1961, Harvard University Press.
10. Weisman, A. D., and Hackett, T. P.: Psychosis after eye surgery, N. Engl. J. Med. **258**:1284, 1958.
11. Leiderman, P. H., et al.: Sensory deprivation: clinical aspects, Arch. Intern. Med. **101**:389, 1958.
12. McKegney, F. P.: The intensive-care syndrome, Conn. Med. **30**:633, 1966.
13. Gellhorn, E., and Kiely, W. F.: Mystical states of consciousness: neurophysiological and clinical aspects, J. Nerv. Ment. Dis. **154**:399, 1972.
14. Gellhorn, E., and Kiely, W. F.: Autonomic nervous system in psychiatric disorder. In Mendels, J., editor: Biological psychiatry, New York, 1973, John Wiley & Sons, Inc.
15. Hess, W. R.: The functional organization of the diencephalon, New York, 1958, Grune & Stratton, Inc.
16. Gellhorn, E.: Principles of autonomic-somatic integrations, Minneapolis, 1967, University of Minnesota Press.
17. Kety, S.: Brain amines and affective disorders. In Ho, B. T., and McIsaac, W. M., editors: Brain chemistry in mental diseases, New York, 1971, Plenum Publishing Corp.
18. Gellhorn, E.: Further studies on the physiology and pathophysiology of tuning of the central nervous system, Psychosomatics **10**:94, 1969.
19. Wise, C. D., Berger, B. D., and Stein, L.: Benzodiazepines: anxiety-reducing activity by reduction of serotonin turnover in brain, Science **177**:180, 1972.
20. Raskin, A., Schulterbrandt, J. G., Reatig, N., Crook, T. H., and Odle, D.: Depression subtypes and responses to phenelzine, diazepam, and placebo, Arch. Gen. Psychiatry **30**:66, 1974.
21. Appleton, W. S., and Davis, J. M.: Practical clinical psychopharmacology, New York, 1973, Medcom Press.
22. Holland, J., Sgroi, S. M., Marivit, S. J., and Solkoff, N.: The ICU syndrome: fact or fancy, Psychiatry Med. **4**:241, 1973.

CHAPTER 5

Therapeutic touch for critically ill patients

Virginia L. Gamble

Touch is perhaps the most vital of human experiences. We came into the world with intense skin hunger, as all the sensations we encounter from our environment are perceived through our skin, the largest organ system of our bodies. Our earliest learning is communicated through the sensory stimulation of the skin, which transmits electrical impulses along neural pathways, activating the development of our brains. So great is the early need for touch that infants may develop illness and die owing to tactile deprivation. This syndrome is termed "marasmus," the Greek word meaning "washing away." The need to be touched is universal and transcultural. Not only is touch an important adjunct of total nursing care, it is a basic requirement in the development and maintenance of optimal health.

Touch has been used by mankind for the purpose of comforting the sick since the dawn of civilization. Primitive man had no scientific methodology or equipment to aid him in the care of the sick and the dying. He had to rely on such natural healing tools as his perception of the universal force that surrounded him and his body, which he used as an instrument of healing. He used his hands for the acquisition and preparation of food, the building and maintenance of his shelter, and the ministering to the sick and dying. Reaching out and touching was an extension of his own being, of his own humanity. His education for helping the sick was obtained by observing the forces of nature surrounding him. Man learned about the universe through direct experience

of his environment. His knowledge of life was mainly intuitive, creative, and instinctual.

As civilization progressed and the division of labor developed, the role of the healer passed into the hands of the spiritual leader of the tribe. His function was to interact with the forces of nature for the purpose of healing the sick. Traditionally, the ruling class was also involved in a healing role. Artwork and writings from the Third Egyptian Dynasty indicate that the Pharaohs used "laying on of hands" to help the sick. Artifacts found in the tomb of Imhotep, who lived in 2980 BC, declared him to be the chief physician of Zoser. In tenth century England and France, the "laying on of hands" was known as the "royal touch" or the "king's touch." History records that King Henry IV held large festivals at which he performed healings. And so, historically, touch has been used by many as a healing or therapeutic modality.

The phenomenon of touch as a healing instrument has been evidenced in many cultures throughout history. Each culture developed its own vocabulary and explanation of this "life force" or "healing force" that it experienced. Hippocrates stated there was "something" that emanated from his hands and had a salutary effect on his patients. He urged young physicians not to disregard this method in their medical practice.

Various cultures developed their own systems for incorporating the principles in the use of touch in healing. A cross-cultural study of these belief systems shows similarities in experiences and uses of touch. In the Chinese culture it is believed that a "life force" or "chi" energy fills and surrounds all living things. Illness, they believe, is caused by an imbalance or blockage in the flow of this "chi" energy in the body. They believe that this blockage can occur in either or all of the physical, mental, emotional, or spiritual bodies. Their method of healing is to restore the balance in the patient and allow the energy to flow freely. Acupuncture and acupressure are the forms of touch used to restore balance and promote healing.

The Hindus believe in the same life force that flows through all living beings. They call this energy "prana," which translated means life breath. It is their belief that it is this same life force that is inhaled and exhaled with the respiratory cycle. A healthy person is filled with "prana" to overflowing, while illness is caused by a deficiency of this life energy. The Hindus and Yogis also describe in their writings a series of energy centers in the subtle body, or "chakras," that correspond in location to the endocrine glands in the physical body. Health is restored by removing blockages in these energy centers. This same life force is known in other cultures as "Tao," "Ki," and "bioplasma" (USSR).

We have noted the polarization of the physician and the spiritual leader into distinct and separate roles. It is interesting to note that Hippocrates was both a physician and a priest. Scientific and technologic advances, especially in the present century, have altered the healing role. As recently as 50 years ago, physicians relied primarily on their own eyes, ears, fingers, and intuition in making diagnoses. The use of these tools necessitated close physical interaction with the patient. Now, health care technicians have very sophisticated instruments and methods used in diagnosis and treatment that prevent them from directly interacting with patients. These include electrocardiograms, x-ray machines, echocardiography, radionucleotide imaging, blood chemistry profiles, invasive monitoring of vital functions, and many others. Direct physical contact of the patient is now minimal in diagnosis and may be nonexistent in treatment. In many instances, especially in critical care units, the patient becomes an

extension of the machinery that is being used to monitor him. The machines begin to be given precedence over the patient, and because of this, the patient suffers depersonalization and dehumanization. The primary care staff, in order to manage the reality of the suffering of its acutely ill patients, may find it easier to manipulate the dials of the machines than to cope with the anxiety, fear, and frustration of the patient.

Having stayed in a critical care unit, the patient may have recovered from an acute physical illness but may continue to experience nightmares and other symptoms of anxiety that are the direct result of having been exposed to a stress-producing environment. Severe psychologic problems, including depression, withdrawal, suicidal ideation, and severed family bonds may all be sequelae to acute illness.

Just as change is the only constant in the evolution of mankind, a change away from the totally mechanistic, scientific approach to patient care is beginning to emerge. Many of the health care professions are beginning to look at man as a total entity, not just as the sum total of his physiologic complaints. We are beginning to discern the interrelationship of mind and body and to understand how an individual's state of mind influences his physiologic functioning. Adjunctive therapies and modalities are beginning to be developed to decrease the depersonalization process begun by the use of technology. One of these modalities is touch and its therapeutic use in patient care. The time has arrived to emphasize the care of patients rather than machines.

■ How does the stress response affect the critically ill patient?

The patient in a critical care unit faces many elements, both internal and external, that cause him acute and chronic stress. The GAS, or general adaptive syndrome, as defined by Hans Selye, is the response of the body to any stressor. Even in positive stress situations such as a promotion or being released from a critical care unit, the organism responds in the same way as it would to a negative situation. In an acutely negative stress reaction such as slamming on one's brakes, we are subjected to a rapid activation of the adrenocortical hormones and their resultant effect to ready the body for fight or flight. This is followed by resolution of the stress in which the body adapts to the stressor and then returns to the physiologic baseline. In a chronic stress situation the source of the stress may be ambiguous or multiple, and resolution never takes place. The patient is caught in a constant state of attempting to cope with multiple stressors, many of which have no instant denouement. This cycle of chronic stress may become self-perpetuating with stress begetting more stress. Constantly high stress levels make increasingly high demands on an already highly taxed organism. If this alarm state is not alleviated, the result is total exhaustion and death. Selye states, "No living organism can be maintained continuously in a state of alarm. If the body is confronted with an agent so damaging that continued exposure to it is incompatible with life, then death ensues during the alarm reaction within the first hours or days." Touch, as a therapeutic tool, may effectively intercede in this stress cycle and reestablish the coping mechanisms that may ultimately result in the patient's survival.

■ What are the elements that cause stress in the critically ill patient?

There are many factors that cause stress in the critically ill patient, including physiologic, environmental, physical, emotional, chemical, spiritual, biologic, and social factors.

Physiologic. Initially there is an assault on the homeostasis of the individual owing to the disease state or trauma, which causes a disruption of body structures and functions. During surgery the manipulation of the patient, such as artificially altering his state of consciousness through anesthesia and the removal or alteration of body structures, is a source of stress. In critical care units procedures such as the insertion of pulmonary artery catheters, arterial lines, temporary pacemakers, or intra-aortic balloon pump lines, the withdrawal of venous and arterial specimens, and the insertion or removal of other catheters and tubes are all sources of acute stress for patients.

Environmental. The physical environment of a critical care area is awesome and frightening. The patient is devoid of all personal belongings, including clothes. The surroundings are entirely new and unfamiliar, resplendent with a formidable array of machinery and tubing. The patient may have never experienced such an environment before. The sounds of the environment are foreign and stress producing: the cycling of the respirators, the alarms and buzzers, the sounds of unfamiliar voices and cries of pain and suffering, and the incessant clicking of the fluid administration units. Unpleasant odors are also stressful and irritating. The touch the patient receives from his caregivers is usually painful. Very often, because of the use of numerous monitoring and lifesaving devices, the patient's hands may be restrained, limiting his kinesthetic movement. Because of intubation, he may not be able to talk or communicate.

Physical. With the lights on in a critical care unit for 24 hours a day, the body experiences a loss of the natural circadian rhythm of a day-night cycle, and this is a source of stress for the individual. Both extremes of cold and heat activate the stress response. We also need to be aware that the patient is forced to endure territorial limits (that is, the confines of his bed). This may also be a source of stress.

Emotional. The awareness of being acutely ill, coupled with the fear of possible death, is one of the common, though unverbalized, sources of stress for the critically ill patient. Because of the nature of intensive care, the patient is separated from family and significant others, who formerly comprised his support system. He is alone and afraid. He may be experiencing pain, either emotional or physical. He may be concerned with the changes in body structure and function that affect his body image. He may be contemplating a life-style change, which may be his only chance of survival, or he may be contemplating survival itself.

Chemical. Medications and their side-effects may be prime sources of stress in the critically ill patient.

Spiritual. The patient may feel a loss of the sense of self and self-worth owing to the acuity of his illness. He may feel that there is no meaning in his life. Many feel that illness is a punishment from God, and the estrangement that they feel from their higher power may be a source of stress.

Biologic. Another source of stress is the assault on the body by pathologic organisms.

Social. The patient experiences many role changes as a result of his illness. In assuming the sick role he may be passive and dependent, which are contrary to his normal role. This may be a source of stress. He may experience powerlessness and loss of control over his own life and environment. Anxiety may occur because of role changes in his family environment caused by illness.

• • •

In examining the average day of a critical care patient you are able to see how many stressors enter his life, and the way he is able to respond and adapt to these stressors, internal and external, has a direct bearing on his ability to survive.

■ **What are the functions of the skin?**

Of all the organ systems the skin is the largest and comprises approximately 16% to 18% of our total body weight. *Gray's Anatomy* describes the function of the skin as: "Covering the surface of the body and sheltering it from the injurious influences of the environment is the skin or integument. It protects the deeper tissues from injury, from drying, and from the invasion by foreign organisms; it contains the peripheral endings of the many sensory nerves; it plays an important part in the regulation of body temperature, and also has limited excreting and absorbing powers." Thus the skin functions as protection, as a barrier mechanism, as a temperature regulator, as an outlet of excretion, and as a sensory organ.

Until recently, very little importance has been placed on the functions of the skin. In nursing education the information on the importance of skin was limited to that of insensible loss and decubitus formation. Nurses learned very little about the function of the skin as a sensory organ. Ashley Montague, in his book entitled *Touching: The Human Significance of the Skin,* tells about the adaptive role of the skin in assessing incoming sensory information and its adaptive role of making adjustments in order to maintain the homeostasis of the organism. He describes the wide variety of information that the skin is capable of sensing and how this information is relayed to the brain to assist it in making the needed ad-

justments. With the development of biofeedback, the role of the skin as a transmitter of information is becoming known. The skin has the potential to conduct electrical current. During a stress reaction there are measurable changes in the skin's electrical activity. As long ago as the 1880's, a scientist named Féré discovered that the resistance of the skin to a small electrical current changed in response to something that aroused and affected the emotions. The skin is a powerful communications medium, with direct connection between brain and skin. Researchers have called this phenomenon "skin talk." As a communicator, the skin gives us much information about the internal physical and emotional condition of the individual.

By becoming increasingly aware of the many functions of the skin, we can begin to use the skin more intensively in the assessment of physical and psychologic states, and we can also learn to use it more therapeutically by means of interventions.

■ **What is therapeutic touch?**

Although there are techniques that can be learned, they are only a part of what can be termed therapeutic touch. It is an approach to patient care and patient care systems in which the individual is viewed as a unified whole, an open system, and not merely the sum of his parts. In this approach the health caregiver is concerned not only with attending to the physical needs of the patient but also to the other aspects of his being, including the emotional and spiritual aspects. Therapeutic touch involves the use of the hands in the giving of patient care, but in a way that differs from routine functions such as taking vital signs, turning patients, and so forth. It is the deliberate and the intuitive use of touch to decrease acute and chronic stress. It is used to comfort and soothe and to eliminate pain. Touch is used for communicating and to alter the effects of sensory deprivation and sensory overload. It may be used to foster positive feelings about self- and body image. Therapeutic relationships may be quickly established owing to touch. Touch is invaluable for assessment of physical and psychologic functions. It can be used to decrease fear at the time of death. It is used to support family members during periods of crisis. At times it may be used to initiate a spark in the patient, which is sometimes referred to as the will to live. Touch is a dynamic force within all interpersonal relationships.

Touch as communication

Touch is an important form of communication in the critically ill. To effectively communicate, it is important to know the different communication patterns. In order to communicate with someone who is visually oriented, you need to verbally construct a clear picture of what you want to communicate. For those who communicate on an auditory level, you have to use words in such a way that what is being heard verbatim is what you want to communicate. Those who have a kinesthetic orientation need to be touched in some way in order for them to understand what is being communicated. To understand the sensory bombardment in the critical care unit, it is sometimes important to use touch to reinforce what is being said. A hand on the shoulder or on the arm with a moderate amount of pressure, coupled with an attempt to maintain eye contact, is very efficient in communicating exactly what you need to relate to the patient. If eye contact is not possible, a touch on the shoulder, or at any other point, reinforces the fact that the verbalization is directed at the patient.

Touch is a nonverbal way of communicating when words are either inadequate or inappropriate. Language is very limited and linear. Touch is a way of communicating caring, love, and concern. Empathy is often best expressed without words. With words, it may be experienced as sympathy. It only requires a short time to stroke an arm and pat or squeeze a hand. This type of touch done in conjunction with other nursing care and procedures communicates that the nurse cares and wants to help. This can also reduce stress for the patient by making him feel that the environment is not entirely hostile.

Touch to decrease sensory deprivation

Touch can also be used to reduce sensory overload and sensory deprivation. Being in a horizontal position and experiencing the lack of meaningful sensory input can cause sensory deprivation.

The patients' sensory awareness states are al-

tered and they may experience a feeling that their body no longer has outlines. As one patient remarked, "I blend in with the sheets. I didn't know where I stopped and the sheets started." With the alteration in sensory awareness comes a loss of orientation and a loss of intellectual functioning.

One way to remedy this is with the use of a technique called a "brush down." Long, quick stroking movements can be made along the sides of the arms, legs, torso, and back. Starting at the top of the shoulder, a long sweeping motion is made with the hand over the entire length of the arm and over the hands and fingers to the fingertips. Both hands may be used on one arm, finishing off with one hand on top of the patient's hand, and the other hand under the patient's hand. It is important that the sweep be terminated at the end of the fingertips. It is also important to shake your own hands vigorously, as if throwing off water, at the end of each sweep. This can be completed three to four times per extremity, and three to four times over each surface of the torso and back. This technique is very efficient in redefining body limits and also has the effect of relaxing them. This technique could also be used to augment the effect of pain medication.

Critically ill patients receive an overwhelming amount of stimulus from their environment, including the large number of physicians, nurses, and ancillary personnel who come into contact with them daily. Many times this stimulus of contact with others is painful. Giving touch in a positive, soothing way, rather than a painful, uncomfortable one can be a way of reducing stress in the patient, thus allowing him to cope more effectively with his environment.

Touch used to relieve stress

The admission to a critical care unit is usually a period of acute stress for the patient. Vital signs taken during admission show an elevated pulse and respiratory rate and increased blood pressure as a result of adrenocortical stimulation, and the resulting effect on the body as the organism prepares to flee or fight. The patient may be hyperalert, exhibit diaphoresis, pallor, and nausea. Blood glucose levels drawn at this time are usually elevated because of the mobilization of glucose for energy and anti-inflammatory defenses.

Part of the admitting procedure should include some form of touch to interrupt the stress reaction and allow for adaptation and resolution. The type of touch used may be dictated by the individual and the situation. Sometimes talking in reassuring tones accompanied by light to moderate stroking of the arm, or a firmer touch applied to the shoulder, or even holding someone's hand may be enough to break the alarm cycle. With adaptation and resolution, a decrease in blood pressure to more normal limits and a decrease in pulse and respiratory rate may be seen.

The interventions for chronic stress are similar to those of acute stress. It needs to be emphasized that the choice of method depends entirely on the situation, the patient, and the health caregiver. After a while, you will be able to intuit what is needed in a given situation. For those in chronic stress, frequent interventions may be needed. Something particularly soothing, such as a back rub may be required to allow the patient to relax enough to sleep. With sleep the patient may be able to allow his body to return to his physiologic baseline and allow his coping mechanisms to function properly.

Touch to relieve pain

Touch is often used to comfort and soothe those who are in pain. In the Lamaze method for labor and delivery, the woman is instructed to do a circular massage on her abdomen. This touch interrupts the sensory message to the brain, and the pain message is altered. Stimulation of another part of the body, other than the part that is painful, is often very effective in relieving pain. A good soothing massage or back rub with cool, not cold, lotion may augment the use of pain medication and in many instances may decrease their usage. Using a light, moderate stroking action on the arm several times before doing venipuncture will decrease the patient's subjective discomfort during the procedure. For a vein in spasm during venipuncture, a light, upward stroking action of the vein above the venipuncture sites will often release the spasm, thus negating the need for an additional venipuncture.

Touch to enhance self-image

Because of his illness, the patient may experience changes in his body image and self-es-teem. He may have guilt feelings about the origins of his illnesses. By using touch, the nursing staff conveys to the patient their feelings of acceptance for who he is. For many, being touched in a warm, human way may increase feelings of self-worth and self-esteem and decrease some of the negative emotions he may be experiencing. A state of positive feelings and emotion promotes healing and decreases stress. This is the spiritual quality of touch. This sometimes awakens new life in a patient, sometimes called the will to live.

Hugging is another example of the spiritual quality of touch. It's like embracing another person's spirit and means "I'm accepting you, and you're accepting me." Not all patients and health caregivers are comfortable about this degree of human contact, but it has beneficial qualities for both the giver and the recipient. The Council of Nurse Healers has prescribed "four hugs a day" as the minimum daily requirement for optimal mental and physical health. A nursing prescription written on paper and given to patients may give patients permission they need to get their affection needs filled. A sample prescription may read, "Hugs qid and prn." This type of intervention is especially good during the recovery phase of an acute illness.

Touch in family intervention

Admission to a critical care unit is a period of stress and crisis both for the patient and the family. For some patients in the critical care unit, the primary threat may be imminent death. For the families waiting outside the doors, the uncertainty and acuteness of the situation generates a high degree of anxiety and fear. During this crisis period, it is very difficult for both patient and families to understand exactly what is happening. The ability to think and to problem solve is affected. All of their available resources are activated in order for them to cope with the immediate situation at hand.

Touch can be used to assist patients and family through the crisis period. Specific interventions for patients have been previously mentioned. When communicating with family members, a firm touch of the hand on the shoulder, while maintaining eye contact, will facilitate the communication of pertinent information. In acute situations people are much more open to being touched by a stranger. Holding their hand often encourages verbalization of feelings, which might have otherwise been kept inside. This is also very therapeutic since it quickly creates a therapeutic and empathetic bond between the caregiver and the family. For more reassurance, both of the nurse's hands can hold the hand of the family member. Stroking the arm with long strokes will also be effective in calming the person in crisis.

When the family member is escorted into the unit for the first time, the scene may be overwhelming and frightening. Touch can be used to support the family member at this time. A hand on or around the shoulders provides the support that is needed. A full hug, or embrace, is sometimes an appropriate intervention during a crisis period or following the death of the patient. The willingness to hug a patient or family member is dependent on how comfortable the caregiver feels with this intimate, personal interaction. The family member in a crisis situation is usually very accepting of this intervention.

The nurse can also use touch to foster interactions between patients and their families. Because of all the tubes and wires, family members are often very reluctant to touch the patient. Families can be encouraged to touch and can be utilized productively in this way. The family of a shock patient on an intra-aortic balloon pump were encouraged to use touch during their visits. The patient's stress was greatly relieved by the physical presence of his family. This decreased the need for tranquilizers, which would have further compromised his hypotensive state. His family were his natural tranquilizers. This intervention, that of encouraging the family to touch, was a significant element in keeping the integrity of the family together during this period of crisis.

Touch as comfort for the dying

Death is a frequent visitor in critical care units. Some of the more common fears of patients facing death are the fear of intractable pain, loss of control, and being abandoned. These fears are not readily verbalized, but all critical care nurses can identify terror in their patients' eyes. Policies in critical care units usually prohibit families from being present at the time of death. The resuscitation of patients precludes having the family present. While the procedures for resuscitation

methods are well defined and priorities established, it is important to realize that amid all the procedures lies a human being whose life is ebbing away. Conscious patients can benefit from touch at this time. Other dying patients readily accept touch for comfort and support. It imparts much stronger communication and feelings than does the spoken word.

Through the ages down to the present time, touch has been used to comfort the sick. It is, in fact, essential to life itself. The indications for the use of touch in a critical care unit are many. The stress that is relieved with therapeutic touch may enhance the chance of survival. Touch humanizes the critical care environment and makes it easier for natural coping mechanisms to come forth.

Touch builds a bond between the patient and the health caregiver to allow them to work as a team. It is through touch that the energy of caring is passed to the patient. Love is demonstrated in the solidarity of touch and may be a key factor in affecting the will to live.

BIBLIOGRAPHY

Blondis, M. N., and Jackson, B. E.: Nonverbal communication with patients, New York, 1977, Wiley Medical Publication.

Brown, B. B: New mind, new body, New York, 1975, Bantam Books.

Gordon, R.: Your healing hands, the polarity experience, Santa Cruz, 1978, Unity Press.

Krieger, D.: Therapeutic touch: the imprimatur of nursing, Am. J. Nurs. **75:**784, 1975.

Krieger, D.: The relationship of touch with intent to help or heal, to subjects in-vivo hemoglobin values: a study in personalized interaction. Paper presented at Ninth American Nursing Associations Research Conference, San Antonio, Texas, March, 1973.

Loomis, E. G.: Healing for everyone, New York, 1975, Hawthorn Books, Inc.

Mayeroff, M.: On caring, New York, 1971, Perennial Library.

Moos, R. H.: Coping with physical illness, New York, 1977, Plenum Publishing Corp.

Oyle, I.: The healing mind, Millbrae, Calif., 1975, Celestial Arts.

Randolph, G.: Therapeutic touch and the regulation of alarm reactions. Paper submitted in partial fulfillment of requirements for matriculation as a candidate for the degree of Doctor of Philosophy, 1976.

Roberts, S.: Behavioral concepts and the critically ill patient, Englewood Cliffs, N.J., 1976, Prentice-Hall, Inc.

Pelletier, K. R.: Mind as healer, mind as slayer, San Francisco, 1977, Delta.

Selye, H.: The stress of life, New York, 1956, McGraw-Hill Book Co.

CHAPTER 6

Pharmacology and fluids and electrolytes in children and adults

Dennis L. Ming and Karin Zenk

This chapter is designed to provide information on some of the more common problems encountered in critical care and will deal with certain key areas wherein the care of the critically ill patient poses certain pharmacologic questions. It is hoped that the reader will be encouraged to seek further knowledge through the use of the bibliography provided and any number of other excellent publications available.

CARDIOVASCULAR DRUGS

■ **Are there any precautions that should be taken when using metaraminol in patients who have been treated with reserpine?**

If an indirect-acting sympathomimetic agent such as metaraminol (Aramine) is given to counteract hypotension in a patient taking reserpine, the pressor response is less than expected. If the patient has been taking large doses of reserpine for a long period of time, the vasopressor, that is, metaraminol, may be completely ineffective. This is caused by the amine-blocking and depleting effects of reserpine. The use of levarterenol (Levophed) would produce a better effect because of its direct stimulating properties.

■ **What are some of the drugs used for the treatment of hypertensive crisis?**

Drugs used in the treatment of hypertensive crisis are summarized in Table 6-1.

■ **Since diazoxide will cause retention of sodium and water, should a diuretic be administered concomitantly?**

Because the repeated administration of diazoxide may cause sodium and water retention, a diuretic should be administered to patients receiving multiple doses in order to achieve maximum hypotensive effects, avoid congestive heart failure, and prevent the development of apparent drug resistance. Although thiazide diuretics prevent sodium and water retention, these drugs may be ineffective or may aggravate the condition of the patient with renal impairment. More potent diuretics such as furosemide and ethacrynic acid are more useful because of the increased action on preventing sodium retention and because they do not lower the glomerular filtration rate. This is important when a hypertensive crisis is associated with acute pulmonary edema or renal failure.

■ **Are there any differences in the digoxin tablets made by various manufacturers that could affect the way patients respond to therapy?**

Digoxin is a drug with a very narrow therapeutic index, that is, a very small range between therapeutic and toxic doses; therefore altering the amount of digoxin that is absorbed can be dangerous. Physicians should be aware that either underdigitalization or toxicity may result from changes in the source or even the lot of the digoxin tablets from the manufacturer. If a particular patient is doing well on a particular brand of digoxin, it should be continued. However, if a change occurs in the patient's response to therapy, serum digoxin concentrations should be measured in blood taken 8 hours or more after the last oral maintenance dose. Doses of 0.25 to 0.5 mg daily of a preparation of good bioavailability usually create serum concentrations between 0.5 and 2.0 ng/ml. This is usually a good therapeutic range for most patients. Toxicity can occur at serum levels over 2.0 ng/ml.

■ What are the indications for intravenous nitroglycerin?

The use of nitroglycerin intravenously has been reported in the literature as a means of: (1) reducing left ventricular filling pressure, (2) improving perfusion to and/or decreasing oxygen demands in the borderline ischemic areas surrounding the central zone of infarction in patients with myocardial infarction, and (3) treating hypertension during or after open-heart surgery.

■ How is intravenous nitroglycerin prepared?

There is no commercial preparation of nitroglycerin available and all compounding of this new dosage form must be performed carefully and aseptically. The solution is prepared by dissolving nitroglycerin tablets in sterile water for injection and then filtering the dissolved solution through a 0.22 μ filter into sterile containers of either 0.9% sodium chloride or 5% dextrose in water. The concentration will depend on the orders from the cardiologist and may vary from 15 to 100 μg/ml. The final solution should be used within 48 hours after preparation. It should be noted that the use of intravenous nitroglycerin is investigational.

■ What is dobutamine (Dobutrex)?

Dobutamine hydrochloride is a new agent that has a direct-acting inotropic effect by stimulating β-receptors of the heart while producing comparatively mild chronotropic effects. It does not cause the release of norepinephrine as does dopamine. The onset of action is 1 to 2 minutes. It is contraindicated in patients with idiopathic hypertrophic subaortic stenosis. Adverse reactions include increases in heart rate, blood pressure, and ventricular ectopic activity; anginal pain; nausea; vomiting; and shortness of breath.

It is used for inotropic support in the short-term treatment of adults with cardiac decompensation caused by depressed contractility resulting from organic heart disease or from cardiac surgery.

Dobutamine should not be mixed with sodium bicarbonate because it is incompatible with alkaline solutions but may be diluted in 5% dextrose in water, saline, or lactated Ringer's solutions. The usual dosage range is 2.5 to 10 μg/kg of body weight/min. Doses above 20 μg/kg/min are more likely to cause tachycardia and arrhythmias.

Table 6-1. Drugs used for hypertensive crisis

Drug	Onset of action	Duration of action	Disadvantages
Diazoxide (Hyperstat), IV	Within 5 min	12-24 hr	Difficulty in control of blood pressure because of bolus injections
Trimethaphan camsylate (Arfonad)	Immediate	About 15 min	Necessary to frequently monitor blood pressure
Sodium nitroprusside (Nipride), IV	Immediate	About 15 min	Necessary to frequently monitor blood pressure and to protect solution from light
Pentolinium (Ansolysen), IM	10-30 min	4-8 hr	May cause severe hypotension, also has parasympatholytic effects
Hydralazine (Apresoline), IV, IM	About 15 min	2-6 hr	Produces cardiac-stimulating effects

■ **What is the difference in action between dobutamine and isoproterenol?**

In patients with depressed cardiac function, both dobutamine and isoproterenol increase the cardiac output to a similar degree. In the case of dobutamine, this increase is usually not accompanied by marked increases in heart rate (although tachycardia is occasionally observed), and the cardiac stroke volume is usually increased. In contrast, isoproterenol increases the cardiac index primarily by increasing the heart rate, while stroke volume changes little or declines.

■ **What are the indications for bretylium tosylate (Bretylol)?**

Bretylium is a new antiarrhythmic agent for the treatment of ventricular fibrillations and ventricular tachycardia that have failed to respond to adequate doses of lidocaine or procainamide. It can be administered intramuscularly or intravenously; however, faster onset of action is seen with the latter route of administration. Some of the adverse effects encountered with this drug include hypotension, bradycardia, increased frequency of premature ventricular contractions, and renal dysfunction. The clinical use of bretylium is for short-term use only, and patients should be observed for postural hypotension. For life-threatening ventricular fibrillation, a starting dose of 5 mg/kg body weight undiluted, IV push, is used. For other ventricular arrhythmias, bretylium should be diluted in at least 50 ml of 5% dextrose in water, or 0.9% sodium chloride, and infused over a minimum of 8 minutes. The dosage of bretylium should be reduced and discontinued in 3 to 5 days under electrocardiographic monitoring. If indicated, other antiarrhythmic drugs should then be employed.

■ **What are some of the drugs used in cardiopulmonary arrest?**
Sodium bicarbonate

Sodium bicarbonate is an alkalinizing agent that is used to combat acidosis in cardiopulmonary arrest. Acidosis occurs rapidly in arrest situations caused by lactic acid accumulation. Vasopressor drugs, if necessary, may be ineffective in acidosis.

Administration. One mEq/kg of body weight, IV push, may be repeated once. Then it is followed at one half of the initial dose, IV push, every 10 minutes while the patient is apneic. Arterial pH should be determined frequently to regulate repeat doses.

Caution. Sodium bicarbonate should not be mixed with epinephrine or calcium salts. Epinephrine will become rapidly deactivated and calcium carbonate will form if mixed with calcium salts. Excess amounts may cause alkalosis, tetany, or pulmonary edema.

Availability. Sodium bicarbonate may be obtained as 3.75 g (44.6 mEq)/50 ml in prefilled syringes.

Lidocaine

Lidocaine reduces irritability of the heart. It is used in recurrent cardiopulmonary arrest caused by ventricular fibrillation and when the heart resumes sinus or nodal beats with frequent ectopic ventricular beats.

Administration. Lidocaine is administered initially in doses of 1 to 2 mg/kg (usually 50 to 100 mg) by IV push. This is followed by starting an infusion of lidocaine containing 1 g in 250 ml of 5% dextrose in water (4 mg/ml). This is usually administered at the rate of 2 to 4 mg/min (30 to 60 microdrops/min). If an IV push is not given, it will take approximately 8 to 9 minutes to achieve a therapeutic blood level after an infusion of lidocaine is started.

Caution. Lidocaine should be withheld if the ventricular rate is less than 60 beats/min or if heart block is present. It will produce hypotension, atrioventricular (AV) block, and CNS stimulation with twitching, fasciculation, and convulsions. The dosage should be reduced in patients with liver and/or renal impairment or congestive heart failure.

Availability. Lidocaine is available as 100 mg/10 ml (1%) in prefilled syringes for IV push. As 1 g/25 ml (4%) in prefilled syringes, it must be diluted before use.

Epinephrine

Epinephrine is an adrenergic agent with alpha (vasoconstrictor) and beta (cardiac-stimulating peripheral-vasodilating, and smooth muscle–relaxing) effects. In cardiopulmonary arrest epinephrine stimulates an asystolic heart to contract and increases the amplitude of fibrillating ventricular waves. This latter effect may increase the success rate of defibrillation, but it may also increase the tendency toward ventricular fibrillation.

Administration. Epinephrine is administered in doses of 0.5 to 1.0 mg by IV push or intracardiac injection (5 to 10 ml of 1 : 10,000 solution).

Caution. Epinephrine must be used as a 1 : 10,000 dilution. It may cause tachycardia or ventricular arrhythmias, including fibrillation; it must not be mixed with or injected into the sodium bicarbonate IV line, since up to 60% of epinephrine's activity will be destroyed on contact with sodium bicarbonate.

Availability. Epinephrine may be obtained as 10 ml of 1 : 10,000 solution in prefilled syringes with a 1½-inch needle for IV push or 3½-inch needle for intracardiac injection.

Atropine

Atropine blocks vagus nerve activity (vagolytic and anticholinergic), thus increasing the sinoatrial (SA) and atrioventricular (AV) nodal activity. It is used in sinus arrest, bradycardia, and AV block.

Administration. Atropine may be given in doses of 0.5 to 1.0 mg by IV push. Frequent smaller doses are preferred if the drug is to be used repeatedly.

Caution. Atropine may cause tachycardia, arrhythmias, and occasionally ventricular fibrillation. Urinary obstruction and acute glaucoma may be initiated or worsened.

Availability. Atropine is available as 1 mg/10 ml in prefilled syringes.

Isoproterenol

Isoproterenol (Isuprel) is a β-adrenergic drug that will increase cardiac rate and contraction (at the expense of increased O_2 requirement) and cause peripheral vasodilation. It is used in complete heart block with slow ventricular rates and in certain forms of shock.

Administration. Isoproterenol is never given by IV push. A 4 μg/ml solution is prepared by adding 2 mg of isoproterenol to 500 ml of 5% dextrose in water. Using a microdrop administration set, the preparation is given by IV infusion at a rate of 1 to 4 μg/min (0.25 to 1 ml/min).

Caution. The blood pressure and ECG should be monitored during infusion. The drug should be stopped or the rate of infusion decreased if the blood pressure exceeds 120/60 or if premature ventricular contractions or ventricular tachycardia occurs.

Availability. Isoproterenol is available as 2 mg/10 ml in prefilled syringes and as 1 and 5 ml ampules of 1 : 5000 solution.

Calcium

Calcium ion is necessary for cardiac muscle contractility. It is sometimes administered in cardiopulmonary arrest to strengthen the contractions of the heart. It is a very short-acting drug, but ectopic calcific deposits may occur.

Administration. From 5 to 10 ml of calcium chloride (supplies 6.8 to 13.6 mEq of calcium ion) or 10 to 20 ml of calcium gluconate is administered by IV push (supplies 4.8 to 9.6 mEq of calcium ion). Note that the chloride salt provides almost one and one-half times the calcium ions that the gluconate salt provides.

Caution. Calcium chloride is very acid and should be avoided in acidosis; instead, calcium gluconate should be used. Calcium ion can also cause hypotension, and if used in excess, it may be cardiotonic. Intracardiac administration of calcium salts is usually not recommended. Calcium should not be used in digitalis toxicity. Calcium salts will precipitate when in contact with sodium bicarbonate; that is, calcium carbonate is formed and may obstruct the IV line.

Availability. Calcium chloride is available as 1 g/10 ml (10%) in prefilled syringes. Calcium gluconate may be obtained in 1 g/10 ml (10%) ampules.

■ **What are some of the ECG changes resulting from quinidine therapy?**

The ECG changes that result from the direct effects of quinidine include a decrease in rate, an increase in the QRS duration, and an increase in Q-T interval. The direct (depressant) effect of the drug on AV conduction is to increase the P-R interval, whereas the antivagal effect, when present, is manifested by a decreased P-R interval.

■ What special caution should be observed when administering digoxin to preterm infants?

The doses of digoxin recommended for loading and maintenance therapy in preterm infants are lower than those used in term infants. In spite of this, high serum levels of digoxin have been noted in some preterm infants. Age-related variations in drug clearance and volume of distribution have been suggested as possible explanations for these high levels; however, the inability to administer accurately such small doses of digoxin to these patients may be a source of considerable error and may contribute to the high serum levels achieved.

The most dilute solution of digoxin commercially available for parenteral administration contains 0.1 mg of digoxin/ml. Therefore a 1 kg neonate receiving 0.01 mg/kg/24 hr of digoxin would receive 0.05 ml every 12 hours. These small volumes of medication are dispensed commonly with a tuberculin syringe. If the syringe is "flushed" with the parenteral fluid solution after its contents are expelled into an indwelling vascular catheter, the infant receives an inappropriately large dose of medication. There is a large size of dead space relative to the size of the calibrated syringe volume. Their study showed that flushing the syringe results in more than twice the calculated amount of medication being delivered to the patient when the syringe is filled to the 0.05 ml mark.

Their report recommends that a special dilution of digoxin be prepared by the pharmacy for these small preterm infants so that larger volumes may be administered. They also recommend that the syringe never be "flushed" after administration of the dose. Preparation of a more dilute digoxin would also minimize the additional amount of digoxin administered if the syringe were inadvertently flushed.

■ What are some of the pharmacokinetic and toxic properties of procainamide?

Similar to quinidine, procainamide (Pronestyl) is well absorbed after oral administration and ex-

creted primarily by the kidneys. About 50% is excreted unchanged. It can be given by IV administration, but it is considerably more depressant than lidocaine when given by this route. The most common side-effects of procainamide when used orally are gastrointestinal disturbances such as nausea and vomiting. Flushing, hypotension, and dizziness may occur. Direct cardiac toxicity may occur as with quinidine; this takes the form of decreased contractility, sinus arrest, and conduction impairment. Severe overdosage may cause cardiac arrest or ventricular fibrillation. These properties have relegated procainamide to the role of quinidine substitute when the latter drug is not well tolerated.

■ When should digitalis treatment precede quinidine therapy?

Quinidine, when used in the treatment of atrial arrhythmias, may occasionally produce an increased ventricular rate caused by a vagolytic effect. Quinidine therapy should then be preceded by digitalization in the treatment of atrial arrhythmias; digitalization may reduce but does not abolish the possibility of increased ventricular rate.

■ What is the role of magnesium in the treatment of cardiac arrhythmias?

In hypomagnesemia both ventricular and supraventricular arrhythmias have been reported. The exact mechanism for the arrhythmias remains speculative but lack of adenosine triphosphate activity as a result of magnesium depletion appears to cause a diastolic leak of potassium from myocardial cells, producing an unstable milieu. A number of studies have shown that magnesium depletion potentiates and promotes digitoxic arrhythmias. Clinical studies have also revealed a higher incidence of hypomagnesemia in patients with digitoxic arrhythmias.

Magnesium was used for digitoxic arrhythmias as early as 1935. Studies, however, have shown that magnesium in doses of 10 ml of 20% $MgSO_4$ is inconsistent and transient in its therapeutic effect, whereas a dosage of 15 to 20 ml of 20% $MgSO_4$ is more consistent in normalizing the rhythm. Arrhythmias not caused by digitalis have also been treated. The results with 10 ml of

20% MgSO₄ solutions were also inconsistent, although 20 ml of the 20% solution is more effective.

A safe and effective dose would be 10 ml of 20% MgSO₄ given IV over a 60-second period followed by 500 ml of 2% solution given over 6 hours. If magnesium deficiency can be established, a second bottle of 500 ml of 2% MgSO₄ can be given during the remainder of the 24-hour period. As much as 70% of the infused magnesium will be excreted if urine production continues, even though the patient is depleted of magnesium.

Toxic effects of magnesium are probably related to serum magnesium levels. Transient symptoms of flushing and increased sensation of heat may occur with the initial IV injection. Prolonged levels above 5 mEq/L should be avoided, since hypotension, bradycardia, and AV blocks are observed in dogs having levels greater than this. Tendon reflexes probably are depressed or abolished when serum levels exceed 6 mEq/L. Respiratory depression, respiratory arrest, and cardiac arrest occur when levels exceed 10 mEq/L.

■ What are the disadvantages of subcutaneous administration of heparin?

The subcutaneous administration of heparin is not recommended unless an IV dose cannot be administered and relatively rapid anticoagulation is desired. Local pain, ecchymosis, and hematoma occur on injection. Absorption may be unpredictable and uncontrollable, depending on the patient's condition. Large doses or frequent injections are required. Clotting times must be determined at certain times relative to when the last dose was given. Neutralization with protamine sulfate is difficult and unpredictable. Hemorrhagic complications include hemorrhage into the rectus abdominis muscle, femoral nerve paralysis secondary to a hematoma in or on the iliac muscle, and retroperitoneal hemorrhage.

■ If a patient receives an overdose of heparin or warfarin, what can be done to control the hemorrhaging?
Heparin

The antedote to heparin is protamine sulfate. It neutralizes heparin by forming a complex that is pharmacologically inert. Protamine is also an anticoagulant and care must be taken to avoid overdosage, since it may cause a continuation of the bleeding. Other side-effects of protamine sulfate include hypotension, bradycardia, dyspnea, nausea, vomiting, and lassitude, Protamine is administered by slow IV injection over a 1- to 3-minute period. Generally 1 mg of protamine sulfate will neutralize 100 to 120 units (USP) of heparin. Since heparin blood levels decrease rapidly after IV administration, the dose of protamine sulfate required also rapidly decreases as time elapses following IV administration of heparin. Not more than 50 mg should be given in any 10-minute period.

Warfarin

Vitamin K₁, also known as phytonadione (Aquamephyton), is the drug of choice for warfarin (Coumadin) overdose. Because of its more rapid, more potent, and more prolonged action, IV administration of phytonadione is preferred to other vitamin K analogues such as menadione in the presence of impending or actual hemorrhage. Following IV administration, the effects of the drug appear within 15 minutes, bleeding is usually controlled within 6 hours, and a normal prothrombin level may be obtained in 12 to 14 hours. Oral administration of the drug generally produces beneficial effects in 6 to 10 hours. It is not effective in reversing the action of heparin. When bleeding is not present or immediately threatening, 2.5 to 10 mg of phytonadione may be administered orally or by IM injection. This dose can be repeated in 12 to 48 hours. When bleeding is present or immediately threatened, 5 to 25 mg of phytonadione may be given by IV injection.

■ What are some precautions to take when administering digoxin to infants or children?

The recommended precautions in using digoxin are as follows:

1. Check the dose given. The average total digitalizing dose for infants or children is 0.03 to 0.05 mg/kg body weight. One half of the total digitalizing dose is given (usually by IM administration) to start. If this is enough, the digitalization may be stopped. If further digitalization is

needed, one fourth of the digitalizing dose is given in 6 to 8 hours. If necessary, in another 6 to 8 hours, the last one fourth of the digitalizing dose is given. The maintenance dose is calculated as one eighth of the effective amount of digoxin used for digitalization and is given orally every 12 hours. The maintenance dose is started 12 hours after administration of the last digitalizing dose. If the patient has renal or liver disease, a smaller maintenance dose of digoxin or a greater interval between doses will be required.

2. Another person who is knowledgeable in this area should calculate the volume of digoxin to be administered before the drug is given to the patient.

3. During digitalization and changes in digoxin dosage, a lead II rhythm strip is run on the ECG machine. This is most useful at the time of maximum effect of the drug, that is, 1½ to 5 hours after administration.

4. Hypokalemia, hypercalcemia, hypermagnesemia, or hypoxia may predispose the patient to cardiac arrhythmias.

5. Digoxin and diuretic should be discontinued at the first suspicion of toxicity and a physician notified.

6. Cardiac toxicity is usually treated by administration of potassium by IV infusion, and the ECG should be monitored frequently. If cessation of digoxin and diuretic and administration of potassium does not control arrhythmia, an antiarrhythmic agent such as phenytoin may be used.

■ What side-effects are seen with furosemide therapy?

Furosemide (Lasix) is a rapid-acting diuretic more potent than the thiazide diuretics and therefore more apt to cause severe adverse effects. As with other diuretics, excessive diuresis may cause water and electrolyte depletion that may result in circulatory collapse or vascular thrombosis and embolism, particularly in older patients. Reversible deafness has been seen in patients who have been given high IV doses (over 1 g), especially in the presence of diminished renal function. Therapy with furosemide can lead to hyponatremia and convulsions. An increase in the excretion of potassium, calcium, and magnesium occurs consistently, and the ensuing fall

in blood level of these electrolytes can cause cardiac and neuromuscular abnormalities. Also, it has in rare instances precipitated attacks of gout, it interferes with carbohydrate metabolism, and it may produce hyperglycemia and glycosuria.

■ How does dopamine exert its action in patients with cardiogenic shock?

Dopamine possesses a variety of useful pharmacologic properties. It functions as an α-adrenergic agonist, causing vasoconstriction of peripheral capacitance and resistant vessels; it also is a β-adrenergic agonist, producing an increase in cardiac rate and an augmentation of myocardial contractility. It also dilates renal and mesenteric vascular beds directly. Recent evidence indicates that dopamine inhibits the renal tubular reabsorption of sodium. Thus dopamine can be used to increase systemic arterial pressure by stimulating the myocardium without compromising renal blood flow and urine output. Dopamine may be the sole drug utilized after volume expansion and therapy with other catecholamines have proved ineffective. In other instances another catecholamine in combination with dopamine may prove efficacious.

Dopamine hydrochloride should be diluted in 5% dextrose and water to a concentration of 800 μg/ml for IV administration. Infusion is usually begun at a rate of 1 to 2 μg/kg body weight/min. This dose is increased by 1 to 4 μg/kg/min every 15 to 30 minutes until an optimal effect is obtained as judged by urine output and systemic arterial pressure. Maintenance doses in surviving patients average approximately 9 μg/kg/min.

■ What are some of the uses for glucagon?

Glucagon has been used in the treatment of insulin-induced hypoglycemia. It may be given by the IV, IM, or subcutaneous route in a dose of 1.0 mg. When it is given subcutaneously for hypoglycemic coma, a return to consciousness should be observed within 20 min; otherwise IV glucose must be administered as soon as possible.

Investigators have shown that small amounts of glucagon released by the pancreas stimulate hepatic glycogenolysis and gluconeogenesis. Large amounts increase adipose tissue lipolysis, stimulate adrenal medulla to release catecholamines, exert inotropic and chronotropic effects on myocardium, and stimulate insulin secretion.

Clinical investigations are being conducted to explore the use of glucagon in cardiac disorders as an inotropic and chronotropic agent that may be less productive of cardiac arrhythmias than are β-adrenergic catecholamines.

■ In what conditions would phentolamine be indicated?

Phentolamine (Regitine) is an α-adrenergic blocking agent used frequently in the diagnosis of pheochromocytoma. In patients with sustained hypertension the ability of the α-adrenergic blocking agents to block circulating catecholamines in smaller doses than are required to block neurally liberated norepinephrine can be utilized.

Phentolamine is also used to prevent the local necrosis that may follow the accidental paravenous injection of norepinephrine during the treatment of shock. The drug is infiltrated locally.

■ How does morphine work in patients with acute pulmonary edema?

Morphine is the drug of choice in the treatment of acute pulmonary edema, and its effectiveness is such that it is often described as a specific treatment. The mechanism by which morphine brings about relief is not clear. Its effectiveness is one of several pieces of data suggesting that acute pulmonary edema, which occurs in association with other than cardiac disease, should not be thought of as a consequence of acute left ventricular failure but as a reflexly generated state that can be interrupted by this central depressant. It does help to allay the anxiety that patients with acute pulmonary edema experience. The drug is usually administered by IV push as a dilution of 1 ml of morphine mixed with 9 ml of normal saline solution to give a dilution of 1 mg/ml. This dilution is pushed slowly to avoid acute depression of respiration.

ANALGESIC AGENTS

■ In what instances would acetaminophen have advantages over aspirin?

Acetaminophen (Tylenol) has some of the pharmacologic properties of aspirin, that is, as an analgesic and antipyretic agent. However, it lacks the anti-inflammatory action for which aspirin finds usefulness in the treatment of arthritis. The side-effects are also different. Acetaminophen is less likely than aspirin to cause gastrointestinal bleeding and irritation, asthmatic attacks in susceptible patients, drug interactions with oral anticoagulants, adverse effects on platelet function, and, in patients with gout, interference with tubular excretion of uric acid.

■ How effective is naloxone in comparison with other narcotic antagonists?

Naloxone (Narcan) is a relatively new addition to the small group of narcotic antagonists. It is available in 0.4 mg/ml and 0.02 mg/ml solutions for IV, IM, and subcutaneous injection. Similar to the other narcotic antagonists nalorphine (Nalline) and levallorphan (Lorfan), naloxone will also antagonize the respiratory, analgesic, miotic, and most other pharmacologic effects of narcotics such as morphine, meperidine, methadone, and heroin. The important contrast between naloxone and the other antagonists is that naloxone, when not preceded by the administration of a narcotic, will not produce respiratory depression, sedation, analgesia, or miosis, which do occur when nalorphine and levallorphan are administered. It is almost completely free of such effects. Unlike the two other drugs, it can counteract the narcotic-like effects of pentazocine (Talwin). It will not, however, counteract the respiratory depression caused by barbiturates, cocaine, and cannabis. Because of its lack of respiratory depressive effects, it is the drug of choice if the diagnosis of narcotic poisoning is in error, as in barbiturate overdose, If large amounts of narcotics have been taken, naloxone can be given by IV administration as 0.01 mg/kg repeated every 5 minutes if required. Its maximum effect occurs 2 to 3 minutes after IV administration; after IM or subcutaneous administration it occurs after 15 minutes.

■ Why are medications, specifically analgesics, given to patients preoperatively?

In order to reduce the patient's anxiety so that the induction and maintenance of anesthesia will be smooth, preanesthetic medications are administered. Some of the broad classifications of drugs used for this purpose are narcotics, anticholinergics, and sedatives.

Narcotics

Narcotic agents are useful for patients who may have pain preoperatively; however, they may cause respiratory depression, hypotension, nausea, vomiting, and constipation. The two most common agents are meperidine (Demerol) and morphine. There is available a fixed-ratio combination of fentanyl, a narcotic, and droperidol, a sedative. This combination, however, has sometimes produced apnea, anoxia, respiratory depression, and death. When pentazocine (Talwin) is used, care must be taken because pentazocine is a narcotic antagonist and may produce problems in unrecognized narcotic addicts, and when narcotics are used during or after surgery, its analgesic effects may be antagonized.

Anticholinergics

Anticholinergic agents are used to control excess respiratory secretions and prevent bradycardia. Examples are atropine and scopolamine.

Sedatives

Sedatives are used to potentiate the CNS-depressing effect of narcotics to achieve the overall desired effect of reducing anxiety for the purpose of easing the induction of anesthesia. Drugs such as barbiturates, diazepam (Valium), and antihistamines such as hydroxyzine (Atarax) and promethazine (Phenergan) have been used. The antihistamines are less likely to cause hypotension or respiratory depression.

■ **Why is morphine sometimes given by IV injection to children?**

The principal reasons for which morphine may be given by the IV route to children are as follows:
1. Morphine exerts an immediate effect on pain and anxiety.
2. It is possible to know promptly what effect has been achieved.
3. There will be no risk of delayed absorption such as could occur with poor peripheral circulation as in shock or with edema of tis-

sue. If circulation is restored, it will then pick up a great deal of drug left in tissue, resulting in an overdose.

In addition to relieving pain and anxiety, morphine may also be used for relief of pulmonary edema in the infant or child with congestive heart failure. When given by IV injection, morphine must be administered slowly over several minutes. The dose in children is 0.1 to 0.2 mg/kg/dose. Overdoses of morphine are treated with a narcotic antagonist such as naloxone, 0.01 mg/kg/dose administered by IM or IV injection.

■ **What are some of the drugs currently being used to treat neonatal withdrawal syndrome?**

Infants born to mothers who are addicted to drugs are often addicts themselves and have withdrawal symptoms shortly after birth. Paregoric, chlorpromazine, and phenobarbital are used to treat this neonatal withdrawal syndrome. The major advantages of paregoric are oral administration and lack of adverse effects (constipation may be seen with excessive doses). Withdrawal from paregoric can take a long time, since too rapid lowering of the dose may lead to recurrence of symptoms. Chlorpromazine (Thorazine) is also effective. If symptoms are controlled, the drug is continued for 5 to 10 days. Discontinuance with dosage tapering can often be accomplished in 2 to 3 weeks, but occasionally a 2-month treatment is necessary in severe cases. Phenobarbital may also control neonatal withdrawal symptoms, especially irritability and insomnia. The dose is maintained for 4 to 10 days and tapered off over 1 to 3 weeks. High phenobarbital doses may sedate the infant and prevent adequate fluid and caloric intake.

■ **What are some of the adverse effects of oxyphenbutazone and phenylbutazone?**

Phenylbutazone (Butazolidin) and oxyphenbutazone (Tondearil) are closely related and are used in the treatment of rheumatoid (ankylosing) spondylitis and acute gout after other first-line drugs have failed. Both drugs can produce such adverse effects as aplastic anemia and agranulocytosis. Other harmful effects include ulceration of the esophagus and stomach, hepatitis, nephritis, serum sickness, purpura, and sodium and water retention. Because the toxic effects of these drugs are believed to be more severe in older patients, these two agents should be used cautiously, and particular attention should be paid to salt and water retention leading to edema, congestive heart failure, and hypertension.

■ What is the treatment for Lomotil poisoning in children?

Lomotil is an antidiarrheal preparation containing diphenoxylate, a narcotic somewhat similar to meperidine, and atropine. The clinical features of toxicity from accidental ingestion include the anticholinergic syndrome caused by atropine with flushing, hallucinations, hyperpyrexia, lethargy, urinary retention, and tachycardia. At the same time or following the atropine effects, respiratory depression, miosis, lethargy, coma, and death have also occurred as a result of the narcotic effects of diphenoxylate. Treatment includes inducing emesis, unless contraindicated by convulsions, coma, or absence of a gag reflex. Naloxone (Narcan), a narcotic antagonist, in a dose of 0.01 mg/kg should be used. Admission for observation in an intensive care unit for 24 hours following ingestion, regardless of clinical status, should be undertaken, because gastric emptying may be significantly delayed by the drug and the onset of symptoms may be retarded. Magnesium sulfate, 250 mg/kg, may be given orally or by lavage with or following the administration of activated charcoal.

■ An asthmatic patient had been on chronic theophylline therapy. In the past week his physician had prescribed erythromycin for a skin infection. The patient now called the physician complaining of nausea, vomiting, and tachycardia. What could be the problem with this patient?

When erythromycin and theophylline are given together, the erythromycin tends to prolong the half-life of theophylline. Therefore, when this patient was given erythromycin, it tended to slow the metabolism of the theophylline, leading to toxic levels of theophylline. Vomiting, nausea,

and tachycardia are signs of theophylline toxicity. Erythromycin should be avoided in patients on theophylline therapy, or serum theophylline levels should be monitored closely if the two are concurrently prescribed and the theophylline dose adjusted accordingly.

■ Aminophylline (theophylline) is now being used in neonatal intensive care units to treat apnea/bradycardia of the newborn. What are the correct dosage and therapeutic serum levels?

Apnea associated with bradycardia (A-B spell) is a common problem in preterm infants in the neonatal intensive care unit. Apnea severe enough to produce cyanosis or bradycardia is a potentially serious threat to the nervous system of infants. The definition of A-B spells varies from institution to institution; apnea as defined by some is cessation of breathing for more than 30 seconds, or cessation of breathing for 20 to 30 seconds if accompanied by bradycardia or cyanosis. Theophylline (aminophylline), a drug commonly associated with its use in asthmatic patients, has been found to be effective in the treatment or prevention of apnea of prematurity. Theophylline may act to increase the sensitivity of the central nervous system to elevations of CO_2 levels and thereby decrease apneic spells. The only significant side-effect is a rise in heart rate. Therapeutic levels are 6 to 11 μg/ml. Theophylline may be administered to preterm infants either as the oral alcoholic elixir, as a nonalcoholic oral syrup, or intravenously as the ethylenediamine salt of theophylline, aminophylline.

Aranda and co-workers suggest a loading dose of 5.5 mg/kg followed by a maintenance dose rate of 1.1 mg/kg/8 hr, given as a constant intravenous infusion over 20 minutes. Parenteral administration of very small volumes of medications such as this at a constant infusion rate requires an infusion pump. Another dosage regimen is recommended by Giacoia and co-workers. They suggest that to achieve a therapeutic serum concentration of about 6 to 8 μg/ml rapidly on the first day, an initial loading dose of 6 mg/kg should be given. They recommend that following administration of the loading dose, the total daily maintenance dose of approximately 2 mg/kg/12 hr would result in a steady state serum concentration of about 8 μg/ml in most infants. These studies were done on small numbers of infants and any dosing regimen should be carefully followed with serum theophylline levels and monitoring of the heart rate. If the serum level exceeds the therapeutic range or if the heart rate exceeds 180 beats per minute, the dose should be reduced. If the heart rate is greater than 200, the drug should be discontinued.

■ **When should corticosteroids be used in the treatment of status asthmaticus?**

When an adequate trial or sympathomimetic drugs and aminophylline have failed and the patient received steroids in the preceding year, a dose of corticosteroids may be warranted. However, the most common errors committed in using corticosteroids are (1) using too small a dose during the acute episode and (2) anticipating a quick response when the usual response time is 4 to 6 hours. Tapering the dose is usually not necessary if the total daily steroid course was 5 days or less.

■ **In the treatment of asthma, are there any differences between isoproterenol and metaproterenol as bronchodilators?**

Isoproterenol (Isuprel) was the first of the synthesized β-receptor stimulants and rapidly became the most commonly used as well as the prototype for future bronchodilators. Most pharmacologists agree that, although isoproterenol is a very rapidly effective bronchodilator, its action is relatively brief and its side-effects many; specifically, tachycardia is a problem when another cardiotonic agent such as aminophylline is being administered concomitantly. For this reason the structural formula of isoproterenol was altered to form metaproterenol (Alupent, Metaprel). The resulting agent has greater selectivity for bronchial activity rather than general action on both cardiac and bronchial muscle. Other advantages of metaproterenol are longer duration of action, minimum side-effects, no tachyphylaxis, and no paradoxical reactions.

■ **What precautions should be taken when aminophylline is being administered by the IV route?**

The principal cautions to be observed are as follows:

1. Aminophylline should be administered slowly to avoid headaches, fall in blood pressure, and subjective awareness of a forceful heartbeat.

2. When used as a rapid infusion, it should be infused over 20 to 30 minutes to minimize the side-effects just mentioned.

3. Adding other drugs to the solution containing aminophylline should be avoided because of the problem of precipitating theophylline crystals.

4. The concomitant administration of cardiotonic agents such as isoproterenol should be avoided. The doses can be staggered in terms of the times of each administration to avoid any cardiac side-effects such as tachycardia.

5. The practitioner should be aware of recent aminophylline treatment to avoid toxicity; for example, the patient may have been given an aminophylline suppository just prior to hospitalization, during which aminophylline is to be administered by the IV route.

■ **Are there any incompatibilities with aminophylline in solution?**

The optimum pH range for stability is above pH 8.0. Crystals of theophylline will deposit below pH 8.0, but probably not unless the concentration is over 40 mg/ml. Therfore this incompatibility is more apt to occur if certain admixtures are made in syringes or small volumes of fluids than if components are added separately to large-volume IV fluids.

■ **What are some of the drugs that should be avoided in the treatment of asthma?**

All respiratory depressants such as narcotics, barbiturates, propoxyphene (Darvon), and tranquilizers should be avoided in the treatment of asthma.

■ **Are there any patients who should not use acetylcysteine?**

N-Acetyl-l-cysteine (Mucomyst) is effective in thinning extremely viscid tracheobronchial secretions. Its clinical usefulness has been limited because it is difficult to administer and will react with most metals, rubber, and to some extent oxygen. It decreases the viscosity of sputum to a much greater extent than does a saline control solution. However, the drug may increase bronchial secretions independent of its effect on sputum, particularly in patients with bronchial asthma. This effect may lead to serious bronchial obstruction; therefore this agent should not be used in asthmatic patients without concomitant bronchodilator treatment. The drug may also produce stomatitis, rhinorrhea, and hemoptysis.

■ **If an asthmatic child cannot take aminophylline orally, could rectal suppositories be used?**

The absorption of aminophylline from rectal suppositories in children is unpredictable. Serious overdosages have occurred when the drug was administered by this route. If a child cannot take medications orally, the IV route should be used.

■ **What physical measurements should be monitored in treating asthmatic patients with bronchodilators?**

Changes in blood pressure, heart rate, and cardiac rhythm must be carefully and frequently observed to establish the maximum acceptable dose of bronchodilator. Measurements of pulmonary function and pulse rate before and 10 minutes after the initial dose of aerosol are important in assessing the maintenance of a therapeutic effect.

■ **What are the differences between epinephrine hydrochloride suspensions and epinephrine solution?**

Acute asthmatic attacks are usually relieved within 3 to 5 minutes after subcutaneous injection of 0.2 to 0.5 mg or epinephrine. Repeated doses can be administered every 15 to 20 minutes. If symptoms occur, massage of the site of injection may produce relief by enhancing absorption of the drug.

For prolonged relief from bronchospasm, usually in chronic asthma, epinephrine in suspen-

sion (Sus-phrine) is sometimes used, and a dose of this may produce relief. Epinephrine in suspension provides both rapid and sustained epinephrine activity. The rapid action results from the epinephrine in solution, whereas the sustained activity is caused by the crystalline epinephrine free base in suspension. Prolonged activity has been found to last for as long as 8 to 10 hours, avoiding the need for constant and repeated injection of aqueous epinephrine (1 : 1000 solution). Caution should be taken to avoid giving epinephrine aqueous solution in addition to the epinephrine in suspension. Additional doses of epinephrine should not be administered within 4 hours of the previous dose.

Whatever drug is chosen, the smallest dose affording relief should be used.

■ **What are some of the drugs used to control respiration?**

The most frequently used drugs are succinylcholine and pancuronium bromide. Neither of these drugs should be mixed with any barbiturate drugs or with diazepam (Valium) in the same syringe or needle because of the possibility of precipitation of either of the latter two drugs.

Succinylcholine

Succinylcholine (Anectine) is an ultra-short-acting depolarizing-type muscle relaxant. When a single effective IV dose of the drug is given, muscular relaxation occurs within 1 minute, persists for about 2 minutes, and returns to normal within 8 to 10 minutes. If a paralyzing IM dose is given, the onset of action may be delayed for 2 to 3 minutes. When given by IV drip, a predetermined degree of muscular relaxation can be closely approximated by adjusting the rate of flow of the infusion. The paralysis following the administration of succinylcholine is generally initially selective and usually appears in the following muscles consecutively; levator muscles of the eyelids, muscles of mastication, limb muscles, abdominal muscles, muscles of the glottis, and finally intercostal muscles and the diaphragm.

The IV drip solution containing 1 mg/ml may be administered at a rate of 0.5 to 10 mg/min to obtain the desired amount of relaxation. The amount required will depend on the individual response as well as the degree of relaxation required. The IV dose for infants and children is 1.0 to 2.0 mg/kg body weight.

Pancuronium bromide

Pancuronium bromide (Pavulon) is a nondepolarizing neuromuscular blocking agent possessing all of the characteristic phramacologic actions of the curariform class of drugs on the myoneural junction and is approximately five times as potent as d-tubocurarine. The onset and duration of action of pancuronium are dose dependent. With the administration of 0.04 mg/kg the onset of action is usually within 45 seconds, and its peak effect is usually within 4.5 minutes; 90% recovery usually takes place in less than 1 hour. Larger doses, more suitable for endotracheal intubation, such as 0.08 mg/kg have a time of onset of about 30 seconds, and a peak effect within 3 minutes. Pancuronium has little effect on the circulatory system. The most frequently reported observation is a slight rise in pulse rate. It also has no known effect on consciousness, the pain threshold, or cerebration. It is therefore useful as an adjunct to anesthesia to induce skeletal muscle relaxation or to facilitate the management of patients undergoing mechanical ventilation.

In adults the initial IV dosage range is 0.04 to 0.1 mg/kg. Later incremental doses starting at 0.1 mg/kg may be used; however, the higher increments will increase the magnitude and duration of the blockage. Experience in children is insufficient at this time to provide a dosage range.

d-Tubocurarine

d-Tubocurarine (curare) is used primarily to produce skeletal muscle relaxation during surgery after general anesthesia has been induced. It may be used to increase pulmonary compliance during assisted or controlled respiration and for facilitating endotracheal intubation.

Following the usual single IV dose of d-tubocurarine, muscle relaxation occurs rapidly and reaches a maximum within 5 minutes. The duration of paralysis is related to the total dosage and the number of doses administered, subsiding in 20 to 30 minutes.

The initial dose of d-tubocurarine as an aid in controlled respiration is 16.5 μg/kg body weight (average 1 mg); subsequent doses should be determined by the requirements and response of the patient.

ANTISEIZURE MEDICATIONS
■ Are there any special precautions to follow when diluting phenytoin for IM or IV use?

The special diluent for sodium phenytoin (Dilantin) injection contains propylene glycol, benzyl alcohol, and water and is buffered to pH 10.0 to 12.3 with sodium hydroxide. Reconstituted, clear solution of sodium phenytoin may be stored at room temperature and should be discarded if haziness or precipitation develops or if the solution is not used within 4 to 6 hours of preparation. Solutions of sodium phenytoin are not compatible with acid solutions; a precipitate may form if the drug is diluted with dextrose or other acidic solutions.

■ Are there any problems associated with the IV administration of phenytoin?

Following IV administration, shock, hypotension, cardiovascular collapse, respiratory depression, bradycardia, partial or complete heart block, and ventricular fibrillation with resultant precipitation or potentiation of heart failure may occur. Therapy should be discontinued if any of these reactions occur. These effects may be minimized by administering the drug at a rate not to exceed 50 mg/min. Repeated IV use may produce a cumulative effect in decreasing the force of myocardial contractions.

■ What drug is considered by many as the drug of choice for most cases of status epilepticus in adults and children?

Diazepam (Valium) given by the IV route is now considered by many as the drug of choice in most cases of status epilepticus. Distinct advantages are its swift effectiveness, sometimes within seconds, and its margin of safety if administered properly as the initial drug. If the patient has already received parenteral barbiturates or other hypnotic agents, blood pressure and respiration should be monitored carefully.

■ **How is diazepam administered safely for status epilepticus in children?**

Diazepam must be administered slowly at a rate of 1 mg every 1 to 5 minutes up to a total, if necessary, of 5 to 10 mg each session in a child 5 years or older. In infants the dose is 0.2 to 0.5 mg up to a total of 5 mg each session. Because of its relative water insolubility, diazepam may also precipitate when administered by the IV route and may occasionally cause thrombophlebitis. Therefore it is important to ensure that the needle does not inadvertently penetrate an artery and that each dose is followed by a thorough flushing of the vein with saline solution.

■ **What is the main disadvantage of diazepam administered by the IV route?**

The swift control of status epilepticus by diazepam can be short lived. It is not unusual that seconds after injection the patient ceases convulsing, only to begin convulsing again. However, a second or third injection may bring lasting relief.

■ **Can paraldehyde be used for status epilepticus in children?**

Some authorities advocate the use of paraldehyde alone or as an adjunct for the treatment of status epilepticus, especially in children. Its volatile mode of excretion and wide margin of safety are indeed points in its favor for use in emergency situations. It can be administered rectally at a dose of 1 ml for each year of age, not to exceed a total of 5 ml regardless of age; this dose may be repeated 1 hour later. Because of its irritative action on the rectal mucosa, a gastric tube should be used if repeated administration is anticipated. Gavage of 2 to 5 ml can be performed at 2- to 4-hour intervals.

■ **What startling reaction can occur when children are given phenothiazines, particularly prochlorperazine?**

The phenothiazines, most commonly prochlorperazine (Compazine), may produce undesirable side-effects, not necessarily related to dosage, characterized by the acute onset of contractions of various voluntary muscle groups with torticollis, trismus, opisthotonus, drooling, and swallowing difficulty. These episodes are sometimes called "pseudotetanus" or "extrapyramidal crisis." They may be mistaken for psychotic episodes, postinfectious encephalomyelitis, or tetanus.

■ **What is the antidote for pseudotetanus or extrapyramidal crisis caused by prochlorperazine?**

The extrapyramidal signs are dramatically alleviated within minutes by the slow IV administration of 1 to 5 mg of diphenhydramine (Benadryl)/kg. No other treatment is usually indicated.

■ **What are some of the drugs used to treat alcoholic delirium tremens, and are any more effective than others?**

It is generally considered that symptoms of the different stages or degrees of severity of the alcohol withdrawal syndrome are best treated by replacing alcohol with a drug pharmacologically equivalent to alcohol in its action on the CNS. Alcohol is unsatisfactory because of its short duration of action. There have been a few well-controlled studies using agents such as paraldehyde, chloral hydrate, the barbiturates, diazepam (Valium), and chlordiazepoxide (Librium). Phenothiazines have been used but have been shown to be less effective than the other drugs previously mentioned. Some consultants regard paraldehyde as more effective than chlordiazepoxide in the prevention and control of delirium tremens; however, the odor of paraldehyde may be intolerable to the patients and hospital personnel, and glass syringes are needed if injected, since paraldehyde will react with plastic syringes. It can also cause sterile abscesses at the site of IM injection. Diazepam may possibly be more effective than chlordiazepoxide and may prove to be as effective as paraldehyde in preventing and controlling delirium tremens by the IM or IV routes of administration. However, more well-controlled trials are needed before any conclusive statements can be made about the relative merits of these drugs.

ANTIBIOTICS

■ For which antibiotics should the doses and dosing intervals be modified in patients with renal impairment?

Since most antibiotics are eliminated by the renal route, severely impaired excretion may result in dangerously high concentrations in the blood and tissues unless the interval between doses is greatly increased or the individual doses are decreased in conjunction with careful, frequent monitoring of renal function and blood level. Modifications should be made in the administration of kanamycin, streptomycin, gentamicin, the polymixins, tetracycline, cephaloridine, and vancomycin. Methicillin in high doses has caused renal nephritis and should be used cautiously in patients with renal impairment. The recommendations of the manufacturers for modifying dosages should be followed.

■ How should gentamicin and kanamycin be administered to a patient with elevated serum creatinine levels?

Since both of these agents have the potential to cause renal toxicity and hearing loss, the doses should be reduced and the interval between doses increased. Many clinicians have developed nomograms to determine dosages for their patients; however, if the nomograms are unavailable, a simple method to calculate the dosage interval can be used. For example, in using gentamicin for a patient with a serum creatinine level of 3, this value is multiplied by 8 to give a rough estimate of the number of hours between each dose:

$$3 \times 8 = 24 \text{ hr}$$

Therefore the dose should be reduced to 1 to 2 mg/kg given every 24 hours.

For kanamycin, if the value of the serum creatinine level is multiplied by 9, this will give a rough estimate of the number of hours between each dose:

$$3 \times 9 = 27 \text{ hr}$$

Therefore the dose should be reduced to 7.5 mg/kg given every 27 hours.

These figures are, again, rough estimates, and efforts should be made to adjust the doses according to available nomograms for each drug. Of course the most ideal way would be to measure the serum concentrations periodically in order to arrive at the proper dose based on renal excretion and blood level data.

■ Why is probenecid occasionally administered with penicillin?

Probenecid is a uricosuric agent that decreases the tubular reabsorption of urates. When administered with penicillin or a cephalosporin, it increases the serum concentration of the antibiotic by inhibiting its tubular secretion; it has proved useful when high antibiotic concentrations are needed. The peak serum levels of either oral or parenteral penicillin are elevated 50% to 300%. The duration of activity in the blood is prolonged, and the cerebrospinal fluid level is raised. The disadvantages are that probenecid can cause nausea and vomiting, can be only administered orally, and can cause a rash, which would make it difficult to judge whether the probenecid or the antibiotic is responsible if an allergic reaction should occur. The dose is 0.5 g/6 hr during therapy.

■ What is the "gray baby syndrome" in relation to the use of chloramphenicol in neonates?

The gray baby syndrome is fatal chloramphenicol toxicity, which may develop in neonates, especially premature babies, when exposed to excessive doses of this drug. The illness usually begins 2 to 9 days (average 4 days) after treatment is started. Manifestations in the first 24 hours are vomiting, refusal to suck, irregular and rapid respiration, abdominal distention, periods of cyanosis, and passage of loose green stools. All infants are severely ill by the end of the first day and in the next 24 hours develop flaccidity, ashen gray color, and a decrease in temperature. Death occurs in about 40% of the patients, most frequently on the fifth day of life. This toxic effect is thought to be caused by failure of the drug to be detoxified by the liver and inadequate renal excretion of the drug. Children 1 month of age or younger should receive chloramphenicol in a daily dose no larger than 25 mg/kg body weight. After this age daily quantities of up to 50 mg/kg may be given without difficulty. The child should be observed very carefully during treatment and the drug discontinued at the first sign of toxicity.

■ **Are there any advantages to using clindamycin rather than lincomycin?**

Clindamycin is a semisynthetic derivative of lincomycin that is available for use in parenteral and oral form. It has a distinct advantage over lincomycin in its lesser incidence of side-effects. The spectrum of action is similar; clindamycin is effective against bacteroids.

■ **What serious systemic reactions could occur when a child is given a pertussis vaccine (alone or as diphtheria-pertussis-tetanus vaccine)?**

Convulsion, severe febrile reaction, or thrombocytopenia are the reactions of greatest consequence.

■ **What type of child is more susceptible to these reactions?**

Children with cerebral damage should not be innoculated with diphtheria-pertussis-tetanus vaccine. In such infants active immunization procedures should be delayed until active cerebral irritation has subsided or until the child has reached 1 year of age. Thereafter single antigens are recommended and pertussis should be administered last. An initial dose of 0.05 or 0.1 ml should be given to test tolerance before the remainder of each dose is administered.

■ **Why are sulfonamides such as sulfisoxazole usually not administered to preterm infants?**

Certain factors predispose an infant, especially a premature infant, to the development of kernicterus at lower serum levels of bilirubin. These factors (acidosis, low albumin levels, sulfonamide administration, elevated free fatty acid, and so forth) mainly result in decreased albumin-binding capacity for bilirubin. In addition, sulfonamides compete with the glucuronide transferase system, the system in the liver of the infant that changes bilirubin to a soluble form so it may be excreted. A marked increase in kernicterus and death has been reported in premature infants receiving sulfisoxazole (Gantrisin).

■ **Are there any advantages that cefazolin sodium has over the other injectable cephalosporins?**

Cefazolin is an antibiotic similar to cephalothin and cephaloridine. It is available for IM and IV administration. It does not produce the severe pain associated with IM doses of cephalothin and, unlike cephaloridine, it does not appear to damage the kidneys. The antibacterial spectrum of cefazolin is similar to that of the other cephalosporins, but it is more active against *E. coli* than cephalothin and somewhat more easily inactivated by penicillinase than other cephalosporins. Organisms resistant to cephalothin are generally resistant to cefazolin. For those infections caused by organisms susceptible to both penicillin and cefazolin, penicillin is still the drug of choice and much less costly to administer.

■ **Why is it unadvisable to change from ampicillin administered IV to using the IM or oral route after several days of treatment of *Haemophilus influenzae* meningitis in a child even though the child is afebrile and seems to be doing well clinically?**

Ampicillin achieves a cerebrospinal fluid (CSF) concentration that is 30% of the simultaneous blood concentration early in the course of the meningitis. Later, as the inflammatory responses subside, the concentration in the CSF may, somewhat surprisingly, fall to 5% of that in blood. Such a dramatic fall might easily reduce the CSF antibiotic concentration to less than that which is antibacterial, a phenomenon that may operate in cases reported as ampicillin failures. As the inflamed meninges heal, less antibiotic can cross into the CSF and thus the last few days of antibiotic treatment are the most critical. Adequate levels of antibiotic can best be assured by using IV therapy throughout the course of treatment.

■ **What are the criteria for discontinuing ampicillin therapy when treating a child who has *Haemophilus influenzae* meningitis?**

A recent review of the diagnosis and treatment of bacterial meningitis suggests the following criteria: (1) therapy should be continued until the patient is afebrile for 5 days and (2) if at that time the spinal fluid contains 50 or less leukocytes per milliliter and the protein concentration is less than 50 mg/100 ml, antibiotic therapy is discontinued. In most infants this means 10 to 14 days of antibiotic therapy.

■ **What are the most important drugs to administer immediately to a child who has just been diagnosed as having *Haemophilus influenzae* meningitis?**

A child who has just been diagnosed as having *Haemophilus influenzae* meningitis should have ampicillin and chloramphenicol administered by IV push. Usually the earlier a child is treated, the better the prognosis will be. Later, when antibiotic sensitivities are known, one antibiotic may be discontinued.

■ **What are the different types of penicillin allergy and what is the recommended treatment?**

Penicillin is the drug of choice for many infections. The drug has a low incidence of toxicity, estimated to be 1% to 5% of the courses of penicillin therapy. Allergic reactions are most common in patients with histories of asthma, hay fever, or atopic dermatitis.

The allergic reactions are divided into three categories based on the time of onset of the allergic reaction:

1. Immediate. These reactions generally occur within 20 minutes with symptoms such as urticaria, flushing, and diffuse pruritus. Less commonly the reactions are anaphylactic and are manifested by shock, cardiac arrhythmias, and laryngeal edema, sometimes with wheezing.
2. Accelerated. Accelerated reactions start between 1 and 72 hours after penicillin therapy and are usually urticarial, although other rashes occasionally appear.
3. Late. These reactions begin from days to weeks after the initiation of therapy, usually with urticaria or other rashes.

Ampicillin is more likely to cause rashes than other penicillins; some rashes are the result of true allergy, others are not.

Treatment of penicillin allergy would be to discontinue the medication and, in cases of anaphylaxis, treat the patient with epinephrine administered by the subcutaneous or IV route. The subcutaneous dose is 0.3 to 0.5 ml of a 1:1000 solution. The IV dose is 0.2 to 0.3 ml diluted in 10 ml of saline solution and injected slowly. IV fluids and plasma expanders should be available to raise the blood pressure.

Care must be taken to avoid the automatic and sometimes routine use of cephalosporins in patients with penicillin allergies, since this series of drugs has been shown to have cross-reactions; that is, certain patients allergic to penicillin have also been allergic to cephalosporins.

■ **What is the use of vidarabine (Vira-A)?**

Vidarabine is an antiviral agent recently released for intravenous administration in the treatment of herpes simplex encephalitis. Its mechanism of action is in inhibiting DNA synthesis. The recommended dosage of vidarabine is 15 mg/kg of body weight/day, given intravenously over 12 to 24 hours and continued for 10 days. It is recommended that 2.2 ml of IV fluid be used for every milligram of vidarabine to ensure solubility. Side-effects include nausea, vomiting, weakness, tremor, ataxia, dizziness, and confusion. This drug has been shown to be very effective if given early in the course of the disease.

■ **What are the current recommendations regarding the use of silver nitrate prophylaxis in newborn infants?**

The occurrence of gonococcal ophthalmia neonatorum in spite of the use of 1% silver nitrate may result from flushing the infant's eyes with water or saline after instillation. The National Society for the Prevention of Blindness, the American Academy of Pediatrics, and the package insert recommend that irrigation (usually done with water or saline) not be done. Many hospitals are irrigating infants eyes, apparently to minimize the chemical conjunctivitis caused by silver nitrate; however, conjunctivitis caused by silver nitrate is usually self-limiting (24 to 48 hours). Silver nitrate should be instilled into newborn infants' eyes and should not be followed by irrigation.

■ **What are the recent cautions with respect to pregnant personnel washing their hands with hexachlorophene-containing soaps?**

Recent data suggest that pregnant hospital personnel who wash their hands frequently (40 to 60 washings per day) with a hexachlorophene-containing soap (such as pHisoHex) may be injuring the fetus. Systemic absorption of hexachlorophene may occur and be distributed across the placenta to the fetus. Pregnant personnel are advised to use hand washing soaps that contain no hexachlorophene.

MISCELLANEOUS DRUGS

■ **What precautions should be taken in changing drug regimens prior to surgery to avoid interactions with anesthetics and/or the surgical procedure?**

Although there are no rigid criteria for the discontinuation of medications prior to surgery, the possible interactions should be considered.

Anticoagulants

Anticoagulants may cause bleeding with spinal, epidural, dental, or other types of regional blocks or with tracheal intubation or other instrumentation. They may also increase bleeding during and after surgery.

Antimicrobials

Tetracyclines predispose to renal insufficiency after methoxyflurane anesthesia. Kanamycin, streptomycin, gentamicin, and neomycin may cause neuromuscular block and apnea and therefore have an additive effect if *d*-tubocurarine or other nondepolarizing neuromuscular blocking agents are used.

Cardiovascular drugs

β-Adrenergic blockers such as propranolol may add to the myocardial depression of general anesthetics, induce bronchospasm, and prevent adequate circulatory response to blood loss. Despite these hazards, it may sometimes be preferable to continue the drug in certain patients. Digitalis and other cardiac glycosides should as a rule be continued, but the possibility of digitalis intoxication during general anesthesia should be kept in mind. Quinidine, procainamide, and lidocaine may aggravate myocardial depression, impair cardiac conduction, and cause peripheral vasodilation. They may also potentiate neuromuscular blocking agents. Diuretics, especially the thiazides, furosemide, and ethacrynic acid, can lead to hypovolemia, hypotension, alteration in sodium and potassium metabolism, and prolonged paralysis when used together with muscle relaxants. Antihypertensive agents may cause additive hypotensive effects.

Corticosteroids

Corticosteroid agents should not be discontinued; sudden withdrawal may cause adrenocortical insufficiency.

Drugs acting on the nervous system

Anticonvulsants should not be tapered off in too short a period before surgery because this may result in convulsions, and sudden cessation may lead to status epilepticus. Phenobarbital can add to respiratory depression. Phenothiazines may add to the hypotensive effects of sedatives, narcotics, and general anesthetics.

Insulin

Dosage should be reduced at the time of surgery. Some anesthesiologists have withheld insulin until the postoperative period.

■ **Are there any rules that should be followed when different insulins are to be mixed in the same syringe?**

Insulins are mixed primarily to modify their action in customizing the insulin requirements to individual needs. This usually results in an intermediate-acting mixture; however, with commercially available intermediate insulins this is less common. If a mixture is needed, the shorter acting insulin should always be drawn into the syringe first. For example, in mixing regular insulin with protamine zinc insulin, if the protamine zinc insulin is drawn first and then injected into the regular insulin vial, the amount of protamine zinc insulin will gradually change the activity of the regular insulin to that of a longer acting compound. Hence the activity curve for the regular insulin is altered and its actions become unpredictable.

Table 6-2. Forms and times of action of insulin

Insulin	On-set (hr)	Peak (hr)	Dura-tion (hr)
Fast-acting preparations			
Regular insulin (crys-talline zinc)	½-1	2-6	5-8
Semilente insulin	½-1	3-9	12-16
Intermediate-acting preparations			
Lente insulin	1-4	6-16	16-24
NPH insulin	1-4	7-12	24-30
Long-acting preparations			
Ultralente insulin	4-8	10-30	34-36
Protamine zinc insulin	1-8	12-24	30-36

■ **What are the different forms of insulin and their hours of activity?**

Data concerning insulin are summarized in Table 6-2.

■ **What are some of the drugs that are commonly abused, and how effective is either forced diuresis or hemodialysis in treating overdosage of these agents?**
Meprobamate

Hemodialysis is effective and appropriate in very severe cases. Good clinical results have also been noted with peritoneal dialysis. Since a small amount of this drug is excreted in the urine and is relatively insoluble in water, forced diuresis may be of little value. The drug is nonionized; therefore pH adjustment of the urine would probably have no effect on excretion.

Ethchlorvynol

Hemodialysis and forced diuresis have been successful in removing ethchlorvynol. Peritoneal dialysis is probably somewhat less effective than forced diuresis. Since the drug is not ionized, there appears to be no reason for alkalinizing the urine.

Methyprylon

This drug is reasonably soluble in water and its excretion should be increased by forced diuresis. Diuresis and peritoneal dialysis are not as effective as hemodialysis.

Benzodiazepines

The benzodiazepines (chlordiazepoxide, diazepam, oxazepam) are strongly bound to tissue protein so that blood levels are very low. Consequently, neither forced diuresis nor dialysis techniques are likely to be of much help in increasing the excretion of these drugs.

Phenothiazines

Chlorpromazine and related psychotropic phenothiazine derivatives are strongly bound to tissue proteins, and the chances of effectively accelerating the metabolism of the absorbed drug appear not to warrant the use of forced diuresis or dialysis techniques.

Dibenzazepines

In relation to the dibenzazepines (imipramine, amitriptyline), as with the phenothiazine derivatives, tissue binding appears to be of such a high degree that dialysis techniques offer little in the way of effective treatment.

Barbiturates

Forced diuresis increases excretion and decreases the duration of coma in patients with long-acting barbiturate intoxication. The removal rate of pentobarbital is increased 20% by osmotic diuresis; phenobarbital removal is doubled. Alkalinization of the urine does not increase the nonionic diffusion of short-acting barbiturates into the urine because the pH of these drugs is above that which can safely be achieved in the urine. Hemodialysis removes barbiturates 10 to 30 times faster than diuresis, depending on the specific drug ingested. The removal of short-acting barbiturates is slower with either method because of protein binding. Barbiturate clearance with diuresis varies from 5 ml/min with short-acting drugs to 17 ml/min with long-acting barbiturates. Hemodialysis is the procedure of choice when renal failure and barbiturate intoxication coexist.

■ **A patient who has been on chronic steroid therapy is scheduled for surgery. What should be done to prevent adrenal crisis?**

Patients who are receiving adrenal steroids currently or who have received adrenal steroids from 4 to 30 days in the past 6 months, or 1 to 3 months during the past year, or 3 months or more anytime in their lives have an unpredictable degree of functional adrenocortical suppression. These patients should be managed as if they have adrenocortical insufficiency. The recommended schedule involves the administration of cortisone acetate in doses of 100 mg IM 12 hours preoperatively, 100 mg in the morning prior to surgery, and 100 mg in the evening postoperatively. The total daily dose can be tapered over several days.

If hypotensive crisis occurs during or following surgery, the patient should be treated with hydrocortisone sodium succinate or phosphate in doses of 100 mg given by the IM or IV route immediately and 100 mg IV infusion every 8 hours for the first day. The same amount is given every 8 hours on the second day, and then the dosage is gradually reduced. The regimen of dose reduction should be judged by clinical status. When the patient can tolerate oral feedings, the drug can be given orally.

■ **What are the different types of oral hypoglycemic agents?**

There are two classes of oral hypoglycemic agents currently used in the treatment of diabetes: the sulfonylureas and the biguanides. The sulfonylureas act by stimulating the release of insulin from the beta cells of the islets of Langerhans.

In the absence of the pancreas or in cases of juvenile diabetes where the pancreas is grossly deficient in its ability to secrete insulin, the sulfonylureas are ineffective. These drugs are of greatest value in the treatment of mild maturity-onset diabetes wherein the pancreas continues to produce insulin.

Examples of these drugs are tolbutamide (Orinase), chlorpropamide (Diabinese), and tolazamide (Tolinase). These drugs differ primarily with respect to their duration of action.

The biguanides, for example, phenformin (DBI), do not activate the release of insulin from the pancreas, nor do they induce hypoglycemia in nondiabetic patients. It appears that phenformin may act by accelerating the intracellular oxidation of glucose, a process that is depressed in the absence of insulin. Phenformin is used alone for the treatment of maturity-onset diabetes and

in combination with insulin in juvenile diabetes. Some physicians can achieve better management of diabetes by concurrently using sulfonylureas and phenformin.

■ **What are some of the toxic effects of cocaine?**

Repeated snorting of cocaine can erode the nasal membranes causing ulcers and/or perforation. In large doses cocaine, like other local anesthetics, can cause convulsions. Deaths from hyperpyrexia or ventricular fibrillation have also been reported. Paranoid states and adverse psychotic reactions, similar to those that occur with amphetamines, have occurred with chronic use.

■ **What are some drugs that have been found to have poor absorption when administered by the intramuscular route?**

The intramuscular administration of a number of drugs results in relatively slow or incomplete absorption. These are phenobarbital, phenytoin (Dilantin), digoxin, chlordiazepoxide (Librium), and diazepam (Valium).

■ **What are the recommendations with respect to the use of vitamin E in preterm infants?**

Preterm infants are born with low serum levels of vitamin E. Feeding these infants diets rich in polyunsaturated acids, particularly when the diet is supplemented with iron, can produce a hemolytic anemia if the vitamin E deficiency is not corrected. Vitamin E is a potent antioxidant, and deficiency of vitamin E appears to enhance damage from oxygen to blood, eyes, and lungs, such as bronchopulmonary dysplasia and retrolental fibroplasia. The administration of parenteral vitamin E at a dose of 125 to 150 mg/kg *total* dose, administered intramuscularly in four divided doses over the first week of life (days 1 and 2 and days 7 and 8), maintained vitamin E sufficiency during the first 6 weeks of life. No serious toxicity has resulted from this dosage; mild erythema and induration have occurred at the injection site if larger amounts are given in a single injection (therefore the four divided doses). One milligram of vitamin E (*dl*-alpha tocopherol acetate) is equivalent to approximately 1 international unit (1 mg = 1 IU) of vitamin E.

■ **Several topical agents may prove hazardous to neonates. What are these agents and their toxic effects?**

Newborn infants, especially if preterm, have very permeable skin; topical agents safe in older children and adults may be harmful to these infants. If the skin is denuded, burned, or inflamed, topical absorption is enhanced even more. Some examples are as follows:

1. Merbromin (Mercurochrome). Neonatal mercury poisoning can occur by topical application of merbromin to an absorptive surface. Clinical signs of mercury poisoning have been reported in 13 neonates with large omphaloceles treated with 2% merbromin. Symptoms included pink urine, progressive oliguria, and central nervous system disturbances.

2. Topical iodine solutions such as povidone-iodine (Betadine). Systemic absorption by neonates of topical iodine solutions (povidone-iodine and others) was also recently reported.

3. Topical sulfa creams. The manufacturers' literature concerning silver sulfadizine cream (Silvadene) warns that, because sulfonamide therapy is known to increase the possibility of kernicterus, the cream should not be used at term pregnancy, on premature infants, or on newborn infants during the first month of life. The manufacturers have found that in the treatment of burn wounds involving extensive areas of the body, the serum sulfa concentration may approach adult therapeutic levels even though the application is topical.

4. Hexachlorophene. Although the efficacy of the use of soap containing hexachlorophene in controlling staphylococcal colonization and disease in newborn infants has been demonstrated, studies indicating neurotoxicity of hexachlorophene (HCP) have led to restriction of its use. Repeated whole-body bathing of premature infants in 3% hexachlorophene-bearing soap (undiluted pHisoHex) is associated with a vacuolar encephalopathy of the brain stem reticular formation. The prevalence of the vacuolar encephalopathy appeared to be related to the number of exposures to hexachlorophene, to the birth weight (gestational age), to the length of survival, and to thoroughness of rinsing. From these observations it is concluded that hexachlorophene should

not be used on neonates under 1400 g birth weight and should be used only sparingly in full-term neonates with thorough rinsing.

FLUID AND ELECTROLYTE SOLUTIONS

■ **In treating hypernatremic dehydration in children, what fluid and electrolyte solutions should be used and at what rate?**

If dehydration is severe, 20 ml/kg of normal saline solution or Ringer's lactate should be given and repeated once if necessary. To calculate liters of water necessary to restore present serum sodium concentration (C_p) to normal, the following formula may be used:

$$\frac{C_p - 140}{140} \times \text{kg body weight} \times 0.6$$

When shock has been corrected, water is given as 5% dextrose and 0.25% saline solution at a rate calculated not to lower serum sodium more than 15 mEq/L/day. The state of hydration and serum sodium concentration should be evaluated every 6 hours to determine the end point of IV therapy.

■ **What severe complication could occur if the sodium concentration dropped too rapidly in the treatment of hypernatremic dehydration?**

The rapid correction of hypernatremia and reexpansion of cells can result in convulsions.

■ **What is the program of management of acute dehydration in children in terms of fluids to be administered and rate of administration?**

Treatment is directed toward the restoration of extracellular fluid by infusion of isotonic solution in the following sequence:

1. Immediately give by IV route 20 ml/kg of 0.9% normal saline solution. This may be repeated once.
2. Replace fluids gradually to allow them to be absorbed and not overload the heart. One way in which this may be done is to give one half of the calculated deficit in the first 8 hours and the remainder in the following 16 hours.

3. Do not add potassium to the IV solution until urine flow is established.

■ Why is it a good idea to include 5% dextrose in all maintenance parenteral fluids?

All maintenance solutions should contain at least 5% dextrose to reduce the caloric deficit that usually occurs in patients who need parenteral fluid and electrolytes. The use of dextrose also minimizes ketosis and the buildup of "starvation solutes" (urea, phosphate, and other protein breakdown products) that increase the excretory load.

■ How can acidosis associated with impaired renal function, starvation, or diabetes be corrected?

Continuous rehydration, which enhances renal perfusion, and, in diabetics, insulin therapy usually suffice to correct acidosis. When the plasma pH is less than 7.2 or carbon dioxide content is less than 10 mEq/L, however, administration of bicarbonate or bicarbonate precursors may be required.

■ What are the maintenance water requirements intended to supply normal daily requirements to patients who are not taking water orally?

These requirements are summarized in Table 6-3.

Table 6-3. Maintenance water requirements based on surface area

Body weight		Surface area	Approximate maintenance water (ml/24 hr)
kg	lb		
3	6.6	0.21	300*
6	13.2	0.30	500
10	22.0	0.45	700
20	44.0	0.80	1300
30	66.0	1.05	1700
40	88.0	1.30	2100
50	110.0	1.50	2400
60	132.0	1.65	2600
70	154.0	1.75	2800
80	176.0	1.85	3000

*Less in the first 2 weeks of life.

■ What could be some manifestations of the accidental IV administration of a toxic dose of potassium and how could they be treated?

The manifestations of hyperkalemia are muscle weakness, tetany, or paresthesias with ascending paralysis. ECG shows elevated T waves, QRS lengthening, and ventricular fibrillation. To treat the patient, if cardiac arrhythmias are present or serum potassium levels are over 8.0 mEq/L, sodium bicarbonate and/or 10% calcium gluconate are given slowly by the IV route. For serum potassium levels over 6.0 mEq/L sodium polystyrene sulfonate (Kayexalate) enemas may be given as necessary. Dialysis is occasionally indicated.

■ When is replacement therapy needed in addition to maintenance therapy with IV fluids?

Replacement therapy is needed when there is a heavy loss of water and electrolytes, as in severe vomiting, diarrhea, nasogastric suction, or fistulous drainage.

■ What is the formula for calculating the amount of replacement IV fluid therapy a patient might need?

A *Medical Letter Review* on parenteral water and electrolyte solutions states that in many instances 70 ml of an electrolyte solution/kg/day in addition to the maintenance water requirements will replace about 70% of the deficit in a 10% dehydrated adult. Thus a 50 kg patient would require 3500 ml of electrolyte solution for replacement plus 2400 ml for maintenance. In order to avoid the consequences of fluid overload, especially in elderly patients and those with renal or cardiovascular disorders, monitoring of the central venous pressure is considered desirable.

■ A patient's urine output has suddenly dropped; however, measurement of the IV fluids indicates that they have maintained the same rate as when the kidneys were functioning well. Later the patient develops tachycardia, tachypnea, and edema. What is wrong and how could it be corrected?

The patient is probably fluid overloaded. The manifestations of this complication are the clinical signs of congestive heart failure (tachycardia, tachypnea, hepatomegaly, venous distention, edema, increased weight, weakness, and cardiac gallop). The patient would be treated as for congestive heart failure through the use of oxygen, sedation, diuretics (furosemide), and rarely, digitalis.

■ **For patients in shock or in the absence of clinical improvement after 2 hours of rapid replacement IV therapy, what IV solutions may be indicated?**

Whole blood, plasma, albumin, plasma protein fraction, or dextran may be indicated if the patient is in shock or if no clinical improvement has occurred after 2 hours of rapid replacement. The patient's central venous pressure should not be elevated and pulmonary congestion should not be present if these solutions are used. Albumin and dextran have the advantage of not transmitting serum hepatitis.

■ **What cautions should be observed in administering sodium bicarbonate to a newborn?**

Sodium bicarbonate is administered by the IV and sometimes oral route to newborn infants for correction of acidosis. The formula used to calculate the dose is:

$$NaHCO_2 \ (mEq) = \text{Body weight (kg)} \times \text{Base deficit} \times 0.35$$

Recent data suggest that excessive sodium bicarbonate administration to newborns with or without hypernatremia may place the infant at a higher risk of intracranial hemorrhage. Thus the newborn's sodium intake from all sources should be carefully controlled, and intakes of more than 8 mg/kg body weight/24 hr should be regarded as excessive.

■ **An irritative substance (such as calcium, hypertonic bicarbonate, or vinblastine) is being administered by the IV route to a child, and the solution has leaked into the surrounding tissue, which appears red and swollen and feels hot. How could this be treated?**

Irrigation with saline solution, aspiration, immobilization of the extremity, application of heat pads, and cutaneous application of 0.1% triamcinolone cream with occlusive dressing may allow adequate steroid absorption to decrease local reaction.

■ **A toxic IM dose of a drug has accidentally been administered to a child. What could be done?**

The potential complications of the toxic dose are drug dependent and must be treated as toxic overdose (specific antidotes if available). When IM or subcutaneous routes are used, the procedure involves the following:

1. Use of proximal tourniquet
2. Local irrigation and aspiration with saline solution
3. Local application of ice
4. Administration of subcutaneous epinephrine into injection site, 0.01 ml/kg of 1:1000 solution

■ **What are some of the precautions that should be taken with patients on parenteral hyperalimentation?**

Parenteral hyperalimentation solutions are usually composed of amino acids, dextrose, vitamins, and minerals to provide the necessary caloric and other nutrient requirements to patients with disorders that prevent them from being fed orally. Formulas have been prepared and are available commercially; however, any formulation must be altered to fit the needs of the individual patient.

Because these solutions are hypertonic, they must be infused into large central veins where rapid dilution prevents damage to vessels. Therefore daily catheter care should include dressing removal, skin cleansing with an antiseptic, and restoration of occlusive dressings. Catheters should be immediately removed and cultured for bacteria and fungus if a patient shows signs of sepsis.

A 0.22 μ in-line final filter should be used to filter the solution and changed every 24 hours or when difficulty is encountered in adjusting the flow rate.

To prevent the accidental infusion of large amounts of fluid, an infusion pump should be used to regulate the flow. Even with the pump frequent checks should be made to verify that the proper rate of infusion is maintained.

It is not advisable to administer antibiotics or other IV medications through the alimentation cannula, since precipitation or other physical or chemical incompatibilities may result, and the chance of bacterial or fungal contamination may also be increased. Drugs that are catabolic such as tetracycline should be avoided if possible, or at least the weight of the patient should be monitored carefully to make sure that a drug interaction is not occurring. Insulin has been added to the solutions with the purpose of increasing the storage of the dextrose; however, insulin has a tendency to adhere to the sides of the IV bottle and to the tubing to an extent of 20% to 40%.

Since the solutions contain large amounts of electrolytes and glucose, dangerous electrolyte imbalances may occur, and frequent determinations of serum electrolyte (especially potassium) levels and glucose concentrations are essential during the first few days of therapy.

Other precautions include watching for fluid overload, especially in small infants, hypophosphatemia, elevation in blood ammonia levels, and acidosis.

Total IV fluid therapy is effective; however, precautions must be taken to ensure safety for the patient. Great care in all phases of the technique should be exercised to reduce the risk of septicemia, and so on. This therapy should be carried out by an experienced team and in areas where frequent monitoring of the patient can be provided.

■ What caution must be observed in correcting hypernatremic dehydration in adult patients?

Water intoxication must be prevented in the correction of hypernatremic dehydration. Serum sodium concentration should be determined after administration of one half of the calculated water deficit. The volume of water necessary to restore the serum sodium concentration to normal (body water deficit) in adults may be estimated by the following calculations (TBW is total body water):

$$TBW \ (L) = 0.6 \times Normal \ body \ weight \ (kg)$$

$$\frac{Normal \ serum \ (Na^+) \times TBW}{Measured \ serum \ (Na^+)} = Current \ TBW$$

Normal TBW − Current TBW = Body water deficit

Correction of the salt deficit is best performed gradually with a sodium-free solution. The patient should be observed for improvement in skin turgor and stabilization of blood pressure and central venous pressure.

■ What is an essential guideline for treatment of dehydration?

Acute change in weight is directly related to change in fluid volume. Just as the amount of water lost in dehydration equals the weight loss, the amount of water gained in the process of rehydration equals the amount of weight gained by the patient. Weighing the patient daily or twice daily is helpful in assessing the progress of the patient in the treatment of dehydration.

■ What are the three main objectives of parenteral therapy?

The three main objectives of parenteral therapy are: (1) to maintain daily requirements for water and electrolytes, (2) to restore any previous losses, and (3) to replace present losses.

■ Why is glucose important for IV therapy?

Glucose, a necessary nutrient in maintenance therapy, is important for the following reasons: (1) it is converted to glycogen by the liver, thereby improving hepatic function; (2) by supplying necessary calories for energy, it spares body protein; and (3) it minimizes the development of ketosis, which occurs when fat is metabolized for energy in the absence of glucose.

■ What is the basic caloric requirement for a 70 kg adult?

Approximately 1600 calories per day is the basic caloric requirement, and the administration of at least 100 of glucose per day is considered sufficient to prevent ketosis.

■ What is osmolality?

Osmolality is the total solute concentration and reflects the relative water and total solute concentration since it is expressed per liter of serum. The osmotic pressure is determined by the amount of solute in solution. The unit of osmotic pressure is the osmole, and the values are expressed in milliosmoles (mOsm). Normal blood plasma has an osmolality of 250 mOsm. The determination of serum osmolality can be used to detect the degree of dehydration or overhydration.

■ What are the normal values for body electrolytes in the adult?

The normal values for body electrolytes in the adult are as follows:
Sodium—135 to 145 mEq/L
Chloride—100 to 106 mEq/L
Potassium—4.0 to 5.5 mEq/L
Magnesium—1.7 to 2.3 mEq/L
Calcium—5 mEq/L
Phosphate—1.7 to 2.3 mEq/L

■ When is a patient considered acidotic or alkalotic?

The acidity or alkalinity of a solution depends on the degree of hydrogen ion concentration. An increase in the hydrogen ion concentration results in a more acid solution, and a decrease results in a more alkaline solution. Acidity or alkalinity is expressed by the symbol pH and refers to the amount of hydrogen ion concentration. A pH of 7 is regarded as normal. The extracellular fluid has a pH ranging from 7.35 to 7.45 and is thus slightly alkaline. When the pH of the blood is higher than 7.45, an alkaline condition exists; when the pH of the blood is lower than 7.35, an acidic condition exists.

■ What is the purpose of body electrolytes?

Electrolytes serve two main purposes: (1) to act in controlling body water volume by osmotic pressure, and (2) to maintain the proper acid-alkaline balance of the body.

■ What are the more commonly used intravenous solutions?

Intravenous solutions are divided into two main categories: crystalloid and colloid. Crystalloid solutions are prepared by dissolving crystals of salts, such as sodium chloride and dextrose, into water. They do not impart oncotic pressure changes but do have the ability to change the osmotic pressures. Colloidal solutions are made up of large molecules—too large to cross the capillary membranes. These solutions will impart a change in oncotic pressure and remain within the vascular compartment for a considerable period of time.

The most commonly used crystalloid and colloidal solutions can be found in Table 6-4.

■ What are the uses for dextran?

Dextran is a plasma volume expander used for the treatment of hypovolemia. It increases the osmotic pressure, draws interstitial fluid into the vessels and increases the blood volume. It is a synthetic product with three advantages: it is less expensive than albumin products; there are no storage problems; and there is no danger of hepatitis (which can occur with albumin). Allergic reactions with dextran are rare; however, the first few millimeters of dextran infusion should be administered slowly and the patient observed for signs of mild urticaria, tightness of the chest, and hypotension. Dextran should be used cautiously in patients with heart or kidney disease, since too rapid an administration rate may cause congestive heart failure and pulmonary edema.

■ What are hypernatremia and hyponatremia?

Hypernatremia is a condition of elevated serum sodium (greater than 145 mEq/L), indicating an increase in body fluid tonicity (a net deficit of pure water). It is seen in patients whose water losses are not replaced because either the patient does not perceive thirst or cannot get water. Elderly patients with strokes are perhaps the commonest cases. Treatment requires replacement of free water with 5% dextrose in water intravenously or orally depending on the patient's physical condition.

Hyponatremia occurs when the serum sodium is less than 135 mEq/L. This condition represents a reduction in serum sodium concentration, indicating hypotonicity of the body water. The symptoms resulting from hyponatremia include anxiety, agitation, cloudy sensorium, convulsions, and coma. Common causes are endocrine disorders such as Addison's disease, hypopituitarism, and myxedema; cirrhosis of the liver; congestive heart failure; hypovolemia caused by gastrointestinal losses and diarrhea; and inappropriate secretion of antidiuretic hormone.

■ What is the treatment for hyponatremia?

Treatment for hyponatremia will depend on the underlying causes; for example, in patients with congestive heart failure and/or cirrhosis of the

Table 6-4. Most commonly used crystalloid and colloidal solutions

Solution	Type of solution	Osmolality (mOsm/L)	pH	Concentration of solutes/L
0.9% sodium chloride	Crystalloid	308	5.0	154 mEq sodium 154 mEq chloride
Lactated Ringer's	Crystalloid	275	6.5	130 mEq sodium 109 mEq chloride 28 mEq lactate 4 mEq potassium 3 mEq calcium
0.45% sodium chloride	Crystalloid	154	5.0	77 mEq sodium 77 mEq chloride
5% dextrose in water	Crystalloid	253	4.5	5 g dextrose/100 ml
5% dextrose in 0.2% sodium chloride	Crystalloid	320	4.0	5 g dextrose/100 ml 34 mEq sodium 34 mEq chloride
5% dextrose in 0.45% sodium chloride	Crystalloid	406	4.0	5 g dextrose/100 ml 77 mEq sodium 77 mEq chloride
5% dextrose in 0.9% sodium chloride	Crystalloid	560	4.0	5 g dextrose/100 ml 154 mEq sodium 154 mEq chloride
5% dextrose in lactated Ringer's	Crystalloid	524	5.0	5 g dextrose/100 ml 130 mEq sodium 109 mEq chloride 28 mEq lactate 4 mEq potassium 3 mEq calcium
10% mannitol	Crystalloid			
5% albumin	Colloidal	300	6.8	5 g albumin/100 ml 140 mEq sodium 120 mEq chloride
25% albumin	Colloidal	7.0	7.0	25 g albumin/100 ml 100-160 mEq sodium Not more than 1 mEq potassium Note more than 120 mEq chloride

Dextran 40, 70, 75
  In 5% dextrose
  In water or 0.9% sodium
    chloride
	Colloidal		3.5-7.0	In 5% dextrose—5 g dextrose/100 ml
				In 0.9% sodium chloride—154 mEq sodium
				      154 mEq chloride

liver there is an excess of body sodium and water. Therapy therefore would be a restriction of water rather than the administration of saline. Patients with hypovolemia are deficient in total body sodium and water. Water restriction is therefore inappropriate. Generally isotonic rather than hypertonic sodium chloride serves to correct hyponatremia. In patients with excess total body water, water restriction constitutes appropriate therapy.

■ **What are the causes of hypokalemia?**

Hypokalemia exists when the serum potassium level falls below 4.0 mEq/L. This condition may be due to inadequate intake of potassium, excessive gastrointestinal losses (diarrhea, bowel fistulas), and excessive urinary losses as a result of diuretic therapy. The latter remains the most common cause of hypokalemia. Diuretics such as furosemide, ethacrynic acid, and hydrochlorothiazide are commonly employed and consequently a main reason for the condition. However, there are diuretics that conserve potassium, which can be administered concomitantly with the potassium-depleting agents. Examples of drugs in this category are triamterene and spironolactone.

■ **How is hypokalemia treated?**

An alkalosis usually accompanies hypokalemia. To correct both the alkalosis and potassium depletion, replacement therapy should be instituted with potassium chloride rather than with potassium acetate, lactate, or citrate. Intravenous replacement in severely depleted patients is hazardous if administered too rapidly. Electrocardiographic monitoring should be available, especially if the patient has impaired renal function and when infusing more than 40 mEq/hour and in concentrations in excess of 40 mEq/L.

If replacement is to be done by the oral route, it should be noted that the enteric-coated preparations of potassium chloride have been associated with a high frequency of small bowel lesions, obstruction, and hemorrhage. The syrup, solution, and effervescent tablet forms have a lesser incidence of these problems; however, the palatability of these preparations is questionable. Foods such as bananas, vegetables, and citrus juices can be used; however, additional supplementation may be necessary.

■ **What are the causes of hyperkalemia?**

Hyperkalemia develops when there is an associated factor such as acute renal failure, excessive potassium load, severe acidosis, potassium-sparing diuretics such as spironolactone and triamterene, and a deficiency of endogenous steroids.

■ **What are the electrocardiographic changes associated with hyperkalemia and at what serum level do these changes usually occur?**

With an increase in serum potassium levels above 7.0 mEq/L, there is a progression of peaked T wave, loss of P wave, and a widening of the QRS complex.

■ **What is the treatment of hyperkalemia?**

In acute emergencies treatment can be aimed at shifting potassium intracellularly or removing potassium from the body.

Shifting potassium intracellularly can be accomplished by the use of insulin and glucose. The amount of insulin will vary; however, a commonly used ratio of 3 to 4 g dextrose per unit of regular insulin has been employed.

The removal of potassium from the body requires the use of cation exchange resins such as sodium polystyrene sulfonate (Kayexalate). If complete exchange is accomplished, each gram of resin exchanges more than 2 mEq of sodium for each milliequivalent of potassium. Therefore sodium levels should also be monitored carefully to avoid hypernatremia.

If these methods are unsuccessful, peritoneal dialysis or hemodialysis may be employed.

■ **What is the usual dose of polystyrene sodium sulfonate (Kayexalate)?**

Polystyrene sodium sulfonate (Kayexalate) can be given orally or administered as an enema.

When used orally, 15 to 20 g can be thoroughly mixed with 30 to 50 ml of 70% sorbitol. The sorbitol aids in preventing constipation and fecal impaction.

If the oral intake is not tolerated, 40 to 50 g polystyrene sulfonate plus 50 ml of 70% sorbitol mixed with 150 ml of tap water can be given as an enema and retained for at least 30 minutes. This can be repeated as necessary to obtain the desired decrease in serum potassium.

■ **How is hypocalcemia treated?**

Tetany and seizures are the major manifestations of hypocalcemia and can be treated by administering various calcium salts, such as calcium gluconate, chloride, or gluceptate, orally or intravenously. The intravenous route should not exceed 2.5 mEq calcium per minute without checking serum calcium levels and monitoring the electrocardiogram. Oral doses of calcium gluconate (1 g) or lactate (300 mg) may be used.

■ **What is the role of mithramycin in treating hypercalcemia?**

Mitramycin is an antitumor agent that acts by inhibiting bone resorption and blocking vitamin D action. When used in doses of 25 μg/kg of body weight, it produces a marked decrease in serum calcium in 48 hours. Side-effects include transient nausea and vomiting. In some patients the serum calcium may rise again in 72 to 96 hours after stopping therapy, but in others the levels may remain depressed.

■ **What are normal serum electrolyte values for infants and children?**

Normal serum electrolyte values for infants and children are as follows:

Chloride—95 to 110 mEq/L
Sodium—138 to 145 mEq/L
Potassium—3.5 to 5.5 mEq/L (may be higher in neonates)

■ **What are the usual maintenance requirements for sodium and potassium in infants and children?**

The usual maintenance requirements for sodium and potassium in infants and children are as follows:

Sodium—2 to 5 mEq/kg/24 hr
Potassium—1 to 2 mEq/kg/24 hr

■ **What is the sodium content of "salt-poor" albumin?**

All 25% normal serum albumin (human) manufactured after February 28, 1978, must have a range of sodium content between 130 and 160 mEq/L. In addition, the labeling for this product may no longer include the term "salt-poor." The changes in the sodium content of normal serum albumin under the new standards are minimal.

In fact, the term "salt-poor" is a misnomer that has persisted since high-salt products containing 300 mEq of sodium chloride/L disappeared from the market over 30 years ago. The FDA's Bureau of Biologicals comments that until the stocks of older material are depleted, hospitals and pharmacists may encounter products having slightly different sodium contents than the new standard, using different units to express the sodium concentration, or bearing the term "salt-poor." They emphasize that there is no therapeutic difference between these older products and those meeting the new regulations.

The product formerly labeled "salt-poor" albumin, 25%, will now be labeled 25% normal serum albumin (human).

■ **What parameters should be monitored to successfully treat an infant with parenteral fluid therapy?**

Fluid and electrolyte balance must be carefully monitored to successfully treat an infant with parenteral fluids. Data such as the following should be regularly followed:

1. Intravenous and/or oral fluid and electrolyte intake
2. Urinary volume, specific gravity, or osmolality and glucose analysis
3. Abnormal losses, such as chest tube or nasogastric tube
4. Body weight
5. Serial serum electrolytes
6. Clinical assessment for the state of hydration

■ **How does the insensible water loss of low birth weight infants, in ml/kg/24 hr, compare to term infants?**

The insensible water loss in low birth weight infants is higher than term infants and is inversely proportional to gestational age. Insensible water loss in term infants is approximately 15 to 20 ml/kg/24 hr, and for an infant who is 28 weeks gestation it is approximately 40 to 45 ml/kg/24 hr.

■ **What are the major characteristics of body composition in low birth weight infants?**

One of the major characteristics of body composition in low birth weight infants is a high body water content with a large extracellular fluid compartment. The total body water and extracellular fluid compartment of a 28-week gestational age infant account for 85% and 55% of body weight, respectively. The other important characteristic in the body composition of these infants is the lower subcutaneous fat content. The low subcutaneous fat content may account for the higher rate of cutaneous heat exchange and insensible water loss.

■ **Why is insensible water loss such an important consideration in calculating the maintenance fluid therapy for low birth weight infants?**

Low birth weight infants have a higher rate of insensible water loss than full-term infants. This may be accounted for by (1) lower subcutaneous fat content, (2) larger body surface area in reference to body mass, (3) relatively undeveloped skin structure, (4) proportionately larger blood supply to the skin than for its tissue mass, and (5) larger water content of the skin.

In addition, factors such as respiratory distress, phototherapy for the treatment of hyperbilirubinemia, use of radiant warmer as a means of maintaining body temperature, and cold stress may further increase insensible water loss in this group of infants.

■ **What precautions should be observed when administering 10% intravenous fat infusion (Intralipid)?**

Intralipid has proved to be safe and useful in children and adults who require parenteral alimentation. It provides a source of essential fatty acids and a high caloric value (1.1 calories/ml). It is used intravenously without a surgically inserted central line and can therefore provide caloric supplement with minimal mechanical difficulty. Most complications that have arisen with this product have been directly related to the rate and duration of fat infusion. Although acute toxic effects with Intralipid are rare (febrile reactions are the most common, occurring in about 2%), four cases of fat embolism in small infants (weight 1.65 to 3.13 kg) receiving prolonged intravenous infusion of fat (Intralipid, 20%) have been reported. The condition is similar to fat em-

bolism following trauma and practitioners must be alert for the following signs in children who are on long-term Intralipid infusion—hypoxia, pyrexia, anemia, thrombocytopenia, fat excretion in the urine, raised serum lipase or macroglobulinemia, "snow storm" chest x-ray films, and neurologic abnormalities such as paresis. Transient rapid infusion rates of Intralipid may be a factor in the etiology of this condition.

BIBLIOGRAPHY

AMA Department of Drugs: AMA drug evaluation, ed. 2, Acton, Mass, 1973, Publishing Sciences Group, Inc.
American Hospital Formulary Service, Washington D.C., 1975, American Society of Hospital Pharmacists.
Arnanda, J. V., et al.: Pharmacokinetic aspects of theophylline in premature newborns, N. Engl. J. Med. **295:**413, 1976.
Barson, A. J., et al.: Fat embolism in infancy after intravenous fat infusions, Arch. Dis. Child. **53:**218, 1978.
Beckman, H.: Dilemmas in drug therapy, Philadelphia, 1967, W. B. Saunders Co.
Bennett, E. J., et al.: Pancuronium bromide: a double-blind study in children, Anesth. Analg. (Cleve.) **52:**12, 1973.
Berman, W., et al.: Inadvertent over-administration of digoxin to low-birth-weight infants, J. Pediatr. **92:**1024, 1978.
Editorial Board: Label changes on albumin—a reminder, FDA Drug Bull. **8:**32, 1978.
Giacoia G., Jusko, W. J., Menke, J., and Koup, J. R.: Theophylline pharmacokinetics in premature infants with apnea, J. Pediatr. **89:**829, 1976.
Goodman, L., and Gilman, A.: The pharmacologic basis of therapeutics, New York, 1968, Macmillan, Inc.
Graeber, J. E., Williams, M. I., and Oski, E. A.: The use of intramuscular vitamin E in the premature infant, J. Pediatr. **90:**282, 1977.
Horowitz, K., and Iseri, L. T.: Drugs used in cardiopulmonary arrest, The Pharmacy Newsletter, Orange County Medical Center **4:**2, 1973.
Hospital formulary monograph on Silvadene cream (micronized silver sulfadiazine), Kansas City, Mo., 1973, Marion Laboratories, Inc.
Iseri, L. T.: Magnesium and cardiac arrhythmias, The Pharmacy Newsletter, Orange County Medical Center **5:**4, 1975.
Karliner, J. S.: Dopamine for cardiogenic shock, J.A.M.A. **226:**1217, 1973.
Kempe, C. H.: Immunization update with a word of caution, Drug Therapy, p. 71, 1974.
Kempe, C. H., Silver, H., and O'Brien, D.: Current pediatric diagnosis and treatment, Los Altos, Calif., 1972, Lange Medical Publications.
Khan, W., et al.: *Haemophilus influenza* type B resistant to ampicillin, a report of two cases, J.A.M.A. **229:**289, 1974.
Lasry, J. E., and Glassner, M. L.: Cardiovascular drugs, 1970, The California Heart Association Publication.
Loeb, H. S., et al.: Acute hemodynamic effects of dopamine in patients with shock, Circulation **44:**163, 1971.
Lombroso, C. T.: The treatment of status epilepticus, Pediatrics **53:**536, 1970.

Lopez, R. I.: Fluid and electrolyte balance. In Graef, J. W., and Cone, T. E., Editors: Manual of pediatric therapeutics, ed. 1, Boston, 1976, Little, Brown & Co., p. 83.

Marion Laboratories, Manufacturer literature on Silvadene cream, 1978.

Melmon, K. L., and Morrelli, H. F.: Clinical pharmacology, basic principles in therapeutics, New York, 1972, Macmillan, Inc.

Meyers, F.: Review of medical pharmacology, Los Altos, Calif., 1972, Lange Medical Publications.

Mitchell, A. A., and Mandell, F.: Hospital variations in the use of silver nitrate prophylaxis, Pediatric Alert (April 13):30, 1978.

Nadas, A.: Pediatric cardiology, Philadelphia, 1963, W. B. Saunders Co.

Oh, W.: Fluid and electrolyte management of low birth weight infants. Development aspects of fluid and electrolyte hemeostasis, Meade Johnson Symposium on Perinatal and Development Medicine No. 10, Florida, December 5-9, 1976, p. 55.

Parenteral electrolyte solutions, 1973, Med. Lett. Drugs Ther. Reference Handbook.

Parker, E. A.: Parenteral incompatibilities, Hosp. Pharm. **4:** 14, 1969.

Pascoe, D., and Grossman, M.: Quick reference to pediatric emergencies, Philadelphia, 1973, J. B. Lippincott Co.

Pediatric Alert, **2:**95, 1977 and March 2, 1978.

Pfeifer, R., et al.: Arch Dis. Child 53:218, 1978.

Pierog, S. H., and Ferrara, A.: Approach to the medical care of the sick newborn, ed. 2, St. Louis, 1976, The C. V. Mosby Co.

Randall, R. J.: Diazoxide, The Pharmacy Newsletter, Orange County Medical Center **5:**2, 1974.

Rumack, B. H., and Temple, A. R.: Lomotil poisoning, Pediatrics 53:495, 1974.

Shirkey, H. C.: Pediatric dosage handbook, Washington, D.C., 1971, American Pharmaceutical Association.

Shirkey, H. C.: Pediatric therapy, ed. 6, St. Louis, 1980, The C. V. Mosby Co.

Shuman, R. M., Leech, R. W., and Alvord, E. C.: Neurotoxicity of hexachlorophene in the human: I. A clinicopathologic study of 248 children, Pediatrics **54:**689, 1974.

Smith, D. H., et al.: Bacterial meningitis, diagnosis and treatment, a symposium, Pediatrics **52:**586, 1973.

Simon, M., et al.: Hypernatremia, intracranial hemorrhage and sodium bicarbonate administration in neonates, N. Engl. J. Med. **291:**6, 1974.

Tomeh, M., et al.: Ampicillin-resistant *Haemophilus influenza* type B infection, J.A.M.A. **229:**295, 1974.

Travenol guide to fluid therapy, Deerfield, ILL, 1970, Traveol Laboratories.

Treatment of neonatal withdrawal syndrome, Med. Lett. Drugs Ther. 15:46, 1973.

Visconti, J. A.: The dialysis of drugs, Philips-Roxan Laboratory White Sheet.

Vswanathan, C. T., et al.: J. Clin. Pharmacol. **18:**100, 1978.

Yeh, T. F., et al.: Mercury poisoning from mercurochrome therapy of infected omphalocele, Lancet 1:210, 1978.

CHAPTER 7

The physical examination

Louis Schwartz

PHYSICAL ASSESSMENT

The role of the examiner in a critical care situation is to reach a swift, accurate diagnosis of the patient's medical problems. This is not a simple project, nor is it an easily attainable goal in many cases. A critical care situation may necessitate truly swift assessment and appropriate action. All medical examiners have been trained to obtain certain items of information regarding their patient (that is, the complete medical history) prior to treating the patient's problem. The initial examiner of the critically ill person may only be able to obtain the sketchiest history and in many cases no history at all. Whether one is the initial examiner of a patient with virtually no medical history available or the examiner of a patient who has had a complete workup and has been hospitalized for many days, the assessment process should remain the same. It must be as systematic, thorough, and accurate as possible under the prevailing circumstances.

If no history is available or none is obtainable from ambulance attendants, relatives, observers, or other appropriate parties, one must proceed with the physical examination somewhat blindly. If the patient or reliable other sources are available for information, one should attempt to obtain as much information regarding the immediate situation as possible and practical. *Time,* because of the illness of the patient, may be a luxury and only the most pertinent questions should be asked during the physical assessment. A more complete history may be obtained when the critical aspect of the situation is over.

THE SYSTEMATIC REVIEW

In any systematic review one must have a starting point. Depending on the illness, the emergence of the situation, and the prior knowledge that one may have of the patient, one must progress with the physical examination in the order that is deemed to be most appropriate. One decides on the order of the examination by individual choice. Many examiners have a completely different order of examination, but all usually agree on a systematic, thorough, and accurate physical assessment that includes all systems of the body. Methods may be different, but the results are very similar. Obviously, any major signs or symptoms should be attended to first and the remaining system or systems attended to at a later time. It is not within the scope of this chapter to individualize patient examination, but rather to provide an overview guideline for the initial assessment of the critically ill individual.

EXAMINATION OF THE INTEGUMENTARY SYSTEM

In any systematic physical examination the skin (including hair and nails), since it is external and obviously highly visible, is usually the first system under investigation. The skin can be an indicator of disease within and of itself and an indicator of many systemic problems. The skin must be examined for its color, any outstanding vascularity, edema, temperature, turgor, lesions, moisture, texture, and thickness. A normal physical assessment would begin by assessment of the skin with the examination of the hands, face, and forearms, but in an examination of a critically ill patient one would begin with examination of the skin of the face, looking for cyanotic changes. The ankles and lower extremities should be examined for any signs of edema, and then the overall remaining skin for the obvious signs of cyanosis, jaundice, pallor, and any other color changes. Examination of the hair is rarely included in a physical examination in an acute situation, but examination of the nails should be included, looking for such well-known signs as the splinter hemorrhages of subacute bacterial endocarditis, the microhemorrhages of vasculitis around the cuticle area, the horizontal ridge depressions in the nails called Beau's lines indicative of major illness of recent origin, and clubbing indicating the possibility of chronic illnesses. Signs of peripheral edema can alert one to the possibility of congestive heart failure and other circulatory problems. Lack of skin turgor may indicate protein deficiencies or dehydration. Skin texture may well reveal the possibilities of endocrine disturbances. Examination of the skin, while perhaps not the first system to be examined in an acute situation, should nonetheless be as thorough and as complete as any of the systematic examinations.

EXAMINATION OF THE EXTERNAL AND INTERNAL EYE

Depending on the situation, the examination of the internal and external eye can be first or virtually last on the agenda of systems examined. If the patient is unconscious, examination of the internal eye may be of prime importance and thus the first examination that one would do. A funduscopic examination can be very rewarding. One should be on the lookout for the obvious signs of increased intracranial pressure, including hyperemia and papilledema and any type of hemorrhage that may indicate the possibility of a vascular accident. The retina should be examined for the signs of diabetic retinopathy, which may be an outstanding clue as to the unconscious status of the patient. The eye should also be examined for the arterial narrowing indicative of hypertension and for any other obvious defect. The inner eye should be examined for problems

such as glaucoma, cataracts, and retinal defects, all of which are important but usually of a chronic nature and treated in a nonemergent situation. The external eye should be examined for signs of illness such as jaundice, causing a yellowing of the sclera; nystagmus, indicating a neurologic problem; pupillary responses, both direct and consensual, indicating a cranial nerve problem, possibly secondary to other neurologic problems; and the palpebral conjunctivae should be examined for signs of anemia.

EXAMINATION OF THE THORAX AND LUNGS

Examination of the thorax and lungs should proceed in a systematic fashion using the techniques of inspection, palpation, percussion, and auscultation. During the examination one should try to form a mental image of the underlying structure and tissues, to begin to get the mental picture that is so important in forming the final diagnosis. Compare the left side of the thorax to the right side, thus allowing the patient to act as his own control, since variations between patients are great and individual problems can be excluded. The main problems, and the obvious ones to look for, are the rate and rhythm of breathing. Are they within normal limits? Does there seem to be impairment in respiratory movement? Is there bulging of the intercostal spaces during expiration or retraction of the intercostal spaces during inspiration? Is there use of accessory musculature during the respiratory cycle? Does there seem to be movement on one side while the other moves to a lesser extent, possibly indicating a pneumothorax? During the examination of the thorax watch for signs of respiratory difficulty such as "pursed lip" breathing, painful expression on the patient's face, clenched fists, and other unusual signs of respiratory difficulty. If the patient is awake, alert, and cooperative, one might try to elicit vocal or tactile fremitus through the usual methods by asking the patient to repeat the words "ninety-nine" over and over again. Identification of fremitus is useful as it is decreased or absent in the presence of an obstructed bronchus or pleural effusion or air in the pleural space. An increase in fremitus may be present near large bronchi and over consolidated lung tissue. If the patient is unable to cooperate, obviously one cannot use this valuable portion of the examination. The same may apply to checking for diaphragmatic excursion. Again, this will depend on the cooperation of the patient. Percussion should be used to determine any areas of consolidation. Auscultation of the lungs is perhaps the most valuable portion of the examination of the thoracic cavity. It is useful in assessing the air flow through the tracheal-bronchial tree, detecting the presence of any fluid or obstruction of the air passages and the general condition of the surrounding lungs and the attendant pleural space. If the patient is cooperative, one might be able to test for the presence of bronchophony or egophony. If the patient is unconscious or uncooperative, then one must be content with listening for any adventitious sound: rales, rhonchi, friction rubs, and wheezes.

EXAMINATION OF THE HEART

The heart, in an emergency situation, is an obvious central focus of examination, especially if there is little or no history obtainable. As this is not a primer on auscultation of the heart, suffice it to say that the heart should be auscultated for murmurs, cardiovascular sounds with components of both systolic and diastolic cycles such as pericardial friction rubs, and venous hums. Splitting of the heart sounds should be noted, and *special attention should be given to the second heart sound*. In conjunction with the examination of the heart, an electrocardiogram is of prime significance and importance. Acute myocardial infarction, usually quite easily diagnosed by history, may also be partially diagnosed by the presence of an S_3, S_4, or paradoxically split S_2, owing to decreased left ventricular compliance. The patient is usually short of breath. Blood gases, if available, would reveal the presence of metabolic acidosis and/or respiratory alkalosis. It is impossible to exclude the examination of the large blood vessels of the body when speaking of examination of the heart. Examination of the large vessels can be helpful in the diagnosis of cardiac tamponade when distended neck veins are present. The arterial pulsus paradoxus is an important finding in tamponade as well as in a few other cardiac problems. The measure-

ment of the arterial blood pressure is indicated in examination of the heart and vascular system and is of vital importance in patient assessment as it is a first-class indicator of the adequacy or inadequacy of organ perfusion. Evaluation of the peripheral arterial pulses is an extremely important component of the examination of the circulatory system. The pulses that should be evaluated are the carotid, brachial, radial, femoral, popliteal, and pedal pulses, along with the apical pulse rate. The peripheral pulses should be compared bilaterally for rate, rhythm, volume, and contour. A pulse deficit should not be present.

In addition to the major arteries, the jugular veins should be examined for distention and abnormal wave patterns.

EXAMINATION OF THE HEAD, EARS, NOSE, AND ORAL CAVITY

Examination of the head, ears, nose, and oral cavity should be accomplished and, depending on the situation, placed in its appropriate rank in the systematic evaluation. Depending again on the circumstances, the head should be observed for any obvious signs of trauma such as frank bleeding, edema of any portion from a blow, structural abnormalities, and any other observable signs. The ears should be examined quickly for signs of intracranial problems, including leakage of blood or cerebrospinal fluid into the canal. Ruptured eardrums can also be easily observed. The nose should be examined for obstruction to the clear passage of air. The mouth should be examined for loose dentures, broken teeth, swallowed blood, and/or mucus and dirt or foreign objects in the mouth occluding the air passageway. The tongue, of course, should be in its normal position and not occluding the air passageway, and the head should be examined for lymph node involvement of any significant nature.

EXAMINATION OF THE GENITOURINARY SYSTEM

Once again, depending on the cooperativeness of the patient, the genitourinary system is examined directly through observation and palpation of the external genitalia, but unless the trauma was almost directly to those areas, the findings will probably be of little significance. What *can* be significant is the possibility of bleeding into the external genital areas such as the vulva, labia, and the scrotal areas. *The possibility of subcutaneous emphysema as a sign of a break in the pulmonary system being evidenced in the genital region has been noted,* although this is usually a delayed development. The urinary tract is usually examined indirectly through urinalysis and appropriate blood chemistry. If the patient is able to cooperate, renal palpation can be of limited help in the evaluation of this system. Dry skin may be of diagnostic significance. Edematous tissue, lack of turgor, or poor texture can be of some help in the evaluation of the renal system, but if pathology is suspected with renal involvement, appropriate x-ray examinations and laboratory analyses are indicated.

NEUROLOGIC SYSTEM

The neurologic system should be one of the first systems examined in the critically ill patient, especially if the patient is unconscious. In that case it should receive priority over all other systems examined. The deep tendon reflexes should be examined as well as the cranial nerves to the extent that they can be examined for intactness, making sure that the major spinal nerves are without damage. Some of the superficial reflexes should also be tested. Hyperactive deep tendon reflexes are suggestive of upper motor neuron disease and, when correlated with other findings, might very well lead to a diagnosis. Superficial reflexes such as the abdominal and cremasteric (in the male) reflexes may be absent in both upper and lower neuron disorders. A sustained reaction or slowed relaxation phase in the Achilles tendon reflex may suggest hypothyroidism as the problem. Positive plantar reflexes, the well-known Babinski responses, indicate upper motor neuron disease; this coupled with sustained ankle clonus may make the diagnosis of upper motor neuron disease a certainty. When checking for meningeal signs, such as deflexion of the patient's leg at the hip and the knee, one should look for resistance or pain that may indicate or suggest meningeal inflammation or possibly spinal disc problems. Certainly, any neurologic deficit is reason for a full and complete investigation. The status of the patient may preclude many of the neurologic examinations that one might like to perform, such as gait; coordination; orientation as to time, place, and person; and muscle strength and coordination. However, enough of the neurologic examination is available even in an unconscious patient to give the astute examiner excellent clues as to the whereabouts of the patient's problem.

SUMMARY

While physical examination of the critically ill patient should be systematic, thorough, and accurate, it is obvious that a complete examination is often precluded because of the status of the patient. Unconsciousness, obtundation, confusion, or other problems may not allow one to obtain the complete history that one would prefer to have. The inability of the patient to answer questions, commands, or the inability to perform voluntary movements obviously prevents some portions of the physical assessment from being accomplished; however, enough of the physical examination can be carried out to make a reasonable diagnosis. Certain adjustments must be made in the examination of the critically ill patient. For example, prostate and rectal examinations are sometimes just not done at the moment of initial assessment. It is important, as soon as it is practical, to complete a thorough and all-inclusive physical examination on the patient. As soon as initial emergent problems have been adequately taken care of, the complete physical should be done. Other problems not apparent at the initial assessment may be found, and they may have a distinct and important bearing on the total management of the patient. A complete history should also be attempted as soon as practical as some portions of patient management may be contraindicated, or changes and modifications of the management program may be indicated. No attempt at explaining a complete physical examination and its ramifications is made in this chapter; merely a brief overview of the essentials of an initial assessment of a critically ill patient is presented. The positive findings that one might encounter are very adequately explained in this and other excellent reference texts.

The initial physical assessment of the critically

ill patient can be compared to a compass. When you are completely lost, a compass is very useful in determining in which direction you should travel. The initial physical assessment, much like the compass, determines the direction in which one should travel; it determines the laboratory tests that would be in order; it determines the x-ray procedures that are essential in diagnosis; it determines whether or not other procedures such as computed tomography, electroencephalograms, and other highly specialized testing are necessary and indicated; it determines whether another specialized examiner should be called in for consultation. The initial assessment is the compass that determines the direction of the patient's management and his hope for eventual return to as much normalcy as possible.

CHAPTER 8

Envenomation: marine injuries and emergencies

Carmen Germaine Warner and James R. Stewart

The potential danger of marine injury infection or even death always poses a threat for those who live near and enjoy the coastal waters of this country. Lack of awareness and recognition of these dangerous marine animals, concomitant with minimal knowledge regarding assessment and intervention, necessitates the formation of this chapter.

Even though specific consultation might be required with certain injuries, it is imperative that the reader initiate treatment as rapidly as possible.

■ What is meant by venomous animals?

For the purpose of this text, the term "venomous animals" will be used when referring to creatures who produce a poisonous substance in a secretory organ or group of cells and are capable of delivering this toxin while biting or stinging. By comparison, poisonous animals are identified as creatures whose tissues as a whole or in part are considered toxic. In essence, all venomous animals are considered poisonous, but not all poisonous animals are venomous.

These animals in delivering the venom possess a sting, spine, jaw, tooth, or fang identified as a venom apparatus. This term has been expanded to denote the gland and duct as well. In discussing various venomous marine animals, the following categories will be addressed in this chapter: marine animals that bite, marine animals that sting, marine punctures, and marine reptiles. Marine animals that pose a problem through ingestion will not be dealt with in this chapter (see Chapter 40).

MARINE ANIMALS THAT BITE
■ What are the dangerous biting marine animals inhabiting the coastal waters of this country?

Those animals of primary concern to practitioners who live in areas bordering Atlantic, Pacific, or Mexican waters include the shark, barracuda, moray eel, wolf eel, octopus, seals, and sea lions. There are other dangerous marine animals, but their natural habitat does not include United States coastal waters.

■ What factors should be remembered regarding assessment and intervention of shark attacks?

The greatest danger of shark attacks occurs in waters located between 30 degrees north to 30 degrees south of the equator. It is not uncommon for attacks to be reported off California and the Eastern seaboard of the United States. The reason for this is because of periodic migratory patterns into near shore waters in quest of food. The great white shark that had long been thought a tropical form is the prime source of attack off central California. The most common temperature range for shark attacks is around 70° F, with the greatest month for recorded attacks being January. The bull shark of the Atlantic and its counterparts throughout the world possess the necessary organs within their bodies to allow

157

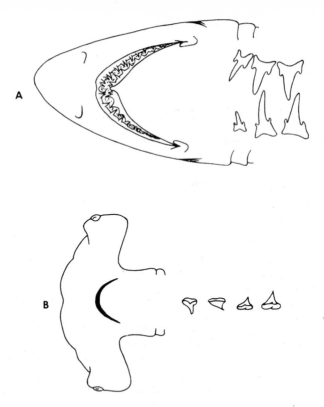

Fig. 8-1. A, Sand snake, *Carcharias taurus* Rafinesque. **B,** Hammerhead shark, *Sphyrna diplana.*

them to range freely into freshwater. These sharks have been found as far as 120 miles into a river.

Despite the dreaded fear of shark attacks, approximately 120 positive cases are reported each year worldwide. Unfortunately, when bites do occur, they are severe. The cause of death is usually due to hemorrhage or shock, with a reported fatality rate of 50% to 80% worldwide (Figs. 8-1 and 8-2).

Bites producing multiple parallel linear cuts, jagged tears, or crushing injuries generally result in the loss of extensive amounts of tissue and massive hemorrhage. However, slashing attacks caused by the raking effect of the upper teeth only may occur, resulting in little or no tissue loss.

Accompanying shock and severe blood loss may be neurogenic shock and exhaustion. The death rate is directly proportional to the number of major blood vessels injured (Table 8-1). Intervention should be concerned with control of hemorrhage and shock through maintenance of body warmth and fluids.

In initiating proper intervention, the patient must be removed from the water immediately and treatment begun on the beach. Prehospital, advanced life-support measures should be instituted, and the patient maintained on NPO. Despite the severity of injuries, the patient should *not* be moved for a minimum of 30 minutes. It has been documented that most patients who die do so as a result of aggressive transport procedures.[1]

Blood, plasma, 5% albumin, normal saline, dextran, or other plasma expanders must be rushed to the patient—not vice versa. Hemostasis and fluid replacement are of primary importance. Sedation may be required depending on the patient's condition. Mobile transport may begin once stabilization has occurred.

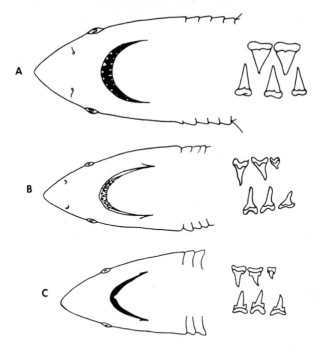

Fig. 8-2. A, White shark, *Carcharodon carcharias* (linnaeus); **B,** Mako shark, *Isurus oxyrinchus* Rafinesque; and **C,** Mackerel shark, *Lamna nasus* (bonnateme).

Table 8-1. Severity of injuries resulting from shark attacks*

Degree of injury	Vessels severed and wound description	Likely prognosis
First degree	Both femoral arteries One femoral and one posterior tibial artery One femoral artery in upper third of thigh	Fatal
Second degree	One femoral artery in lower two thirds of thigh One brachial artery Two posterior tibial arteries Abdominal wounds with major bowel involvement	Should survive if proper treatment rendered on the beach
Third degree	One posterior tibial artery Superficial limb wounds; no vessels cut Superficial abdominal wounds; no peritoneal involvement	Always survive if proper treatment secured at time of injury

*Modified from information by Edmonds, C.: Dangerous marine animals of the Indo-Pacific region, Newport, Victoria, Australia, n.d., Wedneil Publications, p. 20.

Emergency department resuscitation intervention should be the first priority. Following stabilization, x-ray films should be taken to assess bone damage and surgical treatment then evaluated.

Wounds should be debrided and injured vessels ligated as soon as feasible, allowing a 4- to 6-day period for inspection of the wound in case of possible infection. If an infection does not develop, advanced surgical procedures, including primary closure and grafting, should be instituted. Throughout surgical intervention, the wound should be explored for possible teeth particles or other identifying matter. This must be saved and forwarded to the proper authorities.*

Tetanus booster or tetanus antitoxin and antibiotic therapy should be administered immediately. One must note that penicillin-resistant bacteria (paracolon bacillus) have been discovered in shark mouths; consequently, tetracycline or chloramphenicol may be more effective.

No sure prevention of shark attacks is noted. The best advice for swimmers and divers is to remember the following: (1) refrain from carrying speared fish next to the body; (2) dark colors appear to be less attractive to sharks; (3) do not swim with abrasions or bleeding wounds; (4) do not urinate in the water; (5) do not use underwater explosives; (6) move gently and quietly, without panic; (7) if swimming, stay with a group; and (8) *always* dive with a buddy. Careful assessment of one's surroundings, laced with deep respect for the potential devastating effects these animals may cause, is paramount.

■ **What knowledge should practitioners possess regarding the barracuda?**

The great barracuda, which may attain a length of from 6 to 8 feet, is of minor danger to United States coastal residents. The only recorded incidence is in the waters between the West Indies and Florida and in some of the waters surrounding the Hawaiian Islands.

A barracuda's large mouth houses enormous knifelike canine teeth that cause traumatic wounds similar to those of the shark (Fig. 8-3). The difference is in the type of resulting cuts. Shark lacerations leave curve-shaped cuts similar to the shape of their jaws, while injuries from a barracuda bite are straight lined. These lacerations produce a large amount of tissue loss and massive hemorrhage and must be surgically treated similar to the intervention outlined in the treatment of shark bites.

Other points to consider regarding intervention is to keep the patient lying down and quiet, reassuring him continuously. It is wise to maintain

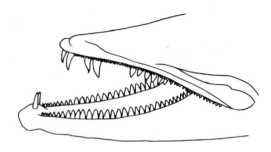

Fig. 8-3. Barracuda.

them on NPO until the extent of surgical repair is assessed. Adequate hemostasis should be assured throughout, and fluid volume must be monitored and corrected as need be.

X-ray films and wound cultures must be taken to clarify the extent of the injury. Neomycin as a topical antibiotic has been applied with success, accompanied with the use of broad-spectrum antibiotics and tetanus prophylaxis.

Awareness and respect of the barracuda's attraction to bright colors or shiny objects is one's best prevention. Appreciation of their pattern of striking any speared fish or flashing light will be valuable preventive action if adhered to.

■ **How should bites precipitated by an eel attack be dealt with medically?**

There are approximately 20 species of moray eels in existence, although the majority are mainly tropical. The California moray is found in the temperate waters of southern California. Although notoriously powerful and vicious biters, morays seldom attack unless provoked (Fig. 8-4).

Wolf eels are located in colder waters and have doglike teeth used for crushing shellfish. Bites are uncommon but do occasionally occur.

In either instance severe lacerations may be sustained from these knifelike or crushing teeth, and eels may retain their bulldog grip until death. Wounds usually are of a tearing, jagged nature, but may also produce a simple puncture. Bleeding may be profuse, and secondary infection is common. It has been reported that an accompanying venomous substance may produce local paralysis.

Treatment principles to be followed are the

---

*All foreign materials should be sent to James R. Stewart, Diving Officer, Scripps Institute of Oceanography, University of California, San Diego, 8602 La Jolla Shores Drive, La Jolla, California 92093, for identification purposes.

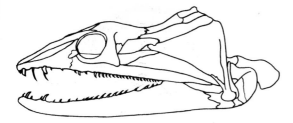

Fig. 8-4. Moray eel.

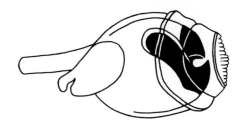

Fig. 8-5. Octopus.

same as for shark bites. Maintenance of body warmth and adequate fluid balance is imperative. The wound should be debrided and injured vessels ligated as soon as feasible. A period of 4 to 6 days should be allowed for the wound to be observed. If infection does not occur, advanced surgical procedures, including primary closure and grafting, should be instituted. Tetanus booster or tetanus antitoxin along with broad-spectrum antibiotic therapy should be administered immediately.

Moray eels, primarily night feeders and bottom dwellers, live in caves or holes under rock ledges. More tropical forms may be found free swimming but are not aggressive. Burrowing eels may also be found, and their habitat and life-style should be respected as they will attack if their domain is intruded upon.

Bites generally occur to individuals who reach under rocks or into holes without first looking. In more tropical areas eels may be seen with only their head protruding from the sandy bottom. Generally, only people who harass these animals or attempt to spear them are bitten. Heavy protective clothing should be worn if contact is possible.

■ How should octopus attacks be assessed and treated?

The hazardous aggressive natures of most octopuses is fictional. For the most part, they are shy and retiring, although their presence might create alarm as some cold water octopuses have a recorded tentacle span of over 25 feet. However, the more commonly found shallow water forms rarely reach over 3 feet in span.

Bites usually consist of two small puncture wounds caused by a parrotlike beak and vary with the size of the animal (Fig. 8-5). They are known to possess some type of venom in salivary secretions, which accounts for a burning, tingling sensation as the initial symptom. This discomfort may radiate from the wound site to encompass the entire appendage. One of the authors (JRS) has been bitten several times by smaller California specimens with no more trauma other than that of the wound itself.

Bleeding may be profuse for the apparent size of the wound, perhaps indicating the presence of an anticoagulant. Swelling, redness, and heat commonly develop in the wound site, and recovery is usually relatively uneventful.

Treatment of octopus wounds is aimed at accomplishing three primary objectives: alleviating pain, combating the effects of the venom, and preventing secondary infection. Pain results from the effects of venom as it is introduced into the wound. The venom, very difficult to remove, often requires incision, suction, and irrigation. Further recommended treatment includes soaking the limb in hot water for from 30 minutes to 1 hour. If a facial wound is sustained, hot, moist compresses should be applied. Antibiotic therapy may be desirable, and tetanus antitoxin is advisable.

In an attempt to prevent these bites, underwater caves of octopuses should be avoided unless one is experienced in the handling of octopuses and then done so only with the use of gloves.

■ What facts should be considered when treating injuries sustained from seals and sea lions?

Wounds produced by these marine animals are similar to those produced by a dog. A puncture rather than a laceration is the usual occurrence.

In addition to the laceration, injuries have been produced by a charging seal bumping a person. Since these animals may attain lengths of 6 feet or more, weights of 250 to 300 pounds, and are capable of swimming at speeds of over 35 miles per hour, the problem is self-evident. Broken bones are frequently sustained as a result of the impact.

Treatment focuses around two areas. In the case of injuries sustained from a bite, specific treatment is identical to that outlined under care of an octopus bite. One addition to be noted is the need for débridement and further cleansing of a laceration following the initial soaking procedure. It may be necessary for the wound to be closed with dermal sutures. However, should the wound be massive, a small drain might be warranted for several days.

During breeding season harem bulls become easily irritated and have been known to bite or physically pursue a swimmer right out of the water and onto the shore. Females with small pups may also pose problems for swimmers. Awareness of this breeding period, with apppropriate distance maintained, is a wise precaution.

MARINE ANIMALS THAT STING

■ **There are a number of stinging injuries caused by marine animals without backbones. What awareness and treatment of them must be noted?**

Numerous marine animals without backbones pose problems as a result of stinging. These animals can be broken down into the following categories representing only those presenting a threat to persons located along the United States coastal waters. They are categorized as follows:

> Coelenterates
> Hydroids
> Jellyfish
> Portuguese man-of-war
> Elk horn coral
> Fire coral or stinging coral
> Sea anemones

The coelenterates, which include hydroids, jellyfish, corals, and sea anemones, possess tentacles equipped with stinging cells known as nematocysts. It is these stinging cells that create the variety of stinging, burning sensations often reported by swimmers and divers (Fig. 8-6).

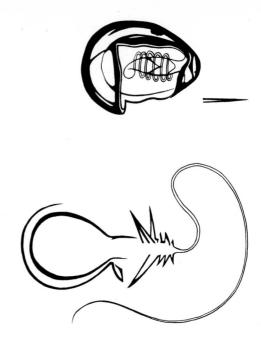

Fig. 8-6. Coelenterates.

Hydroids are generally found growing with a plumelike or feathery appearance and frequently are found attached to rocks, pilings, or seaweed. There are three common stinging members of this group that should be acknowledged—the Portuguese man-of-war, the stinging or fire coral, and the hydroid itself, which may resemble any number of nonstinging gorgonian corals.

The Portuguese man-of-war, a colonial hydroid, is commonly mistaken for a true jellyfish. Floating at the water's surface, this hydroid is found from the Gulf of California throughout the endo-Pacific and Hawaii. It can be recognized by its multiple short, frilled stinging tentacles and a single long "fishing" tentacle that extends for up to 10 meters in length. All the tentacles are suspended from balloonlike floats, usually blue in color.

Jellyfishes of the Scyphozoa class are free-swimming medusae also exhibiting trailing tentacles. Those located along the California coast normally produce only mild skin irritations and do not pose the problems of other species located elsewhere.

In the group Anthozoa only the sea anemone and fire coral are of noteworthy concern. Sea anemones that attach themselves to rocks or other substrata have many growth forms and varying colors. Fire or stinging coral is a coelenterate possessing many growth patterns ranging from upright columnar and fan-shaped designs to encrusting forms. They usually range from mustard brown to light cream in color. Elk horn coral, branches of which might measure 18 inches in length, are found in the Florida Keys, Bahamas, and West Indies and are easily recognized by their whitish, thick, hornlike structure.

Danger from these marine animals occurs on physical contact. When a person brushes against any of the above mentioned, hundreds of stinging cells or nematocysts may either discharge a venom or adhere directly to the skin, resulting in symptoms that vary with the specific species and the affected person. In general, these animals produce only local skin irritations, with commonly occurring symptoms varying from an immediate stinging sensation to a definite burning pain. Although usually localized, the pain may radiate to other parts of the body. The area in contact with the tentacles usually becomes reddened; a blistering skin reaction occurs, and swelling with minute skin hemorrhages may follow. Larger specimens contain a fluid-filled, capsular nematocyst with a hollow, threadlike tube inside. Venom within this capsule is introduced into the skin on contact.

Severe cases may result in shock, muscle cramps, abdominal rigidity, diminished touch and temperature sensation, nausea, vomiting, severe backache, loss of speech, frothing at the mouth, sensation of throat constriction, respiratory difficulty, paralysis, delirium, convulsions, and even death.

Treatment of these patients is focused on relieving pain, alleviating effects of the poison, and controlling primary shock. Direct pressure or freshwater soaks should *not* be applied to the affected areas, as pressure or change in pH will cause the cells that have not discharged to automatically do so. Injuries are best treated with local anesthetic ointment, applications of alcohol, or household ammonia cut to 5% with freshwater. Morphine has been effective in controlling pain, with calcium gluconate being advised in the control of muscle spasms. Oral histamines and topi-

cal preparations may be useful in treating the existing rash. If the eye is affected, a nonaqueous local anesthetic solution should be instilled, followed by a steroid ointment. All aqueous drops should be avoided. Life-support measures may be required should severe reactions occur, recognizing that some patients are more allergy prone than others. To date, no specific antidote has been discovered.

Avoid contact with these types of animals if at all possible. Jellyfish have been known to possess tentacles that trail 50 feet behind the main body, so careful observation is warranted. Some jellyfish that are washed ashore and appear dead still may produce local irritations, although they usually produce no long-term effects. Hydroids and anemones are usually located on the bottom and are not often contacted by swimmers. However, divers should be aware of their presence and should avoid touching them with bare hands. If tentacles adhere to the skin, a towel, rag, seaweed, or sand should be used in assisting with the removal. Swimming on cloudy days or at dusk may hinder one from detecting these animals.

■ **Another category of the venomous marine invertebrates includes annelid worms. What factors are important in the assessment of these injuries?**

Some species within this group have setae that develop into stinging mechanisms, while others possess biting jaws. The bloodworm (Glycera), used by fishermen for bait, is known for its biting jaws and is able to penetrate the skin. Once bitten, the first sensation is much like that of a bee sting. The visible marks from the jaws are oval shaped with a red mark in the center. The area covered by the penetrating jaws is approximately $3/16$ inch in diameter.

The skin surrounding the puncture may develop a whitish appearance. The affected skin often becomes hot and swollen for a day or two, followed by slight numbness and itching that may last up to 1 week. Secondary infection with an increase in swelling and pain and accompanying discharge may develop within hours. There is no specific identification of whether or not a toxin is actually involved. Specific treatment for annelid worms does not differ from that of intervention of fish stings. The bristles are best removed from the skin by use of adhesive tape or by rubbing the area with sand. Calamine lotion, local anesthetic ointments, or steroid cream may relieve the initial discomfort.

Should general reactions become severe, oral antihistamines and systemic steroids may be required. For allergy-prone patients, intravenous hydrocortisone, 100 mg, may be indicated, with adrenaline recommended in allergic bronchospasm and oral antihistamines advised with dermatologic allergies.

Bristles that may be left in the wound have been known to become encapsulated by calcareous deposits and, subsequently, may be scraped out.

The best form of prevention focuses on the avoidance of contact with these animals and cautious awareness when turning over rocks and corals. Protective cotton gloves and clothing should be worn.

■ What venomous marine vertebrates are of notable danger to man?

The specific categories of marine animals with a backbone inflicting injury by stinging include fishes and reptiles. Within this division of fish are included stingrays, of which butterfly rays, California bat rays, and round stingrays are species found off the California coast.

Of additional concern in the fish category noted to be dangerous because of their sting are the following: spiny dogfish, rat fish, sea catfish, toad fish, surgeon fish, star gazer, and scorpion fish. Of all the venomous animals that post a danger to man through their sting, the greatest percentage are attributed to stingrays, with over 1000 stingray wounds occurring in the United States annually. These animals are usually found buried in the sandy, muddy bottoms of coastal shores. It is critical that bathers or persons walking in the water be extremely careful as they are prime victims. Occasionally, abdominal punctures do occur to people while body surfing in shallow water when they are nonobservant of the ocean floor.

Both puncture and lacerated types of wounds occur as a result of stingray contacts. Their barbs vary in length and width, but they all have sawlike edges (Fig. 8-7). In the common round ray the barb may reach a length of 2 inches and a

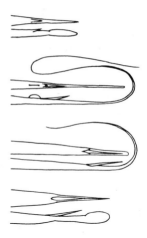

Fig. 8-7. Stingrays (venom organs).

width of ¼ inch. The larger diamond ray, a specimen collected in the San Diego area, possesses a barb 8 inches in length by ⅜ inches in width. The barbs, consisting of a hard, bonelike material, may inflict painful wounds. In most rays the barb lies toward the base of the tail; however, in the round ray, the barb is located toward the tip of the tail. When the tail is lashed upward, the barb is held erect at almost a 90-degree angle to the tail surface and is driven into any object within its reach. As the barb penetrates flesh, its gelatinous sheath tears, allowing venom produced by glands in the barb to enter the wound. It is important to note that rays may possess more than one spine, greatly increasing the danger.

Sharp, intense pain is the primary symptom, manifesting a rapid onset. It is characterized as sharp, shooting, spasmodic, and throbbing in nature, increased over 1 to 2 hours and easing after 6 to 12 hours. More generalized symptoms constitute a drop in blood pressure, nervousness or delirium, vomiting, diarrhea, sweating, vasoconstriction, second- and third-degree atrioventricular block, some respiratory depression, muscle cramps, tremors or paralysis, and even death.

Stingray wounds are identified as either lacerations or punctures. Penetration of the skin produces minimal damage, but withdrawal results in severe tissue damage as a result of the recurved spines. Bleeding may be profuse, followed by a mucoid secretion. Local swelling exists in all cases, accompanied by an ashy appearance that later turns cyanotic and finally reddish in color. Local necroses, ulcerations, and/or secondary infections are common and may produce prolonged incapacity if not treated.

There is no known antidote. Immobilization of the affected part, irrigation of the area, and encouraged minor bleeding from the wound site should be initiated immediately. Immersion of the wound in water as hot as one can tolerate is recommended in order to break down the venom's protein. This process should take 30 to 90 minutes, and Epsom salts may be added during the soaking. All stingray wounds must be investigated to ensure that no portion of the barb or covering sheath is present in the wound. A local anesthetic without adrenaline may be infiltrated into the wound, and systemic analygesics such as codeine or intravenous infusions of 5 ml of 1% procaine in 15 ml isotonic sodium chloride over a 5-minute duration have proved effective.

X-ray films should be taken to assess the area for foreign bodies and bone injury. Surgical intervention is indicated if the injury has involved the pleura, pericardia, or peritoneum. Vital signs including CVP and urinary output must be monitored, and electrolytes, ECG, and EEG recorded as indicated. Débridement, cleansing, and suturing should be carried out as required, depending on the patient's condition. Broad-spectrum antibiotics, along with topical medications, are to be instituted as quickly as possible.

Most wounds occur to careless fishermen who step on a ray, pinning it to the bottom, and allowing it to institute a successful strike. The most effective means of preventing such strikes is for one to shuffle the feet along the bottom or to carry a stick that is used as a probing device.

■ What factors should be remembered when treating catfish wounds?

Catfish in general inhabit freshwater streams of the tropics, but a few species are found along the eastern coast of America. Venomous catfish possess a single, sharp, stout spine located in front of the soft-rayed portion of the dorsal and pectoral fins (Fig. 8-8). These spines are specifically hazardous because they can be locked into an extended position at will. Venom from the cat-

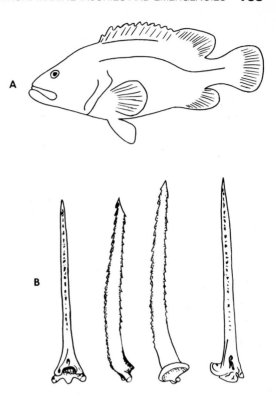

Fig. 8-8. A, Venomous catfish; **B,** fin spines of catfish.

fish is a heat-labile, water-soluble protein that acts as a vasoconstrictor.

The resulting pain, which commences immediately, is characterized as resembling a stinging, throbbing, or scalding sensation that may be localized or radiate up the affected limb. The skin changes from an immediate pallor to cyanotic in appearance, followed by redness and swelling. It has been noted that severe swelling may be accompanied by numbness and gangrene, with shock occurring in some cases. Bleeding has been noted on numerous occasions, and this will reduce subsequent symptoms. In addition, other symptoms might include painful groin or axilla lymph glands; mild anorexia, nausea, or vomiting; shock; and cardiovascular collapse.

A specific antidote is not known, and treatment is directed toward alleviating pain, combating the venomous effects, and preventing secondary infection that may delay healing. Pain persists because of traumatic reactions to the fish spine, venom, and the presence of slime or other irritating materials being introduced into the wound. Considerable soft tissue damage may be present.

Immobilization of the affected limb is recommended, with attempts being made to encourage bleeding. An attempt may be made to incise the wound parallel to the long axis of the limb and to apply suction, but this measure, even though properly executed, at best provides poor results. Prompt irrigation of the wound using sodium bicarbonate is encouraged. Immediate immersion of the body member in extremely hot water (50° C) should be instituted for 30 to 60 minutes in an attempt to break down the protein. Infrared rays may be helpful to replace the heat treatment; 20 minute applications are suggested.

Infiltration of the wound with 0.5% to 2% procaine may prove effective. Should local measures fail, meperidine (Demerol) may be useful. Skin débridement and repeated cleansing might be required. The need for dermal sutures or instillation of a small drain will depend on the severity of the wound. An antibiotic regimen with both local and systemic treatment and a course of tetanus antitoxin is advisable. Primary shock will require life-support measures.

Extreme caution should be taken should these fish require handling. Swimmers or fishermen, when walking in shallow water, should shuffle their feet and always wear protective shoes.

■ **How should scorpion fish injuries be assessed and treated?**

Members of the family Scorpaenidae are found along both coasts, with a wide distribution located off the Pacific coast from central California to the Gulf of California. *Scorpaena phemiera,* one of several closely related species, is found along the Atlantic Coast from Massachusetts to the West Indies. For the most part, these fish are shallow water, bottom dwellers located in bays, along sandy beaches, rocky coastlines, or coral reefs. They appear to be fearless and totally uninterested in their surroundings.

The prime symptom from a scorpion fish sting is pain that is quite severe and may last for several days. Much like that of the stingray in intensity, it is described as being immediate, sharp, and shooting, often radiating from the affected part.

The area surrounding the wound initially appears whitish in color, later turning cyanotic. Tissue becomes swollen, feels hot to the touch, and is often susceptible to secondary infection. Subsequent sloughing of tissues around the wound site may occur. The generalized symptoms produced by the venom may cause nausea, vomiting, malaise, fever, a decrease in arterial pressure, and an increase and then a decrease in CVP, respiratory depression, and abnormal ECG and EEG tracings.

Recommended treatment of scorpion fish stings is the same as has been outlined for the catfish previously, with hot water (50° C) immersion appearing to be the best available treatment. Specific antibiotic treatment with tetracycline has proved effective in treating secondary infections.

The best advice regarding prevention is not to attempt to touch or move these fish and to refrain from placing one's hands in crevices or holes inhabited by these fish. Fishermen should use pliers or hold the fish by its lower jaw.

MARINE PUNCTURES

■ **Echinoderm punctures are fairly common in this country, and their treatment is frequently unfamiliar to practitioners.**

Temperate water West coast sea urchins do not have venom associated with their spines; however, injury frequently occurs from punctures. Most puncture wounds occur to persons walking on urchin-covered rocks, to swimmers who are thrown against urchins by wave action, or to divers either affected by bottom surge throwing them against urchins or persons attempting to lunge for game located in urchin-lined crevices. The injuries that occur are of the puncture type and frequently the spines remain in the wound (Fig. 8-9). In many cases people do not realize the puncture even exists until they leave the water. At that time an intense, burning sensation may occur, followed quickly by redness, swelling, and generalized aching. The ache often extends centrally, involving the entire limb. Lymph glands will then become tender and swollen. Secondary infections may develop with the area sloughing within a few days. In addition to pain a sea urchin sting could possibly cause faintness, numbness, generalized muscular paralysis, loss

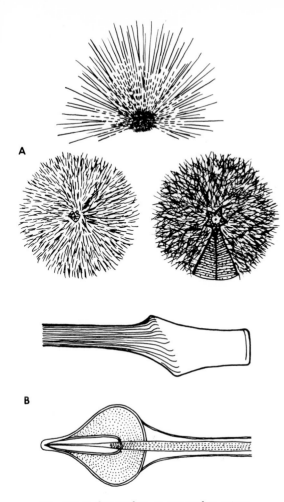

Fig. 8-9. A, Sea urchin; **B,** sea urchin spines.

x-ray assistance is necessary. Additionally, spines not removed may calcify causing long-term discomfort and decreased joint mobility. There frequently is some discoloration surrounding the wound, which is due to the purple dye excreted by the animal and, although cosmetically unpleasant, should not be disturbing. The affected limb should be immobilized, and the spines *must not* be removed. Submersion of the affected part in hot water (50° C) is advised, and advanced life-support measures instituted if breathing or cardiac difficulties develop.

Local anesthesia when administered will result in immediate reduction of pain. X-ray films should be taken to determine foreign bodies, with proper surgical removal following as soon as possible.

Local and broad-spectrum antibiotics will reduce the effects of secondary infections. In the case of respiratory paralysis, proper measures must be taken to maintain normal arterial Po_2, Pco_2, and pH levels. Systemic steroids, adrenaline, or antihistamines are valuable for delayed allergic reactions.

Sea urchins with needlelike spines should not be handled. One must realize that even leather or canvas gloves, shoes, or flippers do not afford protection from these spines.

MARINE REPTILES
■ What marine reptiles are of concern to coastal residents and tourists?

Sea snakes, the most common marine reptile, are primarily found in the tropical Pacific and Indian oceans. With one exception, a single freshwater species found on the Island of Tuzin, Philippines, all the rest are marine reptiles.

The yellow-bellied sea snake has been noted along the Gulf of California, and two specimens have been recorded along the shore islands of the coast of California. Snake bites occur primarily to divers who harass the reptiles, to fishermen while handling their nets, or to people who are wading and accidentally step on the snake.

Sea snakes inflict their wounds with the use of venom fangs, which are maxillary teeth known to be hollow and reduced in size. Most snakes have two fangs on each side of the head located below the eye (Fig. 8-10).

of speech, respiratory distress, and, in some severe cases, death has been recorded. Pain may diminish after 15 minutes, but existing paralysis could last 6 hours or longer. Spines of all temperate-water, West coast species are solid and have blunt ends. Of the four common types, three have smooth spines and one has serrations. If protruding, the spines may be removed gently; however, application of too much force might cause the spines to break off in the skin. When this occurs, urchin spines have been known to migrate inward and to apply pressure to nerves, tendons, or even to enter the area surrounding joints. When this occurs surgical removal with

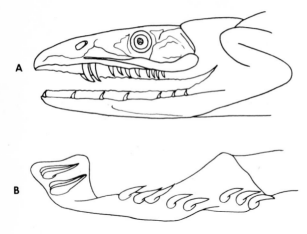

Fig. 8-10. A, Sea snake; **B,** sea snake, right upper jaw.

Symptoms following a bite develop rather slowly, taking from 20 minutes to several hours for full onset. There is usually no pain aside from the initial prick, which causes the victim to dissociate the illness with the bite. The wound site produces no reaction, and initial symptoms include a mild euphoria, some aching, and anxiety. Additional symptoms during this early stage include thickening of the tongue and general muscle stiffness. Paralysis may soon follow and is usually generalized, with lockjaw identified as a predominant accompanying symptom. The pulse may become weak and irregular, and the pupils often may become dilated. Thirst, nausea, and vomiting may be present, accompanied by muscle twitching and spasms. Respiratory distress is pronounced, at which time the victim becomes unconscious. The overall mortality rate is estimated at 25%.

Routine incision with suction is *not* recommended in sea snake bites, and physical exertion, as with all snake bites, is to be avoided. A tourniquet should be applied to the thigh in leg bites and above the elbow in hand bites. This stricture should be released at 30-minute intervals. Snakes should be captured for identification purposes in case they may be found to be harmless.

Sea snake antivenin should be used cautious-

ly and only in the most serious cases. It can be very dangerous to persons who may be allergic to it. Polyvalent land snake antivenin can be used if sea snake antivenin is unavailable.

Bed rest should be maintained throughout the period of time when envenomation is present, followed by close observation for at least 24 hours in case additional antiserum is required. Recommended treatment for possible depressed respirations, renal failure, or cardiovascular shock and convulsions should be adhered to. An adequate fluid and electrolyte balance must be maintained if vomiting or increased diaphoresis is noted. Antibiotic therapy and sedation may be required, and gastric intubation and supportive IV therapy might be required because of lockjaw. Should respiratory paralysis develop, intervention would require intubation, tracheotomy, and respirator support. Once recovery occurs, it is rapid and complete.

Sea snakes are noted to be very docile reptiles, but handling or agitating them should be avoided. While walking along muddy bottoms, one should shuffle the feet in order to provide sufficient escape time for the snake.

SUMMARY

Injuries caused by venomous marine animals, though not frequent, produce severe reactions and concern in the victims. Practitioners confronted with intervention of these problems frequently must seek consultative advice—which requires time. Tissue, limb, and life are all in jeopardy when this occurs. It is the hope of the authors that this information will be of value to the reader in expediting proper assessment and intervention of their patients.

REFERENCE

1. Edmonds, C.: Dangerous marine animals of the Indo-Pacific region, Newport, Victoria, Australia, n.d., Wedneil Publications.

BIBLIOGRAPHY

Halstead, B. W.: Dangerous marine animals, Cambridge, Maryland, 1959, Cornell Maritime Press.
Russell, F. E.: Poisonous marine animals, New York, 1971, Academic Press, Inc.

CHAPTER 9

In-hospital emergency care of the critically injured

Teresa L. Romano and David R. Boyd

The Industrial Revolution began the mechanization of our society; with the greater use of machines there has been an increase in the number of serious injuries from vocational and recreational activities. In 1972 the National Safety Council reported 11 million injuries from all types of accidents. Wage losses, medical expenses, and insurance administrative costs resulting from trauma totaled $13.5 billion. The estimated overall cost of this pandemic is over $30 billion annually. In the United States there are about 100,000 civilian accidental deaths annually, of which one half are the result of vehicular accidents. The one-millionth traffic fatality occurred in 1951 and, if the present rate continues, the two-millionth victim will die by 1976. Accidents are currently the third most common cause of death in the United States, the accidental death rate being only slightly less than those of cardiovascular disease and cancer. Trauma is the leading cause of death in individuals under 40 years of age.[1] There are over 15 million injuries to children under 14 years of age annually, and of these 16,000 are fatal. Trauma is the commonest cause of death in children, the peak incidence occurring in children from 2 to 3 years of age. One third of all hospital admissions, approximately 2 million a year, are the result of accidents. In one study pediatric patients accounted for 47% of all emergency room visits, and of these one fourth were treated for trauma.[2]

The continually increasing incidence and magnitude of serious injuries resulting from high-speed transportation, complex industrial equipment, civil disturbances, and unpredictable mass catastrophes necessitates a reevaluation and reeducation concerning the priorities and techniques of trauma patient care. Changing patterns of traumatic injuries of all types and newer developments in the surgical subspecialties and biomedical disciplines have been responsible for major progress in the field of trauma management.

Trauma care is team care. The functions of the team begin in the prehospital phase and may appropriately be performed by specialized physicians, nurses, and allied health professionals such as emergency medical technicians or paramedics. This chapter elucidates some of the key aspects of resuscitation and initial treatment of the injured patient to be carried out in the emergency department, with emphasis on the team concept.

■ What are the priorities in the emergency management of the trauma patient?

The outcome after severe trauma depends on two basic factors: availability of initial medical care and adequacy of early therapeutic measures. The first objective in examining an injured person is the preservation of life. Resuscitation and proper evaluation of life-endangering injuries are critical to survival. Injudicious or inadequate emergency management can result in unnecessary fatality or permanent disability.

169

When dealing with acute trauma, it is impossible to separate diagnostic and therapeutic measures. Resuscitation is not dependent on an etiologic diagnosis. Airway obstruction, shock, and cardiorespiratory failure often must be treated without knowledge of the precipitating cause of these disorders. Once the patient's functions are stable, rapid and thorough evaluation of the cause of these derangements is in order. Patients with complex, multiple-system injuries often require the skills of many specialists. In these cases it is essential that one practitioner assume the role of the patient's primary physician. This person remains in charge during the entire course of the illness and coordinates the efforts of other consultants utilizing established priorities. This team concept is carried through the operative and acute posttraumatic period. When the patient can be safely managed by one specialist, the individual is then released to that practitioner's care. Patients may need to be moved to a more distant facility or to other remote areas in the hospital, such as the x-ray department, for additional evaluation and treatment. During this period they should be continuously observed by a physician, nurse, or highly qualified emergency medical technician. Once stabilized, the patient can be moved to the intensive care unit for additional monitoring or to the operating room, as indicated. Also, transportation to distant specialty centers can be safely performed when the patient is fully resuscitated.

■ **What are the factors leading to airway obstruction in the injured patient and what are the essential steps in establishing and maintaining an adequate airway?**

Patients with depressed consciousness from intoxication, cerebral injury, or shock have a high risk of aspiration of blood, food, vomitus, and dentures. Insertion of an oropharyngeal airway after aspiration and removal of any foreign bodies is the first consideration. The patient must be observed closely and suctioning performed frequently. The patient must not lie unattended flat on the back or be restrained in this position. A semiprone position is more satisfactory. Two common causes of upper airway obstruction are bleeding of and edema of the mouth, tongue, posterior pharyn-

geal wall, and epiglottis. Penetrating wounds of these parts are particularly dangerous. Cervical spine injuries producing vertebral subluxation and retropharyngeal hematoma can also compromise the upper airway. Severe maxillofacial trauma with obliteration of the nasal passage will contribute to these problems. Respiratory distress with stridor, a contusion of the neck, and a history of steering wheel injury may indicate the presence of a fractured larynx or trachea. Endotracheal intubation will be unsuccessful in such a case, and emergency tracheostomy is necessary. A patient exhibiting only abdominal breathing may have a cervical vertebral dislocation and spinal cord injury. Any manipulation before stabilizing the neck may complete a partial transection of the spinal cord. Vascular injuries in the neck producing hematomas may compress the airway and require intubation. Patients must be examined for evidence of sucking chest wounds, flail chest, tension pneumothorax, hemothorax, simple pneumothorax, or contused lungs. Airway obstruction (suction and intubation) and respiratory insufficiency (oxygen and positive pressure ventilation) must be relieved. Patients who are combative because of hypoxia can be intubated by using a rapidly acting neuromuscular depolarizing agent. Primary tracheostomy is almost never indicated today, except for patients with major upper airway obstruction from severe facial trauma, massive soft tissue trauma, or cervical vertebral dislocation. Although tracheostomy is relatively easy in a nonemergency situation, it is extremely risky in patients who are restless and agitated from hypoxia. Primary endotracheal intubation followed by controlled tracheostomy is the safest approach.

■ **What is the esophageal obturator and what are the in-hospital implications of its use?**

The esophageal obturator is a recently developed apparatus used to establish and maintain a patent airway. The obturator consists of three main parts: the mask, the tube, and the balloon. The mask is used to seal off the nose and mouth and to anchor the airway. The tube, which is blocked at the distal end, contains perforations in the area of the pharynx through which air escapes and is forced into the trachea (the only unblocked opening). The 30 cc balloon when inflated prevents aspiration of vomitus and inflation of the stomach by forced ventilation.

The esophageal obturator is being used primarily in prehospital resuscitations usually by paramedical personnel. It is easily inserted, requiring no special insertion equipment and very little specialized training. It can also be placed in patients with suspected cervical spine injuries without hyperextending or flexing the neck.

It can be inserted in 5 to 30 seconds and allows air intake equal to that found in endotracheal intubation. These advantages make the esophageal obturator ideal for field use by paramedics. Although not as widely used, the obturator would also be an ideal adjunct for airway management by nurses in rural emergency departments without full-time physician staff.

Once the patient arrives in the emergency department with the obturator in place, an endotracheal tube can be inserted around it, facilitating this sometimes difficult task. If the patient has effective spontaneous respirations and the obturator is to be removed, always deflate the balloon *first* by removing the air with a syringe. The patient should be turned on his/her side to avoid aspiration, and suction should be ready.

■ **What can cause cardiac arrest in trauma?**

Severe hypoxia and profound metabolic acidosis are probably the most common causes of cardiac arrest associated with trauma. In addition, direct trauma to the heart may cause cardiac tamponade or cardiac arrest. In rare cases a fatal arrhythmia may be triggered by indirect trauma. Standard cardiac arrest procedures must be instituted immediately if arrest occurs. Mouth-to-mouth resuscitation must be employed immediately, followed by endotracheal intubation. Closed chest massage is preferred and is effective except when the chest wall is unstable, as in flail chest. In such cases, emergency thoracotomy and manual cardiac compression may be necessary. Ventilation with an Ambu (manual ventilator) bag and oxygen are provided while cardiac compression is carried out. Metabolic acidosis is corrected with the IV administration of sodium bicarbonate. Initial and periodic arterial blood gas and pH analyses are essential. ECG monitoring

is mandatory. Cardiac defibrillation may be needed, since a hypoxic and acidotic heart is prone to arrhythmias, fibrillation, and asystole.

■ **What are the acceptable methods of hemorrhage control in the injured patient?**

Direct manual pressure over the bleeding site can control most external hemorrhage. Continued gentle pressure is often all that is necessary until the patient is taken to the operating room, where vascular repair may be necessary. There is no place for the application of tourniquets or clamping and ligation of bleeding vessels, as further injury may ensue. The possibility of loss of blood within the body cavities must be evaluated; thoracentesis and paracentesis will help establish the diagnosis of such hemorrhage.

■ **What is the antishock suit and what is its application for hemorrhage control?**

The antishock suit, popularly known as MAST Trousers or Air Pants, is a three-chambered trouser garment made of double-layered polyurethane. The suit fits over the lower body and once inflated provides external pressure of 104 mm Hg. This external pressure serves to redirect the available circulating blood volume out of the lower extremities and into the central circulation, providing vital organs with needed oxygenated blood. The circumferential pressure of the antishock trousers provides, in essence, an autotransfusion of about 1000 ml of blood within 2 minutes of application. It also immobilizes the lower extremity injuries and reduces further blood loss by direct pressure. The suit contains three separate chambers (two legs and an abdomen). Each can be inflated or deflated independently as necessary.

Antishock trousers are used on patients with major trauma and signs of hypovolemic shock. Their most frequent use has been in the prehospital phase, applied and monitored by specially trained emergency medical technicians or paramedics.

The use of this garment is usually reserved for the management of injuries to the abdomen or lower body but can also be used with upper extremity injuries if bleeding has been controlled. Since it causes an increase in intrathoracic and intracranial pressure, it is contraindicated in such conditions as pulmonary congestion, head injuries, chest trauma, or uncontrolled bleeding from the chest, head, or upper extremities.

However, if hypovolemia exists and is uncontrollable by other measures, the suit might be a lifesaving measure. Its use would therefore override any contraindications. The suit is *not* indicated in shock states where hypovolemia cannot be established as the cause.

Since the suit is a stabilization procedure and does not correct underlying pathology, all routine procedures for the management of a trauma patient should be instituted concurrently. These would include airway management, control of bleeding, replacement of intravenous solutions, and notification of the surgical team.

Removal of the suit causes a prompt drop in circulating blood volume, which can cause sudden circulatory collapse. For this reason, the antishock trousers cannot be removed until the surgical team is ready for the patient. To prevent an uninformed person from removing the suit and injuring the patient, the emergency department nurse must ensure that *all* personnel from the emergency department, radiology, and surgery are oriented to the suit and understand its use.

■ How can blood loss be assessed and appropriate volume replacement and treatment be determined?

Once hemostasis has been obtained, blood volume must be restored. Major blood loss must be replaced by blood. The magnitude of blood loss can be estimated by clinical observation. Keen observation of physiologic signs and an accurate assessment of all potential injuries can provide a working basis for initiating shock therapy and blood replacement. The severity of traumatic hemorrhage can be effectively graded or categorized into minor (I), moderate (II), major (III), and massive (IV) for initial assessment and to anticipate immediate treatments.[3] Subsequent patient improvement or failure of an adequate treatment response can be measured and reassessed in relationship to these shock-hemorrhage categories.

Minor blood loss

The normal circulating blood volume in a 150-pound (70 kg) adult is approximately 5 L. Small injuries with minor (grade I) blood loss of less than 10% to 15% (500 to 750 ml) may cause no apparent physiologic changes. This type of hemorrhage may be caused by blood donation, a laceration, or bleeding into a distal extremity fracture site. The treatment is simply control of further hemorrhage and blood replacement by crystalloid solution (Table 9-1 shown on p. 173).

Moderate blood loss

A moderate (grade II) hemorrhagic loss of 15% to 30% of the circulating blood volume (750 to 1500 ml) should be well compensated for in most individuals who are otherwise healthy. The injured patient with this degree of injury should demonstrate many of the visible signs of physiologic compensation (Table 9-1, grade II): cool skin, slight tachycardia (110 beats/min), tachypnea (24 respirations/min), a fall in pulse pressure, and possibly a small decrease in systolic blood pressure. These effects are caused by significant injuries such as ruptured spleen or a major femoral shaft fracture. Treatment is by hemorrhage control and the rapid infusion of blood substitutes, that is, crystalloid and colloid solutions (plasma or albumin). Oxygen should be administered by mask. If hemorrhage is controlled, blood replacement will not be required, and the infusion of 2 to 3 L of crystalloid and colloid solutions will suffice.

Major blood loss

Major (Table 9-1, grade III) hemorrhage with a loss of 30% to 45% of the effective circulating blood volume (1500 to 2250 ml) will cause marked physiologic decompensation. This classic "shock" patient has cold, clammy skin, is restless, and exhibits tachycardia (120 beats/min), tachypnea (32 respirations/min), and hypotension (less than 80 mm Hg); oliguria and a marked metabolic acidosis will also be present.

Obvious points of external loss from a major vessel or severe internal injuries (lacerated liver or pelvic fractures) should be the suspected lesions. Whole blood replacement for resuscitation must be included in addition to those measures just discussed. Bicarbonate ($NaHCO_3$) must be administered to combat the metabolic acidosis of shock, and these patients will need to have repeated physiologic monitoring of systolic blood

Table 9-1. Classification and treatment of hemorrhagic shock*

Grade	Clinical findings	Etiology		Treatment
		External loss	Internal loss	
I—minor blood loss, 10%-15% of blood volume (500-750 ml)	Well compensated; dizziness; tachycardia (100 beats/min)	Blood donation; laceration	Hematoma; extremity fracture; hemothorax	Control of hemorrhage; crystalloid infusion
II—moderate blood loss, 15%-30% of blood volume (750-1500 ml)	Partial compensation; cool, sweating skin; thirst, anxiety; tachycardia (110 beats/min); tachypnea (24 respirations/ min); slight hypotension (90-100 mm Hg); decrease in pulse pressure	Major laceration	Visceral injury (for example, spleen rupture); fractured femur	Control of hemorhage; crystalloid and colloid infusion; oxygen administration; evaluation of obscure bleeding
III—major blood loss, 30%-45% of blood volume (1500-2250 ml)	Decompensation; pale, cold, clammy skin; restless, agitation; tachycardia (120 beats/min); tachypnea (32 respirations/min); hypotension (80 mm Hg); oliguria (30 ml/hr); metabolic acidosis	Vascular injury	Visceral injuries (for example, liver rupture); pelvic fracture	Control of hemorrhage; crystalloid, colloid, and blood infusion; oxygen and bicarbonate administration; physiologic monitoring
IV—severe blood loss, 45% of blood volume (over 2250 ml)	"In extremis"—marked pallor, cyanosis; semiconscious; tachycardia (over 120 beats/min); respiratory distress; profound hypotension (60 mm Hg); anuria; metabolic acidosis	Traumatic amputation	Vascular (for example, aortic rupture); multiple injuries	Control of hemorrhage; oxygen administration; blood, colloid, and crystalloid infusion; bicarbonate administration; cardiac monitoring; antibiotics

*Modified from Boyd, D. R.: S. Afr. J. Surg. **11:**163-175, 1973.

pressure and central venous pressure (CVP), urinary output, hematocrit, and arterial blood gas concentrations. The seriously ill patient can be effectively resuscitated if therapy is appropriate to a sound diagnosis, a correct interpretation of the physiologic derangements, and those pathophysiologic signs that are readily detectable by the astute clinician.

Massive blood loss

Massive (Table 9-1, grade IV), or severe, blood loss is a catastrophic situation wherein the extent of loss (over 45%) has gone uncorrected and the patient is first seen in extremis. The physiologic compensatory mechanisms have failed, and many have developed pathologic characteristics and are effecting further detriment to the patient.

The patient may be cyanotic with marked pallor, have a severe and irregular tachycardia, experience respiratory distress, exhibit marked hypotension (less than 50 mm Hg), and have complete anuria. Patients with catastrophic losses of over 45% of their effective circulating blood volume are severely prostrated, hypoxic, and unresponsive. These patients, if not vigorously resuscitated, will progress to cardiopulmonary arrest.

Massive trauma and shock are associated with decreased function of the reticuloendothelial system, so that during the early posttraumatic period the ability of the body to clear bacteria from the circulation is depressed. Prophylactic antibiotic therapy may be indicated in these circumstances.

Multiple severe trauma will cause these effects, but more importantly such injuries and even lesser trauma can deteriorate to this state if hemorrhage is not initially controlled and physiologic therapy is not correctly administered. These patients, unfortunately, often represent a "systems failure" or a "patient management failure," wherein the proper trauma care was not given early enough to prevent this deteriorated state.

■ What are important considerations in blood volume replacement in shock?

For initial volume replacement infusion of moderate volumes of a buffered saline solution (Ringer's lactate) is satisfactory. It is necessary to replace approximately two to three times as much of this crystalloid solution as the estimated amount of blood lost. The oxygen-carrying capacity of hemoglobin is diminished by the hemodilution. It is safe in most patients without previous cardiovascular disease to maintain the hematocrit at 30% to 35%. There has been considerable argument about the equilibration period for blood after hemorrhage. The hematocrit determination has certain limitations during acute changes, but serial measurements provide valuable information about hypovolemic shock. No other parameter, including blood volume determinations, has proved to be more helpful during this acute period.[4] The management of shock is facilitated by repeated observations of blood pressure, heart rate, respiratory rate, skin temperature, CVP, and urinary output. An increase in systolic blood pressure and a decrease in pulse and respiratory rates herald successful resuscitation. A return of normal skin temperature and urinary output and improved state of consciousness attests to the restoration of adequate tissue perfusion.

■ How is the CVP used in the patient in shock?

CVP monitoring is one of the most significant advances in the management of shock patients. An IV catheter is inserted into the superior vena cava. A venous blood sample is taken for type, cross match, blood counts, and biochemical tests, and an infusion of Ringer's lactate solution is started. The CVP is monitored intermittently through the catheter in the superior vena cava using a simple water manometer. The pressure readings are not a measure of "blood volume"; instead, they reflect a dynamic state between the adequacy of the venous return and the pumping action of the right ventricle. Absolute values are not as important as relative changes observed over periods of time. Typically in hypovolemic shock the CVP is below the normal values of 4 to 8 cm of saline solution. With adequate volume replacement a rise in CVP and systolic blood pressure is observed. A persistently low CVP after adequate volume replacement should stimulate a search for occult bleeding. Blood losses into fracture sites, especially the major long bones or pelvis, occult rupture of the liver or spleen, and collections in silent areas such as the pleural cavity and the retroperitoneal space must be considered. An elevated CVP and low systemic blood pressure suggest a pericardial tamponade, myocardial infarction, or acute congestive heart failure. Changes in the quality of the heart tones, cardiac rhythm, ECG findings, and the response to volume loading are helpful in this diagnostic dilemma.

All patients with blood loss, chest injury, or major trauma should have a CVP catheter inserted and serial measurements taken.

■ What are the advantages and disadvantages of the commonly employed volume replacement fluids?
Crystalloids

The use of crystalloid solutions in initial volume replacement has become an acceptable clinical practice. Normal saline solution (0.9% NaCl) and buffered salt solutions (Ringer's lactate) are inexpensive, stable in storage, readily available, free of immediate reactions, and do not require any special matching prior to use. There are theoretical advantages to using the buffered salt solutions, and they are preferred even though they contain a small (28 mEq/L) amount of lactate. This small amount of lactate is inconsequential when compared to the massive amounts of lactate produced by the body during shock. As the circulation is restored, the lactate is readily converted by the liver to bicarbonate and excreted as carbon dioxide by the lungs. Noncolloid salt solutions rapidly diffuse out of the circulation to the extravascular extracellular space, so that two and one-half to four times the amount of blood lost must be infused as crystalloid solutions to restore the blood volume.

The effects of dilution on the hemoglobin and plasma protein concentrations are factors limiting the use of crystalloid solutions. It is desirable to maintain the hematocrit above 30% and the total protein in excess of 6 g/100 ml. At these values the oxygen-carrying capacity and oncotic pressure of the blood will protect against further hyp-

oxia and tissue edema. There is no place for salt-free crystalloid solutions (dextrose in water) in primary resuscitation. When given in the early posttraumatic state, the water is retained because of the action of antidiuretic hormone, and hypo-osmolality results.

Colloids

Table 9-2 illustrates the types of colloids currently used in volume replacement and the advantages and disadvantages of each.

Table 9-2. Types of colloids used in volume replacement*

Category/definition	Solution	Advantages	Disadvantages	Use
Colloids: Solutions containing high molecular weight particles; remain in intravascular fluid compartment exerting osmotic pressure to expand plasma volume	Whole blood	Oxygen-carrying capacity Provides plasma proteins Restores some clotting factors if fresh Very fresh blood contains viable platelets	Hepatitis risk Expensive Limited supply 21-day storage life Deficient in clotting factors and platelets High potassium and acid content Degenerated platelets and white blood cells have been blamed for wet lung and disseminating intravascular coagulopathy Cold blood requires warming Citrated stored blood binds ionized calcium Type and cross match necessary except in dire emergencies where O negative uncross matched or type specific uncross matched blood is used. O positive can also be used for men and for women past childbearing age if O negative unobtainable Possible transfusion reactions	To replace blood loss of 1000 ml or more

*From Romano, T. L.: J. Emergency Nurs. **3:**51, 1977.

Continued.

Table 9-2. Types of colloids used in volume replacement—cont'd

Category/ definition	Solution	Advantages	Disadvantages	Use
Colloids—cont'd				
	Active blood component therapy Albumin	No hepatitis risk Easily stored Exerts osmotic pressure	Infuses slowly For massive hemorrhage would require a large amount Nonoxygen carrying Does not provide clotting factors Transient effect is used alone Increases tendency toward respiratory failure	Concurrently with crystalloids as a blood volume expander Increases colloidal osmotic pressure
	Packed cells	More red blood cell mass than white Oxygen-carrying capacity Less acid and potassium load than whole blood Increased hematocrit Minimum antigen-antibody level	Expensive Some hepatitis risk Deficient in clotting factors 21-day storage limitation	To replace red blood cell mass To improve utilization of blood products
	Plasma (single donor or pooled)	Exerts osmotic pressure Physiologically similar to body plasma	Expensive Hepatitis risk is great Deficient in clotting factors Platelet deficient Nonoxygen carrying	Plasma volume expander To replace plasma lost in burns To combat hemorrhage when whole blood is not immediately available
	Fresh frozen plasma	Physiologically similar to body plasma Exerts osmotic pressure Has clotting factors (except platelets)	Expensive Takes 20 min to thaw Decreased factor V levels after 2 mo Hepatitis factor Nonoxygen carrying Thrombocytopenic bleeding can occur	Plasma volume expander To provide clotting factors
	Plasma protein fraction (Plasmanate)	Easily stored Physiologically similar to body plasma A source of protein Prolonged blood volume expansion	Expensive Nonoxygen carrying Platelet deficient	See Plasma

Table 9-2. Types of colloids used in volume replacement—cont'd

Category/definition	Solution	Advantages	Disadvantages	Use
Artificial colloids: Colloid-like solutions of large carbohydrate molecules that stay in the intravascular space exerting osmotic pressure to expand plasma volume	Dextran 70 (Macrodex) Gentran, Expandex Dextran 40, low molecular weight dextran (LMWD), Rheomacrodex	Effective plasma volume expander Shelf storage Inexpensive Some evidence of reducing sludging of red blood cells and increasing blood flow to microcirculation units	May cause clotting deficiencies Possibility of renal toxicity Possibility of allergic reaction Interferes with coagulation and testing for coagulation defects Interferes with typing and cross-matching procedures May cause increased hemorrhage and hematoma formation by reducing platelet aggregation. Should not be used with known bleeding tendencies, clotting factor deficiency, or oliguria Dextran 40 may create fluid overload because of rapid volume expansion. Contraindicated for patients with overhydration or congestive heart failure	Last choice of available blood substitutes As supplement to crystalloid infusion for plasma volume expansion Dextran 40 exerts osmotic pressure for 6-8 hr; dextran 70 for 24 hr Dextran 70 useful to reduce transcapillary fluid leak into interstitial spaces during sepsis; expands volume slightly in excess of volume infused; maximum recommended infusion is 500 cc for 24 hr Dextran 40 expands volume by twice the volume infused. Improves tissue perfusion by expanded intravascular volume and by decreasing blood viscosity

■ **What drugs are commonly needed in treating the injured patient?**

In shock decreased tissue blood flow and oxygenation lead to anaerobic glycolysis. Excess lactic and pyruvic acids are produced and enter the circulation. The metabolism of these organic acids by the liver is depressed, and metabolic acidosis supervenes.

Sodium bicarbonate (5%) is an extracellular buffer effective in combating this acidosis and is available in 500 ml bottles. Rapid changes in blood pH may be induced and cause cardiac arrhythmias, so that patients receiving rapid infusions of buffers must be monitored by continuous ECG's.

Maintenance of adequate urinary output (over 30 ml/hr) is a prime aim in the management of shock and major trauma. In shock sympathetic compensatory mechanisms cause a decrease in renocortical blood flow and a marked elevation of circulating antidiuretic hormone (ADH), promoting increased water reabsorption from the distal tubule. Effective circulating plasma volume is thus conserved. When hypovolemia is inadequately treated, or when circulating tissue debris (hemoglobin and myoglobin) is filtered but not cleared from the tubules because of decreased urine flow, renal shutdown may result. Osmotic or chemical diuretics in addition to volume replacement should be employed early when renal function is precarious or when frank failure is suspected. Mannitol, a monosaccharide that is filtered but not reabsorbed by the kidney, induces an obligate excretion of filtered water that helps maintain renal tubular flow and patency. Up to 100 ml of 20% mannitol solution may be infused rapidly, and the infusion may be repeated within the next hour if diuresis is not established. Mannitol also acts as a plasma expander; the CVP must be monitored during therapy. If no response is obtained to mannitol, ethacrynic acid (50 mg) or furosemide (10 to 20 mg) may be given. These agents also may be repeated within 1 to 2 hours. The effectiveness of diuretic agents is dependent on an adequate circulating blood volume. Neither approach (osmotic or chemical) will be effective in hypovolemia.

Should a urinary output be initiated, an attempt should be made to maintain the hourly volume at over 60 ml/hr. Urine specific gravity, which is simple to measure, or urine osmolality, determined by the freezing point depression method, is a guide to the efficacy of therapy and helps in estimating the functional status of the kidneys. A high urine specific gravity (over 1.025) or osmolality (700 mOsm/kg) indicates persistent hypovolemia; a low specific gravity (under 1.010) or osmolality (150 mOsm/kg) may mean overinfusion. An isosmotic value (specific gravity 1.010 or osmolality 300 mOsm/kg) may represent the effect of diuretics or be the first sign of loss of concentrating function and impending tubular failure. Further fluid or diuretic therapy may be chosen intelligently by comparing serial serum and urine osmolality measurements. Mannitol and chemical diuretics can be given intermittently each 6 to 8 hours as necessary to maintain adequate urine flow.

Release of endogenous catecholamines is maximal after major trauma and hemorrhage. The adrenal medulla secretes large quantities of norepinephrine, causing increased arteriolar tone, increased peripheral resistance, and diminished flow in the vascular beds of the skin and viscera. Administration of vasoconstrictor agents only augments this pathophysiologic state, causing further cellular hypoxia, anaerobic glycolysis, and lactic acid production. The basic defect in traumatic and hemorrhagic shock is a blood volume deficit. Therapy must be directed toward correction of this primary defect. Vasoconstrictors may be helpful in other conditions associated with disturbances in vascular reactivity, for example, neurogenic, cardiac, septic, or anaphylactic shock. Norepinephrine (Levophed), 1 ampule (0.4 mg), or metaraminol (Aramine), 10 ml vial (100 mg), may be given in 1000 ml of crystalloid solution initially infused at a rate of 1 ml/min and titrated to produce a systolic blood pressure of 100 mm Hg. It is mandatory that hypovolemia be entirely ruled out as the cause of hypotension prior to administration of any vasoconstricting agent.

Theoretically the use of drugs to block the intensive sympathetic vasoconstriction observed in shock would allow blood flow to return to previously ischemic, hypoxic, and acidotic tissues. Prior to administering vasodilating agents, blood volume must be restored and volume repletion continued concomitantly with administration of the drug. Without these precautions the patient may develop total peripheral collapse, for as tissue beds are opened up pharmacologically there must be adequate circulating volume available to fill the expanded system. Of the clinically available vasodilating drugs, chlorpromazine (Thorazine) given by the IV route every 2 to 3 hours (5 to 15 mg) will produce an appreciable change in tissue perfusion, at least in terms of skin temperature and color.

In most cases of traumatic shock one is dealing with an otherwise normal myocardium that has become hypoxic. Digitalization is not usually needed, since heart function will improve with successful treatment of the blood volume deficit. However, older patients who may have underlying primary myocardial disease, patients who develop a very rapid tachycardia that persists after volume replacement, and certainly those patients who develop cardiac failure or exhibit a high CVP with a low systemic blood pressure are candidates for digitalis therapy. The serum potassium concentration must be measured before giving digitalis. The rapidly acting cardiac drugs lanatoside C (Cedilanid) and digoxin are preferred. Contraindications to digitalization include the presence of conduction abnormalities (partial or complete heart block) and irritability of the myocardium (ventricular ectopic beats or ventricular tachycardia).

Isoproterenol (Isuprel) has both inotropic and chronotropic effects on the heart, that is, it increases both contractility and heart rate. Isoproterenol also stimulates β-receptor sites in peripheral muscle beds, causing vasodilation and improved flow to these tissues. The total effect is a decreased blood pressure and peripheral resistance and an increased cardiac output. A serious drawback to the use of isoproterenol is that many patients develop a tachycardia (over 140 beats/min) and administration of the drug must be decreased or discontinued.

■ **How much sodium bicarbonate is necessary to reverse the acidosis of shock?**

After major blood loss and shock, tissue anoxia results in an increased concentration of lactic acid in the blood. Accumulation of hydrogen ion causes a fall in blood pH. Usually there is an attempt to compensate for this by increased ventilation, permitting excretion of hydrogen ion from carbonic acid (as water and carbon dioxide). In a typically severe case the arterial blood pH is 7.30 or below, and the Pco_2 is 28 or below. Using standard nomograms (Sigaard-Andersen), the degree of metabolic acidosis is expressed as a base deficit (-10 to -20 mEq/L) (Figs. 9-1 and 9-2). For adequate replacement the milliequivalent of bicarbonate needed is equal to the base deficit (milliequivalents per liter) multiplied by body weight in kilograms by the bicarbonate space factor of 0.30, as in the following formula[5]:

Bicarbonate (mEq) =
    Base deficit (mEq/L) × Body weight (kg) × 0.30

■ **Besides obvious external hemorrhage, what are the possible etiologies of shock in the trauma patient?**

Blood loss from fractures, especially of the long bones or pelvis, occult rupture of the liver or spleen, and collections of blood in "silent areas" such as the pleural cavity and the retroperitoneal space must be considered. Blood loss into tissues around fracture sites may be deceptive. A fracture of the femoral shaft may cause the loss of 2 to 4 pints of blood, but a pelvic fracture may result in the loss of 10 or more pints. Hematuria, hemoptysis, bloody nasogastric suction, or rectal bleeding are other possible sources of blood loss. Most injuries causally related to shock are either obvious on careful inspection or can be diagnosed by simple measures. Paracentesis, thoracentesis, intravenous pyelography (IVP), and endoscopy will indicate most occult bleeding sites. Inability to restore blood pressure and circulating volume in an acutely traumatized patient by adequate blood volume replacement indicates that a source of uncontrolled hemorrhage is present. Continuing major hemorrhage is seen commonly in liver, retroperitoneal, and vascular injuries. Further attempts to stabilize the circulation in such cases will be unsuccessful and may cause the death of the patient. Patients with such injuries often must be taken to the operating room in shock and exploratory procedures performed for direct access to the sources of bleeding.

■ **What are the steps to take following resuscitation of the injured patient?**

After successful resuscitation the critically ill trauma patient must be continually evaluated for the possible deterioration of any vital function. The assessment includes careful observation of the level of consciousness, spontaneous motion of the extremities, chest excursion, abdominal habitus, and injured regions. A total clinical evaluation is performed. All patients are disrobed and totally examined, including a complete physical examination. Deformities or asymmetry of body parts, lacerations, and contusions demand special attention. A rapid assessment of the extent of injuries is performed by gentle but firm palpation of all body parts, especially those areas where injuries are suspected. Palpation of the scalp, facial bones, trachea, and vertebral column as well as gentle compression of the thorax, ribs, pelvis, and extremities will expose hidden fractures and dislocations and lead to intelligent and precise requests for x-ray films to be taken. Local tenderness, crepitation of subcutaneous air, and grating of bony parts will suggest a diagnosis. The chest is auscultated for signs of pleural collapse, rub, and effusion. Changes in heart tones and the occurrence of murmurs in the chest or over extremities will be diagnostic of vascular injuries. A careful abdominal examination for peritoneal irritation and distention is mandatory. Rectal and pelvic examinations are routinely per-

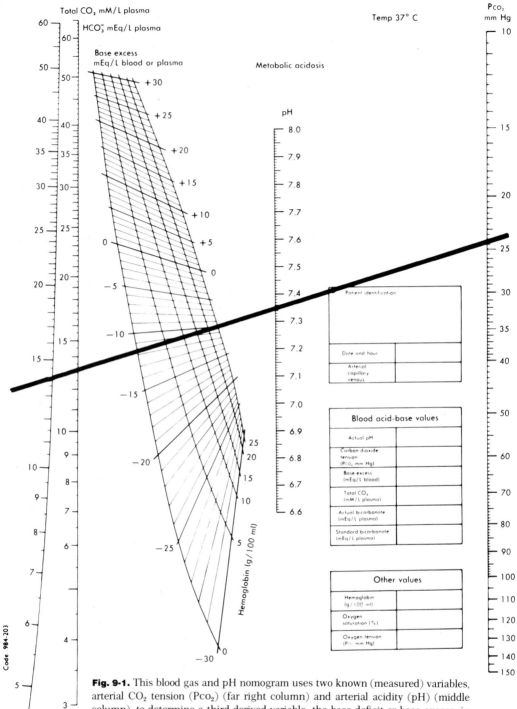

Fig. 9-1. This blood gas and pH nomogram uses two known (measured) variables, arterial CO_2 tension (Pco_2) (far right column) and arterial acidity (pH) (middle column), to determine a third derived variable, the base deficit or base excess, in milliequivalents per liter of blood (middle hatched area). Base changes are affected slightly by hemoglobin levels, hence grid to account for possible effects of hemoglobin in any clinical setting. Alignment of this shock patient's Pco_2 (24 mm Hg) and pH (7.35) results in base deficit of 11 mEq/L (read as −11 at 15 g/100 ml of red blood cell hemoglobin).

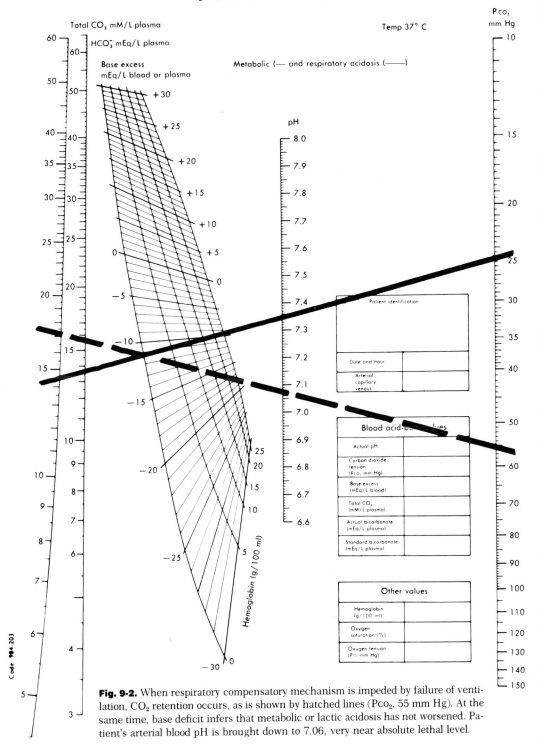

Fig. 9-2. When respiratory compensatory mechanism is impeded by failure of ventilation, CO_2 retention occurs, as is shown by hatched lines (Pco₂, 55 mm Hg). At the same time, base deficit infers that metabolic or lactic acidosis has not worsened. Patient's arterial blood pH is brought down to 7.06, very near absolute lethal level.

formed. Checking palpable pulse, temperature, and neuromuscular tone of all extremities is necessary.

This initial rapid physical examination must be followed by an in-depth evaluation of each regional anatomic area and its relevant physiologic systems. Those with obvious injuries will be carefully scrutinized. This must not divert the examiner to concentrate only on the most apparent injuries, but a continual search for the less obvious hidden occult injuries must complete the examination.

A patient with multiple injuries from an automobile accident will require such a rapid and repeated examination. Much information about this patient can be obtained by simple observation. One can observe cranial, facial, and laryngeal injuries. This observation, along with the respiratory noises caused by blood and aspirated materials, is enough to appraise initially the adequacy of the upper airway. High-pitched and rattling breath sounds will dictate the obvious necessary first resuscitative steps.

A quick appraisal of the state of consciousness, arousal, and pupillary reflexes will afford an advantage in evaluating the frequency, depth, and adequacy of spontaneous ventilatory efforts. Thoracic contusions, bony irregularities, open wounds, asymmetric paradoxical movements, or lack of intercostal muscle activity will provide adequate information for instituting the proper lifesaving measures.

Hemorrhage may be obvious, as from a forearm laceration. However, unexplained shock may be caused by an occult injury, and blood loss may be occurring into the pleural space (hemoperitoneum) or into the soft tissues around fractures or major burn sites.

Obvious external rotation and shortening of a leg provides the necessary preliminary diagnosis; a lesser priority of care is assigned to this situation, although the injured limb is positioned to prevent unnecessary further injury. Simple identification, dressing, and splinting of all soft tissue and extremity injuries of scalp, forearm, and leg is all that is necessary at this initial stage. To attempt more definitive care at this junction would probably give less than optimum results and may detract the practitioner from other and possibly less obvious critical injuries. This initial evalua-

tion and care can and should be performed at the accident scene or in the emergency department prior to transportation of the patient. At this time as much information as possible is obtained from clinical examination and interviewing. All critical information must be gained as soon as possible.

The patient must be observed in an emergency department or trauma care hospital. The airway should be established and maintained by the passage of an endotracheal tube. This is the most direct and sure way and should be among the skills of every practitioner, nurse and physician alike. In many communities rescue emergency medical technicians are becoming skilled in this and other lifesaving techniques.

Additional information can be readily obtained at this time. Clinical findings must be reevaluated and recorded in order to recognize treatment progress or clinical deterioration. Repeated examination should be performed by the same individual or a team of trauma specialists so that reliable and correct management decisions can be made. It is essential that all critical parameters (blood pressure, CVP, pulse, urinary output, and physical findings) be recorded sequentially to detect early pathophysiologic trends.

■ **What essential facts should be obtained from the history?**

As thorough a history as possible is obtained, including health status before the injury, factors causing the accident, and conditions at the scene of the accident. Previous medical problems, allergies, medications, or diseases (for example, coronary disease or hemophilia) must be ascertained. Since this information may be critical to survival, it must be sought from any source possible.

■ **What laboratory and diagnostic tests are indicated in the emergency trauma patient?**

An aggressive diagnostic approach to the trauma patient is necessary for proper evaluation. The decision as to how many x-ray films to order is based on the clinical situation and status of the patient. X-ray films take valuable time and are performed under conditions that are not ideal for continuous observation. Often a few routine views are adequate. The unconscious patient is more difficult to evaluate and may require additional studies. Single views of possible fractures and dislocations and standard views of chest and abdomen are obtained. Special studies such as tomograms of facial fractures can be obtained later. The IVP, cystogram, and arteriography are often useful. The patient with traumatic hematuria from any cause and with suspected renal trauma must have an IVP. To identify injuries to the bladder, pelvic fractures are evaluated by cystography, visualizing the full and empty bladder in the standard and lateral views.

Arteriography is particularly useful when circulation in an extremity is impaired, in abdominal and chest trauma, and in closed head injuries. There is no significant morbidity from these studies, and they are often of great value. An incidental excretory nephrourogram is obtained 15 minutes after the arteriogram.

Paracentesis is helpful for the rapid evaluation of intra-abdominal injuries. If fluid is obtained, it is tested for bile and examined microscopically for white and red blood cells; a portion is sent for determination of amylase concentration. If no fluid is obtained, a plastic catheter may be inserted through the lower abdominal area in the midline and 300 ml of peritoneal dialysis solution slowly infused.[6] The fluid is then aspirated after 5 minutes and tested. A positive tap is a definitive indication for laparotomy.[7] A negative tap cannot be considered evidence of the absence of intra-abdominal injury.

Thoracentesis may be employed for the rapid evaluation of the patient with a possible chest injury. Blood and air, especially if under pressure, are immediate indications for establishment of tube drainage even prior to taking x-ray films. These findings prompt investigation for other underlying visceral injuries.

Direct laryngoscopy and bronchoscopy are performed when injury of the upper airway, trachea, and major bronchi are suspected. Proctoscopy is done in all suspected rectal injuries prior to operation.

Since the introduction of ultrasonic techniques by Leksell,[8] the usefulness of echoencephalography in acute head injuries has been established. Rapid and repeatable examinations are of great value, especially in children. Repeated echoencephalograms and neurologic examinations are effective and reliable ways to observe head trauma patients safely.

Routinely ordered biochemical tests include serial serum and urine amylase determinations, especially in those patients with abdominal injuries caused by a blunt force. A high amylase concentration suggests major injury to the pancreas. Complete blood counts are serially performed. Changes in hematocrit reflect the status of the circulating red cell mass. Leukocyte counts are elevated in those patients with visceral injuries, especially when serosal irritation is present. Determination of osmolality by freezing point depression is useful in the monitoring of fluid and electrolyte problems and in defining the status of renal function after severe injury.[9] It is also more useful than measurements of the specific gravity of the urine.

■ **How are fractures and soft tissue injuries best handled in the emergency trauma patient?**

Gross fractures of an extremity are easily identified by simple inspection and palpation. Grossly deformed limbs should be gently returned to an anatomic position and then adequately immobilized. Pneumatic and Thomas splints should be available in every ambulance and emergency department. Proper care will prevent a closed fracture from becoming an open one. The presence of distal pulses before and after manipulation of a deformed extremity should also be noted. Many times it is not possible to treat soft tissue wounds at the time of injury because other important visceral injuries require attention. In these situations it is best to elevate the wounded part, provide hemostasis by compression, and dress the area to protect it against further injury and contamination. Tetanus prophylaxis and antibiotics must be given. When definitive therapy of a soft tissue wound is to be carried out, it is necessary to provide suitable anesthesia, clean the wounds and surrounding area, remove all foreign matter, debride, repair injured tissues, close the wound if indicated, apply an absorptive bulky dressing, and immobilize and elevate the injured part.

■ **What are significant pathophysiologic events of critical injury?**
Shock

Decreased venous return. The common denominator pathophysiologically basic to all forms of shock is a decrease in venous return. The circulating blood volume is deficient and has either been lost externally or is held out in the body periphery and cannot be effectively redistributed by the heart. Consequently, a decreased venous return is the first defect observed in shock. The CVP is a convenient bedside monitor of this physiologic function.

Decreased cardiac output. Decreased venous return is followed by a decrease in cardiac output, which is normally about 5 L/min. This decreased pumping action is one of the causes of poor circulation in peripheral tissues in the shock state. The cardiac output can be measured accurately electronically by a dye dilution technique. A rough measure of the adequacy of the cardiac output can be quantified clinically by evaluating the systolic blood pressure and the systolic pulse pressure. This important parameter can also be estimated at the bedside by carefully palpating the femoral or radial pulses for rate, rhythm, strength, and fullness. With some practice a good clinician can become quite expert at estimating this important central cardiac function at the bedside.

Arteriolar constriction. A decreased cardiac output stimulates arteriolar vasoconstriction. This arteriolar compensatory mechanism attempts to restrict blood flow in nonvital areas and to make the available blood volume go further. This is a normal physiologic response. However, if sustained for extended time periods, it will create a pathologic condition. The intense vasoconstriction seen in the shock patient is first observed in the skin as it becomes cold, clammy, and loses color, and later may be identified in other organs as a decrease in urinary output or a loss of consciousness. As blood volume is restored, these pathologic events should be reversed, and the changes in these areas can be used as an index of successful treatment.

Decreased tissue perfusion. During these compensatory processes there is a decreased tissue perfusion that will subsequently affect all vascular beds. By this mechanism blood is diverted initially from the skin and muscle and later from the liver and kidneys so that blood flow will be maintained through the vital organs (heart and brain). This decreased blood flow to the muscle beds, skin, and then kidneys results in a decreased skin temperature, decreased muscle motion, decreased urinary output, decreased liver function, and intermediary metabolism. In each organ this diminished blood flow has its specific effects while, in addition, contributing to a developing metabolic acidosis and lactic acid production and accumulation.

Hypoxia and anaerobic glycolysis. Decreased perfusion leads to tissue hypoxia because oxygen and nutrients do not enter the tissues. Cellular metabolism in these tissues then converts to an anaerobic form of glycolysis (hypoxic carbohydrate metabolism). This is a complex process, but essentially glucose is metabolized without efficient consumption of oxygen. In this type of metabolism there is only a small amount of energy produced and the vital energy is generated in a less efficient manner. Under these circumstances energy is produced in much smaller amounts and at a greater cost to the patient. This shift in glucose metabolism from a normal aerobic (oxygen-consuming) to an anaerobic state is a normal compensatory mechanism that is useful in moderate exercise, but when this situation exists for prolonged periods, the patient will deplete existing energy stores necessary for essential cellular work functions.

Lactic acidosis. In the anaerobic glycolytic pathway glucose is not broken down to carbon dioxide and water but to lactic acid. This organic acid is produced normally in exercise, and these circulating lactates are readily metabolized in the healthy body if there is normal muscle and liver perfusion. In the pathologic shock state lactic acid and other metabolic acids accumulate and cause a myriad of problems. These acids decrease the tissue and blood pH and may in themselves be considered a biologic toxin at high levels.

Blood pH can now be easily measured along with oxygen and carbon dioxide tensions in millimeters of mercury. Blood lactates can also be measured, but the time required to do so precludes this parameter from being an emergency department tool. From the pH–blood gas nomogram the base deficit can be extrapolated and used as a fairly accurate indicator of the magnitude of the existing metabolic acidosis. This should be made available for patient management decisions in the emergency department.

Respiratory alkalosis. Early in shock a compensatory respiratory alkalosis occurs in response to changes in blood pH and the lactic acidosis. Shock patients compensate by breathing heavily and blow off carbon dioxide in order to raise the blood pH and to lessen the effects of the metabolic acidosis. Another early sign of shock is hyperventilation caused both by tissue hypoxia and acidosis. As shock patients hyperventilate to improve their oxygen intake, they concomitantly eliminate the metabolite carbonic acid (H_2CO_3) as volatile carbon dioxide (CO_2). This compensatory hyperventilation may become impeded by muscular fatigue or by any cause of mechanical ventilatory dysfunction; this is rapidly associated with CO_2 retention and respiratory acidosis. This final insult will further increase hypoxia and worsen the metabolic acidosis, and the patient will die as a result of the drastic reduction in blood pH (pH < 6.9).

The shock syndrome with its diminished venous return, lowered cardiac output, increased peripheral resistance (arteriolar vasoconstriction), decreased tissue perfusion, metabolic acidosis, and respiratory alkalosis can be observed and measured during the emergency period. A sound knowledge of the pathophysiologic sequelae of shock and skills in interpreting certain critical parameters will result in better shock management and patient survival in these true emergencies.

Ventilatory insufficiency

Pulmonary dysfunction can be caused by direct injury or can be secondary to nonthoracic trauma. Improvements in the treatment of shock, methods of blood procurement and replacement, prevention of renal failure, and control of overwhelming clostridial and other bacterial infections have produced a new form of posttraumatic sequelae in certain patients. Many of these patients develop an insidious and progressive pulmonary insufficiency. This syndrome, which probably has many different etiologic mechanisms, is becoming more readily recognized as a potential hazard to all patients who have had major trauma or surgery. The syndrome has been described by many eponyms that usually relate to the apparent precipitating cause (for example, shock lung, postperfusion lung, congestive atelectasis, or posttraumatic pulmonary insufficiency). The ability to distinguish these entities by clinical comparisons or experimental models has not yet been developed. Similarities in the progression of clinical events and postmortem analysis suggest a common pathophysiologic basis and probably represent the limited nature by which the pulmonary parenchyma is able to react to trauma of varying types.

The commonly associated conditions responsible for the development of this clinical problem have been direct injury, fluid overload, and embolization of microthrombi of fat, fibrin, and cellular debris from peripheral sources. Also, circulating catecholamines, histamine, serotonin, fatty acids, and the vasoactive polypeptides, especially bradykinin, have been implicated because of their known effects on vascular permeability and bronchospasm.

The complex interrelationship of extravascular fluid movements with the lung has received considerable attention. Alterations of pulmonary surfactant production can occur after a wide variety of pathologic conditions, including those that affect the alveolar lining cells, as occurs after aspiration and transudation of fluid into the lung parenchyma. Pulmonary surfactant is a complex phospholipid that is essential for the physiologic stability of the air-liquid phase in each alveolus. The pathologic effects of oxygen toxicity may be caused by direct injury to the alveolar cells that produce this important surface-active agent. Other conditions that are known to be detrimental to the lung include shock, systemic and pulmonary sepsis, prolonged cardiopulmonary bypass, and disseminated intravascular coagulation.

■ What are the clinical features of pulmonary insufficiency?

All patients with a major surgical stress develop some degree of pulmonary impairment and may progress, if not adequately supported, to terminal respiratory failure. The initial phase, which occurs immediately after injury, is characterized by cardiovascular stabilization; after being adequately resuscitated the patient may go on to develop a high cardiac output and lowered peripheral resistance. There is usually associated mild hypoxemia (Pao_2 = 70 to 80 mm Hg), hypocapnia, and hyperventilation. Patients usually show arterial alkalosis, primarily respiratory, and have an adequate oxyhemoglobin saturation level. A patient may improve at this point, at which time these pathophysiologic changes will subside. A satisfactory outcome depends on many factors, including the magnitude of injury, the necessity of extensive resuscitative measures with colloid-poor crystalloid solutions or stored blood, and the length and nature of the surgical intervention.

For reasons not well understood, many patients progress insidiously to a phase of greater pulmonary difficulties. Some of these patients appear surprisingly well at this time but on closer examination will show increased ventilatory effort with tachypnea and shallow breathing. These patients are usually not very cyanotic, and they may even show a rosy complexion. The skin is warm and pink, because the peripheral vessels are dilated and oxygen is less readily released from hemoglobin in the alkalotic state (Bohr effect). The pulse rate is elevated and the cardiac output will remain high. Blood gas concentrations will deteriorate with a fall in arterial oxygen tensions (Pao_2 = 60 mm Hg). Hypocapnia persists ($Paco_2$ = 24 to 30 mm Hg). The alkalosis is now caused by a combination of both metabolic and respiratory components (pH = 7.58, base excess +12 mEq). At this point patients are working harder to breathe, are less able to extract oxygen from the air and, despite increased cardiac action and tissue flow, are less able to release oxygen at the cell level for normal metabolic processes. These patients will soon require some form of enhanced oxygen delivery, including assisted ventilatory support. Those patients who are adequately evaluated, monitored, and sustained during this period can and should survive.

Without intensive management at this point and because of still poorly understood reasons, some patients go on through a phase of progressive pulmonary insufficiency when normal arterial oxygen tensions cannot be maintained even while on assisted ventilation. Carbon dioxide excretion becomes impossible, cellular oxidative metabolism is diminished, and cardiac or respiratory arrest is inevitable. Terminally, blood lactic acid levels rise and the arterial pH falls as hypoxic blood is sluggishly and poorly distributed through the systemic and pulmonary circulatory systems.

■ **What are the essential steps in the evaluation of thoracic trauma?**

Chest trauma may result from penetrating or blunt injury of the chest or its contained viscera. An initial assessment of airway patency is essential. The patient should be observed for signs of obstruction such as stridor, retraction, or wheezing. An evaluation should be made with regard to the possibilities of obstruction from fractures of mandible, maxilla, larynx, or trachea; aspiration of blood; or obstruction by a foreign body. An oral airway and frequent suctioning may be necessary to keep the upper airway patent. As stated previously, endotracheal intubation is preferable to tracheostomy as an initial means of bypassing upper airway obstruction.

Next the adequacy of ventilation must be assessed. This should be done by physical examination and supported by determination of arterial blood gases. The patient should be observed for cyanosis or gasping respiration. Restlessness alone may indicate beginning hypoxia. An examination should be made for failure of chest expansion and for flail or paradoxical motion. Auscultation and percussion of both sides of the thorax should be performed to evaluate the possibilities of pneumothorax and/or hemothorax.

Cyanosis or gasping respiration in a patient who does not have airway obstruction, hemothorax, or pneumothorax means that insufficient oxygen is being absorbed across the alveolar membrane. The cause may be lung contusion, intra-alveolar hemorrhage, or pulmonary edema. Positive pressure ventilation with oxygen enrichment is indicated.

The possibility of respiratory failure must be considered. In massive trauma and shock this may pass undetected while attention is focused on the emergency situation and adequate resuscitation. Fast, shallow respiration may occur early after trauma but may disappear as muscular fatigue progresses. Acute respiratory failure may result from massive atelectasis, lung contusion, simple pneumothorax, hemothorax, tension pneumothorax, flail chest, pneumonia, pulmonary embolism, hemoptysis, or aspiration. Chest tube insertion coupled with positive pressure ventilatory support may be necessary.

■ **What are the consequences of flail chest?**

Flail chest develops when several ribs are fractured on both sides of the point of impact, leaving a portion of the rib cage unstable. Fracture of the sternum in several places may also result in flail chest.

The unsupported chest wall segment behaves in paradoxical fashion, sucking in during inspiration (negative intrapleural pressure) and blowing out during expiration, preventing full lung expansion and adequate oxygen exchange. The lung under the flail segment becomes progressively atelectatic. During expiration end-expired air leaving the unaffected lung is drawn into the affected lung. This to-and-fro movement results in an increase in the dead space and a decrease in arterial oxygen saturation. The failure of the lungs to fill and empty synchronously causes the mediastinum to swing back and forth. This compromises venous return with a resultant decrease in cardiac output. The abnormal movements of the chest wall and the accompanying pain impair effective coughing and result in retention of secretions.

■ **What is the treatment of flail chest?**

Stabilization of the flail segment can be accomplished most effectively by tracheostomy and mechanical volume ventilator support. Less commonly, operative internal fixation of fracture segments with internal wires and plates may be employed when there are multiple fractures of the sternum, a large rib flail segment, or bilateral injury to the thoracic cage.

In the emergency period an endotracheal tube may be used, followed later by tracheostomy. Anywhere from 1 to 4 weeks under this treatment regimen, or until paradoxical motion of the chest has decreased and the patient is able to maintain arterial oxygen saturation without ventilatory support, will be necessary. Ventilatory support must be provided by a mechanical ventilator capable of delivering sufficient volume at whatever pressures are necessary to ventilate the lungs. The patient's pH, Po_2, and Pco_2 must be evaluated frequently. Ventilatory defects secondary to direct lung injury may further affect adequacy of ventilation. The patient can be weaned gradually from the ventilator with close observation of the arterial blood gas concentrations.

Towel clips or hooks passed around the flail segment with the application of external traction is an ineffective method of stabilization and should not be used.

■ **What are the pathologic consequences of hemothorax and pneumothorax and the appropriate clinical intervention?**

Pneumothorax, the accumulation of air in the pleural cavity, can result from both penetrating and nonpenetrating chest injuries. In pneumothorax air is sucked into the pleural space by negative intrapleural pressure during inspiration, gradually accumulating and compromising effective ventilation. Clinically the patient may have diminished or absent breath sounds on the injured side, asymmetry of chest expansion, and subcutaneous emphysema. All major forms of traumatic pneumothorax are treated definitively by insertion of a chest tube connected to underwater seal drainage or to suction. Minimal (under 30%) pneumothorax may be treated conservatively and will reabsorb spontaneously.

A condition warranting immediate attention to prevent rapid deterioration and death is tension pneumothorax. Usually associated with fractured ribs, or less commonly with penetrating injuries such as stab wounds, tension pneumothorax results from the accumulation of air under tension in the pleural space. Unlike pneumothorax, where air enters and leaves the pleural sac with inspiration and expiration, a "valvelike" effect occurs in tension pneumothorax that prevents the release of air and increases pressure in the sac with each inspiration. As pressure builds, the mediastinum is pushed to the contralateral side with progressive impairment of venous return and ventilatory exchange.[10] The clinical picture is severe respiratory distress, cyanosis, and distended neck veins. Breath sounds are absent on the affected side, and tympany is present on percussion. If not recognized and treated immediately by needle aspiration, the patient will experience respiratory arrest. Needle aspiration will bring immediate dramatic results and of course should be followed by definitive thoracostomy and water-seal drainage.

Hemothorax is an accumulation of fluid or blood in the pleural cavity. Laceration of vessels of the chest wall, of intrathoracic great vessels, or of the heart may lead to hemothorax with hypovolemic shock, compression of lung, hypoxemia, and hypercapnia. The clinical picture is similar to pneumothorax. Restoration of blood volume by fluid or blood administration and removal of blood from the pleural cavity should be carried out immediately and simultaneously.

Major hemothorax is drained with a chest tube and suction. The chest tube should be placed in a dependent position, the best location being through the sixth or seventh intercostal space in the midaxillary line, directing the tube posterior to the lung.

Hemothorax may require emergency thoracotomy and operative control of the bleeding source under specific clinical circumstances, for instance, if there is a large clotted hemothorax with a shift in the mediastinum that does not improve on tube drainage, if measured blood loss from the chest tube continues at a rate greater than 250 ml/hr after the first 2 hours, or if the blood loss persists for more than 6 hours.

■ **What is cardiac tamponade and what are the necessary steps for resuscitation?**

Cardiac tamponade is an accumulation of blood in the closed pericardial sac, most commonly caused by a small wound in the heart. As blood is trapped within the inelastic pericardium, blood flow to and from the heart is impeded, resulting eventually in shock and finally cardiac arrest. This cardiogenic shock can occur within several minutes to several hours, depending on the amount of blood accumulated, but may become life-threatening at a volume of as little as 150 ml.

A small puncture wound anywhere on the chest or upper abdomen should arouse suspicion of cardiac tamponade. Characteristic features include muffled or distant heart sounds, a falling

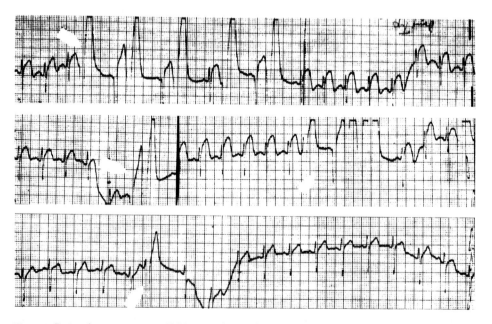

Fig. 9-3. Pericardiocentesis using ECG control. Note large ventricular waves and absence of P waves, denoting ventricular contact and intrapericardial position of needle.

blood pressure, and most importantly, a rising venous pressure. It is essential for this reason that all patients with chest or upper abdominal trauma have a CVP catheter inserted and monitored closely.

Once the diagnosis is made, treatment must be initiated immediately. Needle pericardiocentesis (aspiration) is the initial treatment. The removal of as little as 15 to 20 ml of blood may be sufficient to revive the patient. Pericardiocentesis is accomplished using a No. 21 spinal needle attached to a three-way metal stopcock. A 50 ml syringe is placed on one outlet of the stopcock and the chest lead of a standard ECG monitor is attached to the remaining outlet. The monitor is set to lead II and is closely watched while the practitioner inserts the needle just lateral to the xiphoid process at a 45-degree angle inward and upward (Larrey's point).

An ECG tracing of large ventricular QRS complexes indicates that the needle has traversed the pericardial sac and made contact with the ventricular wall (Fig. 9-3). The needle is then withdrawn slightly with continued aspiration. Any fluid or blood aspirated is from the pericardial cavity. This aspiration may cause relief of symptoms but may only be considered a temporary treatment. The patient must be observed continuously, with the anticipation of subsequent aspiration and possible surgery. The CVP, pulse, and blood pressure must be checked every 15 to 30 minutes because of the possibility of recurrence of tamponade. Continued or massive bleeding will indicate the need for operative intervention.

■ What are the other less obvious consequences of thoracic trauma?

Contusions of the lung, heart, and other thoracic viscera are common sequelae of blunt chest trauma. Contusion of the heart is manifest by ECG changes in epicardial injury or myocardial ischemia. Contusion of the lung reveals itself as an area of increased density in the chest x-ray film, appearing 12 to 72 hours after injury. Areas of lung contusion are associated with hemorrhage; cavitation of the damaged area may occur later.

Tracheal or bronchial rupture or laceration produces pneumomediastinum or pneumothorax. Tension pneumothorax occurs occasionally. Mediastinitis and compression of the trachea are the chief complications. The presence of subcutaneous emphysema, especially in the neck, may indicate the possibility of a serious airway injury. Bronchoscopy may establish the diagnosis. Tracheostomy is used to control respiration, to remove secretions, and to prevent further leakage of air from the high intratracheal pressures that occur with coughing or a Valsalva maneuver. Chest tubes should be inserted if pneumothorax is present. If the volume of air leaking is large, operative repair of the tracheal or bronchial laceration should be done as soon as the patient's general condition permits.

Rupture of the diaphragm is seen after blunt trauma to either the chest or abdomen. The torn diaphragm is totally ineffective and no longer provides a barrier between the thorax and the abdomen. The respiratory impairment caused by diaphragmatic ruptures is very similar to that seen in flail chest. During inspiration (increased negative intrathoracic pressure) abdominal viscera are drawn into the chest, preventing normal inflation of the lung, which then becomes atelectatic. During expiration the involved lung becomes partially filled by the gases being released from the other lung. Compromise of circulation caused by shift of the mediastinum and arterial oxygen unsaturation as a result of shunting are the consequences. A ruptured diaphragm must always be repaired operatively.

Blunt chest trauma, especially of the deceleration type, may lead to aortic injury. The most common point of rupture is just distal to the origin of the left subclavian artery. A widened mediastinum seen on an upright posteroanterior chest x-ray film indicates the possibility of a ruptured aorta and demands diagnostic aortography that, if positive, warrants emergency thoracotomy with cardiopulmonary bypass.

SUMMARY AND CONCLUSIONS

The approach to the multiple injury patient is resuscitative, diagnostic, and finally therapeutic. Airway and ventilatory adequacy are essential to maintenance of resuscitative effort, and subtle respiratory insufficiency can best be detected by measuring the pH and arterial blood gas concentrations. Treatment of hypovolemia and shock should always include adequate volume replacement and only the judicious use of drugs such as mannitol, vasodilators, dextrans, isoproterenol, and digitalis to improve and maintain tissue perfusion after adequate volume replacement has been assured.

Diagnostic evaluation should be limited to necessary procedures and performed with a minimum of delay and patient manipulation. Abdominal trauma resulting in rupture of solid organs (liver and spleen) and/or retroperitoneal vascular injury can only be managed by operative intervention. Physical findings, paracentesis, and evaluation of vital signs will give indications for surgery. All of the resuscitative measures discussed must be performed to adequately prepare such a patient for operative intervention. The team approach to the multiple injury patient is essential to accomplishment of these aims.

REFERENCES

1. National Academy of Sciences–National Research Council, Committee on Trauma and Committee on Shock, Division of Medical Sciences: Accidental death and disability: the neglected disease of modern society, Washington, D.C., 1966, U.S. Government Printing Office.
2. Izant, R. J., Jr., and Hubay, C. A.: The annual injury of 15,000,000 children: a limited study of childhood accidental injury and death, J. Trauma **6:**65, 1966.
3. Boyd, D. R.: A systems approach to improve trauma patient care, S. Afr. J. Surg. **11:**163, 1973.
4. McLean, L. D.: What's new in surgery shock and metabolism? Surg. Gynecol. Obstet. **126:**299, 1968.
5. Shoemaker, W. C., et al.: Sequential oxygen hemodynamic events after trauma to the unanesthetized patient, Surg. Gynecol. Obstet. **132:**1033, 1971.
6. Gumpert, J. L., Froderman, S. E., and Mercho, J. P.: Diagnostic peritoneal lavage in blunt abdominal trauma, Ann. Surg. **165:**70, 1967.
7. Gertner, H. R., Jr., et al.: Evaluation of the management of vehicular fatalities secondary to abdominal injury, J. Trauma **12:**425, 1972.
8. Leksell, L.: Echoencephalography. II. Midline echo from the pineal body as an index of pineal displacement, Acta Chir. Scand. **115:**225, 1958.
9. Boyd, D. R., and Mansberger, A. R., Jr.: Serum water and osmolal changes in hemorrhagic shock: an experimental and clinical study, Am. Surg. **34:**744, 1968.
10. Ballinger, W. F., II, Rutherford, R. B., and Zuidema, G. D.: The management of trauma, Philadelphia, 1968, W. B. Saunders Co.

CHAPTER 10

Orthopedic trauma

Margaret Caldwell

Most orthopedic injuries seen in intensive care units are injuries to long bones and are secondary to other injuries, generally multiple trauma. They have lower care priority because they are of minor importance when compared with increased intracranial pressure, pulmonary injuries, or rupture of abdominal viscera. These injuries are not life-threatening but can result in permanent loss of function if complications are not prevented.

The usual nursing care plan may well consist of "maintain traction" and "assess neurovascular status." Spinal or skull fractures are important only in terms of the resulting neurologic damage—or rib fractures with resulting pulmonary damage.

■ **Are there any fractures that are life-threatening?**

Pelvic fractures can be life-threatening because of the massive damage to bone and blood vessels with resulting blood loss. A pelvic crush may result in massive blood loss. Pelvic fractures have been reported to be second only to head injuries as a cause of traumatic death with a fatality rate as high as 30% from pelvic hemorrhage.

■ **What are the essential points to be considered in the assessment of an orthopedic injury?**

The essential points to be considered in assessing an orthopedic injury are discussed in the following.

General appearance. Look for deformities such as angulation or shortening of the area. It is important to realize that bones support the muscles that surround them and to remember that muscles are contractable. The shortening and angulation can be understood by thinking of a pencil with a rubber band stretched over its length. If you break the pencil, the rubber band will contract and cause angulation or override of the broken ends of the pencil.

Pain. Evaluate the patient's subjective reaction to discomfort. A break in the bone causes pain in and of itself because of the C-fiber pressure. Pain can also be caused by the broken bone fragment encroaching on surrounding muscle, or from the stretching of muscles as a result of deformity. The most common cause of pain at a fracture site is muscle spasm that results from any movement of the limb. It is very important whan a fractured limb is moved that firm support is given to the fractured limb on both sides of the fracture and that movement is slow and firm to avoid putting the muscles into spasm. Pain can be severe enough to cause shock so it is important to prevent pain. Splinting the limb will prevent spasm pain and further injury to surrounding structure.

Crepitus. In assessment of the orthopedic injury, one must consider that the sound and feel is caused by bone fragments rubbing together or by bone in the tissue. Air in the tissues may also give the "tissue paper" sound and feel.

Swelling. To some degree swelling is the result of tissue reaction to injury, but it is primarily caused by actual bleeding into the area. Swelling can result in pressure on surrounding tissues to the point of cutting off the blood supply distal to the injury. Because of this, it is important to elevate the limb to enhance return flow and decrease further swelling. Application of ice to the fracture site encourages contraction of blood vessels, reduced bleeding, and encourages clotting. Ice is effective for the first 16 to 24 hours following injury.

Neurovascular evaluation. Neurovascular evaluation must be done early and often. A set routine of both content and time should be agreed on and done by anyone responsible for this assessment. If subtle changes are missed, permanent damage can result. It is important to remember that neurovascular assessment must be continued until stabilization and healing have occurred. The following parameters are useful in neurovascular assessment: pain, pulse, paresthesia, paralysis, and pallor. Each of these should be checked every 1 to 2 hours for 24 hours, then every 4 hours for 3 days, and every 8 hours during the remainder of the hospital stay.

PAIN. In this context, we are referring to pain distal to the fracture site—what might be described as pressure pain, resulting from impaired blood supply. This pain differs from fracture site pain and must be evaluated separately. Swelling can best be avoided by elevation of the limb and having the patient move the area distal to the fracture, such as fingers and toes. To gain cooperation of the patient, it is often helpful to explain that the blood vessels contain one-way valves and that blood returns to the central circulation as a result of muscle contraction squeezing the blood from valve to valve. Since motion is painful for the patient, support and encouragement by the nurse is very important.

PULSES. Check the entire limb for pulses and document the presence or absence of each. This not only gives a baseline from which to evaluate changes but also gives information as to the site of the vascular damage. Palpated pulses are generally adequate, but if one is having difficulty, a Doppler ultrasound instrument is very useful. The absence of pulses, or diminishing quality, needs to be reported to the physician at once to allow time for further evaluation and prompt intervention. See Fig. 19-1 and the following for the location of pulses.

1. Brachial artery—is best checked high in the arm, medial to the humerus, and again just above the antecubital fossa before it bifurcates into the radial and ulnar arteries

2. Radial artery—is best checked on the radial side of the wrist
3. Ulnar artery—can be checked on the ulnar side of the wrist
4. Femoral artery—can be felt midway between the anterosuperior spine of the ilium and the symphysis pubis; runs down the medial side of the thigh and goes posterior at the knee to form the *popliteal artery*, which can best be felt just above and behind the knee; check pulse on the outer aspect on the top of the foot

PARESTHESIA. Paresthesia is the loss of sensory perception resulting from nerve damage caused by actual severing of the nerve or by pressure on the nerve from swelling. Sensory loss can be tested by pin prick; squeezing the area; light pressure, such as a light touch or brushing with cotton; or temperature, such as using a cold alcohol sponge. This is generally adequate.

PARALYSIS. Paralysis is the inability to move a part. In checking for paralysis it is important to differentiate between "can't" and "won't" move. Pain is frequently a limiting factor in movement so the nurse must encourage the patient to try very hard to move the part and be very alert to even slight movement that would indicate an intact nerve; flexion, extension, flaring, and apposition are all indicators of intact innervation.

PALLOR. Pallor is the most drastic color change. The following is a slight simplification of the total check of color as a reminder of the gradations of problems related to color:

1. Red indicates peripheral dilatation with adequate arterial flow and venous return.
2. Blue generally indicates adequate arterial flow with compromised venous return, oftentimes from swelling, which increases capillary pressure and O_2 deprivation. The need for elevation and muscle activity of the part must be emphasized to prevent or rectify compromised venous return. If the swelling is allowed to increase, the intervascular pressure increases to equal the arterial pressure and no blood can enter the area to oxygenate the tissues.
3. White (or pallor) indicates that no arterial blood is getting into the tissues and they are being deprived of oxygen. This is a grave emergency, and rapid definitive interven-

tion is imperative. The nurse should notify the physician and lower the limb to neutral position to aid the arterial flow.

4. Temperature indicates the blood supply to the area. A cool limb is not being perfused. Compare the temperature of the limb to that of the uninjured limb and to the central temperature. Use the back of the hand as it is generally more sensitive to temperature than the palmar surface of the hand.

■ What symptoms are important to observe in suspected or documented pelvic fracture?

The following symptoms are important to observe in suspected or documented pelvic fracture:

Shock as a result of blood loss (5 units of loss is common)

Back pain from retroperitoneal bleeding

Abdominal distention from intra-abdominal bleeding (*Bedline* to *bedline* measurements over a marked line on the abdomen are easier than trying to get a tape under the patient.)

Urinary output and appearance as an indicator of reduced profusion from hypovolemic shock (Urine must be checked for blood, which may indicate damage to the bladder, ureters, or kidneys. If damage to these structures is suspected, an intravenous pyelogram or cystogram will be done.)

Pelvic injuries, especially multiple fractures, with an unstable pelvis may result in injuries to the bladder, making it imperative that a Foley catheter be in place to check for blood, reduce the size and rigidity of the bladder to prevent further damage, and make it possible to evaluate kidney perfusion on the basis of hourly urine output and specific gravity.

■ How are pelvic fractures treated orthopedically?

Pelvic fractures are generally treated according to the extent of the damage.

WITHOUT DISRUPTION OF THE PELVIC RING: Log rolling is done until the pain becomes too great. Ambulation is begun with a walker progressing to crutch walking. Healing is generally complete in 2 months.

WITH DISRUPTION OF PELVIC RING: These are treated with skeletal traction on the affected side or bilateral hip spica casts. Pelvic traction is generally not used because of the discomfort to the patient.

The patient who is not in a cast must be log-rolled to prevent damage to the internal organs, to reduce pain, and to promote healing by stabilization of the fracture site. Movement along with coughing helps to promote pulmonary toilet and prevent congestion. Skin care of the back must be carried out on a regular basis with massage to stimulate circulation and prevent breakdown of the skin.

■ What blood work is essential in following the status of the orthopedic patient?

Most patients admitted to intensive care units have a multiplicity of laboratory work, but only the implications related to orthopedic conditions will be discussed here. A baseline complete blood count, electrolytes panel, and type and cross match will be drawn in the emergency department before fluids are started. One can assume that this will give an accurate picture of the patient's preinjury status. The hematocrit does not fall as a result of bleeding until the patient is rehydrated. It is important for the unit personnel to ascertain when the initial blood samples were drawn in relationship to starting an IV because of the dilution that takes place.

1. Serial hematocrit—important as a tool to estimate blood loss into the tissue as a result of the fracture (This gives information as to the need for early blood replacement.)

2. Partial thromboplastin time—or other clotting determinations (Stored blood does not supply clotting factor in equal proportion to RBC's.)

3. Potassium—may elevate rapidly as a result of cell breakdown from the crushing injury, from breakdown of RBC's, and with the transfusion of stored blood

4. Urine for fat—as an indicator of impending fat emboli (A full flask should be obtained for proper laboratory analysis.)

5. pH—a decrease in pH increases the solubility of calcium and can result in demineralization of the bone

■ Are dislocations less serious than fractures?

Dislocations often result in more serious damage than fractures because of the gross deformity with stretching and tearing of nerves and blood vessels. The unit nurse seldom sees a dislocation because they are reduced in the emergency room or operating room before the patient's arrival in the unit. However, it is very important to be aware that one is dealing with a patient who has had a reduced dislocation and to be very alert in assessing the neurovascular status of the distal part. This will give the physician ample time for further evaluation with arteriograms and definitive intervention to prevent permanent damage.

■ Is an adequate history important to the unit nurse and physician?

The history is always important in planning nursing care for any patient, but it is extremely important with orthopedic patients. Excessive force is generally involved in fracture of any large bone and may result in injuries to soft tissue or internal viscera. The sequence of events may be extremely important, especially in older patients. The history may state that the patient fell and was found unconscious. The obvious assumption is that the patient fell, sustained a fracture, and "passed out," but one must consider the possibility that the patient had cerebral bleeding or a transient ischemic attack and sustained a fracture from the resulting fall. Pelvic fracture may result from a side collision with a seat belt in place, but it is wise to check the patient's neck for bruises that may have resulted from acceleration forward against the chest belt with a high attachment. If such bruises or abrasions are noted, one must be alert for respiratory distress as the result of damage to the larynx.

■ Is it important for the unit nurse to know the types of fracture?

It is important for the unit nurse to know the types of fractures only as a tool to anticipate the chance for recovery without complications. Closed fractures disrupt the continuity of the bone and may result in bleeding or neurologic damage. Infection at the site of a closed fracture results only from internal seeding of bacteria to the injured area. One must be aware that old blood is an excellent medium for bacterial growth. An open or compound fracture is any fracture in conjunction with an open wound over the fracture site. The skin wound does not have to be the result of perforation by fracture fragment. An open fracture is always considered a site for infection and débridement of the site is carried out in surgery, but the unit nurse will want to pay close attention to the dressing or cast and attempt to prevent wick contamination into the site.

■ How can one best control the pain resulting from orthopedic injuries?

Spasm is a frequent cause of pain in patients with orthopedic injuries. This can be prevented by moving the patient slowly with a firm, gentle grip above and below the fracture site. Any sudden movement of the limb or adjustment in the traction weights will produce spasm and may also cause movement of the healing fracture site; therefore traction weights are never removed or reduced to move a patient because it will result in muscle spasm and, therefore, pain. In the unit small doses of narcotics administered at frequent intervals are often better than large doses administered at 4 to 6 hour intervals. The advantages are that the patient remains relatively pain free and, therefore, does not experience the anticipation of pain but also does not experience the euphoria of large doses of narcotics that may be the forerunner of drug dependency. Emotional support and provision of general physical comfort are extremely important to reduce the need for narcotics.

■ Why are the psychologic aspects of orthopedic care so important?

Orthopedic injuries are very devastating to a person because of the very real concern regarding altered life-style and altered body image. Orthopedic injuries are long-term injuries, and long after the patient has recovered from more severe and life-threatening injuries, the orthopedic condition continues to be incapacitating. Return to a former occupation or life-style may seem unlikely and be very worrisome to the patient. Encouraging the patient to do everything possible for himself is a very constructive method of reducing the "helpless syndrome" and will increase the patient's sense of self-worth.

It is usually faster and easier to do things for

patients with orthopedic injuries, but be very sure you are not meeting your own emotional needs at the expense of the patient. It is also useful to work with the family to encourage this attitude toward the patient.

■ Can casts be comfortable?

Casts are restricting and unyielding but should not be painful. A limb should sit in the center of a cast, which means its edges should not dig into tissue.

This can be accomplished by adjusting the pillow support that elevates the cast until the cast sits evenly around the limb. Support on each side of the cast will reduce muscle strain caused by the patient trying to keep the cast from falling to the side.

Some orthopedic surgeons fold a stockinette back over the raw edge of the cast to pad the sharp edges; others do not. If the edge of the cast has not been covered, it is useful to "pedal" the cast. This can be done with pieces of 4-inch tape cut approximately 3 inches long in chevron strips. The tape is applied to the edges of the cast as shown:

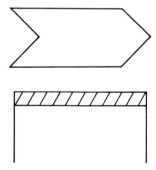

It is also important to keep the skin at the cast edge dry. Powder may help.

If cast edges become bent or were pulled when the plaster was wet, it may be necessary to bend them up away from the skin to prevent pressure areas. This can be done with your fingers on larger casts or with a straight Kelly forceps in more restricted areas such as around the thumb or across the back of the hand. Slight flaring of cast edges to prevent pressure does not reduce the support of the cast and does offer increased comfort of the patient.

Casts should not exert pressure on the underlying soft tissue. If a patient complains of a sustained feeling of pressure, the cast will need to be windowed over the area. It is also useful to feel the cast for "hot spots," which may indicate irritation or infection under the cast. Hot spots need to be investigated. Common trouble spots are heel areas, calf areas that may have been flattened by pressure when the cast was wet, areas over bony prominences, or any place that there is a depression in the cast.

■ What deficit might be expected in a patient who has sustained a spinal injury?

1. Lifting elbow up to shoulder height—C5
2. Bending the elbow—C6
3. Straightening elbow from flexion position—C7
4. Gripping—C-8-T1
5. Lifting leg off or flex hip—L3
6. Extending knee—L4-5
7. Wiggling toes backwards—L5
8. Pushing toes downwards—S1

■ What type of injury can occur to the spine?

The three types of injury that can occur in the spine are as follows:

COMPRESSION FRACTURE: Compression fracture of the cervical spine generally results from a direct blow to the top of the head. Forward flexion of the head frequently occurs, resulting in damage to the anterior body of the vertebra. A "bursting" injury is crushing of the vertebra with displacement into the spinal canal, with resulting cord damage.

DISLOCATION: Dislocation in the cervical area is caused by a sudden rotation of the head with an articular process sliding over the one below. Tearing of the capsule or disc damage may occur. Nerve root damage is more likely than cord damage.

SUBLUXATION: Subluxation occurs when one vertebra slides anteriorly or posteriorly out of line with adjacent vertebra. A facet fracture is generally present to allow the subluxation.

■ Why are injuries to cervical or lumbar vertebrae more common than in the thoracic area?

The thoracic spine is supported by the ribs and associated muscles. The major flexibility of the spine occurs in the cervical and lumbar areas, making these areas more vulnerable. The junction of the fixed thoracic and flexible lumbar region is a common area for compression fracture, resulting from a fall on the bottocks or feet with the trunk in a forward position.

■ **What would make you suspect a patient might develop fat emboli?**

A fracture of a long bone, especially if the limb had been manipulated excessively such as in transport with a nonsplinted fracture, would make one suspect development of fat emboli. Fat from the bone marrow gets into the circulating blood and lodges in the lung. This will generally occur within the first 72 hours after injury.

■ **What symptoms would one look for to indicate the presence of fat emboli?**

The following are symptoms that might indicate the presence of fat emboli.
1. Disturbance of consciousness, probably caused by deprivation of O_2 to the brain (This symptom makes the safety of the patient, as well as protection of the fracture site, a high nursing-care priority.)
2. Difficult breathing, resulting from the shunting and spasm caused by the foreign body in the lung, a Po_2 below 60 mm Hg, and sinus tachycardia with pronounced S waves and depressed ST segment on ECG's
3. Petechiae caused by intravascular coagulation (This will also result in a low platelet count.)
4. Increased serum lipase seen on settled or spun blood as milky appearing serum

■ **How are fat emboli treated?**

Fat emboli may be treated as follows:
1. Corticosteroids to reduce pulmonary inflammation
2. Respiratory support with O_2, possibly requiring intubation with a volume ventilator with PEEP
3. A volume expander to treat shock
4. Diuretics for pulmonary edema
5. Ethanol, 5%, in 5% dextrose and low-dose heparin sometimes recommended

■ **What is the primary nursing goal for patients with spinal injuries?**

The primary nursing goal for patients with spinal injuries is the *prevention of compression or hemorrhage into or transection of the cord*. This is best accomplished with 10 to 15 pounds of traction. A head halter can be used but is very uncomfortable for the patient and may cause skin breakdown under the chin and around the ears. The application of Crutchfield tongs placed into the skull plate makes a much more comfortable and secure attachment for the weights. The scalp wounds created by the insertion of tongs must be cleaned and inspected daily to prevent infection.

■ **Why is careful documentation of major importance when caring for the orthopedically damaged patient?**

The psychologic impact, loss of body image, and long confinement period with incomplete or delayed return of function were discussed previously. These factors make the possibility of legal action very real. Therefore the nursing notes with careful documentation of assessment findings to reflect the nurse's knowledge of possible complications, their presence or absence, and the nursing action for each is paramount. Each nursing action should reflect response to specific assessment data.

It is often better to describe one's observation rather than interpretation. For example, toes of the left foot are swollen and blue rather than: impaired circulation in toes of left foot. The first statement gives data that can be used to formulate an assumption. The second gives only an opinion and leaves the reader with many unanswered questions.

■ **What are the legal ramifications of orthopedic injuries?**

Orthopedic injuries heal slowly, and it takes a long time to regain effective function of the limb after bone healing has taken place. These injuries alter life-style, often to a greater degree than other injuries that are more serious medically. Patients with orthopedic injuries do not feel sick, only restricted, frustrated, and frightened. This is the type of patient who will bring legal action. Nurses can do a great deal to prevent such action by explaining the pathophysiology of an ortho-pedic injury to the patient to give him realistic expectations regarding his recovery and to teach him to do everything possible for himself to lessen his feeling of helplessness.

BIBLIOGRAPHY

Barry, J.: Emergency nursing, New York, 1978, McGraw-Hill Book Co.

Brunner, L. S., and Suddarth, D. S.: The Lippincott manual of nursing practice, Philadelphia, 1974, J. B. Lippincott Co.

Coscriff, J., and Anderson, D.: The practice of emergency nursing, New York, 1975, J. B. Lippincott Co.

Iverson, L. D., and Clawson, D. K.: Manual of acute ortho-pedic therapeutics, Boston, 1977, Little, Brown & Co.

Sharpe, J. C., and Marx, F. W.: Management of medical emer-gencies, New York, 1969, McGraw-Hill Book Co.

CHAPTER 11

Nutritional support in hospitalized patients

George L. Blackburn and Paul A. Thornton

Body cells need constant nourishment in order to keep the total organism in what is commonly referred to as the "healthy state." This is not a problem for most people in our society because of the easy availability of food and the individual's means of adapting to varying dietary habits and patterns of intake. However, for some, especially the sick and/or hospitalized and the aged who are often compromised both nutritionally and physiologically, malnutrition occurs for a number of reasons. For example, some people should not eat because of their medical problem (that is, acute pancreatitis), others cannot eat or cannot eat enough because of bowel obstruction or other conditions, and some people refuse to eat because of psychologic difficulties. Still others have clinical problems that cause them to lose nutrients from the body faster than voluntary food intake can compensate. Also, illness may be associated with changes in metabolism that are characterized by decreased efficiency of nutrient utilization; thus the actual nutritive requirement is increased. Finally, evidence has shown that routine therapeutic procedures followed during hospitalization may contribute to the decline of nutritional status because they often prevent the patient from eating properly. One or any combination of these conditions can result in the loss of protein and calorie reserves. With these losses, the patient becomes increasingly less able to combat stress, to mount an immune response to invading organisms, or to exhibit an optimal healing rate when wounds are involved.

Before the late 1960's many such people died of starvation or from overwhelming infection that prospered in the virtual absence of nourishment with consequent decreased immune resistance. In this context the method of complete nourishment by the intravenous route was developed as a practical procedure. Much of the credit for these early efforts should go to Rhoades, one of the pioneers, who clearly appreciated the essentiality of complete nourishment for reducing morbidity and mortality associated with disease. Under his guidance, Dudrick and co-workers[1,2] made the initial breakthrough in showing that intravenous hyperalimentation was a means of maintaining life in people who otherwise would not have survived. Since that time, the concept has experienced rapid development and expansion, so that we now think more generally in terms of nutritional support. This includes not only intravenous hyperalimentation (IVH), but also enteral tube feeding of defined formula diets, peripheral intravenous feeding, and various combinations of these procedures. Such methods may be used in combination or individually, as supplements to limited oral intake of the usual foods. The term "hyperalimentation" is appropriate for describing both the parenteral and enteral routes, since it means providing nourishment at a level higher than that needed to maintain nitrogen balance.

These developments have made it possible to meet the nutrient requirements of the critically ill patient while staying within the fluid and electrolyte tolerances and the hemodynamic and pulmonary capacities. However, provision of these expanded services requires considerable sophistication and training of the medical personnel involved. Furthermore, a coordinated medical team is essential if best results are to be realized. Such a team should include experienced nutritionists, physicians, and allied health professionals, particularly nurses, dietitians, pharmacists, and physical therapists. Finally, certain facilities and practices are essential, including a 24-hour biochemistry laboratory, rigorous techniques and guidelines to monitor the safety of IVH in the event of complications, and carefully constructed audits of therapy practice to ensure their safety, effectiveness, and scientific basis.

Thus, while the use of a nutritional support service can be ranked in importance with the discovery of antibiotics, heart/lung bypass, and renal dialysis in its influence on survival, its employment should not be undertaken haphazardly. A tragedy can result if IVH of critically ill patients, particularly those with organ failure, is attempted in units where the necessary facilities and medical personnel are not available. Clearly intravenous feeding for the critically ill patient is an evolving medical specialty. Thus the current review will be an effort to summarize the various facets of hyperalimentation, both enteral and parenteral, but by no means should present practices become common without further study.

■ Why is it important to maintain an adequate nutritional state in the patient?

Obviously an adequate nutritional state is important in all individuals, but it is particularly important in sick people for several reasons. For example, a number of independent observations associate the nutritional state with the degree of immune competency. From this it can be surmised that a malnourished person would have a lower degree of immunity and would therefore be more subject to infections and susceptible to more serious infections once the process was initiated. This premise is supported by clinical observations indicating that patients with adequate nutrition have fewer postoperative complications related to infection. Also, wound healing rates are more rapid in well-nourished patients compared to nutritionally compromised patients. In the treatment of cancer the possibility exists that an adequately nourished person has a more favorable response to radiation and chemotherapy. Generally it appear that the better nourished patients can tolerate higher doses and accept more treatment per unit of time, and they appear to have fewer side-effects to treatment. Collectively these various areas of improvement would enhance a patient's prognosis.

It has also been observed that failing organ systems seem to improve when the patient is well nourished via parenteral hyperalimentation. This effect has been seen in renal failure and respiratory support as well as in cardiac and hepatic patients. On the cellular level it has been shown that IVH improved the function of the sodium pump mechanism, causing a reversal of the sick cell syndrome.

From this brief review it follows that maintaining a high nutritional state or providing nutritional support for the malnourished patient has an important bearing on patient prognosis over a broad range of clinical conditions.

■ Is it more difficult to maintain an adequately nourished state in a sick person than in a healthy person?

The answer to this question is an unequivocal yes. There are a number of reasons for this situation. As stated previously, many sick people will not eat. Sometimes conditions preclude their eating or may keep them from eating enough to sustain themselves; thus they may develop malnutrition in an indirect manner. Stress resulting from illness also causes malnutrition to develop indirectly via the changes brought about by hormonal alterations induced by the patient's condition. Perhaps this is best illustrated by comparing fasting in a healthy person to fasting in a sick person. Fasting alone does not cause high mortality rates until a 40% weight loss has occurred, whereas fasting plus illness and/or injury results in high death risks after only a 25% weight loss.

This difference occurs because the body adjusts to starvation by decreasing the metabolic rate and because the body adaptively conserves lean body mass (LBM) via greater central nervous system use of ketones in place of glucose, which is normally generated by gluconeogenic action. However, when noneating is combined with trauma, there is no reduction in the metabolic rate and there is continuing gluconeogenesis, which perpetuates protein catabolism. This response appears to be somewhat proportional to the severity of the condition and lasts as long as the acute phase persists. Thus it is clear that starvation associated with trauma accelerates the rate of weight loss and causes a relatively greater loss of LBM compared to adipose tissue.

Trauma elicits endocrine responses that are activated by a release of catecholamines from the adrenal medulla and sympathetic nerve endings. This causes inhibition of insulin secretion and markedly stimulates glucagon secretion. This total response is accompanied by an increased release of ACTH from the anterior pituitary gland, which in turn stimulates the production and release of adrenal glucocorticoid hormones. This hormonal interplay effects peripheral protein catabolism and subsequent gluconeogenesis. Epinephrine and glucagon provide a strong glycogenolytic stimulus, and the oxidation of fat is increased owing to the lipolytic effect of the catecholamines. The glucocorticoids antagonize the peripheral action of insulin, leading to greater use of lean tissues, which favors the supply of free amino acids for visceral protein synthesis and energy fuel substrates.

From the foregoing it is obvious that nutritional support, at least quantitatively, if not qualitatively, is needed for persons under stress. This increased need, combined with the patient's inability to eat or to eat enough, intensifies the probability of malnutrition development.

■ How does one determine when special nutritional needs are indicated?

Contrary to what was formerly thought and in fact was often the case, classic vitamin deficiencies are no longer commonly observed. Although the possibility of such deficiencies cannot be ignored, it is more probable that protein-calorie malnutrition (PCM) will be found. Thus one needs to become aware of situations in which PCM is most likely to occur. Are there certain clues or clinical conditions that can be related to the condition? A number of clinical conditions are immediately

suspect for precipitating PCM. For example, cancer, particularly of long-standing occurrence, is highly associated with PCM development. Chronic diseases, gastrointestinal problems that influence eating, trauma, and psychic problems all are often associated with this deficiency.

An excellent clue of impending PCM is a recent weight loss of 10% or more, regardless of whether it is associated with one of the previously mentioned conditions or not. However, this requires clarification since the time element and mode of weight loss are important. For example, a 10% weight loss in less than 2 weeks, in the absence of an accompanying infection, is more likely to be a problem of fluid balance than a reflection of either adipose tissue or LBM loss. On the other hand, a similar weight loss over a 1- to 3-month period would be indicative of both adipose and LBM loss, suggesting PCM. The higher the percentage loss of LBM, the more severe the PCM. This presupposes that the patient had not been following a weight reduction dietary regimen.

In examining the patient it is most important to determine the degree of PCM development. This entails a determination of the physiochemical composition of the weight lost, the influence of the weight loss on the visceral protein status, and its effect on immune competency. A means of assessing the nutritional status has been devised in recent years. This procedure requires a profile (index) that includes a diet history and anthropometric, biochemical, and immunologic testing. Complete details of these procedures and their application are available in nutrition journals.[3]

From the foregoing, it appears that a number of clinical conditions cause PCM development, the most easily observed symptom of which is unexplained weight loss. When this occurs, tools are available to gain additional evidence of this obvious change and to quantitate the severity of the development. Apparently a considerable number of hospitalized patients have developed PCM and are in need of nutritional support.[4,5]

Nutritional support of some type is warranted in any individual in whom assessment has indicated a deficiency. It is also needed in those who have suffered recent trauma, contracted a serious illness, or experienced surgical injury, even when their current nutritional status may seem adequate. This is true because nutritional support is directed toward minimizing excessive loss of body cell mass* and preserving host defense mechanisms (Fig. 11-1). Thus, even in the well nourished, it is important to maintain status quo in regard to body energy and protein stores. This is not easily accomplished since the body's response to stress leads to a general trend toward catabolism via changes in hormone secretions, as discussed previously. Briefly, the metabolic changes in this state include increased energy expenditure, mobilization of labile protein reserves, and an elevation in biosynthesis of new protein necessary to ensure recovery. The net result of these changes is a progressive loss of body reserves in order to support sustained organ function, wound healing, and host defense. Thus what was earlier considered to be a "catabolic" response to severe stress, and therefore bad, is now looked on favorably as a functional redistribution of the body

---

*The total mass of living, functioning, energy-exchanging, and mitotically active cells of the body.[6]

cell mass (Fig. 11-2). Nevertheless, the result of such progressive depletion in a setting of critical illness is often death caused by sepsis and sequential organ failure. For this reason the early institution of aggressive nutritional support is indicated for the critically ill person, especially if the illness is accompanied by evidence of moderate to severe malnutrition. The goal in these patients should be to limit the depletion of amino acid pools and body cell mass. Any delay in providing metabolic support will only allow the reserves to be progressively depleted and increase the risk of eventual morbidity and mortality.

■ What are the preferred methods of nutritional support?

The method selected to supply nutrients must be based on patient needs and capabilities. If the alimentary tract is functional, it is always the preferred route. The gastrointestinal tract and liver play important regulatory roles in body protein metabolism in addition to their involvement in more than 50% of the body's normal daily turnover. Forced feeding of critically ill patients via

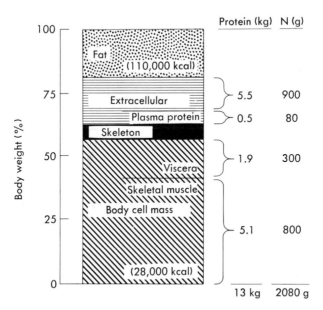

Fig. 11-1. Schematic view of adult man demonstrating endogenous nutrient reserves. Note that body cell mass involves large fraction of body protein content and constitutes a functionally expensive energy source. Nutritional support in critical illness is designed to prevent depletion of this compartment.

Functional redistribution of body cell mass

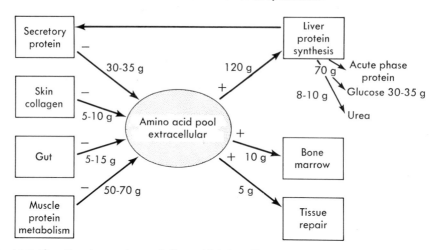

Fig. 11-2. Alterations in protein metabolism with injury. Protein reserves from muscle, gut, and skin are released to support biosynthesis in areas more critical for recovery. Provision of exogenous protein and energy will fortify amino acid pools and support this metabolic response.

nasogastric or nasoduodenal tubes, as well as the use of gastrostomy or enterostomy catheters, constitutes the safest and most efficient form of nutritional support. Comprehensive reviews of the various defined formula feedings and modular supplements are available.[7,8]

Alimentary feeding is an effective means of achieving nitrogen balance; it is a more "physiologic" approach than IVH since the nutrient uptake and utilization are regulated by the gut and liver; and the probability of infection is reduced. As in any therapeutic regimen, certain precautions must be observed; thus there is a need for a policy and procedure outline to ensure safe and effective enteral hyperalimentation. Many concerns and benefits of enteral hyperalimentation have been reviewed.[9] It appears that the method can be used when only small parts of the gastrointestinal tract are functional, and so it provides a means for nourishing patients with a variety of intestinal tract abnormalities.

However, when the intestinal tract cannot or should not be used, it becomes necessary to feed the patient using the intravenous route entirely. Even though less than 5% of the admissions to acute-care hospitals fall into this category, intra-

venous nourishment has made survival possible in many otherwise hopeless cases. However, with its use a number of concerns must be addressed, as discussed at the beginning of this chapter.

Foremost is knowing the amount and composition (particularly the ratio of protein:carbohydrate:fat) of the solution required to optimally benefit the critically ill patient. For example, some carbohydrates are needed to protect the liver from endotoxin, thus aiding host defense. Because carbohydrate is obviously a supplier of calories, however, the question of how much carbohydrate to infuse should be considered. Excessive amounts have been shown to raise the respiratory quotient above 1.0, which could compromise respiratory function in an elderly depleted patient. Since it is known that glucose oxidation in stressed individuals is limited, excessive infusions (more than 4 mg/kg/min) create other serious problems. For instance, with the continuous infusion of large amounts of dextrose and amino acids, an increased need for insulin is generated. Under these circumstances (high plasma insulin levels) appreciable amounts of dextrose are converted to fat, particularly in the liver, the major site for *de novo* synthesis in man. This can lead to excessive triglyceride and glycogen storage resulting in hepatomegaly with impaired structural and secreting function.

One means of avoiding this problem was tested using the techniques of "cyclic hyperalimentation." Cyclic hyperalimentation is a parenteral feeding method in which amino acid infusions are given continuously but administration of hypertonic dextrose is discontinued during part of the day. This permits the development of a postabsorptive state, facilitating the mobilization and utilization of calories stored as fat during the hypertonic dextrose infusion. One study [10] suggests that cyclic hyperalimentation is better tolerated by the liver than continuous hyperalimentation and that it allows recovery of hepatic damage incurred during continuous therapy with hypertonic glucose. Thus it follows that while hyperalimentation has proved to be a valuable tool in medical therapy, there are many problems yet to be solved.

Moreover, many patients requiring intravenous feeding are not only suffering from malnutrition but may also have sepsis. In such cases there may be subclinical deficiencies of vitamins and minerals in addition to the need for increased calories and protein. Little is known, quantitatively, about these needs, particularly when additional factors such as age, sex, and racial origin are also considered. Thus in spite of the success that practitioners of hyperalimentation have enjoyed, much remains to be learned before optimal results will be realized.

Parenteral protein-sparing therapy is yet another option that has been used postoperatively to minimize the loss of body protein.[11] Traditionally dextrose has been used for this purpose since the early observation that glucose reduced the negative nitrogen balance normally seen in fasting people.[12] In practice, nitrogen balance in postoperative patients given dextrose is improved compared to the patients undergoing total starvation. However, it can be argued that the practice of glucose infusion may not be entirely desirable on the following basis. Glucose elevates insulin, which is highly antilipolytic, therefore preventing free fatty acid (FFA) mobilization from adipose tissue and the subsequent formation and release

of ketone bodies (KB's) from the liver. Thus glucose, via insulin, reduces the supply of circulatory energy substrates by inhibiting the use of adipose tissue, a relatively unimportant tissue. Secondly, insulin is important in causing amino acids to be taken up by muscle and converted into protein, thus reducing the supply of essential building blocks that are needed for the new protein synthesis so critical to the body during the response to stress. In essence, glucose may be a detrimental force in inhibiting the usual body response to trauma.

Conversely, the peripheral infusion of amino acids plus vitamins and minerals, but without dextrose, has been shown to be more effective in improving nitrogen balance,[13,14] and it also enhances visceral protein synthesis. Most importantly, it allows the body to adapt in a manner very similar to that seen in simple starvation. That is, it does not cause plasma insulin elevation, as does 5% dextrose, and therefore body fat stores are mobilized and used for energy. Subsequently KB's become elevated in the plasma and are used for neural tissue energy supply, thereby sparing body protein.

Unlike glucose infusion, peripheral amino acid infusion therapy is compatible with those expected metabolic changes seen during stress response. These changes represent the animal organism's never-ending quest to survive in a hostile environment by evolving mechanisms most suited to counter undesirable change, including trauma. Amino acid therapy seemingly does not interfere with any of those "natural" responses to stress. More importantly, it largely prevents the depletion of body protein reserves that does occur "naturally" in long-term stressful situations.

CONCLUSIONS AND PROJECTIONS

Proper nutritional support is essential for the recovery of the critically ill patient. Surveys have indicated that the nutritional status of hospitalized patients in the United States is often compromised, with a relatively high percentage suffering from moderate to severe malnutrition. This type of malnutrition is frequently not recognized and therefore remains untreated. Fortunately the medical community is becoming increasingly aware of the problem. We now have adequate tools to gain a reliable index of patient nutritional status rapidly. Further, we have a variety of means to implement nutritional support procedures, even for the most vulnerable patients. However, we have not arrived at the apex of this development because we know very little about the actual nutritional needs for the many different clinical cases.

For the future it seems axiomatic that considerable efforts will be made to learn more about the quantities and qualities of nutrients required for each situation. This is important because we know that trauma response is associated with a change in protein and energy requirements. Perhaps other changes are also effected by trauma but remain symptomatically subtle. The fact that infections are associated with a change in the plasma amino acid profile and that mineral concentrations (including iron, zinc, and copper) in the plasma vary simultaneously is of possible importance. Does this mean that patients need more or less of these various nutrients to best support their response to trauma? It is hoped that many of these concerns can be investigated so that nutritional support of patients can become increasingly optimized.

ACKNOWLEDGMENTS

The work on which this chapter is based was performed pursuant to Contract GM-22691-04 awarded by the National Institute of General Medical Sciences, DHEW. Data organization and analysis were performed on the PROPHET system, sponsored by the Chemical/Biological Information Handling Program, National Institutes of Health. This is article 665 from the Cancer Research Institute of the New England Deaconess Hospital.

REFERENCES

1. Dudrick, S. J., Wilmore, D. W., Vars. H. M., and Rhoades, J. E.: Can intravenous feeding as the sole means of nutrition support growth in the child and restore weight loss in an adult? An affirmative answer. Ann. Surg. **169:**974, 1969.
2. Dudrick, S. J., Wilmore, D. W., Vars, H. M., and Rhoades, J. E.: Long-term total parenteral nutrition with growth, development, and positive nitrogen balance, Surgery **64:**134, 1968.
3. Blackburn, G. L., et al.: Nutritional and metabolic assessment of the hospitalized patient, JPEN **1:**11, 1977.
4. Bistrian, B. R., Blackburn, G. L., Hallowell, E., and Heddle, R.: Protein status of general surgical patients, J.A.M.A. **230:**858, 1974.
5. Bollet, A. J., and Owens, S. L.: Evaluation of nutritional status of selected hospitalized patients, Am. J. Clin. Nutr. **26:**931, 1973.
6. Moore, F. D., et al.: Body cell mass and its supporting environment, Philadelphia, 1963, W. B. Saunders Co.
7. Heymsfield, S. B., et al.: Enteral hyperalimentation, Ann. Intern. Med. **90:**63, 1979.
8. Shils, M. E., Bloch, A. S., and Chernoff, R.: Liquid formulas for oral and tube feeding, Clin. Bull. **6:**151, 1976.
9. Kaminski, M. V., Jr.: Enteral hyperalimentation, Surg. Gynecol. Obstet. **143:**12, 1976.
10. Maini, B., et al.: Cyclic hyperalimentation: an optimal technique for preservation of visceral protein, J. Surg. Res. **20:**515, 1976.
11. Blackburn, G. L., Flatt, J. P., and Hensle, T.: Pheripheral amino acid infusions. In Fischer, J. E., editor: Total parenteral nutrition, Boston, 1976, Little, Brown & Co., p. 363.
12. Gamble, J. L.: Harvey Lect. **42:**247, 1946.
13. Blackburn, G. L., Flatt, J. P., Clowes, G. H. A., and O'Donnell, T. E.: Peripheral intravenous feeding with isotonic amino acid solutions, Am. J. Surg. **125:**447, 1973.
14. Blackburn, G. L., et al.: Protein sparing therapy during periods of starvation with sepsis of trauma, Ann. Surg. **177:**588, 1973.

BIBLIOGRAPHY

Fischer, J. E., editor: Total parenteral nutrition, Boston, 1976, Little, Brown & Co.
Johnston, I. D. A., editor: Advances in parenteral nutrition, London, 1978, M.T.P. Press Ltd.
Shenkin, A., and Wretlind, A.: Parenteral nutrition, World Rev. Nutr. Diet. **28:**1, 1978.

CHAPTER 12

Electrocardiographic changes

Allan Pribble and Thomas A. Preston

ELECTROPHYSIOLOGY

ECG changes in critically ill patients result from a wide variety of metabolic, pharmacologic, ischemic, and inflammatory influences. Changes in heart rhythm, in QRS, T, and P complexes, and in S-T and Q-T segments are commonly seen in the intensive care unit, both as a result of disease and from therapeutic intervention. Arrhythmias may compromise cardiac function but are even more important as clinical signals of underlying metabolic or hemodynamic changes. Alterations of the Q-T and S-T segments and of the various waveforms do not interfere with cardiac function but may provide clues to underlying metabolic problems.

Before discussing specific problems a brief review of the electrophysiology of cardiac electrical activity and its relation to rhythm and conduction is necessary. General mechanisms that alter these electrophysiologic events and their ECG implications will be explained.

■ How is cardiac electrical activity generated?

Cardiac electrical activity is generated by the movement of charged particles—sodium (Na^+) and potassium (K^+) ions—across cell membranes. Fig. 12-1 relates the sequence of these events in a single cell to the electrical forces recorded on the surface ECG.

Depolarization (phase 0)

An electrical stimulus conducted to the cell membrane causes the resting potential to move toward 0 mv (become less negative). When the transmembrane potential reaches the threshold potential (approximately -70 mv), a sudden change in membrane permeability allows instantaneous movement of positively charged Na^+ into the cell. This sudden inrush of positively charged particles changes the intracellular potential to nearly $+20$ mv.

As the wave of depolarization spreads through the heart muscle, the action potentials generated are recorded on the ECG as the QRS complex. Although depolarization of a single cell requires only 1 millisecond, sequential depolarization of the entire ventricular muscle mass requires 0.06 to 0.12 second.

Depolarized state (phases 1 and 2)

Following depolarization, the transmembrane potential quickly decreases to 0 (phase 1) and establishes a new steady state (phase 2). Normally no change in transmembrane potential is recorded during phase 2 so the ECG is recorded as a baseline potential, the S-T segment.

Repolarization (phase 3)

Return to the original resting state requires repolarization (phase 3) of the cell membrane, which begins after a brief pause (S-T interval) in the depolarized state. Repolarization is equal in electrical magnitude to depolarization but occurs more slowly. For this reason the ECG manifestation of repolarization, the T wave, is longer in duration than the QRS complex of depolarization. During repolarization K^+ flows out of the cell, causing inscription of the T wave. When repolarization is complete, ionic steady state is achieved, with the transmembrane potential at -90 mv.

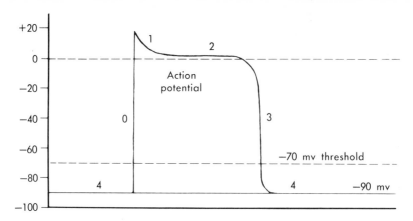

Fig. 12-1. Cardiac cell membrane potential.

Baseline potential (phase 4)

During diastole (phase 4) the muscle cell membrane is fully polarized with a transmembrane potential of -90 mv, the inside of the cell being negative in relation to the outside. Intracellular K^+ concentration is 30 times higher than extracellular concentration, and extracellular Na^+ concentration is 10 times higher than intracellular concentration. Net ionic motion is prevented by the cell membrane, so that no current is generated, and the ECG is recorded as a baseline potential.

■ What function does cardiac electrical activity serve?

Cardiac electrical activity regulates the timing of cardiac contraction and the synchronization between atrial and ventricular contractions. Three major types of heart tissue participate in cardiac electrical activity: pacemaker, or automatic, tissue, conduction tissue, and myocardium. Pacemaker, or automatic, cells originate the electrical impulses that begin muscular contraction. Normally the dominant pacemaker area is the sinoatrial (SA) node, which depolarizes rhythmically approximately 80 times/min. Pacemaker cells in the atrioventricular (AV) junctional area have a slower intrinsic rate of 40 to 60 beats/min. Conduction cells rapidly transfer electrical impulses from pacemaker sites to myocardium. Myocardial

contraction is initiated by depolarization of myocardial cell membranes. Only myocardial electrical activity is visible in the surface ECG, because its bulk is relatively much greater than that of the conducting and pacemaking tissue. Although the cells of each of these tissues have distinctive electrical characteristics and functions, the basic sequence of depolarization and repolarization described in Fig. 12-1 is common to all.

■ How do pacemaker cells initiate impulses?

Pacemaker cells are called automatic cells because they depolarize spontaneously. Fig. 12-2 illustrates the basic characteristic of automatic cells; that is, the presence of slow, spontaneous depolarization during phase 4. When this slow diastolic depolarization reaches threshold, spontaneous depolarization occurs. An external current applied during diastolic depolarization can cause the automatic cell to depolarize before it reaches threshold spontaneously. In this way pacemaker cells of the SA node, with rapid diastolic depolarization, dominate other automatic cells by depolarizing them before they reach threshold spontaneously. If the SA cells fail to depolarize, the next fastest depolarizing cells, located in the atrium or AV node, "escape" the dominance of the SA node and assume pacemaking duties at their slower intrinsic rates. Safety valve

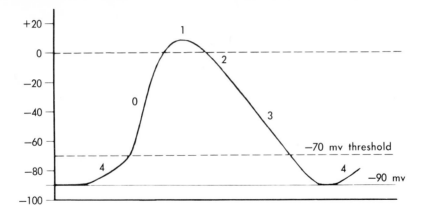

Fig. 12-2. Spontaneous but slow depolarization during phase IV allows cell membrane to reach threshold for depolarization and to generate spontaneous action potential. Pacemaker cells depolarize more slowly than Purkinje and muscle cells, and resulting action potential is of lower amplitude.

automatic cells in the ventricular conducting system can initiate contractions at a rate of approximately 40 times/min if AV conduction fails (complete heart block).

■ What ECG changes correlate with changes in phases of the action potential?

Decreased rate of rise of the action potential (phase 0) results in slowed conduction that can be manifested by widened P and QRS complexes, AV block, and fascicular or bundle branch block.

Phase 2 corresponds to the S-T interval, and therefore shortening (during digitalis therapy) or prolongation (in response to hypocalcemia) of phase 2 is reflected in the duration of the S-T segment. Since the duration of the Q-T interval is more conveniently measurable, phase 2 changes are expressed as shortening or prolongation of the Q-T interval. Damage to the cell membrane may render it incapable of normal regulation of ionic flow during the normally isoelectric phase 2, resulting in a "current of injury" reflected by elevation or depression of the S-T segment (see Fig. 12-18).

Rapid repolarization during phase 3 is represented by the T wave. Prolongation of phase 3 (caused by hypokalemia) causes lower amplitude and longer duration of the T waves.

Phase 3 terminates with a period of supernor-mal excitability that coincides with the U wave. Hypokalemia exaggerates the prominence of the U wave by prolonging phase 3.

■ How do arrhythmias result from alterations of action potential characteristics?

Stimuli that increase the rate of diastolic depolarization (phase 4 of automatic cells) can result in the appearance of ectopic beats from the atria, junctional area, or ventricles. Prolongation of repolarization (phase 3) or of depolarization (phase 0) provides special circumstances favoring the development of reentry circuits that are manifested as repetitive tachycardias (atrial or ventricular tachycardia) and as isolated extrasystoles.

■ How do metabolic abnormalities influence cellular electrical activity?

Since cellular electrical impulses are generated by ionic movement across the cell membrane, alterations in ionic activity and in the membrane itself can alter the shape and duration of the action potential.

Certain electrolyte abnormalities exert specific and identifiable effects on the ECG through alterations of the action potential (Table 12-1). Many drugs, particularly antiarrhythmic agents, alter phases of the cellular action potential and result in changes in the ECG (Table 12-2).

Automaticity (spontaneous phase 4 depolarization) can be increased by many stimuli, such as hyperadrenergic states, hypoxemia, acidosis, and alkalosis. Acidosis and alkalosis may influence cellular electrical activity only indirectly by causing hyperkalemia and hypokalemia, respectively. Hyperkalemia and certain antiarrhythmic drugs are particularly important causes of slowed conduction, because they decrease the rate of rise and the amplitude of phase 0.

Common metabolic problems

Major illness, trauma, and the postoperative state are almost invariably attended by metabolic abnormalities. The combination of hypoxemia and respiratory alkalosis, with or without metabolic acidosis, occurs in more than 60% of postsurgical patients and is common during acute myocardial infarction, shock, and other trauma.

Endogenous serum catecholamines, which are potent stimuli to automaticity, are elevated in many illnesses, especially acute myocardial infarction, congestive heart failure, and shock.

Abnormalities of serum electrolytes, particularly serum potassium and calcium, accompany many illnesses, either as primary illness-related problems or as consequences of therapy. Many

Table 12-1. Influence of serum potassium and calcium abnormalities on the ECG

Serum electrolyte abnormality	Effect on action potential	Effect on ECG
Hypokalemia	Prolonged phase 3, shortened phase 2	Prolonged low-amplitude T wave and prominent U wave with normal Q-T interval
	Increased rate of spontaneous (phase 4) depolarization	Ectopic beats
Hyperkalemia	Decreased slope phase 0	Slowed conduction with intra-atrial, AV, and intraventricular block
	Shortened phases 2 and 3	High-amplitude "peaked" T waves
Hypocalcemia	Prolonged phase 2	Prolonged Q-T interval
Hypercalcemia	Shortened phase 2	Shortened Q-T interval

Table 12-2. Commonly used medications and ECG changes

Preparation	Serum level	
	Therapeutic	Toxic
Antiarrhythmic drugs		
Quinidine, procainamide	QRS complex prolonged up to 25%, prolonged Q-T interval, depressed S-T segment, low-amplitude or inverted T wave, prominent U wave	QRS complex prolonged 25% to 50%, AV block, SA block, asystole
Phenytoin, lidocaine	Shortened P-R and Q-T intervals	AV block
Propranolol	Slowed AV conduction and sinus rate	Sinus bradycardia, AV block
Digitalis	S-T segment depressed, short Q-T interval, T wave changes	Arrhythmias, AV block
Mood changers		
Phenothiazines	Shortened P-R interval, prolonged Q-T interval, flattened and notched T waves	Arrhythmias, including ventricular fibrillation
Tricyclic amines	Prolonged Q-T and P-R intervals, prolonged QRS and P complexes	Ventricular and supraventricular arrhythmias, AV block
Catecholamines	Sinus tachycardia, shortened P-R interval	Subendocardial infarction pattern, supraventricular and ventricular arrhythmias

therapeutic agents, including bronchodilator and pressor catecholamines, anesthetic agents, digitalis and other cardioactive drugs, and even tranquilizers, have direct or indirect effects on the ECG. Intelligent interpretation of arrhythmias, conduction abnormalities, and changes in ECG complexes and intervals in critically ill patients requires understanding these basic facts.

The following case histories illustrate ways in which metabolic derangements can complicate the care and alter the ECG's of critically ill patients.

■ Fig. 12-3 is an ECG monitor strip from a 21-year-old female with aspiration pneumonia following spontaneous ventricular fibrillation. What is abnormal, what phase of the action potential is implicated, and what is the metabolic cause of the abnormality?

Referral to Table 12-3 reveals that the Q-T interval is prolonged for a heart rate of 125 beats/min in a female. Prolongation of the Q-T interval means that repolarization, (phases 2 and/or 3 of the action potential) is prolonged. Blood gas analysis revealed a Po_2 of 55 mm Hg. When normal oxygenation was restored, the Q-T interval returned to normal.

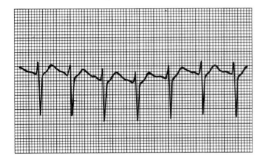

Fig. 12-3. Sinus tachycardia at 125 beats/min with Q-T interval at 0.36 second.

Table 12-3. Upper limits of the normal Q-T interval

Heart rate (beats/min)	Men and children (sec)	Women (sec)	Heart rate (beats/min)	Men and children (sec)	Women (sec)
40	0.49	0.59	70	0.40	0.40
43	0.48	0.49	75	0.38	0.39
46	0.47	0.48	80	0.37	0.38
48	0.46	0.47	86	0.36	0.37
50	0.45	0.46	92	0.35	0.36
52	0.44	0.46	100	0.34	0.35
54	0.44	0.45	109	0.33	0.33
57	0.43	0.44	120	0.31	0.32
60	0.42	0.43	133	0.29	0.30
63	0.41	0.42	150	0.27	0.28
66	0.40	0.41	172	0.25	0.26

Table 12-4. Upper limits of the normal P-R interval

| Heart rate (beats/min) | Adults | | Children | | |
	Large (sec)	Small (sec)	14-17 yr (sec)	7-13 yr (sec)	1½-6 yr (sec)
Below 70	0.21	0.20	0.19	0.18	0.16
71-90	0.20	0.19	0.18	0.17	0.165
91-110	0.19	0.18	0.17	0.16	0.155
111-130	0.18	0.17	0.16	0.15	0.145
Above 130	0.17	0.16	0.15	0.14	0.135

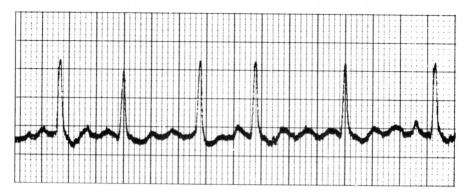

Fig. 12-4

■ **During therapy for bacterial pneumonia with mild respiratory failure, the patient's pulse rate suddenly became rapid and irregular. The rhythm strip shown in Fig. 12-4 was obtained. What does it show, and what are the clinical and electrophysiologic implications?**

This rhythm strip demonstrates atrial fibrillation with a ventricular rate varying from 100 to 150 beats/min (see later discussion of arrhythmias).

The development of arrhythmias in respiratory failure often results from increased automaticity, that is, more rapid rate of diastolic (phase 4) depolarization of ectopic pacemakers caused by metabolic abnormalities. Blood gas analysis of this patient revealed moderate hypoxemia and respiratory alkalosis from overventilation. The combination of hypoxemia and respiratory alkalosis is particularly arrhythmogenic and is a common metabolic problem in the critically ill patient.

■ **The ECG shown in Fig. 12-5 was recorded after diuretic therapy for acute pulmonary edema had caused a 6 L diuresis over a period of 8 hours. What abnormalities are present, and what action potential abnormalities do they represent?**

This ECG implicates prolongation of phase 3 of the action potential manifested by prolonged, low-amplitude T waves and prominent U waves. Rapid diuresis frequently causes rapid loss of body potassium stores, resulting in significant

hypokalemia. Replacement of potassium quickly corrected these abnormalities.

■ **During the initial evaluation of a patient in diabetic ketoacidosis, the ECG shown in Fig. 12-6 was obtained. What does it illustrate?**

This ECG reflects the characteristic high-amplitude, peaked T waves of early hyperkalemia caused by shortening of phases 2 and 3 of the action potential.

Administration of insulin and appropriate IV fluids rapidly corrected this potentially dangerous situation. Fig. 12-7 graphically illustrates the progressive changes associated with increasing serum potassium levels, culminating in ventricular fibrillation or asystole. Recognition of hyperkalemia from the ECG can alert the critical care worker to a life-threatening danger for the patient.

■ **During treatment with IV aminophylline for acute asthma, the rhythm strip shown in Fig. 12-8 was obtained from a 24-year-old male. What may be seen?**

A normal sequence of electrical activity is followed by a ventricular ectopic beat. (See discussion of arrhythmia analysis.) This patient was mildly hypoxemic and was receiving the catecholamine aminophylline, thus being subjected to two potent stimuli of phase 4 depolarization. Careful monitoring and cautious dose reduction allowed the continued use of aminophylline without progression to a more serious arrhythmia.

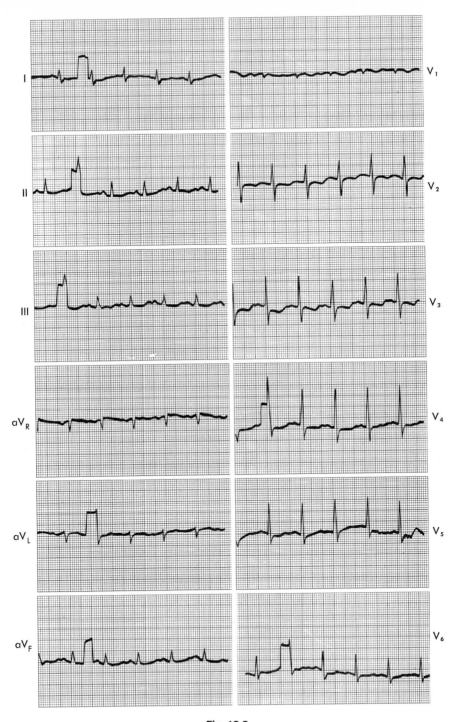

Fig. 12-5

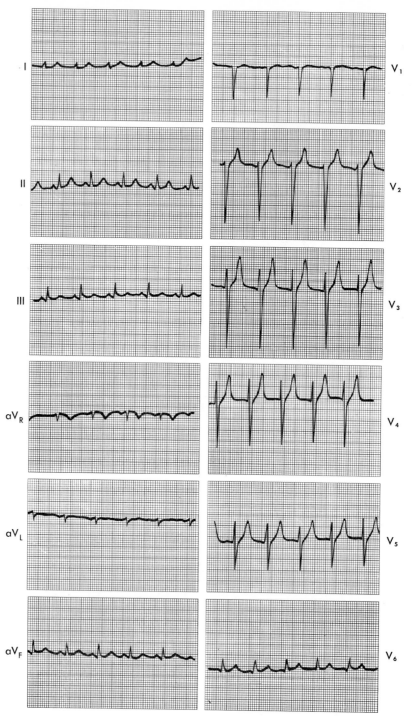

Fig. 12-6

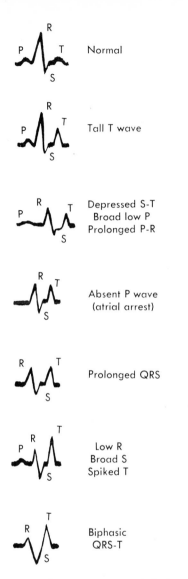

R
P T   Normal
S

R
P T   Tall T wave
S

R
P T   Depressed S-T
S   Broad low P
     Prolonged P-R

R
T   Absent P wave
S   (atrial arrest)

R T   Prolonged QRS
S

T
P R   Low R
S   Broad S
     Spiked T

T
R   Biphasic
S   QRS-T

Fig. 12-7. QRS-T changes at progressively increasing serum potassium levels.

■ **During dialysis for acute renal failure a routine ECG** (Fig. 12-9) **was obtained. What abnormalities are present, and what is their significance?**

This ECG demonstrates marked prolongation of the Q-T interval consistent with the increased duration of phases 2 and/or 3 of the action po-tential. Determination of serum electrolyte concentrations demonstrated hypocalcemia, a frequent abnormality during renal failure.

ARRHYTHMIAS

■ **When are arrhythmias dangerous?**

Arrhythmias are dangerous if they reduce cardiac output or if they predispose to ventricular fibrillation.

Rapid supraventricular tachycardias can reduce cardiac output by limiting diastolic filling time. Elderly patients may experience significant decreases in cardiac output at ventricular rates above 150 beats/min. The absence of coordinated atrial contraction, as with atrial fibrillation or ventricular tachycardia, also impairs ventricular filling and can decrease cardiac output. When the atrial contribution to ventricular filling is lost, rapid heart rates that limit diastolic filling time are particularly deleterious to cardiac output.

Premature contractions force the ventricle to eject blood before adequate diastolic filling has occurred, thus limiting stroke volume. Cardiac output can be reduced by premature contractions when they are very frequent.

Progression to ventricular fibrillation is the major danger of any ventricular arrhythmia during acute myocardial infarction and acute respiratory failure. Certain types of ventricular arrhythmias are traditionally considered to be signs of advanced heart disease and predictive of subsequent sudden cardiac death. Fig. 12-10 illustrates these phenomena.

■ **What is the clinical approach to arrhythmia interpretation?**

Interpretation of the clinical significance of arrhythmias includes the following:

1. Assessment of the hemodynamic impact. Does the patient exhibit signs of inadequate cardiac output?
2. Assessment of prognostic significance. Will this arrhythmia predispose to a more serious one such as ventricular fibrillation?
3. Assessment of the reason for its appearance. What underlying hemodynamic or metabolic changes prompted its appearance?
4. Assessment of the relationship of digitalis therapy to the arrhythmia. The possibility of digitalis toxicity is enhanced in critical

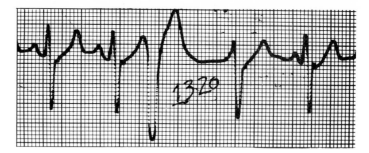

Fig. 12-8

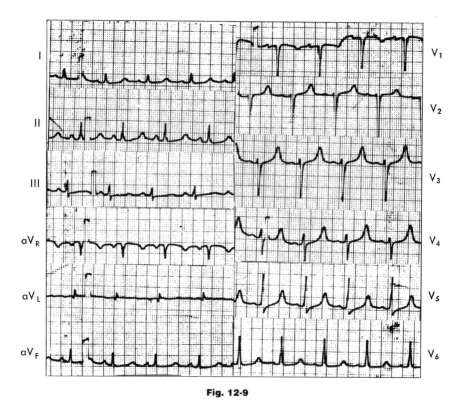

Fig. 12-9

care situations and is an important and frequent cause of arrhythmias.

5. Diagnosis of the specific type of arrhythmia. Recognition is necessary in evaluating the overall significance of the condition.

■ How are arrhythmias diagnosed using the ECG?

Most of the commonly observed arrhythmias can be rapidly diagnosed by using the following five simple checkpoints:

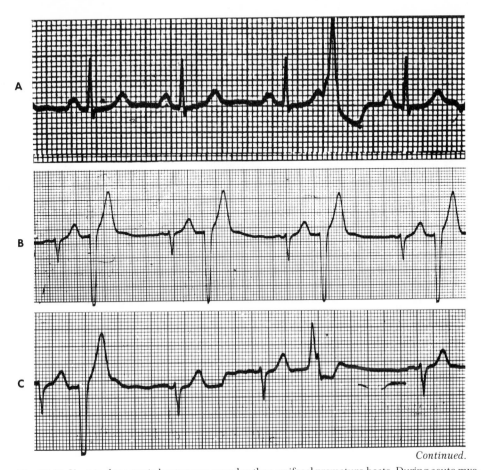

A

B

C

Continued.

Fig. 12-10. Ventricular ectopic beats more complex than unifocal premature beats. During acute myocardial ischemia these abnormal beats may rapidly progress to ventricular fibrillation. When seen during routine evaluation of asymptomatic individuals, they correlate with subsequent sudden cardiac death. **A,** "R-on-T" phenomenon. T wave following third QRS complex is interrupted by premature ventricular QRS complex. **B,** Ventricular bigeminy. Each normal QRS complex is followed at consistent interval by premature ventricular beat. Abnormal beats are identical in form and thus presumably originate from same focus. **C,** Multifocal ventricular premature beats. Two abnormal premature ventricular complexes are seen. Both QRS forms and coupling intervals are different, suggesting two different foci of origin. **D,** Ventricular tachycardia. A premature ventricular beat is followed by four ventricular beats at a rate of approximately 150 beats/min. This arrhythmia is nearly always indicative of serious underlying heart disease. **E,** Repetitive premature ventricular beats. Two premature ventricular complexes, possibly from different foci, occur without intervening normal complexes. **F,** Ventricular fibrillation. There is total absence of definable QRS complexes. This random, disorganized electrical activity reflects totally disorganized ventricular muscle activity. During ventricular fibrillation there is essentially no blood flow, and instantaneous loss of consciousness ensues.

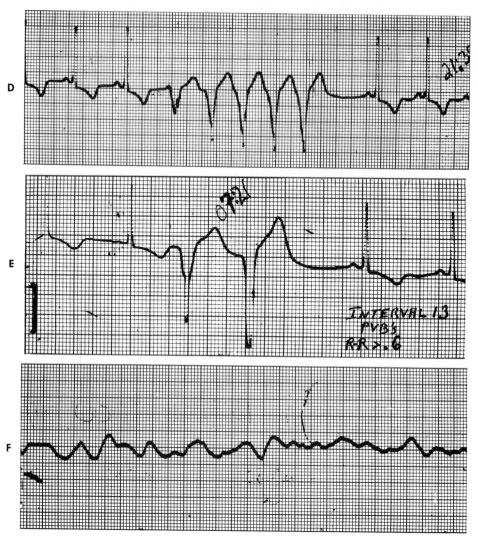

Fig. 12-10, cont'd. For legend see p. 215.

1. Ventricular rate. Ventricular rates above 150 beats/min are commonly associated with paroxysmal supraventricular tachycardia, atrial flutter or fibrillation, or ventricular tachycardia. Ventricular rates below 50 beats/min suggest sinus bradycardia, junctional escape rhythm, or complete heart block with idioventricular rhythm.

2. Ventricular rhythm. Ventricular response to supraventricular arrhythmias may be regular or irregular. Totally irregular ventricular response is found with atrial fibrillation and chaotic atrial tachycardia, as well as with random unifocal and multifocal atrial and ventricular ectopic beats. Group beating, or repetitions of a series of irregular beats, characterizes the Wenckebach phenomenon, trigeminy, and bigeminy.

3. QRS analysis. QRS analysis helps determine whether the arrhythmia is ventricular or

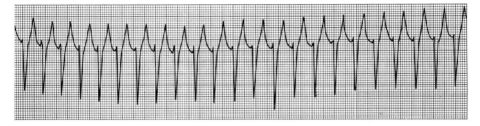

Fig. 12-11

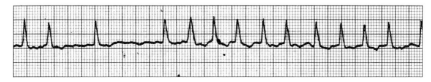

Fig. 12-12. From Conover, M. H.: Cardiac arrhythmias, ed. 2, St. Louis, 1978, The C. V. Mosby Co.

supraventricular. Normal-width (less than 0.12 second) QRS complexes always denote an atrial or junctional (supraventricular) focus. Arrhythmias of ventricular origin always have wide (0.12 second or more) QRS complexes. Aberrant conduction of supraventricular impulses frequently causes wide QRS complexes, leading to confusion with ventricular arrhythmias.

4. P wave analysis is crucial to identification of supraventricular arrhythmias. If P waves are not visible in the 12-lead ECG, then esophageal, right atrial, or Lewis leads should be employed to identify them. Carotid sinus massage may slow a rapid ventricular rate enough to expose atrial activity otherwise obscured by QRS complexes.

5. Observation of the onset and termination of sustained tachycardias can yield valuable diagnostic information. Supraventricular tachycardias are nearly always initiated by a premature supraventricular beat with an abnormal P wave. Ventricular arrhythmias are not preceded by ectopic P waves. Following termination of a supraventricular arrhythmia, there is a period of sinus pause, or abnormal P waves, occurring before resumption of normal sinus rhythm. Ventricular tachycardias may be followed by a full compensatory pause.

■ **Is the arrhythmia shown in Fig. 12-11 supraventricular or ventricular?**

The ventricular rate is 175 beats/min, immediately placing the arrhythmia in the category with paroxysmal supraventricular tachycardia, atrial flutter or fibrillation, or ventricular tachycardia. Because the QRS complexes are normal in duration, this is a supraventricular tachycardia. The rate and regular rhythm make this paroxysmal atrial tachycardia.

■ **What commonly encountered arrhythmia is shown in Fig. 12-12?**

The ventricular rate of approximately 130 beats/min is not specific for any particular arrhythmia, but the normal QRS duration identifies a supraventricular origin. In this case the rhythm is the leading indicator of the arrhythmia, as it is totally irregular and therefore must indicate atrial fibrillation. Multifocal or chaotic atrial tachycardia could also give an irregular rhythm, but no definite P waves are seen, affirming that this is atrial fibrillation.

■ **What is perhaps the most commonly misdiagnosed serious arrhythmia?**

Since the QRS complexes are normal in duration, the arrhythmia shown in Fig. 12-13 is of

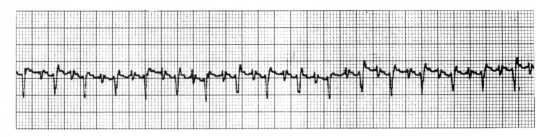

Fig. 12-13

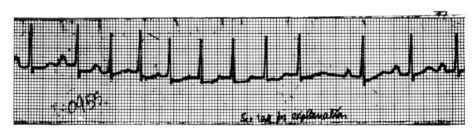

Fig. 12-14

supraventricular origin, and the possible diagnoses based on the rate of 130 beats/min are sinus tachycardia, paroxysmal supraventricular tachycardia, and atrial flutter. Careful inspection reveals that what appears to be a terminal positive QRS deflection is actually a P wave. Atrial flutter with 2:1 conduction frequently occurs this way, with every other P wave (flutter wave) hidden or buried in the QRS complex. Untreated atrial flutter usually has 2:1 conduction, and therefore the ventricular rate is between 140 and 160 beats/min. That is the case in this example, and the diagnosis is confirmed by gentle carotid sinus massage, increasing the block at the AV node and unmasking a series of two or more consecutive flutter waves, by which the diagnosis can be made.

■ **What is the mechanism of the onset of the arrhythmia shown in Fig. 12-14?**

In this case the tachycardia was initiated by an atrial ectopic beat (sixth complex from left) followed by a supraventricular tachycardia. After termination of the arrhythmia sinus rhythm resumes without a full compensatory pause. It is

always helpful to analyze the onset of a sustained tachycardia for clues as to its origin.

■ **What might cause a relatively long pause in the P wave?**

P wave analysis could show an absence of one P wave at a time when it should have occurred. The P wave terminating the long pause would occur at the expected time; thus the arrhythmia would consist of one missed atrial depolarization and one QRS complex. Had a P wave occurred during the pause, but with no QRS complex following it, the diagnosis would have been AV block; with no atrial activity occurring, it is an SA node block. The block may be in the tissue surrounding the SA node, thus preventing escape of the impulse into the atria.

■ **Are the atria and ventricles associated or dissociated in Fig. 12-15?**

In this example there is one P wave with every QRS complex, and a constant relationship exists between them. Therefore there is association between the ventricles and atria; in this example, however, the P waves follow the QRS

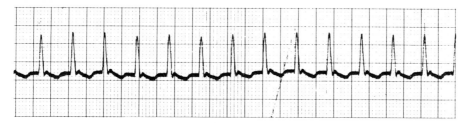

Fig. 12-15

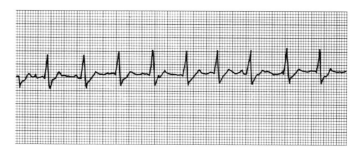

Fig. 12-16

complexes rather than preceding them. This is typical of an AV junctional rhythm. The diagnosis is based on the occurrence of the P wave after each QRS complex and on an abnormal P wave configuration, representing retrograde conduction from the AV junction through the atria.

■ **On the basis of the QRS configuration, what are the two possible reasons for the arrhythmia illustrated in Fig. 12-16?**

With large, wide QRS complexes this is either ventricular tachycardia or a supraventricular tachycardia with aberrant conduction (intraventricular conduction defect). In this case the presence of P waves occurring at a different rate and unassociated with the QRS complexes confirms that this is ventricular tachycardia. With a supraventricular tachycardia there would be a 1 : 1 relationship between the P waves and the QRS complexes.

■ **What is the nature of the wide, abnormal-looking QRS complexes in Fig. 12-17?**

This is an example of aberrant conduction of supraventricular impulses. The abnormal beats

are conducted with a right bundle branch block configuration. In most patients the right bundle branch remains refractory slightly longer than the left bundle branch, resulting in a brief period during which a premature supraventricular impulse conducted through the ventricles travels through the left bundle branch but is blocked at the right bundle branch. This results in a QRS complex with a right bundle branch block configuration. Occasionally the phenomenon occurs with left bundle branch block, but in the majority of cases the aberrant conduction is of the right bundle branch variety.

Three general rules help to identify aberrant conduction:

1. If a P wave precedes the anomalous QRS complex, it is probably supraventricular.
2. The period during which aberrant conduction can occur is at the end of the refractory period following the previous impulse. Therefore a beat that comes at a relatively short interval following a beat that was preceded by a relatively long interval is likely to undergo aberrant conduction. The general rule favoring aberrant conduction is a short

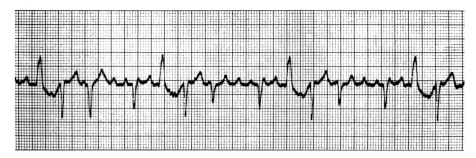

Fig. 12-17

R-R interval following a longer R-R interval.

3. In most cases, aberrant conduction is of the right bundle branch block variety.

HEART DISEASE

■ What ECG changes are caused by coronary artery disease?

Heart damage from coronary arteriosclerosis is caused by obstruction to coronary blood flow leading to myocardial hypoxia. Three degrees of hypoxic damage are associated with specific ECG changes. *Ischemia* refers to reversible myocardial damage leading to altered repolarization. Deep, symmetric T wave inversion is the ECG sign of epicardial ischemia, and a large, peaked T wave is the sign of subendocardial ischemia. *Injury* is a more severe form of damage, in which cell membrane abnormalities result in a *current of injury* that displaces the normally isoelectric S-T segment. This electric current is registered as elevation or depression of the S-T segment. Subendocardial injury causes S-T segment depression, and subepicardial or transmural injury causes S-T segment elevation. Areas of injury can recover or proceed to infarction. *Infarction* is irreversible death of myocardium leading to absence of normal electrical forces and is manifested by a negative initial QRS deflection called the *Q wave*. Q wave duration must be 0.04 second or greater to correlate significantly with infarction. (Many normal individuals have initially negative QRS deflections of 0.02-second duration in left ventricular leads that represent septal depolarization.)

Coronary artery disease is clinically manifested as myocardial infarction, which causes ECG changes in 80% to 90% of incidents, and as angina pectoris, which is associated with less frequent and less specific changes.

■ What ECG changes result from acute myocardial infarction?

Myocardial infarction can be *transmural*, that is, involving at least the outer two-thirds of the ventricular wall, or *subendocardial*, that is, limited to the inner one third or endocardial surface of the ventricular wall.

Acute transmural infarction causes the appearance of the Q wave. An accompanying S-T segment elevation (epicardial injury) and T wave inversion (epicardial ischemia) indicate that the event is probably recent.

■ Why does a Q wave result from transmural infarction?

Dead tissue is unable to generate a depolarization current; it is electrically silent. Leads monitoring the depolarization current from an infarcted area will record an initial negative deflection caused by depolarization of the opposite heart wall. The Q wave is the ECG sine qua non of transmural infarction and represents dead tissue.

■ Why are S-T segment and T wave changes present?

Surrounding the infarction area is a zone of injury and around that a zone of ischemia. Since transmural infarction involves the epicardial surface of the heart, epicardial injury occurs and an elevated S-T segment results. S-T segment elevation usually resolves within a few days and

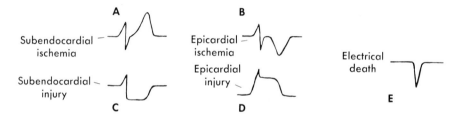

Fig. 12-18. Schematic ECG forms of ischemic events. **A,** Tall T waves of subendocardial ischemia. **B,** Inverted coved T waves of epicardial ischemia. **C,** RST segment depression of subendocardial injury. **D,** RST segment elevation of epicardial injury. **E,** QS wave of electrical death.

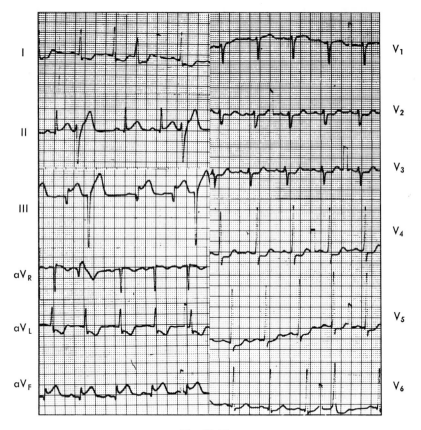

Fig. 12-19

therefore is considered necessary for ECG diagnosis of *acute* myocardial infarction.

Symmetrically inverted T waves indicate the presence of an ischemic zone of altered repolarization. Transmural myocardial infarction usually causes epicardial ischemia as well as injury,

and therefore T wave inversion is usually present at some time during the event.

Fig. 12-18 schematically illustrates typical S-T segment and T wave changes.

Infarction of the subendocardial layer, which includes the inner third of the ventricular wall, causes only S-T segment and T wave changes. Healthy tissue in the overlying epicardium is still capable of generating a normal QRS complex and no Q waves appear. However, the ischemia and injury associated with the infarction are manifested by the S-T segment and T wave changes. S-T segment depression reflects endocardial injury, contrasting with the S-T segment elevation of epicardial injury normally seen in transmural infarction. Deep symmetric T wave inversion occurs if the endocardial ischemia extends to the epicardial surface.

■ **The ECG shown in Fig. 12-19 was taken after the patient had been resuscitated from ventricular fibrillation. What is the diagnosis?**

Compared with a prior normal ECG, this one demonstrates the recent appearance of 0.04-sec-

ond duration Q waves in lead III, plus S-T segment elevation in leads that monitor the inferior or diaphragmatic surface of the heart—II, III, and aV_F. Reciprocal S-T segment depression appears in leads I and aV_L. The pattern is typical of acute diaphragmatic (inferior) transmural myocardial infarction. Premature ventricular contractions are also present, and with acute myocardial infarction, might lead to ventricular fibrillation.

■ **Shortly after a 58-year-old man developed crushing precordial chest pain and severe weakness, the ECG shown in Fig. 12-20 was obtained. What abnormalities are present, and what is the location of the infarction?**

Leads I, aV_L, and V_1 through V_6 exhibit striking S-T segment elevation, and reciprocal S-T seg-

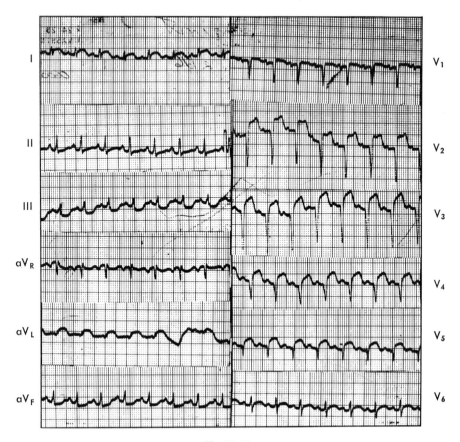

Fig. 12-20

ment depression is found in leads II, III, and aV$_F$. The absence of initial R waves, that is, the presence of Q waves, in precordial leads V$_2$ through V$_4$ designates this as an anterolateral myocardial infarction. T wave inversion has not yet developed.

■ What are the earliest ECG findings of acute myocardial infarction?

Fig. 12-21 displays precordial leads from a patient whose myocardial infarction developed in the hospital. The tracing in Fig. 12-21, *A*, is the normal admission record. In the tracing in Fig. 12-21, *B*, there is a dramatic increase in T wave amplitude associated with S-T segment elevation in leads V$_1$ through V$_3$ and reciprocal depression in leads V$_4$ through V$_6$. One day later, 0.04-second Q waves appear in leads V$_2$ through V$_4$, with S-T segment elevation and T wave inversion in leads V$_2$ through V$_6$.

Initial epicardial injury (S-T segment elevation) and endocardial ischemia (tall, peaked T waves) characterize the "hyperacute" myocardial infarction. Within hours or days the more familiar Q waves of transmural infarction and T wave inversion of accompanying epicardial ischemia evolve.

■ How long does the ECG remain changed after an acute myocardial infarction?

S-T segment changes can disappear within hours or may persist for days. S-T segment elevation present months after an infarction may signal the presence of a ventricular aneurysm. T waves may remain inverted for months, and Q waves usually remain permanently. Q waves may regress or disappear after months or years as the myocardial scar contracts and decreases in size.

■ How does the ECG localize infarctions anatomically?

Areas of infarction are localized by determining which leads display pathologic Q waves. Leads II, III, and aV$_F$ best display changes from the in-

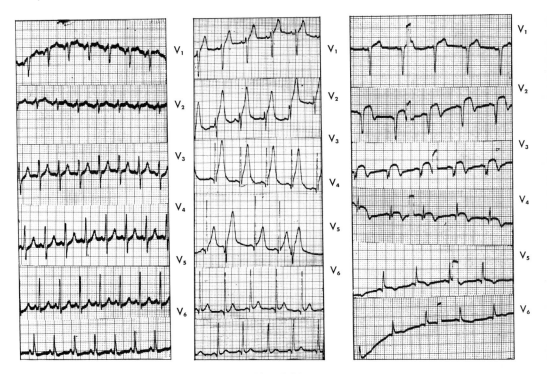

Fig. 12-21

ferior surface of the heart, whereas the anterior and lateral walls of the left ventricle are monitored by I, aV_L, and V_2 through V_6. Lead V_1, over the right ventricle, senses changes in the posterior left ventricular surface. Table 12-5 lists anatomic sites of infarcts relative to the ECG leads in which Q waves appear.

■ What ECG changes accompany angina pectoris?

Three syndromes of angina pectoris exist, and all three can be associated with ECG changes. Approximately 50% of the episodes of stress-induced angina pectoris result in subendocardial injury with S-T segment depression. Specific criteria have been developed to separate the stress-induced subendocardial injury pattern of S-T segment depression caused by coronary disease from

Table 12-5. ECG localization of infarction

Anatomic type of infarction	ECG leads affected
Inferior (diaphragmatic)	II, III, aV_F
Anteroseptal	V_1-V_3
Anterior	V_2-V_4
Anterolateral	I, aV_L, V_4-V_6
Apical	V_3, V_4
Posterior*	V_1, V_2

*The truly posterior infarct is sensed only reciprocally by V_1, since there are no leads over the back. If an esophageal lead is used, Q waves, S-T segment elevation, and T wave inversion are found—the reciprocal changes of which are reflected in V_1 as a broad (0.04-second) R wave, S-T segment depression, and upright T waves.

that caused by metabolic and nonspecific changes. Reliable correlation with the presence of coronary disease requires that the S-T segment be depressed at least 1 mm below the baseline (P-R interval) for at least 0.06 second after the junction point between the QRS complex and the S-T segment is written (Fig. 12-22).

Preinfarction angina is clinically a more severe form of angina pectoris with a high rate of progression to myocardial infarction. ECG changes of typical angina pectoris are often observed in this syndrome. Prinzmetal, or "variant," angina pectoris is a syndrome of angina occurring at rest associated with S-T segment elevation.

■ What other problems cause S-T segment depression?

Many nonspecific metabolic and inflammatory processes cause S-T segment depression. These can create confusion by imitating subendocardial "injury." Adherence to the criteria described previously for stress-induced injury patterns will usually resolve the confusion.

Common causes of S-T segment depression not associated with subendocardial injury in critically ill patients include the following:

1. Digitalis therapy can cause a smoothly "scooped-out" concave S-T segment depression (Fig. 12-23).
2. Hyperventilation can cause mild S-T segment depression and T wave inversion.
3. Rapid heart rates can result in artifactual depression of the initial part of the S-T segment (Fig. 12-24).

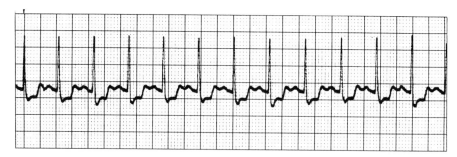

Fig. 12-22. S-T segment remains depressed more than 1 mm below baseline (P-R or T-P interval) 0.06 second after the "J" point is inscribed. This pattern correlates with underlying coronary artery disease.

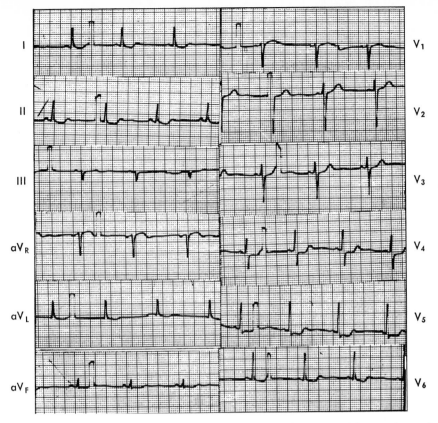

Fig. 12-23. Digitalis causes a nearly unique smoothly "scooped" depression of the initial part of the S-T segment.

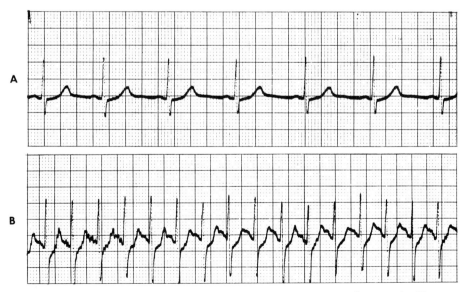

Fig. 12-24. Depression of S-T segment for less than 0.06 second is commonly seen in healthy persons when the heart rate increases.

■ **What cardiac problems other than coronary artery disease cause ECG changes?**

Myocarditis, endocarditis, and pericarditis are encountered in critically ill patients either as primary problems or as complications of other diseases.

Myocarditis and endocarditis are relatively uncommon diseases and cause nonspecific S-T segment and T wave changes. Myocarditis with acute rheumatic fever often causes transient first-degree AV block with P-R interval prolongation. Vegetations from endocarditis can embolize to a coronary artery and cause acute myocardial infarction with associated ECG changes.

Pericarditis is a common clinical event associated with specific ECG changes. Pericarditis complicates hemodialysis for renal failure, chest trauma, open-heart surgery, pulmonary embolism, disseminated bacterial or fungal infections, metastatic malignancies, collagen-vascular diseases, and allergic reactions to drugs. "Idiopathic" pericarditis can occur spontaneously in healthy individuals and often creates confusion with myocardial infarction.

■ **Both pericarditis and myocardial infarction can complicate hemodialysis for renal failure. How can the ECG help distinguish acute pericarditis from acute myocardial infarction?**

Acute pericarditis and acute myocardial infarction both cause epicardial injury leading to S-T

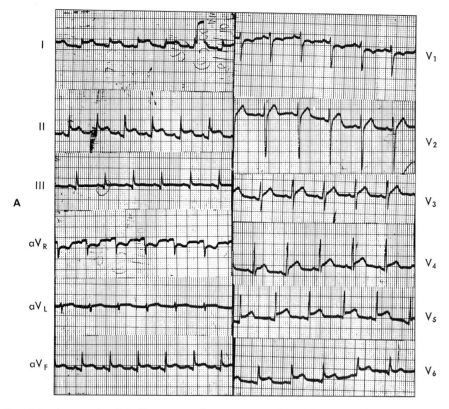

Fig. 12-25. Acute pericarditis. Tracing in **A** demonstrates striking S-T segment elevation in limb leads I, II, III, and aV$_F$ and in all precordial leads except V$_1$. Reciprocal S-T segment depression is apparent in leads aV$_R$ and V$_1$, the "right ventricular" leads. Tracing in **B** documents return of S-T segment to baseline and development of T wave inversion in leads I, aV$_L$, and V$_2$ through V$_6$.

segment elevation in the left ventricular leads. Myocardial infarction, however, is a focal event involving one discrete area of the heart, whereas pericarditis often involves the entire surface of the left ventricle. Consequently, pericarditis classically causes S-T segment elevation in nearly all left ventricular leads, whereas infarction involves only a few. Reciprocal S-T segment depression occurs in leads opposite those reflecting a myocardial infarction but is usually absent in pericarditis because all leads are recording epicardial injury.

Pericarditis also causes a progression of changes differing from that of acute myocardial infarction (Fig. 12-25). The sequential ECG changes of pericarditis are as follows:

1. Diffuse S-T segment elevation

2. Return of S-T segment to baseline potentials
3. Inversion of T waves
4. Return of T waves to normal

Q waves do not evolve in pericarditis. S-T segment elevation and T wave inversion usually do not occur simultaneously in pericarditis but often do in myocardial infarction. Unfortunately 75% of patients with pericarditis display nonspecific ECG changes because of the limited extent of the inflammation or simply because one or more of the typical sequential changes was missed or did not occur. These patients may have only mild S-T segment and T wave changes.

Arrhythmias of all kinds frequently complicate pericarditis but those of ventricular origin do not lead to ventricular fibrillation, in contrast to the situation in acute myocardial infarction.

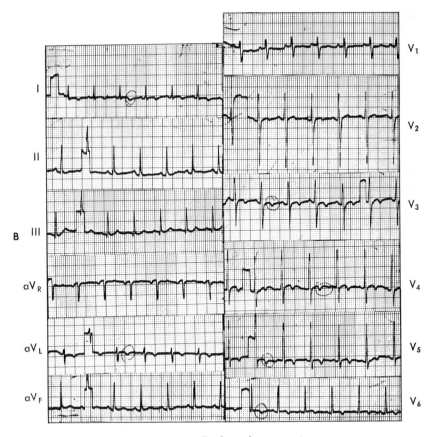

Fig. 12-25, cont'd. For legend see opposite page.

■ What ECG changes occur in patients following open-heart surgery?

Open-heart surgery patients represent an increasingly numerous population in the critical care unit. In addition to the metabolic and pharmacologic influences common to all patients during recovery from major surgery, special cardiac problems are observed.

Pericardiectomy is a necessary maneuver for exposing the heart and results in pericarditis, manifested by appropriate ECG changes, during healing.

Acute myocardial infarction occurs in up to 15% of coronary artery bypass operations and presents with Q waves with or without S-T segment and T wave changes.

Arrhythmias are the most frequent ECG abnormalities after heart surgery. Although any type of arrhythmia may complicate this situation, some general rules are useful:

1. Supraventricular arrhythmias commonly complicate mitral valve surgery, particularly when atrial dilatation is present.
2. Complex ventricular arrhythmias (other than unifocal premature ventricular contractions [PVC's]) occurring after coronary artery bypass procedures should be treated with the same vigor as those complicating

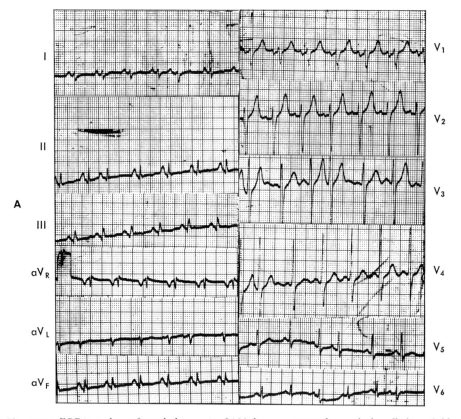

Fig. 12-26. ECG in **A** shows frontal plane axis of 100 degrees, incomplete right bundle branch block, and P waves 3.5 mm high in lead II with P wave axis at 60 degrees. Occasional PAC's are noted. Changes would represent acute pulmonary hypertension, or chronic cor pulmonale. Comparison with previous ECG, **B,** demonstrates that rightward axis shift, abnormal P waves, and incomplete right bundle branch block are all recent changes. Pulmonary angiography confirmed acute pulmonary embolism.

acute myocardial infarction; ventricular tachycardia or fibrillation in the postoperative coronary artery bypass patient is associated with 50% mortality.

ECG CHANGES AND PULMONARY DISEASE

■ How does respiratory failure alter the ECG?

Arrhythmias and alterations of the ECG waveforms and intervals frequently accompany respiratory failure.

Most of the ECG effects of acute and chronic respiratory failure result from the metabolic and hemodynamic effects of hypoxemia. Hypoxemia with or without hypercapnia is an invariable result of respiratory failure. Besides its metabolic effects on automaticity and repolarization, hypoxemia causes pulmonary hypertension by stimulating the vasoconstriction of pulmonary arterioles. Pulmonary hypertension can cause acute right atrial and ventricular dilatation, and if sustained, will eventually cause right atrial and ventricular hypertrophy.

Arrhythmias can also be stimulated by the use of β-adrenergic bronchodilators in hypoxemic patients, by overventilation with respirators, causing respiratory alkalosis, and by hypercapnia. Endotracheal suction frequently induces ar-

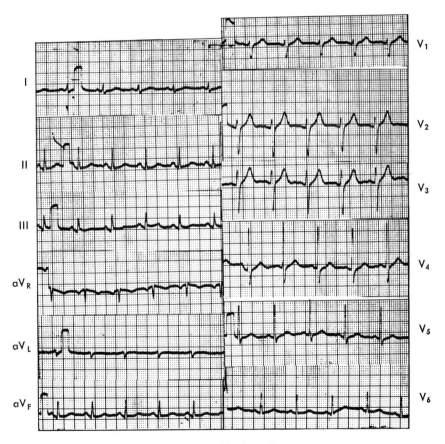

Fig. 12-26, cont'd. For legend see opposite page.

rhythmias, both by transient hypoxemia from interrupted ventilation and by vagal stimulation.

■ Do acute and chronic respiratory failure differ in their ECG effects?

Arrhythmias are frequent in both acute and chronic respiratory failure. The major ECG difference between the two is the development of right atrial and right ventricular hypertrophy with chronic respiratory failure. Chronic hypoxemia causes sustained pulmonary hypertension and results in right ventricular hypertrophy (eventually causing right atrial hypertrophy), which in the absence of left ventricular disease is called cor pulmonale. Acute hypoxemia occurring in an otherwise healthy person, such as when respiratory arrest results from barbiturate overdose, may cause arrhythmias and Q-T interval prolongation but does not usually cause P wave or QRS complex alterations. Acute pulmonary embolism is associated with ECG changes thought to represent the effects of sudden acute pulmonary hypertension (Fig. 12-26), as demonstrated by the following example.

Thirty-six hours after an abdominal hysterectomy a 47-year-old patient experienced the sudden onset of pleurisy and dyspnea and was found to be wheezing and hypotensive. An emergency chest x-ray film demonstrated right lower lobe atelectasis, arterial oxygen tension was 55 mm Hg, and the ECG shown in Fig. 12-26, *A*, was obtained for comparison with the preoperative ECG (Fig. 12-26, *B*).

Large, acute pulmonary embolism causes sudden pulmonary hypertension, which may force dilatation of the right atrium and ventricle, This sudden dilatation may be observed electrocardiographically as P pulmonale, transient right bundle branch block (complete or incomplete), a rightward and posterior shift of the mean QRS axis, clockwise rotation with QS or rS complexes in leads V_1 to V_4, and S-T segment deviation and T wave inversion in right precordial and inferior limb leads. P pulmonale is manifested by P waves at least 2.5 mm high in leads II, III and aV_F, denoting inferior shift of the P wave vector. QRS vector alterations can result in the S_1, S_2, S_3, or S_1Q_3 patterns in the limb leads. Chest leads may demonstrate smaller amplitude R waves in leads V_1 to V_5 as the QRS axis shifts posteriorly.

Acute cor pulmonale of pulmonary embolism can resemble diaphragmatic myocardial infarction if the S_1Q_3 pattern occurs (Fig. 12-27). Lack of appropriate S-T segment changes and failure of Q waves to develop in other inferior leads (II, aV_F) are helpful differential clues.

Rarely, S-T segment elevation and T wave inversion in lead V_2 may occur, simulating anterior myocardial infarction. Lack of Q wave development and rapid resolution of this pattern help exclude anterior myocardial infarction as a diagnosis.

Arrhythmias can complicate major pulmonary embolism, especially when underlying heart disease is present, but they are usually of no clinical significance.

Although these "classic" ECG changes are helpful when they occur, most large pulmonary emboli cause nonspecific changes, and medium-sized and smaller emboli usually cause no changes. ECG changes in patients experiencing major acute pulmonary embolism who did not have prior cardiac or pulmonary disease are listed in Table 12-6. These changes are transient and usually disappear within 2 weeks.

Acute ECG changes have also been described with large (30% to 100%) spontaneous pneumothorax. This syndrome of sudden pleurisy, dyspnea, and apprehension clinically mimics acute pulmonary embolism and acute myocardial infarction. Since ECG changes accompany all these entities, care must be given to interpretation of these changes in arriving at a correct diagnosis. Spontaneous and induced pneumothorax can cause a rightward shift in the mean frontal QRS axis, diminution of the precordial R wave voltage, decreased QRS amplitude, and precordial T wave inversion (Fig. 12-28). Since these changes can also accompany acute pulmonary embolism, differentiation of these two entities requires a chest x-ray study. Acute transmural myocardial infarction is easily differentiated when Q waves and S-T segment elevation are present. Subendocardial infarction manifested only by inverted precordial T waves does not cause a rightward shift of the frontal plane axis or a decrease in precordial R wave and QRS amplitude.

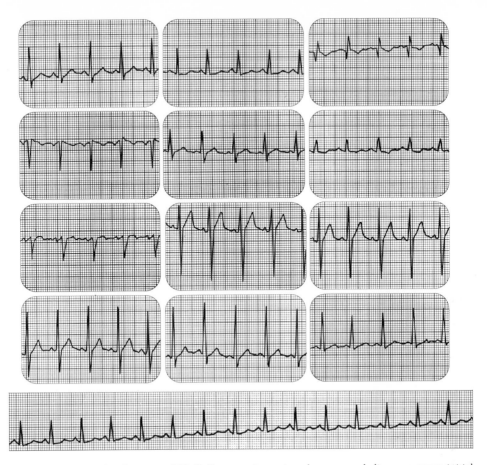

Fig. 12-27. Sudden development of "S_1,Q_3" pattern in acute pulmonary embolism can cause initial confusion with acute myocardial infarction.

Table 12-6. ECG changes with major pulmonary embolism*

ECG changes	Percentage of patients affected
Nonspecific S-T segment changes	41
Nonspecific T wave changes	42
"Acute cor pulmonale" (one or more of the following: $S_1Q_3T_3$ or right bundle branch block or P pulmonale or RAD)	26
Low voltage	6
Normal ECG	6
Left axis deviation	7
Right axis deviation	7

*Applies to patients not having had prior cardiac or pulmonary disease.

■ What are the ECG changes of chronic pulmonary disease?

Two factors influence the ECG in patients with chronic pulmonary disease: (1) hyperinflation of the chest and (2) hypertrophy of the right atrium and ventricle.

Chest hyperinflation increases the distance between the heart and the chest leads and can result in low-amplitude QRS complexes in these leads.

Right atrial hypertrophy is reflected by tall (greater than 2.5 mm) P waves in leads II, III, and aV_F, and a P wave axis greater than 75 degrees in the frontal plane. Right ventricular hypertrophy is manifested in lead V_1 by a dominant

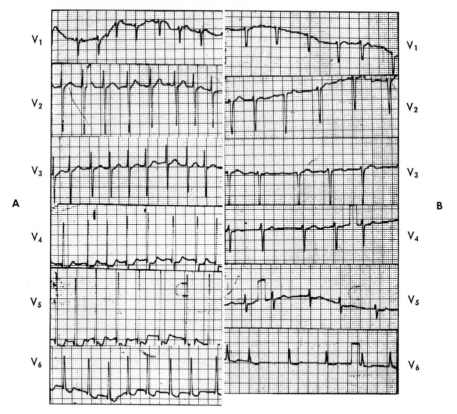

Fig. 12-28. Tracing in **A** represents chest leads of admission ECG from patient with fever and pleural effusion. Shortly after diagnostic thoracentesis he complained of severe shortness of breath, and tracing in **B** was obtained. Significant posterior shift in QRS axis has caused much reduced amplitude of precordial R waves. Chest x-ray film demonstrates large left pneumothorax.

(greater than 7 mm) R wave in lead V_1, with an R:S ratio greater than 1. Because the increased muscle mass of the hypertrophied right heart requires more time to depolarize and generates more electrical force, the QRS axis may be shifted toward the right and anteriorly. Prolongation of depolarization prolongs the terminal QRS complex, resulting in a S wave of greater than 0.02-second duration in leads I, II, and III (the $S_1S_2S_3$ pattern) and/or "incomplete right bundle branch block" with normal QRS duration and an rsR′ pattern in lead V_1. Fig. 12-29 demonstrates some of these changes. Unfortunately cor pulmonale usually causes only nonspecific changes in the S-T segment and T wave and remains difficult to detect.

■ **Ventricular and supraventricular arrhythmias of variable severity can be detected in more than 80% of patients with chronic stable pulmonary disease. What arrhythmias complicate acute respiratory failure?**

Both ventricular and supraventricular arrhythmias occur during acute respiratory failure. Supraventricular arrhythmias other than premature atrial contractions are seen in nearly 50% of these patients. Any supraventricular arrhythmia can occur, but chaotic or multifocal atrial tachycardia and paroxysmal atrial tachycardia are the most common arrhythmias.

Ventricular arrhythmias more complex than PVC's are common and include ventricular bigeminy, tachycardia, and fibrillation. Ventricular

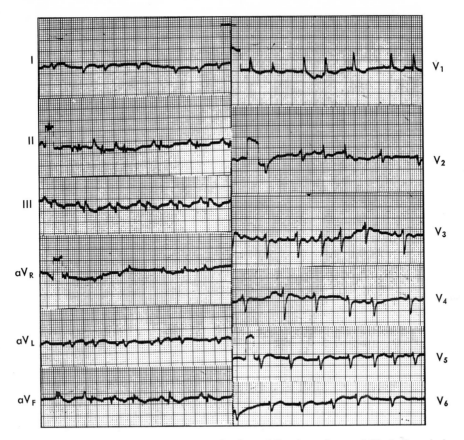

Fig. 12-29. Right axis deviation, low QRS amplitude, and P pulmonale are visible in frontal plane leads. Incomplete right bundle branch block and posterior QRS axis are present in chest leads. Sinus arrhythmia and frequent premature atrial contractions are also demonstrated.

fibrillation is reported to occur in up to 25% of patients with acute respiratory failure. Ventricular arrhythmias carry grim prognostic implications for the patient, probably because they reflect severe underlying pulmonary disease. Nearly 70% of patients having acute respiratory failure who develop PVC's die during that hospitalization.

Table 12-7 lists the arrhythmias developing during acute respiratory failure in one study.

■ How should arrhythmias be treated during acute respiratory failure?

Treatment for arrhythmias during respiratory failure is based on correction of hypoxemia and other metabolic abnormalities and discontinu-

ance of β-adrenergic bronchodilators if possible. If these drugs must be used, careful monitoring is essential. The following example illustrates a common occurrence in the critical care unit.

During treatment for an episode of acute respiratory failure a patient developed the rapid, irregular supraventricular arrhythmia shown in Fig. 12-30, *A*, after receiving an aminophylline suppository. The arrhythmia appears to be atrial fibrillation. An alert consultant recorded P waves from a transvenous right atrial electrode in order to document the diagnosis and presented the rhythm strip shown in Fig. 12-30, *B*. The right atrial recording shows P waves of variable configuration with variable P-R interval and a ventricular rate above 120 beats/min, thus satisfying the diagnostic criteria for multifocal (chaotic) atrial tachycardia (MAT).

This arrhythmia mimics atrial fibrillation when the surface ECG does not record recognizable P waves. Treatment of MAT with digitalis, a drug normally recommended to slow AV conduction in atrial fibrillation, is usually not helpful, because this arrhythmia is associated with advanced pulmonary disease and its attendant metabolic abnormalities. In addition, patients with pulmonary insufficiency are highly susceptible to digitalis toxicity.

Similar to PVC's in respiratory failure, MAT has a poor prognosis because of its association with severe underlying pulmonary disease. Fortunately this arrhythmia is transient and usually does not cause serious hemodynamic deficiencies. Correction of the underlying pulmonary abnormalities is the best therapeutic approach.

Table 12-7. Arrhythmias during acute respiratory failure in 70 patients*

Arrhythmia	No. of patients affected
Sinus tachycardia	43
Sinus brachycardia	2
Sinus arrhythmia	3
Ectopic atrial pacemaker	9
Wandering atrial pacemaker	5
Atrial tachycardia	11
Atrial flutter	7
Atrial fibrillation	6
MAT	12
AV junctional arrhythmia	5
Ventricular bigeminy	5
AV dissociation	4
Idioventricular rhythm	4
Ventricular tachycardia	4
Ventricular fibrillation	15

*Most patients experienced more than one arrhythmia.

MISCELLANEOUS ELECTROGRAPHIC ABNORMALITIES—CASE HISTORIES
Case 1. Respiratory arrest

A 38-year-old male with acute ascending paralysis (Guillain-Barré syndrome) was being monitored while completely dependent on a respirator for ventilation. An alert practitioner noted a sudden change in the ECG monitor pattern and obtained the rhythm strip shown in Fig. 12-31.

Sinus bradycardia was diagnosed because each normal QRS complex was preceded by a normal P wave and the rate was 32 beats/min.

Acute hypercapnia, particularly in the presence of hypoxemia, causes intense vagal stimulation, which can result in sinus bradycardia or

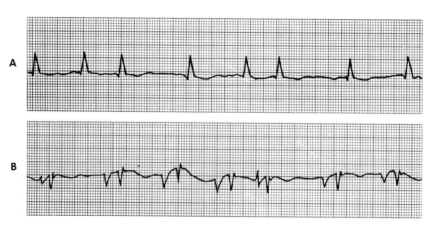

Fig. 12-30. Tracing in **A** reveals irregular supraventricular arrhythmia mimicking atrial fibrillation. Tracing in **B,** from an intra-atrial lead, clearly demonstrates definite P waves of variable configuration preceding each QRS complex.

arrest. This patient had become separated from the respirator when a connecting tube broke. Rapid restoration of ventilation restored sinus rhythm by lowering the arterial Pco_2 and improving oxygenation.

Case 2. Hypothermia

A 45-year-old male chronic alcoholic was found unconscious in a city park. On admission his rectal temperature was less than 30° C and the ECG shown in Fig. 12-32 was recorded.

Hypothermia has both reflex and direct effects on cardiac automaticity and conduction. Induction of hypothermia, such as for cardiac surgery, is relatively arrhythmia free, but rewarming can be hazardous. During rewarming the core temperature, including that of heart, lags behind the peripheral temperature. As the peripheral temperature increases, peripheral oxygen demand increases, but if the heart is still hypothermic, cardiac output cannot increase adequately to meet this demand. Both peripheral and myocardial hypoxia can result, and ventricular fibrillation may ensue. Slow rewarming with careful cardiac monitoring will help to avoid this complication.

Table 12-8 lists the effects of hypothermia on the ECG.

Sinus bradycardia and an abnormal deflection of the terminal QRS complex (Osborn wave) suggest hypothermia. Marked slowing of repolarization is reflected by the low-amplitude T waves and Q-T interval prolongation.

Case 3. Tricyclic amine overdose

A 44-year-old female was found comatose after telephoning a friend that she had just taken a bottle of "tranquilizers." Shortly after admission she suffered a grand mal seizure. The rhythm strips shown in Fig. 12-33 were obtained.

The initial postictal tracing demonstrates markedly prolonged intraventricular conduction followed by development of wide-complex tachycardia. This combination of coma, grand mal seizures, and arrhythmias is characteristic of tricyclic amine overdoses. These commonly used antidepressants slow depolarization and thus slow intra-atrial, AV, and intraventricular conduction. Supraventricular and ventricular arrhythmias commonly occur and may progress to ventricular fibrillation. Treatment with phenytoin

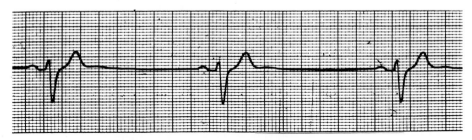

Fig. 12-31. Rhythm strip from respirator-dependent patient.

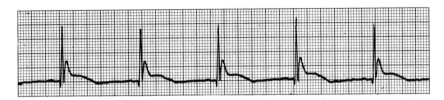

Fig. 12-32. ECG from patient with hypothermia. (From Conover, M. H.: Cardiac arrhythmias, ed. 2, St. Louis, 1978, The C. V. Mosby Co.)

successfully reversed the ECG abnormalities of this patient.

Case 4. Subarachnoid hemorrhage

The ECG shown in Fig. 12-34 was obtained from a 49-year-old female admitted to the inten-

Table 12-8. ECG effects of hypothermia

Temperature (°C)	ECG results	Physiologic abnormality
35-37	Sinus bradycardia	Increased vagal tone, cooling of SA node
30-35	Prolongation of P-R interval, QRS complex, Q-T interval	Slowing of depolarization and repolarization
27-30	Ventricular arrhythmias	?Myocardial ischemia
25	"Osborn wave"— positive deflection of terminal 0.04 sec of QRS complex	Unknown

sive care unit because of sudden onset of severe headache followed by a rapid loss of consciousness and the development of acute pulmonary edema.

This ECG demonstrates striking T wave inversion and minor S-T segment depression consistent with subendocardial injury and epicardial ischemia, but no Q waves are apparent. This pattern is consistent with subendocardial infarction. A diagnosis of subarachnoid hemorrhage was documented by lumbar puncture and arteriograms.

ECG changes associated with subarachnoid hemorrhage are transient and reflect spotty subendocardial and intramural myocardial necrosis. S-T segment and T wave changes reflecting subendocardial infarction are most commonly seen, but the Q waves of transmural infarction are also occasionally observed. In many instances only Q-T interval prolongation or arrhythmias occur. A sudden increase of serum catecholamine levels is thought to be the reason for myocardial necrosis in these patients.

Although subarachnoid hemorrhage is the most common neurologic cause of ECG changes,

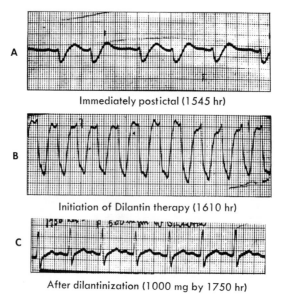

A

Immediately postictal (1545 hr)

B

Initiation of Dilantin therapy (1610 hr)

C

After dilantinization (1000 mg by 1750 hr)

Fig. 12-33. A, Abnormal intraventricular conduction followed by ventricular tachycardia, **B, C,** Dilantin therapy corrected both conduction defect and arrhythmia.

they are also seen with status epilepticus, intracranial mass lesions, meningitis, cerebral infarction, and diagnostic procedures, including pneumoencephalography. Similar ECG changes have been reported following carotid endarterectomy.

Case 5. Pericardial tamponade with electrical alternans

A 63-year-old woman had been admitted for treatment of cardiomegaly and dyspnea with the provisional diagnosis of congestive heart failure. She failed to respond to conventional diuresis and 2 nights after admission became hypotensive with a sudden increase in dyspnea and orthopnea. Physical examination revealed distended neck veins and an inspiratory decrease in systolic arterial pressure from 110 mm Hg to 80 mm Hg. Her electrocardiogram is illustrated in Fig. 12-35.

There is a change in QRS amplitude in alternate complexes. This phenomenon is *electrical alternans* and is indicative of pericardial tamponade. When alternation of voltage affects only the QRS amplitude, it is referred to as "partial" electrical alternans. Total electrical alternans is a rare ECG finding in which alternate or every third P, QRS, and T complex is inverted.

Electrical alternans represents a rhythmic change in electrical axis of the heart caused by motion of the heart within a distended fluid-filled pericardium. Thus the heart "swings" back and forth with each alternate contraction, no longer held in place by the normal restraint of the pericardial sac. This change in position causes a change in electrical axis, which is manifested by changes in amplitude of ECG complexes on the surface electrocardiogram.

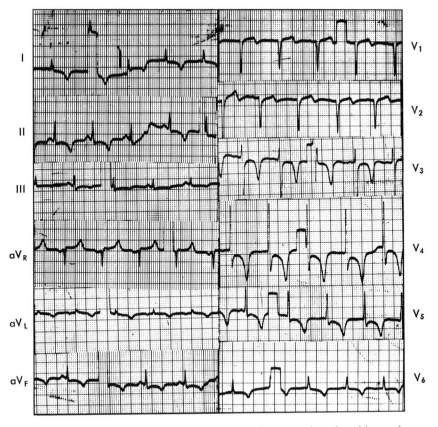

Fig. 12-34. Striking T wave inversion in a patient with acute subarachnoid hemorrhage.

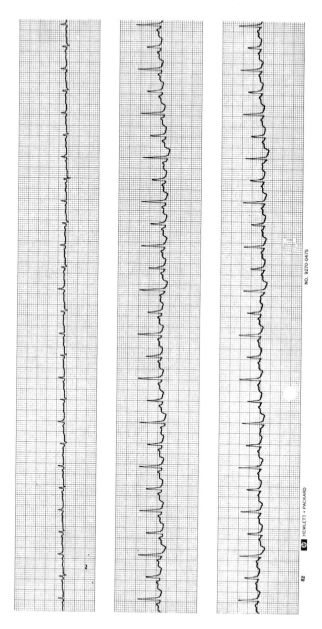

Fig. 12-35. Electrical alternans consistent with pericardial tamponade.

Shortly after this ECG was taken, an echocardiogram confirmed massive pericardial effusion. Emergency pericardiocentesis yielded 450 ml of hemorrhagic pericardial fluid (hematocrit 33) and corrected the pulsus paradoxus, electrical alternans, and dyspnea.

SUMMARY

Cardiac electrical activity recorded by the ECG is generated by ionic motion across the myocardial cell membrane. Ionic motion and the membrane itself are altered by changes in the metabolic environment. Critically ill patients experience frequent and varied metabolic, inflammatory, and hemodynamic abnormalities that can alter the ECG. Many therapeutic maneuvers and pharmacologic agents can also alter the ECG. Intelligent interpretation of the ECG of the critically ill patient requires thorough knowledge of the extent and meaning of these changes.

BIBLIOGRAPHY

Ayres, S. M., and Grace, W. J.: Inappropriate ventilation and hypoxemia as causes of cardiac arrhythmias, Am. J. Med. **46**:495, 1969.

Bellet, S.: Essentials of cardiac arrhythmias, Philadelphia, 1972, W. B. Saunders Co.

Bhargava, R. K.: Cor pulmonale, Mount Kisco, N.Y., 1973, Futura Publishing Co., Inc.

Hoffman, B. F., and Cranefield, P. F.: The physiological basis of cardiac arrhythmias, Am. J. Med. **37**:670, 1964.

Hudson, L. D., Kurt, T. L., Petty, T. L., and Genton, E.: Arrhythmias associated with acute respiratory failure in patients with chronic airway obstruction, Chest **63**:661, 1973.

Lipman, B. S., Massie, E., and Kleiger, R. E.: Clinical scalar electrocardiography, Chicago, 1972, Year Book Medical Publishers, Inc.

CHAPTER 13

Clinical management of common cardiac abnormalities*

Robert E. Ingham, Theodore B. Berndt, and Donald C. Harrison**

Abnormalities of the heart and great blood vessels frequently produce emergencies that necessitate the admission of a patient to a critical care unit. The large number of conditions that may be present and their diagnosis and management can be discussed only briefly in this chapter; therefore those syndromes that occur most commonly have been selected for emphasis. In each instance the syndrome is defined, its diagnosis outlined, classic examples presented, and the prognosis discussed. The following specific syndromes are presented: cardiac arrhythmias, congestive heart failure and pulmonary edema, cardiogenic shock in acute myocardial infarction, acute valvular lesions, acute pericarditis, acute myocarditis, infective endocarditis, and dissecting aneurysm of the aorta.

CARDIAC ARRHYTHMIAS
■ What is a cardiac arrhythmia?

An arrhythmia is an abnormality of the formation or conduction of an electrical impulse so that a portion of the heart beats abnormally fast, abnormally slow, or the rhythm is irregular. In the normal heart an electrical impulse originates in the sinoatrial (SA) node, and from there the impulse spreads throughout the right and left atria, eventually reaching the atrioventricular (AV) node. After spending some time traversing the AV node the impulse emerges to be conducted

through the bundle of His to the right and left bundle branches. These main bundle branches arborize throughout the ventricular myocardium. This normal conduction sequence is represented in Fig. 13-1. If a sinus impulse results in a heart rate slower or faster than normal, if an impulse arises from some location other than the SA node, or if a normal impulse is conducted through the heart in an abnormal fashion, an arrhythmia results.

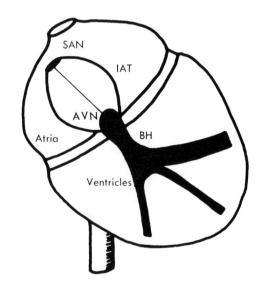

Fig. 13-1. Normal conduction sequence. *SAN*, Sinoatrial node; *IAT*, intra-atrial tracts; *AVN*, atrioventricular node; *BH*, bundle of His.

*Supported by NIH Grants No. HL-5866 and HL-15833-01.
**With the assistance of Lela Manley, R.N.

■ What is the clinical importance of cardiac arrhythmias?

The appearance of an arrhythmia has little significance in itself, but it must be considered in relation to the clinical situation it accompanies. Sinus bradycardia in a 65-year-old male is a very different situation from sinus bradycardia in a 22-year-old distance runner. Similarly, paroxysmal supraventricular tachycardia in an 18-year-old female has a different significance from such a tachycardia occurring in a 48-year-old male with severe aortic stenosis. The approach to take and the degree of significance to be attached to an arrhythmia may be determined by answers to the following questions:

1. What is the nature of the arrhythmia?
2. What are the hemodynamic effects of the arrhythmia, as manifest by mental status and renal, respiratory, and myocardial function?
3. What is the prognosis of the arrhythmia in this patient?
4. Will the patient be symptomatically or physiologically improved with therapy for this arrhythmia?

In attempting to answer each of these questions in an individual clinical situation, the relative importance of any arrhythmia to a patient's general condition will become clearer.

Table 13-1 summarizes the common arrhythmias that may be encountered in a critically ill patient. Table 13-2 summarizes the common antiarrhythmic medications used in the therapy of these conditions.

■ What are the important tachycardias?
Paroxysmal supraventricular (atrial) tachycardia

Common causes of paroxysmal supraventricular tachycardia (PSVT) in the ill patient include digitalis intoxication, rheumatic heart disease, acute myocardial infarction, pulmonary embolism, and chronic obstructive pulmonary disease. PSVT also occurs relatively frequently in persons with the preexcitation syndrome and may occur in otherwise normal people. The ECG's of patients with PSVT show an atrial rate generally between 150 to 250 beats/min, although faster or slower rates may occur. During the tachycardia P waves are difficult to identify, and conduction through the ventricles may be in an aberrant fashion. The ventricular response depends on the

Table 13-1. Common arrhythmias (with usual rates in the absence of treatment)*

Arrhythmia	Atrial rate (beats/min)	Ventricular rate (beats/min)	Rhythm
Sick sinus syndrome—brady-tachy syndrome	40-60, 100-200	40-60, 100-200	Regular
Atrial flutter	250-350	75-150	Regular with constant block, irregular with varying block
Atrial fibrillation	300-500	140-175	Grossly irregular
Paroxysmal supraventricular (atrial) tachycardia	150-250	150-250	Regular
AV junctional tachycardia	100-180 (retrograde depolarization of atria)	100-180	Regular
Ventricular tachycardia	Variable (AV dissociation)	150-200+	Regular (usually slightly irregular)
Sinus bradycardia	40-60	40-60	Regular
Escape rhythms†			
AV junctional rhythm	Variable	40-60	Regular
Idioventricular rhythm	Variable	30-40	Regular

*From Coltart, D. J., and Harrison, D. C.: Primary Care **1:**123, 1974.
†The term "escape rhythms" refers to those rhythms originating in lower centers when SA rhythmicity is depressed or when marked AV block occurs.

Table 13-2. Commonly used antiarrhythmic drugs: pharmacologic principles*

Drug	Therapeutic range	Dosage	Elimination	Absorption			Toxic reactions
				Orally	IV	IM	
Quinidine	2-8 µg/ml	200-400 mg 4-6 times daily	Renal, decreased in alkaline urine	Maximum effect 1-3 hr, duration 6-8 hr		Maximum effect 30-90 min	Cinchonism, nausea, vomiting, diarrhea
Procainamide	4-8 µg/ml	6 mg/kg every 3 hr IV, 100 mg/5 min until 1 g given	60% excreted by kidney	Maximum effect 15-60 min	Maximum effect 5-10 min		Agranulocytosis, lupus-like syndrome
Propranolol	20-120 ng/ml	20-80 mg 4 times daily orally, 0.15 mg/kg IV	Hepatic metabolism	Maximum effect 1-2 hr	Maximum effect 10-30 min		Respiratory, hypoglycemia
Disopyramide	Unknown	150 mg 4 times daily	Hepatic and renal	Maximum effect 2-4 hr enhanced after several initial doses			Anticholinergic (constipation, dryness of mucous membranes), depressed myocardial function
Lidocaine	1-6 µg/ml	20-60 µg/kg/min	Hepatic metabolism		Maximum effect 2-5 min	Maximum effect 30 min	Muscle fasciculation, drowsiness, convulsions
Phenytoin	10-20 µg/ml	0.5-0.6 g daily orally, 100 mg every 15 min IV	Hepatic metabolism	Maximum effect 8-12 hr	Maximum effect 30-60 min		Nystagmus, lethargy, ataxia

*From Coltart, D. J., and Harrison, D. C.: Primary Care **1:**123, 1974.

degree of AV block, but is frequently 1:1, with a ventricular response equal to the atrial rate. Various degrees of AV block exist when there is excessive digitalis present (Fig. 13-2).

Episodes of PSVT may precipitate angina pectoris, myocardial infarction, syncope, or frank congestive heart failure with pulmonary edema or shock and, as such, require urgent measures. Electrical cardioversion at 50 to 200 watt-seconds is the treatment of choice in any situation requiring emergency measures, although if digitalis intoxication is the probable cause, other therapy should be attempted first. Carotid sinus massage, edrophonium (Tensilon), 10 mg, given by the IV route, Valsalva's maneuver, or pressor agents such as methoxamine (if there are no contraindications to pressor agents) may be attempted individually. Digitalis is a preferred therapy if the patient has not been taking the drug. If digitalis intoxication is the probable cause, digitalis should be discontinued and blood drawn for a serum digitalis level determination. Phenytoin may be useful if digitalis intoxication is suspected, and if the serum potassium level is low, IV fluids contain-

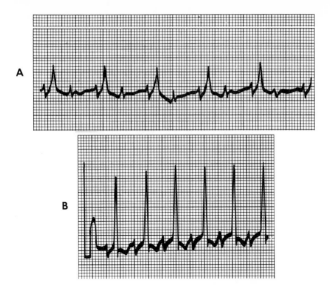

Fig. 13-2. A, Paroxysmal atrial tachycardia with block. **B,** Sinus tachycardia. Serum digoxin level was in toxic range when the ECG in **A** was taken but had dropped to therapeutic levels on trace in **B.**

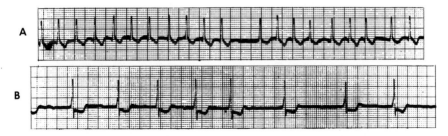

Fig. 13-3. A, Untreated atrial fibrillation with rapid ventricular response. **B,** Atrial fibrillation well treated with digoxin. Ventricular response is slow and irregular. Atrial fibrillatory waves can be seen.

ing potassium chloride should be administered. Propranolol has proved useful in slowing and terminating episodes of PSVT.

Patients may find recurrent episodes of PSVT very incapacitating, and in such a situation chronic medical therapy may be required. Digitalis is useful if PSVT is not caused by digitalis intoxication. Other medications that may be tried on a chronic basis are propranolol, quinidine sulfate, procainamide, reserpine, and guanethidine. The patient should also be advised to stop smoking and to eliminate caffeine and other stimu-lants. It should be emphasized that PSVT in and of itself is not an indication for chronic medical therapy, but when there is evidence of hemodynamic compromise, as often occurs when other abnormal cardiovascular conditions exist, it should be treated aggressively.

Atrial fibrillation

Atrial fibrillation is a common arrhythmia that can be associated with a number of conditions such as rheumatic heart disease, pericarditis, hyperthyroidism, ischemic heart disease, hypertension, or chronic obstructive pulmonary disease. The ECG of a patient in atrial fibrillation shows total disorganization of atrial activity and is represented by fibrillatory waves along the baseline (Fig. 13-3). The ventricular response to this chaotic atrial activity is irregularly irregular, and the rate can span the range from slow to very fast. The loss of atrial contraction may be an important contributing factor to a low cardiac output state, and when combined with a rapid ventricular response, there may be a serious hemodynamic compromise that requires urgent therapy.

When a patient has atrial fibrillation, the goals of therapy must be determined; that is, would the patient be significantly improved by returning to sinus rhythm, or would the patient be improved simply by slowing the ventricular response to allow better diastolic filling of the ventricles? If the goal of therapy is sinus rhythm and the patient has not received digitalis, the treatment of choice is electrical cardioversion. When a patient is acutely ill with atrial fibrillation exhibiting shock, pulmonary edema, or other signs of cardiac decompensation, electrical cardioversion should be undertaken without delay in an attempt to restore sinus rhythm. When a patient has chronic atrial fibrillation and is not significantly compromised by the arrhythmia, then there is more time for medical therapy, and control of the ventricular response can be the primary goal of therapy. Digitalis is the drug of choice because it slows conduction through the AV node, thereby allowing fewer of the atrial impulses that constantly bombard the AV node to gain entrance to ventricular conducting tissues. The result is a slowing of the ventricular rate. Propranolol is also a useful agent in slowing the ventricular rate. Quinidine sulfate, in combination with digitalis, has previously been used in an attempt to "medically cardiovert" a patient from atrial fibrillation to normal sinus rhythm; however, episodes of ventricular fibrillation have been reported, and this is not a recommended procedure.

Atrial flutter

The causes of atrial flutter are much the same as those of atrial fibrillation. The ECG features of atrial flutter include an undulating, wavy baseline with regular flutter waves at a rate commonly between 250 and 350 waves/min (Fig. 13-4). The ventricular rate is some fraction of the atrial rate, usually one half, one fourth, or one third, expressed as 2:1, 4:1, and 3:1 AV block, respectively, and is typically very regular. There may be confusion between atrial flutter with 2:1 block, PSVT, and atrial fibrillation, because each may have similar ventricular responses. Carotid sinus massage, Valsalva's maneuver, or edrophonium may slow the ventricular response sufficiently to allow characterization of the atrial mechanism. Atrial flutter can be a source of difficulty to the patient when there is no AV block (a 1:1 atrial-ventricular response) or only 2:1 AV block, so that the ventricular response is very rapid. The treatment of atrial flutter is much the same as that of atrial fibrillation and requires a clinical judgment as to the urgency of the situation. If the rapid rate is compromising the hemodynamic status of the patient, then electrical cardioversion is the treatment of choice. This can usually be ac-

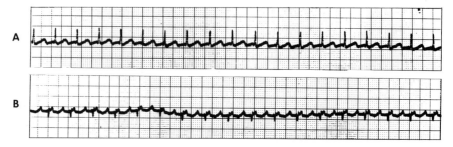

Fig. 13-4. Atrial flutter. **A,** Lead II. **B,** Lead V_1. Leads in this combination best show flutter waves as characteristic undulations with no isoelectric interval.

complished at low energies (25 to 100 watt-seconds). If more time is available, digitalis will produce AV block and slow the ventricular rate to a level that is better tolerated. Propranolol may also produce AV blockage and thereby slow the ventricular rate. Not infrequently the result of such medical therapy is atrial fibrillation.

Sick sinus syndrome — "brady-tachy syndrome"

The sick sinus syndrome falls in the general category of a "brady-tachy syndrome," a term that describes episodes of sinus bradycardia interrupted by bursts of supraventricular tachycardia that are not necessarily sinus in origin. In the brady-tachy syndrome the tachycardia episodes may be PSVT, atrial flutter, rapid atrial fibrillation, or sinus (in which case the term "sick sinus syndrome" is applied). The brady-tachy syndrome is characterized by episodes of very fast heart rate alternating with very slow heart rate, and the patient may develop symptoms from either of these aberrations. The sinus P waves are characteristically normal but are very irregular. Either syndrome may be a result of ischemic heart disease or generalized cardiomyopathy, or it may also occur without other evidence of cardiovascular disease. The dilemma in therapy for these patients comes in treating episodes of tachycardia with medications that may be detrimental during the phase of bradycardia. Therapy is therefore aimed at minimizing the effect of bradycardia with a transvenous pacemaker and treating the tachycardia episodes with such medications as digitalis, propranolol, quinidine sulfate, and procainamide. It should be noted that there is significant incidence of disease of other portions of the conducting system of the heart in patients with sick sinus syndrome, or brady-tachy syndrome, giving added importance to the need for a pacemaker before medical therapy is undertaken.

Ventricular tachycardia

Ventricular tachycardia is defined as three or more consecutive ventricular ectopic beats. Paroxysms of such beats may begin with an appropriately timed ventricular premature contraction that falls in the vulnerable period of a sinus beat and can then initiate a repetitive response of ventricular tachycardia. An irritable ventricular focus can also initiate a series of impulses at a rapid rate and produce ventricular tachycardia.

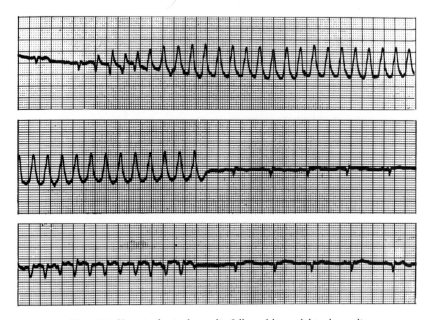

Fig. 13-5. Ventricular tachycardia followed by nodal tachycardia.

Such repetitive episodes are most common in diseased hearts and cause a severe hemodynamic compromise because of disorganized ventricular depolarization and lack of effective stroke volume. Common settings for ventricular tachycardia are acute myocardial infarction, cardiomyopathy, and digitalis intoxication. The ECG features of ventricular tachycardia include broad bizarre-appearing ventricular complexes, usually at a rate of over 100 beats/min (Fig. 13-5). If untreated, ventricular tachycardia frequently degenerates into ventricular fibrillation. Electrical counter-shock is the treatment of choice, and lidocaine may be given in an attempt to suppress ectopic activity after conversion has been completed. If lidocaine fails to suppress subsequent runs of ventricular tachycardia or frequent ventricular ectopic beats, then procainamide by slow IV injection may be attempted. Other medications that could be considered are quinidine sulfate, phenytoin, potassium chloride (especially if the serum potassium level is low), and propranolol. Occasionally cardiac pacing has been successful in overdrive suppression of the ventricular focus. All other potentially reversible conditions that may predispose to ventricular tachycardia, such as hypoxia, acidosis, heart failure, and hypotension, should be treated.

Ventricular fibrillation

Ventricular fibrillation constitutes a cardiac emergency, and immediate therapy with elec-

trical defibrillation should be undertaken at 400 watt-seconds. Cardiopulmonary resuscitation should be instituted, and simultaneous attention should be given to correcting situations that may cause ventricular fibrillations, such as ventricular ectopy, shock, hypoxia, bradycardia, and digitalis intoxication. Rapid ECG recognition of ventricular fibrillation is mandatory; the ECG exhibits a waving baseline without evidence of ventricular depolarization (Fig. 13-6).

■ What are the important bradycardias?
Sinus bradycardia

Sinus bradycardia has already been mentioned as a component of the sick sinus or brady-tachy syndrome (Fig. 13-7). It may also be a normal response in the physically fit. When sinus bradycardia appears to compromise hemodynamic status, as is most commonly the case in older patients with some degree of coronary artery disease, it warrants therapy with a permanent cardiac pacemaker.

Heart block

Heart block is an abnormality in the conduction of sinus beats to the ventricles. The most common site for such an abnormality is in the AV node, and the conduction disturbance may be of several types. First-degree heart block consists simply of a prolongation of the P-R interval to greater than 0.20 second and rarely requires therapy. Second-degree heart block is a condition

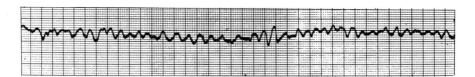

Fig. 13-6. Ventricular fibrillation.

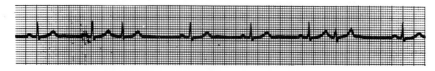

Fig. 13-7. Sinus bradycardia with atrial extrasystoles.

wherein some, but not all, sinus impulses are transmitted to the ventricles. Mobitz type I second-degree heart block (Wenckebach's phenomenon) is characterized by progressive prolongation of the P-R interval in successive sinus beats, with subsequent block of a sinus beat (Fig. 13-8). The net effect is a "grouping" of QRS complexes on the surface ECG and varying P-R intervals. Common causes of Wenckebach's phenomenon include digitalis intoxication, increased vagal tone, and inferior myocardial infarction. Wenckebach's phenomenon rarely causes hemodynamic compromise, and hence rarely does the arrhythmia itself require treatment.

Another type of second-degree heart block is termed Mobitz type II and is characterized by the occasional lack of propagation of sinus beats through the AV junctional area to the ventricle. The patient is in sinus rhythm with regular P waves, but occasional P waves are not followed by a QRS complex. Mobitz type II heart block itself does not require therapy unless the dropped beats are so frequent as to result in a bradycardia that is a source of difficulty for the patient. Atropine or isoproterenol may result in lessening of the degree of the block, but pacing may be required to restore an adequate ventricular rate. The major importance in recognizing Mobitz type II heart block is that it commonly progresses to third-degree heart block and severe bradycardia with frequent hemodynamic compromise. This progression occurs most often in conjunction with acute myocardial infarction of the anterior wall, degen-

eration of the ventricular conducting system, or a cardiomyopathy.

When third-degree (complete) heart block is present, there is a slow ventricular rate from a junctional or ventricular pacemaker (less than 60 beats/min), and there is frequently a lack of response of this low rate to various physiologic stresses. Therapy in the form of a pacemaker is usually required. Complete heart block is identified on the ECG by a lack of relationship between P waves and QRS complexes (Fig. 13-9). Patients with either ischemic heart disease or cardiomyopathy are generally less able to tolerate this slower-than-physiologic heart rate, and therapy is required more urgently. Isoproterenol given by IV drip may temporarily increase the heart rate to levels better tolerated by the patient, but this requires close monitoring because a ventricular rhythm may degenerate into ventricular tachycardia or fibrillation. Temporary transvenous pacemakers also increase the heart rate in complete heart block. Temporary pacing is accomplished by inserting a unipolar or bipolar electrode percutaneously into a peripheral vein (usually subclavian or internal jugular) and positioning it in the right ventricle under fluoroscopic and ECG monitoring. A pacemaker is then attached to this electrode and ventricular pacing instituted.

■ What is an "ectopic" rhythm?

An ectopic beat is one that originates outside the usual site of impulse formation, which is lo-

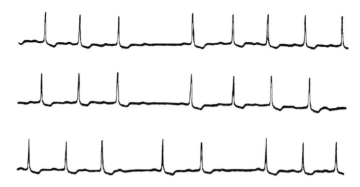

Fig. 13-8. Mobitz type I (Wenckebach) second-degree AV block. Note progressive prolongation of P-R interval until no ventricular response follows a P wave. Cycle is then reset.

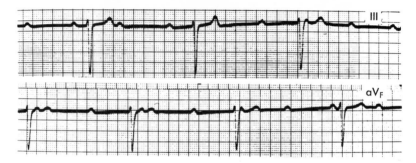

Fig. 13-9. Complete heart block. Note absence of any association between P waves and QRS complexes.

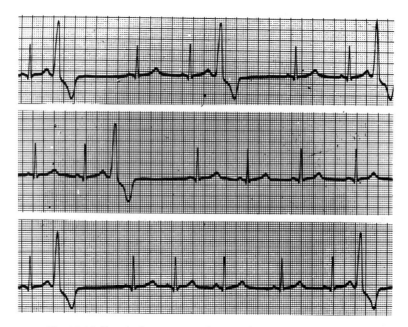

Fig. 13-10. Ventricular premature beats with compensatory pauses.

cated in the SA node; this beat may originate in the conduction system, the ventricle, atria, or elsewhere.

Ventricular premature beats (VPB's) are ectopic beats that originate in the ventricle and produce broad, bizarre QRS complexes and T waves that are markedly different from the patient's sinus QRS complexes and T waves (Fig. 13-10). VPB's may occur in otherwise normal people, or

they can be caused by myocardial ischemia, hypoxia, digitalis intoxication, pulmonary emboli, ventricular aneurysm, or hypotension. They may also be parasystolic in origin, or they may be related to a sinus bradycardia.

The hemodynamic effect of VPB's relates to the following: (1) the duration of time after the preceding sinus beat that allows for ventricular filling and (2) the degree of disorganization of ventricular contraction as a result of an abnormal sequence of ventricular depolarization. If the ventricles are not allowed to fill, as occurs with an early VPB, or if there is a large degree of asynchrony in the depolarization of the ventricles so that there is ineffective ventricular contraction, frequent VPB's may cause hypotension, pulmonary vascular congestion, and other signs of low cardiac output. An additional situation that demands attention even in the absence of hemodynamic compromise is when VPB's occur on the peak or early downsloping portion of the T wave (R-on-T phenomenon). These VPB's fall in the vulnerable period of ventricular repolarization and are associated with ventricular tachycardia and fibrillation.

VPB's that are multifocal, that is, that have a number of broad bizarre configurations in any given ECG lead, and are also considered malignant and predispose to ventricular tachycardia and fibrillation. VPB's in conjunction with myocardial ischemia or infarction should be observed closely, and if the frequency is greater than 3 to 5 VPB's/min, they should be treated.

Given these situations that demand therapy for VPB's, the first step is to diligently search for reversible underlying causes. If this is not successful in eliminating the VPB's, medical therapy should be instituted. Useful drugs include a lidocaine bolus followed by lidocaine by drip infusion, procainamide, or quinidine sulfate; Table 13-2 offers a guide to the therapeutic blood levels of the most useful antiarrhythmic preparations. If frequent VPB's occur in the setting of sinus bradycardia, ventricular pacing may serve to suppress the irritable ventricular focus.

CONGESTIVE HEART FAILURE AND PULMONARY EDEMA
■ **What is congestive heart failure and associated pulmonary edema?**

Congestive heart failure is a clinical state in which the heart is unable to maintain an adequate cardiac output in relation to the venous return and tissue metabolic needs at that particular moment. Symptoms result from the secondary inadequate tissue perfusion and organ congestion. Pulmonary edema is the acute accumulation of fluid within the pulmonary interstitial spaces and alveoli, usually caused by severe left heart failure.

A common cause of congestive heart failure and pulmonary edema is myocardial infarction, which is an acute insult to the heart often associated with severe two- or three-vessel coronary artery disease. Scars from an old myocardial infarction may also be present. Furthermore, reflex mechanisms from the acute myocardial injury, reaction to the severe pain, and drugs used to control symptoms or arrhythmias may further compromise the normal circulation.

Recently the hemodynamics of congestive heart failure and pulmonary edema associated with acute myocardial infarction have been defined. Cardiac output is usually maintained, and total peripheral resistance is not significantly increased. Heart rate is increased and stroke volume index and stroke work index are significantly decreased, whereas left ventricular filling pressure is increased. On rare occasions, usually in association with inferior wall myocardial infarction, there may be a predominance of right ventricular damage and right ventricular failure. With an acute myocardial infarction the left ventricle also appears to become "stiffer," with altered compliance that may last several days. When the high left ventricular filling pressure is transmitted to the lungs and the pulmonary capillary hydrostatic pressure exceeds the oncotic pressure, fluid exudes into the intra-alveolar and interstitial space. Secondary right ventricular failure may follow and other hormonal homeostatic mechanisms are set in motion, causing further fluid retention.

Depending on the criteria used, some form of heart failure occurs in 23% to 71% of patients hospitalized with acute myocardial infarction. Severe congestive heart failure or pulmonary edema occurs in only about 12% of patients hospitalized with acute myocardial infarction. The incidence of congestive heart failure appears to be greater with anterior wall myocardial infarction and to increase with age and with a history of previous myocardial infarction. In some cases congestive heart failure or pulmonary edema may be the presenting manifestation of a recent myocardial infarction. At other times an acute arrhythmia such as rapid atrial fibrillation may precipitate pulmonary edema in patients with acute myocardial infarction.

■ What are the signs and symptoms of congestive heart failure?

The signs, symptoms, and abnormal laboratory studies in congestive heart failure reflect organ dysfunction secondary to poor perfusion and fluid congestion. Dyspnea and orthopnea are common. Paroxysmal nocturnal dyspnea may occur with intermittent left ventricular dysfunction. Right upper quadrant pain from liver congestion, with or without ascites, and peripheral edema occur with progressive heart failure as fluid is retained.

Physical examination usually reveals a sinus tachycardia with or without a complicating arrhythmia contributing to the congestive heart failure. A ventricular filling sound (S_3) is usually heard, as may be an S_4. An S_3, however, may occur without ventricular decompensation, especially when there is associated mitral regurgitation. Jugular venous distention may be present in cases of right ventricular congestive heart failure or after a right ventricular myocardial infarction. Inspiratory rales are usually heard over the lung fields.

Chest x-ray films show pulmonary venous distention, loss of definition of pulmonary vessels, pulmonary clouding, prominent septal lines, pleural effusions, increased diameter of the right pulmonary artery, and almost invariably some increase in cardiac size. Pulmonary edema is recognized when excessive intra-alveolar fluid accumulation produces a characteristic butterfly-shaped pattern in the pulmonary vascular markings.

The clinical signs of congestive heart failure often correlate poorly with roentgenographic findings and hemodynamics. Furthermore, chest x-ray films often show subtle changes of congestive heart failure (interstitial edema, pulmonary venous congestion) before overt clinical signs of congestive heart failure develop, Similarly, clinical signs of congestive heart failure may resolve before the x-ray signs. Generally there is some correlation between the left ventricular filling pressure and the degree of congestive heart failure noted on chest films.

Arterial hypoxemia is common following an acute myocardial infarction, and the degree generally correlates with the severity of left ventricular dysfunction. This is secondary to pulmonary arteriovenous shunting, and its degree generally correlates with the pulmonary artery diastolic pressure.

The myocardial damage from the acute myocardial infarction, the altered ventricular geometry from areas of akinesia and dyskinesia, the mitral regurgitation secondary to loss of integrity of the mitral valve apparatus, the metabolic acidosis secondary to poor tissue perfusion, the arterial hypoxia from pulmonary arteriovenous shunting, in addition to complicating arrhythmias, and the use of drugs that may further suppress the heart all contribute to congestive heart failure with acute myocardial infarction.

The prognosis of congestive heart failure with acute myocardial infarction is variable. Mortality rates range from 8% to 44% and correlate with the degree of congestive heart failure. Very high left ventricular filling pressures and a low cardiac work level indicate a poor prognosis.

■ What is the usual therapy for acute myocardial infarction?

Bedrest, oxygen, pain relief, sedation, and correction of metabolic abnormalities should be instituted in these patients. Hemodynamically significant arrhythmias and significant hypertension should receive prompt attention. Since the incidence of pulmonary emboli is higher with congestive heart failure, many advocate short-term anticoagulation therapy in this clinical setting. Mild congestive heart failure—rales, apical S_3, early interstitial edema on chest x-ray films—often respond to diuretics such as furosemide administered by the IV route. Potassium losses and severe hypovolemia must be avoided. The administration of digitalis to patients with acute myocardial infarction is controversial. There is some evidence that hearts suffering recent myocardial infarction do not respond to digitalization with increased inotropism and that myocardial injury may actually increase when digitalis is given. Furthermore, the toxic threshold to digitalis decreases in animals having recent myocardial infarction. Many practitioners, however, have noted generally good clinical response to digitalis in patients with congestive heart failure from an acute myocardial infarction. They therefore advocate cautious IV digitalization when there are signs and symptoms of significant congestive heart failure that have not responded to salt restriction and diuretics. Blood levels of the digitalis preparation should be monitored.

■ **What measures may be taken to relieve pulmonary edema?**

Pulmonary edema is an emergency condition and requires prompt attention. Patients with pulmonary edema are usually extremely anxious and suddenly develop dyspnea and cough productive of frothy sputum; they literally drown in their own secretions. Treatment requires a rapid reduction of the left ventricular filling pressure. This is accomplished by IV morphine sulfate, which causes venous pooling and relieves anxiety; rapid-acting and potent diuretics such as IV furosemide; phlebotomies; and the use of oxygen. Cautious use of digitalis, especially with PSVT's, may be beneficial. Intermittent positive pressure breathing will often improve the arterial oxygen saturation.

Recently experimental and clinical evidence has resulted in a new dimension in the treatment of severe congestive heart failure. "Afterload reduction" is the reduction of stress on the left ventricular myocardium by reducing the resistance against which the ventricle expels blood. By cautious use of such vasodilators as nitrates, prazosin, or nitroprusside, left ventricular emptying is augmented, ventricular filling less impeded, and pulmonary vascular congestion relieved.

Usually these measures will relieve the signs and symptoms of congestive heart failure and pulmonary edema. However, not uncommonly these patients progress to further ventricular dysfunction manifested by a shock state.

CARDIOGENIC SHOCK IN ACUTE MYOCARDIAL INFARCTION

■ **What is cardiogenic shock in acute myocardial infarction?**

General concepts regarding shock are presented in detail in Chapter 41. Thus only a brief consideration of the pathophysiology, diagnosis, and therapy of cardiogenic shock in acute myocardial infarction will be presented here.

Shock may be defined as a critical fall in capillary perfusion that reduces oxygen delivery to levels below the tissues' nutritional requirements to maintain cellular viability. This may be caused by inadequate venous return to the heart, inadequate ejection of blood from one of the cardiac chambers, or an abnormality of the peripheral circulation so that the capillary beds receive inadequate circulation. In cardiogenic shock secondary to myocardial infarction the problem is usually major with irreversible damage to the left ventricle, which is unable to eject enough blood. In a few cases there may be an inadequate response of the peripheral systemic resistance in the face of a relatively normal cardiac output. Severe coronary artery disease with two- or three-vessel involvement is common, especially in the case of the left coronary artery that has suffered recent damage involving at least 40% of the left ventricle. Anteroseptal wall infarction and surrounding areas of borderline viability are noted. There may be an associated interventricular septal perforation and/or papillary muscle dysfunction and/or rupture. Hemodynamics usually show a diminished cardiac output with increased total peripheral resistance, increased left ventricular filling pressures, a diminished ejection fraction and stroke volume, and increased sympathetic nervous tone. The mean aortic pressure is reduced, further impairing coronary blood flow. Metabolic acidosis and compensatory hyperventilation follow inadequate tissue perfusion. This is reflected by elevated blood lactate levels and arterial blood gases that show hypocapnia initially and acidosis and hypoxia as the shock state progresses. These metabolic changes further suppress already critically depressed myocardial function.

Recognition of the clinical state of shock involves signs and symptoms reflecting poor tissue and organ perfusion and increased sympathetic tone modified by associated factors such as fever and arrhythmias. The clinical setting is usually a recent myocardial infarction (0 to 5 days old). There may be persistent or recurrent major arrhythmias and/or chest pain. The heart rate is rapid and the blood pressure is low, usually less than 90 mm Hg systolic. Auscultatory brachial blood pressure determinations may be inaccurate estimators of the central aortic pressure when there is peripheral vascular constriction, and intra-arterial pressures may be required. The skin is cool and clammy. The peripheral pulses are small or absent. Mentation is altered with states of agitation, restlessness, confusion, and somnolence. Heart examination may reveal a diffuse cardiac impulse with secondary impulses, an S_3 or S_4, and murmurs of an interventricular septal defect or mitral regurgitation from papillary muscle dysfunction or rupture. Urine flow is diminished (less than 20 ml/hr) with high specific gravity and osmolality in the early phase.

It is important to emphasize that the shock syndrome associated with recent myocardial infarction is not uniformly caused by pump failure secondary to myocardial necrosis. The following lists other etiologies of the shock syndrome that may occur in conjunction with myocardial infarction.

Shock with myocardial infarction; other considerations
Arrhythmias—marked tachycardias or bradycardias
Iatrogenic causes
   Analgesics
   Sedatives
   Diuretics—hypovolemia
   Other drugs—antiarrhythmic drugs and beta blockade therapy (propranolol)
Other cardiopulmonary causes
   Cardiac tamponade
   Pulmonary embolism
   Aortic dissecting aneurysm

The appropriate diagnosis and therapy of these alternatives may correct the shock state and prevent further myocardial necrosis and death. These causes should be excluded in any person with shock and myocardial infarction.

The aim of therapy is to restore tissue perfusion as soon as possible and minimize further cardiac damage. Appropriate therapy requires continuous monitoring of the cardiac rhythm and central venous pressure. If possible, pulmonary artery and intra-arterial blood pressures should be monitored with a Swan-Ganz catheter in the pulmonary artery and with a brachial artery or femoral artery catheter. Urine output, total fluid balance, electrolytes, and arterial blood gases should be measured frequently. If hypovolemia is present as manifested by a decreased central venous pressure and/or pulmonary artery wedge pressure, appropriate fluid should be administered so that left ventricular filling pressure is in the optimum range of 14 to 18 mm Hg. Hypoxia and hypercapnia should be treated with oxygen and, if required, endotracheal intubation with positive pressure ventilation. Sodium bicarbonate may be required to correct acidosis, but volume overloading should be avoided.

Various drugs that raise cardiac output, heart rate, and peripheral resistance or redistribute blood flow have been utilized in the treatment of cardiogenic shock. This is usually accomplished at the expense of increased myocardial oxygen consumption and possible extension of myocardial injury. Norepinephrine increases total peripheral resistance and arterial blood pressure. Metaraminol causes similar changes. Isoproterenol increases cardiac output and heart rate and decreases total peripheral resistance with little change in blood pressure. Dopamine increases cardiac output and arterial blood pressure with fewer chronotropic effects than isoproterenol. Digitalis has little inotropic effect on an acutely infarcted heart and probably should be avoided unless there are associated arrhythmias or signs of overt congestive heart failure. The role of glucagon and corticosteroids in cardiogenic shock remains controversial. More recently the use of left ventricular afterload reduction by nitroprusside and use of intra-aortic balloon counterpulsation in cardiogenic shock have shown some encouraging results. Despite the use of all these measures, the mortality for shock caused by acute myocardial infarction continues to be in the range of 80% to 100%. During the last few years coronary artery bypass grafting and infarctectomy have been tried in this clinical setting, usually with disappointing results. Surgical correction of a ruptured papillary muscle or repair of a ruptured interventricular septum may, however, be lifesaving.

Because of the continuing high mortality of cardiogenic shock in acute myocardial infarction, various devices coming under the heading of assisted circulation have been used when other medical measures fail. Basically these are devices that increase tissue perfusion without increasing myocardial oxygen demands. Of these, the intra-aortic balloon pump has received the greatest clinical trial. The effect these devices have on mortality remains uncertain. They may buy time and allow studies so that the patient may eventually reach surgery.

ACUTE VALVULAR LESIONS

The left side of the heart, being the systemic, high-pressure system, is subjected to much greater forces than the right side, low-pressure system. Abnormalities of valvular structures of the left side therefore have a greater impact on the efficiency with which the heart performs than do abnormalities of valves of the right side. Two valvular lesions, acute mitral insufficiency and severe aortic stenosis, are most likely to produce an acute illness in a cardiac patient. Other valvular diseases tend to follow a protracted course over several years marked by progressive symptoms, and the patient is less likely to seek medical aid for an acute illness.

■ What is the etiology of acute mitral insufficiency?

The rupture of chordae tendineae results in a flail mitral leaflet that is free to prolapse into the left atrium. This may occur in conjunction with chronic mitral regurgitation secondary to rheumatic heart disease, or it may result in an acute form from infective endocarditis. Less common causes of ruptured chordae include traumatic blows to the chest, myxomatous degeneration of valve structures, or simply nonspecific thinning and stretching of chordae. The amount of regurgitation produced depends on the extent of mitral leaflet tethered by the ruptured chorda; rupture of small chordae close to the leaflet produces less regurgitation than does rupture of large chordae close to the papillary muscle.

If mitral regurgitation suddenly develops in a patient who has coronary artery disease or has recently had myocardial infarction, it is most likely caused by papillary muscle dysfunction of rupture of a papillary muscle. These muscles are particularly susceptible to ischemic injury and abnormal function can produce varying degrees of mitral regurgitation. Rupture of a papillary muscle represents the most severe form of this spectrum and commonly occurs in a very dramatic fashion in association with recent infarction. The patient becomes acutely ill with intractable congestive heart failure and often dies

within 24 hours. The combination of acute severe mitral regurgitation and an infarcted ischemic myocardium apparently dictates the patient's fate rather than either of these factors alone.

■ What treatment is recommended for acute mitral insufficiency?

Digitalis glycosides are often useful when severe mitral regurgitation is present and serve to help the ventricle pump more efficiently as well as to control the PSVT's that are frequently present. Potent diuretics such as furosemide or ethacrynic acid also help relieve pulmonary congestion. If the patient is in shock, pressor agents are of little benefit and will most likely cause increased mitral regurgitation. Significant advances have been made recently in the use of afterload-reducing agents such as nitroprusside and hydralazine when shock is associated with the acute mitral regurgitation. These agents appear to decrease the regurgitant fraction and increase the forward cardiac output as a result of reducing afterload. If afterload reduction is attempted, adequate measures must be taken to monitor arterial pressure (preferably with an intra-arterial line), central venous or pulmonary artery pressure, urine flow, and heart rhythm. It should become apparent early in the course whether medicine alone will stabilize the patient's condition. Surgical replacement of the mitral valve should not be delayed for the patient who does not respond to medical therapy.

In an effort to assess the risks of surgery, patients with severe mitral regurgitation should undergo hemodynamic evaluation and left ventricular angiography. The angiogram will help quantitate the degree of mitral regurgitation as well as general myocardial dysfunction. The greater the degree of myocardial abnormalities, the greater is the risk of surgery and the less likely is the possibility that mitral valve replacement alone will alter the patient's course.

■ What factors should be considered in the diagnosis of severe aortic stenosis?

When a patient with aortic stenosis complains of angina-like chest pain, episodes of faintness or symptoms of heart failure such as shortness of breath or orthopnea, it is likely that a severe degree of stenosis has developed. These symptoms may signal a rapid deterioration in the patient's condition and survival is usually limited to less than 3 to 4 years after the onset of these symptoms. Congestive heart failure appears to be the most ominous sign and generally heralds a rapidly deteriorating condition developing over a period of 2 to 3 years.

There are several indications on physical examination that there is severe stenosis. If the stenosis is severe, the crescendo-decrescendo murmur tends to peak late in systole and actually may become softer. The second heart sound becomes diminished or even absent. Fourth heart sounds are most common with severe degrees of aortic stenosis, and a third heart sound is indicative of some degree of left ventricular failure in older patients with aortic stenosis. Evidence of left ventricular hypertrophy on the ECG is often present when lesions are severe, and the chest x-ray film commonly reveals calcium in the aortic valve. If a patient with stenosis complains of ominous symptoms or has these physical findings, cardiac catheterization should be undertaken without delay in an effort to assess the severity of the aortic disease. Coronary angiography should be performed in anyone with signs or symptoms of ischemia, even though this may occur without coronary artery disease. It has been our general practice to perform coronary angiography in any patient undergoing aortic valve replacement for aortic stenosis, even if symptoms of angina are not present.

■ **In the management of end-stage aortic stenosis, what modalities should be considered?**

Acute decompensation in severe aortic stenosis may take the form of pulmonary edema, shock, or syncope. Arrhythmias, especially atrial fibrillation, are poorly tolerated in patients with thick, hypertrophied, noncompliant left ventricles and should be managed in a critical care unit. If the patient is hypotensive, inotropic agents such as isoproterenol should be administered promptly. Digitalis glycosides may be administered. If pulmonary edema is present, rotating tourniquets and opiates should be utilized, but a vigorous diuresis is to be avoided. Time should not be lost in

medical therapy that is not promptly effective. The patient should undergo cardiac catheterization as soon as possible, and a decision should be made regarding valve replacement. Although the risks of aortic valve replacement in the acutely ill patient are considerable, the risks of ongoing medical management are greater, and many reports of successful acute aortic valve replacement are available.

ACUTE PERICARDITIS
■ **What is acute pericarditis?**

Acute pericarditis is an inflammatory process involving the visceral and parietal pericardium, usually with associated fluid accumulation in the pericardial sac.

The following is a list of some of the well-recognized etiologies of acute pericarditis.

Etiology of acute pericarditis
Connective tissue disorders—rheumatoid arthritis, acute rheumatic fever, disseminated lupus erythematosus
Infections
  Viruses—coxsackie B virus, echovirus, influenza
  Bacterial infections
  Fungi—histoplasmosis
Neoplasm—especially lung and breast
Uremia
Radiation—to the chest
Drugs—procainamide, hydralazine
Postmyocardial infarction syndrome (Dressler's syndrome)
Postthoracotomy
Traumatic—penetrating and nonpenetrating injuries to the chest
Iatrogenic—cardiac catheterization, central venous pressure lines
Idiopathic

Many infectious agents that cause myocarditis may also cause pericarditis, often during the same illness. In the United States the most common etiologies of acute pericarditis are probably viruses and uremia. In many cases no cause can be identified.

■ **What are the signs and symptoms of acute pericarditis?**

The signs and symptoms are those of the primary systemic illness and the inflammatory process of the pericardium. Often a viral upper respiratory infection has occurred in the preceding week. Complaints may be restricted to those of the systemic illness such as fever, arthralgia, myalgia, fatigue, or symptoms of uremia. Usually there is substernal chest pain radiating to the neck and left arm that increases on sudden turning of the thorax, deep inspiration, or lying flat on the back and is relieved by sitting forward. Physical examination will often show tachycardia, fever, a pericardial friction rub that may have from one to three components, distended neck veins, and a diffuse cardiac impulse if there is significant pericardial fluid. With pericardial tamponade a paradoxical pulse (greater than 8 mm Hg drop in systolic pressure during quiet inspiration) and on occasion inspiratory neck vein distention (Kussmaul's sign) will be found.

The ECG will usually demonstrate generalized S-T segment elevation followed by T wave inversion. Low voltage and electrical alternans (of the P wave and QRS complexes) can be seen if there is significant pericardial fluid accumulation. The chest x-ray film is often normal. There may be an associated pleural effusion and pulmonary infiltrate and cardiomegaly if significant pericardial fluid accumulates or associated myocarditis is present. Radioisotope and contrast studies will often demonstrate an increased pericardial space. Currently the best technique to demonstrate pericardial fluid accumulation is echocardiography. Fig. 13-11 shows the records of a typical case of acute pericarditis with large accumulation of pericardial fluid.

An etiologic diagnosis will depend on a complete medical evaluation and appropriate stains and cultures of various body fluids, including pericardial fluid. Serologic studies may also be of aid.

■ What treatment modalities are indicated?

Treatment is directed at the underlying systemic illness and the relief of symptoms caused by the pericardial inflammatory process. Bed rest with the head of the bed elevated 30 to 45 degrees is recommended. Fever and pain should be relieved with aspirin. Indomethacin is also beneficial. In some cases stronger analgesics will be required. If symptoms persist and are severe, and bacterial, fungal, and tuberculous etiologies have been excluded, adrenal steroids may give dramatic symptomatic results in idiopathic, postradiation, postmyocardial infarction, and postthoracotomy pericarditis. If a bacterial, fungal, or tuberculous agent has been identified, appropriate therapy for the infection should be started immediately. Uremic pericarditis usually responds to hemodialysis, and lupus erythematosus is susceptible to steroids and/or antimetabolite preparations.

In a small percentage of patients with pericardial inflammation or injury pericardial tamponade results secondary to rapid fluid accumulation in the pericardial sac. Usually this is marked by rapidly progressive cardiorespiratory distress and classically by a rising central venous pressure, a falling arterial blood pressure, and a small,

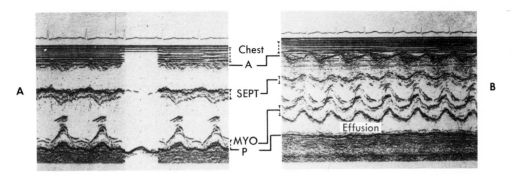

Fig. 13-11. A, Normal echocardiogram. **B,** Echocardiogram depicting pericardial effusion. *A,* Anterior heart wall; *SEPT,* intraventricular septum; *MYO,* myocardium of posterior left ventricle; *P,* pericardium. Space between left ventricular myocardium and pericardium represents pericardial effusion.

quiet heart. The primary problem is resistance to cardiac filling secondary to increased intrapericardial pressure. On physical examination there is a low blood pressure with a reduced pulse pressure and increased paradoxical pulse, with or without a positive Kussmaul's sign, tachycardia, high central venous pressure, and a quiet precordium with distant heart sounds. An ECG may show generally low voltage and/or total electrical alternans. Cardiomegaly may or may not be present on chest x-ray films. Echocardiography provides more specific diagnostic information. The final diagnosis and treatment requires immediate needle aspiration of the pericardial fluid, usually with dramatic results. If pericardial fluid rapidly reaccumulates, further consideration must be given to a pericardiectomy or repair of an associated cardiac lesion. If facilities for a pericardial tap and/or further cardiac surgery are not immediately available, temporary support may be given by providing optimum filling pressures (maintaining a central venous pressure in the range of 14 to 18 ml H_2O) and by the use of inotropic agents such as isoproterenol that augment left ventricular emptying.

ACUTE MYOCARDITIS
■ What is acute myocarditis?

Myocarditis may be defined as an inflammatory process involving the myocardium. Many bacteria, viruses, rickettsia, fungi, and parasites may cause the syndrome. Acute myocarditis can occur with exposure to certain toxic agents, radiation therapy to the chest, and coronary vasculitis. However, the leading causes are the postviral syndromes that occur following infection with many viral agents. The incidence and agent involved vary with age, location, and criteria used to describe the disease. In some cases the myocarditis may be secondary to a vasculitis or an immunologic phenomenon following an infection. Myocarditis may occur in 10% to 25% of patients with diphtheria, usually during the second week of illness as a result of the metabolic disturbances caused by the diphtheria toxin. Typhoid fever may be associated with peripheral vascular collapse and myocarditis, usually in the second or third week of illness. A β-streptococcus infection may of course be followed in 3 weeks by

a pancarditis involving the myocardium. Meningococcemia, especially fatal cases, may involve an interstitial myocarditis and associated circulatory collapse. Any cause of endocarditis can include small infarctions, microabscesses, and myofiber swelling. Other less common bacterial causes may be found on p. 257. Rickettsial infections such as Rocky Mountain spotted fever and Q-fever may cause myocarditis. In the United States coxsackie B virus and influenza virus have been the best documented etiologic agents of clinical myocarditis. Often, however, no specific etiologic agent can be identified by bacteriologic, serologic, or fluorescent techniques.

Pathologically the heart is usually large and flabby. Microscopically there may be areas of focal hemorrhage, interstitial edema, myocardial degeneration and necrosis, a mononuclear or polymorphonuclear cellular infiltrate, small abscesses, areas of vasculitis, gumma, or tuberculous nodules, depending on the agent involved. In many cases an inflammatory process also involves the endocardium and/or pericardium. Mural thrombi can often be seen in both ventricles.

Clinical recognition involves signs and symptoms reflecting the primary infectious process with its unique features, inadequate cardiac output, and associated congestive heart failure. Often there are associated signs and symptoms of an inflammatory process of the endocardium and/or pericardium. There may have been previous upper respiratory or enteric symptoms. Typically the patients complain of dyspnea, fatigue, palpitations, and chest discomfort. On physical examination there may be fever, hypotension, tachycardia, an enlarged heart with a diffuse PMI, distended neck veins, soft heart sounds with an associated S_3 and/or S_4, murmurs of tricuspid and/or mitral regurgitation, and other symptoms of congestive heart failure. A pericardial friction rub is often heard. The ECG will often show diffuse ST-T wave changes, occasional QRS abnormalities, various degrees of heart block, and all the known types of atrial and ventricular arrhythmias. Final diagnosis depends on appropriate cultures and serologic tests. The entire course may conclude in sudden death, systemic or pulmonary emboli, severe heart failure, partial resolution with a persisting chronic congestive cardiomyopathy, or total and complete recovery.

Appropriate treatment requires an early etiologic diagnosis so that appropriate antibacterial, antirickettsial, or antifungal agents or antitoxin are utilized. Bedrest, oxygen, salt restriction, ECG monitoring, and control of fever are essential, since there is experimental evidence that hypoxia and exercise can enhance viral myocarditis in animals. Hemodynamically significant arrhythmias should be treated with antiarrhythmic agents, although these drugs should be used with caution in such patients so as to prevent further myocardial depression. Heart failure should be treated with diuretics and digitalis, although increased sensitivity to digitalis in myocarditis requires the use of lower doses. Patients should receive anticoagulants if there have been any systemic or pulmonary emboli; however, vigilance should be applied to avoid any development of hemopericardium. The use of steroids and other anti-inflammatory agents in rheumatic myocarditis or vasculitis appears to be of significant benefit, but the role of steroids in acute viral or idiopathic myocarditis is controversial. Other inflammatory reducing agents such as aspirin, indomethacin, and cyclophosphamide may be indicated. The preventive role of immunization and vaccination should always be emphasized.

INFECTIVE ENDOCARDITIS
■ What is infective endocarditis?

Infective endocarditis is a bacterial, fungal, or possibly viral infection of cardiac structures that destroys or damages these structures and makes them incompetent. Virtually any bacteria or fungus can cause endocarditis, but some organisms are more common than others and can infect heart valves. Frequently they accompany congenital defects or contaminate prosthetic materials placed at the time of heart surgery. The organisms invade the tissues, resulting in inflammatory and immunologic reactions that then destroy these tissues. Holes in valve cusps and leaflets, ruptured chordae, myocarditis, myocardial abscesses, or communications between chambers may develop. The mass of organisms, fibrin, col-

lagen, and debris as they collect and organize on a valve or prosthetic structure can impede the motion of a valve, rendering it stenotic or incompetent. As a result, there are a number of possible ways the heart may exhibit infection and hence a myriad of ways a patient may be seen with endocarditis.

Endocarditis also produces a classic but atypical syndrome involving practically every system in the body. Neurologic, hematologic, renal, musculoskeletal, peripheral vascular, and integumentary manifestations of infective endocarditis may all appear. With such a variety of possible systemic manifestations it is not uncommon for a patient to be treated for a number of the peripheral manifestations of infective endocarditis rather than to have the primary process itself discovered or even considered.

■ What is the differentiation between "acute" or "subacute" infective endocarditis?

Endocarditis may be either acute or subacute. The term "acute infective endocarditis" is applied to the disease in patients who, without treatment, would not survive for a length of time (6 to 8 weeks), while the term "subacute infective endocarditis" refers to the disease in patients who experience a longer and more indolent course. This distinction originated in the preantibiotic era when the natural course of the disease could be observed unaltered by the administration of antibiotics. Acute infective endocarditis affects and destroys cardiac structures before more chronic manifestations can develop, whereas in subacute infective endocarditis there is more time for immunologic and inflammatory factors to evolve the full-blown, classic syndrome. Certain organisms such as staphylococcus and pneumococcus are more commonly associated with the acute form of the disease, whereas less virulent organisms such as *Streptococcus viridans*, fungi (particularly *Candida*), or enterococcus usually cause subacute endocarditis. The rapid appearance of extensive damage such as acute aortic regurgitation or tricuspid regurgitation in a setting suggestive of endocarditis, signals the probability that a more virulent process exists. This classification is useful in characterizing the tempo of an episode of endocarditis, but it is not useful in dictating early management of a given patient. Pragmatically each case of endocarditis should be considered to be "potentially acute" and deserves prompt attention.

■ What factors should be considered in the diagnosis of endocarditis?

Fever is the most common presenting symptom of a patient with infective endocarditis, and fever in a person with acquired valvular abnormalities or congenital heart disease should always signal the possibility of an infectious cardiac process. Although rheumatic heart disease is still the most common underlying cardiac abnormality, the relative incidence of other abnormalities such as mitral valve prolapse or calcific or atheromatous lesions of the aortic or mitral valves has been increasing in frequency. The incidence of infective endocarditis in normal hearts has increased recently as well, particularly in conjunction with heroin abuse or chronic hemodialysis when vascular manipulations are common or in the patient taking immunosuppressive agents. Therefore any fever even without cardiac abnormality suggests the possibility of endocarditis. The absence of fever does not, however, rule out a cardiac infection, particularly in aged or uremic patients. The empiric use of antibiotics is a common disguise for a fever.

The most significant laboratory tests pinpointing the diagnosis of infective endocarditis are positive blood cultures. One positive blood culture does not determine the diagnosis, but its occurrence should stimulate further blood cultures and suggest the possibility of infectious endocarditis. Some organisms such as diphtheroids or *Staphylococcus albus* are common contaminants in routine blood cultures, but the practitioner should also be aware that these organisms have been implicated in infectious endocarditis as well and should not totally dismiss them as contaminants.

Generally five to six blood cultures, appropriately obtained under strict conditions of asepsis, will be sufficient to recover an organism if endocarditis is present. The timing of the cultures may be important. Blood obtained just prior to a temperature elevation is likely to be most productive, but as a temperature rise may not be anticipated, the next best yield will be obtained as the fever rises. A volume of 10 ml of venous blood obtained after thoroughly cleansing and sterilizing the venipuncture site should be planted in both aerobic and anaerobic culture medium. Cultures are frequently negative when infection is present on the right side of the heart, if antibiotics have been administered, or if the responsible organism, such as a rickettsia, simply will not grow on the culture media.

■ What therapeutic approach is recommended in the management of endocarditis?

Adequate therapy for infective endocarditis requires characterization of the causative organisms. Once this information is available from the microbiology laboratory, the most logical course of therapy is often clear. It may be reasonable to delay therapy until these antibiotic sensitivities are determined, particularly if the clinical course appears to be that of a subacute infection, and symptoms have been present for some time. If the symptoms of acute endocarditis are present, or the patient appears acutely ill, has had symptoms for a relatively short period of time, and does not have any murmurs or has murmurs of tricuspid or pulmonic insufficiency, no time should be lost in instituting therapy on a presumptive basis. If staphylococcus is suspected to be the causative agent, the regimen should include large doses of a penicillinase-resistant semisynthetic penicillin. The initial regimen should cover the most likely organisms against each serum dilution. A serum dilution of $1:8$ that impedes multiplication of the organism is considered effective therapy.

The duration of recommended therapy has been somewhat empiric, and it is generally accepted that at least 4 weeks of therapy are required. Although there is no statistical evidence, some practitioners prefer to prolong treatment for 6 weeks. There is the theoretical consideration that with the broad spectrum of coverage gained by high doses of antibiotics and with a longer treatment period, there will be some predisposition to superinfection.

■ What factors should be considered during the follow-up evaluation of the patient?

Signs of early or increasing heart failure must be carefully sought. Heart failure may be caused by myocarditis but more often is a result of progressive valvular destruction or disruption of the valvular mechanism by vegetation. Such valvular disturbances are usually marked by murmurs that may change as valvular damage increases. The heart size and contour on chest x-ray films is important in demonstrating cardiac enlargement, which may result from either congestive heart failure or insufficiency of aortic or mitral valves. The appearance of a pericardial friction rub indicates the possibility of the extension of infection, particularly in acute bacterial endocarditis, through cardiac structures to involve pericardial surfaces. Such an extension can rapidly develop into purulent pericarditis or pericardial tamponade, and the echocardiogram is a sensitive tool for early detection of accumulating pericardial fluid. Jugular venous pulse waves, as visualized at the bedside and recorded on the phonocardiogram, may be of importance in evaluating competence of the tricuspid valve in the presence of endocarditis of the right side. The evolution of new infiltrates in the lung fields associated with supposedly adequate antibiotic therapy of endocarditis of the right side points toward an ongoing infectious valvular process. ECG's should be obtained occasionally, as the evolution of new conduction defects support an ongoing infectious process.

Two-dimensional echocardiography yields a dynamic picture of intracardiac structures and has been helpful in localizing the vegetations of endocarditis. Follow-up echocardiograms can be useful in assessing valve abnormalities, myocardial function, and the appearance of shunts as therapy progresses.

■ **Under what circumstances would aggressive surgical intervention be indicated, and what complications might be anticipated?**

Progressive and intractable cardiac failure as a result of infective endocarditis destroying valve mechanisms is the most common indication for surgery, and congestive heart failure secondary to mitral regurgitation is the most common lesion.

Valve surgery in patients with infective endocarditis is associated with a high mortality rate that must be contrasted to the 100% fatality rate of progressive cardiac failure if surgery is not performed. Failure can also result from rupture of

the interventricular septum and can require surgical repair. When one course of antibiotic therapy has not eradicated the infection, a second course should be attempted; little is gained, however, by trying a third or fourth course, and surgical excision should be considered. Such a situation is most common with fungal infections of valves on the right side. The resistant nature of fungal endocarditis and the very toxic nature of the therapeutic regimens required for treatment raise the issue of surgery whenever endocarditis caused by a fungus is documented.

With the abundance of prosthetic materials placed in the heart during cardiac surgery over the past decade, the significance of positive blood cultures in the setting of these prostheses has become a frequent issue. Positive blood cultures in the early postoperative period (less than 25 days), considering the many complicating factors and modes of entrance to the bloodstream available in the surgical patient, are generally not regarded as indicative of infection of prosthetic material. Bacteremia occurring more than 25 days after surgery has more significance, and should suggest the probability of infected prosthetic materials. There is a high incidence of fungal (particularly *Candida*) antibiotic-resistant gram-negative organisms (*Staphylococcus epidermitis* and *Staphylococcus aureus*) in the postoperative patient. In view of the very poor results in treating infections of prosthetic materials by medications alone and the bizarre nature of the organisms usually involved, time should not be wasted in attempting repeated courses of antibiotics; early surgery is the preferable course of action.

DISSECTING ANEURYSM OF THE AORTA
■ **What is a dissecting aneurysm of the aorta?**

Dissecting aneurysm of the aorta is a cleavage of the layers of the aortic wall by blood and hematoma that gains access through a tear in the intima of the aorta. The dissection may spread both proximal and distal to the initial tear. Dissection occurs in people who are hypertensive but may occur in Marfan's syndrome or when there has been trauma to the chest. The danger involved in a dissecting aneurysm is rupture of the aorta and most often occurs into the pericardial sac with acute tamponade and death. A dissection may also occlude any of the major branches of the aorta with subsequent ischemia or infarction of end-organs. Dissecting aneurysms of the aorta is a medical-surgical emergency and requires prompt aggressive therapy with close monitoring.

■ On what basis is the diagnosis made?

The most frequently seen symptom of a patient with a dissecting aneurysm is commonly described as a "ripping" or "tearing" chest pain located in the substernal region or in the interscapular area. It commonly radiates down the back as the hematoma dissects along the aortic wall. Shortness of breath, orthopnea, or symptoms of frank pulmonary edema result from involvement of the aortic root and resultant aortic regurgitation. Shock as a result of leakage into a body cavity or the pericardium with tamponade may occur. Signs of occlusions of major branches of the aorta such as stroke or bowel ischemia are seen.

The impressive chest pain suggests a myocardial infarction. However, the ECG in uncomplicated dissections is normal, and when myocardial infarction is eliminated after normal enzymes and the absence of ischemic patterns on the ECG, a dissecting aneurysm should be suspected.

Physical examination is not very helpful in diagnosing a dissecting aneurysm. Pressure differentials in the arms, pulseless lower extremities, signs of pericardial effusion or tamponade, and shock are all relatively nonspecific but when seen together are highly suggestive of a dissecting aneurysm. Chest x-ray films classically demonstrate a wide mediastinum that is the result of dilatation of the ascending aorta, descending aorta, or both. The heart may be enlarged and bottle shaped if pericardial fluid is present.

The definitive diagnosis of a dissection is made by aortography, and this should be undertaken as soon as possible after the diagnosis is suspected. The study should define the intimal tear, the extent of the aneurysm, and any occluded blood vessels to aid in the surgical corrections.

■ What treatment may be considered when the presence of a dissecting aneurysm is suspected?

The initial therapy of any patient exhibiting the signs of a dissection, that is, hypertension and severe chest or back pain, should consist of immediate blood pressure control with the goal of maintaining a systolic blood pressure of 100 to 120 mm Hg. The medication most useful in achieving this are trimethaphan (Arfonad) or nitroprusside (Nipride) in combination with propranolol (Inderal). Propranolol will decrease the force with which blood is ejected from the heart. Pain must be controlled, and opiates are required in most cases. Urine flow, state of mentation, blood pressure (preferable with an arterial line), and central venous or pulmonary artery pressure should all be monitored.

After the diagnosis has been confirmed and adequate blood pressure control achieved, a decision regarding surgery must be made. Generally surgery is the therapy of choice when the aneurysm originates in the ascending portion of the aorta. Aneurysms from this location are associated with a higher risk of death and occlusion of major vessels than aneurysms from the descending portion of the aorta. Medical therapy as outlined may be attempted for aneurysms occurring in the descending aorta, but any signs of progression such as ongoing pain or leakage should be indications for surgery.

■ What is the prognosis?

The percentage of survival from a dissecting aneurysm of the descending aorta has been reported to be about 70% in patients medically treated and at least 75% when a combination of medical and surgical therapy is applied to an ascending aortic aneurysm. Aortic valve replacement is often required if there is severe aortic regurgitation. The basic pathologic process of cystic medial necrosis is obviously still present in a patient who has recovered from the acute stages of a dissecting aneurysm. Continued blood pressure control and diminution of the force with which blood is ejected from the left ventricle (dp/dt) are therefore imperative. Reserpine and propranolol are probably the best medications for these purposes. Blood pressure should be monitored with the patient in a supine position and should be less than 130 mm Hg systolic. Chest x-ray films should be followed routinely for further discrete dilatations. Any report by the patient of renewed pain or symptoms referable to new major arterial branch occlusions indicates an ongoing dissection process, and surgical therapy is warranted.

BIBLIOGRAPHY
Arrhythmias

Coltart, D. J., and Harrison, D. C.: Office management of arrhythmias, Primary Care 1:123, 1974.

Marriott, H. J. L., and Myerberg, R. J.: Recognition and treatment of cardiac arrhythmias and conduction disturbances. In Hurst, J. W., and Logue, R. B., editors: The heart, New York, 1970, McGraw-Hill Book Co.

Congestive heart failure and pulmonary edema

Karliner, J. S., and Braunwald, E.: Present status of digitalis treatment of acute myocardial infarction, Circulation 45: 169, 1972.

Lassers, B. W., George, M., Auderton, J. L., Higgins, M. R., and Philip, T.: Left ventricular failure in acute myocardial infarction, Am. J. Cardiol. 25:511, 1970.

Ramo, B. W., et al.: Hemodynamic findings in 123 patients with acute myocardial infarction on admission, Circulation 42: 567, 1970.

Wolk, M. J., Scheidt, S., and Killip, T.: Heart failure complicating acute myocardial infarction, Circulation 45:225, 1972.

Cardiogenic shock in acute myocardial infarction

Haddy, F. J.: Pathophysiology and therapy of the shock of myocardial infarction, Ann. Intern. Med. 73:809, 1970.

Page, D. L., Caulfield, J. B., Kastor, J. A., DeSanctis, R. W., and Sanders, C. A.: Myocardial changes associated with cardiogenic shock, N. Engl. J. Med. 285:133, 1971.

Perlroth, M. G., and Harrison, D. C.: Medical therapy for shock in acute myocardial infarction. In Yu, P. N., and Goodwin, J. F., editors: Progress in cardiology, Philadelphia, 1973, Lea & Febiger.

Scheidt, S., et al.: Intra-aortic balloon counterpulsation in cardiogenic shock, N. Engl. J. Med. 288:979, 1973.

Shubin, H., and Weil, M. H.: Practical considerations in management of shock complicating acute myocardial infarction. A summary of current practice, Am. J. Cardiol. 26:603, 1970.

Acute valvular lesions

Cobbs, B. W.: Clinical recognition and medical management of rheumatic heart disease and other acquired valvular disease. In Hurst, J. W., and Logue, R. B., editors: The heart, New York, 1970, McGraw-Hill Book Co.

Acute pericarditis

Connolly, D. C., and Burchell, H. G.: Pericarditis: a ten-year survey, Am. J. Cardiol. 7:7, 1961.

Fowler, N. O., and Manitsas, G. T.: Infectious pericarditis, Prog. Cardiovasc. Dis. 16:323, 1973.

Grist, N. R., and Bell, E. J.: Coxsackie viruses and the heart, Am. Heart J. 77:295, 1969 (editorial).

Shabetai, R., Fowler, N. O., and Guntheroth, W. G.: Hemodynamics of cardiac tamponade and constrictive pericarditis, Am. J. Cardiol. 26:480, 1970.

Spodick, D. H.: Differential diagnosis of acute pericarditis, Prog. Cardiovasc. Dis. 14:192, 1971.

Acute myocarditis

Abelmann, W. H.: Virus and the heart, Circulation 44:950, 1971.

Abelmann, W. H.: Viral myocarditis and its sequelae, Annu. Rev. Med. 24:145, 1973.

Gardiner, A. J. S., and Short, D.: Four faces of acute myopericarditis, Br. Heart J. 35:433, 1973.

Gerzen, P., Granath, A., Holmgren, B., and Zetterquist, S.: Acute myocarditis, a follow up study, Br. Heart J. 34:575, 1972.

Wenger, N. K.: Infectious myocarditis, Cardiovasc. Clin. 4: 167, 1972.

Infective endocarditis

Weinstein, L., and Schlesinger, J.: Treatment of infective endocarditis, Prog. Cardiovasc. Dis. 16:275, 1973.

Dissecting aneurysm of the aorta

Daily, P. O., et al.: Management of acute aortic dissection, Ann. Thorac. Surg. 10:237, 1970.

Wheat, M. W., Jr.: Treatment of dissecting aneurysms, Prog. Cardiovasc. Dis. 16:87, 1973.

CHAPTER 14

Current concepts and mechanisms of acid-base disorders

Orhan Muren, William Richard Smith, and Frederick L. Glauser

■ How are acid-base terms defined?

Deviation of the arterial pH beyond its normal limits is called acidemia if the pH falls below 7.35 or alkalemia if the pH is above 7.45.

Acidosis is a physiologic disturbance that can lead to acidemia. It is usually indicated by a decreased serum HCO_3^- when of metabolic (non-respiratory) origin and by hypercapnia when of respiratory origin. There may or may not be associated acidemia.

Alkalosis is a physiologic disturbance that can lead to alkalemia. It is usually indicated by an increased serum HCO_3^- when metabolic in origin and by hypocapnia when respiratory in origin. Alkalemia may or may not be present.

Hypocapnia (hypocarbia) is a reduced arterial Pco_2.

Hypercapnia (hypercarbia) is an increased arterial Pco_2.

■ What are the various acid-base disturbances?

The four simple or primary acid-base disorders are respiratory acidosis, respiratory alkalosis, metabolic acidosis, and metabolic alkalosis. In addition, mixed or combined disorders exist and are indicative of two or more independent or primary acid-base abnormalities going on simultaneously.

■ What is respiratory acidosis?

Respiratory acidosis is characterized by hypercapnia, that is, a primary increase in Pco_2. It re-

sults when CO_2 production in the tissues exceeds the rate of its removal by the lungs.

■ How does the body defend pH against acute hypercapnia?

The defense of pH during acute hypercapnia depends on the generation of HCO_3^- by non-bicarbonate buffers, particularly hemoglobin. When Pco_2 increases acutely, from 40 mm Hg to 90 mm Hg, plasma HCO_3^- increases less than 3 to 4 mEq/L. On the average, plasma HCO_3^- concentration rises 0.8-1 mEq/L for every 10 mm Hg rise in the Pco_2. Because of this limited HCO_3^- generation, the body defense mechanism against acute hypercapnia is limited.[1] For example, in uncomplicated acute hypercapnia (with a sudden increase in Pco_2 to as high as 90 mm Hg) the plasma HCO_3^- concentration should fall between 25 and 30 mEq/L. Plasma HCO_3^- concentrations below 25 mEq/L show the coexistence of a metabolic acidosis.[1] In humans the bicarbonate level appears to have a curvilinear response to hypercapnia and tends to be more horizontal (less HCO_3^- is generated as Pco_2 rises) at 80 mm Hg.[1]

Blood H^+ increases linearly as Pco_2 increases. For each millimeter of mercury rise in Pco_2 that occurs acutely, plasma H^+ concentration rises 0.75 nmole/L. These physiologic response curves or "95% significance bands" can be helpful in appraising the acid-base status of patients with acute hypercapnia. Thus in a patient with hypercapnia, if the response falls in the "95% significance band," the response is considered appropriate and indicates acute uncomplicated hypercapnia. On the other hand, if the response is out of the significance bands, it indicates the presence of a mixed acid-base disorder. However, the clinical information (history, physical examination, laboratory findings, medications taken, and so on) is vitally important in evaluating the mixed acid-base disorders.

■ What is the body defense against chronic hypercapnia?

The defense of pH in chronic hypercapnia is accomplished by renal compensatory mechanisms. An augmented renal tubular sodium-hydrogen ion exchange mechanism is responsible for increased acid excretion. Therefore more HCO_3^- is generated and returned to the blood. Coincidental with this augmented cation-exchange mechanism during chronic hypercapnia, chloride is rejected by the renal tubular cells and increased chloride excretion takes place. The usual electrolyte pattern in uncomplicated chronic hypercapnia is characterized by a reduced plasma chloride and increased bicarbonate, with no change in the "measurable anions" in the plasma (chloride + bicarbonate).[2-10] However, increased generation and absorption of HCO_3^- from the kidneys during chronic hypercapnia is not sufficient to restore the arterial pH to normal, and thus patients with chronic CO_2 retention have either acidemia or a low-normal pH.[4]

Chronic uncomplicated hypercapnia in man produces a curvilinear rise in plasma HCO_3^- with incremental increases in Pco_2.[8] As a rule of thumb, for every 3 mm Hg rise in Pco_2 the plasma HCO_3^- concentration can be expected to increase by 1 mEq/L. Blood H^+ increases linearly as Pco_2 increases. For each millimeter of mercury rise in Pco_2 that occurs chronically, plasma H^+ concentration rises 0.25 nmole/L.[9] If the acid-base status of a patient with chronic hypercapnia is outside the physiologic response curve, a mixed acid-base disorder is present or insufficient time has elapsed for maximal renal compensation (usually 3 to 5 days is required). The most important aspect of intelligent interpretation of the acid-base status of the patient is still the clinical assessment of the patient and prior knowledge of the pH and HCO_3^- concentration appropriate to

the given degree of uncomplicated hypercapnia.[10]

In summary, body buffers play the major role in the defense of pH against acute hypercapnia by generating HCO_3^-, but this is usually insufficient to prevent acidemia. On the other hand, the renal generation of HCO_3^-, which occurs over a period of 3 to 5 days, defends the arterial pH to the maximal degree in chronic hypercapnia.

■ How do we recognize respiratory acidosis clinically, and what are some causes?

The signs and symptoms of CO_2 retention are nonspecific and in general have no predictable relationship to the level of arterial Pco_2. Patients may have confusion, irritability, flapping tremor, somnolence, or coma.[3] The only diagnostic sign of respiratory acidosis is an elevated arterial blood Pco_2.

The following are causes of respiratory acidosis:

1. Chronic obstructive pulmonary disease (COPD)
2. "Stiff" lungs and thorax
3. Central nervous system depression by drugs or medullary respiratory center disorders
4. Motor system disorders (spinal cord, motor nerves, neuromuscular junction, and so on)
5. Obstruction of upper airways
6. Acute pulmonary edema
7. Marked obesity
8. Deep sleep
9. Metabolic alkalosis (compensatory hypoventilation)

■ How do we treat respiratory acidosis?

The treatment of respiratory acidosis should be directed at the cause of the CO_2 retention. Therapeutic measures to improve effective alveolar ventilation should be utilized, that is, bronchodilators, tracheobronchial toilet to improve the patency of the airways, antibiotics if indicated, removal of central nervous system depressants, and ventilatory support if needed. In acute respiratory acidosis Pco_2 can safely be reduced to normal levels rapidly. However, in chronic respiratory acidosis, if the Pco_2 is reduced rapidly, severe alkalosis can occur that may cause cardiac arrhythmias, central nervous system dysfunction, seizures, or coma. As a general rule, Pco_2 probably should not be reduced more than 5 to 10 mm Hg/hr. Once the Pco_2 is within the normal range, the plasma bicarbonate will slowly return to normal as a result of bicarbonate diuresis. Keep in mind that a posthypercapnic alkalosis will persist if the patient is not given adequate chloride replacement during the hypercapnic episode and after correction.

■ **What is respiratory alkalosis?**

Respiratory alkalosis is characterized by a primary decrease in arterial Pco_2. When CO_2 elimination by the lungs exceeds CO_2 production in the tissues, the result will be a lowering of arterial Pco_2. During acute hypocapnia HCO_3^- in extracellular fluid is reduced by nonbicarbonate buffers, whereas the renal excretion of HCO_3^- plays only a minor role. Approximately one third of the extracellular fluid HCO_3^- reduction associated with acute hyperventilation is due to blood buffers, principally hemoglobin. The remaining two thirds are due to tissue buffers.[11] During acute hyperventilation there is a small increase in blood lactate and, to a lesser degree, pyruvate; the buffer role of these two organic acids is small. When Pco_2 falls acutely from 40 to 20 mm Hg, the average plasma HCO_3^- fall is 7.5 mEq/L.[11-14]

■ **What is the response to acute hypocapnia?**

The response to acute hypocapnia in man has been described.[11] A reduction in Pco_2 from 40 mm Hg to 15 mm Hg results in prompt reduction in H^+ concentration from 40 to 20 mEq/L (pH 7.70). There is a linear reduction in H^+ concentration and a curvilinear decline in HCO_3^- concentration.[11] In the acute hypocapnic state, a plasma HCO_3^- level less than 15 mEq/L indicates the presence of a complicating metabolic acidosis. In acute respiratory alkalosis, the plasma HCO_3^- concentration falls approximately 2.5 to 3 mEq/L for each 10 mm Hg reduction in Pco_2, but usually not lower than 18 mEq/L and rarely to levels as low as 15 mEq/L.

■ **What is the response to chronic hypocapnia?**

There are no studies of chronic hypocapnia in man. However, one study in dogs indicates that HCO_3^- concentration is further reduced as a result of suppression of net acid excretion, and

there is a tendency toward hyperchloremia.[15] Chronic hypocapnia reduces the renal HCO_3^- threshold and leads to retention of Cl^- by the kidneys. Bicarbonate levels may be reduced to levels as low as 12 mEq/L. On the average, the plasma HCO_3^- concentration falls 5 mEq/L for each 10 mm Hg reduction in the Pco_2.

Patients with chronic respiratory alkalosis do not appear to have increased lactate in the plasma, and the pH tends to be slightly high but may be normal. In chronic respiratory alkalosis low plasma HCO_3^- is associated with hyperchloremia. Interestingly, the same electrolyte composition is seen in patients with hyperchloremic metabolic acidosis. However, the pH tends to be high in chronic respiratory alkalosis and low in hyperchloremic metabolic acidosis.

■ **How do we recognize respiratory alkalosis clinically, and what are some causes?**

Many patients can tolerate a significant reduction in arterial Pco_2 with little clinically obvious respiratory effort.[16] However, some complain of paresthesias of the extremities and circumoral region, light-headedness, irritability, and sometimes carpopedal spasms. These manifestations may be related to pH changes in body fluids, decreased blood flow in the brain, and reduced ionized calcium in the plasma.[17] The definitive diagnosis of respiratory alkalosis is made primarily by arterial blood gas studies. The following are common causes of primary respiratory alkalosis:

1. Psychogenic hyperventilation
2. Hypermetabolic states (fever, thyrotoxicosis, and so on)
3. Significant degrees of hypoxemia (pulmonary congestion and edema, diffuse interstitial pneumonitis or fibrosis, high-altitude living, and so on)
4. Salicylate intoxication
5. Disturbances of the respiratory center caused by central nervous system disease
6. Gram-negative septicemia
7. Assisted mechanical ventilation
8. Cirrhosis of the liver
9. Reflex hyperventilation (pulmonary hypertension, pneumothorax, pulmonary embolism, and so on)

■ How do we treat respiratory alkalosis?

The treatment of respiratory alkalosis is directed at the cause of the disorder. However, rebreathing into a paper bag, sedation, and reassurance may be utilized to increase Pco_2 levels in some patients with psychogenic hyperventilation. In some severe cases mixtures of CO_2 and O_2 can be administered.

■ What is metabolic acidosis, and what are the usual causes?

Metabolic acidosis is characterized by an increased H^+ activity or reduced pH in the extracellular space. There is a primary reduction in plasma HCO_3^- concentration. The resulting pH depends on the severity of the metabolic abnormality, the buffering capacity of body fluids, and effective alveolar ventilation. Metabolic acidosis occurs whenever HCO_3^- is lost or destroyed in the body fluids. The following mechanisms are usually responsible for the development of metabolic acidosis:

1. Administration of large amounts of exogenous acid or increased production of endogenous acid
2. Failure of the kidneys to secrete the normal endogenous acid load or to reabsorb filtered HCO_3^-
3. Loss of significant amounts of alkali from the body, such as might occur in severe diarrhea or draining pancreatic or duodenal fistulas
4. Rapid dilution of the extracellular space with a solution (that is, normal saline) that does not contain HCO_3^-

■ How does the body respond to metabolic acidosis?

The pH of the body is defended by buffers in both the extracellular and intracellular compartments, respiratory compensation, and renal compensation.[18]

Buffers are the first defense line against metabolic acidosis. During intracellular accumulation of H^+, electroneutrality is maintained by forcing K^+ and Na^+ out of the cells. If renal function is impaired or extracellular volume is depleted, K^+ will be retained, thereby leading to potentially harmful serum K^+ levels.

Respiratory compensation begins promptly in response to the development of metabolic acidosis. Increases in both frequency and depth of respiration reduce the arterial Pco_2. However, the respiratory compensation is never sufficient to return the pH to normal. As a maximal compensatory response to the most severe metabolic acidosis, a normally functioning respiratory system can reduce the Pco_2 to levels as low as 8 to 10 mm Hg. Arterial Pco_2 does not fall below 8 to 10 mm Hg because the effort required to increase alveolar ventilation further results in a CO_2 production that increases out of proportion to alveolar gas exchange. At this point a slight reduction in HCO_3^- concentration would produce a significant decrease in pH.

In an uncomplicated metabolic acidosis, the ventilatory response is probably the most predictable. For each decrease of 1 mEq/L in plasma HCO_3^-, the Pco_2 should be reduced by 1 to 1.5 mm Hg. If lesser or greater change in Pco_2 is seen, a mixed acid-base disorder should be suspected.

The lack of appropriate respiratory compensation for metabolic acidosis indicates an improper ventilatory response and thereby suggests an underlying disorder such as chronic obstructive pulmonary disease, central nervous system depression, or respiratory muscle weakness.

Renal compensation is the final defense against metabolic acidosis. However, 3 to 5 days are required to increase the excretion of NH_4^+ and titratable acid sufficiently to regenerate the HCO_3^- necessary to restore plasma HCO_3^- concentration to normal levels.

The in vivo response to primary acute and chronic metabolic acidosis has been described in man, and "significance bands" have been designed.[18,19] However, clinical assessment of the patient, along with the appropriate laboratory data, is essential to the proper use of these bands.

■ How do we recognize metabolic acidosis?

The signs and symptoms associated with metabolic acidosis are variable and nonspecific. They are primarily related to the underlying disorder responsible for the metabolic acidosis. Frequently patients have hyperpnea. However, mild to moderate chronic hyperventilation may not be detected in clinical observation. The definitive diagnosis of metabolic acidosis is made by finding a reduced plasma HCO_3^- level, with an associated reduction of Pco_2. With an incomplete respiratory compensation, the pH would be acidotic.

■ **What is the anion gap and how does it relate to causes of metabolic acidosis?**

The calculation of unmeasured anions (known as the anion gap) gives information regarding the possible causes of metabolic acidosis. The anion gap is determined by subtracting the sum of the plasma Cl^- and HCO_3^- from the plasma Na^+. Normally this "anion gap" is approximately 10 to 12 mEq/L. The presence of any fixed acid, other than HCl, in the extracellular fluid produces a widening of the anion gap.

Some causes of metabolic acidosis with a normal anion gap include diarrhea and draining fistulas, renal tubular acidosis, carbonic anhydrase inhibition, ammonium chloride, arginine HCl, chronic pyelonephritis, obstructive uropathy, hyperalimentation, and ureterosigmoidostomy.

Some causes of metabolic acidosis with an increased anion gap include diabetic ketoacidosis, lactic acidosis, azotemic renal failure, salicylate intoxication, methanol ingestion, paraldehyde ingestion, ethylene glycol poisoning, and ketoacidosis associated with alcoholism.

A reduced anion gap may be caused by: (1) reduced concentration of unmeasured anions, which may be seen in dilutional states and hypoalbuminemia; (2) systemic underestimation of serum sodium, which may occur in hypernatremia and hyperviscosity syndromes; (3) systemic overestimation of serum chloride, which may be present in brominism; or (4) retained nonsodium cations such as paraproteins, calcium, and lithium.

■ **How is metabolic acidosis treated, and what precautions are necessary?**

Treatment of metabolic acidosis should be directed toward any correctable underlying disorder such as severe hypoxemia or ketosis. However, if the acidosis is life-threatening or the underlying disorder cannot be corrected, administration of alkali will be required. Since acidosis depletes both extracellular and intracellular buffer stores, calculation of the amount of alkali to be given must consider both fractions of the total body buffers. Estimates of alkali requirements assume a distribution for HCO_3^- in a volume of approximately 40% to 50% of body weight. Thus the amount of HCO_3^- required for complete correction can be calculated by the following formula:

$$25 \text{ mEq/L} - \text{Actual plasma } HCO_3 \text{ concentration} \times$$
$$0.50 \times \text{body weight (in kilograms)} =$$
$$\text{mEq of } HCO_3^- \text{ required for correction}$$

However, the change in HCO_3^- concentration expected from the above calculation does not always occur. The patient losing alkali in severe diarrhea or the acidotic patient with continued endogenous acid production may require greater amounts of alkali in order to obtain a given incremental increase in the serum HCO_3^- level. This phenomenon may also be seen with drug ingestion. In these patients arterial blood gas studies and pH should be obtained frequently. For instance, some patients with severe lactic acidosis may require 600 to 800 mEq of HCO_3^- over 12 to 24 hours in order to maintain plasma HCO_3^- at a level of 10 mEq/L.[20] Since an accurate assessment of the HCO_3^- deficit is difficult to obtain, only one half of the calculated deficit should be replaced initially; then the patient should be reevaluated. Fifty percent of the calculated deficit may be replaced in 3 to 4 hours or sooner if the acidosis is extreme, provided congestive heart failure is absent. In most patients with severe metabolic acidosis, prompt correction of the total alkali deficit is usually not necessary. If the plasma HCO_3^- level is increased to 15 mEq/L, the arterial blood pH will be increased to an acceptably safe level. The treatment of the underlying disorder and renal compensation can restore plasma HCO_3^- concentration and pH to normal levels. A large and rapid increase in HCO_3^- concentration can lead to severe alkalosis, which in turn can be responsible for further acidification of the spinal fluid with alterations of consciousness and even a deterioration of the clinical condition in some patients.[21]

In general, sodium bicarbonate is the drug of choice for metabolic acidosis. Although sodium lactate is an alkalinizing agent, it must first be metabolized to bicarbonate in order to be effective. Also, lactate administration may be ineffective or even harmful in patients with lactic acidosis. Tris(hydroxymethyl)aminomethane (THAM or TRIS) is an organic buffer that has been used in metabolic acidosis. The effect of THAM is due partly to the removal of carbonic acid and partly to bicarbonate generation, as shown below:

$$CO_2 + H_2O \rightleftharpoons H_2CO_3 + THAM \rightleftharpoons H\ THAM + HCO_3^-$$

As a result of the reduction of Pco_2, ventilation can be depressed and hypoxemia can become more severe in patients with chronic obstructive pulmonary disease. Even if the patient is on a ventilator, huge amounts of THAM are necessary to neutralize the CO_2 produced during metabolism. One mmole of THAM buffers only 1 mmole of CO_2 (about 13,000 mmoles of CO_2 are produced in 24 hours). THAM has no advantage over bicarbonate and has several side-effects that can be harmful to the patient. Since a solution of THAM is very alkaline, intravenous use can cause phlebitis. Therefore it must be given slowly into a central vein.[22]

Patients with cardiac or renal failure may develop volume overload or hypernatremia when given sodium bicarbonate. These patients can benefit from peritoneal dialysis or hemodialysis. Since dialysis solutions contain lactate or bicarbonate, these anions are a source of bicarbonate. Also, the contraction of plasma volume produced by dialysis with hypertonic solutions can be very helpful in these patients.

Finally, the correction of metabolic acidosis without correcting the K^+ deficit may lead to fatal hypokalemia. K^+ replacement should not be undertaken until the acidosis has been partially corrected and a falling serum K^+ concentration has been observed.

■ What is metabolic alkalosis?

Metabolic alkalosis is characterized by a primary increase in plasma HCO_3^- concentration. It results from either an abnormal loss of acid or an excessive retention of alkali.

■ How does the body respond to metabolic alkalosis?

The pH is defended by buffers, exchanges of ions between extracellular and intracellular com-

partments, and respiratory compensation. The action of buffers is prompt. In alkalosis H^+ moves from within cells to the extracellular space in exchange for Na^+ and K^+, thus minimizing the severity of the alkalosis.

Respiratory compensation is quick but somewhat incomplete. The Pco_2 does not usually rise above 50 mm Hg even in severe metabolic alkalosis. However, in an occasional patient with severe metabolic alkalosis the Pco_2 may exceed 65 mm Hg. On the average, the Pco_2 rises 0.6 mm Hg for every 1 mEq/L increment in the plasma HCO_3^- concentration. The most extreme increments in Pco_2 are 0.5 to 1 mm Hg for every 1 mEq/L increase in plasma HCO_3^- concentration.

Renal excretion of excess alkali is necessary and is ultimately responsible for the correction of this acid-base disorder. Normally, the kidneys reabsorb approximately 25 mEq of HCO_3^-/L of glomerular filtrate, and when plasma HCO_3^- is increased above normal by HCO_3^- administration, the excess HCO_3^- is rapidly excreted. Therefore even administration of a massive dose of HCO_3^- (or endogenously generated HCO_3^-, for example, by vomiting or gastric suctioning) produces only a temporary metabolic alkalosis. If plasma HCO_3^- is increased from 25 mEq/L to 45 mEq/L by HCO_3^- administration, 20 mEq HCO_3^- will be lost in the urine whenever a liter of glomerular filtrate is formed. At a glomerular filtration rate of 180 L/day, maintenance of plasma HCO_3^- concentration of 45 mEq/L would necessitate the administration of 3600 mEq of HCO_3^-/day (180 × [45 − 25]) or a daily loss of 36 L of gastric juice containing 0.1N HCl. These conditions are rarely observed in clinical practice. However, chronic sustained elevations of plasma HCO_3^- concentrations occur frequently in patients who are neither receiving HCO_3^- nor losing acid gastric juice. This observation indicates that the renal reabsorption of HCO_3^- in these subjects must be very large. The urine of an alkalotic patient characteristically has an acid pH and is free of bicarbonate. It is essential that the cause of metabolic alkalosis be identified so that defects in bicarbonate excretion can be corrected by the proper therapeutic measures. It is known that reabsorption and generation of bicarbonate take place by a process involving sodium-hydrogen exchange in renal tubules. Any stimulus that augments the sodium-hydrogen exchange mechanism will concurrently increase HCO_3^- reabsorption and generation and thus produce metabolic alkalosis.

■ **What are the causes of metabolic alkalosis, and what mechanisms are active?**

The following are causes of metabolic alkalosis:
1. Loss of acid gastric juice (vomiting, gastric suction)
2. Excessive alkali administration
3. Chloride depletion
4. Diuretic therapy
5. Contraction alkalosis (volume depletion)
6. Severe potassium depletion
7. Posthypercapnic alkalosis
8. Mineralocorticoid excess syndromes (administration of mineralocorticoid, ectopic ACTH syndromes, Cushing's syndrome, Bartter's syndrome, licorice ingestion)
9. Chloride-rich diarrhea[23]

In clinical medicine more than one factor is generally responsible for metabolic alkalosis; for instance, a patient with pyloric stenosis with persistent vomiting is not only losing H^+ and Cl^-, but also losing K^+ in addition to being volume depleted.

The mechanisms leading to metabolic alkalosis during vomiting or gastric suction can be explained as follows: As a result of loss of HCl, HCO_3^- is generated and plasma HCO_3^- is increased. Sodium, previously filtered with chloride in the kidney, is now filtered with HCO_3^-. Since HCO_3^- is not as easily reabsorbed as chloride, large amounts of $NaHCO_3$ are delivered to the distal tubules. The distal exchange mechanism cannot reabsorb this large sodium load, and therefore some $NaHCO_3$ is lost in the urine. Because of this increased cation exchange mechanism, some K^+ is also lost in exchange with sodium. As a result of sodium loss and volume depletion, sodium reabsorption is stimulated and sodium-hydrogen exchange is augmented. These events lead to the conservation of sodium and subsequent generation of HCO_3^-, thus maintaining an elevated HCO_3^- concentration in the plasma. Therefore chloride depletion is primarily responsible for a chronic sustained elevation of

plasma HCO_3^- during persistent vomiting or gastric suctioning.

Chloride depletion is the most common cause of metabolic alkalosis.[21-26] Sodium is reabsorbed from the renal tubules either with Cl^- or in exchange for H^+ and K^+. If serum Cl^- is reduced, either Na^+ must be excreted in greater amounts in the urine or the cation exchange mechanism for Na^+ absorption must be augmented. In fact, in Cl^- depletion the amount of Na^+ reabsorbed in the exchange for H^+ and K^+ (cation exchange mechanism) is stimulated. When Na^+ is filtered with a nonpermeant anion and reabsorbed, in order to maintain electrical neutrality additional H^+ and K^+ are secreted into the lumen of the renal tubules. Thus the additional H^+ ion secretion is responsible for more HCO_3^- generation.

It should be remembered that for every mEq of H^+ secreted into the renal tubule lumen, an equivalent quantity of HCO_3^- enters the blood, either by indirect reabsorption of filtered HCO_3^- or by generation of new HCO_3^- in the renal tubular cells. During the increased cation exchange, some K^+ will also be lost. This will result in a hypochloremic, hypokalemic metabolic alkalosis. The same basic mechanism is responsible for diuretic-induced metabolic alkalosis. Diuretics such as furosemide and ethacrynic acid block NaCl absorption in the proximal tubules and are responsible for delivery of greater amounts of Na^+ and Cl^- to sodium-avid exchange sites. As a result of this augmented cation exchange, H^+ is lost in the urine with Cl^- and an equivalent quantity of HCO_3^- is generated. As with alkalosis caused by gastric suction, two conditions are necessary for sustained augmented sodium-hydrogen exchange in distal tubules: continued marked stimulus to Na^+ absorption and persistent Cl^- depletion.

Patients with chronic hypercapnia lose Cl^- in their urine. If Cl^- deficits are not corrected when the arterial Pco_2 becomes normal, there will be a continuous increase in the plasma HCO_3^- concentration associated with the augmented hydrogen-sodium exchange mechanism.[27]

The sudden reduction in arterial Pco_2 in patients with chronic CO_2 retention, as a result of assisted mechanical ventilation, is also a common cause of metabolic alkalosis. Prompt reduction of

Pco_2 should be avoided to prevent marked increases in pH. Arterial Pco_2 and pH should be monitored. Patients should also be given KCl to prevent the development of metabolic alkalosis.

The exact mechanism resulting in a rise in HCO_3^- concentration in Cushing's syndrome and primary aldosteronism remains to be clarified. However, K^+ depletion and increased Na^+ reabsorption associated with augmented cation exchange may be responsible for the metabolic alkalosis.[28]

Sustained metabolic alkalosis can be divided into two major groups: (1) In NaCl-responsive metabolic alkalosis, urinary chloride is usually less than 10 mmoles/L. Vomiting, gastric drainage, diuretic therapy, and rapid correction of chronic hypercapnia are usually responsible for this type of metabolic alkalosis. (2) NaCl-resistant metabolic alkalosis is usually characterized by a urine Cl^- greater than 20 mmoles/L. These cases are usually due to excess mineralocorticoid activity as in hyperaldosteronism, Cushing's syndrome, Bartter's syndrome, and excessive licorice intake.

■ How do we diagnose metabolic alkalosis?

There are no specific signs or symptoms of metabolic alkalosis. Arterial blood gas studies interpreted in the light of clinical information are necessary for definitive diagnosis.

■ What is the therapy for metabolic alkalosis?

The treatment should be directed toward correction of any fluid and electrolyte disturbances, or any abnormality such as pyloric obstruction that may be responsible for the alkalosis. Persistent Cl^- deficiency in the presence of increased Na^+ absorption is basically responsible for the abnormally large HCO_3^- generation and reabsorption from the kidneys. This type of fluid and electrolyte abnormality can be corrected by administration of NaCl and water.[25] KCl is useful in edematous patients with metabolic alkalosis, since Na^+ administration is in general contraindicated.

Metabolic alkalosis associated with mineralocorticoid excess syndromes can be treated by the administration of KCl, or, if possible, the surgical elimination of the hormonal stimulus for enhanced cation exchange. Patients with Bartter's syndrome and hypokalemic metabolic alkalosis are usually resistant to correction with KCl. In these patients spironolactone may be a useful adjunct to therapy. Metabolic alkalosis caused by administration of excessive alkali usually responds to discontinuation of the alkali, provided there is no associated severe depletion of Cl^- and K^+.

In severe metabolic alkalosis mineral acid is the therapy of choice. L-arginine monohydrochloride intravenously, lysine monohydrochloride orally, or ammonium chloride orally or intravenously is effectively used in metabolic alkalosis to provide H^+ and Cl^-. However, the amount of ammonium chloride that can be given is limited because of the possibility of central nervous system toxicity. Not more than 40 mEq of NH_4Cl over a period of 4 hours should be given to an adult. This is especially true in the presence of liver disease. Dilute HCl (0.1N) can also be given intravenously.[29] However, dilute HCl is irritating and must be infused through central venous catheters.

The amount of H^+ required to reduce the plasma HCO_3^- should be calculated on the basis of 50% of body weight. Thus the number of mEq of mineral acid required equals kg body weight $\times$ 0.5 $\times$ desired decrement in HCO_3^- concentration.

Correction of diuretic-induced metabolic alkalosis, which is primarily caused by chloride depletion and volume contraction, merely necessitates administration of Cl^- and volume.

■ What are mixed acid-base disorders, and how may they be recognized?

A mixed acid-base disorder indicates the presence of more than one simple or primary acid-base disorder.

In simple acid-base disorders, HCO_3^- and $Paco_2$ always change in the predictable direction. If they are out of the predicted range for one simple disorder, a mixed disorder is probably present.

In mixed respiratory acidosis and metabolic alkalosis, compensation for either disturbance alone will be inappropriately high. HCO_3^- and $Paco_2$ will be elevated. However, the pH may be high, low, or within normal limits.

In mixed respiratory alkalosis and metabolic

acidosis, compensation for either disturbance alone will be inappropriately augmented. HCO_3^- and $Paco_2$ will be reduced. The pH may be high, low, or within normal limits.

In mixed respiratory and metabolic acidosis, compensation will be impaired. HCO_3^- and $Paco_2$ may be high, low, or within normal limits. However, the pH will be significantly reduced.

In respiratory and metabolic alkalosis compensation will be impaired. HCO_3^- and $Paco_2$ may be high, low, or within normal limits. However, the pH will be inappropriately increased.

In cases of high anion gap metabolic acidosis, superimposed upon metabolic alkalosis, the increase in anion gap is much greater than the reduction in plasma bicarbonate. However, in patients with normal anion gap metabolic acidosis who develop superimposed metabolic alkalosis, acid-base values may be entirely within normal limits. In these cases only clinical information and the evaluation of previous arterial gas studies can give the correct diagnosis.

■ **What are some special facts regarding acid-base disturbances?**

In simple or primary acid-base disturbances, the stimulus for compensation is the change in pH caused by the primary change in Pco_2 or HCO_3^-. Since abnormal pH is the stimulus, normal compensation should not overcorrect or overcompensate and should not even return the pH to control level.

A pH value opposite to that expected for the initial disturbance indicates a mixed acid-base disorder.

If there is a marked disturbance in a primary acid-base disorder, there will be less likelihood of a normal pH. A normal pH, in this instance, strongly suggests the presence of a mixed acid-base disorder.

The lack of any compensatory response to a marked acid-base disturbance strongly suggests a mixed acid-base disorder. However, there are two exceptions: Little, if any, increase in plasma HCO_3^- concentration occurs in acute respiratory acidosis, and only a slight or moderate rise in arterial Pco_2 occurs in acute or chronic metabolic alkalosis.

No definite conclusion can be drawn from serum total CO_2 content alone. At least two unknown factors in the Henderson-Hasselbalch equation should be measured so that the third can be calculated. For instance, in acute respiratory acidosis the total CO_2 content may be entirely normal. For example, a serum total CO_2 content of 24 mEq/L may suggest normal acid-base status. The pH might be found to be 7.2, which is equal to (H^+) = 63 nmoles/L. If one uses a rearranged Henderson's equation,

$$Pco_2 = \frac{H^+ HCO_3^-}{24}$$

In the above example:

$$Pco_2 = \frac{63 \times 24}{24} = 63 \text{ mm Hg}$$

Intelligent interpretation of the acid-base status requires that the following points be checked: (1) clinical assessment of the patient, which should include a history and physical examination, noting previous medication and therapeutic measures such as assisted mechanical ventilation, limited salt intake, and so on; (2) serum electrolytes and other routine laboratory tests such as blood urea nitrogen, serum creatinine, blood sugar, and liver function tests, urinalysis, and so on.

In a patient with metabolic alkalosis (provided no diuretic is being administered), a low urinary Cl^- is virtually diagnostic of metabolic alkalosis following Cl^- depletion.

Serum CO_2 content in mmoles/L is almost identical to serum HCO_3^-.

The anion gap should be calculated, whereas Pco_2 and pH should be measured.

In chronic azotemic renal failure alone, the anion gap seldom exceeds 25 mEq/L. Undetermined anion fractions above 25 mEq/L are usually observed in salicylate, methanol, and ethylene glycol poisoning and lactic or diabetic ketoacidosis.

Serum K^+ levels may be useful in predicting arterial pH. In acidosis there is a tendency for serum K^+ to rise unless there is underlying K^+ depletion, which occurs in diarrhea, renal tubular acidosis, and administration of carbonic anhydrase–inhibiting agents.

Remember, arterial blood gas studies and pH

determinations can be vitally important in the management of patients with a variety of serious medical and surgical problems. These studies should be interpreted in the light of clinical findings and necessary laboratory tests. Therefore a good basic knowledge of the mechanisms of the acid-base disorders is essential for proper management of these disturbances.

REFERENCES

1. Brackett, N. D., Jr., Cohen, J., and Schwartz, W. B.: Carbon dioxide titration curve of normal man, N. Engl. J. Med. **272:**6, 1965.
2. Cohen, J. J., and Schwartz, W. B.: Editorial: evaluation of acid-base equilibrium in pulmonary insufficiency, Am. J. Med. **41:**163, 1966.
3. Dulfano, M. J., and Ishikawa, S.: Hypercapnia: mental changes and extrapulmonary complications, Am. Intern. Med. **63:**829, 1965.
4. Eichenholz, A. A., Blumenthal, S., and Walker, F. E.: The pattern of compensatory response to chronic obstructive pulmonary disease J. Lab. Clin. Med. **68:**265, 1966.
5. Polak, A., Haynie, G. D., Hays, R. M., and Schwartz, W. B.: Effects of chronic hypercapnia on electrolyte and acid-base equilibrium. I. Adaptation, J. Clin. Invest. **40:**1223, 1961.
6. Refsum, H. E.: Acid-base status in patients with chronic hypercapnia and hypoxemia, Clin. Sci. **27:**407, 1964.
7. Sapir, D. G., Levine, D. Z., and Schwartz, W. B.: The effects of chronic hypoxemia on electrolyte and acid-base equilibrium, J. Clin. Invest. **46:**369, 1967.
8. Brackett, M. D., Jr., Wingo, C. F., Muren, O., and Solano, J. T.: Acid-base response to chronic hypercapnia in man, N. Engl. J. Med. **280:**124, 1969.
9. Schwartz, W. B., Brackett, N. C., Jr., and Cohn, J. J.: The response of extracellular hydrogen ion concentration to graded degrees of chronic hypercapnia, J. Clin. Invest. **44:**291, 1965.
10. Van Ypersele deStrihou, C., Brasseur, L., and deConick, J.: The 'carbon dioxide response curve' for chronic hypercapnia in man, N. Engl. J. Med. **275:**117, 1966.
11. Arbur, G. S., Herbert, L. A., Levesque, P. R., Etsten, B. E., and Schwartz, W. B.: Characterization and clinical application of the "significance band" for acute respiratory alkalosis, N. Engl. J. Med. **280:**117, 1969.
12. Sykes, M. K., and Cooke, P.: Effect of hyperventilation on "excess lactate" production during anesthesia, Br. J. Anaesth. **37:**372, 1965.
13. Prys-Roberts, C., Kelman, G., and Nunn, J. F.: Determination of in vivo carbon dioxide titration curve of anaesthetized man, Br. J. Anaesth. **38:**500, 1966.
14. Eldridge, F., and Salzer, : Effect of respiratory alkalosis on blood lactate and pyruvate in humans, J. Appl. Physiol. **22:**461, 1967.
15. Gennari, F. J., Goldstein, M. B., and Schwartz, W. B.: The nature of the renal adaptation to chronic hypocapnia, J. Clin. Invest. **51:**1722, 1972.
16. Saltzman, H., Hezman, A., and Sieker, H.: Correlations of clinical and physiological manifestations of sustained hyperventilation, N. Engl. J. Med. **268:**1431, 1963.
17. Okel, B., and Hurst, J.: Prolonged hyperventilation in man: associated electrolyte changes in subjective symptoms, Arch. Intern. Med. **108:**747, 1961.
18. Lennon, E. J., and Lemann, J., Jr.: Defense of hydrogen ion concentration in chronic metabolic acidosis: a new evaluation of an old approach, Ann. Intern. Med. **65:**265, 1966.
19. Albert, M. S., Dell, R. B., and Winters, R. W.: Quantitative displacement of acid-base equilibrium in metabolic acidosis, Ann. Intern. Med. **66:**312, 1967.
20. Oliva, P. B.: Lactic acidosis, Am. J. Med. **48:**209, 1970.
21. Posner, J. B., Swanson, A. G., and Blum, F.: Acid-base balance in cerebrospinal fluid, Arch. Neurol. **12:**479, 1965.
22. Bleich, H. L., and Schwartz, W. B.: Tris buffer (THAM): an appraisal of its physiologic effects and clinical usefulness, N. Engl. J. Med. **272:**782, 1966.
23. Evanson, J. M., and Stanbury, S. W.: Congenital chloridorrhaea or so-called congenital alkalosis with diarrhea, Gut **6:**29, 1965.
24. Kassirer, J., Berkman, P., Lawrencz, D., and Schwartz, W.: Critical role of chloride in correction of hypokalemic alkalosis in man, Am. J. Med. **38:**172, 1965.
25. Kassirer, J., and Schwartz, W.: Correction of metabolic alkalosis in man without repair of potassium deficiency: re-evaluation of role of potassium, Am. J. Med. **40:**19, 1966.
26. Schwartz, W., Van Ypersele deStrifou, C., and Kassirer, J.: Role of anions in metabolic alkalosis and potassium deficiency, N. Engl. J. Med. **379:**630, 1968.
27. Schwartz, W. B., Hays, R., Polak, A., and Haynie, G.: Effects of chronic hypercapnia on electrolyte and acid-base equilibrium. II. Recovery, with special reference to the influence of chloride intake, J. Clin. Invest. **40:**1238, 1961.
28. Kassirer, J. O., et al.: Aldosterone in metabolic alkalosis, J. Clin. Invest. **46:**1558, 1967.
29. Frick, P. G., and Senning, A.: The treatment of severe metabolic alkalosis with intravenous N/10 or N/5 hydrochloric acid, Ger. Med. **9:**242, 1964.

CHAPTER 15

Respiratory management

Bernhard A. Votteri and Jacqueline F. Wade

The recognition and treatment of respiratory dysfunction in critically ill patients makes up a major part of the work load of intensive care units. Advances in resuscitative methods and the treatment of acute renal failure have resulted in the survival of many patients through the early stages of acute disorders such as shock. In the later phases of resuscitation, respiratory failure has emerged as a leading cause of morbidity and mortality. Respiratory failure in such patients is usually a result of an acute derangement of ventilatory function and is thus distinguished from the general deterioration of pulmonary function seen in patients with chronic respiratory disease. The critically ill patient is often noted to have progressive failure of pulmonary gas exchange, which can be defined as failure to add oxygen to or remove carbon dioxide from venous blood. In such patients respiratory failure develops over a time frame of approximately moments to 24 or 48 hours. The goal of this chapter is to provide an introduction to the appropriate ventilatory management of such patients.

Multiple reports now attest to the efficacy of mechanical ventilatory support in acute respiratory failure. Mortality among patients treated for acute respiratory failure in critical care units has declined from 70% to as low as 20%.[1-4] Such increases in survival have been attributed to the development of well-equipped, well-staffed intensive care units where the systematic evaluation of patients for the detection of respiratory failure and the monitoring of cardiorespiratory function has permitted early comprehensive treatment of the critically ill patient.[1-10]

■ **What are the most common causes of acute respiratory insufficiency in intensive care units?**

Acute respiratory failure is usually caused by one of the following disorders: adult respiratory distress syndrome, drug-induced ventilatory depression, impaired chest wall function caused by chest wall trauma or neuromuscular disorders, exacerbations of chronic obstructive pulmonary disease, and status asthmaticus.[2,7,11]

Respiratory distress syndrome is the most common disorder requiring intensive pulmonary care. It has been conservatively estimated that 150,000 patients each year demonstrate this syndrome in the United States.[4] Although there is considerable discussion over the precise name for this pulmonary disorder, it is generally agreed that the syndrome may follow surgical or accidental insults and is commonly associated with shock, cardiopulmonary bypass, fat embolism, viral and aspiration pneumonia, septicemia, inhaled or ingested toxins, oxygen toxicity, and CNS injury.[12-18] Ashbaugh and associates[14] stated that patients with respiratory distress syndrome usually had severe dyspnea, tachypnea, and grunting respirations. Intercostal and suprasternal retractions were usually present, and cyanosis and hypoxemia responded poorly to oxygen administration. Progressive differences between alveolar and arterial oxygen tension (A-a ΔPo_2) could be demonstrated and were attributed to air space closure in areas where blood flow continued. This space closure resulted from alveolar epithelial injury, reduced surfactant, altered surface tension, pulmonary capillary injury, and interstitial edema

272

formation. Such closed air spaces could not be reopened and ventilated without generating high transpulmonary pressures and increasing inspiratory force.[19] The resultant increase in the work of breathing required to maintain lung inflation ultimately leads to patient exhaustion; this was followed by generalized air space closure and increased shunting of blood that was reflected by progressive hypoxemia.

Most cases of the adult respiratory distress syndrome present the clinical picture of pulmonary edema, and increased lung water has been recognized in patients with this disorder. Indeed, the clinical separation of acute respiratory distress syndrome from left ventricular failure may be most difficult.[20] Pulmonary edema formation in adult respiratory distress syndrome usually develops in the presence of normal capillary wedge pressure and is not a result of cardiac dysfunction.[21] The pulmonary edema appears to result from a diffuse alteration of the pulmonary vasculature with a resultant increase in pulmonary capillary permeability and loss of plasma and fluid into the interstitial space.[22,23] Recent reviews of the mechanisms of pulmonary edema point out that rapid protein losses into the interstitial space may follow pulmonary capillary and alveolar insults.[24,25] Such alteration could readily explain the fulminant pulmonary edema often seen in adult respiratory distress syndrome.

■ What are the clinical signs of respiratory failure?

Although the signs of respiratory failure are frequently nonspecific and may simply involve restlessness and disorientation, other signs are frequently present, such as changes in the rate or pattern of breathing. Breathing may be rapid, shallow, labored, or associated with cough. The skin may be moist and appear cyanotic. Hypertension and tachypnea are often noted. Irritability, restlessness, sleeplessness, and/or coma may be present. It is now recognized that hypoxemia and acidemia are the major determinants of such symptoms and signs. The finding of any of the clinical signs just discussed is an urgent indicator for a more definitive diagnosis that can be achieved only by blood gas analysis. Without such studies, unrecognized hypoxic restlessness

may lead to the administration of a sedative that may hasten progressive respiratory failure.

■ What is the definition of respiratory failure?

It is difficult to set forth a single definition of respiratory failure that is acceptable to all clinicians and physiologists. However, the following findings are most frequently accepted as evidence of respiratory failure: an inability to oxygenate arterial blood as shown by arterial oxygen tension (Pao_2) of less than 50 torr while breathing room air with or without an impaired elimination of carbon dioxide as demonstrated by an elevation of arterial carbon dioxide tension ($Paco_2$).[2,26,27]

■ Do all patients having respiratory dysfunction require mechanical ventilation for the control of respiratory failure?

Identifying respiratory failure does not invariably indicate a need for mechanical ventilatory assistance. Many patients who are in respiratory failure can be adequately supported by applying the full spectrum of respiratory care, consisting of the administration of controlled oxygen and humidified gases, intermittent positive pressure breathing (IPPB) treatments accompanied by chest physiotherapy and postural drainage, the use of bronchodilators, nasotracheal suctioning, bronchoscopy, and careful administration of IV fluids and diuretics.[6,26] Despite such complete supportive care, as many as 50% of severely ill patients will nonetheless require prolonged artificial ventilation.[28,29]

■ What are the criteria used in deciding to provide mechanical respiratory assistance?

Although attempts have been made to establish criteria for the use of continuous mechanical ventilation, these criteria are often modified to describe a specific pulmonary disorder in an individual patient.[2,30] The need for mechanical ventilation is, however, obvious when sudden hypoventilation or prolonged apnea is demonstrated. More often the development of acute respiratory failure is not heralded by apnea. Instead, acute respiratory failure will usually be associated with progressive respiratory dysfunction, and arbitrary values must be established at which juncture intervention with airway control and mechanical ventilation will be undertaken. Such intervention is determined by reviewing serial objective measurements, including respiratory rate, tidal volume, vital capacity, maximum inspiratory force, A-a ΔPo_2, and $Paco_2$.[2,3,6] The A-a ΔPo_2 has been particularly useful in assessing the severity of deranged gas exchange.[15] Serial assessment of the chest x-ray film and intermittent measurement of tidal volume and airway pressure relationships during IPPB, or so-called effective compliance (V_T/P), is also useful.[3,6] Progressive worsening of all of these values despite full supportive respiratory care measures usually indicates the need for mechanical ventilatory support. Other measures that provide additional information about the adequacy of spontaneous ventilation and oxygenation include the measurement of the dead space:tidal volume ratio, lung compliance, and work of breathing.[3,6] Automated pulmonary measurement systems have recently been developed that permit rapid serial measurement of these variables. The use of such devices has made possible the early identification of the patient who will ultimately progress to overt respiratory failure.[30-33] Mechanical ventilation with control of the airway by endotracheal intubation will usually be required in the following situations: (1) acute respiratory failure associated with coma or progressive obtundation, (2) inability to raise Pao_2 above 40 torr in a cooperative patient who is breathing 100% oxygen, (3) drop in vital capacity to 15 cc or less/kg and maximum inspiratory force to less than 25 cm H_2O, and (4) progressive rise in $Paco_2$.[2,9]

Although the prophylactic use of mechanical ventilation has been promoted, its advantage over the initiation of mechanical ventilation after the monitoring of deteriorating pulmonary status has not been clearly established.[34,35] Some experimental models of pulmonary aspiration and other forms of shock lung in animals suggest that morbidity and mortality may be reduced when mechanical ventilation is used prior to or during the induction of lung injury.[36,38] Many respiratory care units have applied prophylactic mechanical ventilation in situations where a high incidence of alveolar collapse, pulmonary shunting, reduced cough, and impaired secretion removal is expected.[16,35,39] Thus prophylactic mechanical ventilation has been recommended in the postop-

erative care of patients with cardiovascular or neuromuscular disorders.[40-42] It has also been used in the care of the severely traumatized patient, especially when flail chest or pulmonary contusion is demonstrated.[15,43] Mechanical ventilation in the postoperative care of chronic obstructive pulmonary disease patients has also been effective in avoiding the development of acute respiratory failure.[3,6,39]

■ **What are the initial measures to be employed when sudden hypoventilation or prolonged apnea develop?**

Immediate steps must be taken to improve alveolar ventilation and oxygenation. The mouth is cleared of secretions and foreign bodies, then mouth-to-mouth, mouth-to-airway, or bag mask resuscitation is immediately started, employing supplemental oxygen if available. Immediate attention is given to the observation of the chest for symmetric movement with each bag mask inflation. It is unwise for the inexperienced worker to spend much time trying to insert an endotracheal tube, since most patients are well ventilated with a bag mask device. When the patient's ventilation has been stabilized, a definitive airway is established, and use of a ventilator is then started.[44]

■ **Is endotracheal intubation required to ventilate patients mechanically?**

Endotracheal intubation is required whenever compromise of airway patency is recognized and in particular whenever the normal protective cough is diminished or inadequate tidal volume and vital capacity are demonstrated. When continuous mechanical ventilation is necessary, endotracheal intubation is employed to secure a protected airway.

■ **Can intubation and mechanical ventilation be avoided by the use of narcotic antagonists and respiratory stimulants?**

The action of narcotic antagonists such as naloxone is clearly defined.[45-49] When given in single, repeated doses or as continuous IV infusions, such antagonists reverse the effects of opiates such as morphine and reduce the level of respiratory depression. However, such drugs have transient action, and the effects of morphine frequently reappear. As a result, careful monitoring of the patient and judicious readministration of the drug antagonists are required. Nonetheless, such antagonists offer great value in drug-induced respiratory depression when the depressing agent is known. Unfortunately many episodes of ventilatory depression are a result of the abuse of multiple agents, and in such instances the depression is often ineffectively antagonized by naloxone. The use of respiratory stimulants has received renewed interest in the management of such drug-induced respiratory depression. It has been suggested that agents such as doxapram may reduce the duration and depth of such depressions; however, the need for definitive control of the airway is frequent nonetheless. Intensive nursing treatment and supportive care remain the treatment of choice in the management of multiple drug–induced ventilatory depression. Adequate provision for a definitive airway and a method to provide mechanical ventilation remain essential in treating such patients. The judicious use of specific antagonists offers an important adjunctive role. Respiratory stimulants such as doxapram may even be of value in reducing the duration of mechanical ventilation. However, further assessment of this drug is necessary before its proper role in the management of such patients is established.[50]

■ Which is the initial airway of choice?

A cuffed endotracheal tube is preferred over tracheostomy as the initial airway in almost all patients requiring respiratory support. In most patients tracheostomy will be performed over a previously placed endotracheal tube if the period requiring mechanical ventilation is expected to be greater than 2 to 5 days. With meticulous care endotracheal tubes may be left in place for a much longer period without serious sequelae.[51] Tracheostomy may be employed as an initial airway when facial burns or trauma makes an oral airway undesirable or impossible to pass.[52]

Nasotracheal intubation is frequently preferred by the patient and is better tolerated when it is anticipated that tracheal airway control will be required for greater than 12 to 24 hours, particularly in the patient who is alert. A properly placed nasotracheal tube can be more readily stabilized with less danger of accidental extubation and still permits appropriate mouth care. Nasotracheal intubation is technically slightly more difficult, and the additional length of the tube may lead to kinking as well as greater difficulty in tracheal and bronchial suction.[53,54] Orotracheal intubation is usually employed in comatose patients, in short-term postoperative ventilatory management, and in cardiopulmonary emergencies, where it provides a quick and definitive airway.

■ What precautions should be observed during endotracheal tube placement?

Intubation is a period of great stress. It is usually accompanied by hypoxemia and increased catecholamine release. These factors lead to a high incidence of cardiac irregularities. Preparation of the patient with appropriate description of the method, local anesthetic, and application of the tube by experienced personnel with avoidance of laryngeal stimulation are essential to avoid complications. Prior to and during intubation, ventilation with high concentrations of oxygen is essential. The period of intubation itself should require less than 45 to 60 seconds. The tip of the endotracheal tube should be located 2 cm proximal to the carina in order that intubation of the right mainstem bronchus is avoided. If placement of the endotracheal tube tip is at or just below the carina, suctioning of the left mainstem bronchus is precluded, regional ventilation to the left lung is reduced, and accumulation of secretions and subsequent atelectasis soon follow.[8,55]

■ How can endotracheal tube placement be assessed?

Both lung fields should be regularly auscultated to detect inadvertent endobronchial intubation. Auscultation should be repeated following movement of the patient, particularly flexion of the neck, which may advance the end of the tube beyond the carina. Unfortunately normal breath sounds and normal chest movement may be demonstrated despite right mainstem intubation with incomplete occlusion of the left bronchus. For this reason a postintubation chest x-ray film to determine tube position is mandatory. Regular evaluation of the tube should be undertaken to detect tube displacement and to identify obstruction against the tracheal wall. Patency of the tube can usually be assured by passing a large-bore catheter through the endotracheal tube. Definitive confirmation of satisfactory placement can, however, be achieved only by portable chest x-ray film or bronchoscopic evaluation.[56]

■ **How can patency of the airway be maintained?**

Following placement of an endotracheal tube, aseptic endotracheal suctioning is necessary to remove secretions in order that inspissated secretions do not coat and block the endotracheal tube and airway. The inspired gas is heated and humidified and the airway temperature is monitored in order to provide water content equivalent to 100% relative humidity at body temperature. The patient is turned regularly and chest percussion, vibration, and postural drainage are used to prevent the accumulation of secretions in dependent airways.[57-59] The volume and viscosity of sputum are assessed at the bedside. Tenacious secretions in the airway are a clue to infection or inadequate airway moisture. Although tracheal lavage with 2 to 4 ml washings of normal saline solution may be used to liquify secretions, this is rarely necessary if a heated humidifier is continuously used. The use of curved-tip catheters with fluoroscopic visualization permits the evacuation of persistent secretions. If patency of the airway cannot be maintained as evidenced by loss of breath sounds and radiographic demonstrations of atelectasis or volume loss of the lung despite the use of frequent turning, chest percussion, and sighing, it may be necessary to perform fiberoptic bronchoscopy during continuous ventilation and thereby remove such secretions under direct visualization.[60,61] These maneuvers are often accompanied by regional disturbances of ventilation that may increase the alveolar-arterial oxygen difference. Thus most workers will provide supplemental oxygen during the procedure and some will monitor oxygenation.[62,63]

■ **What are the hazards of endotracheal suctioning?**

Hypoxemia produced by suctioning may be followed by cardiac irregularities and cardiac arrest. Oxygen supplementation and hyperin-flation of the patient before and after suctioning is now practiced in many units and has markedly reduced the incidence of tachycardias.[64,65] Lung collapse, alveolar hypoventilation, and hypoxemia can be avoided if the vacuum does not exceed 100 torr and application is limited to 15 seconds each time. In addition, the catheter diameter must not exceed half of the diameter of the endotracheal lumen; otherwise the vacuum would be applied directly to the peripheral airway.

■ **How frequently should endotracheal suctioning be performed?**

Suctioning should be performed only when necessary. Clinical assessment such as evaluation for the presence of breath sounds and/or the presence of coarse rales or rhonchi will frequently give a clue to the presence and location of airway secretions. Routine and frequent suctioning without indication is not recommended because of the risk of producing traumatic tracheal lesions as well as the need for the interruption of ventilation and the reduction in mean airway pressure with possible production of atelectasis. In addition, suctioning frequently intensifies the patient's apprehension and feeling of helplessness.

■ **What are the major hazards in the use of endotracheal tubes?**

The hazards of tube displacement and bronchial intubation have already been mentioned. In addition, laryngeal and/or pharyngeal injury at the time of insertion should be considered.[66,67] Late developments include granuloma formation at the cords and tracheal cuff site. The pathogenesis of this injury has been attributed to endotracheal cuff–induced pressure necrosis of the mucosa, submucosa, and tracheal cartilage.[68-75]

■ **Can complications from prolonged tracheal intubation be prevented?**

Although recent workers have demonstrated the predictable appearance of mucosal and ciliary alteration following careful intubation and meticulous cuff management, others have found that clinically significant cuff injury is rare when properly inflated high-compliance endotracheal tube cuffs are used in intubated patients.[69,70] The cuff should be inflated only to the volume that provides a minimum leak at the required peak airway pressure. The use of the minimum occlusive volume (MOV) techniques and the monitoring of cuff volume inflation with maintenance of intracuff pressures of less than 30 cm H_2O have proved to be important in reducing injury to the trachea.[69,71,75,76] It should be recognized that intracuff pressures are transmitted directly to the tracheal wall by the compliant cuff. Thus monitoring of cuff pressure is clearly essential.[69] When cuff pressure monitoring with a manometer and MOV is employed, continuous cuff inflation may be maintained without tracheal injury.[77,78] Careful fixation of the endotracheal tube and avoidance of traction remain essential in avoiding traumatic tracheal injury. The use of flexible tubings and rotating joints as well as support of the inspiratory ventilator tube is necessary to achieve such protection.[3,5]

■ Is periodic cuff deflation necessary?

If proper cuff inflation technique is practiced, periodic cuff deflation is avoided and in fact condemned by some workers because deflation introduces the risk of tracheal-bronchial secretion aspiration, movement of tube, and reduced ventilation.[74] Cuff deflation would not appear to be necessary when high-compliance cuffs are employed or MOV inflation techniques are used.[78] If intermittent deflation is practiced, laryngeal secretions must be aspirated before deflation and tracheal-bronchial secretions immediately after deflation.[74] Cuff deflation during the positive pressure phase of inspiration may be of value in that the forcefully escaping gas expels oropharyngeal secretions that have collected above the cuff. Intermittent cuff reinflation also provides an opportunity to reevaluate intracuff volume, pressure, and MOV.

■ What are the acceptable levels of Pa_{O_2}?

Although Pa_{O_2} is an important factor, it must be emphasized that the major factor in maintaining the integrity of cellular metabolism is adequate oxygen transport. Therefore the Pa_{O_2} must be considered in conjunction with cardiac output and ultimately tissue perfusion. When cardiac output and tissue perfusion are normal, it can be demonstrated that a Pa_{O_2} below 40 torr leads to marked changes in cerebral metabolism.[79] In critically ill patients with reduced cardiac output and compromised ability to increase cerebral blood flow caused by arteriosclerosis or heart disease, cerebral injury might be expected despite a Pa_{O_2} of 40 torr. Therefore a Pa_{O_2} less than 50 torr should be considered undesirable. In general a Pa_{O_2} of 60 to 80 torr is sought, since such a Pa_{O_2} provides adequate saturation of normal hemoglobin. In addition, if sudden major changes in ventilation-perfusion relationships created by suctioning or turning are expected, a Pa_{O_2} of 80 to 100 torr is desirable to provide some margin of safety.

Whereas the Pa_{O_2} defines the adequacy of arterial oxygenation, oxygen delivery to the tissues is assessed by measuring the saturation of mixed venous blood ($S\bar{v}_{O_2}$), the arteriovenous oxygen difference, and blood lactate levels.[80,81] A Sv_{O_2} of 60% or a $P\bar{v}_{O_2}$ of 35 torr or higher is desirable. The blood lactate level should be maintained below 2 mmoles/L.

■ What fraction of inspired oxygen (FI_{O_2}) will provide a Pa_{O_2} between 80 and 100 torr in a critically ill patient?

Recently multiple physiologic parameters that determine Pa_{O_2} have been reviewed.[82-86] It was shown in critically ill patients that if hypoventilation, severe anemia, and reduced cardiac output were excluded as factors, the addition of unoxygenated venous blood, or so-called shunted blood, to the circulation was the most frequent and severe cause of hypoxemia.[2] In acute respiratory failure this shunting of blood was usually caused by venous blood passing through the capillaries of nonventilated or severely underventilated alveoli.[87] Such shunting can be estimated by Pa_{O_2} determinations in the patient who is breathing a known concentration of oxygen. Often the magnitude of the shunt is assessed by determining the A-a ΔP_{O_2} while the patient is breathing 100% oxygen.[2,15] Several investigators have recently reviewed the relationship between FI_{O_2} and Pa_{O_2} in acute respiratory failure and have offered graphic simplification that aids in the selection of appropriate FI_{O_2} values after a shunt determination has been made. Such diagrams offer a practical approach to oxygen therapy and are regularly used in our unit.[88,89]

To use such nomograms, an initial FIO_2 is arbitrarily chosen if previous blood gas determinations are not available. About 15 to 20 minutes later an arterial blood gas analysis is performed. The shunt diagram is then rechecked to rapidly select the next FIO_2 that will provide a Pao_2 of 70 to 90 torr. Thereafter regular arterial blood gas determinations are done to confirm the maintenance of an adequate Pao_2 during continuous mechanical ventilation. Meanwhile every effort is made to provide the optimum patterns of ventilation that will permit decreases in the FIO_2. The goal of therapy is to inflate collapsed air spaces and increase lung volume in order that the oxygenation of the blood can be achieved at a low inspired concentration of oxygen. It has been suggested that the use of high tidal volumes provides the optimum pattern of ventilation. Tidal volumes of 12 to 15 ml/kg delivered at a frequency of 10 to 14 respirations/min are usually recommended.[2,90] In patients with disorders such as pulmonary edema and adult respiratory distress syndrome, peak airway pressures of greater than 40 cm H_2O would often be required to achieve such high tidal volume. Webb and Tierney[91] have cautioned against the use of high inspiratory pressure, since such ventilatory patterns have produced pulmonary edema and increased hypoxemia in animal studies. They have recommended that low frequency ventilation at peak inspiratory pressures of less than 30 cm H_2O be employed when possible. The avoidance of high airway pressures is especially indicated when low end-expiratory lung volumes are expected. If hypoxemia progresses with such a ventilatory pattern and compliance decreases, they have favored the early use of positive end-expiratory pressure (PEEP) instead of progressive increases in tidal volume, airway pressure, and FIO_2.

That increases in lung volume and oxygenation can be achieved by the use of PEEP is now widely recognized.[14,15,17] It can be anticipated that the use of PEEP ventilation, or so-called continuous positive pressure ventilation (CPPV), will be widely applied to stabilize air spaces and thereby reduce the frequency with which high concentrations of inspired oxygen will be required in critically ill patients.

■ Can oxygen saturation or tension be monitored by noninvasive devices?

The ear oximeter is a noninvasive device that assesses oxygen saturation by transillumination of the ear. The device is well tolerated by patients and is easily operated by nurses or pulmonary therapists. Several investigators have demonstrated the value and accuracy of the Hewlett-Packard 47201 Ear Oximeter in monitoring oxygen saturation.[92,93] We have confirmed these findings in our intensive care unit where monitoring of oxygen saturation by ear oximetry is regularly performed on patients who require mechanical ventilation. The major advantage of the device is that immediate feedback of information is available to the critical care team members, which permits them to make appropriate adjustments in inspired oxygen. Ear oximetry has the additional advantage of requiring no blood drawing, and it provides a continuous display of the dynamic changes in oxygenation. The use of the following physician's orders at Sequoia Hospital has led to the delivery of predictable oxygen saturation and reduced the need for frequent arterial blood gas sampling in monitoring of oxygen tension or saturation:

1. Adjust FIO_2 to provide Sao_2 by ear oximeter of 91% to 95% saturation.
2. Repeat arterial blood gas when Sao_2 is stable or in 30 minutes.

Such adjustments of FIO_2 are made by the nurse or pulmonary therapist and the adequacy of the Sao_2 is checked by drawing an arterial blood gas sample when the desired ear oximetry value is reached. The wider clinical application of the ear oximeter is probably limited at the present time by the high purchase price.

Another noninvasive approach to monitoring oxygenation has been provided by the transcutaneous oxygen monitor. This device has been extensively tested and used with great success in infants for assessment of arterial oxygen tension.[94,95] There has been limited experience with the use of the device in monitoring critically ill adults.[96] The major disadvantage of the transcutaneous monitor is the need for careful assembly of the sensor to ensure accurate results. In addition, a variable equilibration period is required before reliable values are displayed. Other problems include the need for a separate sensor for each patient application, the requirement of a skin adhesive to seal the sensor, the risk of thermal skin injury, and the high cost of the device.

If the technical features can be improved and more extensive clinical experience with the equipment is gained in the care of the critically ill patient, wider application of these devices in noninvasive monitoring of oxygen tension may be anticipated.

■ Does oxygen administration produce pulmonary injury?

High concentrations of oxygen are commonly used for extended periods of time in the care of critically ill patients with respiratory failure. In the past 10 years much attention has been directed to the finding that high partial pressures of inspired oxygen have a deleterious effect on the lung. Best known is the development of interstitial and alveolar edema during the breathing of pure oxygen. Weibel[97] has suggested that such lung abnormalities are a result of damage to alveolar epithelial and capillary endothelial cells, which are the cells that are directly exposed to the oxygen-rich atmosphere. When animals breathed pure oxygen for 48 hours, pronounced damage of the endothelial cells with marked thinning was evident. Such endothelial and alveolar alterations could permit an increased leakage of plasma protein and water into the interstitial and alveolar areas.[98-100]

The precise action of oxygen toxicity on lung function in the critically ill patient has been difficult to define, since shock and nonpulmonary trauma produce pulmonary lesions anatomically similar to the lesions of oxygen toxicity. Nonetheless, studies in man have revealed that significant lung dysfunction occurs in critically ill patients who are ventilated with 100% oxygen for long durations.[101] Barber and co-workers[102] showed increased shuntlike effect, greater wasted ventilation, and heavier lungs in 100% oxygen–ventilated patients when compared to patients ventilated with air. Dysfunction became more evident with increasing exposure and was particularly marked for 40 hours of 100% oxygen breathing. Hyde and Rawson[103] described the development of patchy pulmonary infiltrates and progressive hypoxemia in patients who were ventilated with 83% to 91% oxygen. A reduction of

inspired oxygen concentrations to less than 50% led to improvement as seen by chest x-ray films, pulmonary compliance and oxygenation. Although such lung dysfunction was in part attributed to the ventilators that delivered the oxygen, recent laboratory studies in animals reveal that fatal pulmonary edema would develop in animals exposed to 100% oxygen irrespective of whether the animal was breathing spontaneously or was being mechanically ventilated.[104] Many other aspects of lung function and structure appear to be harmed by oxygen administration. Lung units that are distal to areas of airway closure become air free or atelectatic within 15 minutes of beginning 100% oxygen breathing.[105] Huber and co-workers[106] have shown that bacterial inactivation by alveolar macrophages is inhibited by the administration of pure oxygen for 48 hours. In addition, surfactant formation and mucus transport systems may be impaired by oxygen administration.[107,108]

These problems created by exposure to oxygen dictate that patients should not be given unnecessarily high oxygen concentrations. However, fear of oxygen toxicity should not prevent the use of sufficiently elevated inspired oxygen concentration to provide adequate oxygenation. Withholding oxygen when the patient is severely hypoxemic for fear of oxygen damage may lead to the fatal complications of hypoxemia long before oxygen toxicity could become a real danger. The short-term administration of 50% to 75% oxygen to patients with cardiovascular failure has not been associated with major adverse effects on lung function.[109] Oxygen concentrations should be titrated to provide a Pao_2 of 70 to 100 torr at the lowest FIO_2.[110] If long-term oxygen administration proves to be necessary at an FIO_2 of greater than 0.5 to 0.6, attention must be directed to improved patterns of ventilation and/or the use of PEEP.

■ What minute ventilation is required to provide adequate ventilation?

The minute ventilation required to maintain a given $Paco_2$ depends on the carbon dioxide production and the efficiency of ventilation.[6] Acute hypercapnia indicates that ventilation is not keeping pace with the metabolic production of carbon dioxide. When this happens, rapidly profound respiratory acidemia may occur. This situation requires therapeutic intervention to improve alveolar ventilation. In the critically ill patient increased carbon dioxide production and inefficient ventilation may demand twice the minute ventilation predicted for a normal man.[111,112] In the critically ill patient an initial tidal volume (V_T) of 12 to 15 ml/kg of body weight delivered at a frequency (f) of 10 to 14 respirations/min has been recommended.[16,113] Large tidal volumes are chosen to improve the distribution of ventilation and reopen collapsed air spaces as well as increase alveolar ventilation. Such high minute ventilation may, however, lead to severe respiratory alkalosis unless alveolar ventilation is promptly controlled by appropriate adjustments of mechanical dead space, tidal volume, and breathing frequency.[114,115] Proper adjustment of dead space to provide the desired alveolar ventilation and $Paco_2$ can be established by the use of the Suwa nomogram.[90,116] Some workers prefer to add 6-inch lengths of inspiratory tubing at 15-minute intervals and recheck end-tidal carbon dioxide or $Paco_2$. Within 15 to 20 minutes of such adjustments a repeat arterial blood gas analysis should be obtained.

Selecky and associates[117] have also developed a ventilation nomogram that accurately predicts the change in $Paco_2$ induced by alterations in minute ventilation. This nomogram has been used for over 2 years in our unit and has permitted smooth control of the $Paco_2$ in a wide range of respiratory disorders. An alternate method of controlling $Paco_2$ is to blend 1% to 3% carbon dioxide into the inspiratory line of the mechanical ventilator while monitoring expired Pco_2 or $Paco_2$.[118,119]

The rapidly progressive acidosis of acute respiratory failure must be distinguished from the slow elevation of $Paco_2$ compensated by renal generation of bicarbonate in patients with chronic obstructive lung disease states. Such hypercapnia may be regarded as a physiologically adaptive response to severe airway obstruction.[120] The treatment of patients with such compensated states of hypercapnia is largely centered on the use of controlled oxygen therapy. Artificial ventilation is usually delayed as long as possible while supportive measures are used. Only when progressive hypercapnia cannot be controlled by other measures is continuous ventilatory therapy applied.[121] In this instance hypercapnia should be reduced slowly, preferably at less than 10 torr/hr. Arterial pH should be monitored in order that alkalemia produced by the sudden removal of carbon dioxide can be prevented.[122] In order that acid-base derangements are rapidly identified, blood gas determinations should be performed within 30 minutes of initiating mechanical ventilation and within minutes of major alterations of ventilatory settings. Whenever the patient's condition deteriorates as evidenced by changes in heart rate, respiratory frequency, alterations in effective compliance, and so on, repeat blood gas determinations are also appropriate.[114] In the patient who is stable using mechanical ventilation, blood gas determinations may be reduced to every 12 hours. At a minimum, daily reassessments of blood gas levels should be performed for patients on continuous mechanical ventilation. The boxed material on p. 281 lists some of the orders required for initiating mechanical ventilation at Sequoia District Hospital. The guidelines prescribed by the primary physician are carried out by the critical care team, which consists of registered nurses experienced in respiratory care, respiratory therapists, laboratory technicians, and physical therapists. The team effort is coordinated by the head nurse and medical director who work closely with the primary physician.[123]

Monitoring of the alveolar ventilation has largely depended on serial arterial blood gas sampling; however, accurate control may eventually be achieved by continuous monitoring of intra-arterial Pco_2. Safe, stable, intra-arterial Pco_2 electrodes and pH and Po_2 sensors have not been available. When sensors are developed, they could readily be coupled with an electronically equipped ventilator such as the Servo-Ventilator 900 to provide smooth control of $Paco_2$.

■ What are the complications of arterial puncture for obtaining blood gas samples?

The most common complications of arterial puncture are pain at the puncture site and hematoma formation. This is particularly noted in patients who are receiving anticoagulants.[124,125] Less common problems resulting from radial artery cannulation consist of peripheral embolization with Osler node formation, hand discomfort,

SEQUOIA DISTRICT HOSPITAL INITIAL VENTILATION ORDERS

1. Ventilation
   a. Establish minute ventilation, $(V_T \times f) = (10 - 14 \text{ ml/kg})$, at 10-14 respirations/min.
   b. Adjust $(V_T - V_{DM})$ f using V_D/V_T nomogram to provide a $Paco_2$ of _____ to _____ torr and a pH of _____ to _____.
2. Oxygenation
   a. Initial $FIO_2 = 0.70$.
   b. Adjust FIO_2 using shunt diagram to provide Pao_2 of 60-100 torr.
   c. Adjust FIO_2 to provide Sao_2 of 90%-95%. Repeat arterial blood gas determination when Sao_2 is stable or 30 minutes after adjustment.
   Repeat blood gas determinations after each adjustment to provide stable values as previously.
3. Parameters to be monitored
   a. Continuously: ECG, rhythm and respiratory rate and pattern.
   b. Hourly: V_T, f, V_t/P, FIO_2, inspiratory:expiratory ratio, cuff pressure, temperature.
   c. Every 20 minutes: blood pressure and pulse.
4. Restrain hands until otherwise ordered.
5. Use upright portable chest x-ray films to visualize postintubation tube placement.
6. Perform continuous intake and output check and measure urine specific gravity every 8 hours.
7. Take daily weight: Yes _____ No _____
8. Use postural drainage and turn from side to side every 2 hr.
9. Submit tracheal aspirate for sputum Gram stain and culture.
10. Perform suctioning and tracheal care as per Sequoia District Hospital guidelines.

and major ischemic episodes.[126] Up to 20% of the patients who are clinically free of arterial injury develop thrombosed radial arteries that recannulize.[124,127] Despite these occasional complications from arterial blood sampling, it is generally agreed that arterial blood samples are essential in providing safe ventilator care.[128,129] Other sampling sites do not provide equivalent information. Central venous catheter blood samples are not suitable substitutes for arterial samples.[130] Arterialized capillary blood sampling. although safe and convenient, is relatively unreliable in assessing the Pao_2 in patients with reduced perfusion. The insertion of plastic catheters into the radial artery either percutaneously or by direct exposure has facilitated both intermittent and continuous sampling of arterial blood and the monitoring of systemic arterial pressure.[127] This arterial cannula should be kept patent by the continuous infusion of heparinized solution. If flushing is done, this should be limited to a 3 ml bolus or less and the infusion should be slowly administered. Rapid infusions of 6 ml or greater cause predictable retrograde flushing to the subclavian ar-

teries, a maneuver that may lead to cerebral embolization.[131] In order that the results of blood gas determinations yield the greatest information, a record of the tidal volume, respiratory rate, and FIO_2 should be made at the time of sampling. All samples must be obtained under anaerobic conditions, and the sample should be stored in ice water if a delay is anticipated before analysis. Frequent calibration of the analytic equipment is necessary to ensure accurate results.

■ What is the purpose of the mechanical ventilator?

The goal of positive pressure mechanical ventilation is to improve the distribution of gas within the lungs, to reinflate partially collapsed segments of the lung, to maintain patency of the small airways, and to avoid disrupting pulmonary blood flow, thereby promoting adequate gas exchange. The basic principles underlying the use of ventilators have been provided by reviews.[37,132-134] However, the crucial test of a mechanical ventilator is its ability to provide adequate ventilation under conditions of increased airway resistance and reduced lung compliance in the patient.

■ What feature should be sought in a mechanical ventilator?

The type of ventilator to be used is largely a matter of personal preference and should be chosen in consultation with individuals knowledgeable in the use of mechanical ventilation devices. The ventilator should have an adequate driving force to permit the ventilation of patients with markedly increased airway resistance and reduced compliance. In critically ill patients it may be necessary to provide long-term ventilation at pressures exceeding end-tidal pressures of 50 cm H_2O and minute ventilation of up to 20 L/min. The ventilator should be capable of delivering accurate tidal volume as well as providing measurement of the expired and inspired volumes. An airway pressure monitoring device that can identify disconnection or excess pressure is a mandatory feature. Mechanical ventilators that are not self-monitoring cannot be recommended for the modern respiratory care of the critically ill patient, since accidents caused by ventilator malfunction and tubing disconnection continue to occur.

Currently available ventilators that possess the necessary performance and monitoring features include the Bennett Volume Ventilator-MA-1, MA-2, Bourns BEAR, Ohio 560, Searle Adult Volume Ventilator, and Servo-Ventilator 900 (Elema-Schnonander). Several of these ventilators include desirable features such as removable patient circuits that are disposable or that can be autoclaved. Some of these devices can be controlled by servomechanisms. The Servo-Ventilator 900 can be programmed to adjust minute ventilation in response to alterations of PE_{CO_2} or $Paco_2$. The place of this latter feature in continuous ventilation therapy awaits further clinical evaluation.

■ Why are volume-cycled ventilators frequently employed?

A volume-cycled ventilator is frequently chosen because it delivers a preset tidal volume despite marked variation in airway resistance or compliance. In addition, most volume ventilators can be adjusted to provide automated sighing. Pressure-cycled ventilators are less desirable because inspiratory gas flow delivery is limited by a preset pressure. In such ventilators tidal volumes show wide variations as a result of changes in airway resistance or compliance. Routine measures such as turning, suctioning, and coughing may be followed by marked reductions in tidal volume. Such unpredictable reductions in alveolar ventilation may then lead to significant hypoventilation with respiratory acidemia. Dangerous increases in alveolar ventilation may suddenly appear if compliance improves while a patient is ventilated in the control mode on a pressure-limited volume ventilator.[114,129,135]

■ What ventilator settings are first selected?

When the patient is first placed on a ventilator, an effort should be made to provide small tidal volumes, low inflationary pressure, and rapid inspiratory gas flows, so that the inspiratory time occupies no more than one third of the entire respiratory cycle. If the patient shows no deleterious cardiovascular response to such initial settings, progressive increases in inspiratory volume and pressure as well as sustained pressure plateaus as necessary to achieve the desired distribution of ventilation can be chosen. If a clear reduction in arterial pressure, skin temperature, and urine flow suggest reduced cardiac output, it is likely that a circulatory deficiency exists. In such patients the repletion of intravascular volume may be necessary before increases in mean airway pressure and tidal volume can be undertaken.

■ Should the mechanical ventilator be set on the assist or the control mode to adequately ventilate the patient?

The administration of IPPB may be achieved either by setting the ventilator to follow the patient's spontaneous ventilatory effort and augment the tidal volume (assisted ventilation) or by cycling the ventilator automatically and thereby establishing a predetermined respiratory pattern for the patient (controlled). The assist mode is used on conscious or comatose patients who have normal, regular, and vigorous breathing patterns and who thereby maintain the $Paco_2$ in a desirable range. When complete apnea is present, the choice is obviously simple, in that controlled ventilation is necessary to ensure predictable gas exchange. Controlled ventilation is used in patients who are conscious or in a coma but who have apnea or are breathing very slowly or irregularly. Excessive tachypnea and flail chest are additional situations in which controlled ventilation should be undertaken.[43] The conversion from assisted to controlled ventilation can usually be accomplished by increasing the Pao_2 and lowering the $Paco_2$. Verbal reassurance of the patient is also important in these adjustments. If a rapid respiratory rate persists in the face of an adequate Pao_2, Pvo_2, and modest respiratory alkalemia, it may be necessary to employ drug therapy to control ventilation.

■ How is the patient who is fighting the ventilator managed?

When the mechanical ventilator cannot be synchronized with the patient's breathing, an immediate search should be undertaken to identify the presence of a mechanical derangement in the ventilatory inspiratory tubing or patient's airway. Factors such as kinked airway, airway obstruction, or displacement of the airway should be immediately excluded by clinical assessment. Observation should be made of chest wall movement, and the presence of breath sounds should be ascertained. Inspired oxygen concentration should be checked as well as tidal volume and airway pressures. Arterial blood gas analysis should be undertaken. During such assessment the patient should be supported by bag mask ventilation until the problem is identified. If hypoxemia is present, it should be relieved by appropriate adjustment of supplemental oxygen or ventilatory pattern. Other factors such as pain, confusion, or apprehension should be allayed, and slight increases in alveolar ventilation to appropriately adjust the $Paco_2$ should be made. Periodic sighing maneuvers or an increase of tidal volume with added mechanical dead space to stabilize the $Paco_2$ may ease the patient's fighting. If sedation is still necessary after these measures and a chest x-ray film has excluded mechanical factors such as pneumothorax, sedation can be achieved by the IV administration of 5 mg of diazepam over

a 1- to 5-minute period while monitoring the patient's clinical and blood pressure response.[136] Many workers prefer the IV use of morphine sulfate, 2 to 10 mg, infused at 2 mg/min until adequate synchronization with the ventilator is achieved. If the use of opiates or diazepam is considered undesirable, nondepolarizing relaxants without ganglionic blocking activity such as pancuronium may be employed.

■ What airway pressures are maintained during mechanical ventilation?

The airway pressure employed is the airway pressure that will provide a predetermined tidal volume. This pressure, which is measured in the ventilator or can be measured at the mouth, will reflect alterations in airway resistance and lung compliance. In patients with low lung compliances airway pressures greater than 40 to 50 cm H_2O would be required to deliver high tidal volume. On the other hand, in patients with high total compliance such as in emphysema, airway pressures as low as 10 to 15 cm H_2O may be sufficient to provide the desired tidal volume.

■ When should negative phase ventilation be used?

The application of subatmospheric pressure to the airway (negative phase ventilation) reduces lung volume.[137] Reduced lung volume alters surface forces, makes alveolar units unstable, and leads to the collapse of alveolar units and terminal airways. These changes impair ventilation-perfusion matching and result in shunting of blood and progression of hypoxemia. Such adverse effects of negative phase ventilation preclude its use in the care of critically ill patients.

■ What is the purpose of the sighing maneuver?

Deep breathing, or sighing, maneuvers act to restore lung volume, reopen collapsed air spaces, and reduce hypoxemia produced by monotonous low tidal volume ventilation.[137,138] In addition, sighing maneuvers frequently relieve the patient's complaint of inadequate chest expansion.[139] Many ventilators are equipped with automatic devices that provide a deep breath at fixed intervals. Sighing volumes of 15 to 20 ml/kg are often administered at 15- to 30-minute intervals. Sighing can, however, be dangerous in patients with high lung volumes or in patients who require high mean airway pressures during tidal breathing. When sighing maneuvers are applied to such patients and in patients who are already receiving PEEP ventilation, increases in mean airway pressure may lead to alveolar rupture.[140] Webb and Tierney[91] have pointed out other risks of high pressure ventilation. Such observations call for a reexamination of the role of sighing maneuvers. Sighing is particularly hazardous and best avoided in patients with obstructive airway disorders who breathe at high lung volumes and utilize only the easily communicating airways.

■ Which variables should be monitored during mechanical ventilation?

Close clinical monitoring of the ventilated patient is mandatory. In addition, when patients are mechanically ventilated, the most useful variables to be measured include respiratory rate, expired tidal volume, airway pressure, inspired oxygen concentration, and end-expiratory Pco_2 or $Paco_2$. The end-expiratory Pco_2 has been found to be a useful rapidly available guide to the patient's $Paco_2$.[31] Recently the identification of altered lung compliance has been used as an early indicator of atelectasis, pneumothorax, pulmonary edema, or pulmonary emboli. Serial assessment of lung compliance has been of further use in the application of PEEP. During incremental increases in PEEP the lung volume expands until elastic limits are approached, at which point further increases in PEEP result in a sharp reduction in compliance. Such observations may indicate that the upper limits of PEEP have been reached.[31] Since mechanical ventilation may decrease cardiac output, hemodynamic measurements should also be assessed. Fluid balance must also be regularly monitored. The assessment of so many parameters plus hemoglobin, plasma, and urine osmolality, serum bicarbonate, base excess, and so on, rapidly leads to the accumulation of an unmanageable data base. In order that the clinical events, drug administration, and objective measurements can be promptly assimilated and applied to clinical care, appropriate flow sheets should be developed for bedside use. Fig. 15-1 shows the flow sheet used in the care of

critically ill patients at Sequoia District Hospital. This chart is mounted at the foot of the bed and subsequently folds and is accommodated by a standard-sized hospital chart. This single sheet replaces five or six redundant nursing and respiratory sheets, permits the entry of data at the bedside, and assures immediate accessibility to the patient's medical record. The continuity of nursing, respiratory therapy, and physician management is enhanced by such records.[141-142]

■ What is the goal of PEEP ventilation?

The goal of PEEP is to improve systemic oxygen transport while delivering lower inspired oxygen concentrations. It is not sufficient to provide an increase in arterial oxygen alone. If arterial oxygen is increased by PEEP but cardiac output is reduced, less oxygen is in fact delivered to the tissues. An index of tissue oxygenation is obtained by examining mixed venous blood obtained from the pulmonary artery.[143] Such sampling has been considerably simplified by the advent of the Swan-Ganz catheter.[143,144] The determination of the Svo_2 before and after the onset of PEEP is of distinct value in assessing changes in cardiac output as a result of the application of PEEP.[145,146] Falls in Svo_2 during PEEP administration suggest either reduced cardiac output or increasing shunt as a result of the treatments. An optimum response to PEEP application will reveal increased Pao_2 and Svo_2 in the face of FIO_2 reductions.[2,144,145,147]

■ How is PEEP applied?

PEEP is produced in the airway by placing an impedance to outflow of the expired air. This can easily be achieved by attaching a large-bore tube to the exhalation port of the ventilator and then immersing the free end of the tubing in water to create the desired pressure of 2 to 15 cm H_2O. The airway pressure at end-expiration will therefore be determined by the column of water that must be displaced by the escaping gas. Accessory devices are now available on most ventilators to permit the application of variable pressures to the exhaled gas. In such cases airway pressure described by the manometer at end-expiration will be used as the guide for PEEP adjustment.

Increases in transpulmonary pressure achieved

Age: _____

Hemodynamic status

	ECG
Systemic	Radial
	Cuff
	Gage S/D
	Gage mean
LA	cm H_2O / mm Hg
Venous	cm H_2O / mm Hg
PA	S/D
	Mean
	C.O. (CI)

Preoperative weight: _____ — Weight

Output
- Urine
- Shift total

Fluid intake
- Shift total

Respiratory status
- Airway
- Ventilation equipment
- V_T/P
- Respiratory rate
- Inspiration:expiration
- Cuff volume
- F_1O_2/O_2 LPM
- P_{O_2}
- pH
- P_{CO_2}
- Base excess
- Sampling time
- Sampling site
- Hemoglobin/Hematocrit
- Sputum

Neurologic status
- Level of consc.
- Motor

Blood chemistry
- Time drawn
- Test and result

Medications

Nursing notes

Fig. 15-1. Critical care flow sheet.

by the devices just described lead to the reinflation of previously underinflated or closed alveoli and terminal airways. In patients with decreased lung compliance and reduced lung volumes, increases in lung volume usually follow incremental increases in PEEP.[144,145]

■ **When is PEEP used?**

PEEP is employed when the Pao_2 is less than 60 torr or showing a progressive decline while the patient is receiving FIO_2 of 0.6 or higher by a closed system or when the functional residual capacity is less than half of normal despite appropriate adjustment of tidal volume and inspiratory:expiratory ratio, treatment of bronchospasm and cardiac failure, proper adjustment of fluid balance, frequent positional changes, and vigorous tracheal toilet.[19,145,147,148]

■ **What is the optimum level of PEEP?**

The optimum level of PEEP is determined by the cardiopulmonary response to increases in end-expiratory pressures. A Pao_2 of 65 to 75 torr and Svo_2 of 60% on a FIO_2 of 0.6 is desirable. The appropriate level of PEEP is provided by the gradual application of increments of pressure at 2 to 4 cm H_2O while reassessing the adequacy of cardiac output by monitoring blood pressure, pulse, skin temperature, and urine output and by analyzing $P\bar{v}o_2$ and content, and lactate blood levels.[143] Suter and co-workers[149] demonstrated that the best PEEP level could be selected by monitoring compliance, a simple and nonintrusive measurement.[149] Careful attention to airway pressure is necessary to confirm that the desired end-expiratory pressure is indeed achieved. PEEP effect is often lost if the patient inhales or exhales out of phase with the ventilator. In such instances the control of ventilation may be achieved by a temporary increase in oxygenation, reduction in $Paco_2$, or increases in sedation or neuromuscular block. If the first three measures are carefully applied, there will rarely be a need for neuromuscular blockade. In patients with low lung compliance, low lung volumes, adequate intravascular volume, and good cardiac function, a progressive rise of Pao_2 is usually noted within minutes of the application of PEEP. Pvo_2 and Svo_2 and blood lactate usually remain

the same or improve.[143] Recent work suggests that measurements of "best PEEP" alone may not provide an adequate indication of oxygen transport, and regular reassessment of the previously noted parameters is indicated in choosing the "best PEEP" level.[150] Occasionally it may be necessary to apply a PEEP of greater than 20 cm H_2O in order to increase the Pao_2.[151] In such patients it is frequently necessary to reduce tidal volumes in order to avoid the need for excessive high inspiratory airway pressures. The use of PEEP in a patient with obstructive airway disease is best avoided because of the risk of creating pneumothorax and decreasing cardiac output.[140]

If cardiac output falls during PEEP administration, PEEP should be reduced to the level best tolerated.[150] The reapplication of PEEP may be done later after the tidal volumes have been reduced and IV fluids, especially plasma, are administered. Supplemental measures to correct underlying disorders such as atelectasis, pneumonia, congestive heart failure, and/or fluid overload may subsequently permit the reduction of PEEP. If arterial oxygen tension has been improved by PEEP, priority should then be given to reducing the inspired oxygen to less than 60% oxygen. Once this is achieved, PEEP can slowly be reduced in increments of 1 to 2 cm H_2O. Arterial blood gas determinations should be monitored during the removal of PEEP, since lung volume reduction, air space closure, and hypoxemia may recur if the underlying disorder has been inadequately repaired. In particular the removal of PEEP in the hypervolemic patient may result in sudden increases in venous return, which may embarrass cardiac function in the patient with preexisting diminished myocardial contractility. The identification of left ventricular failure as a complicating factor in acute respiratory failure has been much facilitated by the use of the Swan-Ganz catheter.[20,152] Once recognized and appropriately treated, rapid clearing of the left ventricular failure will permit reductions in PEEP and FIO_2.

■ **What are the circulatory effects of employing IPPB or CPPB?**

Reduced cardiac output commonly occurs when high airway pressure is transmitted to intrathoracic blood vessels.[153] This may occur with IPPB or CPPB.[154,155] The more compliant the lungs, the more profound will be the effect of airway pressure on the pulmonary and systemic circulation. If, in addition, intravascular volume has been depleted by blood loss, dehydration, or antecedent diuretic therapy, further decreases in cardiac output should be expected. Patients with compromised peripheral venous tone, such as those with idiopathic polyneuritis, spinal cord injury, or pretreatment with antihypertensives, ganglionic blocking medications, and opiates, will be particularly subject to reduction in cardiac output with increasing mean airway pressure. Reduction in cardiac output associated with the initiation of IPPB is most often seen when high inflation pressures are combined with a prolonged inspiratory phase of ventilation.[153] If, on the other hand, low tidal volumes, low mean airway pressures, and short duration of inflation are applied during the initiation of ventilation, circulatory adjustment may occur and may later permit marked changes in mean airway pressure without serious circulatory depression. The excessive elevation of PEEP may similarly produce reductions of cardiac output. However, careful incremental application of PEEP often increases output and may produce less circulatory disturbance than IPPB alone.[156]

■ Is there a risk of pneumothorax occurring in patients receiving PEEP?

Pneumothorax frequently occurs when patients receive mechanical ventilation, particularly when mean airway pressures are elevated and/or PEEP is applied.[55,140,157] Patients who run the highest risk of developing pneumothorax are those patients with underlying chronic obstructive pulmonary disease and/or emphysema in whom large tidal volumes and high inflation pressures are used. In such patients tidal volumes above 12 to 15 ml/kg and inflation pressures greater than 45 cm H_2O are commonly associated with pneumothorax. The incidence of pneumothorax has been estimated to be approximately 15% to 30% in patients who are also receiving PEEP.[55,140,157] Some workers have observed subcutaneous emphysema and pneumothorax in 50% of patients who have been ventilated with

PEEP.[28,157] To reduce such complications, measures to lessen the need for high airway pressures must be exploited. Such measures include the removal of secretions and the use of bronchodilators when airway obstruction is evident. The selective use of sedation and/or neuromuscular paralysis may reduce the need for high airway pressure in the struggling patient. Since pneumothorax occurs so commonly in ventilated patients, immediate recognition of this disorder is *essential*. The development of pneumothorax is frequently attended by the development of subcutaneous emphysema, tachycardia, diminished breath sounds, increased resonance to percussion, cyanosis, diaphoresis, and irregularities of the pulse.[140] Asynchronous chest movement and tracheal deviation may also be present. When these signs and symptoms are associated with rising peak airway pressure and sudden difficulty in ventilation of the patient, one should first conclude that a pneumothorax has developed. Since pneumothorax in the ventilated patient can lead to sudden death, a plan should be drawn up in advance to ensure prompt placement of the chest evacuation tubes, suction, and continuous decompression of any pneumothorax that may develop. As prolonged air leakage and delayed sealing of the pneumothorax may occur during PEEP ventilation, precautions should be exercised prior to the removal of tubes if the patient continues to require mechanical ventilation. Tubes should be patent, air leaks should have ceased, and the lungs should remain fully expanded for 48 hours prior to discontinuing the chest tubes. During the period of tube thoracostomy every attempt should be made to reduce mean airway pressures or to discontinue PEEP.[140]

■ When can the mechanically ventilated patient be returned to spontaneous breathing?

Techniques for assessing the patient's readiness for removal from the mechanical ventilator have recently been reviewed by Hodgkin and coworkers.[158] It is generally agreed that the patient should be hemodynamically stable, reasonably alert, and coughing effectively. A spontaneous vital capacity of 15 cc/kg and a maximum inspiratory force of greater than 25 cm H_2O are the most predictive indicators in assessing the patient's preparedness for the discontinuation of mechanical ventilation.[2,158-160] These measurements offer a useful means at the bedside for predicting the ability of the patient to be removed from the ventilator. Although arterial blood gas determinations are useful in establishing the stability of gas exchange while the patient is receiving mechanical ventilation, such stable values are not an accurate or good predictor of the ability of the patient to maintain adequate ventilation while breathing spontaneously. It is essential that oxygen supplementation be continued while the patient is off the ventilator to be certain that arterial hypoxemia does not supervene. In addition, deep breathing, chest physiotherapy, and tracheobronchial suctioning must be continued. Patients who develop progressive hypoxemia during spontaneous breathing may benefit from continuous positive airway pressure (CPAP). CPAP, a method of providing impedance to expired gas, has been employed to increase lung volume and thereby prevent alveolar collapse in infants with acute respiratory distress syndrome.[161] This same method has been used in spontaneously breathing, intubated adults where it has been effective in reducing the alveolar-arterial oxygen gradient and increasing vital capacity in patients who have developed rapid alveolar collapse during weaning from ventilation.[162]

■ Does intermittent mandatory ventilation simplify weaning?

Intermittent mandatory ventilation (IMV) has been recommended as an alternate method of assuring smooth weaning from mechanical ventilation.[163] The IMV system design permits the patient to breathe humidified, oxygen-enriched gas at ambient pressure spontaneously. The ventilator is preset to provide the desired number of breaths, which are delivered to the patient regardless of his spontaneous breathing rate. The IMV rate is usually set slower than the patient's spontaneous breathing rate. The IMV frequency is then progressively reduced until the patient initiates all breaths spontaneously at ambient pressure. At that point the ventilator can be entirely removed from the breathing circuit. Our observations to date agree with those of Dr. Feeley and

his associates that IMV adds no substantial advantage in weaning the "difficult-to-wean" patient.[162] In addition, the IMV method creates the potential hazard of delivering a preset breath at a time when the patient has spontaneously inspired. Since the IMV breaths are usually set at an appropriate tidal volume, this problem should not create excessive barotrauma. However, if PEEP or high tidal volumes were being applied, then a real hazard of pneumothorax could be created. Because of the latter problem, recent workers have suggested that intermittent demand ventilation (IDV) would minimize the risk of increased thoracic pressure and provide additional advantages over conventional weaning methods.[164] The IDV system is designed to permit the patient to breathe humidified, oxygen-enriched gas at the rate chosen by the patient. In addition, however, mechanical breaths are delivered at a preset rate by the ventilator as the patient initiates inspiration. Thus excessive intrathoracic pressure can be theoretically avoided. No adequate scientific evaluation of IMV or IDV has clearly established that these methods are superior to the conventional methods of weaning. Nonetheless, such methods may be applicable in occasional patients who have become dependent on mechanical ventilation.

■ What place does extracorporeal oxygenation have in the management of respiratory failure?

Increasing attention has been directed to the use of extracorporeal oxygenation in the support of patients with acute respiratory failure who cannot be adequately oxygenated by the use of 100% oxygen employing volume-limited ventilation with PEEP incorporated into the circuit. The goal of therapy is to gain time for pulmonary recovery to occur. Current problems that need to be further explored before the efficacy of this method is clear include better guidelines for the selection of patients with potentially reversible pulmonary disorders and measures to control coagulation disorders and sepsis during prolonged bypass use.[165] The need for the total commitment of professional and technical staff and ancillary services for days to weeks at a time limit this method to use by a small number of well-equipped centers.[166] It should be remembered that improvement in oxygenation is often outstanding with CPPB alone, and this mode of respiratory therapy should always be tried prior to consideration of the institution of extracorporeal oxygenation. Marked improvement in arterial tension without significant increases of the arterovenous oxygen content difference may preclude the need for membrane oxygenator support.

■ What are common complications of continuous mechanical ventilation?

Alterations of alveolar ventilation frequently occur during continuous mechanical ventilation. Alveolar hypoventilation is usually a result of ventilator malfunction or changes in lung mechanics. Alveolar hyperventilation is also a hazard and is particularly noted in the patient who is being ventilated by a pressure ventilator that is set on a control mode. In this situation the improvement in pulmonary mechanics leads to marked increases in tidal volumes. Since the frequency of breathing is fixed, minute ventilation rapidly increases and respiratory alkalemia, dangerous cardiac arrhythmia, seizures, and death may follow.[114,119,129]

The accumulation of body and lung water is another frequent problem in acute respiratory failure. This syndrome has been characterized by positive water balance, radiographic changes suggestive of pulmonary edema, and impaired blood gas exchange in patients receiving prolonged artificial ventilation.[167] X-ray film changes of the lungs vary from localized to diffuse densities of the lungs. Positive water balance in acute respiratory failure is often unaccompanied by recognizable cardiac failure or elevated central venous or pulmonary artery wedge pressures. When left ventricular failure does supervene in respiratory failure, diagnosis by Swan-Ganz catheterization is useful in directing specific therapy.[20,21,152] Frequent and careful weighing as well as special attention devoted to fluid and salt intake and output are essential to avoid water imbalance. Regular assessment of plasma and urine osmolality will lead to early detection of this disorder. It should be recognized that a daily weight loss of approximately 500 g is expected in critically ill patients.

It is frequently necessary to limit fluid administration for daily maintenance to 20 to 25 ml/kg/24 hr in patients who are mechanically ventilated to avoid positive water balance.[2,167]

Although contributions from humidifiers are not routinely measured, it should be understood that the humidifier is an additional source of water intake that may contribute up to 400 ml of water/day. The supplementary use of diuretic drugs may frequently prove necessary to maintain water and salt balance. Frequent changes of position are important in preventing the formation of pulmonary edema in dependent lung segments. Side-to-side changes are performed hourly.

■ What are the causes of infection during mechanical ventilation?

Hospital-acquired infection during ventilator therapy has been attributed to contamination of the humidifiers, respiratory tubing, and cleaning solutions. Cross contamination between patients by breaks in sterile tracheal suction apparatus has also been reported. The regular cleansing and sterilization of the patient's circuits and particularly humidifiers are important in preventing bacterial contamination of the airway from the ventilator circuit.[168] The use of aseptic suction techniques is important in preventing the inoculation of organisms into the airway. Despite meticulous techniques being employed, tracheal colonization by gram-negative bacilli frequently occurs. The development of fever, pulmonary consolidation defined by chest x-ray, and the identification of gram-negative organisms in the sputum suggest the appearance of a hospital-acquired gram-negative pneumonia.[169] Appropriate antibiotic treatment will frequently need to be started on a clinical basis, as the danger of septicemia with shock from these organisms is a major risk in the management of acute respiratory failure.

■ Is mental dysfunction encountered in the ventilated critically ill patient?

Mental dysfunction is often demonstrated in the ventilated patient and may appear as drowsiness, confusion, and inappropriate behavior with or without hallucinations.[170,171] Such behavior may be more difficult to anticipate or to control than many of the complications that were discussed earlier. Inappropriate behavior may endanger the patient by leading to premature self-extubation with tracheal injury, fighting the ventilator, and other such complications. A plan for the early recognition of delirium has been suggested.[170] Investigation and correction of underlying metabolic abnormalities such as acidemia, hypoxemia, and electrolyte derangement should always be considered in patients demonstrating delirium. Environmental factors that deprive patients of sleep and remove patients from familiar contact should be avoided. The reassurance of seriously ill patients is important and is provided in large part by the constant presence of a careful, receptive, and knowledgeable staff. A nurse: patient ratio of 1:1 should be provided during continuous ventilation. Explanations and reassurance are given during suctioning, changing of tracheostomy, chest physical therapy, and other such bedside procedures. The use of a call bell or clicking mouth noises should be encouraged for use as signals to attract the staff's attention. Writing pads or laryngeal vibrations and periodic cuff deflation should be used to permit communication. Visits with the staff, psychiatric nurse, and family often permit and promote verbalization or expression of fears or hallucinations.[172]

■ What is the most important component of respiratory care?

Although specialized equipment and monitoring devices are important, it should be recognized that these are merely supplementary tools to be used by a knowledgeable staff. Attendants must be constantly present when a patient is on controlled ventilation, since transient disconnection of the tube, tube occlusion or displacement, or failure of the ventilator may prove to be rapidly fatal.

The respiratory care unit should be staffed with well-qualified critical care practitioners who have had clinical experience in respiratory care and cardiac monitoring. Ongoing critical care in-service education should be available to all personnel, and in addition, closely supervised bedside clinical experience should be provided to all new personnel.

Respiratory care protocols should be regularly reviewed with the staff and revision made during hospital joint practice committee meetings (meetings with physicians, nurses, and other allied health care personnel).

REFERENCES

1. O'Donohue, W. J., Jr., Bake, J. P., Bell, G. M., Muren, O., and Patterson, J. L., Jr.: The management of acute respiratory failure in a respiratory intensive care unit, Chest **58:**603, 1970.
2. Pontoppidan, H., Geffin, B., and Lowenstein, E.: Acute respiratory failure in the adult, N. Engl. J. Med. **287:**690, 743, 799, 1972.
3. Hedley-Whyte, J., Burgess, G. E., Feeley, T. W., and Miller, M. G.: Applied physiology of respiratory care, Boston, 1976, Little, Brown & Co.
4. Respiratory Diseases Task Force: Report on problems, research approaches and needs, DHEW Pub. No. NIH 73-432, Washington, D.C., 1972, Department of Health, Education, and Welfare.
5. Bates, D. V.: Organization of intensive care units: results in cases of respiratory failure, Anesthesiology **25:**199, 1964.
6. Bendixen, H. H., et al.: Respiratory care, St. Louis, 1965, The C. V. Mosby Co.
7. Bigelow, D. B., et al.: Acute respiratory failure, experiences of the respiratory care unit, Med. Clin. North Am. **51:**323, 1967.
8. Safar, P.: Respiratory therapy, Philadelphia, 1965, F. A. Davis Co.
9. Seriff, N. S., Khan, F., and Lazo, B. J.: Acute respiratory failure: current concepts of pathophysiology and management, Med. Clin. North Am. **57:**1539, 1973.
10. Campbell, D., Reid, J. M., Telfer, A. B., and Fitch, W.: Four years of respiratory intensive care, Br. Med. J. **4:**255, 1967.
11. Scoggin, C. H., Sahn, S. A., and Petty, T. L.: Status asthmaticus—a nine year experience, J.A.M.A. **238:**1158, 1977.
12. Murray, J. F.: The adult respiratory distress syndrome (may it rest in peace), Resp. Dis. **111:**716, 1975.
13. Petty, T. L.: The adult respiratory distress syndrome (confessions of a "lumper"), Resp. Dis. **111:**713, 1975.
14. Ashbaugh, D. G., Bigelow, D. E., Petty, T. L., and Levine, B. E.: Acute respiratory distress in adults, Lancet **2:**319, 1967.
15. Moore, F. D., et al.: Post traumatic pulmonary insufficiency, Philadelphia, 1969, W. B. Saunders Co.
16. Pontoppidan, H., Laver, M. B., and Geffin, B.: Acute respiratory failure in the surgical patient, Adv. Surg. **4:**163, 1970.
17. Safar, P., Grenvik, A., and Smith, J.: Progressive pulmonary consolidation: review of cases and pathogenesis, J. Trauma **12:**955, 1972.
18. Blaisdell, F. W., and Lewis, F. R.: Respiratory distress syndrome of shock and trauma; post traumatic respiratory failure, Major Probl. Clin. Surg. **21:**1, 1977.
19. Ashbaugh, D. G., Petty, T. L., Bigelow, D. B., and Harris,

T. M.: Continuous positive pressure breathing (CPPB) in adult respiratory distress syndrome, J. Thorac. Cardiovasc. Surg. **57:**31, 1969.

20. Unger, K. M., Shibel, E. M., and Moser, K. M.: Detection of left ventricular failure in patients with adult respiratory distress syndrome, Chest **67:**8, 1975.

21. Karliner, J. S.: Non-cardiogenic forms of pulmonary edema, Circulation **46:**212, 1972.

22. Robin, E. D., Carey, L. C., Grenvik, A., Blouser, F., and Gaudia, R.: Capillary leak syndrome with pulmonary edema, Arch. Intern. Med. **130:**66, 1972.

23. Katz, S., Aberman, A., Frand, U., Stein, F., and Faloys, M.: Heroin pulmonary edema: evidence for increased pulmonary capillary permeability, Am. Rev. Respir. Dis. **106:**472, 1972.

24. Robin, E. D., Cross, C. E., and Zelis, R.: Pulmonary edema, N. Engl. J. Med. **288:**239, 1973.

25. Staub, N. C.: State of the art review. Pathogenesis of pulmonary edema, Am. Rev. Respir. Dis. **109:**358, 1974.

26. Sykes, M. K., McNicol, M. W., and Campbell, E. J. M.: Respiratory failures, ed. 2, Oxford, 1976, Blackwell Scientific Publications, Ltd.

27. Weg, J. G., and Alexander, J. G.: Acute respiratory failure, clinical challenge in cardiopulmonary medicine with self assessment, Am. College Chest Physicians **1**(4):1, 1978.

28. Olcott, C., Barber, R. E., and Blaisdell, F. W.: Diagnosis and treatment of respiratory failure after civilian trauma, Am. J. Surg. **122:**260, 1971.

29. Safar, P., and Grenvik, A.: Multi-disciplinary intensive care, Mod. Med. **39:**92, 1971.

30. Peters, R. M., Hilberman, M., Hogan, J. S., and Crawford, D. A.: Objective indications for respiratory therapy in post-trauma and postoperative patients, Am. J. Surg. **124:**262, 1972.

31. Osborn, J. A.: Monitoring respiratory function, Crit. Care Med. **2:**217, 1974.

32. Turney, S. Z., McAslan, T. C., and Cowley, R. A.: The continuous measurement of pulmonary gas exchange and mechanics, Ann. Thorac. Surg. **13:**229, 1972.

33. Peters, R. M., and Hilberman, M.: Respiratory insufficiency: diagnosis and control of therapy, Surgery **70:**280, 1971.

34. Macklem, P. T.: The indications for artificial ventilation are limited: controversies in internal medicine II, Philadelphia, 1974, W. B. Saunders Co.

35. Singer, M. M.: The advantages of an aggressive prophylactic approach: controversies in internal medicine II, Philadelphia, 1974, W. B. Saunders Co.

36. Camerson, J. L., Sebor, J., Anderson, R. P., and Zuidema, G. D.: Aspiration pneumonia; results of treatment with positive pressure ventilation in dogs, J. Surg. Res. **8:**447, 1968.

37. Stallone, R. J., Herbst, H., Cafferata, H. T., Blaisdell, F. W., and Murray, J. F.: Pulmonary changes following regional ischemia; response to treatment, Am. Rev. Respir. Dis. **98:**144, 1968.

38. Uzawa, T., and Ashbaugh, D. G.: Continuous positive-pressure breathing in acute hemorrhagic pulmonary edema, J. Appl. Physiol. **26:**427, 1969.

39. Lecky, J. H., and Ominsky, A. J.: Postoperative respiratory management, Chest **62**(suppl.): 50S, 1972.

40. Copperman, L. H., and Mann, P. E.: Postoperative respiratory care; a review of 65 consecutive cases of open-heart surgery on the mitral valve, J. Thorac. Cardiovasc. Surg. **53:**504, 1967.

41. Lefemine, V., and Harken, D. E.: Postoperative care following open-heart operations; routine use of controlled ventilation, J. Thorac. Cardiovasc. Surg. **2:**207, 1966.

42. Norlander, O. P.: The use of respirators in anesthesia and surgery, Acta Anaesthesiol. Scand. **30**(suppl.):5, 1968.

43. Roscher, R., Bittner, R., and Stockman, U.: Pulmonary contusions, clinical experience, Arch. Surg. **109:**508, 1974.

44. Standards for cardiopulmonary resuscitation (CPR) and emergency cardiac care (ECC), J.A.M.A. **227**(suppl.): 833S, 1974.

45. Buchner, H., Cimino, J.A., and Raybin, H. W.: Naloxone reversal of methadone poisoning, N.Y. State J. Med. **72:**2305, 1972.

46. Martin, W. R.: Drugs five years later: naloxone, Ann. Intern. Med. **85:**765, 1976.

47. Longnecker, D. E., Grazis, P. A., and Eggers, G. W., Jr.: Naloxone for antagonism of morphine-induced respiratory depression, Anesth. Analg. **52:**447, 1973.

48. Foldes, F. F., Duncalf, D., and Kuwabara, S.: The respiratory circulatory and narcotic antagonistic effects of nalorphine levallorphan and naloxone in anaesthetized subjects, Can. Anaesth. Soc. J. **16:**151, 1969.

49. Hasbrouck, J. D.: The antagonism of morphine anesthesia by naloxone, Anesth. Analg. **50:**954, 1971.

50. Fritz, H. W., and Rochester, D. F.: Respiratory stimulants and obstructed airways, N. Engl. J. Med. **288:**464, 1973.

51. Klaustermeyer, W. B., Winn, W. R., and Olson, C. R.: Use of cuffed endotracheal tubes for severe exacerbations of chronic respiratory airway obstruction, Am. Rev. Respir. Dis. **105:**268, 1972.

52. Selecky, P. A.: Tracheostomy: a review of present day indications, complications and care, Heart Lung **3:**272, 1974.

53. Haberman, P. B., et al.: Determinants of successful selective tracheobronchial suctioning, N. Engl. J. Med. **289:**1060, 1973.

54. Shapiro, A. G., and Walker, C. G.: Respiratory intensive care, Med. Clin. North Am. **55:**1217, 1971.

55. Zwillich, C. W., et al.: Complications of assisted ventilation; a prospective study of 354 consecutive episodes, Am. J. Med. **57:**161, 1974.

56. Amikan, B., Landa, J., West, J., and Sackman, M.: Bronchofiberoscopic observation of the tracheobronchial tree during intubation, Am. Rev. Respir. Dis. **105:**747, 1972.

57. Bushnell, S. S., Bushnell, L. S., Reichle, M. J., and Skillman, J. J.: Respiratory intensive care nursing, Boston, 1973, Little, Brown & Co.

58. Gaskell, D. V., and Webber, B. A.: The Brompton Hospital guide to chest physiotherapy, ed. 3, Oxford, 1977, Blackwell Scientific Publications, Ltd.

59. Rie, M.: Physical therapy in the nursing care of respiratory disease patients, Nurs. Clin. North Am. **3**:463, 1968.
60. Sackner, M. A.: Bronchofiberoscopy, Am. Rev. Respir. Dis. **111**:62, 1975.
61. Wanner, A., Landa, J. F., Nieman, R. E., Vevaina, J., and Delgado, I.: Bedside bronchofiberoscopy for atelectasis and lung abscess, J.A.M.A. **224**:1281, 1973.
62. Dubrawsky, C., Awe, R. J., and Jenkins, D. E.: The effect of *bronchofiberscopic* examination on oxygenation status, Chest **67**:137, 1975.
63. Albertina, R. E., Harrell, J. H., and Moser, K. M.: Management of arterial hypoxemia induced by fiberotic bronchoscopy, Chest **67**:134, 1975.
64. Shim, C., Fine, N., Fernandez, R., and Williams, M. H., Jr.: Cardiac arrhythmias from tracheal suctioning, Ann. Intern. Med. **711**:1149, 1969.
65. Urban, B. J., and Weitzner, S. W.: Avoidance of hypoxia during endotracheal suction, Anesthesiology **31**:473, 1969.
66. Hawkins, D. B., Seltzer, D. C., Barnett, T. E., and Stoneman, G. B.: Endotracheal tube perforation of the hypopharynx, West. J. Med. **120**:282, 1974.
67. McGovern, F. H., Fitz-Hugh, G. S., and Edgeman, L. J.: The hazards of endotracheal intubation, Ann. Otol. Rhinol. Laryngol. **80**:556, 1971.
68. Blanc, V. F., and Tremblay, N. A.: The complications of tracheal intubation; a new classification with a review of the literature, Anesth. Analg. **53**:202, 1974.
69. Lewis, F. R., Schlobohm, R. M., and Thomas, A. N.: Prevention of complications from prolonged tracheal intubation, Am. J. Surg. **135**:452, 1978.
70. Klainer, A. S., et al.: Surface alterations due to endotracheal intubation, Am. J. Med. **58**:674, 1975.
71. Bryant, L. R., Trinkle, J. K., and Dubilier, L.: Reappraisal of tracheal injury from cuffed tracheostomy tubes; experiments in dogs, J.A.M.A. **215**:625, 1971.
72. Geffin, B., Grillo, H., Cooper, J., and Pontoppidan, H.: Stenosis following tracheostomy for respiratory care, J.A.M.A. **216**:1984, 1971.
73. Grill, H. C., Cooper, J. D., Geffin, B., and Pontoppidan, H.: Low-pressure cuff for tracheostomy tubes to minimize tracheal injury, J. Thorac. Cardiovasc. Surg. **62**:898, 1971.
74. Harley, H. R.: Laryngeal tracheal obstruction complicating tracheostomy or endotracheal intubation with assisted respiration, Thorax **26**:493, 1971.
75. Shelly, W. M., Dawson, R. B., and May, I. A.: Cuffed tubes as a cause of tracheal stenosis, J. Thorac. Cardiovasc. Surg. **57**:623, 1969.
76. Cox, P. M., and Schatz, M. E.: Pressure measurement in endotracheal cuffs: a common error, Chest **65**:84, 1975.
77. Ching, N., and Nealon, T. F.: Cuff pressure measurements, Chest **66**:604, 1974.
78. Jenicek, J. A., Danner, C. A., and Allen, C. R.: Continuous cuff inflation during long term intubation and ventilation: evaluation of technique, Anesth. Analg. **52**:252, 1973.
79. Cohen, P. J., Alexander, S. C., Smith, T. C., Reivich, M., and Wollman, H.: Effects of hypoxia and normocarbia on cerebral blood flow and metabolism in conscious man, J. Appl. Physiol. **23**:183, 1967.
80. Lee, J., et al.: Central venous oxygen saturation in shock; a study in man, Anesthesiology **36**:472, 1972.
81. Krauss, X. H., Pieter, D., Verdou, W., Hugen-Holtz, P. G., Nauta, J.: On-line monitoring of mixed venous oxygen saturation after cardiothoracic surgery, Thorax **30**:636, 1975.
82. Mithoefer, J. C., Holford, F. D., and Keighley, J. F.: The effect of oxygen administration on mixed venous oxygenation in chronic obstructive pulmonary disease, Chest **66**:122, 1974.
83. Tenny, S. M.: A theoretical analysis of the relationship between venous blood and mean tissue oxygen pressure, Respir. Physiol. **20**:283, 1974.
84. Barrocas, M., et al.: Gas exchange abnormalities in diffuse lung disease, Am. Rev. Respir. Dis. **104**:72, 1971.
85. Snider, G.: Interpretation of the arterial oxygen and carbon dioxide partial pressure. A simplified approach for bedside use, Chest **63**:801, 1973.
86. West, J. B.: Ventilation/blood-flow and gas exchange, ed. 2, Philadelphia, 1970, F. A. Davis Co.
87. Hedley-Whyte, J., Laver, M. B., and Bendixen, H. H.: Effects of changes in tidal ventilation on physiologic shunting, Am. J. Physiol. **206**:891, 1964.
88. Benatar, S. R., Hewlett, A. M., and Nunn, J. F.: The use of iso-shunt line for control of oxygen therapy, Br. J. Anaesth. **45**:711, 1973.
89. Druger, G. L., Simmons, D. H., and Levy, S. E.: The determination of shunt-like effects and its use in clinical practice, Am. Rev. Resp. Dis. **108**:1261, 1973.
90. Suwa, K., Geffin, B., Pontoppidan, H., and Bendixen, H. H.: A nomogram for dead space requirement during prolonged artificial ventilation, Anesthesiology **29**:1206, 1968.
91. Webb, H. H., and Tierney, D. F.: Experimental pulmonary edema due to intermittent positive pressure ventilation with high inflation pressures, protection by positive end-expiratory pressure, Am. Rev. Respir. Dis. **110**:556, 1974.
92. Scoggin, C., Nett, L., Pettey, T.: Clinical evaluation of a new ear oximeter, Heart Lung **6**:121, 1977.
93. Flick, M. R., and Block, A. J.: Continuous in vivo measurement of arterial oxygen saturation by oximetry, Heart Lung **6**:990, 1977.
94. Huch, A., and Huch, R.: Transcutaneous noninvasive monitoring of pO_2, Hosp. Pract. **2**:43, 1976.
95. Peabody, J. L., Gregory, G. A., Willis, M. M., and Tooley, W. H.: Transcutaneous oxygen tension in sick infants, Am. Rev. Respir. Dis. **118**:83, 1978.
96. Al-Diaidy, W., Skeates, S., Hill, D. W., and Tinker, J.: The use of transcutaneous oxygen electrodes in intensive therapy, Intens. Care Med. **3**:35, 1977.
97. Weibel, E. R.: Oxygen effect on lung cells, Arch. Intern. Med. **128**:54, 1971.
98. Kapanci, Y., Weibel, E. R., Kaplan, H. P., and Robinson, F. R.: Pathogenesis and reversibility of the pulmonary lesions of oxygen toxicity in monkeys. II. Ultrastructural and morphometric studies, Lab. Invest. **20**:101, 1969.
99. Kaplan, H., Robinson, S., Kapanci, Y., and Weibel, E. R.: Pathogenesis and reversibility of the pulmonary lesions of oxygen toxicity in monkeys, clinical and light microscopic studies, Lab. Invest. **20**:94, 1969.

100. Kistler, G. S., Caldwell, P. R. B., and Weibel, E. R.: Development of fine structural damage to alveolar and capillary lining cells in oxygen poisoned rat lungs, J. Cell. Biol. **32:**605, 1967.

101. Nash, G., Blennerhassett, J. B., and Pontoppidan, H.: Pulmonary lesions associated with oxygen therapy and artificial ventilation, N. Engl. J. Med. **276:**368, 1967.

102. Barber, R. E., Lee, J., Hamilton, W. K.: Oxygen toxicity in man; a prospective study in patients with irreversible brain damage, N. Engl. J. Med. **283:**1478, 1970.

103. Hyde, R. W., and Rawson, A. J.: Unintentional iatrogenic oxygen pneumonitis—response therapy, Ann. Intern. Med. **71:**517, 1969.

104. Nash, G., Bowen, J. A., and Langlinais, P. C.: Respiratory lung, a misnomer, Arch. Pathol. **91:**234, 1971.

105. West, J. B.: Pulmonary gas exchange in the critically ill patient, Crit. Care Med. **2:**171, 1974.

106. Huber, G., La Force, M., and Mason, R.: Impairment and recovery of pulmonary antibacterial defense mechanisms after oxygen administration, J. Clin. Invest. **49:**47a, 1970. (Abstract 149.)

107. Morgan, T. E., Finley, T. N., Huber, G. L., and Fiaklow, H.: Alterations in pulmonary surface active lipids during exposure to increased oxygen tension, J. Clin. Invest. **44:** 1737, 1965.

108. Gamsu, G., Singer, M., Vincent, J., Berry, S., and Nadel, J.: Postoperative impairment of mucus transport in the lung, Am. Rev. Respir. Dis. **114:**673, 1976.

109. Singer, M. M., Wright, F., Stanley, L., Roe, B., and Hamilton, W. K.: Oxygen toxicity in man; a prospective study in patients after open-heart surgery, N. Engl. J. Med. **283:** 1473, 1970.

110. Pontoppidan, H., and Berry, P. R.: Regulation of the inspired oxygen concentrations during artificial ventilation, J.A.M.A. **201:**11, 1967.

111. Pontoppidan, H., Hedley-Whyte, J., Bendixon, H. H., Laver, M. B., and Radford, E. P.: Ventilation and oxygen requirements during prolonged artificial ventilation in patients with respiratory failure, N. Engl. J. Med. **273:**401, 1965.

112. Radford, E.: Ventilation standards for use in artificial respiration, J. Appl. Physiol. **7:**451, 1955.

113. Bendixen, H. H.: Rational ventilator modes for respiratory failure, Crit. Care Med. **2:**225, 1974.

114. Ayres, S. M., and Grace, W. J.: Inappropriate ventilation and hypoxemia as causes of cardiac arrhythmias. The control of arrhythmias without antiarrhythmic drugs, Am. J. Med. **46:**495, 1969.

115. Lipton, B., and Kahn, M.: Carbon dioxide and large volume ventilation in the management of patients undergoing cardiac surgery, Can. Anesth. Soc. J. **19:**49, 1972.

116. Stoyka, W. W.: The reliability and usefulness of the Suwa nomogram in patients in respiratory failure, Can. Anaesth. Soc. J. **17:**119, 1970.

117. Selecky, P. A., Wasserman, K., Klein, M., and Ziment, I.: A graphic approach to assessing interrelationships among minute ventilation, arterial carbon dioxide tension, and ratio of physiologic dead space to tidal volume in patients on respirators, Am. Rev. Respir. Dis. **117:**181, 1978.

118. Breivik, H., Grenvik, A., Millen, E., and Safar, P.: Normalizing low arterial CO_2 tensions during mechanical ventilation, Chest **63:**525, 1973.

119. Mazzara, J. T., Ayres, S. M., and Grace, W. J.: Extreme hypercapnia in the critically ill patient, Am. J. Med. **56:** 450, 1974.

120. Barach, A. L.: Hypercapnia in chronic obstructive lung disease—an adaptive response to low-flow oxygen theraphy, Chest **66:**112, 1974.

121. Kettel, L. J., Diener, C. F., Morse, J. O., Stern, H. F., and Burrows, B.: Treatment of acute respiratory acidosis in chronic obstructive lung disease, J.A.M.A. **217:**1503, 1971.

122. Safar, P., Nemota, E. M., and Severinghaus, J. W.: Pathogenesis of central nervous system disorder during artificial hyperventilation in compensated hypercarbia in dogs, Crit. Care Med. **1:**5, 1973.

123. Levine, B. E., Kravetz, H. M., Spotnitz, M., and Westfall, R. E.: The role of the community hospital in acute respiratory failure management, Chest **62**(suppl.):10S, 1972.

124. Bedford, R. F., and Wollman, H.: Complications of percutaneous radial artery cannulation; an objective prospective study in man, Anesthesiology **38:**228, 1973.

125. Mortensen, J. E.: Clinical sequela from arterial needle puncture, cannulation and incision, Circulation **35:**1118, 1967.

126. Matthews, J. I., and Gibbons, R. B.: Embolization complicating radial-artery puncture, Ann. Intern. Med. **75:** 77, 1971.

127. Gardner, R. M., Schwartz, R., Wong, H. C., and Burke, J. P.: Percutaneous indwelling radial artery catheters for monitoring cardiovascular function. Prospective study of the risk of thrombosis and infection, N. Engl. J. Med. **290:**1227, 1974.

128. Petty, T. I., Bigelow, D. B., and Levine, B. E.: The simplicity and safety of arterial puncture, J.A.M.A. **195:**693, 1966.

129. Kilburn, K. H.: Shock, seizures and coma with alkalosis during hyperventilation, Ann. Intern. Med. **65:**977, 1966.

130. Phillips, B., and Peretz, D. I.: A comparison of central venous and arterial blood gas values in the critically ill, Ann. Intern. Med. **70:**745, 1969.

131. Lowenstein, E., Little, J. W., and Hing, H. L.: Prevention of cerebral embolization from flushing radial-artery cannulas, N. Engl. J. Med. **285:**1414, 1971.

132. Egan, D. F.: Fundamentals of respiratory therapy, ed. 3, St. Louis, 1977, The C. V. Mosby Co.

133. Mushin, W. W., Rendau-Baker, L., Thompson, P. W., and Mapelson, W. W.: Automatic ventilation of the lungs, Philadelphia, 1969, F. A. Davis Co.

134. Rattenborg, C., and DeBorde, R.: Lung ventilation: function and principles, Inhalation Ther. **12:**48, 1967.

135. Fitzgerald, L. M.: Mechanical ventilation, Heart Lung **5:** 939, 1976.

136. Knapp, R. B., and Dubow, H. S.: Diazepam as an induction agent for patients with cardiopulmonary disease, South. Med. J. **63:**1451, 1970.

137. Mead, J., and Collier, C.: Relation of volume history of lungs to respiratory mechanics in anesthetized dogs, J. Appl. Physiol. **14:**669, 1959.

138. Hedley-Whyte, J., Pontoppidan, H., and Laver, M. B.:

Arterial oxygenation during hypothermia, Anesthesiology **26:**595, 1965.

139. Opie, L. H., Smith, A. C., and Spalding, J. M.: Conscious appreciation of the effects produced by independent changes of ventilation volume and end-tidal PCO_2 in paralyzed patients, J. Physiol. (Lond.) **149:**494, 1959.

140. Steier, M., Ching, N., Roberts, E. B., and Nealon, T. F.: Pneumothorax complicating continuous ventilatory support, J. Thorac. Cardiovasc. Surg. **67:**17, 1974.

141. Hilberman, M., and Peters, R. M.: A data collection system for intensive care, Crit. Care Med. **3:**27, 1975.

142. Kramer, S. G., and Lipson, C. S.: Intensive care unit flow sheet, Surgery **67:**590, 1970.

143. Kausnitz, P., Druger, G. L., Yorra, F., and Simmons, D. H.: Mixed venous oxygen tension and *hyperlactaternia,* J.A.M.A. **236:**570, 1976.

144. Nicotra, M. B., Stevens, P. M., Viroslav, J., and Alvarez, A. A.: Physiologic evaluation of positive end-expiratory pressure ventilation, Chest **64:**10, 1973.

145. Stevens, P. M.: Positive end-expiratory pressure breathing, Am. Thor. Soc. Basics of RD **5:**1, 1977.

146. Swan, H. J., et al.: Catheterization of the heart in man with use of a flow-directed balloon-tipped catheter, N. Engl. J. Med. **283:**447, 1970.

147. Sugerman, H. J., Rogers, R. M., and Miller, L. D.: Positive end-expiratory pressure (PEEP) indications and physiologic considerations, Chest **62**(suppl.):86S, 1972.

148. Kumar, A., et al.: Continuous positive-pressure ventilation in acute respiratory failure, effects on hemodynamics and lung function, N. Engl. J. Med. **283:**1430, 1970.

149. Suter, P. M., Fairley, H. B., and Isenberg, M. D.: Optimum end-expiratory airway pressure in patients with acute pulmonary failure, N. Engl. J. Med. **292:**284, 1975.

150. Tenaillon, A., Labrousse, J., Gateau, D., and Lissac, J.: Optimal positive end-expiratory pressure and static lung compliance, N. Engl. J. Med. **299:**774, 1978.

151. Kirby, R. R., et al.: High level positive end expiratory pressure (PEEP) in acute respiratory failure, Chest **67:**1975.

152. Nicotra, M. B.: The value of flow directed intravascular catheters in cardiorespiratory failure, Am. Rev. Respir. Dis. **107:**1111, 1973.

153. Cournand, A., et al.: Physiologic studies of the effects of intermittent positive pressure breathing on cardiac output in man, Am. J. Physiol. **152:**162, 1948.

154. Powers, S. R., et al.: Physiologic consequences of positive end-expiratory pressure (PEEP) ventilation, Ann. Surg. **178:**265, 1973.

155. Schapiro, M., and Daum, S.: Hemodynamics of the pulmonary circulation in patients on intermittent positive pressure breathing with a bird respiratory, Anesth. Analg. **53:**31, 1974.

156. Colgan, F. J., Nichols, F. A., and DeWeese, J. A.: Positive end-expiratory pressure, oxygen transport and the low-output state, Anesth. Analg. **53:**538, 1974.

157. Kumar, A., Pontippidan, H., Falke, K. J., Wilson, R. D., and Laver, M. B.: Pulmonary barotrauma during mechanical ventilation, Crit. Care Med. **1:**181, 1973.

158. Hodgkin, J. E., Bowser, M. A., and Burton, G. G.: Respiratory weaning, Crit. Care Med. **2:**96, 1974.

159. Sahn, S. A., and Lakshminarayan, S.: Bedside criteria for discontinuation of mechanical ventilation, Chest **63:**1002, 1973.

160. Feeley, T. W., and Hedley-Whyte, J.: Weaning from controlled ventilation and supplemental oxygen, N. Engl. J. Med. **292:**903, 1975.

161. Gregory, G. A., Kitterman, J. A., Phibbs, R. K., Tooley, W. H., and Hamilton, W. K.: Continuous positive airway pressure with spontaneous respiration: a new method of increasing arterial oxygenation in the inspiratory distress syndrome, Pediatr. Res. **4:**469, 1970.

162. Feeley, T. W., Saumarez, R., Klick, J. M., McNabb, T. G., and Skillman, J. J.: Positive end-expiratory pressure in weaning patients from a controlled ventilation: a prospective randomized trial, Lancet **2:**725, 1975.

163. Downs, J. B., Klein, E. F., Desautels, D., Modell, J. H., and Kirby, R.: Intermittent mandatory ventilation; a new approach to weaning patients from mechanical ventilators, Chest **64:**331, 1973.

164. Shapiro, B. A., Harrison, R. A., Walton, J. R., and Davidson, R.: Intermittent demand ventilation (IDV): A new technique for supporting ventilation in critically ill patients, Respir. Care **21:**521, 1976.

165. Divertie, M. B.: Extracorporeal oxygenation: a flower before the spring, Chest **66:**343, 1974.

166. Mortensen, J. D.: Extracorporeal membrane oxygenation for pulmonary assist in patients with ARF, Chest **67:**129, 1975.

167. Sladen, A., Laver, M. D., and Pontopiddan, H.: Pulmonary complications and water retention in prolonged mechanical ventilation, N. Engl. J. Med. **279:**448, 1968.

168. Sanford, J. P.: Infection control in critical care units, Crit. Care Med. **2:**211, 1974.

169. Benner, E. J., Munzinger, J. P., and Chan, R.: Superinfections of the lung; an evaluation by serial transtracheal aspiration, West. J. Med. **121:**173, 1974.

170. Katz, N. M., Agle, D. P., DePalma, R. G., and DeCossee, J. J.: Delirium in surgical patients under intensive care, utility of mental status examination, Arch. Surg. **104:**310, 1972.

171. Hale, M., Koss, N., Kerstein, M., Camp, K., and Barash, P.: Psychiatric complications in a surgical ICU, Crit. Care Med. **5:**199, 1977.

172. Fuhs, M., Rieser, M., and Brisbon, D.: Nursing in a respiratory intensive care unit, Chest **62**(suppl.):14S, 1972.

CHAPTER 16

Management of the patient with atherosclerotic peripheral vascular disease

Perry M. Shoor and Thomas J. Fogarty

Although its complications were recognized during ancient times and the term "atherosclerosis" itself was coined in the early nineteenth century, only during the last 30 or so years have we been able to offer surgical intervention in the treatment of symptomatic atherosclerotic vascular disease. From the early pioneering works performed in the mid-1940's as treatment of congenital cardiovascular abnormalities, the field of vascular surgery has grown both in complexity and scope. The variety of different surgical procedures being performed has grown markedly during the last 15 years and there are now over 75,000 major arterial vascular reconstructions performed yearly in the United States.

The development and growth of vascular surgery has presented a unique challenge to the critical care specialist. As the benefits of peripheral vascular surgery are being extended to an even larger patient population, the care of these critically ill patients can be expected to become even more commonplace throughout the intensive care units of the country. To provide the type of optimum care that allows these patients to undergo reconstructive vascular surgery with minimum morbidity and mortality, the critical care specialist must have an understanding of the nature of the atherosclerotic disease process and the procedures used to counteract its sequelae, as well as the specifics of postoperative care that

apply to the different types of arterial vascular reconstructions. This chapter will attempt to present the pertinent facets of the atherosclerotic disease process, as well as general principles concerning the evaluation, treatment, and rehabilitation of the patient with atherosclerotic peripheral vascular disease.

ATHEROSCLEROSIS
■ What is atherosclerosis?

Atherosclerosis is a disease process affecting primarily the large and medium-sized arteries. The wall of these arteries is comprised of three layers: the innermost intima, the media, and the outermost adventitia. Atherosclerosis can be thought of as a pathologic process that is superimposed on the normal age-dependent degenerative changes of the arterial wall. The World Health Organization defined atherosclerosis as "a variable combination of changes of the *intima* of arteries consisting of a focal accumulation of lipids (fatty substances), complex carbohydrates, blood elements, fibrous tissue and calcium deposits."

Patients become symptomatic relatively late in the disease process, as it has been shown that the earliest changes, fatty streaks (the accumulation of lipids in the intimal layer), are commonly found in the aorta of youngsters by the time they reach puberty. It then usually takes several decades for

295

Stage I asymptomatic	Stage II symptomatic	Stage III complications

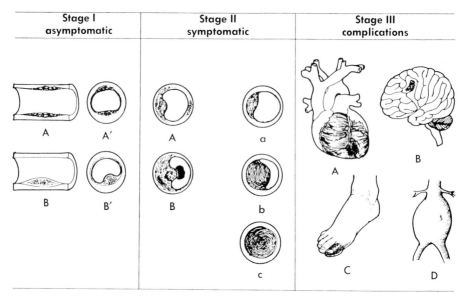

Fig. 16-1. Diagram of natural history of atherosclerosis. Stage I, asymptomatic: *A* and *A'*, fatty streaks; *B* and *B'*, fibrous plaque. Stage II, symptomatic: *A*, fibrous plaque and medial calcification; *B*, enlarged fibrous plaque with thrombus formation; *a*, asymptomatic arterial stenosis; *b*, significant hemodynamic stenosis; *c*, complete occlusion. Stage III, complications: *A*, myocardial infarct; *B*, brain infarct; *C*, gangrene; *D*, aneurysm. (From Vascular surgery principles and techniques by H. Haimovici. Copyright © 1976 McGraw-Hill Book Co. Used with permission of McGraw-Hill Book Co.)

the fatty streaks to "mature" into the next stage of the atherosclerotic process: the fibrous plaque (Fig. 16-1). At this stage the patient is in his or her 40's and is usually still asymptomatic, the fibrous plaque causing minimal narrowing of the arterial lumen. It is on this matrix of fibrous plaque that progression to symptom-causing lesions may occur. Calcification of the intimal plaques leads to further narrowing of the lumen and makes the now irregular plaque a likely site for superimposed thrombosis. Aggregates of platelets and fibrin from the flowing blood accumulate on the surface of the plaque and may result in thrombotic occlusion of the artery, already narrowed by the atherosclerotic process. It is then a combination of atherosclerosis of the vessel wall and secondary thrombosis that leads to occlusion of the arterial lumen. Because the lumen of the vessel may be narrowed by up to more than one half and not result in decreased blood flow, often the patient first becomes

markedly symptomatic at the time of the thrombotic occlusion.

Besides occlusion, the atherosclerotic process may result in other symptom-producing lesions. If the intimal thickening results in a thinning out and weakening of the media (which by virtue of its smooth muscle and elastic fibers lends strength to the arterial wall), aneurysmal dilatation may result. Aneurysms may lead to symptoms by nature of their propensity to rupture (with subsequent hemorrhage), thrombose (resulting in occlusion), and act as a source of embolization of atheromatous and thrombotic debris into the arterial circulation.

Finally, as the intimal plaque grows thicker, nourishment from the blood flow may become insufficient. The subsequent ischemic necrosis and local mechanical stresses result in degeneration of the intimal surface of the plaque, resulting in the so-called ulcerative plaque, which may act as a source of further arterial embolization.

■ Who is at risk for atherosclerotic vascular disease?

Although atherosclerosis can affect anyone, there are several factors that indicate an increased propensity toward the development of atherosclerotic vascular disease. One might imagine the hypothetical person at maximal risk as follows: a 60-year-old hypertensive, diabetic male who smokes heavily, exercises little, consumes a diet high in saturated fats and cholesterol, and has a strong family history of atherosclerotic vascular disease.

Age and gender

Although there are exceptions to the rule, the atherosclerotic patient usually becomes symptomatic during the fifth and sixth decades of life, and premenopausal women are infrequently affected by symptomatic atheromatous disease.

Hypertension

Hypertension appears to be an independent risk factor, and in many studies a significant correlation between the level of hypertension and the extent and severity of the atherosclerotic process has been demonstrated.

Diabetes

Although the strong association between adult onset diabetes and premature and extensive atherosclerotic disease has been recognized for some time, it has recently been recognized that there is also an association between both abnormal glucose tolerance and asymptomatic hyperglycemia and the development of symptomatic atherosclerotic lesions in the cerebral, peripheral, and coronary arteries.

Smoking

There is a wealth of information available attesting to the fact that a significant and direct correlation exists between the quantity of cigarettes smoked and the following: the risk of cerebrovascular disease, the development of premature atherosclerotic lesions of the extremities, and the mortality rates from coronary artery disease. Thus it appears that cigarette smoking is one of the more significant risk factors yet identified, both by virtue of its presumed etiologic role in the development and progression of the atherosclerotic process and its potential for reversibility by quitting the smoking habit.

Exercise

Although it has been hard to document a significant protective effect of exercise on the development of atherosclerosis, many people believe that there is one. It has been shown, however, that a regular plan of exercise may decrease the symptoms produced from lesions already present, by stimulating the development of collateral arterial channels.

Dietary cholesterol and saturated fats

Based on population studies, a positive relationship between the development of premature and extensive atherosclerosis and an excessive dietary intake of saturated fats and total calories has been shown. This type of diet leads to obesity, but whether obesity is itself an independent risk factor is not clear. In addition, it has been demonstrated that there is a very strong correlation between the serum β-lipoprotein fraction (which contains most of the cholesterol) and the incidence of atherosclerotic peripheral and coronary artery disease.

Heredity

Atherosclerotic involvement of the peripheral and coronary arteries has often been recognized to run in families; however, the mechanisms responsible for these hereditary associations have not yet been discovered.

■ Are all segments of the vascular system affected with equal frequency?

Although atherosclerosis is a systemic disease, there are certain areas of the arterial tree that are usually affected earliest and with increased severity. The propensity for some of these sites may be explained by chronic intimal damage secondary to turbulent flow at areas surrounding branches and bifurcations. Chronic arterial compression or bending secondary to nearby ligaments is thought to predispose other sites to premature lesions. Since the atherosclerotic process often follows certain predictable anatomic patterns, we are often able to identify the sites of

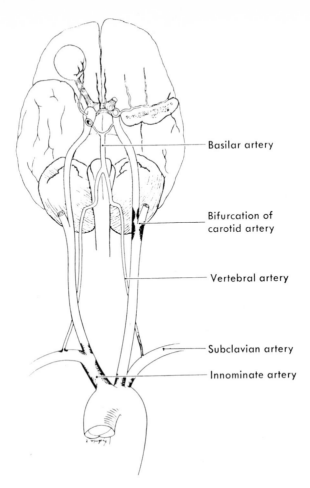

Basilar artery

Bifurcation of
carotid artery

Vertebral artery

Subclavian artery

Innominate artery

Fig. 16-2. Usual sites of extracranial occlusive disease affecting cerebral circulation. (From Hershey, F. B., and Colman, C. H.: Atlas of vascular surgery, ed. 3, St. Louis, 1973, The C. V. Mosby Co.)

involvement, predict future sequelae, and plan the general operative approach by the signs and symptoms present.

The carotid bifurcation and the origin of the arch vessels are the sites of common predilection in the extracranial cerebrovascular circulation (Fig. 16-2). The axillary and upper extremity arteries are infrequently involved in the absence of local arterial trauma. The thoracic and supra-renal abdominal aorta are also usually remarkably free of significant atherosclerotic lesions, and when present, they most frequently affect just the origins of the mesenteric and renal arteries.

On the other hand, the terminal aorta and proximal iliac arteries are among the sites most frequently affected by significant stenosis. Lesions are also frequently found throughout the arteries of the lower extremity, the proximal and distal portions of the superficial femoral artery being affected with greatest frequency (Fig. 16-3). It should also be understood that the patient with significant atherosclerosis in one area, that is, aortoiliac, can be expected to have lesions in the coronary and extracranial cerebral systems as well. However, the severity of these concomitant lesions is not easily predictable.

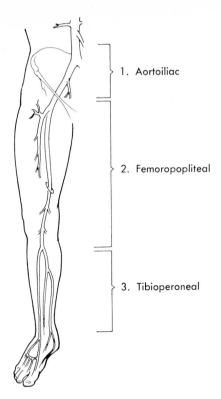

1. Aortoiliac

2. Femoropopliteal

3. Tibioperoneal

Fig. 16-3. Diagram depicting the three major areas of atherosclerotic involvement of the lower extremity. (From Vascular surgery, principles and techniques by H. Haimovici. Copyright © 1976 McGraw-Hill Book Co. Used with permission of McGraw-Hill Book Co.)

■ **What kinds of symptoms are produced by advanced atherosclerosis?**

When the atherosclerotic process results in aneurysm formation, a palpable mass usually results, and rapid enlargement or rupture usually produces significant pain. If the process results in stenosis of a major artery, a significant reduction in blood flow (oxygen and nutrient supply) may be produced. A severe stenosis may result in a resting decrease in blood flow; however, if less severe, the blood supply may be insufficient only during periods of increased blood flow requirement, such as during muscular exercise. Insufficient blood flow results in either decreased function (a transient ischemic attack in the case of the cerebral circulation) or pain (muscle clau-

dication) in the tissue afflicted. Finally, if the atherosclerotic process results in the thrombotic or embolic occlusion of a significant portion of the arterial tree, nutritional flow may be so compromised that tissue necrosis occurs. Common examples of this complication are cerebral and coronary infarcts and gangrene of the toes or feet.

EVALUATION OF THE PATIENT WITH PERIPHERAL VASCULAR DISEASE
■ **What are the pertinent aspects of the patient's history?**

A carefully taken history will, by itself, reveal much regarding the extent of the patient's disease. Generally, there is a correlation between the severity of symptoms and the extent of atherosclerotic lesions present. Those patients with the most severe symptoms often have significant stenoses present at two or more levels (such as both aortoiliac and femoropopliteal lesions).

Patients with ischemic peripheral vascular symptoms often suffer from other manifestations of atherosclerosis, as well as varied other systemic disease states. The critical care specialist should be able to identify these conditions, as they may significantly alter patient management. The patient should be specifically questioned for history of diabetes, arterial hypertension, hyperlipoproteinemia, myocardial infarction or angina, and stroke. The patient should be questioned regarding smoking history, and the duration, severity, and progression of any symptoms present should be ascertained.

Common symptoms associated with cerebrovascular insufficiency include transient ischemic attacks (TIA's), reversible ischemic neurologic deficits (RIND's), completed stroke, and amaurosis fugax.

A TIA is a temporary neurologic deficit that completely resolves within 24 hours; usually within the first 60 minutes. TIA's are thought to result from either embolism of small platelet, cholesterol, and fibrin aggregates or from momentary decreases in cerebral flow secondary to atherosclerotic plaque in the extracranial cerebrovascular system. The TIA may manifest by unilateral extremity weakness, paralysis or paresthesia, and periods of aphasia may accompany the lateralizing signs or occur independently.

A RIND can be thought of as a TIA that takes greater than 1 day but less than 3 days for complete recovery and implies a more significant cerebral insult. The patient with a frank stroke usually has a fixed neurologic deficit that remains relatively stable. The presence of a frank stroke implies cerebral damage, and although some recovery can be expected with time, a residual deficit often remains. Another symptom of extracranial atherosclerosis, amaurosis fugax (transient monocular blindness), results from showers of minute emboli to the retinal arteries. The lesions most commonly associated with this symptom are ulcerated (irregular) plaques at the carotid bifurcation.

The patient with atherosclerotic involvement of the aortoiliac or femoropopliteal system usually has symptoms of discomfort or pain secondary to deficient muscle blood flow. Claudication, a crampy pain in the calf or foot often associated with fatigue and brought on by exercise, is the most frequent manifestation of peripheral atherosclerosis. Typically the pain subsides rather quickly on cessation of exercise, only to recur on resumption of a similar amount of effort. If progression of disease leads to further impairment in blood supply, rest pain may result. Usually localized to the foot, this pain occurs without the added stress of exercise and is often only relieved with dependency by hanging the foot over the edge of the bed or by sitting up in a chair. The presence of rest pain implies very serious compromise in nutritive blood supply and often just shortly precedes the occurrence of gangrene. The patient should be questioned regarding claudication as to frequency of occurrence, level of stress necessary to precipitate an attack, as well as the duration and progression of symptoms. The presence or absence of rest pain should be ascertained, and episodic night cramps in the legs should be differentiated from true ischemic symptoms as just described.

■ What should the critical care specialist look for during the physical examination?

The critical care specialist should be able to perform a detailed evaluation of the peripheral circulation. This is important not only during the initial evaluation of the patient but also during the postoperative period. The status of the surgical repair may then be checked and any complications quickly noted. Palpation of peripheral pulses is the mainstay of the physical examination. A simple but effective system for grading pulses uses a scale of 0 to 2: 0 = no palpable pulse; 1+ = pulse present but diminished; and 2+ = a normal pulse. The so-called supranormal pulse is a manifestation of the cardiac abnormality, such as aortic valvular insufficiency, and not part of the evaluation of the arterial tree.

A complete evaluation should include examination of pulses over the following arteries: carotid, superficial temporal, brachial, radial, ulnar, femoral, popliteal, posterior tibial, and dorsalis pedis arteries. In addition, bruits (the sound produced by turbulent blood flow across a stenosis) should be listened for over the carotid, iliac, and femoral arteries. A bruit may be produced by narrowing, yet insufficient to produce a significant decrease in palpable pulse and can therefore be a more sensitive indicator of mild to moderate stenosis.

Assessment of the color, temperature, and condition of the skin can add information as to the severity of the underlying vascular disease. Patients with mild to moderate inflow obstruction usually have normal appearing feet. When the process is more advanced, a cool, pale foot with atrophic skin and absent toe hair will often be found. These patients often demonstrate extreme blanching of the skin on elevation of the extremity and a marked rubor when in a dependent position. Areas of ischemic skin necrosis (ulceration) and frank gangrene of the toes and foot attest to the severity of the occlusive process.

■ What laboratory tests are pertinent for the vascular patient?

Specific tests offering potential of adding to the initial evaluation of the vascular patient include urinalysis, hematocrit, platelet count, uric acid, fasting blood sugar, creatinine, fasting cholesterol, and serum triglycerides. When cholesterol and triglyceride values are elevated, a serum lipoprotein electrophoresis should be obtained. A chest x-ray film and ECG are also indicated as concomitant pulmonary and atherosclerotic coronary artery disease are quite common. These laboratory tests are utilized to screen out those patients with gout, diabetes, uremia, and hyperlipidemia—conditions often known to be associated with potentially preventable and extensive atherosclerotic vascular disease.

If the patient is scheduled for surgery, the clotting system should be checked with prothrombin time (PT) and partial thromboplastin time (PTT) determinations in addition to an inquiry as to the presence of previous bleeding problems. The blood bank should prepare an adequate number of units for the operation planned, and if the patient has been on aspirin-containing medication within the preceding 10 days, platelet function might be expected to be compromised and fresh platelet concentrates should be available if needed.

■ What radiologic techniques are utilized during the workup of the atherosclerotic patient?

The modern era of angiography was ushered in by Seldinger in the early 1950's. His technique of percutaneous catheter angiography has been widely accepted and is the most commonly utilized method today. An artery, usually the femoral, is punctured with a needle, and the return of pulsatile blood confirms proper placement. A soft flexible guide wire is inserted for a short distance up the arterial lumen. The needle is then pulled back out over the guide wire, leaving the wire within the artery. After an appropriate angiographic catheter is threaded over the guide wire and advanced into the arterial lumen, the guide wire is then removed. The catheter is then positioned under fluoroscopic control to the desired location, and angiograms are taken. Utilizing percutaneous femoral technique, catheters can be easily manipulated into the aortic branches for selective arteriograms or left in the aorta for flush studies.

An optimal angiographic examination requires the use of serial filming, preferably in two planes, and an adequate volume of contrast media injected rapidly just upstream from the area under study. The presently used angiographic contrast media contain iodinated salts that absorb the x-rays, and although quite safe, both allergic and dose-related toxic manifestations are occasionally seen with these agents. Allergic reactions may be manifest by urticaria, bronchospasm, and even anaphylactic shock. Dose-related toxic manifestations may affect the heart (myocardial depression and vasodilatation), kidneys (renal failure), and central venous system (convulsions and depression of level of consciousness).

At the completion of the study, the catheter is withdrawn from the artery and firm pressure is exerted directly over the puncture site for about 15 minutes. This pressure should tamponade the small arterial puncture site and result in hemostasis without completely occluding the arterial lumen. Complications directly related to the arterial puncture such as periarterial hematoma, pseudoaneurysm, peripheral embolization of atherosclerotic debris, and arterial occlusion occur infrequently (about 1%) when procedures are performed by well-trained and experienced angiographers.

The patient is kept flat in bed for the first 6 hours following percutaneous femoral angiography, and the critical care specialists should check the groin area for hematoma and the extremities for evidence of acute arterial insufficiency at frequent intervals (every 30 minutes for 2 hours, every 1 hour for 4 hours, then every 4 hours overnight). In addition, because the contrast media acts as an osmotic diuretic, the patient should be watched closely for signs of bladder distention or hypovolemia. It is imperative that the patient is maintained in a well-hydrated state during the periangiographic period.

■ What is the noninvasive vascular laboratory and how does it help in the evaluation of the vascular patient?

Although a careful history and physical examination will reveal a great deal of information regarding the vascular patient, documentation of the severity of these findings is often quite subjective. The quality of the patient's arterial pulse may be graded differently by two observers at the same time and even differently by the same observer at different times. The noninvasive laboratory allows a level of quantification (and hopefully objectivity) to both the initial evaluation and follow-up of the patient with peripheral vascular disease. In addition, there are areas of the body where the noninvasive laboratory can supply information not obtainable by physical examination alone. It must be remembered by both the surgeon and the critical care specialist that the noninvasive laboratory examination supplements the physical examination but does not replace it.

The basic tools used for the evaluation of the arterial vascular system are the Doppler velocity meter and the oculoplethysmograph. The Doppler velocity meter can be utilized for the evaluation of patency and quality of blood flow in any superficial artery. Clinically, it has proved to be of particular value during the evaluation of extracranial cerebral insufficiency and arterial insufficiency of the extremities. Oculoplethysmography (OPG) is used exclusively for the evaluation of the extracranial cerebral circulation.

Doppler velocity meter

These instruments all function based on the Doppler principle: the frequency of a sound wave "bounced" off a moving object will be reflected back slightly altered, and the amount of change in frequency will be proportional to the speed of that moving object. Therefore by measuring the change in sound (ultrasound) frequency, the velocity and direction of the moving object can be estimated. The Doppler instrument is used to send high-frequency sound toward an artery. The sound is reflected off the moving red cells within the artery and returns to the Doppler instrument at a slightly different frequency, which is interpreted as blood flow. If the vessel is thrombosed, there will be no movement of red blood cells, ultrasound will be reflected back with the same frequency, and no Doppler signal will be produced. It should then be clear that the Doppler instrument measures presence of flow within the artery and is not analogous to hearing the "pulse" that is palpated with the fingertips.

Doppler ultrasound produced by the commonly used instruments will penetrate tissue to a depth of about 3 cm, and subsequently only arteries fairly close to the surface can be examined. With the Doppler instrument, large arteries such as the femoral and small arteries such as the ul-

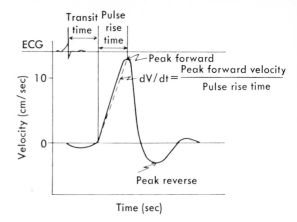

Fig. 16-4. Transcutaneous recordings of arterial velocity profile are routinely obtained at femoral, posterior tibial, and dorsalis pedis levels, with analysis of parameters indicated. Directionally sensitive Doppler device permits quantitation of such tracings. (From Fronek, A.: Am. J. Surg. **126**:207, 1973.)

nar can be easily examined. The high-frequency sound is not transmitted efficiently through air and therefore a gel is utilized as a conducting medium to provide effective transmission of sound waves between the instrument and the patient.

Normal arterial blood flow is pulsatile, with the great majority of forward flow occurring during cardiac systole. During systole, the arterial wall is stretched by the force of the blood and then during diastole returns to normal size secondary to recoil of the elastic fibers in the arterial wall. This elastic recoil of the arterial wall produces a further propulsive force to blood flow. Finally, during cardiac diastole there is a short period of time when there is actual reversal of flow in the large and medium-sized arteries. This triphasic blood velocity pattern is normal and results in the triphasic sound heard with a Doppler velocity meter over a normal large or medium-sized artery (Fig. 16-4). When atherosclerotic narrowing results in reduction in blood flow, the triphasic (flow reversal component) character is lost. With further narrowing and flow reduction, the Doppler signal becomes less intense and the separate components less crisp. Finally with collateral flow, the signal becomes faint and loses its pulsatile character to become a relatively constant "hiss." By practicing for a short time on a young person, one can gain familiarity with the normal Doppler velocity signal, and all critical care specialists should be able to recognize the difference between normal and abnormal flow patterns.

Oculoplethysmography and carotid phonoangiography (OPG-CPA)

The arterial pulse originates within the heart secondary to cardiac systole and is propagated rapidly throughout the arterial tree and generally will arrive simultaneously at two sites equidistant from the heart. However, an area of significant stenosis will slow down the velocity of pulse propagation and result in a delay in pulse arrival to a site beyond the stenosis. The pulse reaches the eye via the carotid and ophthalmic arteries and usually arrives simultaneously at each eye since they are equidistant from the heart. A significant stenosis in one carotid artery will result in a delay in pulse arrival to the eye on that side when compared to the more normal side (Fig. 16-5).

The most commonly utilized OPG instruments measure these ocular pulse arrival differences, which are only on the order of 5 to 30 msec, and thereby detect the presence of a hemodynamically significant carotid artery stenosis. The eye is numbed with a topical anesthetic and small plastic cups are placed on the sclera of the eye and held there by minimal suction. The cups then transmit the ocular pulsations to the instrument for analysis. The test can be performed in a few minutes with minimal patient discomfort and essentially no risk.

Carotid phonoangiography (CPA) utilizes a microphone to pick up sounds over the carotid arteries and an oscilloscope to display them visually. The microphone is sequentially positioned over the upper, middle, and lower portions of the cervical carotid artery and will localize any bruits present. Since the first and second heart sounds are also picked up, the duration of the bruit can be determined as well as its intensity. Utilizing recordings from all three locations, bruits originating from the carotid bifurcation can be differentiated from those originating within the me-

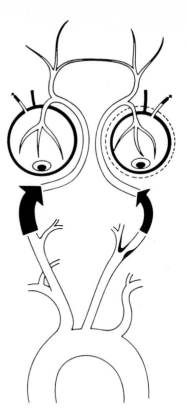

Fig. 16-5. Conceptual representation of slower expansion of left ocular globe during early systole owing to reduced arterial inflow secondary to proximal arterial stenosis. (From Bernstein, E. F., editor: Noninvasive diagnostic techniques in vascular disease, St. Louis, 1978, The C. V. Mosby Co.)

diastinum, such as from the aortic valve. Bruits associated with hemodynamically significant stenoses usually extend throughout systole and are often of considerable loudness. However, it should be remembered that with an occluded or extremely stenotic artery there may be no associated bruit secondary to insufficient blood flow velocity.

The noninvasive arterial examination

The Doppler instrument can be utilized to examine the blood velocity waveform in both auditory and graphic representation over various arterial sites. A complete peripheral arterial study would include bilateral examinations of the brachial, radial, and ulnar arteries as well as the common femoral, superficial femoral, popliteal, dorsalis pedis, and posterior tibial arteries. By comparing the waveform obtained with normal standards, as well as to the waveform from the same location on the other extremity, information regarding the state of the vascular tree can be obtained.

In addition, the Doppler instrument may be utilized for the determination of sequential arterial occlusion pressures. When a standardized pneumatic (blood pressure) cuff is placed around an extremity and inflated to suprasystolic pressure, it acts as an arterial tourniquet to stop the flow of blood. As pressure is slowly released from the cuff, the Doppler probe (positioned over the artery beyond the cuff) will record the instant that blood starts to flow again. That cuff pressure is a measure of the intra-arterial systolic pressure. If there is a significant narrowing in the artery, the systolic pressure will be decreased in the arterial segments beyond the stenosis in proportion to the severity of the stenosis present.

Cuffs are usually placed at upper thigh, lower thigh, and calf levels, and the arterial flow is measured by a Doppler instrument over arteries distal to the cuffs. The occlusion pressures obtained relate to the level of the cuff and not the site of the Doppler probe, except in the lower leg where separate occlusion pressures can be obtained for the dorsalis pedis and posterior tibial arteries. If no significant stenoses are present in the arterial tree, the segmental arterial occlusion pressures will show no decrease when sequentially measured from upper thigh to ankle. In fact, there is normally a slight increase of occlusion pressure as one measures proximally to distally in an extremity. Therefore any significant drop in occlusion pressure points to a hemodynamically significant stenosis located in the intervening arterial segment.

The absolute value of the arterial occlusion pressure at any level is not as informative as the relative pressure between that level and the "central" arterial pressure. Because upper extremity atherosclerosis is much less common than lower extremity involvement, the higher arterial occlu-

sion pressure between the two brachial arteries is taken as the reference central pressure. The occlusion pressure at any level can then be expressed as a ratio comparing it to the brachial pressure. If no stenoses are present, the ratio (that is, ankle/brachial pressure) should fall between 1.0 and 1.1. Significant stenosis results in decreased occlusion pressures and thereby lowers the segmental pressure index as well. A drop in the index of greater than 0.15 between any two adjacent levels is considered significant, and the magnitude of the index drop is proportionate to the severity of the stenosis.

At bedside, the critical care specialist can use the Doppler probe to check the normalcy of flow in palpable arteries as well as document the presence or absence of flow in arteries lacking a palpable pulse. Since a strong palpable pulse is almost always associated with a normal artery and good arterial inflow pressures, the Doppler instrument has the greatest utility in those situations where the pulse is weak or not palpable at all. Therefore, when assessing the arterial circulation, an attempt is first made to palpate the arterial pulse. Then the area where the artery was palpated or is expected to be is covered with an acoustical gel, and the Doppler probe is slowly moved across the skin with gentle pressure. The Doppler signal is monitored with a speaker or headset, and the probe is positioned directly over the artery by identifying the site of maximum Doppler signal.

GENERAL ASPECTS OF THE OPERATIVE TREATMENT OF THE VASCULAR PATIENT

In order to provide optimum acute and long-term care for the vascular patient following surgery, it is necessary to have an understanding of the fundamental aspects of anesthetic and operative techniques utilized. Only when the critical care specialist has knowledge of the specific details of the anesthetic and surgical approach, can he or she play an integral part in the patient's recovery. This knowledge allows the critical care specialist to compare the patient's progress against that expected for the specific operative procedure as well as anticipate the more commonly occurring complications.

■ What types of operative procedures are commonly performed?

The atherosclerotic lesions resulting in the need for surgical intervention are stenosis, ulcerative plaque, occlusion, aneurysm, and dissection; the operative procedure chosen depends on the type and severity of the lesion and its location. Although operative intervention is usually used for symptomatic patients, certain lesions such as a large abdominal aortic aneurysm require operation even in the absence of symptoms. The commonly performed operations include endarterectomy, angioplasty, arterial replacement and bypass grafting, and embolectomy.

Endarterectomy

When the atherosclerotic process results in a stenosis that is relatively localized to a limited arterial segment, endarterectomy may be the procedure of choice to restore normal lumenal diameter and flow. As mentioned previously, the atherosclerotic process is mainly limited to the intimal layer with occasional involvement of the inner third of the media. The remainder of the media may become somewhat atrophic, possibly as a result of compression from the thickened intima.

A natural separation is often present within the medial layer of the arterial wall and can be uti-

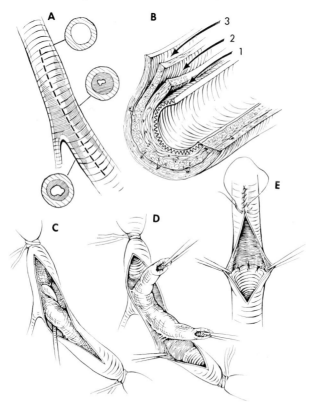

Fig. 16-6. Principles of endarterectomy. **A,** Longitudinal arteriotomy extending beyond occluding core and three cross sections at different levels of arterial lesions. **B,** Planes of cleavage: *1,* subintimal; *2,* transmedial; *3,* subadventitial. Note the two muscular fiber layers of the media, circular (internal) and longitudinal (external). **C,** Dissection and mobilization of atherothrombotic occluding core. **D,** Excision of core. **E,** Distal intimal edge reattached to arterial wall with interrupted stitches. (From *Vascular surgery principles and techniques* by H. Haimovici. Copyright © 1976 McGraw-Hill Book Co. Used with permission of McGraw-Hill Book Co.)

lized to dissect the diseased intima and media away from the remainder of the arterial wall. This technique, first successfully performed in 1946 by Cid dos Santos, is still utilized frequently today. Open thromboendarterectomy is performed by first opening the diseased arterial wall in a longitudinal manner over the lesion present. Then a small, blunt instrument is used to separate and remove the constricting plaque from the remaining wall. After completing the endarterectomy, the arterotomy (arterial incision) is closed with fine sutures (Fig. 16-6). If the procedure is carefully performed, a smooth, non-thrombogenic surface is produced, and long-term patency of the segment can be expected. The advantages of endarterectomy are maintenance of normal blood pathways and the absence of foreign (graft) material, with subsequent increased risk of infection. The disadvantages of endarterectomy, as compared to arterial bypass grafting, are the increased time needed to perform an endarterectomy and the more meticulous and exacting technique required. Endarterectomy is most commonly utilized for operations on the carotid bifurcation as the lesions are almost always segmental in extent at that location. Other sites occasionally suitable for endarterectomy are the aortic bifurcation, the proximal deep femoral artery, and the origins of the visceral branches of the abdominal aorta.

Angioplasty

Another technique utilized to increase blood flow through a relatively short stenotic lesion is patch angioplasty. The artery is opened in a longitudinal manner across the stenotic segment, but the atherosclerotic plaque is not removed. Rather, the arterotomy is closed by suturing a patch of vein or synthetic material to the margins of the arterotomy so as to expand the arterial lumen at that site. Patch angioplasty may be utilized alone or combined with endarterectomy or bypass grafting to increase lumenal diameter over an arterial segment.

Arterial bypass and replacement grafting

The most commonly utilized technique for dealing with an extensive area of atherosclerotic stenosis involves the insertion of a tissue or synthetic graft. This conduit carries blood from a more proximal segment, which has good arterial inflow, to an arterial segment beyond the area of stenosis. Presently, grafting techniques commonly utilize either venous autografts or conduits of various synthetic materials. The graft may be inserted as a replacement for a segment of the arterial tree that has actually been removed or the graft may provide a bypass route around an area of narrowed artery. Bypass grafts are frequently placed adjacent to and follow the course of the normal artery in which case they are referred to as anatomic bypasses, as opposed to extra-anatomic bypass grafts, which follow a route other than the native artery.

Arterial grafts are generally easier to insert and less time-consuming than endarterectomy, particularly when the stenotic segment is extensive. Operative procedures employing grafts may be performed on almost any segment of the arterial tree, but are most commonly utilized in aorto-femoral and femoropopliteal locations. The extra-anatomic routes most commonly used are the femorofemoral crossover graft and the axillofemoral bypass graft.

Embolectomy

When a piece of thrombotic or atherosclerotic debris becomes dislodged from an atherosclerotic plaque, it is washed downstream until it becomes lodged secondary to narrowing of the distal arterial lumen. This event may result in the acute onset of ischemia to a limb, particularly if the embolus occludes a major limb artery. The removal of an embolus required a relatively extensive procedure until 1963 when Fogarty developed a balloon tipped catheter for retrieval of arterial emboli. Utilizing the Fogarty technique, a small arterotomy is made in a normal segment of artery proximal to the embolus, and the deflated catheter is passed down within the lumen past the emboli. The balloon is then inflated and gently removed, retrieving any embolic material present. The small arterotomy is then sutured closed (Fig. 16-7).

Sympathectomy

The sympathectic fibers innervating the wall of medium and smaller arteries belong to the autonomic nervous system. They supply the

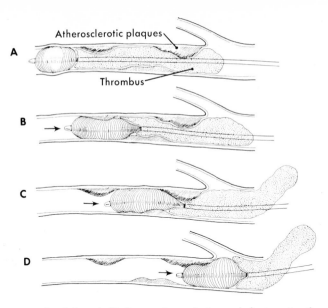

Fig. 16-7. Progression of withdrawal of balloon catheter during embolectomy in atherosclerotic artery. Note changes in degree of balloon inflation matching luminal diameters. (From Vascular surgery principles and techniques by H. Haimovici. Copyright © 1976 McGraw-Hill Book Co. Used with permission of McGraw-Hill Book Co.)

smooth musculature of these arterial walls and act to regulate and maintain vasoconstrictive tone. Although sympathectomy (sectioning of these nerves) has been performed for over five decades, there is still considerable uncertainty regarding both the acute and chronic physiologic effects produced and the proper indications for its use.

Sympathectomy is most frequently performed as part of the operative approach to severe lower extremity ischemia and consists of section and removal of a portion of one or both lumbar sympathetic chains. The left and right sympathetic chains supply fibers to the ipsilateral lower extremity and lie in the retroperitoneum adjacent to the aorta and vena cava, respectively. Section of the lumbar sympathetic chain results in vasodilatation of arterioles in the skin and muscles of the leg, with an associated increase in blood flow to those areas. However, it appears that the increase in muscle blood flow is only temporary and although augmentation of skin blood flow is of long duration, the nutritional benefit of this type of flow has been questioned. Some investigators believe sympathectomy increases the rapidity of development and extent of collateral circulation and utilize it to this end. In spite of the controversy, it is generally agreed that sympathectomy is at best a supplement to direct arterial reconstruction and may have a role when there is extensive atherosclerotic involvement of the smaller vessels distal to the popliteal trifurcation.

■ What are bypass grafts made of?

The commonly utilized synthetic grafts are made of woven or knitted Dacron or Teflon. Dacron grafts have been in use for over two decades and are the standard with which newer synthetic graft materials are compared. The grafts are manufactured in straight tube and bifurcation configurations and come in assorted diameters and lengths. Once implanted, the graft becomes adherent to the surrounding tissues secondary to ingrowth of connective tissue into the interstices of the graft, and the lining of the graft eventually becomes coated with a living neointima. Improvements, such as velour surfaces, are constantly being made in graft design in an attempt to increase the speed with which a living nonthrombogenic lining develops. Knitted grafts are more porous than woven grafts and are therefore felt to result in more rapid tissue ingrowth and neointimal foundation. However, because of this porosity, the graft needs to be preclotted before it will become "watertight." The preclotting process consists of flushing a quantity of fresh nonheparinized whole blood through the graft prior to its implantation, which results in the deposition of fibrin and platelets in the graft interstices and the production of a nonleaking blood conduit. Another synthetic material utilized for graft fabrication is Gortex (expanded polytetrafluoroethylene—PTFE), a plastic that is extruded and promises to be especially useful as an arterial substitute for small caliber arteries.

Autogenous vein is the most commonly utilized natural arterial substitute, and because of its size and availability, the greater saphenous vein is most frequently chosen. Its durability and patency are among the highest of all arterial substitutes in use, and it is the material of choice (when available) for grafts in the 4 to 6 mm range. The greater saphenous vein is carefully removed from the leg and each venous branch ligated with fine suture material. It is then rotated 180 degrees prior to implantation so that the end previously proximal is now distal. This maneuver is necessary to counteract the presence of valves within the venous lumen.

■ **What type of suture material is utilized on arteries and grafts?**

Only nonabsorbable suture material is used to suture arterial and graft wall. This is particularly important when a graft-to-graft or graft-to-arterial anastomosis is made as no true healing develops, and the integrity of the suture line is permanently dependent on the suture material. During the early years of vascular surgery, silk was the suture material most widely used. However, silk suture has proved to be inadequate for this application as it tends to lose tensile strength with time, and there was an unacceptably high incidence of late suture line disruption and pseudoaneurysm formation.

Presently, vascular sutures are either made of Dacron (braided) or Prolene (a monofilament

fiber), and both are available in a wide variety of sizes for use on both large and minute vessels. Vascular suture material is manufactured already mounted (swedged) on a needle so as to produce the smallest possible hole in the graft or vessel wall during suture and result in minimal bleedings from those needle holes.

Operative treatment for extracranial cerebrovascular disease

Until the 1950's there was little impetus for the development of surgical techniques directed at the extracranial cerebral arteries. Cerebrovascular symptomatology, such as transient ischemic attacks and stroke, had been considered almost uniformly a result of intracranial pathology and thus not accessible to a direct surgical approach. The development and increasing use of cerebral angiography during the 1950's resulted in a reappraisal of the situation. It rapidly became clear that a large portion of the patients with cerebral ischemic symptomatology (TIA, amaurosis fugax, and stroke) had at least one significant atherosclerotic lesion in the *extracranial* circulation located at a surgically accessible site. With the realization of the segmental nature and extracranial location of the majority of these atherosclerotic occlusive lesions, surgical efforts at carotid reconstruction soon followed. The first successful carotid endarterectomies were performed in 1953 and 1954 by DeBakey and Eascott.

By far the most common location of symptomatic atherosclerotic stenosis in the cerebral circulation is at the carotid bifurcation area. Other sites of lesions responsible for symptoms of cerebrovascular insufficiency are the origins of the great vessels off the aortic arch and the origins of the vertebral arteries (Fig. 16-2). It is quite rare for atherosclerotic narrowing to extend up the internal carotid for more than a few centimeters, and the intracranial portion of the cerebral circulation is frequently normal although lesions may be found at the carotid siphon.

Because these lesions are commonly localized to the area of the carotid bifurcation, carotid endarterectomy (CEA) is the operation most frequently performed for cerebrovascular symptomatology. The remainder of this section will be mainly concerned with the patient undergoing carotid endarterectomy; however, many of the fundamental aspects also pertain to endarterectomy and bypass procedures performed on the innominate, subclavian, and vertebral arteries.

■ What are the indications for carotid endarterectomy (CEA)?

The great majority of patients undergoing CEA have symptoms attributable to atherosclerotic lesions at the carotid bifurcation. Intimal plaques result in stenosis, usually at the origin of the internal carotid artery and thereby reduce blood flow to the ipsilateral cerebral hemisphere. Depending on the amount of cross-collateral blood flow from the contralateral carotid artery (via the circle of Willis) and the ipsilateral external carotid system, the patient may be symptomatic. In spite of highly stenotic lesions, the patient is often only intermittently symptomatic, as only at times of decreased cardiac output or diminished blood pressure is cerebral flow insufficient to supply brain oxygen needs. These mild and intermittent periods of cerebral insufficiency appear as transient ischemic attacks with unilateral paresthesia, weakness, and paralysis. If the dominant hemisphere (left for right-handed person) is affected, speech difficulties (expressive aphasia) may be encountered as well. More severe narrowing or arterial occlusion may produce a sufficient decrease in blood flow to result in a stroke.

Symptoms may also be produced by plaque that undergoes surface necrosis, resulting in the so-called ulcerative plaque. Aggregates of platelets, fibrin, and cholesterol form there and are subsequently washed from these ulcers by the flowing blood. If these small emboli travel to the eye via the ophthalmic artery, amaurosis fugax (transient monocular blindness) may result. If they lodge in the cerebral hemisphere, a more classic transient ischemic attack or stroke may be produced.

Occasionally there is sufficient narrowing in both carotid arteries to result in deficiency of total cerebral blood flow and subsequent decreased mental function without focal neurologic deficits. These patients suffer from chronic cerebrovascular insufficiency and often have a history of progressive difficulty with memory, mentation, and orientation.

It is well accepted that patients with the aforementioned symptoms and significant lesions at surgically accessible sites should be treated by carotid endarterectomy. When compared to surgical therapy, trials of medical management with anticoagulants and antiplatelet drugs have generally resulted in less favorable outcomes over extended periods of observation. In some of these studies the frequency of transient ischemic attacks was decreased somewhat by these drugs; however, no significant lowering in stroke rate was noted.

The management of the patient with an asymptomatic carotid bruit is more controversial but has been made somewhat easier secondary to developments in the noninvasive laboratory. A significant proportion of the elderly population of this country have carotid bruits. However, not all are the result of potentially troublesome internal carotid plaques. Lesions in the external carotid artery may also result in a cervical bruit but without the same significance. Although carotid angiography is relatively safe, it is not without risk and is both time-consuming and expensive. These factors limit the usefulness of angiography as a screening tool for patients with asymptomatic bruits, as far too many negative studies would result for the risk and time expended. The use of OPG-CPA testing will identify those patients with hemodynamically significant stenoses of the common or internal carotid artery. This is the subgroup of patients with bruits at significant risk of future stroke and therefore who might likely benefit by angiography and a surgical approach. If angiography demonstrates a highly stenotic bifurcational lesion, many feel surgery is indicated in spite of the lack of symptoms. Patients with negative OPG studies and those who show mild atherosclerotic involvement on angiography are not offered surgery but are followed by OPG on a routine basis. It should be emphasized that all patients with cerebrovascular symptoms should have a full workup, including angiography, regardless of the presence of a bruit or OPG findings. The patient with a nonstenotic ulcerated plaque may have a stroke or TIA symptoms even in the absence of a bruit or OPG delay.

Finally, there is mounting evidence that OPG screening is of value in the patient with known symptomatic atherosclerotic involvement of the coronary arteries or the peripheral circulation. The frequency of significant carotid stenosis is substantial and "prophylactic" carotid endarterectomy in these patients with angiographically proven severe stenosis has been shown to lower the stroke rate during major reconstructive surgery such as coronary artery bypass.

■ How is a carotid endarterectomy (CEA) performed?

Even though the critical care specialist need not know all the technical aspects of the operative procedure, a general understanding will make the postoperative course and potential complications following CEA clearer. Although CEA can be performed under local anesthesia and was frequently done this way in the past, general anesthesia with controlled endotracheal ventilation is almost universally utilized today.

Povidone-iodine complex (Betadine) showers with special attention to the face, neck, chest, and head are ordered twice on the day prior to operation. The patient is placed supine on the operating table with the neck extended and rotated to the opposite side. A cervical incision is made in front of the sternocleidomastoid muscle and the dissection is carried down to the carotid artery (Fig. 16-8). Carefully, the common, external, and internal carotid arteries are dissected free from surrounded tissues. Care is taken to identify and spare the vagus and hypoglossal (motor to the tongue) nerves during the dissection. The patient is then given intravenous heparin to prevent thrombosis while the artery is occluded during the performance of the endarterectomy. Three minutes later the clamps are applied and a longitudinal incision is made in the com-

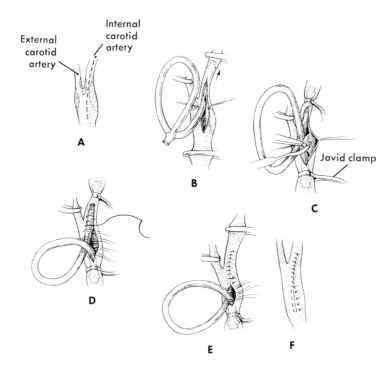

Fig. 16-8. A, Carotid arteriotomy. **B,** Placing internal shunt. **C,** Beginning endarterectomy. **D,** Beginning closure of arteriotomy. **E,** Removing shunt. **F,** Endarterectomy completed. (From Crane, C., and Warren, R.: Procedures in vascular surgery, ed. 2, Boston 1976, Little, Brown & Co.)

mon carotid artery and extended up the internal carotid artery just beyond the plaque. A plastic tube may then be placed to shunt blood from the common carotid to the internal carotid artery in order to maintain cerebral perfusion while the artery is open. Most patients tolerate a limited cerebral ischemic period without sequelae, and the use of a shunt depends on the surgeon's preference and the specific conditions present during each operation.

The intimal plaque is then carefully separated from the remaining arterial wall with a small blunt dissecting tool and removed. After ascertaining that no loose plaque or intimal flap has been left in the internal carotid artery, the incision in the artery is closed. The distal internal carotid artery is palpated to check for the presence of a strong pulse and the absence of a thrill (which would indicate residual stenosis), and the neck incision is closed by layers. Depending on the heparin dose used, protamine sulfate may be given to promote clotting prior to wound closure. Some surgeons leave a small plastic drain in the wound overnight, but others drain only under specific circumstances such as after reoperative surgery or if the tissues appear "wet" (slow generalized oozing of blood) in spite of efforts at hemostasis.

■ What is the usual condition of the patient on arrival at the ICU?

In many hospitals following carotid endarterectomy, the patient goes directly from the operating room to the ICU where he recovers from anesthesia and is followed for the first 24 hours. Although the patient is often still intubated and under relatively deep anesthesia at this time, some anesthesiologists begin decreasing anesthetic depth early enough to have the patient extubated and fairly awake on arrival at the ICU.

The patient will have a central or peripheral intravenous catheter for administration of medications, fluids, or blood products. Depending on the underlying medical history, the patient may arrive with a radial arterial line for continuous monitoring of the blood pressure. There will usually be a modest dressing on the patient's neck and "ECG" leads applied to the chest for continuous monitoring of heart rate and rhythm.

■ What specific parameters should be monitored following carotid endarterectomy?

The majority of patients have a quite benign and uncomplicated postoperative course. However, the potential problems are numerous and only by monitoring the patient closely can these potential problems be detected early and corrected.

Ventilation

If the patient is intubated and on a ventilator, the oxygen concentration, tidal volume, and respiratory rate should be adjusted to maintain a Po_2 of 90 to 120 mm Hg and a Pco_2 of approximately 35 mm Hg. Initial settings for a person with relatively normal pulmonary function would likely be an inspired O_2 concentration (FIO_2) of 50%, tidal volume of 12 to 15 ml/kg (950 ml/70 kg man), and a respiratory rate of 10/min. Further adjustments would be made based on arterial blood gas determinations.

If the patient is extubated, the primary concern would be maintenance of an adequate airway. If still somnolent, a nasal or oropharyngeal airway is often of benefit as is elevating the head of the patient's bed about 20 degrees (blood pressure permitting). The patient should be kept on low flow oxygen for the first few hours after surgery and longer if there is reason to expect pulmonary problems and hypoxia. The combination of laryngeal edema secondary to the endotracheal tube and cervical swelling at the operative site can lead to significant upper airway obstruction. If excessive bleeding occurs postoperatively, a hematoma will collect at the operative site. Because the skin and subcutaneous tissue of the neck are relatively nonelastic, the hematoma may exert considerable force on and result in significant compression of the trachea without alarming external findings. For this reason, the critical care specialist must listen frequently for evidence of early airway obstruction. If present, the surgeon should be notified immediately and if of significant degree, the patient should be taken back to the operating room and the hematoma evacuated. Life-threatening upper airway obstruction following unilateral CEA is almost always the result of an expanding hematoma, and the treatment should be *immediate* opening of the neck incision in the

ICU. Time should not be spent initially at attempts at endotracheal intubation, as they are usually unsuccessful secondary to displacement and compression of the trachea and larynx.

Blood pressure

The blood pressure must be closely followed during the early postoperative period. During the operative procedure, manipulation about the carotid bifurcation often leads to carotid sinus dysfunction (baroreceptor mechanism located there) with subsequent postoperative blood pressure lability. Significant hypertension and hypotension are not uncommon in the immediate postoperative period and must be rapidly recognized. Injection of the carotid sinus nerve with local anesthetic at the time of operation is felt to diminish the likelihood of significant blood pressure fluctuation during this period.

It is important to note whether the patient has a history of significant hypertension, as is frequently the case. Generally the patients do best when their blood pressure is maintained near preoperative values but usually tolerate reasonably wide fluctuations in arterial pressure. However, if marked systolic hypertension occurs, pharmacologic control is warranted. Besides the deleterious systemic effects of marked hypertension, such as myocardial strain and hemorrhagic cerebral infarct, local cervical complications may also be precipitated. Postoperative hematomas are more frequent in the markedly hypertensive patient, particularly when the systolic pressure is greater than 180 mm Hg. Disruption of the arterial suture line with resultant massive hemorrhage is a rare but catastrophic complication, occurring most often in patients with marked hypertension during the first few days.

The drug of choice for controlling marked hypertension during the early postoperative period is nitroprusside. Administered as a slow intravenous infusion at a concentration of 1 mg/5 ml (50 mg/250 ml 5% dextrose in water), the rate of administration is titrated to lower arterial pressure to an appropriate level for that patient. Resulting in blood pressure lowering secondary to a direct vasodilatory effect, nitroprusside is relatively safe as its effect is reversible within minutes by decreasing or discontinuing the drug. Care must be taken that inadvertent rapid administration of nitroprusside, particularly when beginning the drug, does not occur as severe hypotension may be produced.

Significant hypotension following carotid endarterectomy is fortunately rare, particularly if the patient has not been given nitroprusside. Hypovolemia is uncommon since usually little blood is lost during the procedure. However, treatment to raise the pressure must be instituted immediately with the standard measures (elevation of the lower extremities, intravenous fluids, and the administration of vasopressors and cardiotonic agents if needed). If a normotensive state is not reestablished rapidly, myocardial infarction or stroke are not infrequently encountered.

Heart rate

Like arterial pressure, abnormalities in cardiac rhythm are seen in the early postoperative period and are likewise attributed to operative carotid sinus manipulation for the most part. The most common abnormality seen is sinus bradycardia, and it should be treated if the heart rate is below 50/min or if the arterial pressure is affected (lowered). Reflex sinus bradycardia is rapidly and effectively treated by the intravenous administration of 0.4 mg of atropine. The dosage may be repeated if needed, but the bradycardia is usually transient and a more normal rate soon prevails.

Neurologic status

It is extremely important that the critical care specialist follow the patient's neurologic status during the early postoperative period. The incidence of new perioperative temporary and permanent neurologic deficit with carotid endarterectomy is about 3%. Some deficits result from periods of cerebral ischemia and others from embolic events. Although the majority of deficits are present as the patient awakes from anesthesia, some are first seen during the early postoperative period and may result from a technical problem at the operative site. For this reason, close attention to the patient's neurologic status must be maintained. A brief neurologic evaluation, including pupil size, level of consciousness, speech, and motor strength of all four extremities should be performed at frequent intervals along with vital signs. Any adverse change in the neurologic status should be immediately reported to the surgeon.

■ What is the status of the patient during the first 24 hours following carotid endarterectomy?

As the patient awakens from anesthesia, the head of the bed is raised 20 to 30 degrees, blood pressure permitting. This helps lower venous pressure in the neck and decreases the likelihood of significant hematoma, and the semiupright position encourages more efficient pulmonary function. The patient is kept NPO for the first 8 to 12 hours and thereafter is allowed sips of clear liquids if awake, alert, and without neurologic deficit. The following morning, the patient's diet is advanced as tolerated. The patient is also kept in bed during the first day but is allowed up in a chair the following morning to take breakfast. Ambulation is both permitted and encouraged at that time. Assuming the postoperative course has been uneventful and there is no evidence of significant cervical hematoma, the patient is usually transferred out of the intensive care unit on the first postoperative day.

Patients are not usually placed on antibiotics following carotid endarterectomy, as the infection rate about the neck is extremely low secondary to the excellent vascularity there. In addition, no graft material is used that might act as a foreign body and encourage infection. Similarly, no anticoagulant or antiplatelet drugs are used on a routine basis during the postoperative period. Excellent long-term patency can be expected if a good technical result was obtained, and the complications of chronic anticoagulation are greater than the potential benefits from their use.

It is a good idea to significantly limit the amount of analgesic and sedative medications given during the early postoperative period. Cervical incisions are not relatively painful and minimal medication allows one to closely follow the patient's neurologic status during this critical period.

OPERATIVE MANAGEMENT OF PERIPHERAL VASCULAR INSUFFICIENCY

Atherosclerotic lesions leading to symptoms of peripheral vascular insufficiency may be located anywhere between the abdominal aorta and the tibial arteries. Although there is much overlap, these lesions frequently fall into one of the following general patterns: aortoiliac, femoropopliteal, and tibioperoneal involvement (Fig. 16-3). The symptoms produced will be dependent on the specific location and severity of the lesions present.

Recognition of the relationship between severe aortoiliac stenosis and ischemic lesions of the lower extremities dates back to the early nineteenth century. In 1940 the French surgeon Leriche described the classic association of intermittent claudication and sexual impotence with atherosclerotic occlusion of the aortoiliac segment. However, it was not until more than 10 years later that specific operative treatment became possible. The initial approach of resection of the diseased aortoiliac segment and replacement with an aortic homograft (taken from human cadavers) was utilized for several years. Problems with availability of homograft tissue and the nearly universal development of late degenerative changes, provided the impetus for the development of synthetic fabric grafts, which have become the mainstay of peripheral vascular reconstructive surgery. In specific situations, however, operative approaches other than replacement or bypass with synthetic grafts have proved to be effective, and both endarterectomy and autogenous tissue bypass grafting are important tools in the vascular surgeon's armamentarium.

The majority of patients undergoing surgery for symptoms of lower extremity ischemia have hemodynamically significant arterial stenosis located proximal to the groin and undergo aortic reconstruction carried down to the iliac or femoral arteries. Lesions are also frequently found in the superficial femoral and popliteal arteries and bypass from the common femoral artery to popliteal artery is performed with some regularity. This section will address the basic aspects of the operative management of lower extremity ischemia using aortobifemoral and femoropopliteal bypass as focal points for the discussion.

■ What are the indications for reconstructive arterial surgery?

Generally the patient being considered for vascular surgery is troubled by significant ischemic symptomatology of the lower extremities. This may range from claudication to ischemic tissue necrosis. The decision of whether or not a patient should be offered an operative approach depends not only on his symptoms and the location and severity of his lesion but also on the patient's level of activity and projected lifespan. For example, an elderly patient may have moderately advanced disease resulting in claudication after 400 yards of walking. If he had been leading an active life and the claudication was limiting his ability to work or participate in recreational activities, surgical therapy might be appropriate. If, however, he had rarely been required to walk farther than around his house and yard and his claudication was not limiting his ability to participate in his routine activities, subjecting him to the risks of surgery might not be appropriate.

On the other hand, there are conditions that almost always require operative intervention, regardless of the level of symptomatology or the patient's age. Examples of such conditions are a large or expanding abdominal aortic aneurysm or impending gangrene of an extremity. The indications for surgical intervention are discussed in the following for several different patterns of atherosclerotic involvement.

Aortoiliac occlusive disease

The patient with sequential atherosclerotic narrowing of the distal abdominal aorta and or iliac arteries usually has symptoms of intermittent claudication of mild to moderate severity. In the absence of embolic complications, gangrene is very uncommon as there is usually adequate collateral blood flow via the lumbar and mesenteric arterial circulation to support lower extremity tissue viability.

Although *much* individual variability exists, the typical patient with significant stenosis of the aortoiliac segments experiences calf claudication when walking 1 to 4 blocks on level ground and is stopped by leg fatigue or calf, thigh, and occasionally buttock pain at about twice that distance. Usually a short rest results in disappearance of symptoms and the patient can resume walking for a like distance before symptoms again occur. If the atherosclerotic process results in significant bilateral reduction in internal iliac arterial flow, impotence in men may result as well.

Since operative intervention in this group of patients is often undertaken to relieve symptoms and not to save life or limb, it is the severity of symptoms and the limitations these symptoms produce in the patient's daily activities on which the decision to operate is made. Elective reconstructive procedures on the abdominal aorta can be carried out with an overall mortality of under 5%. The aortobifemoral and aortobi-iliac bypasses are warranted in a reasonably healthy person whose symptoms limit his ability to "enjoy" life. The patient with significant disease involving the cardiac, pulmonary, or renal systems has an increased perioperative mortality and usually must have a reasonably severe limitation in his level of activity to warrant operative intervention. Since atherosclerosis is a systemic disease, concomitant coronary artery and extracranial cerebrovascular disease are reasonably frequent in these patients. In order to decrease the perioperative morbidity and mortality of aortic reconstructive surgery, the patient should be screened by history, physical examination, and noninvasive testing (stress ECG and oculoplethysmography) for the presence of coronary and cerebrovascular disease. Appropriate angiographic studies should be carried out and significant lesions repaired prior to elective abdominal aortic reconstruction.

Abdominal aortic aneurysmal disease

Abdominal aortic aneurysms may be seen alone or along with concomitant occlusive disease. The aneurysm usually produces no symptoms itself other than a pulsatile abdominal mass. The infrarenal abdominal aorta is normally about 2 cm in diameter and when increased to greater than 3 cm is usually considered aneurysmal. Statistically, it has been shown that the larger (diameter) the aneurysm, the more likely it is to rupture and that the small aneurysms (4.5 cm) rupture very infrequently. The operative mortality for elective repair is like that of aortoiliac occlusive disease, under 5%. However, it is estimated that only between one third and one half of the patients with ruptured aortic aneurysms live long enough to be brought to a hospital and the perioperative mortality for ruptured aneurysms remains about 50%.

The extremely lethal nature of ruptured abdominal aortic aneurysms dictates that all aneurysms greater than 5 cm occurring in the otherwise healthy younger atherosclerotic patient be repaired. Large aneurysms (greater than 6 or 7 cm) should be repaired regardless of the patient's general condition, since they are at a very substantial risk of rupture at any time. Finally, the patient with an aneurysm who has abdominal or back pain or a tender pulsatile abdominal mass must be presumed to have a rupturing aneurysm and be immediately taken to the operating room for abdominal exploration.

The patient with the small aneurysm who is not operated on should be closely followed for evidence of aneurysm growth. The small aneurysm is difficult to palpate and estimates of size are notoriously inaccurate. The ultrasound scan has proved to be the most useful tool for quickly and accurately following aneurysm "growth."

Femoropopliteal occlusive disease

The patient with atherosclerotic narrowing in the femoropopliteal segment may have ischemic symptoms of the lower leg of varying severity. Generally, the more extensive the stenotic process and the poorer the collateral circulation present, the more severe the symptoms. When the narrowing or occlusion extends over a relatively localized arterial segment and collateral arterial channels have developed fully (such as with segmental superficial femoral artery occlusion), only intermittent claudication might be present. With more extensive disease and a less well-developed collateral circulation, one could expect more advanced ischemic symptoms such as rest pain and ischemic ulcerative and gangrenous changes to be present. Ischemic skin breakdown is usually first manifested on the toes, heel, and lateral malleolar areas. Seemingly insignificant trauma in this setting often quickly leads, with or without local infection, to areas of gangrene.

Within the femoropopliteal segment, the distal superficial femoral artery (SFA) at the adductor hiatus is frequently the first area to occlude. Later, significant stenotic and occlusive lesions may develop at the origin of the superficial and deep femoral arteries and within the popliteal artery. Usually there is relatively abundant collateral circulation in the leg with the deep femoral artery carrying blood to the lower leg in the face of SFA occlusion and the geniculate arterial arcade acting as a collateral route beyond the knee in the presence of popliteal occlusion.

When patients suffer SFA occlusion, they often experience an abrupt exacerbation of ischemic symptoms such as an increase in claudication or the onset of a somewhat cool and painful leg. The natural history of this lesion is, in the majority of patients, that the symptoms abruptly worsen but then over the next several days improve significantly. Often, if the patient embarks on a progressive exercise program, the claudication will lessen markedly over the next 2 to 3 months. If, however, the patient has simultaneous narrowing of the aortoiliac segment or the deep femoral system, insufficient collateral circulation will develop and little if any improvement will be noted.

Bypass procedures that carry blood from the common femoral artery to the popliteal or proximal tibial arteries do not require laparotomy and therefore can be carried out with significantly less morbidity and mortality than abdominal aortic reconstruction. However, because of the smaller diameter and greater length of these grafts, resulting in lower blood flow, grafts in the femoropopliteal position have a much less favorable long-term patency rate. As a result of the likelihood that many of these grafts will fail during the first several years following implantation, these procedures are usually reserved for those patients with more advanced ischemic symptoms.

The patient having recent onset of intermittent claudication owing to femoropopliteal disease is treated conservatively and started on an exercise program with the expectation that some improvement in symptomatology will occur.

■ How are arterial vascular reconstructive procedures performed?

An understanding of the basic principles and techniques utilized during arterial surgery will allow the critical care specialist to play a more significant role in the care of the vascular patient. Physiologic changes secondary to the operative trauma will be more easily understood and potential complications can be anticipated.

Abdominal aortic reconstruction

Preoperative preparation for these procedures usually consists of twice daily showers with an antimicrobial soap, such as Betadine, during the 2 days prior to operation. Special attention is directed to cleaning the groin area, as the normally abundant bacterial flora there increase the risk of wound infection. Patients in whom implantation of prosthetic graft material is anticipated are started on prophylactic antibiotics just prior to the operative procedure. Antibiotics given in these situations have been shown to significantly lower the incidence of wound and graft infection. Cephalosporin antibiotics are often used in these circumstances for their broad-spectrum coverage against both the gram-negative coliform and gram-positive cocci bacteria and their relatively low toxicity. Antibiotic coverage is continued intraoperatively and for 3 or 4 days postoperatively as well.

In order to make operative exposure of the aorta easier and the patient's postoperative course more pleasant, a program of gentle bowel preparation is utilized including cathartics, enemas, and a clear liquid diet on the day prior to surgery. If possible, the patients should be prepped and shaved just prior to surgery on the day of the operation. Small macroscopic as well as microscopic nicks and scratches are produced by even the most careful body shave and can become sites of potential infection when the patient is shaved the evening prior to surgery.

General anesthesia with endotracheal intubation is universally utilized for these major procedures. The patient is positioned supine on the operating table and ECG leads, a Foley catheter, nasogastric tube, and an esophageal or rectal temperature probe is inserted. Two large intravenous lines (one in the central venous system) and an arterial line are usually placed by the anesthesiologist. A surgical scrub with an iodine-containing solution is then performed from the chest to the ankles.

If the reconstructive procedure is to be carried down to the femoral arteries, the groin incisions are made first and the femoral arteries are exposed. The abdomen is entered via a midline or transverse incision and the intestines are gently displaced to the patient's right to expose the ab-

dominal aorta. The infrarenal aorta is dissected free and a tunnel for graft placement is created bluntly in the retroperitoneum along the path of the iliac artery to connect with the femoral artery in the groin. Blood is then withdrawn to "preclot" the relatively porous Dacron prosthesis prior to systemic anticoagulation with intravenous heparin. After heparin has been given and allowed to circulate, the aorta and distal arteries are occluded with special noncrushing clamps. The aorta is opened just below the renal arteries and the previously prepared Dacron graft is sutured to the aorta at that site. The aorta and graft may be

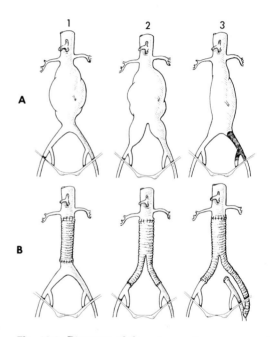

Fig. 16-9. Diagrams of three types of aneurysms and corresponding methods of graft replacement after excision of lesions. *1* **A,** Aneurysm is situated between renal arteries and bifurcation. *1* **B,** Excised aneurysm is replaced with tubular graft between renal arteries and aortic bifurcation. *2* **A,** Aneurysm involves abdominal aorta and two common iliac arteries. *2* **B,** Aortoiliac graft was inserted between renal arteries and bifurcation of iliac vessels. *3* **A,** Abdominal aortoiliac aneurysm is associated with occlusion of left iliac artery, requiring right aortic graft and left aortofemoral bypass procedure, *3* **B.** (From Vascular surgery principles and techniques by H. Haimovici. Copyright © 1976 McGraw-Hill Book Co. Used with permission of McGraw-Hill Book Co.)

connected by either end-to-end or end-(of graft) to-side (of aorta) types of anastomoses. The limbs of the graft are then either sutured to the iliac arteries or carried through the previously created retroperitoneal tunnels and anastomosed to the side of the femoral arteries in the groin (Fig. 16-9). After checking for adequacy of arterial pulsation distal to the graft implantation sites, the wounds are irrigated with antibiotic solution, hemostasis is obtained, and the incisions are closed.

Femoropopliteal reconstruction

The goal in arterial reconstructive surgery for femoropopliteal occlusive disease is the restoration of pulsatile blood flow, under normal pressure at the origin of the tibial and peroneal arteries. If this objective can be achieved, adequate perfusion of the feet via the tibioperoneal system or its collateral arterial channels will usually result. The most commonly performed procedure in these circumstances is the femoropopliteal bypass utilizing a segment of reversed greater saphenous vein. If an acceptable segment of vein is not available, other arterial substitutes such as Gortex (PTFE), bovine heterograft, or Dacron tubular grafts may be utilized as second choices (Fig. 16-10).

When the area of significant disease is localized to a limited arterial segment, endarterectomy of that segment may be the procedure of choice. However, this is uncommon, as the superficial femoral artery is usually diseased throughout its length.

Because these procedures often utilize foreign graft material and involve groin incisions, preoperative depression of skin bacterial flora with twice daily showers for several days proceding surgery is of benefit. Prophylactic antibiotic coverage, as used with aortic reconstructive surgery, is also given during the perioperative period. However, no specific bowel preparation is required and the patient is shaved from the costal margin to the ankles just prior to the surgical procedure.

A general principle of vascular surgery, particularly applicable to femoropopliteal bypass procedures is that both good inflow and runoff are needed to maintain long-term graft patency.

Therefore the proximal anastomosis of the graft must be placed at a site of good arterial flow and pressure. This usually necessitates that the graft originate from the common femoral artery. Equally important to graft patency is the arterial runoff bed; the bypass graft must be attached to a relatively normal arterial segment with an adequate arterial runoff.

Often aortoiliac and femoropopliteal occlusive disease coexist. In this circumstance reconstruction of the more proximal lesions must be carried out either simultaneously or prior to the more distal procedure if the distal bypass is to remain patent. In recent years the importance of the deep femoral artery has been recognized. A patent deep femoral system will supply sufficient collateral flow to the lower leg to support both tissue viability and a moderate level of activity in most patients. Therefore in the setting of occlusive lesions in the SFA, a lesion in the deep femoral ar-

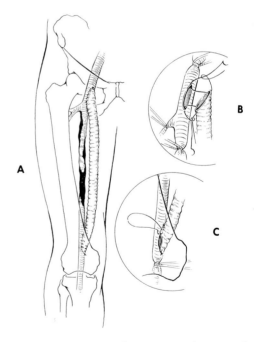

Fig. 16-10. Diagram illustrating synthetic prosthesis femoropopliteal bypass graft above knee. (From Vascular surgery principles and techniques by H. Haimovici. Copyright © 1976 McGraw-Hill Book Co. Used with permission of McGraw-Hill Book Co.)

tery becomes of great clinical significance. Since atherosclerotic lesions are usually limited to the origin and most proximal segments of the deep femoral artery, it is relatively simple to reestablish normal deep femoral flow by the performance of a profundoplasty. This usually entails the opening of the artery from the common femoral artery down onto the deep femoral artery beyond the diseased segment. Then either an endarterectomy may be performed or the lumen of the stenotic segment may be enlarged with a vein or synthetic patch.

Since femoropopliteal reconstructive procedures often take several hours to complete, general endotracheal anesthesia is preferred. The patient is positioned supine on the table, with the affected leg externally rotated and slightly flexed at the hip and knee (frog leg position). After prepping the patient from the costal margin (in case the abdomen has to be entered) to the ankles, incisions are made over the common femoral artery and on the medial (inner) aspect of the knee. The femoral artery and the area of its bifurcation into the superficial and deep femoral arteries are dissected free of surrounding structures. The popliteal artery is also exposed at the knee area at an appropriate location for bypass. The greater saphenous vein is then harvested. Starting at the groin, all branches are carefully ligated and divided and a sufficient length of vein is prepared to reach from the groin to the distal bypass site. If the vein is thrombosed or too small in diameter, a synthetic graft may be used as a second choice.

The vein is reversed so that valves within the vein will not hinder blood flow and is then pulled through a tunnel connecting the femoral and popliteal arteries, generally following the route of the diseased superficial femoral artery. The patient is anticoagulated with heparin and the anastomoses are then carried out to the popliteal and femoral arteries using fine suture material. After "flushing" the graft, flow is established to the distal extremity. When the circumstances preclude anastamosis to the popliteal artery secondary to disease there, the bypass graft may be carried down to the tibial or peroneal arteries with some measure of success. After completion of the anastamosis, the wounds are irrigated with antibiotic irrigating solution and closed. Occasionally,

a closed wound drainage system, such as a Hemovac or Jackson-Pratt, is left in to evacuate any accumulated blood from the popliteal space during the early postoperative period.

■ **What is the usual condition of the patient on arrival at the ICU?**

The aortofemoral bypass patient will be used as a model for a discussion of the postoperative care of peripheral vascular surgery patients in general. Having spent 3 to 5 hours in the operating room, the patient can be expected to arrive in the ICU still intubated and under anesthesia. Mechanical ventilation with a volume cycled respirator is preferred and is usually continued until the following morning. The patient will usually have a catheter in one radial artery for continuous monitoring of blood pressure and withdrawing blood gas samples. A central venous pressure catheter, inserted via either the subclavian or internal jugular vein, and one or two peripheral venous catheters can also be anticipated. If the patient has significant concomitant cardiopulmonary disease, a Swan-Ganz pulmonary artery catheter may have been placed in order to better evaluate the patient's intravascular fluid volume status. The remainder of monitoring equipment will usually consist of ECG electrodes and a rectal temperature probe. Occlusive dressings will be in place over both abdominal and extremity incisions and should be left in place for the first 48 hours providing they remain dry and unsoiled. Wet dressings should be changed using sterile technique by either the critical care specialist or the surgeon according to hospital policy.

The patient will often be relatively hypothermic on arrival in the ICU. During the operative procedure, heat is lost from the peritoneal cavity both directly and secondary to the evaporation of water from the exposed serosal surfaces. Depending on the effectiveness of the efforts of the anesthesiologist (blood transfusion warmer, heating pad on operating table, and so forth), the patient's core temperature may be as low as 32° to 34° C. As a consequence, there is often marked peripheral vasoconstriction and resultant coolness and cyanosis of the hands and feet. Until the patient warms up to more normal temperatures, peripheral pulses may not be palpable, even in patent arteries. However, even in the face of this vaso-constriction patency of these vessels can be con-firmed with the use of the Doppler flowmeter.

■ **What specific parameters should be moni-tored following major vascular reconstruc-tive surgery?**

Rather than discuss the total postoperative management of a patient having undergone ma-jor intra-abdominal surgery, attention will be focused on those aspects that particularly pertain to the vascular patient.

Ventilation

Patients who have had major vascular recon-structive surgery are usually maintained on con-trolled endotracheal ventilation for the first 12 to 18 hours. This allows a period of guaranteed ade-quate oxygenation and optimum pulmonary toi-let. A chest x-ray film should be obtained to check endotracheal tube placement. Arterial blood gas measurements are followed, and appropriate ven-tilator adjustments are made as required. Assum-ing adequate alertness and arterial oxygenation while on the ventilator overnight, the patient is given a short trial of spontaneous respiration with a T-piece in the early morning. If "blow-by" ar-terial blood gasses and respiratory mechanics (tidal volume and forced vital capacity) are ade-quate, the patient is extubated and placed on oxy-gen by mask. Vigorous pulmonary toilet is con-tinued during the postoperative period.

Temperature

As stated previously, following aortofemoral by-pass surgery the patient is often quite hypother-mic. Unless core temperature is below 32° C, the patient should be only covered with blankets and allowed to warm spontaneously. Active measures such as heating blankets and administration of warmed intravenous fluid are rarely required. As the temperature rises, the peripheral vasculature begins to dilate and the effective intravascular space increases. At this point, adequate intra-venous fluid must be given to prevent significant hypovolemia and resultant decreased cardiac out-put and blood pressure. Colloid solutions such as blood or 5% albumin solution are best utilized to

compensate for this vasodilatation, which may in-crease the intravascular space as much as 10%.

Within 3 to 6 hours the temperature has usual-ly returned to normal and often supranormal lev-els. The increased metabolic demands of the fe-brile state are deleterious, and acetaminophen (Tylenol) suppositories are given if the rectal temperature rises above 38° C. This immediate postoperative fever is secondary to the metabolic consequences of the operative and anesthetic trauma and does not usually have a pulmonary etiology as it does later in the postoperative pe-riod.

Fluid balance

Besides ventilation, the maintenance of an ap-propriate intravascular fluid volume is the most critical and demanding aspect of early postopera-tive care. Only by understanding the sources of fluid loss and the degree of transcompartment fluid shifts can the patient's volume status be smoothly managed. To this end the arterial blood pressure (systolic, diastolic, and mean), heart rate, central venous pressure, intake and output (urine, nasogastric drains, and so forth), and he-matocrit are closely followed.

Optimal fluid management actually begins in the operating room. Blood loss should be esti-mated as accurately as possible and replaced in like amount. In addition, the patient will usually require about 1000 ml of crystalloid solution for each hour the peritoneal cavity is opened in or-der to compensate for both intraoperative evapo-ration losses and fluid shifts. During the opera-tive procedure and the early postoperative period, a much greater volume of fluid is sequestered in the retroperitoneum, mesentery, and intestinal wall than is generally recognized. This "third space" loss occurs directly from the intravascular compartment and remains sequestered there for several days before returning to the circulation. This reinfusion of third space losses is the source of the diuresis that occurs on the second to fourth postoperative day.

Even if these losses are replaced during the op-erative procedure, further shifts can be expected during the first 24 postoperative hours. During this period as a result of the operative trauma, large amounts of antidiuretic hormone and aldosterone are released, which act to maintain intravascular volume by decreasing urinary sodium and fluid output. For this reason, little additional sodium is required during the first few days. Blood pressure and heart rate are watched closely and volume (as colloid) is given to maintain urinary output (30 to 50 ml/hr) and central venous pressure at adequate levels.

Renal function

Patients with advanced atherosclerotic vascular disease often have in addition either subclinical or clinically evident renal impairment. Cross-clamping the aorta, even below the renal arteries, may lead to a transient deterioration in renal function in some patients. For this reason, the serum potassium should be followed closely for the first few days and the serum creatinine should be checked on postoperative days 1 and 2. In the face of worsening renal function, additional potassium should be withheld and the volume of intravenous fluid given limited.

Abdominal girth

The abdominal girth should be measured frequently during the first 24 hours. Since almost all patients will require considerable quantities of the fluid during this period, a falling hematocrit and an increasing abdominal girth are often the only evidence for retroperitoneal or intra-abdominal hemorrhage present.

Peripheral pulses

Soon after the patient returns to the ICU, the extremities should be checked for color, temperature, and presence of palpable peripheral pulses. The surgeon should have a good idea of whether or not palpable pulses are to be expected and should communicate this information to the critical care team. If pulses are not palpable, the Doppler flowmeter should be used to confirm vessel patency and characterize the blood flow present. The femoral, popliteal, dorsalis pedis, and posterior tibial pulses should be examined frequently during the first several days. A loss of, or significant decrease in, strength or character of a *previously present* pulse or Doppler signal may signal graft occlusion and should be brought to the attention of the surgeon.

Body position

The patient should be kept at bed rest for the first 24 to 48 hours following major vascular reconstructive surgery. Then ambulation should be encouraged, even though assistance is often required. While in bed, the patients head should be elevated about 20 to 30 degrees to improve respiratory mechanics, but the patient should not be flexed at the hips. Sitting and flexion of the hips or knees are discouraged as kinking of the graft as this stage predisposes it to thrombosis.

BIBLIOGRAPHY

1. Crane, C., and Warren, R.: Procedures in vascular surgery, ed. 2, Boston, 1976, Little, Brown & Co.
2. Bernstein, E. F.: Noninvasive diagnostic techniques in vascular disease, St. Louis, 1978, The C. V. Mosby Co.
3. Haimovici, H.: Vascular surgery principles and techniques, New York, 1976, McGraw-Hill Book Co.
4. Hershey, F. B., and Calman, C. H.: Atlas of vascular surgery, ed. 3, St. Louis, 1973, The C. V. Mosby Co.
5. Jones, R. J., editor: Atherosclerosis: proceedings of the second international symposium, New York, 1970, Springer-Verlag, New York, Inc.
6. Seldinger, S. I.: Catheter replacement of the needle in percutaneous angiography: a new technique, Acta Radiol. **39:** 368, 1953.
7. Strandness, D. E., Jr.: Techniques in the evolution of vascular disease. In Cooper, P., and Nyhus, L., editors: Surgery annual, New York, 1971, Appleton-Century-Crofts, p. 181.
8. Wylie, E. J., and Ehrenfeld, W. K.: Extracranial occlusive cerebrovascular disease: diagnosis and management Philadelphia, 1970, W. B. Saunders Co.

CHAPTER 17

Preoperative care of the adult cardiac surgical patient

Robert A. Steedman

It was not unusual in the mid-1950's to read medical publications relating to the cardiac surgical patient and to note that the mortalities occurring subsequent to this surgery centered around the fiftieth percentile. Now, over 25 years later, large university centers and community hospital cardiac teams are striving in many areas of cardiac surgery to decrease the mortality rate below 1%.

Intraoperative technical advances and the refinements of surgical skills have aided markedly in decreasing mortality in this group of patients. However, the progressive sophistication and medical regimentation of the preoperative, operative, and postoperative care teams have played a major role in the rapid *decline* of *mortality* and *morbidity*. This team sophistication entails the continual and progressive education of all members as well as the concentration on even the minute practical details that are so often of critical significance. This chapter will deal with these minute details of critical care and is intended as a review for all members of the critical care team.

INDICATIONS FOR SURGERY
■ **Which conditions generally require cardiac surgery in adults?**
Congenital defects

The majority of significant cardiac birth defects require surgery during infancy or childhood as a critical necessity for the prevention of complications. However, some of these disorders are undiagnosed for one reason or another until early or occasionally even late adult life. Surgery for congenital defects is usually undertaken early in life to prevent the development of endocarditis, reversed shunting, irreversible pulmonary hypertension, cardiac decompensation, peripheral embolic phenomena, or even cerebrovascular accidents. Examples of the congenital defects requiring prompt surgery include *patent ductus arteriosus, coarctation of the aorta, ventricular septal defects, atrial septal defects* (with or without partial anomalies of the pulmonary venous return), *aortic stenosis*, varying types of *pulmonary artery stenosis, coronary artery anomalies*, and various *anomalies of the aortic arch*.

In some institutions the mere presence of certain congenital cardiac defects indicates surgical correction; these defects include *patent ductus arteriosus, atrial* and *ventricular septal defects, coarctation of the aorta, anomalies of venous return,* and other miscellaneous anomalies.

Contraindications to the performance of surgery on the adult patient with cardiac anomalies include the presence of irreversible pulmonary hypertension and right-to-left shunting, especially when the patient has polycythemia or is cyanotic. Simple closure alone of certain defects or shunts should not be performed when these anomalies are compensating for defects in which the pulmonary blood flow is decreased, such as in tricuspid atresia, tetralogy of Fallot, and pulmonary atresia. In adult life certain other associated disease processes not infrequently contraindicate surgical intervention. The ultimate decision as to which individuals should or should not undergo surgery for congenital lesions is based on the final analysis of each individual case.

Acquired valvular defects

The group of acquired valvular defects includes mitral, aortic, and tricuspid valve stenosis and/or insufficiency, most commonly resulting from rheumatic endocarditis. Acquired pulmonary valvular stenosis and insufficiency caused by rheumatic endocarditis occasionally requires surgical treatment. Recently in the literature numerous cases of *Pseudomonas* endocarditis of the pulmonary valve have been reported to occur in the addict using IV drugs; this defect eventually requires surgery.

Adhesive pericarditis or calcification of the pericardium with pericardial constriction

These cases can occur after inflammatory pericarditis or traumatic hemopericardium and frequently require extensive pericardiectomy.

Conditions developing from coronary artery disease

These indications are becoming more standardized; however, there are still many diversified opinions as to the specific indications for surgical intervention. Cases in which there is little question as to the need for surgery include patients with crescendo angina or angina uncontrollable by medications associated with a major obstructive lesion in the left coronary artery system as proved by catheterization. Other indications include intractable angina in any patient with severe obstruction in multiple vessels, repeated myocardial infarctions, refractory ventricular irritability, ventricular aneurysms with congestive failure or unstable arrhythmias, postinfarction ruptured chorda tendineae and progressive refractory failure, and postinfarction intractable cardiogenic shock. Much controversy centers today around the patient in the younger age group who has suffered a *single* myocardial infarction or who has *controllable angina* with a flow-limiting stenotic lesion in one of the major coronary arteries. The commercial airline pilot or executive presents an even greater problem. Any such patient is a candidate for a cardiac workup, and

if a major stenosis (70% or more) is demonstrated by arteriography in the left main or left anterior descending coronary artery proximal to the first perforating branch, coronary bypass surgery should be performed.

Traumatic cardiac lesions

Depending on the location of the cardiac surgical center, cardiac injuries from knife wounds, bullet wounds, or blunt chest trauma account for a respectable volume of injuries leading to surgery. The majority of the stab wounds of the heart require intervention for cardiac tamponade and hemorrhage and involve simple closure of the chamber lacerations. Occasionally coronary artery bypass to a transected or partially transected coronary artery is also necessary.

Blunt chest trauma with rupture of one of the four major chambers of the heart usually causes immediate death; however, with better paramedic facilities and faster cardiac surgical team efforts, it is possible to institute surgical therapy and to repair the ruptured cardiac chamber. Rupture of the various heart valves and chorda tendineae and/or papillary muscles can now be successfully repaired.

Probably the most common of the vascular blunt trauma injuries requiring surgery is *traumatic dissection of the aorta.* The unquestionable indications for surgery in these injuries include the presence of cardiac tamponade, refractory failure, or cardiac shock (refractory); however, in most situations the diagnosis itself is an indication for surgery.

PREPARATIONS FOR SURGERY
■ **What methods are used to emotionally and psychologically prepare the patient and the family?**

The patient should develop confidence in the cardiac surgical team; this can be done in several ways. Usually the patient has been referred by a physician who knows the capabilities of the cardiac team, and this knowledge should reassure the patient. In addition, the patient has usually met someone in the community who has had a similar surgical procedure. Frequently the patient hears encouraging comments from the nursing staff as to the results of the operating team.

All of the foregoing situations are important and beneficial. However, direct exposure to a patient who has had a similar operation is one of the most satisfactory methods of decreasing the patient's anxiety or apprehension. A patient who has undergone the surgery 3 to 5 days previously is often pleased to discuss the surgery with the surgical candidate.

A member of the *Mended Hearts Association* should be invited to meet the patient and family during the preoperative period. The Mended Hearts Association is composed of county, state, and national chapters of individuals who have previously undergone cardiac surgery. The organization was formed explicitly for the purpose of providing service to individuals who are about to undergo similar operations. The group's function is to help one another after surgery or to help any patient who might have postoperative financial, emotional, or even medical difficulties. One or more representatives of the organization should be invited to meet with the patient, at which time the patient may seek answers to questions related to the coming surgery. All members of the association have been schooled in the techniques of visitation and are careful not to increase the patient's apprehension by the visit.

It is recommended that the operating surgeon and/or other members of the critical care team meet preoperatively with the patient and the family to explain the procedure and to answer any questions. In addition, nursing members of the *cardiac intensive care unit* should meet the patient prior to surgery and conduct a tour of the critical care unit. The patient should be acquainted with the various monitoring devices, endotracheal intubation, and positive breathing equipment and techniques. A detailed explanation relative to the multiple procedures necessary during the coming stay in the unit should be provided.

The anesthesiologist should meet with the patient, usually the night before surgery, to reemphasize certain procedures such as use of IV lines and the probable use of endotracheal respiratory assistance postoperatively.

A valuable adjunct to the cardiac surgery team effort is the incorporation of a liaison practitioner or nurse who would be available at any time to answer questions from the patient or the family. This person should have completed an apprenticeship through the preoperative, operative, and postoperative phases and would be expected to make multiple daily pre- and postoperative visits. This clinician should attend a portion of the cardiac surgery and should serve as a valuable communication link between the operating room and the waiting family and as a major communication vector between the operating surgeon and the hospital critical care unit staff during the postoperative period.

All of the preceding modes of introducing the patient to the surgical procedure have produced marked beneficial insight in our patients undergoing preparation for surgery. However, in recent years there has been an increasing tendency to overinform the interested public with regard to cardiac surgery. This has included the presentation on national television of actual operating room visualizations of cardiac surgeries in progress; these have been detailed to the point of even showing near-catastrophic occurrences in surgery such as bleeding problems, delayed defibrillation in fibrillated hearts, and other complications. This public participation, so to speak, has created great apprehension, especially among patients who visualize television documentary dramas immediately prior to their own surgery. In attempting to ease the patient's apprehension by providing information about the surgical procedure, it is possible that the patient is becoming too deeply involved in a situation for which he is unprepared.

■ **What type of room is ideal for the intended cardiac surgical patient?**

The patient probably understands his own personality best; therefore if he specifically desires a private room and it is possible, such accommodations should be provided. It is generally better for patients to be in a semiprivate room with a relatively well room partner, preferably not a patient undergoing surgery performed by the same surgeon. Short-term exposure to patients with similar physicians is good, but long-term exposure is not always advantageous.

Selection of the patient's room is of extreme importance and should be considered carefully by the staff. For example, placing a smoking patient with a cardiac surgical candidate is a poor selection; an extremely hyperactive or uncooperative patient is a poor room companion; a patient who has an incurable disease or a condition with a poor general outlook is also a poor companion. It is extremely important to obtain a room companion for the cardiac surgical patient who will allow plenty of rest, not cause undue anxiety, and not be critical of the operating team or the hospital.

■ What medications should be used for preoperative showers and how often should they be used?

Many hospitals still utilize hexachlorophene solutions (pHisoHex) for the preoperative showers. However, because of its wide use in commercial preparations, proof that *Pseudomonas* can grow on the periphery of hexachlorophene containers, desensitization of many bacteria to this preparation, and reports of allergic reactions in infants, we now use preparations of povidone-iodine (Betadine).*

Patients are usually admitted 1 day before surgery and are given a Betadine shower at least once daily, including the morning of surgery.

If the patient has been scheduled for cardiac surgery prior to being discharged after catheterization, an attempt should be made to administer at least two preoperative showers or scrubs.

If the patient has recently undergone cardiac catheterization or any other surgical procedure, local scrubbing of the anticipated surgical areas are utilized instead of full-body showers.

■ What diets are recommended for the patient admitted for cardiac surgery?

If the patient has been admitted for myocardial revascularization procedures such as aorto-coronary-saphenous vein or internal mammary artery bypass and has not had congestive failure or diet restrictions for other conditions such as diabetes or gouty arthritis, a patient-select regular diet is recommended. The food is more palatable, nutri-

tion is maintained during the period of expected apprehension, and for the short period of 2 to 3 days no complications should develop.

If the patient was admitted for valvular surgery, has received digitalis preparations and diuretics, and has been maintained on a low-salt diet, then a similar or even more stringent diet should be continued until surgery. This patient will not be disturbed at this restriction because this is probably similar to the preadmission diet.

Overweight patients should be allowed to select their diet, as they probably have been on a weight control regimen for a period of time prior to the operation unless the surgery is urgent; even then the 2 or 3 days prior to surgery will not add any more hazard in contrast to the mental anguish and apprehension produced by calorie restriction.

■ How often should the patient be weighed preoperatively?

It is our policy to weigh the patient daily, both on the standing and bed scales. This gives a correlation between the two scales and introduces the patient to bed-scale weighing, which will be the method of weighing in the immediate postoperative period. This is necessary in routine postoperative cases and especially for patients undergoing rapid diuresis or "drying out."

■ Should respiratory therapy be utilized routinely, even for the patient who does not have pulmonary disease or problems?

It is essential for the cardiac surgical patient to be introduced to inhalation therapy techniques prior to the postoperative period. This preoperative instruction entails two or three visits from personnel of the respiratory therapy department to establish the pulmonary modalities in preparation for the immediate postoperative period. If the patient is not educated preoperatively, apprehension and air swallowing may result, producing gastric distention, diaphragm elevation, basilar atelectasis, and possibly even regurgitation and aspiration.

The patient should be instructed in postural drainage and percussive postural therapy, either by respiratory or physiotherapy department personnel or by the bedside critical care practitioner.

---

*Occasional blister formation has occurred when tape is placed over Betadine preparation solutions that were not washed off prior to the application of dressings.

The preoperative therapy for the patient with pulmonary disease includes an extremely diligent regimen and frequent treatments with intermittent positive pressure breathing, often using one of the mucolytic agents to loosen secretions, followed two or three times a day with percussive postural drainage. The secretions obtained are cultured so that appropriate antibiotic therapy can be instituted preoperatively or be ready for postoperative use. Bronchodilators are only selectively utilized, as they may produce arrhythmias in patients with ischemic or sensitive myocardium.

Better therapeutic results can be obtained if the patient has refrained from smoking during the several weeks before the surgery. However, some benefit is obtained even if smoking has been suspended for the 3 to 7 days preceding the surgical procedure. This often requires some form of tranquilization; we prefer diazepam (Valium), 2 mg, given four times a day.

The specific and usual orders for respiratory therapy would include the following:

1. Administer 0.5 ml of 20% acetylcysteine (Mucomyst) with 3 ml saline solution.

2. In patients with bronchospasm or demonstrated improvement of pulmonary functions with bronchodilators, add 0.25 ml of Bronkosol (preferred) or 4 drops of isoproterenol (Isuprel) to the combination just mentioned.

3. For the patient with nonallergic history who becomes anorexic or nauseous with acetylcysteine, substitute 100,000 units of pancreatic dornase (Dornavac) for acetylcysteine.

4. Use postural drainage either two or four times a day, especially following the early morning and late evening treatments. Any local lung areas to be drained are specified in the orders (for example, left lower lobe or right middle lobe).

In addition, the patient is instructed in the use of incentive spirometer.

■ What preoperative precautions are taken against the development of infection?

It is recommended that patients be placed on sterile linen from the time they enter the hospital and instructed in appropriate hygienic and modified aseptic room procedures. These procedures are enforced more with the infection-prone (diabetic) patient or patients who will receive prosthetic devices.

Preoperative cultures are obtained on the day of admission from the sputum, skin, blood, and urine of patients scheduled for valve surgery. Positive pathogenic cultures have been obtained in 2% to 3% of surgical patients. Positive yields have occurred in each of the mentioned culture sites, including pathogenic *Staphylococcus* from the sputum and skin, *Serratia marcescens* in the blood, and various gram-negative organisms in the urine. Positive cultures and indications of sensitivities frequently are identified the day of or the day following surgery and treatment may be initiated immediately.

The utilization of preoperative antibiotics has been a point of controversy for many years; however, there is general agreement that prophylactic antibiotics should be used in the patient who is destined to have valve surgery, especially if insertion of a prosthetic valve replacement is anticipated. The antibiotic regimen has varied almost semiannually with the introduction and advent of newer synthetic penicillins and newer antibiotics for gram-negative organisms. Each cardiac team seems to have its own preoperative, operative, and postoperative antibiotic regimen; therefore this will not be discussed in detail here.

Adjunctive IM cefazolin sodium (Kefzol) is administered 12 hours and 2 hours prior to surgery for myocardial revascularization procedures, and 1 g of Kefzol is placed in the pump preparation at the time of surgery. The utilization of cephalosporins in numerous patients with a history of penicillin allergy has demonstrated no evidence of cross sensitivity in our cases.

■ What surgical preparation is ordered for the cardiac surgical patient, when is the best time for it to be performed, and who should do it?

In most patients the entire chest, both axillae, the abdomen, the pubic area, and the groin are prepared before surgery. In cases where the saphenous vein is to be harvested, the preparation is extended to the toes, totally circumscribing the legs. In cases in which other than midsternotomy incisions are used, the side of the chest is prepared similar to preparation for thoracotomy and is specifically described by the operating surgeon, who should be contacted if there are any questions.

There remains controversy as to the ideal time to prepare the patient because of reports suggesting that if the patient is prepared too early prior to surgery, there is the potential for instigating infection in abrasion sites and hair follicles. We also believe that if prepared too early, for example, the day or evening before surgery, the patient may have increased apprehension and anxiety; however, this time schedule is occasionally necessary because of personnel reasons.

Immediately after the surgical preparation the patient should have a Betadine shower as well as on the morning of surgery. However, the showers are not ordered for patients with unstable or crescendo angina. It is recommended that the patient be prepared the morning of surgery before going to the amphitheater.

The individual performing the preparation must be professionally oriented; unfortunately it is not uncommon in some hospitals to assign this responsibility to the least experienced member of the surgical team. As a result, the patient may appear to be in need of a blood transfusion or develop additional anxieties as a direct consequence of an inappropriate comment or attitude demonstrated by the individual in attendance. Occasionally patients are inadequately prepared for the surgical procedure, creating complications for the waiting surgeon or assistant who finds the patient is incompletely shaved after having already undergone the surgical scrubbing or partial draping.

■ **Who should obtain the surgical consent for operation, and how should it be worded?**

Today with the more practical approach of enthusiastic introduction of the patient to the preoperative, operative, and postoperative phases by the surgeon, anesthesiologist, Mended Hearts representatives, critical care practitioners, and a cardiac team liaison person, the patient can be more than duly informed of the procedures to be performed. It is recommended that the operating surgeon make note, on the surgeon's order sheet, of the specific wording to be used and note that the patient has been informed, following which it is appropriate for another critical care team member to actually obtain the patient's signature on the consent-for-operation form.

■ **Should the patient be confronted with the legally recommended fully informed consent form?**

This question, we believe, fits into the category of the aforementioned overly dramatized television exposure for the patient. Preparation and presentation to the cardiac surgical patient of a complete informed consent form inclusive of all the minor and major problems or complications and their associated implications could require nearly 3 days of the patient's awake hours and still create confusion or the feeling of not being fully informed. It is not uncommon today in certain subspecialty fields (such as vascular radiology) for practitioners to approach the patient with a most vivid and extensive informed consent form, resulting in a number of patients refusing the crucial procedure recommended. The patients become confused when told of the multiple (however improbable) sequelae that can occur, and it has now been demonstrated that a practitioner can be held liable for complications occurring as a result of a diagnostic or therapeutic procedure not having been performed (for example, the patient was prevented from having the procedure by being frightened or improperly influenced).

We attempt to establish a general agreement and understanding with the patient that the procedure selected is best, and there is the possibility of complications despite the fact that they are not expected. If the complication potentials are higher in a specific patient and if the discussion of these potential complications might endanger the patient's successful outcome in surgery, these factors are usually discussed at length with the members of the family.*

■ **Is preoperative bowel control necessary?**

The majority of patients are allowed oral intake between 12 and 36 hours after the operative pro-

---

*It has become a cold and treacherous professional community when in some circumstances a surgeon is prompted and even advised to possibly sacrifice the patient's successful mental and/or physical outcome to prevent injudicial legal morbidity or assassination.

cedure; therefore complete evacuation of the bowel contents is not necessary. Patients should receive bisacodyl (Dulcolax) suppositories for two nights preceding surgery, and if this is not successful, a rectal sodium biphosphate (Fleet) enema should be utilized for evacuation of the sigmoid and descending colon the evening before surgery. If the patient has a history of chronic constipation, oral cathartics and/or stool softeners are utilized from admission throughout the preoperative period.

■ What medications should be discontinued on admission?

The routine use of a preadmission brochure or mimeographed instruction sheet designed to inform the patient to bring all present medications to the hospital on admission is an important policy. These medications are further verified by the admission medication checkoff sheet obtained by the admitting ward or unit.

The specific times for discontinuing certain medications prior to surgery vary; however, it is recommended that certain medications be discontinued.

Anticoagulants

Anticoagulants such as warfarin (Coumadin) or dicoumarol (Dicumarol) (and occasionally dipyridamole [Persantine]) are discontinued 2½ to 3 days prior to surgery, depending on the admission prothrombin, bleeding, clotting, and partial thromboplastin times. The reason for discontinuing these drugs is evident as an unnecessary nuisance, possibly causing even life-endangering bleeding during the preliminary and early phases of the operation. The timing and discontinuance of anticoagulants in some cases are varied according to individual patients needs. Long-term or chronic use of acetylsalicylic acid (aspirin) products or phenylbutazone (Butazolidin) can also produce bleeding problems postoperatively.

Digitalis preparations

Digoxin (Lanoxin), digitoxin, and so forth are discontinued 3 days prior to the surgical procedure unless the patient is absolutely dependent on them (for example, if the patient has severe congestive heart failure). The period of 2½ to 3

days is an adequate time for discontinuance in the faster acting and rapidly excreted forms of digitalis. The major reason for discontinuing digitalis preparations is to prevent cardiac irritability and arrhythmias, which are especially prone to occur in the overly digitalized patient during and after pump perfusion. Pump perfusion alters the extra-and intracellular concentrations of potassium, which, in conjunction with large digitalis stores, can produce these dangerous arrhythmias. Some authors have advocated the evaluation of patients preoperatively with the injection of 2 ml of meralluride theophylline (Mercuhydrin), and if a diuresis of 3 to 4 pounds of fluid occurs within a short period of time, they believe the patient should be given digitalis preoperatively or maintained on digitalis. We have used this technique in thoracic surgical candidates rather than in cardiac surgical candidates. Publications have indicated increased cardiac irritability associated with the use of digitalis preoperatively in younger thoracic and cardiac surgical patients.[1]

Diuretics

Diuretics such as furosemide (Lasix) and ethacrynic acid are preferably discontinued 3 days prior to surgery to prevent an increased loss of potassium. If maintenance of an extremely dry weight is necessary, these drugs can be continued but with careful daily monitoring of the serum potassium concentration. Restriction of sodium intake is preferred over use of excessive diuretics in the immediate preoperative period. The reason for discontinuing these medications is again the concern of cardiac irritability in the digitalized and even nondigitalized patients with hypokalemia.

Antihypertensive agents

Preparations such as guanethidine sulfate (Ismelin), reserpine (Serpasil), and methyldopa (Aldomet) are discontinued at least 3 days prior to surgery, as they can produce severe induction and operative and postoperative hypotension. These drugs produce their hypotensive effects by facilitating a decrease in circulating catecholamine (epinephrine and norepinephrine) concentrations.

Tranquilizers

Certain tranquilizers such as the phenothiazine derivatives (Thorazine, Stelazine, Compazine, and Combid) can also decrease circulating catecholamine concentrations and produce profound hypotension at various stages of the operation. We now use diazepam (Valium) for control of preoperative anxiety and apprehension and have observed no operative or postoperative complications. Diazepam dosages range from 2 mg four times a day to 10 mg four times a day, but we have been successful in the majority of the patients with only 2 mg four times a day. This can usually be given until the night preceding surgery.

Antidiabetic preparations

Antidiabetic drugs and oral hypoglycemic agents such as tolbutamide (Orinase), chlorpropamide (Diabinese), or phenformin hydrochloride (DBI) should be discontinued 24 hours preoperatively. Subcutaneous or IV regular insulin should not be given later than 12 hours preceding surgery, and long-acting insulins should not be utilized after the patient's admission to the hospital. Better control can be maintained using a sliding scale with regular insulin. Discontinuing these drugs at the recommended times prevents their optimum effects from occurring in the immediate preoperative or operative phase, at which time moderate hypoglycemia may produce severe hypotension with all its complications (myocardial infarction, stroke, and so forth).

Propranolol

Propranolol (Inderal) is reduced to the lowest dosage that will control the patient's symptoms. This reduction is begun 2 to 3 days before surgery and care is now taken to prevent total elimination of the drug as a result of others and ourselves having witnessed hypertension and tachycardia, with resultant ischemic signs that we believe are rebound (hyperadrenal) responses to discontinuation of the drug earlier than 12 to 24 hours before bypass surgery.

This drug has β-adrenergic blocking properties and has demonstrated blockage of both chronotropic and inotropic actions of such drugs as isoproterenol (Isuprel), epinephrine, and norepinephrine; therefore total discontinuation of its use can allow epinephrine- and norepinephrine-like rebound. This recent approach is nearly a total reversal from previous methods of discontinuing the drug anywhere from 3 to 21 days before surgery.

Phenoxybenzamine

Phenoxybenzamine (Dibenzyline) is used infrequently today but has effects similar to propranolol.

• • •

For many patients who have been on multiple medications prior to admission to the hospital it is frequently safer to consider which drugs can be safely continued rather than which drugs should be discontinued.

■ Are there medications that should be continued and, if so, why?
Potassium

Potassium supplementation is continued or instituted until the night before surgery. Potassium is given in some form of palatable liquid in dosages of 10 to 30 mEq three or four times a day. In most cases any excess dose will be excreted by the kidneys. The reason, prevention of hypokalemia, has previously been discussed.

Other preparations

Some anemic patients continue to take oral iron supplements until the night before surgery. Diabetic patients continue to take insulin until approximately 12 hours before the operative procedure. Patients with severe regurgitant esophagitis or gastric hypersecretion are maintained on antacids or coating agents such as Gelusil or Gaviscon Foamtabs until the night before surgery. Continuation of diazepam (Valium) when necessary has been mentioned.

Many incipient complications have been averted by the diligent evaluation of the patient's preoperative medication by the admitting practitioner.

■ When and how are premedications given?

Premedication orders are specifically tailored to each patient and are based on the anesthesiologist's evaluation of the patient's disease, physical findings, and laboratory data. A sedative is usually given the evening preceding surgery. An analgesic agent is given in conjunction with an agent to decrease mucous secretion and block vasovagal responses approximately 45 minutes to 1 hour prior to surgery. It is important to administer this premedication early so as to make the patient relaxed and possibly sleepy for the trip to the amphitheater and to prevent complications in performing endotracheal intubation and induction.

One of the conditions that has markedly improved in most hospitals is the competent but relaxed approach used in giving patients the premedication. In the past it has not been uncommon for the staffing to be less than ideal on the 11 PM to 7 AM shift when the majority of premedications are required. The premedicating personnel have been disproportionately busy at this time. It is important that the staff appear relaxed and efficient in administering the premedication, even though this may entail giving one premedication, smiling, appearing relaxed, and then leaving the room and running down the hall to administer the next premedication injection. If the staff appears rushed or flustered, the patient may assume that this is a reflection of the surgical encounter to follow.

■ **How detailed should the bedside practitioner's preoperative evaluation of the patient be?**

The purpose of publications and texts on intensive care includes stimulation to increase the knowledge of all concerned; therefore I believe that in addition to the principal practitioner's overall evaluation of the patient, the critical care team members should also make their own evaluations. It is of definite advantage to team and patient alike for each team member to perform the following:

1. Read and be acquainted with the patient's history and physical condition on admission.

2. Evaluate the returning laboratory results and be sure the principal practitioner is aware of abnormal reports.

3. Appropriately determine the vital signs, with special care to include both apical and radial pulses. (The bedside practitioner may be the first to pick up an essential variation in peripheral pulses.)

4. Always take the blood pressure in both arms, as it is not uncommon in the patient with advanced atherosclerosis to have a partial block of one subclavian or innominate vessel, with a difference of 10 and possibly even 40 mm Hg between the two determinations. This can be a salient factor in monitoring in the operative and postoperative period. It can also be significant in patients previously undergoing catheterization through upper extremity vessels.

5. Evaluate preoperative pulses. All practitioners should know how to find and evaluate the carotid, brachial, radial, ulnar, femoral, popliteal, posterior tibial, and dorsalis pedis pulses. These should be evaluated before surgery and recorded on the chart as to their intensity (as absent, weak, or strong, or 0, 1+, or 2+, or occasionally 0, 1+, 2+, 3+, or 4+). This evaluation and record can aid in the detection of arterial clots or peripheral dissection and initiate prompt successful intervention. The patient often can also be saved an unnecessary return to surgery by the notation of certain pulses being absent preoperatively. These recordings serve to confirm the principal practitioner's findings.

6. A most important adjunct to the overall preoperative evaluation of the surgical patient is the "complete look" procedure. Many times when patients are examined in the office, in an examining room, or in the hospital their gowns will be brought down to the groin or their trousers will be brought up from the feet, possibly missing or avoiding an area between the limits of the clothing. Occasionally in sitting up in bed or turning over, small areas of the back or the back of the head are missed. In attempting close scrutiny during the examination, a gross asymmetry of body structure can be missed. However, if the patient is evaluated at a distance completely unclothed from the front, back, and side, major factors might be noticed that could even preclude the indication for surgery or could avoid complications at the time of surgery; for example, a large squamous cell tumor of the skin or a metastatic growth, a pulsatile mass in one of the peripheral vessels, a large local varicosity with a thrombus, a local or disseminated area of pyo-

derma or possibly even an ecchymotic area suggesting coagulation problems may suggest other modes of therapy. For individuals who might be embarrassed during this examination, it frequently can be accomplished during the routine weighing procedures, which are performed with the patient nude or in scanty undergarments. In this day of medicolegal infringements any bruises, contusions, or gross deformities should be noticed and recorded before surgical intervention.

■ **What preoperative laboratory work is necessary for the cardiac surgical patient and why?**

With the sophisticated patient monitoring systems, computerized laboratory tests, and increasing numbers of patients in critical care units, it becomes the responsibility of each and every member of the team to evaluate all laboratory work. The majority of laboratories today have a mechanism for bringing to the attention of the supervising personnel those laboratory tests that are abnormal (separate columns, encircling, or recording in differently colored inks). Emphasis is placed in the laboratory on notifying the appropriate critical care personnel of any grossly abnormal laboratory results.

The following are the baseline laboratory tests ordered for preoperative cardiac surgical patients:

1. A routine complete blood count is done to determine if the patient is anemic, has an abnormal platelet count, or exhibits signs of infection or other blood disorders.

2. Urinalysis should be performed primarily to demonstrate any spill of protein or sugar or any signs of tissue breakdown as demonstrated by the presence of acetone. In addition, it is important to note any casts or abnormal pus cells, which might suggest a tendency toward renal failure or postoperative infection.

3. Fasting blood sugar levels are measured routinely to rule out the need for further diabetic workup. In proved diabetic patients they are measured at least daily in correlation with the urine sugar evaluation performed four times each day as a baseline for control. In diabetic patients a fasting blood sugar level is determined the morning of surgery because marked hypoglycemia can

be associated with hypotension, gastric hypersecretion, and other complications in the operative and postoperative period.

4. Blood urea nitrogen (BUN) concentrations are obtained as a preliminary evaluation of renal function and also as a baseline indication of dehydration or possible gastrointestinal bleeding.

5. Serum creatinine levels are a better baseline determination of renal function, and if elevated, prompt a more thorough evaluation, including creatinine clearance, intravenous pyelogram, and urologic consultation. When the creatinine and BUN levels are above normal, dosages of certain nephrotoxic antibiotics such as gentamicin sulfate are lowered accordingly.

6. The VDRL serology test is performed on admission in a majority of hospitals as routine. (However, because of certain administrative and financial dictums associated with state and federal health plans, ECG's and chest x-ray films [even in certain age groups] cannot be routine admission requirements.)

7. Electrolyte determination is performed routinely. Sodium and chloride levels are measured initially to establish sodium loss and/or water retention, and if abnormal, correlation must be made with the patient's physical findings and appropriate balances established. Potassium levels are extremely important in the preoperative phase, as numerous patients take potassium-eliminating medications, and the increased arrhythmias and ventricular irritability associated with digitalis preparations and hypokalemia are well known. Occasionally in patients with chronic renal infection hyperkalemic states can herald a major incipient problem prior to surgery.

Calcium and phosphorus concentrations are obtained for baseline studies and occasionally may indict parathyroid abnormalities, metabolic bone disorders, or possibly disseminated malignant disease.

8. Arterial blood gas measurements should be obtained in conjunction with pulmonary function studies and are important adjuncts to rule out hypoxemia, hypercapnia, and *both* respiratory and metabolic derangements. *With the frequency of utilization of this modality, every graduating critical care practitioner should be able to interpret blood gas evaluations.* Critical care person-

nel must ensure that arterial puncture is not made in femoral vessels in patients with poor leg pulses or questionable peripherovascular insufficiency. The radial artery, which most often is used for the arterial monitoring at the time of surgery, should not be abused when utilized for blood gas sample. Appropriate hemostatic techniques must be utilized when blood gases are drawn, especially in the patient who has been on anticoagulant therapy. It is important that pressure be maintained directly over the puncture site for a minimum of 10 minutes after obtaining a sample and that a modified pressure dressing then be applied. Pressure dressings over the wrists are composed of a small sterile 2 × 2 inch folded pledget, rolled so that it is approximately

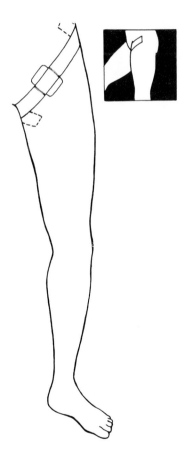

Fig. 17-1. Pressure dressing for femoral artery puncture sites.

1 cm in height, and applied firmly with tape, being sure that the tape does not totally encircle the wrist (complications have occurred with totally encircling constrictive dressings on the extremities). If the blood gas measurement must be obtained in the groin, this pressure dressing is applied using tincture of benzoin spray on the medial aspect of the thigh just below the pelvis and above the iliac crest; when dry, tape is applied well under the medial aspect of the thigh and stretched across to the iliac crest, firmly fixing a ¾-inch wad of sterile dressing over the arterial puncture site (Fig. 17-1). *These dressings are left on no longer than 2 hours and then removed.* If this procedure is followed, there is seldom any extravasation found at surgery.

9. Baseline coagulation screens are routine and include bleeding and clotting time tests performed using one of the accepted methods, partial thromboplastin and prothrombin time tests, fibrinogen level determinations, platelet counts, euglobulin lysis tests, and clot retraction evaluations.

10. The ECG is obtained on admission and compared by the cardiologist with previous ECG's. If the patient has not had previous ECG's in the admitting hospital, attempts are made to obtain previous recent ECG's. The ECG is repeated just prior to surgery and compared with the previous interpretation, which is recorded on the chart. A major change in the cardiac rhythm, development of ischemia, or possibly even a silent infarct has been known to occur in the time elapsing between admission and surgery.

11. Cardiac enzyme levels are also measured. If the patient has daily or crescendo-type angina, appropriate enzyme levels are obtained to eliminate the possibility of acute infarction, which could precipitate immediate surgery or postponement. If the patient's condition is relatively stable and angina does not occur ar rest, enzyme levels are measured on admission and on the day preceeding surgery. The basic cardiac enzymes obtained include creatine-phosphokinase (CPK) and lactic dehydrogenase (LDH). If these enzymes are elevated, then their isoenzyme components are obtained to determine if myocardial muscle damage has recently occurred.

12. Posteroanterior and lateral chest x-ray

PREOPERATIVE ORDERS

ON ADMISSION CALL PHYSICIAN REGARDING:

1. Diet _____

2. Privileges _____
3. V S q shift (Record BP in both arms.)
4. Check all pulses and record.
5. Betadine shower daily AM and PM and AM of surgery.
6. Have all previous charts on ward.
7. Have on ward all medications the patient has been taking within the past 3 weeks and record. Call physician regarding medications to continue.
8. Critical care to be notified of patient's admission.
9. Mended Hearts representative may visit patient.

MEDICATION

1. Antibiotics _____

2. prn sedation _____

3. Nitroglycerin _____ gr (at bedside) prn chest pain.

4. hs sedation _____
5. Laxative: if constipated, Senokot granules, 2 drams, each hs or laxative of choice. If no results, call physician.

LABORATORY WORK ON ADMISSION

1. Urinalysis, CBC, VDRL, cholesterol, uric acid, alkaline phosphatase, calcium, phosphorus, ttl. bilirubin, albumin, Na^+, Cl^-, K^+, creatine, glucose, and BUN
2. C & S of sputum and urine (If preoperative valve surgery, do C & S of blood and skin also.)
3. SGOT, LDH, CPK (Do isoenzymes if elevated.)
4. Cardiac surgery coagulation screen: platelet count, fibrinogen index (FI), prothrombin time, partial thromboplastin time (PTT), activated clotting time, Lee-White bleeding and clotting times
5. ECG, PA and lateral chest film (upright)

LABORATORY WORK DAY PRECEDING SURGERY

1. Pulmonary screen with arterial blood gases
2. Respiratory therapy introduction and instruction on postoperative use of IPPB and incentive spirometer

3. Type and cross match _____ units whole blood and/or _____ units packed cells

EVENING BEFORE SURGERY

1. Surgical consent to read _____
2. Consent for photograph
3. Prep: entire trunk, including both axillae, abdomen, pubis to toes, and completely around legs
4. Check all pulses and record; if different from admission, call physician.
5. NPO at midnight
6. hs and "on call" medications as per anesthesiologist

films are obtained at the time of admission regardless of the time of the last film because a small pneumothorax, pulmonary infiltrate, or signs of failure might have recently developed. If this is the first admission for the patient, special roentgenograms are obtained with and without barium in the esophagus to establish enlargement of the various cardiac chambers.

13. A liver profile includes the prothrombin time test, which reflects hepatic parenchymal function; SGOT and SGPT determinations, which are raised in parenchymal injury; alkaline phosphatase determination, the value of which is elevated with intraductal or postductal obstruction; and bilirubin level determination, the value of which is elevated in biliary obstruction and conditions in which red blood cells are broken down or destroyed. If any of the foregoing tests reveal elevated values, a sulfobromophthalein (Bromsulfthalein, BSP) test is performed, especially in individuals who drink excessively, have a history of hepatitis, or have been subjected to hepatotoxic anesthetics such as halothane. If any of these tests are abnormal, it is essential for the anesthesiologist and cardiac team to avoid potentially hepatotoxic agents.

14. Pulmonary function is evaluated. As previously mentioned, the patient is introduced to the pulmonary therapist, and if history or laboratory and physical findings suggest pulmonary disease, it is essential to obtain a complete evaluation of pulmonary function, including vital capacity, lung volume, expiratory flow rate, forced expiratory volume (FEV_1, FEV_3), and maximum ventilatory volume (MVV or MBC). Consideration of total pulmonary function should also include determination of arterial gas concentrations, as previously mentioned. Some laboratories include measurement of dynamic arterial gases (arterial gas levels during various activities). Very young patients or those without any pulmonary problems are subjected simply to a pulmonary function screening test.

15. The EEG is performed as a baseline only in patients with a positive history or symptoms and/or signs of neurologic involvement.

• • •

The boxed material on p. 332 is a typical example of the preoperative orders for each patient admitted for cardiac surgery.

■ What procedure should be followed once the patient is en route to surgery?

First, the patient should be allowed a short visit from the family the morning of cardiac surgery.

Ideally the individual responsible for the transport of the patient should give the impression of being in control and fully aware of the patient's surgery to be performed. It can be extremely upsetting for a patient to hear an orderly or pickup team arrive at the ward and ask the ward practitioners, "Where is the heart?" or "Where is Mr. What's his name?" or mispronounce the name. The poor patient could be fearful of arriving in the wrong amphitheater and undergoing another patient's surgery. Such considerations may sound trivial; however, when discussing the hospital stay with patients, *these* are examples of what is remembered most about the surgery, as well as the feelings of insecurity or anxiety these thoughts produced.

The patient should be transported to the operating room, hopefully, well covered and warm and securely strapped to the gurney. Ideally operating amphitheaters should have anterooms so that it would be unnecessary for a patient to remain on a gurney in the hallway (possibly listening to nonprofessional chatter or observing other patients en route to other operating rooms). The cardiac patient especially should have an escort or a constant attendant until the anesthesiologist is present.

REFERENCE

1. Juler, G. L., Stemmer, E. A., and Connolly, J. E.: Complications of prophylactic digitalization in thoracic surgery patients, J. Thorac. Cardiovasc. Surg. **58:**352, 1969.

CHAPTER 18

Operative care of the adult cardiac surgical patient

Robert A. Steedman

Following transportation of the patient to the operating room or to an induction room, anesthetics should be administered and monitoring devices preferably inserted by the anesthesia department personnel. If there is difficulty in the percutaneous establishment of the monitoring equipment, the surgical staff should be solicited for appropriate surgical (cutdown) insertion of the required devices. In many hospitals such procedures are performed in the operating room under anesthesia or, in "poor risk" patients, insertion of monitoring catheters as well as femoral artery and vein cannulation for temporary bypass may be performed under local anesthesia prior to the patient's induction. This is especially true in patients undergoing surgery for massive pulmonary embolization or patients with left main coronary artery disease with instability requiring preinduction insertion of the intra-aortic balloon.

ANESTHESIA

In articles concerning the care of the cardiac surgical patient the role of the anesthesiologist is frequently underplayed. His or her role is most important during the operative phase in maintaining the confidence of the patient before induction and establishing stable vital signs during surgery, utilizing a combination of muscle relaxants, anesthetic agents, and pain medications. The anesthesiologist must guarantee that the patient does not receive any toxic insult to the cardiac, pulmonary, renal, CNS, or hepatic systems and must ensure against the development of

critical hypotensive or hypertensive events, therefore having a very tedious but extremely major role in the care of the cardiac surgical patient.

MONITORING
■ What vessel is used for arterial monitoring?

An attempt is usually first made with a percutaneous puncture using one of the large-bore plastic-sleeve needles; once the artery is entered, the sharply pointed needle is removed, and the noncutting plastic sleeve is manipulated for 3 to 4 cm up the radial artery. It is stabilized to the skin by suturing to prevent pullout (Fig. 18-1).

If the percutaneous method is not successful or not facilitated easily, a small incision is used, the vessel is isolated, the needle and cannula are inserted without incising the artery, and recannulation and preservation of the artery after removal is more probable. Special notches are carved in the plastic hub of the needle to which sutures are secured. If the radial arteries cannot be utilized, a cutdown can be performed over the ulnar artery.

If there are poor radial pulses, prior to the ulnar artery cutdown the patient is evaluated with the Allen test to be sure that there is adequate collateral circulation; this test is performed by compressing both the ulnar and radial arteries while the patient repeatedly makes a fist to establish claudication in the hand (pale blanching and tingling) and then either the radial or the ulnar artery is released. If the palm fails to blush after the release of either one of these arteries, this

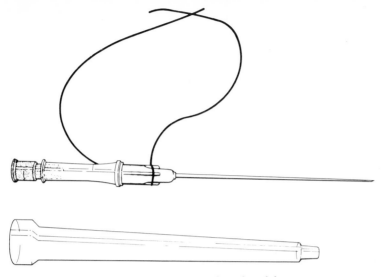

Fig. 18-1. Intra-arterial monitor needle with stabilizing sutures.

suggests decreased vascular supply to the palmar arch from that vessel and the remaining vessel should probably not be used.

In the literature it is extremely rare for digit or hand loss to complicate use of these arteries; however, there have been local areas of necrosis reported. Occasionally these areas of necrosis are caused by frequent irrigation or partial blockage of collaterals from the plastic cannula. There have, however, been recent verbal communications of digit loss from harvesting the radial artery for use in aortocoronary artery bypass.

■ **What other vessels can be utilized for arterial monitoring?**

The nonperfused femoral artery can be used by means of a percutaneous puncture or direct cutdown isolation.

Once described was a small transverse incision made in the antecubital space (at the time of isolating the basilic and cephalic veins for central venous pressure monitoring and venous infusion) with isolation of the brachial artery for arterial monitoring; no complications have been reported. In experienced hands this appears to be a good technique.

A modification of a technique described by Hegeman, Rappaport, and Berger[1] involves the use of the superficial temporal artery. This artery has been used in young adults and children who are burn victims with no accessible extremity arteries. This artery can be interrupted without consequence, the scar can be hidden later by normal sideburn growth in males and usual hairdos in females. The only drawback is the occasional cannulation in a tortuous thin-walled artery.

When the aorta is to be clamped in cases of resection or surgical repair of dissection, it becomes necessary to have an upper extremity (preferably the right) and a lower extremity arterial monitor, so the left heart bypass apparatus can be adjusted to prevent brain and upper extremity hypertension but maintain abdominal visceral perfusion.

■ **What complications can occur as a result of the insertion of arterial monitors?**

In the radial artery small dissections of the intima can occur when attempting to thread the plastic cannula; this causes thrombosis, but if the occlusion is very distal and the ulnar artery is open, there will be no major complications. Recently we have had an increased number of pseudoaneurysms develop at the radial artery puncture sites where the anterior and posterior walls have been violated by multiple punctures.

Either by midjudgment or error, medications can be injected into this cannula and cause severe spasm and thrombosis with resultant skin slough. No medications other than heparinized solutions should be given in arterial lines.

Overenthusiastic irrigations in wrist arteries can produce necrosis and local skin slough.

With femoral artery monitoring, peripheral clots, embolized atheroma, intimal dissection, posterior wall perforations, hematomas, and hemorrhage can occur and occasionally require surgical correction. Some investigators are more skilled than others at performing this procedure.

In the hands of those who use the brachial artery routinely morbidity is probably extremely low; however, because of reports of complicating thrombosis resulting in partial limb loss occurring in young patients monitored by this method, its use is usually avoided.

The cannulation and monitoring procedure that best fits the situation and is most successful in the critical care team's experience should be used.

■ **What are the reasons for using arterial monitors?**

Accurate cuff pressures are extremely difficult to obtain during perfusion when the nonpulsatile mean pressures range between 50 and 70 mm Hg. The arterial monitor decreases the frequent need of wrapping a cuff around the arm when there might be multiple infusion lines in that arm. It also provides a withdrawal line for arterial gas determination, electrolyte levels, and other blood tests during the critical operative and postoperative period.

■ **Can the pressures vary from arm to arm?**

There can be variances as high as 75 mm Hg between the right and left arm if subclavian stenosis from atherosclerosis or brachial artery narrowing from heart catheterization exists; again, this is a valid indication for determining blood pressures in both arms (possibly even simultaneously) as well as evaluating and reporting the quality of each pulse in the preoperative period.

■ **What techniques are utilized and what is the purpose of central venous pressure monitors?**

Any major peripheral vein that will allow manipulation of a catheter into the central venous system (right atrium and superior or inferior vena cava) will usually suffice for central venous pressure monitoring. This can be performed through the external or internal jugular or subclavian veins by percutaneous puncture, through the basilic or cephalic veins percutaneously or by cutdown, or via a branch of the greater saphenous vein.

The cephalic or basilic veins, with attempted manipulation of the catheter into the subclavian, innominate, and finally into the superior vena cava, may be used, but frequently the catheter cannot be passed beyond the peripheral valves or deviates into the veins of the neck or head.

Many anesthesiologists have become skilled at performing percutaneous punctures of the subclavian or internal jugular veins, but problems with hematoma, pneumothorax, and complicating infections have been reported.

Occasionally the external jugular system can be approached by the anesthesiologist through the use of a percutaneous puncture and manipulation of the cannula down into the superior vena cava (similar to passing a transvenous permanent or temporary electrode), but this procedure is more often successful with a cutdown approach. The purpose of the central venous pressure monitor is to establish a guide for fluid replacement to indirectly assess ventricular function. It is more accurate in assessing the need for fluid replacement than it is for monitoring overhydration. There are multiple reports wherein the central venous pressure monitor reflected overhydration, but a left atrial cannula demonstrated hypovolemia; occasionally the opposite has also occured.

■ **What other methods of measurement of hydration and cardiac function or left ventricular function are available?**

Some institutions routinely utilize a left atrial line. This can be placed in the left atrium at surgery by manipulating a plastic catheter through a No. 20- or 18-gauge needle and removing the needle, leaving the catheter in place and stabilized by a small purse-string suture. Problems with this technique include dislodgment of the catheter during the operative and immediate postoperative period, possible air and clot embolization to the brain, intrapericardial bleeding on removal, and where the catheter is brought out a separate puncture site in the anterior chest wall, it can become kinked or plugged. Despite these problems, use of the left atrial cannula is a more accurate means of evaluating left ventricular function and hydration.

When there is dire need of better left ventricular and left atrial assessment, a Swan-Ganz pulmonary artery catheter with an inflatable small balloon tip can be floated from a peripheral vein through the right atrium and right ventricle into the pulmonary artery. The catheter can be manipulated into a peripheral pulmonary artery branch and wedged; this "wedge pressure" reflects the left atrial pressure. It is most often positioned by a cardiologist via a right antecubital vein, but other veins can be used.

Urinary output is a prime reflection of cardiac output and renal perfusion. A catheter is placed aseptically after the other monitor lines have been stabilized. When personnel other than surgeons place these catheters, it is of utmost importance that free-flowing urine be obtained before inflation of the balloon and that the accurate positioning of the catheter be confirmed. If these measures are not followed, creation of a false channel or intraurethral inflation of the balloon can produce a critical situation.

Another parameter of appropriate perfusion during use of the pump is the body temperature, and rectal and esophageal temperature probes are placed prior to induction. These are essential in patients requiring systemic cooling and rewarming.

THE OPERATION
■ What scrub and preparation technique is utilized?

For most cardiac operations today, especially the revascularization procedures, the patient is scrubbed from the chin down to and including the toes. A 10-minute Betadine surgical soap scrub followed by drying, application of the Betadine preparation solution, and redrying is used. The standard techniques of working away from the incision sites to the periphery are followed.

■ Are there any special adhesive coverings utilized?

Most institutions today use various forms of plastic drapes over the intended incision sites; these drapes serve a twofold purpose: they decrease incision contamination from surrounding skin areas, and they are nonconductible, thus preventing possible skin burns.

■ How often is the electrical cautery used and are there any special precautions to be taken?

The electrical cautery apparatus is utilized in the majority of open-heart surgeries performed, but many surgeons will not utilize this apparatus if a temporary or permanent pacemaker is in place for fear of electrical mishaps associated with either intraventricular or epicardial electrodes.

Special nonconductive containers for the individual electrocoagulation units are essential so that patients and/or personnel are not burned or shocked with an exposed primary or secondary unit. Hand-operated units are preferred so that both surgeon and assistant can utilize a unit independently and replace each unit into a separate nonconductive container.

■ What incisions are utilized for cardiac surgery?

The most commonly used incision is the midsternotomy, especially for myocardial revascularization procedures, many of the valve procedures, and most of the adult congenital defect repairs.

Occasionally for the closed valve techniques a right or left inframammary incision is used for cosmetic reasons and technical convenience.

For surgery involving the descending aorta (coarctation, aneurysm, dissection, and so forth) the posterior lateral thoracotomy incision is used, frequently requiring two separate intercostal entrances (for example, at the fourth and seventh intercostal junctions).

Transsternal and thoracoabdominal incisions are only used in exceptionally difficult exposure cases, and the parasternal approach is used for local pericardiectomy, placements of temporary epicardial electrodes, and occasionally evacuation of pericardial tamponade.

■ Which incisions are least painful and less difficult to care for postoperatively?

The incisions that are least painful, most stable, and easiest to care for are as follows in respective order: midsternotomy, parasternal, subxiphoid, inframammary, transternal, posterior lateral thoractomy, and the troublesome and frequently complicated thoracoabdominal incision.

■ What precautionary measures are taken prior to making the skin incision?

Usually 1 or 2 units of blood are in the operating room refrigerator prior to splitting the sternum in case any undue bleeding is encountered, and the pump technician should be in the room and ready in the event immediate perfusion is necessary.

■ What are the routine steps in the cannulation procedure?

The sternotomy incision is completed and electrocoagulation is utilized to control bleeding. Bone wax is applied to control oozing from the divided sternum. The pericardium is carefully cleared of the pleura, thymus, and fatty tissue, taking care not to injure the innominate vein. The pericardium is then opened while a leg incision is made simultaneously for harvesting the saphenous vein. Frequently, the saphenous veins from the ankle to the knee are used as the caliber of the vessel is more equal to that of the coronary artery.

After the pericardium is opened and retracted with stay sutures, a purse-string suture is placed into the right atrium and the patient is then given heparin. The anticoagulation dose is usually 3 mg of heparin per kilogram of body weight. The heparin dosage in the vial from which it is obtained is always verified by the anesthesiologist or surgeon; it is administered by the surgeon directly into the right atrium.

Approximately 3 minutes after heparin infusion, aortic cannulation is completed and then through the previously placed atrial purse-string

sutures a single two-stage cannula is positioned into the right atrium and the inferior vena cava. Occasionally for valve replacement surgery and whenever it is anticipated that the tricuspid valve must be approached, two single cannulas are used, one in the inferior vena cava and one in the superior vena cava.

■ What other methods of arterial cannulation for pump perfusion are available?

Arterial return is usually established through the use of aortic cannulation through a double purse-string suture with the tip directed into the arch of the aorta. Occasionally it is necessary to utilize the femoral route for return of arterial blood. This decision is frequently made when the aorta is dangerously dilated or extensively diseased with atherosclerosis with extensive calcification.

■ What is the pump and how does it work?

The pump, or cardiopulmonary bypass apparatus, is the mechanical substitute for the heart and lungs. There are a variety of models used, but the mechanism of action consists basically of draining unoxygenated blood by gravity from the atrial cannula to a reservoir and oxygenator where the blood is filmed over or through plastic and exposed to high concentrations of inflow oxygen. The blood, now oxygenated, is pumped back to the aortic cannula by means of a rotating modular roller head. The revolving rollers partially occlude or compress the plastic tubes containing the oxygenated blood and force it back to the body through the arterial cannula.

■ With what are the pump and oxygenator primed?

Most oxygenators today are plastic, disposable units initially prepared or primed (filled) with crystalloid solutions, blood, electrolyte solutions or a combination of these solutions. The all-blood solution was the most common prime until approximately 10 to 13 years ago when conversion to the use of more crystalloid solutions began.

When low blood or nonblood primes are initially pumped into the patient, the patient's hemoglobin level and hematocrit are diluted. The hemoglobin content is usually maintained between 7 and 10 g under average circumstances, probably decreasing rouleaux formation of blood cells and preventing sludging and peripheral clotting problems.

When utilizing nonblood primes, protein is frequently added in the form of albumin, plasma substitutes, and occasionally mannitol, which is considered a prophylactic measure against renal shutdown.

The recommended prime solution is between 1½ to 2 L of electrolyte replacement solution (Plasma-Lyte), 50 mg of heparin (25 mg/L of diluent), 200 ml of 25% albumin, frequently 200 ml of 25% mannitol (Osmitrol), and 1 g of cefazolin sodium (Kefzol). In patients who are allergic to the cephalosporins, 2 g of lincomycin (Lincocin) are substituted for Kefzol. Blood may be added if the hemodilution effect lowers the hemoglobin content below 7 g/100 ml, and corticosteroids are added in the form of methylprednisolone (Solu-Medrol). The hemodilution occasionally appears to initially lower the mean pressure to around 50 mm Hg for about 5 minutes, but this can be immediately counteracted by minimum IV doses of phenylephrine hydrochloride (Neo-Synephrine).

■ What are the specific techniques utilized in revascularization?

The patients' cardiac functions are usually maintained by the bypass apparatus and stabilized for a period of 2 to 3 minutes. The patient is then cooled to approximately 30 C and the heart is either fibrillated electrically or placed in standstill by injection into the aortic root of a potassium-containing solution or a cold blood solution containing extra potassium. The aorta is then cross-clamped, the coronary vessel is isolated and opened beyond the obstruction or stenosis with a 0.8 to 1.0 cm vertical slit, determination is made of antegrade and retrograde flow, and cannulation can be performed proximally and distally with special sizing probes (1.0 to 2.5 mm). The saphenous vein (which has been harvested and prepared to avoid leakage) is reversed and anastomosed distally to the coronary artery with very fine (6-0) nonabsorbable (Prolene) suture. In some selected cases the left internal mammary artery is dissected from the chest wall and anastomosed to the left anterior descending coronary artery as an in situ end-to-side graft. When distal anastomoses are completed, the aortic cross-clamp is removed, the heart is defibrillated or allowed to resume contractions, a partial

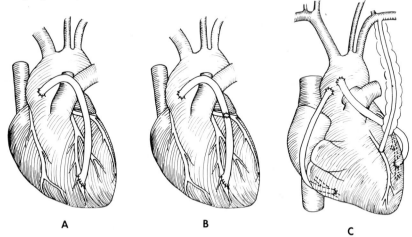

| A | B | C |

Fig. 18-2. Coronary artery revascularization. **A,** Left anterior descending (LAD) saphenous vein bypass. **B,** Sequential (jump) saphenous vein graft to diagonal branch and LAD. **C,** Internal mammary artery in-situ bypass to LAD in conjunction with saphenous vein bypasses to right and circumflex coronary arteries.

occluding clamp is then placed on the aorta, and the proximal vein anastomoses are completed (Fig. 18-2).

■ What is potassium cardioplegia and why is it used?

The ability of potassium solutions to totally arrest the ventricular activity of the heart has been known since 1955. However, the original utilization of this material was as a solution externally applied around the heart in the pericardial cavity, and there was a suspicion that it created focal areas of myocardial necrosis. Recent studies have demonstrated that infusion of potassium-containing solutions into the aortic route, which flows into the coronary arteries and branches, can create total arrest of ventricular activity of the heart and appears to markedly reduce the tendency of the myocardium to be damaged or injured even during prolonged periods of anoxic arrest. This technique of cardioplegia also allows one to work on a totally still and flaccid heart and with repeated injections allows the surgeon to perform all the distal anastomoses or complete a valve replacement without intermittent periods of perfusion in the beating heart.

Additional studies have suggested that cardioplegia effected by injection of potassium-containing blood into the aortic root may be more physiologic and even afford more protection of the myocardium. We are presently using this technique on all cardiac surgical cases. The cardioplegic solution is blood containing the following constituents per 500 ml of blood volume: 15 mEq of potassium chloride, 25 ml of THAM (0.3 molar solution)—a buffering solution to bring the pH to 7.6, 10 ml of citrate phosphate dextrose (CPD) to decrease the ionic calcium to 0.6 mEq, and methylprednisolone sodium succinate (Solu-Medrol) if same is not already being used in the usual priming solution. As the patient is placed on cardiopulmonary bypass, 500 to 1000 ml of blood is withdrawn and placed into a separate reservoir and the previously mentioned proportionate constituents are added. This blood is then cooled to between 10° and 12° C, and then at the time of desired cardioplegia it is injected into the aortic root and within seconds induces total cardiac arrest.

Immediately after this infusion, temperatures are obtained in various areas of the myocardium and ventricular chambers, with the preferred temperature in the aorta and ventricular chambers being between 10° and 14° C and that of the myocardium between 15° and 20° C. The cardioplegic solution is reintroduced every 20 to 30 minutes until the surgical procedure has been completed and there is no further need for arrest.

It has been unofficially reported that in some institutions this technique has been utilized for periods of 4 hours without evident myocardial damage.

There are many other cardioplegic solutions being evaluated and utilized at the present time with the specific advantages of each being investigated. It appears evident at this stage of cardiac surgery that some form of cardioplegia is here to stay.

■ How is the heparin dosage determined during the pump run and how is it reversed at completion?

If the total time of the pump run is 1 hour or less, the total amount of heparin used is the same as the initial heparinizing dose (3 mg/kg of body weight); when the pump time extends beyond 1 hour, approximately one half of the original anticoagulating dose is administered, but this is all dependent on the results of the activated clotting time (ACT), which is run at 20- to 30-minute intervals during the bypass procedure. The ACT is preferably kept at between 450 and 600 seconds (7½ to 10 minutes). At the completion of the perfusion and when the cannulas have been removed, the total reversing dose of protamine sulfate is then titrated according to the final activated clotting time. Evidence of adequate reversal is demonstrated by the formation of small clots with decreased oozing as well as a normal activated clotting time between 1½ and 2 minutes, and this is usually witnessed within a period of 2 to 5 minutes after the administration of the protamine sulfate is completed.

■ Are there any precautions to be taken with the administration of protamine sulfate?

Rapid IV administration of protamine sulfate has been known to cause hypotension, and sensitivity to IV administration has been demonstrated in some patients; therefore protamine sulfate is given by slow micro drop administration over a period of 10 to 15 minutes so that any hypotensive episodes can be recognized and corrected.

■ **At what temperature is the cardiac patient maintained, and how is this controlled?**

During cardiac procedures in which only short-term clamping of the aorta or ventricular fibrillation is used, normothermic temperatures can be maintained; however, it is preferable for the patient's temperature to be 28° to 30° C, as this allows the myocardium to tolerate decreased perfusion for longer periods of time. In some cases of congenital cardiac surgery (especially in infants and children) deep hypothermia can be used (10° to 20° C), which allows total body perfusion to be suspended for periods of as much as 1 hour. Localized cooling of the heart can be accomplished by packing it in iced slush.

Cooling and warming are accomplished by use of an oxygenating system with an integral heat exchange; however, most of these commercial products do not warm the patient as rapidly as is desired by most surgeons.

■ **What technique can be used to prevent air embolization?**

Air bubbles are carefully manipulated out of all arterial lines prior to beginning the perfusion process in the patient. A left ventricular or atrioventricular vent, when used, prevents air accumulation in the left ventricle; prior to removal of this vent the left ventricle is elevated to allow the air to rise to the highest point and be removed by suction. If a vent has not been utilized, the ventricular apex is raised and decompressed with an 18-gauge needle.

During the perfusion run some pulmonary positive pressure is maintained at all times; just prior to removal of vents and cannulas the lungs are hyperinflated with applied pressures to 35 to 40 cm, and the left atrial appendage is manipulated so that air will flow toward the elevated left ventricular apex.

During all these procedures the patient remains with the head down or in the modified Trendelenburg position so that air bubbles passing the aortic valve will be trapped in the aortic root, and an 18-gauge needle or special vent is used to evacuate the air from the aorta. During mitral valve and congenital septal defect surgery an aortic "tack" may be sutured directly to the aorta for continual venting during the cardiac procedure and when the patient is released from the pump.

■ **When are pacemaker wires inserted?**

Pacing wires are sutured to the atrium and myocardium, or myocardium alone, whenever there appears to be increased risk of heart block or any other arrhythmia involving poor cardiac output. These temporary wires can be easily removed in the postoperative period.

When heart block was present prior to the surgery requiring a temporary pacemaker, permanent suture electrodes are placed at the completion of surgery using Medtronics sutureless corkscrew electrodes.

■ **How many chest tubes are utilized, why are they used, and where are they placed?**

If only the mediastinum or pericardium has been violated, two No. 36 or No. 40 argyle plastic chest tubes are sufficient to drain the pericardium, one placed in an anterograde and the other in a retrograde position with regard to the heart for evacuation of blood and clots. When the pleura has been violated on either the left or right side, chest tubes also are placed to evacuate air and allow reexpansion of the lung. The specific placement of the tubes varies with each practitioner. In cases where the pleura has not been violated, some individuals place both chest tubes in a position anterior to the heart; others place one chest tube in an anterior position and the other in a posterior position, hoping to prevent the development of cardiac tamponade.

If either chest cavity has been entered, one chest tube is usually placed in the area of the costovertebral groove to drain blood spilled over from the mediastinum and also to evacuate air. If there is any question of lung perforation, a second tube can be placed near the apex of the lung to ensure air evacuation. In cases where both pleural cavities are entered, it is not uncommon to use as many as four tubes, and when four chest tubes are necessary, it is preferable not to connect them all to the same suction apparatus if maximum efficient suction and drainage is to be obtained.

■ **What parameters are measured during the operative procedure?**

Arterial pressures and pulse wave contours are monitored continuously during the procedure as well as the central venous or left atrial pressure.

Arterial gas determinations should be obtained at least every 20 to 30 minutes to maintain expected gas tensions. The levels strived for are as follows: Po_2 of 100 to 150 mm Hg, Pco_2 of 32 to 40 mm Hg, pH of 7.35 to 7.45, O_2 concentration of 95% to 99%, and a base excess near zero.

The serum potassium levels are obtained every 30 to 45 minutes because, as previously mentioned, hypokalemia can lead to serious arrhythmias, and hyperkalemia can prevent return of ventricular contractility.

The hemoglobin and hematocrit levels are evaluated every 30 to 45 minutes to maintain hemodilution with a hemoglobin concentration between 7 and 10 g and a hematocrit between 22% and 30% until the pump run is completed, when additional blood is added to obtain more normal levels.

Urinary output is measured every 15 minutes and used as an indication of adequate renal perfusion or possible impending renal shutdown. During perfusion outputs greater than 100 ml/hr are desired, and color concentration is noted to evaluate the amount of red blood cell hemolysis. When moderate hemolysis is evident by pink or reddened urine, a higher urinary output is induced to protect against renal failure; with the higher output the serum potassium levels must be carefully observed.

All of these parameters are recorded on an intraoperative flow board (Fig. 18-3) so that the condition of the patient can be evaluated by members of the operating team at any time.

Urine	P_{CO_2}	P_{O_2}	pH	O_2 saturation	HCO_3^-	Hematocrit	Potassium	Time
15 ml	41	120	7.39	98 %	29	43 CVP 16	5.1	8 AM
30 ml	39	104	7.41	97 %	31			8.30 AM
				On bypass ————————→				9 AM
100 ml	33	140	7.48	99 %	24	32	4.6	
60 ml	39	160	7.43	99 %	32	29	4.0	9 30/AM
54 ml	35	130	7.46	97 %	26	27	3.7	10 00/AM
				Aorta cross-clamp → On ————→				10 10/AM
				Aorta cross-clamp → Off ————→				10 24/AM
75 ml	39	170	7.43	98 %	27	29 CVP 12	3.1	10 30/AM
				Off bypass ————————→				10 30/AM
100 ml	33	130	7.49	97 %	24	35	4.0	11.00/AM
25 ml	39	100	7.43	96 %	27	37	4.4	11 15/AM
				To critical care ————————→				11 15/AM

Fig. 18-3. Intraoperative flow board.

■ What are the common intraoperative arrhythmias?

Intraoperative arrhythmias associated with ventricular irritability during periods of myocardial ischemia or immediately after defibrillation are frequently seen and consist of premature ventricular beats (PVB's) and ventricular tachycardia.

Atrial ectopic beats occur often during the period of atrial cannulation, but usually cease spontaneously after manipulation. Atrial fibrillation and flutter occur occasionally after the patient is released from the bypass apparatus, but these can usually be electrically converted during surgery. Sinus bradycardia as a vasovagal or vagovagal response during induction or postperfusion periods with varying degrees of heart block can also occur.

Control of these arrhythmias in the intraoperative period is similar to control in the coronary care units, for example, intravenous lidocaine (Xylocaine) is used for ventricular arrhythmias and ectopic beats; the cautious administration of potassium is employed in hypokalemic-associated ventricular arrhythmias; atropine is utilized in the treatment of severe sinus bradycardia associated with vasovagal or vagovagal response; and occasionally isoproterenol hydrochloride (Isuprel) is used for the hypotensive nonvolume-depleted bradycardia patient.

■ How are episodes of intraoperative hypotension and hypertension controlled?

Hypotension during bypass procedures occurs with imbalance of arterial perfusion and venous return and is frequently associated with hypovolemia. Marked angulation of the atrial cannulas can decrease venous return, but on recognition this is easily corrected. Dampening of the arterial monitor cannulas can give false low readings, and simple irrigation of the peripheral arterial line will rapidly correct this pseudohypotension.

Mild periods of hypotension associated with high cardiac output or the suggestion of collapse of peripheral vascular resistance can be controlled with small doses of phenylephrine hydrochloride (Neo-Synephrine), phenylephrine, norepinephrine, or, for short periods of time, metaraminol (Aramine).

Persistent periods of hypotension after multiple attempts to terminate the use of the bypass apparatus may require drug assistance. When adequate volume is demonstrated by a normal or elevated central venous or left atrial pressure, isoproterenol (Isuprel) or dopamine (Intropin) is administered using a titrated micro drop infusion. Elevation of the blood pressure without tachycardia is the desired effect and the reason for drug titration. Isoproterenol has the advantage of producing an inotropic effect on the heart without constricting the peripheral arterial bed.

The use of drug combinations has been reported in the literature concerning the treatment of hypotension with varying results; these preparations include combinations of epinephrine and isoproterenol, isoproterenol and glucagon, or glucagon or epinephrine solutions alone.

Dopamine (Intropin) has been shown to be very effective in these situations without causing peripheral vascular constriction, uncontrollable tachycardias, or renal complications.

Uncontrollable postoperative hypotension or low cardiac output occasionally requires more radical measures or cardiac assistance. The most common cardiac assistance device used today is the intra-aortic balloon developed as a result of the work of Dr. Adrian Kantrowitz. These apparatuses can be a major asset to the postoperative low cardiac output patient; however, they are not without potential hazards or complications.

Hypertension during the period immediately before using the pump can be extremely hazardous and can cause intracerebral complications or increase the potential for aortic dissection or vascular tears during cannulation or when instituting perfusion. If the hypertension is associated with tachycardia, it may precipitate myocardial ischemia or infarction. This can usually be controlled by the anesthesiologist in maintaining appropriate depths of anesthesia, by the temporary use of halothane (Fluothane) gas, with frequent doses of IV morphine sulfate, or with the administration of IV Inderal.

In situations where the peripheral arterial bed appears to be constricted as evidenced by severe pallor, lack of capillary blanching, and bluish mottling of the skin, 1 or 2 mg of slowly administered IV chlorpromazine (Thorazine) can be given and repeated as necessary.

If the hypertension occurs during the pumping period, IV chlorpromazine or the sublingual or IV use of one of the nitrate preparations is recommended; titration with IV nitroprusside (Nipride, 100 mg in 1000 ml 5% dextrose in water) can be used.

The patient with postoperative refractory hypertension may require treatment with one of the peripheral vasodilating drugs such as trimethaphan camsylate (Arfonad). This requires very diligent second-by-second bedside monitoring and can be most hazardous to the patient if the appropriate monitoring is not utilized. It is recommended only when other means of control are unsuccessful or for patients with labile aortic vascular repairs. Nipride is preferred because of its dependability.

■ How is the sternum closed after it has been divided surgically?

The sternum is reapproximated with No. 20 heavy stainless steel wire attached to a special cutting needle or brought up through the sternum on each side with the use of a sternal awl. The awl looks like a large hand-driven needle or ice pick with a hole in the tip. The wire, once through the sternum on each side, is tightly twisted and cut off so that a length of approximately ¾ cm remains. The end of this twisted wire is then bent flush with the sternum and the muscle and fascia are approximated over the wire.

Approximately 1% or less of patients will have some irritation from the sternal wires requiring removal at a later date; this relatively simple procedure can be done under local anesthesia.

Patients should be advised after their surgery not to receive any deep heat treatment (such as microthermy or diathermy) over the area with the sternal wires as this can cause discomfort and tissue damage. The patient should be informed that the sternum has been closed with wires so that presence on future chest x-ray films will not cause him or his attorney to think that multiple pieces of hardware were left in his chest.

Another technique for closing the sternum utilizes a heavy nonabsorbable plastic suture circumscribing the sternum, with care taken not to injure the internal mammary artery and vein.

■ How is blood loss decreased in the operating room?

The more sophisticated techniques of titrating the administration of heparin and reversal with protamine sulfate, which has greatly decreased the amount of postoperative bleeding and oozing, have been extremely satisfying. In addition, for the last 18 months an apparatus that reprocesses the residual blood left in the perfusion lines, reservoir, and oxygenator by rewashing and automatically packing these cells while the patient is still in the operating ampitheater has been used. Therefore, if the patient appears to need a blood transfusion for stabilization, these washed and refreshened packed cells can be administered back to him or her. Thus the patient is receiving his own blood and some platelets without fear of blood reaction and cutting down the total number of units of blood necessary in the postoperative period.

In the past 10 years all surgical teams have come a long way as evidenced by their ability to decrease total blood needed from 10 to 15 units down to 1 to 2 and frequently no blood transfusions.

TRANSPORT OF THE PATIENT
■ What specific measures are necessary prior to the transport of the patient from the operating room to the critical care unit?

Chest tubes, central venous pressure lines, and arterial lines are sutured to the patient during insertion to prevent pullout. The arterial and venous lines are disconnected from the monitors and for transport are connected to large heparinized syringes with three-way stopcocks.

The chest tubes are secured to the skin with tincture of benzoin and tape. All chest tube connections are taped to prevent any leakage or disconnection during the transfer procedure.

The Emerson suction apparatus is unplugged from its electric energy source or the Pleurevac is disconnected from wall suction, but the tubes are still connected to "underwater seal." *At no time are the chest tubes clamped for transfer.* There still appears to be a major misconception in many hospitals that chest tubes should be clamped during transfer.

The patient is connected to a portable bedside or gurney monitor so the ECG can be observed continually during the transport process.

Oxygen apparatus and an Ambu bag are also connected to the transfer apparatus. A modified shock cart is utilized for the transfer of the patient from the operating room to the critical care unit.

Prior to beginning transport, arterial gas, potassium level, hemoglobin, hematocrit, vital signs, and central venous pressure readings are obtained to establish that the patient's condition is stable.

In the majority of patients the endotracheal tube should be left in place, and the patient should be ventilated with an Ambu bag and 100% oxygen. Transport should be swiftly and carefully accomplished, with at least five members of the cardiac team accompanying the patient during the transfer; this should include the anesthesiologist, at least one surgeon, an operating room practitioner to manage the chest suction device, and two other individuals to assist with the battery-powered defibrillation equipment and to precede the group in order to clear any obstacles between the operating room and the critical care unit.

The family should be escorted to a private waiting room to prevent any undue apprehension associated with seeing the patient enroute with multiple tubes and IV bottles, as well as the professional entourage.

Approximately 20 to 30 minutes prior to completion of the operative procedure and again when the patient is being prepared for transfer, the critical care unit personnel should be notified so that appropriate preparation for the patient's arrival can be carried out.

■ **How many practitioners should be in attendance in the unit when the patient arrives?**

A 2:1 or more nursing care ratio is recommended during the initial phase of postcardiac surgery care.

REFERENCE

1. Hegeman, C. O., Rappaport, I., and Berger, W. J.: Superficial temporal artery cannulation, Arch. Surg. **99**:619, 1969.

CHAPTER 19

Postoperative care of the adult cardiac surgical patient

Robert A. Steedman

Once the cardiac surgical patient has been appropriately placed in the critical care unit, members of the transporting team should step back, remaining prepared to assist if necessary, and observe until all appears stable. Then the postoperative team will take over the patient's care. Needless to say, the patient's overall recuperation from this point on should be primarily the responsibility of the highly skilled critical care unit personnel. The basic routine orders are given in the boxed material on pp. 347-349.

■ **What items are attended to on the arrival of the patient?**

First, attention should be given to providing ventilation and establishing a clear airway. The bedside practitioner and inhalation therapist immediately suction the endotracheal tube, connect the patient to the ventilating apparatus with 100% oxygen, and obtain an arterial gas measurement. Once the first blood gas measurement has been obtained (usually within a period of 5 minutes or less), the tidal volume, respiratory rate, and oxygen concentrations are adjusted appropriately. The original respiratory adjustments are made on the recommendations of the anesthesiologist and surgeon and are based on the patient's needs in surgery. Ventilation adjustments are made every 10 minutes until satisfactory control and gas measurements are obtained. Desired gas concentrations consist of a Po_2 from 100 to 130 mm Hg, a Pco_2 from 35 to 40 mm Hg, a pH from 7.35 to 7.45, and a relatively normal base excess.

Connection of the ECG and arterial and venous monitor lines is performed simultaneously with or immediately following establishment of the airway, but a cuff blood pressure is obtained immediately after the patient is connected to the respirator to guarantee the patient's stabilization while all other lines are being connected.

Continuous pressure infusion of heparinized saline solution is started in both the arterial and the venous lines to prevent clotting. With the equipment now available this requires less than 250 to 400 ml of solution in a 24-hour period. The solution is prepared with a maximum of 5000 units of heparin/L of saline solution, but in some institutions the heparin added is as little as 1000 units/L or as much as 10,000 units/L. The amount of heparin utilized depends on the proficiency and the constant infusion devices.

Attention is given to the chest tubes and urinary catheters, and drainage is ensured.

■ **Who is responsible for the primary care of the patient in the critical care unit?**

The operating surgeon or assistant is primarily responsible for all decisions and usually stays with the patient until conditions are stable or until the endotracheal tube has been removed.

It is the responsibility of the critical care staff to know how to contact the surgeon or assistant at any time, and it is imperative that the staff and the hospital telephone operator be able to contact the cardiologist, anesthesiologist, and pump perfusionist immediately and to set in progress the recall of the complete team.

BASIC POSTOPERATIVE CRITICAL CARE ROUTINE*

MEDICATIONS

1. Follow routine cardiac (coronary) care orders and medications.
2. Morphine sulfate. Mix 30 mg in 30 ml saline solution. Give 1 to 5 mg (or ml) every hour as needed for pain or respiratory control and Demerol IM once the patient is off the respirator.
3. Cefazolin (Kefazol). Give 0.5 g by IV route (PB) every 4 hours. If the patient is allergic or if valve surgery was performed, contact principal practitioner.
4. Acetylsalicylic acid. Give 20 grains rectally for rectal temperature above 101° F. If no results after 2 hours, repeat; if still no results, initiate treatment by cooling blanket and notify principal practitioner.
5. If the patient is allergic to acetylsalicylic acid, give acetaminophen (Tylenol), 20 grains, rectally, in place of acetylsalicylic acid.
6. Use hyperthermia treatment if rectal temperature is below 97° F. Use hypothermia treatment if there is a persistent rectal temperature above 101° F.

RESPIRATORY THERAPY

1. Connect the patient to the MA-I volume respirator set at tidal volume as directed by the anesthesiologist or surgeon to administer 100% O_2 until the results of the first blood gas analysis are obtained (approximately 10 to 15 minutes).
2. Give routine endotracheal tube care, with irrigation (using 3 to 5 ml saline solution) and suction every 30 minutes or more often as needed. Sigh patient every 15 to 30 minutes (hand or machine).
3. Perform deep breathing and cough routine every 30 minutes of the patient's waking hours when the endotracheal tube is removed.
4. Administer O_2 by rebreathing mask at 4 to 6 L after endotracheal tube is removed. Titrate Po_2 at 75 to 100 mm Hg and Pco_2 at 35 to 45 mm Hg.
5. Administer ultrasonic nebulization as needed to control thick secretions 10 minutes prior to IPPB therapy.
6. Turn the patient every 2 hours side to side. If lateral thoracotomy and pulmonary resection were performed, do not turn on unoperated side.
7. Connect chest tubes to 20 cm suction. Milk and strip tubes every 10 minutes or as needed for 4 hours, then every hour or as needed.
8. If the chest drainage measured over 400 ml total in first 4 hours, or if more than 150 ml drains in any 1 hour, contact principal practitioner.
9. Perform nasotracheal suction as indicated by poor cough, preferably after sedation.

FLUIDS AND MONITORS

1. Give 1 L 5% dextrose in water every 12 hours (or a total of 2000 ml/24 hr), with 30 mEq of potassium chloride/L. Recheck this order after first electrolyte determination is made.
2. Keep central venous pressure (CVP) line open with administration of heparinized saline solution. If more than 500 ml is required in 24 hours, contact surgeon.
3. Keep arterial line open with heparinized saline solution; if more than 500 ml is required in 24 hours, contact surgeon.
4. Attach Foley catheter to overside drainage and obtain hourly measurements.
5. Connect ECG, CVP, arterial, pulmonary artery pressure (PAP), and left atrial pressure (LAP) monitors.

*See pp. 377-378 for an example of actual written orders.

Continued.

BASIC POSTOPERATIVE CRITICAL CARE ROUTINE—CONT'D

VITAL SIGNS AND MONITORS

1. Check vital signs every 5 to 10 minutes during the first 2 hours; then if stable, check every 15 minutes for 4 hours, and if stable, every 30 minutes.
2. Notify principal practitioner if:

   Blood pressure above _____ or below _____ mm Hg

   Pulse above _____ or below _____ /min

   Respirations above _____ or below _____ /min

   Temperature above _____ or below _____ °F

   CVP above _____ or below _____ cm H_2O or mm Hg

   LAP above _____ or below _____ mm Hg

   PAP above _____ or below _____ mm Hg

   Wedge pressure above _____ or below _____ mm Hg

   Urinary output above _____ or below _____ ml/hr

   ECG abnormal

3. Perform neurologic check at least every 2 hours for the first 12 hours.
4. Evaluate pulses every hour for 12 hours, then every 4 hours.

LABORATORY DATA

1. Check arterial gas concentrations 10 minutes after the patient is connected to MA-I volume respirator (or mask), then as needed under direction of principal practitioner until condition is stable.
2. Obtain hemoglobin and hematocrit determinations on arrival in unit. Repeat every 4 hours for 8 hours (or as needed), then check each morning before 7 AM for 5 days.
3. Evaluate electrolytes, blood urea nitrogen (BUN), and creatinine on arrival. Repeat in 8 hours or as needed, then in the morning before 7 AM for 5 days.
4. Obtain chest x-ray film 15 minutes after arrival in unit. Repeat in 8 hours, then daily before 7 AM until chest tube is out, and then as ordered.
5. Measure specific gravity and protein, sugar, and acetone concentrations in urine every 8 hours for 16 hours, then daily for 3 days.
6. Obtain ECG on arrival and daily for 4 days.
7. Evaluate cardiac enzymes on the first thru the fifth postoperative day.
8. Check calcium, magnesium, and phosphorus levels on the third postoperative day.
9. Complete postoperative cardiac surgery coagulation panel when ordered.
10. Perform culture and sensitivity test of endotracheal tube secretions on removal of endotracheal tube.

■ How much information does the critical care team need to have regarding the patient's surgery?

The unit staff is entitled to know all of the particulars of the procedures performed, and if necessary, diagram illustrations should be utilized for adequate explanation. The staff should be informed of any possible or potential complications that are expected by the surgeon so that pertinent signs and symptoms will be promptly recognized.

If there are any questions as to where certain monitors, tubes, or drains are located, this should be clarified immediately on the patient's arrival in the unit. Although this may seem rather basic, various cardiac teams place and connect monitoring devices and tubes differently. Those who have seen cases in which oxygen was connected to the nasogastric tube and suction to the nasal cannula can attest to the importance of the need for the proper identification of tubes, drains, catheters, and so on.

BASIC POSTOPERATIVE CRITICAL CARE ROUTINE—CONT'D

DIET

Give nothing orally for 12 to 18 hours, then allow the patient the full liquid bland diet for 12 hours. If this is well tolerated, progress to the soft select diet for 36 hours and then the select diet until further orders of rehabilitation diet.

OTHER

1. Elevate the head of bed 30 degrees. The upright position (if tolerated) is used for x-ray examination or eating.
2. Obtain daily weight measurements, using bed scales until tubes are out, then, if tolerated, using the standing scales.
3. Use elastic wraps from toes to groin. Rewrap as needed when wraps become loose or bind in popliteal space.
4. When possible, place antithromboembolic stockings (TED's) under elastic wraps.
5. Do not allow bending of bed or pillows under popliteal areas.
6. With nasogastric tube, if in place, perform low intermittent suction. Irrigate every 2 hours with 30 ml Gastrolyte solution.
7. Record *all* intake and output, including diaphoresis estimate, bowel elimination, vomitus, nasogastric output, all irrigations that do not return, and drainage from dressings.

DRESSING AND WOUND CARE

1. Clean all Foley, IV, and monitor line entrances daily or as needed and apply antibiotic ointment.
2. If there is progressive drainage in dressings, call principal practitioner.
3. After practitioner performs first dressing removal, cleanse daily with Betadine and sterile saline solution, drying and reapplying dry sterile dressing until orders are received to leave open. Then cleanse and dry three times a day. If the patient is allergic to Betadine, use 3% hydrogen peroxide.

■ What other immediate laboratory work is obtained?

When the first arterial gas determination is made, blood is drawn to evaluate hemoglobin concentrations, hematocrit, electrolyte levels, and, in diabetics, blood sugar levels.

If the patient has bled excessively and there is the possibility of coagulation defects, a coagulation screening test is obtained early, as certain portions of this test require moderate time for completion. This test includes platelet counts, prothrombin, bleeding and activated clotting times, fibrinogen levels, and evaluation for fibrin split products.

■ How often are the patient's vital signs checked and what are considered normal values?

When the patient first returns to the unit, the vital signs should be checked every 1 to 3 minutes until the patient's condition is stabilized, even though the patient may be connected to arterial pressure lines giving readouts and pressure curves. When the electrical readouts are stable, the vital signs can be checked every 5 minutes; however, monitor readouts of the arterial pressure, central venous pressure (CVP), and ECG are visualized continually.

The critical care unit staff is encouraged to evaluate the preoperative chart and anesthesia record in order to know what vital signs are expected with this patient; however, it is most helpful if the operating surgeon writes in the orders the vital signs parameters expected and what deviations merit notification. This is usually written in the manner shown in the boxed material on pp. 377-378.

Although such detail may seem unnecessary, it is extremely important that certain patients not become hypertensive; others who have been chronically hypertensive might exhibit pressures that are normal for most but are inadequate for perfusion of their vital organs. Slower or more rapid heart rates and lower or higher than normal CVP's *are expected* in some patients; thus preliminary written communication can prompt necessary or eliminate unnecessary calls.

■ How important are minimum variations of normal vital signs?

Today it is easy for practitioners to disregard the simple standard evaluations of vital signs because of the sophisticated techniques of monitoring and the numerous laboratory determinations available. But the proper evaluation of vital signs correlated with physical findings can often yield a diagnosis more readily than the finest monitoring equipment or the most advanced laboratory tests.

A falling blood pressure below normal can be a reflection of pain and apprehension, CNS depression caused by oversedation, low output associated with varying arrhythmias, drug-induced peripheral vasodilatation, hypovolemia and impending shock, or low cardiac output for any one of many reasons (poor contractility as a result of infarction, cardiac tamponade, myocardial depression caused by medications, and so on).

Blood pressure elevation can be a sign of peripheral vasoconstriction, pain and apprehension, hypercapnia, CNS insult, or overzealous use of inotropic drugs.

Increases in pulse rate can be associated with hypovolemia, atrial or ventricular irritability, pain and apprehension, sepsis, or the use of any one of many medications.

Slowing of the pulse to under 60 can signify CNS involvement or partial or complete heart block, or it can reflect cardiac response to certain medications such as digitalis, procainamide hydrochloride (Pronestyl), or propranolol.

Temperature elevation in the very early postoperative period most often indicates some degree of atelectasis, but in the later postoperative phase this can be the result of wound or cavity infection, pulmonary embolization, certain medications, blood reactions, or even damage to the CNS. Persistent subnormal temperatures frequently occur when cooling procedures have

been used during surgery, but they can also be indicative of CNS injuries, adrenal insufficiency, or early nonseptic shock.

Respiratory rates increase with pain, apprehension, fever, metabolic acidosis, and any form of sepsis.

Depressed respiration can occur with oversedation, extremely painful chest or abdominal incisions, and not infrequently as a result of certain anesthetic respiratory center depressants such as fentanyl-droperidol combinations (Innovar).

Marked variations of the aberrant vital signs just discussed can occur with any metabolic acid-base imbalances and should stimulate a methodical investigation. Careful observation of vital signs by critical care staff can frequently yield information relating to an established trend or an impending problem and allow correction before the reception of a computer analysis or laboratory test returns.

For example, if the pulse rate is slowed to around 50 beats/min without ECG evidence of heart block, the systolic blood pressure is above 170 mm Hg, and the temperature is subnormal, one could look immediately at the possible causes for these variances and come up with the probable etiology. The bradycardia could be caused from drug depression of the heart rate; however, if this is true, the blood pressure should not be elevated. The blood pressure can be elevated in cases of carbon dioxide retention (hypercapnia), but if this were true, the pulse rate should be more rapid. If sepsis or pain is the cause of the increased blood pressure, then again a rapid heart rate should be expected. Thus with the subnormal temperature one would suspect an overmedication effect (digitalization, and so on) or, more likely, CNS injury.

■ What volume of urine output is expected?

In most shock units the basic minimum of urine output per hour considered adequate to eliminate body waste and demonstrate perfusion of the kidneys averages around 20 ml/hr. For this reason most urine outputs are measured every hour for at least the first 24 to 36 hours postoperatively.

It is not uncommon for patients in the immediate postoperative period to produce large urine volumes as a result of IV colloid, blood, and other fluids coadministered with mannitol or furosemide (Lasix) during surgery.

Occasionally urinary outputs in the range of 13 to 15 ml/hr will be seen after mitral valve surgery, and yet the patient demonstrates no other signs of perfusion deficit or evidence of low cardiac output, and when given small doses of diuretic the urinary output increases respectively. This has been suspected to be the result of a pressure receptor in the left atrial wall that can stimulate the increased production of antidiuretic hormone. The left atrium is distended and tense in severe mitral valvular regurgitation or stenosis, but after correction of the stenosis or insufficiency the pressure is decreased and the body response can be similar to that in hypovolemia, with retention of fluids in an attempt to increase circulating volume. After the body has adjusted to the lower atrial pressures and the initial stress of surgery, there can be a diuretic phase occurring from 36 to 96 hours postoperatively.

Increased urinary outputs obtained on the second to fourth day after surgery are also not uncommon. This postoperative diuretic phase is associated with the reentry of the interstitial and other third-space fluids into the circulating volume and their subsequent elimination through the urinary system. In the past many practitioners attempted to replace this diuresis volume and encountered understandable overhydration complications; thus carefully titrated fluid replacement should be emphasized. The most important facet in this phase is to maintain a constant evaluation of the *electrolyte concentrations* in order that appropriate replacement may be undertaken.

Another important evaluation of the urine includes measurement of the amount of discoloration associated with hemolysis from the bypass procedure. This can result in a urine color comparable to a "vin rosé" and hopefully not a "Burgundy red" wine. If this discoloration occurs but does not begin to clear within a couple of hours after the operative procedure, there is the possibility of frank bleeding from the urinary system. This can be elevated and correlated with plasma and urine hemoglobin levels and microscopic evaluation of the urine for red blood cells.

The specific gravity of the urine is determined every 1 to 2 hours and aids in evaluating hydration, diuresis, renal function, and antidiuretic hormone activity. Sugar, acetone, and protein determinations are routinely obtained as for any intensive care surgical patient.

■ Which specific pulses should be evaluated and why?

Critical care practitioners as well as general ward personnel should be able to evaluate most of the major pulses in the body (Fig. 19-1). Radial and ulnar pulses are most accessible, easily palpated, and most familiar to bedside practitioners. It is extremely important to evaluate the upper extremity pulses when any aortic arch surgery has been performed or when catheters have been utilized previously. With experience this will provide a means of obtaining a palpatory blood pressure in individuals in whom it is difficult to place the cuff and where correlation with the monitors is necessary. These pulses, as well as the others to be described, should all be evaluated shortly after the patient arrives in the unit. Again, it should be stressed that occasionally the blood pressure palpated in the radial or ulnar artery can be lower in one arm than in the other if there is any proximal obstruction (subclavian artery stenosis or brachial artery narrowing from catheterization). These pulses can be absent or nonpalpable as a result of previous arteriotomies or use of monitoring catheters.

Femoral pulses are more often evaluated today; the importance of determining differences of intensity of one pulse as compared to the other is stressed. It is difficult, however, to palpate these pulses through the dressings or after groin incisions have been utilized for perfusion or harvesting of veins, but with simple, careful pressure this can be done without causing the patient too much discomfort. If there is any question as to the integrity of the lower extremity as demonstrated by color, pallor, blotchiness, pain, or motor function, the ability to determine simply the presence of a pulse is important, as well as to compare the intensity of an existing pulse to that recorded preoperatively.

The popliteal pulse reflects patency of the superficial femoral artery. Palpating this pulse re-

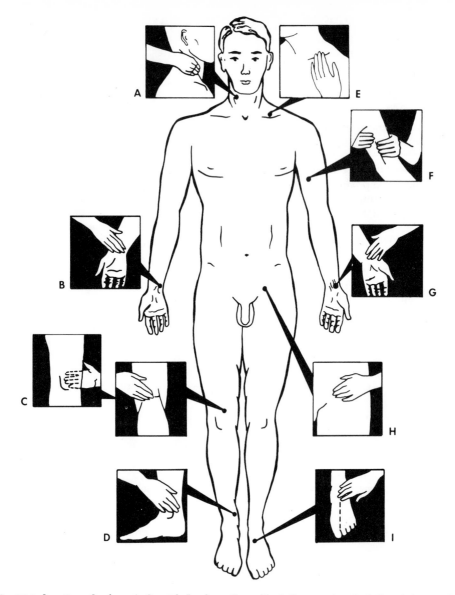

Fig. 19-1. Location of pulses. *A*, Carotid; *B*, ulnar; *C*, popliteal; *D*, posterior tibial; *E*, subclavian; *F*, high brachial; *G*, radial; *H*, femoral; *I*, dorsalis pedis.

quires experience and multiple rehearsals in the normal patient. It is best palpated by placing the right hand behind the popliteal space approaching from the medial aspect with the leg relaxed and in a normal anatomic position or minimally rotated externally; then gentle compressive pressure is applied until a pulse is obtained. Another technique is to compress the popliteal space with either one or both hands until resistance is noted from the fascial and bony structures and then to release the pressure slowly until a palpable pulse is noted. The right hand is utilized for evaluating the right popliteal pulse and the left hand is usually used to document the left popliteal pulse. Again, practice and experience are recommended for evaluation of these pulses.

The dorsalis pedis pulse is the pulse of the lower extremity and has been recently emphasized. It is the superficial continuation of the anterior tibial artery and is best located near the instep of the foot extending between the area of the second tarsometatarsal junction and coursing toward the interphalangeal web between the large and the second toe. A decrease or absence of this pulse frequently signifies an obstruction of the femoral artery or one or all of its branches.

The posterior tibial artery is best palpated by placing the fingers just posterior to the medial malleolus; it is somewhat more difficult to palpate than the dorsalis pedis pulse and again requires pressure to be applied until resistance from bone and fascia is encountered and then slowly released until the pulse is noted. In patients with increased fat pads, edema of the lower extremities, or any body structural abnormality, this pulse becomes very difficult to palpate. It reflects the status of the posterior tibial artery and/or more proximal vessels.

Careful evaluation of all of these pulses, but especially the last two described, is most important in the immediate postoperative phase, especially when the patient has been perfused through, or is being monitored from one of the femoral arteries. Subsequent decrease or disappearance of these pulses without a drop in blood pressure can signify a possible remedial vascular obstruction, but a delay in detection can cause loss of limb or life. It is not uncommon for the pedal and tibial pulses to be present and the popliteal pulses to be weak or absent as a result of long-term obstruction of the superficial femoral artery and excellent collateralization from the deep femoral artery.

The practitioner should also be acquainted with the subclavian and brachial artery pulsations, as these can be used for evaluation when there are dressings or infusion lines at the wrists.

Occasionally palpated and noted by practitioners is a pulse located just anterior and slightly distal to the external or lateral malleolus. This pulse is palpable only 5% to 10% of the time, and it is called the external malleolar artery pulse. It is produced by a branch of the anterior tibial artery but can be dominantly formed from branches of the peroneal, the posterior tibial, or the anterior tibial artery singly or in combination. It is often present when the dorsalis pedis pulse is congenitally absent or small or in cases of long-term obstruction.

Carotid pulses should be easily located not only by professional personnel, but also by lay persons working in the hospital environment. It is well known that youth organizations such as the Brownies, Girl Scouts, Cub Scouts, and Boy Scouts are becoming well versed in the techniques of cardiopulmonary resuscitation and are aware of the presence of the femoral and carotid pulses. Disappearance of the carotid pulse after surgery can be associated with a major catastrophe such as cardiac arrest, aortic arch dissection, or acute occlusion of the common carotid vessels. Practitioners must be well aware of this pulsation point for use in the assessment of cardiopulmonary resuscitation measures. The carotid pulse is best located halfway between the clavicle and the base of the jaw (angle of the jaw) just anterior to the prominent sternocleidomastoid muscle.

It is highly recommended that ward, critical care, and operating room personnel become accustomed to evaluating these pulses on all patients admitted, so that when their evaluation is of critical necessity, these persons are prepared for the task (Fig. 19-2).

■ How are the chest tubes managed postoperatively?

In transport and during most phases of postoperative care the chest tubes *are not clamped*, because if there is an air leak in one or the other part of the chest cavity and the tubes are clamped, no exit is available for the air, thus causing progressive collapse of the lung on the involved side with creation of tension pneumothorax. Eventually alteration of the cardiac output, arrhythmias, and death can occur. In addition, if the chest tubes are clamped for any period of time, the evacuation of blood or clots is impeded and could precipitate cardiac tamponade. Chest tubes should be clamped only when

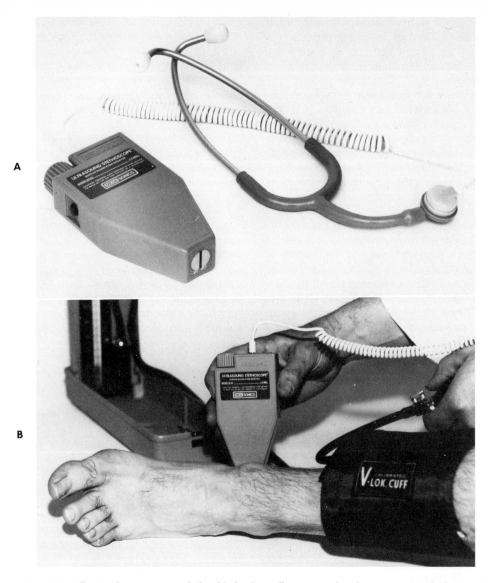

Fig. 19-2. All critical care personnel should also be well acquainted and competent with the use of Doppler instruments for evaluation of nonpalpable pulses (vessels in spasm, low flow, or obstruction).

evaluation for leaks is necessary and when changing the chest suction bottles.

Once the patient has arrived from the operating room, the chest tubes should be evaluated to ensure that they are in an underwater trap (underwater seal). Suction should be applied at a pressure of 60 cm H_2O for 15 to 20 seconds and then reduced to 20 cm H_2O.

There are multiple apparatuses utilized for applying suction to the chest tubes. The *Emerson* suction apparatus (Fig. 19-3), which operates by means of two large bottles connected to a suc-

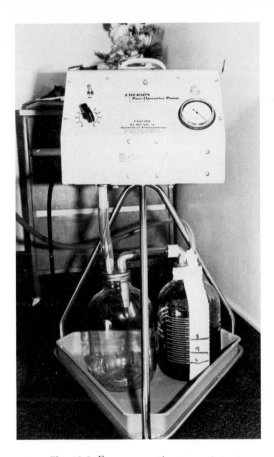

Fig. 19-3. Emerson suction apparatus.

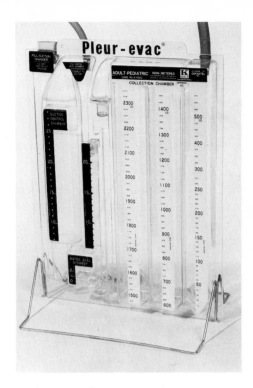

Fig. 19-4. Pleur-evac suction apparatus.

tion machine that is portable and electrically powered, is quite easy to assemble and the fluid levels are easily visualized close up or at a distance. Suction can be increased or decreased continuously or intermittently with simple valve control. The *Pleur-evac* self-contained suction apparatus (Fig. 19-4) connects directly to wall suction and does not require any electricity for function. However, the maximum amount of suction is determined by the fluid levels in the various containers and cannot be altered without changing these volumes. The Pleur-evac apparatus is a disposable unit constructed so it can be placed at any level without fear of fluid backing up into the chest tubes.

The chest drainage is measured when the pa-

tient first arrives in the unit and at least every 5 minutes for the first few hours or until output has markedly decreased or is stable. After that period evaluations every 15 minutes are adequate (Fig. 19-5).

The chest tubes should be milked or stripped whenever there are clots visible or whenever the tubes are completely free (suggesting that there might be intrathoracic clots). They should be stripped at least every 5 to 10 minutes for the first 2 hours, then the frequency should be decreased to not less than once every 30 minutes (Fig. 19-6).

Inspection of the continuity of the chest tubes to the connection with the suction bottles or disposable units should be performed frequently, as it is not uncommon for kinks or twists to develop and prevent needed drainage. Careful scrutiny of bulky chest dressings and chest films may be necessary to recognize kinks or twists at the chest wall or in the thoracic cavity.

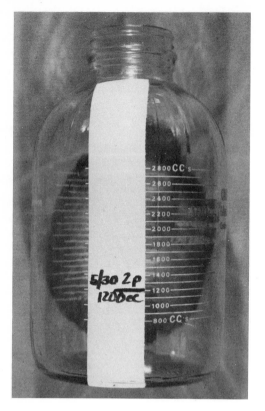

Fig. 19-5. Chest drainage noted on wide cloth tape. Date, time, and amount recorded.

Usually the chest tubes are stabilized in the operating room with nonabsorbable sutures and external dressings, but the critical care unit personnel must *ensure this stability* with additional tape and benzoin if necessary. All connections should be enforced with *nonporous* tape to prevent leakage.

The chest drainage is measured by using the standard attached scale on the bottles or chest apparatus or using a scale prepared by the critical care unit personnel (Fig. 19-5). The drainage is recorded every shift and also marked on a wide piece of cloth tape on the bottle. The tape should record the time, date, and if there is enough room, the total drainage to that time and level.

Two chest tube clamps are kept with the suction apparatus for each tube exiting from the patient; if plastic tubes are placed, rubber or plastic covers on the jaws of these clamps should not be used. Again, the chest tubes are clamped only when examining for air leakage or when changing the suction apparatus.

■ What is the significance of bubbling or non-bubbling in the chest tubes?

Bubbling in the chest drainage bottles on suction suggests an air leak. The source can be the lung, the stab wound for the chest tubes, a non-

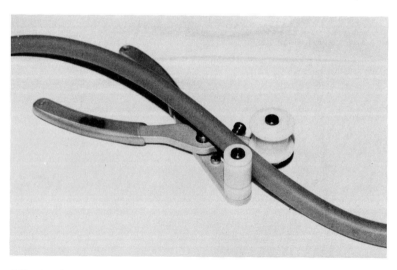

Fig. 19-6. Pilling's tube stripper. Hand tube stripper is designed for effectively milking tubes and conserving effort. (Courtesy Pilling Co., Los Angeles, Calif.)

airtight connection, or a crack or perforation in the drainage tubes.

Early lack of bubbling simply signifies that no pleural or lung violation occurred during the procedure and an airtight continuity of all tubes and connections exists. If some air leakage is expected by the surgeon or if bubbling abruptly stops, the tubes must be evaluated for *plugging clots.*

Any acute increase or decrease in bubbling should be reported immediately to the surgeon.

■ How are the chest tubes checked for leakage?

When a moderate amount of bubbling occurs in the chest bottles, a single clamping procedure can be performed for detection of air leaks. It is necessary to place *two* clamps across plastic tubes to adequately seal against leakage. These clamps should be placed at 180-degree angles from one another, as demonstrated in Fig. 19-7. The tubes are first clamped just outside the chest cavity, and if bubbling decreases markedly or stops, the leakage is probably from the thoracic cavity. If bubbling continues, it suggests that the leakage is more distal, and the second clamping is performed just above the level where the tube is connected to the suction bottle; if bubbling stops at this time, it confirms a leak between the chest cavity and the bottles. The clamps can then be progressively reclamped proximally until the exact area of leakage is located. Bubbling continuing with this lowest clamping usually signifies the lack of an airtight seal at the tube-bottle connection. Critical care practitioners should be aware of this technique and should also be able to set up quickly a complete chest suction apparatus and tray for emergency tube thoracostomy.

■ When are the chest tubes removed and how?

When there are no further clots and minimum drainage, when bubbling has ceased, or when the chest tubes are plugged and the chest appears stable on x-ray film, the chest tubes are removed. In most cardiac cases this occurs between the first and third postoperative days.

Removal of the chest tubes usually requires one or two assistants, depending on the technique utilized. It is recommended that two assis-

tants be available when there are two or more tubes and only one when a single tube is present.

The dressings are removed, any stabilizing sutures are cut, the chest wall around the chest tubes is sprayed with tincture of benzoin, and an encircling pursestring suture around the chest tube incision site (previously placed at surgery) is held taut. The chest suction is increased to 60 cm H_2O (in the hope of sucking back any air that might start to enter the chest cavity), and a double thickness 4×4 inch gauze sponge that has been partially divided is utilized to compress the skin around the chest tube to be removed. The tube is quickly withdrawn as the pursestring suture is cinched. The ties are completed, the redundant strands of the suture are cut, and firm tape is applied over the 4×4 inch gauze sponge that is being applied compressively to ensure against leakage.

If the tubes are connected to Y suction, the tubes are clamped prior to removal so that air entering the removed tube will not simply bypass the Y and go into the chest cavity through the remaining tube. The second and third tubes are removed in a similar manner, and the patient is reassured that the acute discomfort will be relieved within 1 or 2 minutes.

There is a great variance between practitioners as to whether the tubes are removed when the patient is inhaling or exhaling. Some utilize sterile petrolatum (Vaseline) gauze under the 4×4 inch gauze to seal the wound; however, petrolatum gauze can slip and allow a loss of purchase of skin, and air can reenter.

■ How often does pneumothorax occur during chest tube removal and how is it treated?

Minimum pneumothorax occurs after removal of the chest tubes in approximately 3% to 4% of patients, and even then it is usually so minimal (<5%) that it does not require tube replacement.

After chest tube removal a chest x-ray film is immediately obtained; if a small pneumothorax is present, the patient is observed very carefully for any respiratory distress or change in vital signs, and a repeat chest x-ray film is obtained in 1 hour. If the chest appears to be stable over that hour period, another chest x-ray film is obtained in approximately 8 hours, and then a daily chest x-ray film is ordered. Simple pneumothorax, if

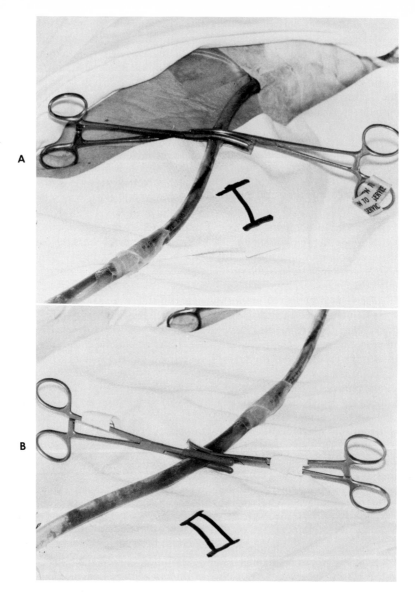

Fig. 19-7. Clamping of tubes. **A,** Tubes clamped adjacent to chest. **B,** Clamp placed beyond first connection. **C,** Tubes clamped above chest suction bottle. **D,** Composite of **A, B,** and **C.**

not accompanied by an air leak, will resolve at a rate of 1% to 3% a day if under 10% and if the patient's condition is stable with no other complications.

If the pneumothorax produced by chest tube removal is 10% to 20% or more and the patient has a suspected air leak, borderline pulmonary functions, or CNS involvement, tube replacement and underwater seal should be instituted immediately.

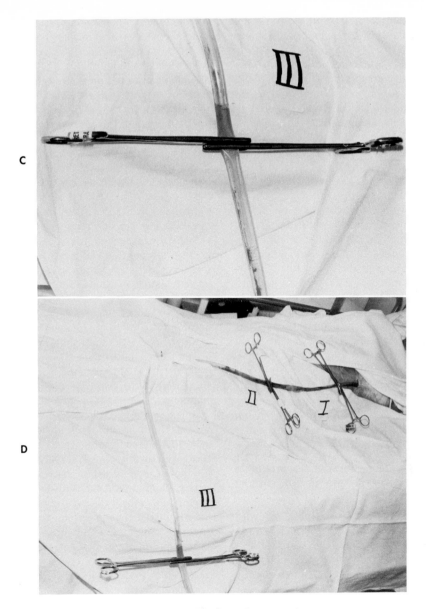

Fig. 19-7, cont'd. For legend see opposite page.

■ How is the arterial pressure monitored and what apparatus is utilized?

The patient is monitored in the postoperative period by use of the intra-arterial line placed during surgery. This artery cannula is connected to an electronic measuring system by a transducer. The transducer is a small intricate electro-manometer or electronic pressure sensor that converts mechanical pressure into electrical impulses that can be read on the bedside monitor by either an appropriately standardized and scaled arterial pulse wave or by direct readout (digital or sweep gauge).

Setting up and connecting this arterial pressure line with the transducer and monitor is one of the most intricate procedures performed in the immediate postoperative period and should be done only by a person experienced with this system, as it is not uncommon for the transducer to become flooded with blood or to leak. This apparatus is a vital measuring device used to assess the patient's cardiovascular status and must be accurate and functional at all times.

A quality electronic intra-arterial monitor and pressure transducer should be utilized. A pressure infuser with an intraflow filter irrigating device should be connected to the arterial line.

The saline solution in the 500 ml bag is heparinized with as much as 2500 units of aqueous heparin, because of the small volume of solution now required to irrigate the arterial line over a 24-hour period (seldom over 250 ml). Some units use a smaller concentration of heparin but a larger volume of irrigating solution.

A major reason for utilizing arterial pressure lines, transducers, and electrical monitoring has been to reduce and eliminate the cuff errors found in patients with pressures below 90 mm Hg, as well as for the convenience and in order to observe the pulse pressure waveform.

■ What complications or specific problems can be expected with the use of arterial monitors?

Despite the excellent results obtained with electrical arterial monitoring devices, it cannot be overemphasized that this is an artificial unit that can fail and give inaccurate results and must be standardized and corrected frequently with cuff pressures. It is not uncommon for a patient to return from the operating room and have a moderately higher blood pressure reading on the arterial monitor than by cuff measurement. Frequently, this is a result of oversensitive transducers, rigid and lengthy tubing, and other parameters, and we have always labeled this condition the "spike," "overshoot," or "fling" phenomenon. It is usually recognized on the monitor by an additional impression suggesting a second

dicrotic notch. Above the uppermost or accessory notch is usually seen a spike contour at the apex of the pulse wave (Fig. 19-8), and the difference from the top notch to the peak of the spike is usually identical to the pressure difference from the cuff and arterial monitors and reflects the sensitive error.

The technique I use for correlating the arterial monitor pressure with the cuff pressure is to have one practitioner inflate the mercury manometer blood pressure cuff until the pulse wave or contour is totally obliterated on the scope; then the cuff is slowly deflated, observing the mercury manometer reading. At the instant the arterial pulse wave returns on the scope or screen (noted verbally by a second person), the manometer reading is noted and that is the patient's blood pressure. If the pressures are different, multiple investigational methods may be required to resolve the difference.

The "spike" or "overshoot" phenomenon is very frequently seen in patients who return to the operating room in a slightly hypertensive state or with a somewhat irritable myocardium, as is not infrequently seen in patients who have increased circulating catecholamines (epinephrine or norepinephrine).

When the "spike" or "overshoot" phenomenon occurs, there are multiple areas to investigate, too numerous to describe specifically here. However, some of the considerations are to decrease the length of rigid tubing between the patient's arterial cannula and the transducer, the best arrangement probably being the transducer at the wrist immediately connected to the cannula; frequent recalibration of the monitoring modules and replacement whenever necessary; utilization of appropriate antihypertensive medications and medications to decrease hypercontractility; standardization of transducers and monitoring equipment in operating rooms and critical care units; and so on.

Problems with plugging of the arterial line are prevented by frequent and appropriate irrigation. Small clots can be dislodged by forceful irrigation or by reinserting the metal stylet into the cannula, but these procedures can cause peripheral small artery occlusions. Troublesome bleeding around the incision site or the percutaneous

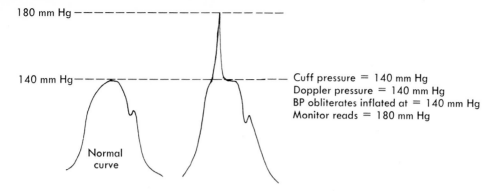

180 mm Hg

140 mm Hg

Cuff pressure = 140 mm Hg
Doppler pressure = 140 mm Hg
BP obliterates inflated at = 140 mm Hg
Monitor reads = 180 mm Hg

Normal
curve

Fig. 19-8. Illustration of the not uncommonly seen "spike" or "overshoot" phenomenon responsible for false high readout pressures.

puncture site can occur but is most often controlled by simple pressure and then a firm dressing (but the tape should not totally encircle the wrist). The main pressure should be applied directly at the entrance site of the catheter. Whenever pressure dressings are applied, the area must be observed frequently for continued excessive bleeding or blanched ischemic areas indicating impending necrosis. The cannula and pressure tracings must be checked frequently to ensure continued intra-arterial positioning. Arterial cannula dislodgment occurs occasionally in very active or agitated patients, and the simple application of continued pressure over the site for 7 to 10 minutes is the recommended procedure followed by placement of a pressure dressing.

Any of the minor problems or complications just discussed might occur and indicate the need for notification of the principal practitioner.

Accurate records should be kept of the amount of blood withdrawn or discarded each time samples are obtained for the evaluation of arterial gases or electrolytes, as this can contribute to the continual hemoglobin concentration and hematocrit drop in a patient requiring frequent determinations. This blood in critical cases can be immediately readministered to the patient, but otherwise this is not recommended. Also, the lines from the patient to the withdrawing syringe can be shortened, therefore decreasing the amount of withdrawn blood to be discarded.

In withdrawing samples for coagulation screens or for bleeding and clotting studies, the blood should be obtained from a separate vein puncture or a source not potentially contaminated with heparin, as this can give abnormal results and prolong recovery.

Arterial cannulas are removed between the first and third days, depending on the stability of the patient's condition. On removal, all stabilizing sutures are cut and carefully removed, and the cannula is withdrawn, with steady pressure being applied directly over the percutaneous or incision puncture sites. This pressure is applied for a minimum of 7 to 10 minutes followed by placement of a nonencircling pressure dressing.

■ What is normal for CVP readings and what does this reflect?

The CVP line is placed in one of the peripheral veins and manipulated up toward the inferior or superior vena cava or right atrium. CVP is a fair reflection of the competency of the pumping mechanism of the heart and a guide to blood volume replacement. The normal values are from 6 to 15 cm H_2O.

A line is connected from the patient through one of the usual CVP measuring devices or is connected to a transducer and subsequently to a sophisticated electrical monitor with either digital or calibrated CVP wave readout. It is wise to connect to a manual CVP measuring device in addition to the transducer monitor, as this low-pressure system reliability is labile and requires frequent checks.

Fluid is infused in the CVP line continually by

slow drip, again with a pressure bag apparatus or with an electrically controlled Ivac fluid administration unit. Because of the usual higher doses of fluid given through the CVP catheter, the solution is heparinized with only 1000 units of heparin/500 ml of fluid. With the larger volumes of fluid given through the CVP line, if larger doses of heparin were used in the irrigation solution, bleeding problems could occur. CVP and atrial pressure measurements should be conducted with the patient supine and the zero point located at the midpoint of the right atrium, usually considered the midaxillary line or half the distance between the front and back of the chest. CVP should be measured with the patient on and off the respirator, and fluctuating and mean pressures not associated with respiration should be noted.

Most practitioners want to be notified whenever the CVP exceeds the 15 to 20 cm H_2O mark or drops below 4 cm H_2O.

The complications or problems with CVP lines are similar to those of arterial lines, with bleeding around the puncture or incision site (especially after removal), intermittent plugging of the line, or dampened readings as a result of clot formation at the tip of the cannula. Inappropriate measurements are reflected by low pressure variations on inspiration and expiration and may signify a kinked, bent, partially plugged, or even misplaced line. The CVP line can inadvertently follow an alternate route and end up in the venous tributaries of the neck or leg during initial placement in surgery. When placed in deep veins, these lines are easily stabilized with an encircling stitch around the vein branch in which it has been placed, and on removal of the catheter, steady, even tension is applied to prevent fracture of the line with possible dislodgment and pulmonary embolization of the plastic remnant. All of these lines or cannulas should be carefully inspected on removal, and it is recommended that only radiopaque CVP lines be used so correct placement and, if necessary, embolization sites can be determined by x-ray examination.

CVP line removal also requires the application of pressure until the "ooze" has stopped. Where the CVP line has been placed in the arm, it is quite simple to apply a minor pressure dressing; however, when the CVP line has been placed in the groin, it not uncommonly requires a groin pressure dressing as previously described (Chapter 17 and Fig. 17-1).

■ **What is the left atrial pressure and how does it differ from the CVP?**

The left atrial pressure (LAP) line is placed by suturing a small cannula into the left atrium and bringing it out through a separate stab incision in the chest wall. The line can be cared for and the pressure monitored in a manner similar to that described for the CVP line.

LAP is a more accurate assessment of the circulating volume and the functional capacity of the left ventricle to handle volume load, with normal measurements ranging from 8 to 18 cm H_2O. Of consequence are readings below 5 cm H_2O and those above 25 cm H_2O. When pressures approach 30 cm H_2O, signs of pulmonary edema are not infrequently seen; these will almost always be manifest with pressures above 35 cm H_2O.

Accidental dislodgment of the cannula requires the simple application of pressure over the percutaneous or stab wound site. The same problems occur with this line as with the CVP line except that it is somewhat more difficult to maintain in place during the immediate closing of the chest and mediastinum. Atrial tears, inability of removal, or arterial embolization of the catheter are conceivable complications.

The LAP line is in the left side of the heart, and with irrigating procedures the introduction of small amounts of air or clot can result in complications from arterial embolizations to the coronary arteries, brain, or peripheral vessels.

The use of this catheter in some institutions has also been described postoperatively for dye injections and x-ray visualization of the mitral valve or its replacement, as well as for evaluation of cardiac output by injection of indicator dyes. This usually requires a somewhat larger cannula than is required for simple LAP monitoring.

■ **What is the Swan-Ganz catheter and how is it used with reference to the CVP and arterial pressures?**

The Swan-Ganz catheter is a No. 5 or 7 French balloon-tipped catheter used for measuring the pulmonary artery pressure (PAP) as well as the pulmonary artery wedge pressure. The direct measurement of the PAP can be obtained and reflects left heart function, which may indicate intrapulmonary congestion and/or blockage.

The pulmonary artery wedge pressure is obtained by advancing the catheter into one of the peripheral branches of the pulmonary artery and inflating the balloon tip for a reflection of the LAP. Pulmonary artery gas concentrations can also be obtained from this cannula for comparison with the arterial gas concentrations. Since these are *venous* gases, they should never be confused with arterial blood gas concentrations.

The Swan-Ganz catheter is usually inserted into either the basilic or cephalic vein at the elbow (other veins can be utilized when necessary) and floated by means of the balloon tip through the major veins into the right atrium and then by the tricuspid valve into the right ventricles (similar to the pathway of the transvenous electrode). It is then carefully manipulated out into the pulmonary artery. The determination of catheter tip position when placed in the operating room and in the ward is on the basis of visualized pressure tracings on the connected monitor during manipulation. It can then be advanced into a peripheral pulmonary artery branch, wedged appropriately with balloon partially inflated, and thus give a wedge pressure tracing. Deflation of the balloon, depending on the placement of the catheter, can give a PAP measurement. Again, its placement is determined on the oscilloscope or monitoring device by the pressure waves and tracings. The normal values obtained are shown in Table 19-1.

The care of this catheter requires irrigation and continuous infusion with solutions similar to those used with a venous line. Complications include catheter plugging, dampening, perforation of the pulmonary artery or its branches, and thrombosis of a peripheral vein. This catheter can bend back on itself, withdraw into the right ventricle, or occasionally even entwine and form an intracardiac knot. Another infrequent but possible complication includes rupture of the balloon with dissemination of small fragments into the pulmonary vascular tree.

The Swan-Ganz catheter is placed by the cardiologist when physiologic cardiac measurements

Table 19-1. Normal values for right ventricle, pulmonary artery, and pulmonary artery wedge pressure*

	Normal values (mm Hg)	
	Average	Range
Right ventricle pressure		
Peak systolic	25	17-32
End diastolic	4	1-7
Pulmonary artery pressure		
Mean	15	9-19
Peak systolic	25	17-32
End diastolic	9	4-13
Pulmonary artery wedge pressure		
Mean	9	4.5-13

*Modified from Yang, S. S., Bentivoglio, L. G., Maranhao, V., and Goldberg, H.: Cardiac catheterization data to hemodynamic parameters, Philadelphia, 1972, F. A. Davis Co.

are required, and the procedure of removal is similar to that used with CVP lines.

The original discouragement with the use of this cannula was associated with the intricate mechanism necessary to maintain patency and obtain readings; however, these procedures have been simplified in the past few years. Experienced maintenance and critical care personnel must be available in the hospital or on an immediate "on call" basis for any problems that might arise with the intricate monitoring setups. Responsibility rests with the critical care unit practitioner and electrical engineer to maintain appropriate function. Critical care personnel must learn by repetitive practical experience how to handle the original setting up and any problems that might arise. Reference protocols must be readily available and spelled out in great but simplified detail for if these systems fail and cannot be restored to normal function, the patient's life could be in jeopardy.

■ **What routine laboratory work is obtained?**

Electrolyte determinations should be made immediately after the patient arrives; if normal, these are thereafter obtained daily, with the exception of potassium. If there are any arrhythmia problems, if there is moderate urinary output, or if the original potassium concentration was abnormal, repeat potassium levels are obtained every 4 hours until the level is stable, and then daily thereafter.

In cases where the use of a nephrotoxic drug such as gentamicin sulfate (Garamycin) is necessary, the blood urea nitrogen (BUN) and creatinine tests are also run daily. If these levels increase at any time, the use of the nephrotoxic drug is decreased or discontinued.

Hemoglobin and hematocrit levels are obtained initially, then every 4 to 6 hours until they are relatively stable, and then daily.

Arterial gas concentrations are obtained as needed to titrate the patient's initial respiratory needs, but once the patient's pulmonary status is stable and the arterial cannula is removed, arterial gas evaluations are not usually necessary. If the need again arises, the opposite radial, brachial, or femoral artery can be used. Whenever an arterial gas measurement is obtained, pressure is applied over the puncture sites and a pressure dressing placed for a period of 1 to 2 hours.

■ What abnormal laboratory tests are of major concern?

Potassium is the cation of major concern, because hypokalemia can lead to dangerous arrhythmias, especially with concomitant digitalis administration. When arrhythmias persist even in the presence of low normal potassium concentrations, the patient will be given a continuous IV drip solution containing potassium, as it has been well documented that in the immediate postoperative period the patient can have high serum potassium levels with low intracellular potassium concentrations. Hyperkalemia occurs less often, but when recognized, no potassium supplements are given; if renal failure is suggested, a means of decreasing the levels can be instituted.

The sodium levels can drop with excessive diuresis, moderate diaphoresis, or when salt replacement is withheld. Daily and continuous decrease in the serum sodium concentration is seen in the patient who retains water, but most clinicians are not concerned until the sodium level drops below 125 mEq/L, and then careful replacement and/or diuresis is needed. A regular full diet appears to be the single most important factor in rebalancing electrolyte concentrations; thus it is necessary to place the patient on a full oral regimen as soon as it is safe.

The chloride concentration can drop with the overzealous administration of nonelectrolyte solutions and also with excessive nasogastric suction. This can be replaced with a number of the commercial IV solutions available, but cessation of suction and institution of oral intake are again essential.

The BUN and creatinine levels are of major concern when elevated in a patient who is not bleeding or dehydrated, especially if nephrotoxic agents are being administered or if any abnormalities of urinary output are present. If these two factors progressively increase with increasing potassium levels or poor response to diuresis, a nephrologist should be consulted for evaluation of early renal failure.

Blood is not administered after the second postoperative day if the patient appears to be stable and if the hemoglobin concentration and hematocrit stay above 10 g/100 ml and 30%, respectively. If these measurements continue to drop without evidence of retained fluids or overhydration, blood is administered in the form of packed cells (to decrease the incidence of hepatitis and prevent added volume load). The point at which blood is added is arbitrary, and in some patients with specific religious convictions blood and blood derivatives are refused. It is not uncommon to see the condition of these individuals finally stabilize with a hemoglobin concentration of 6 or 7 g/100 ml and a hematocrit of 18% to 21%. This leaves the attending practitioner uneasy, as these low levels narrow the time available for any successful emergency resuscitation when the oxygen-carrying capacity is markedly decreased. Total body healing is probably slower and resistance to infection poorer with low red cell and hemoglobin counts. On reviewing the cases occurring in volume in some institutions, the nonuse of blood probably carries a higher morbidity and mortality among cardiac patients.

■ What additional laboratory tests are performed and why?

Daily cardiac enzyme tests are performed starting the day of surgery and repeated daily for 3 to 4 days, even though it is common for most of these values to be elevated in the immediate post-operative period. This is especially true when vents and pursestring sutures have been placed in the left ventricle. If the concentrations of these enzymes or their isoenzymes remain markedly elevated on the fifth day with abnormal ECG's, infarction is considered, and if established, the patient is treated as for acute myocardial infarction with extended care in the unit. The cardiac enzymes can be elevated in conditions other than acute myocardial infarction; therefore the combinations, times, isoenzymes, and duration of elevations are important in substantiating postoperative infarction. The serum glutamic-oxaloacetic transaminase (SGOT), hydroxybutyric dehydrogenase (HBD), and lactic dehydrogenase (LDH) levels are all usually elevated in myocardial infarction at varying times, but they are also frequently elevated in acute liver damage such as hepatitis, hepatic drug injury, and even passive congestion. They are even moderately elevated in other muscle cell damage situations such as burns, crushing injuries, and IM injections. They can all be elevated in ischemia or infarction of the kidney, spleen, or bowel. The HBD and LDH levels can be moderately elevated even when red blood cell hemolysis occurs as a result of using the pump, but this is not usually true of the SGOT level. The creatinine phosphokinase (CPK) concentration, on the other hand, is elevated more in acute muscle injury (as in acute myocardial infarction), but also in dermatomyositis and muscular dystrophy. With computations of times, degree, and combination of elevations a fairly substantial determination of infarction can be established. More specific assessment of myocardial damage can be made with the use of the CPK and LDH *isoenzymes*. Isoenzymes are multiple molecular forms of a particular enzyme that differ in certain physiochemical properties such as electrophoretic mobility. The organ specificity of the various isoenzymes allows detection of myocardial damage even in the presence of active disease in other organs.

Daily albumin and globulin studies are occasionally run starting on the second postoperative day, when the hemoglobin and hematocrit levels continue to drop in association with a blanket lowering of the electrolyte, BUN, and creatinine levels with normal or low specific gravity. Usually after the second postoperative day the albumin and globulin levels remain stable (if whole blood or albumin has not been administered recently) and can be used as an indication of the patient's hydration. Evaluation of all these factors along with the daily weight of the patient can decrease the unnecessary administration of more electrolyte solutions or blood and possibly fluid restriction or diuresis.

ECG's are run daily; there is, however, the need for more emphasis on ECG interpretation.

Daily chest x-ray films are usually obtained until the patient leaves the critical care unit to evaluate adequacy of chest drainage and rule out any residual atelectasis, fluid, or pneumothorax. During endotracheal intubation a major value of the chest x-ray film is to establish tube placement and ensure against blockage of a mainstem bronchus. Chest x-ray film evaluation by all critical care members is encouraged, and immediate reading by the surgeon or radiologist with written interpretation is imperative and is the responsibility of the nursing personnel.

Calcium, phosphorus, and magnesium levels when indicated are obtained on the fourth or fifth day and appropriate administration performed when low levels are found. If there is any suggestion of parathyroid disease or malnutrition, these studies are obtained sooner and repeated more frequently.

POSTOPERATIVE VENTILATION

In the past 10 years better mechanical respirators, frequent use of arterial gas determinations, and coordination of intensive care nursing and respiratory therapy teams have influenced the marked decrease in postoperative morbidity and mortality.

■ Who is responsible for the respiratory care of the patient?

The primary responsibility still rests with the operating surgeon, but there are times when this responsibility may be shared with the cardiologist and/or the pulmonary internist.

Equally as important in the coordinated care of the patient's pulmonary needs are nursing and respiratory services. With the continued subspecialization and training of respiratory therapists, minor conflicts occasionally develop as to the areas of responsibility. Regardless of designated duties of subspecialty departments, the unit practitioner is the overseer of all aspects of the patient's care, and if the mechanical manipulation and management of the respiratory assistance devices are under the auspices of the respiratory therapy department, the nursing staff must be aware of any changes of the inhalation modalities, gas concentrations, or volumes. The unit practitioner *must* be familiar with the respiratory equipment, and it is the responsibility of the respiratory therapy department as well as the nursing supervisors to guarantee familiarity with each apparatus used. I recommend the continued education of respiratory and nursing personnel in an integrated, coordinated program.

■ **What are some of the specifics regarding the use of endotracheal tubes?**

Endotracheal tubes are usually left in place after the operative procedure until the patient is fully responsive and able to cough appropriately on demand. The purpose of the endotracheal tube is to establish a means for adequate assisted or controlled respiration in the sedated patient during the immediate postoperative period when a decreased effort in breathing and a lower work load for the heart are sought.

Endotracheal tubes are usually equipped with adaptors that easily and quickly fit the majority of mechanical respirators, but there must be an absolute *guarantee* that all connectors will appropriately connect. It is essential to have equipment with universal connectors.

Immediately on reaching the unit, the patient is suctioned, the airway cleared, then connection is made to a mechanical respirator after ventilation with an oxygen-supplied Ambu bag operated by the anesthesiologist is discontinued.

The endotracheal tube should be suctioned and cleared of secretions on an "as needed" basis and at least every half hour, even if retained secretions are not suspected. Suction should not be applied for more than 25 to 30 seconds at a time. This is the average time a healthy person can comfortably hold his breath.

A sterile catheter is utilized every time the patient is suctioned, and sterile gloves are worn.

Respiratory precautions are used in any patient who has had a prosthetic valve placed.

A chest x-ray film should be obtained using a portable machine after arrival in the unit in order to evaluate expansion of the lung, detect the presence of atelectasis, and determine placement of the endotracheal tube. Interpretation of the x-ray film may be shared with the entire critical care team. Once the x-ray film has been obtained and the positioning of the endotracheal tube appears to be satisfactory, appropriate restabilization of the tube is accomplished.

The mechanically ventilated patient's oxygen administration should be titrated according to the results of serial blood gas measurements. Chest auscultation should be utilized by critical care personnel as the patient's ventilatory status is evaluated. Visual observation of the patient cannot be overemphasized, since decreased chest excursion may indicate inadequate ventilation.

■ **What can be done to help the patient tolerate the endotracheal tube?**

During the trip from the operating room to the unit the patient is often manually hyperventilated, which decreases carbon dioxide and any hypercapnic drive toward spontaneous respiration. In addition, any low metabolic pH is corrected in the last few minutes of the operation with IV sodium bicarbonate, and this decreases respiratory drive from metabolic acidosis. The 100% O_2 used until the first blood gas determinations are obtained decreases the hypoxemic drive to respiration. If all these measures are not adequate to prevent the patient from fighting the respiratory or to allow spontaneous control, then the IV use of morphine sulfate is advantageous. The usual dose of IV morphine sulfate is 3 to 5 mg (1/20 to 1/12 grain) initially, followed by 1 to 3 mg/hr as needed to decrease agitation from the endotracheal tube. IV morphine sulfate used in this manner usually does not exhibit myocardial depressive action and usually alleviates pain without severely depressing normal respiration. However, after extubation, morphine sulfate is administered subcutaneously or conversion is made to meperidine (Demerol)I.M.

Intubated patients may need extra relaxation for respiratory control, and *d*-tubocurarine, gallamine triethiodide, and/or succinylcholine (Anectine) can be utilized in a repeated dosage or by titrated continuous IV drip. With the use of these paralyzing agents the patient must be under absolutely constant observation by the unit practitioners, as accidental disconnection can result in a respiratory fatality.

Occasionally the IV administration of 5 to 10 mg of diazepam (Valium) may be useful in readjusting respiratory control or assistance. However, as in the use of all such drugs, careful and slow administration must be used, and at the same time the patient must be observed carefully for any hypotensive episodes.

■ **What medications are used with respirator nebulizers?**

Often only simple saline nebulization is used, but in patients with thick, difficult-to-suction secretions mucolytic agents are added every 4 to 6 hours. Acetylcysteine (Mucomyst), 0.25 to 0.5 ml, is mixed with 3 ml of saline solution, but once excessive secretions are obtained, the mucolytic agents are stopped. Another mucolytic agent is pancreatic dornase (Dornavac), usually given in dosages of 100,000 units every 4 to 6 hours.

Nausea can occur with use of acetylcysteine, especially in patients who cannot usually tolerate the odor of hard-boiled eggs, and an occasional case of bronchospasm may be attributed to an allergic response to a specific mucolytic agent, that is, pancreatic dornase.

Isoetharine-phenylephrine (Bronkosol-2) and isoproterenol (Isuprel) combinations are usually avoided in the immediate postoperative period unless absolutely necessary (for bronchospastic problems, and so on), as they can potentiate cardiac arrhythmias. When absolutely necessary, they are used in minute dosages, such as 4 to 10 drops mixed with 3 to 4 ml of saline solution.

Nebulized antibiotics are not rewarding, are possibly associated with complications (such as allergies and resistance of bacteria), and are seldom used.

■ **Why is endotracheal intubation preferred over tracheostomy in cardiac surgical patients?**

The endotracheal tube placed during the operative procedure can simply be left in place in the immediate postoperative period, whereas the continuity of tracheal secretions from a tracheostomy into the mediastinum (midsternotomy incisions, and so on) is subject to the dangers of infection, mediastinitis, sternal disruption, and even death.

An endotracheal tube can be more easily manipulated with respect to placement in the trachea and can safely be left in place for a period of 36 hours or less, but seldom over 3 to 4 days.

If prolonged ventilation becomes necessary or if there are mechanical reasons why nasotracheal or oral tracheal intubation cannot be instituted or continued, tracheostomy becomes a necessity. After multiple days of endotracheal intubation, complications such as late tracheal stenosis, erosion with hemorrhage, and inappropriate cord function are more apt to occur. During endotracheal intubation the patient cannot talk, and thus valuable communication is prevented.

Bilateral cord paralysis following aortic arch and thoracic aortic surgeries have been reported, and in such cases tracheostomy also becomes a necessity. It can be said that tracheostomy is usually performed as a last resort or when the endotracheal tube has been utilized beyond its safe period.

■ **What complications can occur during the routine care of endotracheal tubes and how are they controlled?**

The irritation and agitation of the patient produced by the endotracheal tube has previously been described, and this is usually controlled with appropriate sedation and relaxation.

Occasionally thick mucous secretions will partially occlude the end of the endotracheal tube; this manifests the need for increased ventilation volumes and is evidenced by difficulty in passing the suction catheters. Total obstruction of the end of the endotracheal tube can occur, causing cyanosis, severe agitation, and inability to breathe or obtain ventilation. The lack of chest excursion, the inability to pass the suctioning catheter, and severe patient distress command the immediate removal of the endotracheal tube. If an error has been made and the tube is not blocked, the tube can be replaced or the patient can be ventilated by mask and oral airway until help arrives. Occlusion of the end of the endotracheal tube has occurred with overinflation of a balloon cuff, producing similar findings; simple deflation of the cuff will usually remedy the situation.

Displacement of the endotracheal tube below the carina into one of the major bronchi can easily occur and result in obstruction of the remaining bronchus and total atelectasis of that lung. The endotracheal tube should be marked with india ink or at the lip level after the first x-ray film is taken, so that advancement can be recognized. Failure of chest excursion to occur or evidence of decreased breath sounds on one side is suggestive, but x-ray films provide confirmative proof.

Active bleeding can occur as a result of irritation of the endotracheal tube and repeated suctioning. This bleeding requires repeated irrigation of the endotracheal tube with saline solution followed by frequent suctioning; evaluation and supervision by the principal practitioner is paramount.

The majority of the complications resulting from the use of the endotracheal tube can be eliminated by alertness and frequent evaluation of the patient's respiratory status by the entire team, especially the nursing and respiratory team members.

■ **When is the endotracheal tube removed and are there any special techniques to follow?**

Extubation is performed at some time within the first 12 hours after surgery, but the time of removal depends on the patient's alertness and the overall general respiratory status as confirmed by arterial gas determinations. When possible, it is best to extubate the patient before 8 PM so that if minor problems develop, they will not develop during the 11 PM to 7 AM shift.

The T tube connection, an apparatus for the patient to breathe humidified oxygen off the respirator at concentrations of 40% or 70%, is connected to the patient, and after 10 to 15 minutes an arterial gas determination is obtained. If blood gas concentrations are adequate and the patient is fully awake, the cuff is deflated and the endotracheal tube is removed after the tube and posterior pharynx have been suctioned. This is performed when the patient is exhaling to prevent inhalation of any mucus plugs connected to or in the end of the tube. A large mucus accumulation

in the posterior pharynx or trachea is almost always present and must be immediately suctioned or coughed out. It is wise to have tissues ready.

A firm-fitting facial or rebreathing mask is then placed on the patient to deliver oxygen at the same concentration that was used with the T connection. After 10 minutes an additional arterial gas determination is obtained. From this point the patient undergoes titration with arterial gases until stable and until the right concentrations of oxygen and humidity are being used to maintain an arterial Po_2 of 80 to 95 mm Hg, a Pco_2 of 35 to 40 mm Hg, a pH of 7.35 to 7.45, and an oxygen saturation near 90%. If there is any question of agitation or unavoidable hypoventilation, the patient is reintubated. It is much better to reintubate within a short time after extubation than to wait until the patient is having respiratory difficulties (possibly at 2 to 3 AM).

■ **What are the ventilation and respiratory care recommendations once the endotracheal tube has been removed?**

If the patient's respiratory drive (excursion) is poor using the tight-fitting mask (30% to 40% O_2), a rebreathing mask is substituted with similar O_2 concentration but with the patient's own exhaled CO_2 and moisture. Humidified oxygen is used to prevent drying of secretions.

Instructions are given to frequently breathe deeply and cough at least every 30 to 60 minutes. For this the patient is placed in an upright sitting position utilizing folded pillows. An alternate method would be to have the patient stand while an intensive care staff member provides support to splint or brace the anterior chest wall, decreasing pain and allowing a better cough.

Inhalation therapy treatments when indicated are used with either the mask or the oral tube and administered as necessary after removal of the endotracheal tube. The frequency is increased or reduced depending on the x-ray findings, patient cooperation, and arterial gas concentrations.

Patients who cough poorly, show evidence of retained secretions, and have difficulty in cooperating or utilizing inhalation therapy properly may require appropriate nasotracheal suction. This can be performed in various ways; however, it is recommended that a sterile catheter be carefully passed through the nose and down to the glottic area. The patient's tongue is grasped with a clean sponge and pulled forward. The patient is then asked to inhale, and as he does so, the tube is gently passed down to or beyond the cords, which most often stimulates a cough. Occasionally the tube can actually be passed into the tracheal or bronchial area with aspiration of heavy mucus secretions. The points of pulling out the tongue and having the patient take a deep breath are essential to placement of the tube. Turning the head opposite to the bronchus to be aspirated has been recommended in many articles; however, probably more important is manipulation of the tip of the catheter toward the bronchus to be aspirated.

It is extremely difficult to utilize nasotracheal suction in patients with accentuated gag and vomit reflexes, and it may become necessary to loosen secretions by instituting careful but definitive postural drainage techniques. Patients with sternotomy incisions can tolerate these procedures surprisingly well.

A very frequently used pulmonary modality is the incentive spirometer. This apparatus is constructed in such a way as to stimulate the patient to take progressively increased deep breaths and thus inflate any small areas of local or patchy atelectasis. It is both a prophylactic and a therapeutic mechanism. It stimulates the patient to improve by providing a challenge. It is relatively simple to operate and appears to have very pro-

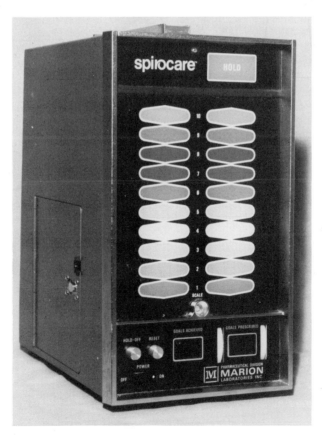

Fig. 19-9. Incentive spirometry unit with multicolored scale lights of patients' prescribed goal and patients' actual level achieved.

ductive results, especially with some of the newer multicolored scale models. (Fig. 19-9).

Personnel in respiratory, cardiac, and general intensive care units today should be as versatile and learned in the interpretation of arterial gas measurements as in understanding ECG's, electrolyte determinations, vital signs, and blood counts.

GENERAL POSTOPERATIVE EVALUATIONS

Monitors, laboratory work, and computerized analysis are all very important assets in patient care; however, general physical evaluation of a patient is essential to an uneventful postoperative recovery.

■ **What can be determined on simple visual and palpatory evaluation?**

The patient's color is frequently a guide to the progress being made. Marked pallor associated with unstable vital signs may indicate the need for repeat hemoglobin and hematocrit determinations to establish the presence of bleeding or hidden hemorrhage. Pallor may be attributed to peripheral vasoconstriction and suggest poor tissue perfusion, indicating the need for a peripheral vasodilating drug. Cyanosis can indicate poor ventilation, major arteriovenous shunting associated with massive pulmonary embolization, or simply be a reflection of the patient's being cold with vascular pooling or sludging.

Palpable coolness with moist diaphoresis can indicate drug reaction or hypovolemic, neurogenic, or cardiogenic shock, whereas coolness without diaphoresis may be caused by the inappropriate warming of the patient after surgical procedure pump cooling. Palpable warmth with diaphoresis associated with hypotension and tachycardia suggests infection or septic shock.

The appearance of urticaria and shaking chills with fever can indicate a blood incompatibility or drug allergy.

A simple look can reveal drainage areas from the chest incision, monitoring sites, or chest tube stab wound. Acquired paraphimosis resulting from retracted foreskin at the time of the initial urinary catheterization in surgery could cause major complications if not recognized in the op-

erating room or intensive care unit. A simple look may result in a major salvage, a happy patient, and no litigation.

Observation (looking, touching, feeling, and palpation) of the patient is stressed so as to avoid missing a correctable problem that could lead to the patient's death. Basic situations can occur such as separation of an arterial line from the patient's wrist under the sheets, disconnection of a chest tube at either the chest tube or the bottle site, or moderate drainage into the dressings.

Visual notes and recordings should be made of any change of consistency of the chest drainage, such as progression from nonclotting bright red blood to clotting darker blood or conversion to serous fluid. In the period following surgeries performed for severe trauma, chest tube drainage may reveal discolored secretions or bubbling only after the patient eats, suggesting rupture of the esophagus.

■ **How often should the patient be weighed, what is the weighing procedure, and what is the value of daily weight records?**

Weighings are completed either once or twice daily with bed scales in the immediate postoperative period. Preoperative bed scale weights are obtained for appropriate comparison. If the patient's weight varies over 2 pounds, this suggests a variance of 1 L of fluid. A gain of 4 pounds or more correlated with peripheral edema, pleural effusion, conjunctival edema (chemosis), or auscultation of fine rales in the lung fields signifies moderate overhydration or fluid retention. After the patient has most of the equipment involved in intensive care, such as monitoring lines and chest tubes, removed, the daily weight can also be measured on the standing scale, but always at the same time of day and with the patient wearing the same clothing.

■ **What simple evaluations can be utilized to evaluate neurologic status?**

In the immediate postoperative period it is essential to determine the patient's level of consciousness and whether or not all extremities can be moved successfully. In addition, the pupillary responses and equalities are determined, as well as the ability to cooperate. Any variations could indicate major stroke or minor brain injury associated with embolization of fine particulate matter or air during the pump run.

Agitation, restlessness, and convulsive-like activity can reflect CNS damage from any of the previously mentioned causes or can possibly indicate drug toxicity or simply reflect the patient's response to pain. In the later stages of the postoperative period agitation, confusion, and psychotic behavior occur and can be associated with sleep deprivation, protein and electrolyte imbalances, or low serum or magnesium either alone or in conjunction with preoperative anxiety, drug or alcohol dependency, or preexisting organic brain involvement.

It is becoming more common for the family or nursing staff to recognize irregular behavior suggestive of symptoms of minor withdrawal from alcohol. The critical care unit staff should notify the principal practitioner initially so that appropriate evaluation and possible therapy can be instituted.

Incidents have been reported in which patients were apparently awake for portions of the operative procedures. These individuals experience nightmares in the postoperative period usually relating to dreams of being stabbed or tortured or undergoing painful situations. These nightmares seem to follow a typical pattern and frequently can be abated by a simple explanation to the patient that he might be recalling certain portions of the operation in his subconscious and assuring him that this situation will pass.

■ **What outputs should be measured, listed, and recorded in easy-to-read form?**

Urinary output should be appropriately recorded whenever a urinary catheter is in place; however, it is also most important to record output when the catheter is removed. If the patient is incontinent, estimated guesses as to the amount of urine lost in the sheets are essential.

Notation should also be made of moderate diaphoresis, as a patient who perspires profusely or who has an elevated temperature can lose as much as 100 ml for each degree of elevation in temperature over a 24-hour period. Thus patients who are undergoing diaphoresis and who are moderately febrile (up to 103° to 104° F) can lose

from 500 to 1000 ml of low-concentration salt solution each day.

Each *individual* chest tube drainage should be recorded; as previously emphasized, the consistency of the drainage should be noted.

Any vomitus or nasogastric suction aspiration must be recorded accurately and should be replaced with electrolyte solutions similar in composition to gastric contents.

A close approximation of liquid or diarrheal bowel movements should be listed in milliliters; the former terminology of small, medium, or large is not accurate enough for scientific recordings or measurements.

■ **What intakes should be listed?**

On the patient's arrival in the unit records should be made of all fluids if they are to be maintained. When many units of blood or fluid are required, a numbering system (written on each bottle) facilitates better record-keeping.

Intakes should include not only the volume of fluid given in each IV infusion but also the consistency of that fluid, such as 5% dextrose in water, 0.45N saline solution, albumin, plasma, or blood. Trade name solutions such as Osolyte M and Gastrolyte solution should also be listed.

Any irrigation fluid that is utilized and not returned, such as those in urinary catheters, endotracheal tubes, or venous lines, should be represented in a separate column or area on the intake and output record sheet.

The fluids utilized to keep the arterial and venous pressure lines open must also be listed. Ice chips and water sips should be recorded accurately, as complications caused by excessive ingestions of ice chips can occur in both young and old postoperative or posttrauma patients.

It is extremely important that appropriate communication between nurses and physicians exists, so that when on postoperative orders the total of all fluids a patient is to receive is listed, this should mean *all* fluids including intravenous, CVP, oral, and nasogastric administrations and the fluids that are utilized to administer piggy back solutions. If there are any questions as to whether "all" means only total IV's or the total of all fluids, this must be clarified with the managing physician, as it is very easy otherwise to overload the patient with anywhere from 1 to 2 L of fluid in a 24-hour period.

Dressings and incision care
■ **What special care is utilized for dressings?**

Separate dressings are recommended for the sternotomy incision and the chest tube wound; thus when the chest tubes are milked in the immediate postoperative period and removed on the second or third postoperative day, the sternotomy incision is not disturbed or contaminated.

All monitor sites (CVP, arterial line) and percutaneous pacemaker wire exit sites are covered with an antibiotic dressing of povidone-iodine (Betadine) or bacitracin ointment. The value of placing an antibiotic ointment on the skin at the time of the original dressing is questionable; however, it appears to enhance the psychologic security of the intensive care practitioner and frequently the physician, and it is still recommended by many.

Dressings are removed on the second or third postoperative day or sooner if they have become saturated with drainage. Incision sites are then cleansed daily with hydrogen peroxide or with Betadine solution and completely dried; a lighter sterile dressing is reapplied or the incisions are left open to the air. If no bleeding occurs after the dressings are removed on the second or third day, natural lines of defense and resistance have been established, and the incisions can be safely left open to the air.

If Betadine is used for preoperative showering and surgical preparation but not washed off well after the surgical procedure, tincture of benzoin and tape application can produce blistering.

Any suspicious drainage is cultured immediately and abnormal discolorations or odors are immediately reported to the principal practitioner.

Diet and oral hygiene
■ **When is the patient allowed liquids or food by mouth, and what diet is appropriate in the immediate postoperative period? Can oral hygiene be instituted immediately on arrival at the unit; if not, why not?**

It is recommended that postoperative patients be given absolutely nothing orally for 12 to 18 hours for the following reasons:

1. The patient given ice chips in the immediate postoperative period sucks on the chips. This is accompanied by a moderate amount of air swallowing, which accumulates air and distends the stomach, elevating the diaphragm, possibly producing basilar atelectasis, and increasing the tendency to vomit.
2. Techniques for oral hygiene such as astringent rinses of the mouth and lemon and glycerin on the lips, aside from possibly nauseating the patient, stimulate licking of the lips and, again, swallowing air.

Gastric distention is one of the most, if not the most, common postoperative complications of cardiac surgery. With the use of nasogastric tubes and/or the absolute prohibition of oral intake it is believed that the incidence of postoperative atelectasis and aspiration pneumonia is decreased.

Start of the postoperative diet is not recommended for 12 to 18 hours (sooner only if bowel sounds and flatus develop); this diet consists of a full liquid bland regimen, including gelatin (Jello), custard, cooked Cream of Rice cereal with milk, and very liquid boiled eggs. The majority of these items do not stimulate increased gastric secretion and create less gastric irritation than most of the clear liquids, such as tea, apple juice, cider, or the clear but salty and frequently spicy hospital bouillon broths.

Bronchial aspiration in the immediate postoperative period can be of critical consequence to any patient, but especially to a borderline cardiac surgical patient. Many of the clear liquids previously mentioned (and occasionally the patient may receive coffee with this order) cause increased gastric and hydrochloric acid secretions, which, when aspirated into the lungs, can produce serious pneumonitis. These gastric juices seem to be neutralized by the full liquid bland substances.

A majority of the patients operated on in the United States are by no means in nutritional deficit at the time of surgery, and it is frequently safer to err on the side of feeding the patient later than feeding him too soon. One of the trite but frequently appropriate quotes we utilize is, "When the bowel will growl, there is need to feed," meaning that when there is good bowel activity and audible bowel sounds, it is probably safe for the patient to begin oral intake.

Patients with cardiac decompensation or those who require no salt, are diabetic, or are following low-calorie or other special diets can be placed on these diets again after an 18- to 24-hour trial on this liquid bland or "super soft" diet.

Intravenous fluids (fluid and electrolyte management)

■ **Which IV solutions are administered and what are the limitations imposed during the immediate postoperative period?**

Between 1500 and 2000 ml of 5% dextrose in water is given during the first 24 hours to most patients, but younger patients without pre- or immediately postoperative cardiac decompensation or renal problems are occasionally administered half of this volume as 5% dextrose in a 0.2 N saline solution.

Acute blood loss as determined from the chest output, pulse wave configuration, arterial pressures, CVP, and/or atrial pressures, hemoglobin determination, and hematocrit is replaced by packed cells and Plasmanate if the patient demonstrates no volume overload or cardiac decompensation. Rapidity of replacement depends on the monitoring factors and clinical manifestations. Except in crisis situations I prefer not to administer blood using the hand pumps, as this can predispose to air embolization and increase fractionization of the red blood cells and platelets. The pressure bag administering devices allow a steady rapid inflow of blood with less damage.

■ **What electrolyte imbalances most frequently occur in the postoperative cardiac surgical patient?**
Hypokalemia

A low serum potassium level is a frequently encountered electrolyte abnormality occurring after cardiac bypass. It can be associated with diuretic regimens and inadequate potassium replacement before surgery. The hemodilution effect from cardiopulmonary bypass and diuresis that occurs during the surgical procedure with the use of mannitol or other diuretics further lowers the serum potassium. Since hypokalemia associated with digitalis administration predis-

poses to dangerous arrhythmias, when low serum potassium levels are noted, IV administration is started immediately. It should be stressed that the bottle should be well marked, or "flagged," when high concentrations of potassium are used.

In moderate depletion or when hypokalemia is suspected as the cause of troublesome arrhythmias, as much as 40 and sometimes 60 mEq of potassium can be placed in 250 ml of fluid and given over a 90-minute period; however, if allowed to infuse at a more rapid rate, cardiac standstill or asystole can occur. Some reports have stressed never administering more than 20 mEq of potassium over a 1-hour period; however, when life-endangering arrhythmias are present, potassium should be given in these larger concentrations, with constant bedside attention to the specific IV solution. It should also be given through a large vein, preferably via the CVP line and never via the arterial line.

Hyperkalemia

Hyperkalemia is not infrequently seen immediately postoperatively when potassium cardioplegia has been used during surgery, and on the second or third postoperative day as the result of overzealous IV administration. Occasionally a marked laboratory error occurs when laboratory personnel mistakenly draw a blood sample from a vein above an infusion line administering potassium solution. Abnormally high levels of serum potassium are found in hemolyzed serum and after the administration of numerous units of old stored blood. If levels above 5.5 mEq/L are obtained, added potassium administration is stopped and potassium levels are measured frequently. If true serum potassium levels reach 6 mEq/L or greater, hypertonic glucose and insulin solutions can be administered to drive the potassium to an intracellular position. However, if there are signs of hyperkalemia on the ECG, this is not a recommended procedure, as it is probably better to maintain the high level of potassium in the serum rather than drive it to an intracellular position. Frequent diuresis with IV furosemide (Lasix) can be utilized to facilitate potassium excretion; in acute situations 1 g of IV calcium chloride can be slowly administered to help counteract the effects of the hyperkalemia. If the potassium level continues to rise, exchange resins may be given by enema, or peritoneal dialysis or hemodialysis may be required. Frequent potassium monitoring during these procedures must be utilized. If, in association with the hyperkalemia, there is increased BUN or creatinine levels, a nephrologist should be consulted.

Hypernatremia and hyponatremia

Hypernatremia is usually not a problem for the postoperative patient; however, hyponatremia occurs and is most often caused by previous preoperative salt restriction, loss with diuretics, dilutional effects from the cardiopulmonary bypass, and use of nonsaline fluids during recovery. Administration of salt for excessive diuresis is not usually necessary until the sodium levels drop below 125 mEq/L. The most successful mechanism of reestablishing normal sodium balance once gastrointestinal function is reestablished is by instituting oral feedings. However, when nondiluted hyponatremia persists with levels below 120 mEq/L, the administration of normal saline solution and occasionally hypertonic salt solutions is necessary.

Hypocalcemia

Hypocalcemia is encountered with dilution, administration of large volumes of acid citrate dextrose blood, and occasionally in patients with hyperventilation. This can easily be corrected with direct IV infusion of 10 ml of a 10% solution of calcium chloride (1 g) given over a 10-minute time span.

Hypercalcemia

Hypercalcemia is seldom seen but can occur in previously unrecognized malignant conditions and other metabolic disorders. When present, it can be treated with a low calcium diet, slow infusion of sodium and potassium phosphate mixtures, corticosteroids, or administration of mithramycin, a calcium-reducing antibiotic. Peritoneal dialysis has also been used in severe cases of hypercalcemia.

Hypomagnesemia

Magnesium deficiency may be noted in patients who have been on long-term administration of IV fluids or are nutritionally depleted; this condition is more common in the cachectic or alcohol-dependent patient. It has been noted that the signs and symptoms of hypocalcemia and hypokalemia can be accentuated with low magnesium levels. Depletion can be treated by IM injection of a 50% solution (1 g) or by slow IV infusion of 500 mg of magnesium sulfate.

Body positions, wraps, and early postoperative activities

As teams have become more experienced, it has been interesting to note progressive change in the orders for body positions, certain wraps, and activities allowed.

■ What body position is preferred for the postoperative cardiac surgical patient?

Sternotomy and also thoracotomy patients obtain more relief from pain when in a low Fowler position as compared to being perfectly flat. This allows the diaphragm to drop for better respiration, decreases fluid return to the heart, seems to allay some apprehension, and is an aid in preventing cerebral edema.

The legs are usually kept extended and straight; under no circumstances is the lower end of the bed bent under the patient's knees, as this contributes to venous stasis in the popliteal veins and potentiates phlebothrombosis and pulmonary embolization.

Commencing 2 to 3 hours after the surgical procedure, the patient should be allowed to turn onto the right or left side if the chest tubes do not impede the turn. All monitor or IV lines are protected against bends or twists. Turning from side to side benefits pulmonary function, prevents pulmonary stasis, and improves lung drainage; it also helps establish better drainage of fluid from the pericardial and thoracic cavities. During the first 2 days the patient is turned every 2 to 3 waking hours.

During the first oral feedings the patient is placed in an upright position; this usually decreases the tendency toward regurgitation and thus aspiration.

When arterial bypass lines have been used in the lower extremities or saphenous veins have been harvested, the legs are wrapped from toes to groin with elastic bandages. When a single long incision has been used for procuring the saphenous vein, a Hemovac drain is left in a subcutaneous position for 12 to 24 hours and may necessitate frequent dressing changes. Occasionally antiembolic stockings are placed from the toes to the groin over or under the Ace wraps; when the drains have been removed and there is no need for the wraps, thromboembolic stockings alone are used.

The patient's activities are quite limited for the first 12 to 18 hours after the surgical procedure with simple turning from side to side, slight increases or decreases in the semi-Fowler position, and upright positions allowed occasionally for the chest x-ray films taken by the portable unit. However, the day (24 to 36 hours) after surgery, the patient is allowed to sit upright for intake of fluids or semisolids (as previously described) and is encouraged to use a footboard for flexion and extension of the toes in order to maintain calf activity for better venous return from the legs.

During the period between 24 and 48 hours after surgery the patient is positioned upright on the bedside with the legs semiextended (to prevent binding in the popliteal space). This is performed three to four times on the second postoperative day.

Depending on the progress made, by the first or second postoperative day the chest tubes and urinary catheter have been removed, most monitoring and IV fluid devices have been discontinued, and the patient is allowed to sit in a chair at the bedside, again with the legs extended. Getting the patient out of bed and into the chair satisfies the activity requirement for patient and personnel, especially when recommended three to four times daily for 15- to 30-minute intervals.

The third or fourth postoperative day the patient is allowed ambulation with assistance. It is recommended that those individuals assisting the patient be strong enough to hold the patient in case he becomes weak. *It is essential that the patient be walked and not dragged,* for studies are conclusive that venous return from the legs is much less in the patient who is upright and motionless than that of a patient even lying in bed. It is common to see patients supposedly being ambulated by very strong aides or physiotherapy technicians with the patient's feet hardly ever touching the floor, of it they touch, they are limply dragging. The purpose of early ambulation is to increase arteriole circulation, improve venous drainage, and retrain muscle groups.

Activity is progressive from this point, depending on the patient's cardiac enzyme levels, ECG, chest x-ray film, other laboratory data, and response to the first simple ambulation. By the sixth or seventh postoperative day, when the patient is usually ready for discharge, the staff members have prepared him for usual home activities such as caring for himself in the bathroom and getting into and manipulating from bed status to sitting in a chair, on a couch, or at a dining table.

When the patient is discharged, it is recommended that home activities be similar to the last hospital day activities.

■ What specific recommendations are made for body positioning at home, activities, and leg wraps?

The patient is advised that it is preferable to sleep alone or with a simple pillow separation from his or her bed partner for 5 to 7 days in order to avoid irritating the multiple tender incisions.

An incline pillow made of sponge rubber can usually be obtained at one of the various department stores or medical supply houses. This allows the patient to sleep at a 15- to 20-degree incline and frequently avoids the need for a surgical bed.

Instructions are given to avoid any heavy lifting and not to indulge in any active walking or strenuous exercise.

Because of late pulmonary embolic phenomena that too often occur after discharge, strict adherence to the use of antiembolic stockings *whenever* upright, in sitting positions, or ambulating is forcefully recommended for at least 3 weeks. The patient at home, as in the hospital, is to avoid crossing the legs, exerting any pressure on or bending in the popliteal space, or assuming any position where the legs just hang without activity. Activities that are allowed are walking (slowly), sitting (moving the legs and ankles), or lying supine rather than simply standing in one position. But in all cases, the support or antiembolic stockings (leotard type preferred over groin length) should be worn.

Medication, routes of administration, and precautions

Because of the frequent acute crises that can occur in critical care units, a very broad variety of medications must be immediately available, and mixtures and dosages must be committed to memory. It is paramount for all personnel, but especially critical care practitioners, to be familiar with the dosage of the common drugs used in critical care and to be reacquainted frequently with the indications, contraindications, methods of preparation, and techniques of administration.

■ **What special precautions should be taken with respect to the dosages and administration of medications?**

All units should have accessible and easy-to-read lists of the most commonly used medications, the various effects, and the modes of administration.

The administration of antibiotics is usually preempted by an evaluation of the patient's record as well as repeated questioning of the patient regarding any allergies. Infrequently used antibiotics are rechecked as to routes of administration, because these change intermittently (for example, in the use of chloramphenicol [Chloromycetin]). Certain antibiotics (gentamicin and kanamycin) are nephrotoxic and must be given in dosages determined by the BUN, creatinine, and creatinine clearance levels, and others (certain tetracyclines) should not be given to individuals who have jaundice or a history of severe hepatic disease. Some antibiotics are restricted to · absolute emergency situations because of depressing or altering effects on certain white blood cells. A point to remember is that most IM antibiotics should be placed *deep* in the muscle for better absorption and to prevent subcutaneous accumulations, fat necrosis, or abscess.

The administration and mixing of certain solutions such as lidocaine, isoproterenol (Isuprel), metaraminol (Aramine), levarterenol (Levophed), and dopamine (Intropin), as well as digoxin (Lanoxin), lanatoside (Cedilanid), procainamide (Pronestyl), quinidine, sodium bicarbonate, and propranolol (Inderal) should be committed to memory and nearly automatic.

The administration of blood can be associated with multiple problems. In order to prevent such problems, blood should be administered following Ringer's lactate or saline solution rather than after dextrose and water. It should be warmed, if possible, to room temperature to prevent chills and to prevent cold agglutinin reactions. Multiple micropulmonary emboli can be prevented with special microfilters to eliminate the large blood platelet aggregates so often present in stored blood. It is uncommon today to have incompatible blood administered to a patient; however, the blood should be quadruply checked: first, by asking the patient's name; second, by verifying the armband of the patient; third, by comparing the patient and donor blood types; and fourth, by rechecking all of these factors with another person. If a blood reaction develops, appropriate measures such as discontinuing the blood infusion and notifying the principal practitioner should be carried out. A urine sample and another blood sample should be sent to the laboratory for retyping and cross matching. The patient should be closely observed for further signs of blood reaction.

The techniques of the IV use of analgesics such as meperidine hydrochloride (Demerol), 10 to 25 mg/hr, and IV morphine sulfate, 1 to 5 mg every 30 to 60 minutes, should be well known to all critical care unit personnel.

IV paralyzing agents such as succinylcholine (Anectine) and *d*-tubocurarine are used for intubation procedures and respiratory control. All critical care personnel should be familiar with these agents and capable of monitoring patients undergoing such therapy.

Any time large doses of IV potassium are being given, the lines should be set up so that rapid administration greater than 60 mEq/hr cannot possibly occur and cause cardiac standstill. IV calcium chloride (usually 500 to 1000 mg) should be given over a 5- to 10-minute period and never into a line containing acid citrate dextrose blood, as it will precipitate coagulation. Magnesium can be given by the IV route for slower pickup with less danger of acute side-effects. When concentrated electrolytes are given by the IV route, the CVP lines are preferred, as many of these solutions cause chemical phlebitis of peripheral veins.

IV heparin can be given by "piggyback," push, or (less preferred) diluted in large volumes of

POSTOPERATIVE ROUTINE CARDIAC SURGERY ORDERS

MEDICATIONS

1. M.S., _____ mg q _____ hr IV; After patient off respirator, Demerol, _____ mg q 2-3 hr IM
2. Antibiotic _____
3. ASA or Tylenol, gr 20, rectally q 3-4 hr for temp above 101° F

RESPIRATORY

1. ET tube irrigation with 3-5 ml N.S. q 30 min or prn
2. Sign pt q 15-30 min (hand or machine)
3. Turn from side to side q 2 hr, HOB (head of bed) elevated 30 degrees

AFTER EXTUBATION

1. O_2 @ _____% by heated mist aerosol with rebreathing mask
2. Cough and deep breath q 30 min of waking hours
3. Nasotracheal suction prn
4. Incentive spirometer q 1 hr 5-10x's—omit from MN (midnight) to 6 AM

FLUIDS

1. IV's—1 L D/W with 30 mEq KCl q 12 hr (2000 ml/24 hr)
2. Foley to gravity, with hourly output; specific gravity, as per routine
3. Intake and output
4. Daily weights (bed scale until tubes out, then standing scale)
5. Chest tubes to 20 cm suction; *report* drainage over 400 ml first 4 hr, or if greater than 150 ml in any 1 hr
6. NG (nasogastric) if in place, to low intermittent suction. Irrigate q 2 hr with 30 ml Gastrolyte solution

VITAL SIGNS

1. V S q 5-10 min × 2 hr; then if stable, q 15 min × 4 hr; then if stable, q 30 min
2. Notify physician if:

    BP above _____ mm Hg or below _____ mm Hg

    Respirations above _____ min or below _____ min

    Temperature above _____ or below _____

    CVP above _____ cm or below _____ cm

    Pulmonary artery pressure above _____ or below _____

    Wedge pressure above _____ or below _____

    Left atrial pressure above _____ or below _____

    Urine output above _____ ml/hr or below _____ ml/hr

3. Neuro checks q 2 hr × 12 hr; pulse evaluation q 1 hr × 12, then q 4 hr

LABORATORY

1. ABG's 10 min after any respiratory mode change, then q 4 hr, until 8 AM day after surgery, and then prn
2. H/H, SATCH-6 on arrival to unit, repeat in 4 hr, or prn, then q AM × 5
3. SGOT, CPK, LDH, 1st through 5th postop days
4. Calcium, magnesium, phosphorus on 3rd postop day
5. Chest x-ray on arrival in unit, then daily until chest tube out and then q 2 days
6. ECG *daily* × 3 and thereafter q 3 days
7. C & S of ET tube secretions on extubation

Continued.

POSTOPERATIVE ROUTINE CARDIAC SURGERY ORDERS—CONT'D

DIET

1. NPO for 12-18 hr, then full liquid bland for 12 hr. If tolerated well, soft select × 36 hr, then select diet or rehab diet

DRESSING AND WOUND CARE

1. Ace wrap from toe to groin on surgical leg; TED's bilaterally
2. Clean all Foley, IV, and monitor line entrances daily prn and apply antibiotic ointment
3. If progressive drainage in dressing, change PRN—don't reinforce
4. After first dressing removal by physician, cleanse daily with Betadine

CARDIAC REHAB TO SEE PATIENT WHEN STABLE

---

fluid. When given by subcutaneous injection, a short (½ inch) No. 25- or 26-gauge needle should be used and the heparin injected in folded fat but never into muscle or subfascia, as this is how large complicating hematomas occur.

Protamine sulfate is required at times to reverse additional heparin effects, but it can produce marked hypotension when given rapidly. It should be diluted and administered over a 10- to 20-minute period.

Chlorpromazine (Thorazine), as well as other phenothiazine agents, can also be responsible for moderate hypotension, especially when given by the IV route. Chlorpromazine is often administered by IV route to correct peripheral vasoconstriction with resultant hypertension and poor perfusion. When needed in the immediate postoperative period, 1 to 2 mg are diluted in 5 to 10 ml of saline solution and administered over a period of 2 to 3 minutes, with repeat doses (up to 10 mg) given as needed. Severe hypotension can occur when larger doses are given in labile postoperative patients.

The reader is encouraged to pursue more in-depth information through independent study and the use of reference material.

CHAPTER 20

Postoperative complications in the adult cardiac surgical patient

Robert A. Steedman

Multiple potentially critical complications can occur in the immediate postoperative period. Prior to the era of critical care units, postoperative mortality rates were high. Early recognition and prompt therapeutic intervention in the minor phases can prevent progression to the major phase with its high toll of life.

CARDIAC COMPLICATIONS
Postoperative bleeding
■ **What is considered excessive postoperative bleeding?**

Increased output in the chest bottle drainage with volumes in excess of 100 ml/hr for more than 5 hours should stimulate major concern, but it is not uncommon. If this rate continues for the first 12 hours (a loss of 1200 ml) or if there is no trend toward decreasing output after 10 to 12 hours, reexploration is recommended.

Any patient who demonstrates blood loss between 150 and 300 ml/hr for more than 4 hours is also a candidate for relatively urgent reexploration procedures.

The signs of cardiovascular instability associated with this bleeding include the following:

1. Tachycardia (rates of 100 to 130 beats/min) that responds to administration of any fluid volume and/or blood
2. Labile blood pressure, the hypotensive aspects of which also respond to the administration of blood or other fluid
3. An adequate pulse or pressure wave despite hypotension and tachycardia
4. Continually dropping central venous pressure (CVP) or left atrial pressure (LAP) that also responds favorably to fluid administration
5. Labile vital signs associated with the intended or accidental use of the "tilt" test, evidenced when simple elevation of the patient's torso for the purpose of taking a portable chest x-ray film or administering respiratory therapy is followed by a moderate to marked drop in blood pressure, the temporary decrease in pulse rate proceeding to a compensation tachycardia and frequently associated with moderate pallor, agitation, and diaphoresis

These findings, in conjunction with dropping hemoglobin and hematocrit levels, indicate blood loss out of proportion with blood replacement and are not usually present unless a deficit of 500 to 1000 ml exists.

Hemoglobin and hematocrit determinations are of value in determining the amount of blood loss, but they should never be taken as the primary or single factor determining need for replacement. The hemoglobin and hematocrit levels in the first few hours postoperatively can be falsely high and not adequately reflect the total blood loss; with hemodilution they can even be falsely low. However, if a patient in the immediate postoperative period presents evidence of deterioration by the signs previously mentioned, the hemoglobin and hematocrit determinations can be of critical importance, especially if very low (hematocrit below 25% and hemoglobin below 7 g/100 ml) during this period of false high readings (especially if hemodilution is not suspected).

Any sudden volume increase in chest drainage over a short period of time after surgery is indicative of major hemorrhage. For example, if the chest tubes have been draining a stable amount (for example, 35 to 50 ml/hr), and then shortly after moving the patient or milking the chest tubes, an output of 200 to 500 ml/hr occurs in a matter of 5 to 30 minutes, activation of a new bleeding site or disruption of a suture line must be considered, and rapid evaluation for surgical intervention must be made.

A sudden decrease or cessation of chest tube output may also herald a problem of serious consequence, as continued bleeding without evacuation of the blood can produce pericardial tamponade or compressive hemothorax with complications of mediastinal shift.

Certain anatomic, physiologic, and technical factors associated with some patients or their surgery predispose to bleeding problems. The patients more prone to postoperative hemorrhage are those with preexisting pericarditis or pleuritis requiring more adhesion division and dissection, those having repeat cardiac operations (again through adhesions and scar), patients requiring multiple bypasses (each additional suture line increasing the potential of another bleeding site), patients with anatomically deep vessels in which isolation precludes deep dissection in fatty and muscular tissue, and any patient with generally poor vascular tissue (caused by generalized debility, ischemia, and advanced atherosclerosis in the aorta and coronary vessels). Incidental minute tears and fragmentation of the tissues with simple suturing, or removal of the atrial or ventricular vents or aortic perfusion cannulas are much more common in debilitated patients, or those undergoing a repeat surgery. When the patient arrives in the unit, these factors are still very fresh in the surgeon's mind, and the postoperative team should be alerted to expect increased bleeding.

■ **What nontechnical factors can be involved in postoperative bleeding?**

Patients who preoperatively demonstrate abnormal clotting studies or present a history of clotting problems with simple tooth extraction and minor cuts and bruises should be evaluated preoperatively by a hematologist so that appropriate measures can be instituted preoperatively and postoperatively to replace clotting factors or prepare for postoperative control.

Any heart-lung apparatus basically damages the red blood cells and insults the clotting mechanisms in the blood. Clotting mechanisms are altered as a result of general protein denaturation, destruction of platelets, and activation of certain fibrinolysins. The longer the pump is run, the more likely it is that these factors will occur.

Either inadequate neutralization of the heparin or "heparin rebound" can be responsible for postoperative bleeding. Heparin used in surgery is reversed as determined by the activated clotting time (ACT) with protamine sulfate. At the time of closure the anticipated clots from neutralization of the heparin are usually evident, but occasionally as the skin is being closed moderate general ooze is evidenced, suggesting that the heparin effect is still present. When this occurs, the activated clotting time or partial thromboplastin time is repeated; if altered, additional protamine sulfate is administered, often with dramatic results. The careful and slow administration of protamine sulfate has been mentioned.

The patient with excessive oozing and blood loss during surgery has received multiple units of acid citrate dextrose (ACD) blood; if this blood has been stored for over 3 to 5 days, it is deficient in all clotting factors. The added ACD anticoagulant binds the calcium needed for coagulation, and when multiple units are administered, functional calcium is depleted in the patient's own blood. Thus 1 g of calcium chloride is administered slowly in a nonblood line for every rapid 3 units of ACD blood used.

Circulating fibrinolysins can be demonstrated with bedside tests and by failure of clot formation or evidence of lysis of the clot after it is formed. It is a less common form of coagulopathy; however, at one time in various institutions it was considered to contribute to postoperative bleeding to the extent that an antifibrinolysin agent, aminocaproic acid (Amicar), was administered routinely during or on completion of every pump perfusion. It is now used only if fibrinolytic activity is suspected or evident.

Bleeding associated with chronic liver disease and/or superimposed acute hepatic insult can occur and not infrequently results in death.

■ What measures are utilized to evaluate the cause of the bleeding?

Most surgeons, when an early bleeding problem is recognized, order the coagulation screening test, which, as previously mentioned, includes evaluation of platelet count, prothrombin time, partial thromboplastin time, thrombin time, fibrinogen assay, Ivy bleeding time, activated clotting time, Lee-White clotting time, euglobulin clot lysis, clot retraction studies, and fibrin split products.

While waiting for the laboratory returns, it is frequently advantageous for the surgeon to place 3 to 5 ml of the patient's blood into two or three nonheparinized tubes and set them at the bedside. The first of these three tubes can be used to determine if any clot forms, and if it forms, the time required for formation and the integrity of the clot can be noted. Certain other bedside evaluations can be performed with the administration of fresh blood, fibrinogen, platelets, or protamine sulfate to the nonclotting blood to see if a good clot is obtained. If the original blood specimen clots without additives but within minutes undergoes lysis, fibrinolysin activity is suggested. These bedside tests are unsophisticated, but frequently will give some information as to cause.

Equally as important is evaluation of the patient's incision, the chest tubes, and venous puncture sites to see if any clotting or lack of clotting is present.

■ How are the various causes of postoperative bleeding managed?

Mechanical causes of postoperative hemorrhage are best handled prophylactically at the time of surgery with appropriate hemostatic suture control and, if necessary, with the use of Teflon pledgets placed for reinforcement of suture lines on the atria, aorta, or ventricle. Diligent electrocoagulation is used on all potential bleeding areas such as the pericardial edges, superior mediastinal areas, substernal musculature, and perichondrial and periosteal edges. Bone wax is used on the divided sternal edges, and all areas are evaluated when the patient's

blood pressure is at normal levels. The incidence of reoperation for hemorrhage may be decreased with the use of sponge (Gelfoam) pledgets soaked in thrombin and placed over various oozing operative sites or the occasional use of Avitene.

The majority of the coagulopathies can be treated with the initial administration of very fresh whole blood or fresh frozen plasma (ffp) During the early phases of cardiac surgery only fresh whole blood or fresh frozen plasma (ffp) cross matched the evening before or the morning of surgery was used; however, this is not presently feasible.

When severe bleeding problems occur and appear refractory to customary treatment, one of the best modes of therapy for patient salvage is administering multiple units of fresh frozen plasma or whole blood (having been obtained within 30 to 90 minutes prior to administration). Regardless of the tedious, time-consuming procedure needed for obtaining fresh whole blood from donors, the efficacy of its use cannot be disregarded.

Fibrinolysis problems can usually be treated effectively with IV aminocaproic acid (Amicar). The patient is usually given 5 g over a 30- to 60-minute period; this is followed by 1 g hourly for the subsequent 4 to 5 hours. Some improvement should be noted after 2 to 3 hours of therapy, and if it is not evident, complete reevaluation with a new coagulation screening test should be performed. Fibrinolysis and intravascular coagulation can occur simultaneously and may require the use of heparin in addition to an antifibrinolysin agent.

Heparin effect is not uncommonly seen in the immediate postoperative period as "heparin rebound." This can usually be determined by the activated clotting time, the partial thromboplastin time, and in cases of moderate overheparinization or inadequate reversal, the prothrombin time can frequently be very low. Slow administration of and titration with protamine sulfate usually reverses all these abnormal tests.

Thrombocytopenia can be detected by microevaluation and platelet counts. When the counts are below 70,000, the situation should be corrected by giving fresh platelet packs; usually a minimum of 4 to 8 packs is necessary with frequent reassessment. Platelet packs are occasionally difficult to obtain after 3 PM but when the need for them is suspected, they should be ordered immediately.

In cases where numerous units of ACD blood have been administered or when hypocalcemia is evident, calcium chloride is given, but never in a line containing blood. It is probably true that adequate calcium can be mobilized from the patient's own bones to supplement the needed calcium. However, this takes time, and frequently in cases of heavy bleeding, time is of the essence.

■ What is DIC and how is it treated?

The letters "DIC" refer to a syndrome with many titles such as "consumption coagulopathy," "diffuse intravascular clotting," "disseminated intravascular clotting," "intravascular coagulation syndrome," and "disseminated intravascular coagulopathy." A simple explanation would be to tag DIC as a syndrome in which excessive coagulation occurs in the peripheral capillaries and occasionally the precapillary arterioles and postcapillary venules, thus blocking these end vessels and producing decreased tissue perfusion and increased arteriovenous shunting. The extensive peripheral coagulation pulls necessary clotting factors from the plasma, basically reducing it to serum, and thus normal hemostasis can no longer be maintained. Uncontrollable hemorrhage begins and can be visualized from simple needle punctures, incision sites, or from the respiratory, gastrointestinal, genitourinary, and integumentary areas, among other regions. Conditions predisposing to the development of this syndrome include traumatic perfusions (long-term pump runs with excessive suctioning of blood); preoperative, operative, or postoperative hypotension or shock syndromes; infection; severe acidosis and other metabolic imbalances; and severe drug or blood transfusion reactions. In its severe and advanced stages generalized poor tissue perfusion with severe hypoxia, acidosis, hepatic and renal failure, subcutaneous ecchymoses and hemorrhage, and digital and extremity gangrene can occur.

DIC is best identified by appropriate evaluation of the coagulation screening test, although it is occasionally difficult to differentiate from primary fibrinolysis. The laboratory findings in DIC include prolonged prothrombin, partial thromboplastin, and thrombin times. The platelet count and fibrinogen and antithrombin factor III levels are low, and the euglobulin lysis time is shortened or decreased. The levels of fibrin degradation products, or *fibrin split products,* are *elevated;* this is one of the most significant of all the tests mentioned in differentiating DIC from the other coagulopathies. In comparing DIC and primary fibrinolysis, it should be noted that in both conditions the thrombin time is prolonged and the fibrinogen level is low (usually much lower in DIC). Thrombocytopenia can be present in both after a pump run, but the platelet count is lower in DIC than in primary fibrinolysis. The euglobulin lysis time is abnormally short in both conditions, but reduction is much greater in primary fibrinolysis.

The primary *treatment* of this syndrome is controversial, but when primary organ failure such as kidney or lung is suspected, most still recommend *heparin* administration. The heparin is administered in an attempt to stop the microscopic thrombosis; since heparin exerts antithrombin activity, it hopefully neutralizes free circulating thrombin. Its other anticoagulant principles are even more important in the treatment of this disease. Heparin should be administered by the IV route and frequently given in therapeutic doses with the initial amount sufficient to induce total anticoagulation in the patient (similar to undergoing cardiopulmonary bypass procedures). The therapeutic administration sometimes requires dosages as high as 20,000 units every 2 hours; however, in cases where both renal and hepatic impairment are present, heparin dosage must be markedly decreased, as the heparin half-life is prolonged. (Heparin is eliminated by renal excretion, and heparinase is produced by the liver.)

Needless to say, once uncontrollable bleeding problems are encountered, recruitment of the hematopathologist and/or the hematologist is essential, with immediate investigation into the possibilities of obtaining fresh whole blood.

Occasionally reexploration procedures are necessary when the patient exhibits signs of mechanical bleeding or when the available blood is extremely limited. Patients with rare blood types and those who through their religious beliefs

(Jehovah's Witnesses) refuse blood or blood derivatives cannot be treated with long waiting or procrastination when bleeding continues and must be returned to the operating room for mechanical hemostasis with use of the cell saver where feasible and if acceptable.

■ **What are the complications involved in transfusion of whole blood or blood components, and how are they treated?**

Hepatitis can occur from 3 to 20 weeks after the administration of blood, and the incidence increases with the number of units of blood transfused. Renal shutdown can occur any time from the initial transfusion until 7 days later. Allergic reactions with urticaria most often occur within hours after a transfusion, as do febrile reactions with chills and fever.

Those symptoms that can occur in the acute stages of transfusion reactions include chills, fever, urticaria, pruritus, tachycardia, chest pain, dyspnea, nausea and vomiting, back pain, hematuria, and icterus.

When a reaction is suspected, the transfusion should be immediately stopped, and all factors on the blood bag or bottle should be rerecorded and the following steps taken:

1. Return the unit of blood to the blood bank for re-cross matching and retyping with the patient's original clot and with a recently obtained sample.
2. Send a specimen of anticoagulated blood or determination of plasma hemoglobin.
3. Send a sample of urine for hemoglobin determination.
4. Institute therapy with chlorpheniramine maleate (Chlor-Trimeton) or diphenhydramine hydrochloride (Benadryl), and if the allergic reactions involve bronchospasm or signs of angina or ankle edema, the use of epinephrine compounds as well as aminophylline and possibly even hydrocortisone or dexamethasone may be necessary.

In cases where moderate hemolytic reaction is suspected as a result of moderate increase in the plasma and urine hemoglobin, the administration of an osmotic diuretic such as mannitol or the use of furosemide (Lasix) is indicated to prevent pigment deposition in the renal tubules

with possible anuria. Sodium bicarbonate can be given in acidotic reactions and aids in creating an alkaline urine in which hemoglobin precipitates less freely. Severe bleeding problems may ensue; these can be a manifestation of DIC. If renal shutdown is a reality, care must be instituted as discussed later in this chapter and in Chapter 24.

Low cardiac output syndrome and hypotension

In the immediate postoperative period the low cardiac output condition can develop; this is characterized by low arterial pressure with normally elevated CVP or atrial pressure, cool and possibly cyanotic skin and extremities, a narrowing pulse pressure with tachycardia, poor to nonobtainable peripheral pulses, changes in the sensorium, and suppression of urine formation. Thus a condition exists wherein the central pump mechanism (left ventricular action) for one reason or another is inadequate to maintain appropriate tissue perfusion and satisfy metabolic body requirements.

■ **What are the etiologies to be considered when the hypotension or low cardiac output syndromes occur?**

In all categories of cardiac surgery a mechanical problem such as cardiac tamponade must always be initially considered. In cases of repair of cardiac defects incomplete repair of that defect and/or residual aortic, subaortic, pulmonary valvular, or infundibular stenosis, or disruption of a surgical repair must also be considered.

When valves have been replaced, the possibility of breakdown and leakage around the prosthetic valve must be excluded, and consideration should be made regarding various types of obstruction to inflow and outflow associated with the replaced valves, such as simple clot obstruction of the valve, surgical mishaps (such as sutures impeding appropriate function of the disc or ball components), or placement of a valve cage that is too large for a small ventricle.

Possible additional causes are left atrial thrombosis, pulmonary embolization, pulmonary atelectasis, or severe pulmonary hypertension.

Multiple nonmechanical causes of low cardiac output exist and include the following:

1. Myocardial insult may result from anoxia

during the time of surgery such as aortic valve replacement or myocardial revascularization with long periods of cardiac arrest and inadequate coronary perfusion or cooling.

2. Low cardiac output may occur in cases wherein left or right ventriculotomies are performed with resultant repair or in which left ventricular vent tears occur and require extensive suture and pledget reconstruction or support.

3. Some patients who develop this syndrome are prone to myocardial insult; they are usually older or have had chronic strain on the myocardium from cardiac valvular disease, coronary artery obstructive disease with years of poor myocardial perfusion, or associated myocardiopathies of one type or another.

4. Various arrhythmias can produce low output; these include tachycardias, atrial fibrillation or flutter (which does not allow adequate atrial filling or emptying), bradycardia, and certain types of heart block.

5. Other causes include metabolic acidosis or occasionally even respiratory alkalosis, electrolyte imbalances with hyperkalemia, hypocalcemia, and arrhythmias associated with hypokalemia.

6. Numerous drugs can be associated with decreased myocardial contractility in the postoperative period; some of these have been previously mentioned, such as propranolol, large doses of barbiturates, large doses of morphine derivatives, and multiple antiarrhythmic agents.

■ What is the treatment for low cardiac output syndrome?

If the etiology of the syndrome is mechanical, return to surgery is necessary for appropriate repair of the mechanical defect (evacuation of clots in pericardial tamponade, completion of the repair for aortic or pulmonary stenosis, rerepair of any suture line disruptions, and possible additional valve replacement or repair).

In conditions where electrolyte depletion is suspected, calcium and potassium can be replaced as previously mentioned. In hyperkalemia diuretics, exchange resins (oral or rectal), or the other methods of lowering potassium can be used.

Respiratory alkalosis can simply be corrected with attention to proper respiratory mechanics; metabolic acidosis can be frequently corrected by the instillation of sodium bicarbonate by IV push or infusion of a 5% bicarbonate solution.

The treatment of the various arrhythmias has been described elsewhere in this text, but emphasis should be placed on the critical care practitioner's responsibility for understanding causes such as infarction anoxia, ischemia, or hypokalemia.

The use of certain inotropic agents after adequate hydration or volume replacement is the most common mode of therapy for this syndrome, and the drug frequently used is isoproterenol (Isuprel) titrated until the inotropic effect is evidenced. This drug works moderately well in patients appropriately hydrated and when the cardiac rate is below 70 beats/min. In hypovolemia its use can aggravate the hypotension, and when the heart is irritable or tachycardia persists, it can precipitate critical arrhythmias. Metaraminol (Aramine) can be used in a concentration of 100 to 300 mg in 500 ml of solution and titrated to the desired pressure; however, sustained use has been indicated as causing constrictive ischemia to the kidneys with irreversible renal damage. Phenylephrine (Neo-Synephrine) can be utilized intermittently as a direct IV bolus or in intermittent piggyback solutions; however, refractory reactions to this drug occur in a very short period of time. Other drugs used alone or in combination have been epinephrine, epinephrine and isoproterenol, isoproterenol and glucagon, and epinephrine and glucagon.

Combinations of the previously mentioned inotropic and vasoconstricting drugs with peripheral vasodilating drugs such as phenoxybenzamine (Dibenzyline) or chlorpromazine (Thorazine) have been described. I have seen marked reduction in the systolic blood pressure with very minimum amounts of these vasodilating drugs even in hypotensive states, and I use them with a maximum of caution.

As a last resort it may be necessary to rely on levarterenol (Levophed), which is a very potent vasoconstricting agent and is known to cause decreased peripheral perfusion and to predispose to renal failure, especially when used in high concentrations or for long periods of time. This drug also can be used in combination with one of the peripheral vasodilating agents, but I limit its use.

A now frequently used drug is dopamine hydrochloride (Intropin). This drug is a naturally occurring catecholamine precursor of norepinephrine that exerts an inotropic effect on the myocardium to effect an increased cardiac output. It is most commonly used by adding 5 ml or 200 mg to 250 or 500 ml of any one of the commonly used solutions (5% dextrose in water, 5% dextrose and 0.45N saline solution, and so forth). These dilutions yield a final concentration for administration of 800 μg/ml (200 mg in 250 ml dilution) or 400 μg/ml (200 mg in 500 ml). In most of my patients the increase in cardiac output has paralleled an increase in urine output and has occurred without the nuisance of tachycardia during short-term use. Recent articles have reported that long-term and increased dosage use where 50 μg/min is necessary for relatively long periods of time result in annoying tachycardia. Other reports have also been promising as to the combined usage of dopamine hydrochloride and isoproterenol, with smaller concentrations of each.

The use of steroids in massive doses (10,000 to 20,000 mg of hydrocortisone, 3000 mg of methylprednisone, and 300 to 400 mg of dexamethasone) has been reported in cases of low cardiac output syndrome, and during the past 13 years numerous articles have appeared regarding this technique. It is common to see the effects of peripheral vasodilatation (warm skin, improved color, and so forth), but often these effects are associated with a further drop (10 to 30 mm) in systemic pressure and usually without any significant major improvement in the patient's overall outcome. Most have since ceased the use of this regimen.

All sophisticated modes of monitoring and measuring are necessary at this time of low cardiac output and an extremely diligent search for the specific etiology of this life-endangering condition is continued. LAP, pulmonary, and wedge pressure measurements are invaluable at this time.

■ What are cardiac assistance devices and when are they used?

Certain devices have been developed to decrease cardiac work load and support mean aortic pressure. The use of these instruments is usually restricted to cases wherein all conventional measures have resulted in failure and the patient is otherwise destined to die.

The most commonly used apparatus today, the counterpulsation or diastolic augmentation device, consists of an intra-aortic balloon that is usually inserted through the femoral artery and then connected to a carbon dioxide (CO_2) or helium-filled inflating device. Once inserted and connected, the balloon is appropriately inflated during diastole and deflated during systole. This apparatus reportedly reduces the myocardial oxygen demand, decreases cardiac work, and increases coronary flow when it raises the diastolic aortic pressure during inflation. The balloon is usually passed through a Dacron graft connected to the femoral artery and positioned in the thoracic aorta just distal to the left subclavian artery. It can be placed preferably in surgery or when necessary in the unit.

■ Are there any problems associated with the use of the intra-aortic balloon?

The use of this apparatus usually requires heparin anticoagulation and/or use of dextran and carries the usual inherent complications of any anticoagulation and/or intravascular foreign body. Manipulation of the catheter beyond the aortoiliac junction is often very difficult, and loss of the lower extremity has occurred with difficult placement and long-term use. Difficult placement has required more extensive retroperitoneal dissection for common iliac or lower abdominal placement with bleeding and infection problems. If the balloon migrates or is malpositioned, it can occlude the major vessels to the arm or head with limb loss or death.

■ Can this apparatus be used at an earlier time rather than as a last resort?

Investigators have recently developed the means of earlier detection in cases that will require such support, and it is possible that the judicial use earlier will increase survival in these specific patients.

■ Are there any other support devices?

For very short-term intervals (3 to 10 hours) some of the partial cardiac bypass procedures can be used, but the continual need for heparin creates problems. Encouraging are the results of a left ventricular bypass apparatus devised by Wakabayashi and Connolly, which, because of simple construction and a nonthrombogenic polyurethane-polyvinyl graphite coating, requires no heparin and has been used as an assistance for as long as 8 days.

Pericardial tamponade

Increased collection of blood and/or clots in the pericardium with impedance of ventricular expansion and contraction, pressure compression of the atria, and tight constriction of the venae cavae impedes cardiac filling and output and produces the characteristic pericardial tamponade syndrome. The potential salvage of the patient depends on prompt recognition.

■ What are the factors leading to pericardial tamponade?

Any surgical intervention that has resulted in moderate bleeding without appropriate drainage or evacuation of blood and clots predisposes to tamponade. A typical condition is one in which moderate to massive bleeding has been occurring, with an acute cessation of the bleeding once the coagulopathy or bleeding problem has been controlled, resulting in rapid deterioration or development of low cardiac output.

The CVP continues to rise rapidly, the arterial systemic pressure drops with a noticeable decrease in the pulse pressure (pressure difference between the systolic and diastolic levels), cyanosis of the head and neck develops with evident venous distention of the neck and arm veins, and the patient is severely apprehensive and anxious. Auscultation of the heart reveals distant cardiac sounds, and paradoxical pulse is usually present.

Paradoxical pulse is described as an abnormal inspiratory fall in systolic blood pressure, a normal fall being 6 and 10 mm. A drop in the systolic blood pressure during inspiration of greater than 10 mm Hg is considered accentuated or paradoxical. It is detected by inflating a cuff pressure to a level greater than the expected systolic pressure, having the patient slightly accentuate the depth of respiration, and as the cuff pressure is slowly released, auscultating the blood pressure

on expiration and then on inspiration. The difference between expiration and the re-pickup during inspiration, if greater than 10 mm Hg, is considered paradoxical.

■ How is pericardial tamponade treated?

Giving an inotropic drug such as isoproterenol (Isuprel), epinephrine, or dopamine will frequently increase the systolic pressure without change in the CVP and is probably indicative of pericardial tamponade. However, if the findings just discussed regarding CVP and paradoxical pulse are found, there is need for a diagnostic two-directional echocardiogram, radioactive heart-lung scan, and/or pericardiocentesis. If positive, or even suggestive, the patient should be immediately returned to surgery for pericardial evacuation.

It is necessary in these cases to do as much as possible of the evacuation procedure under local anesthesia, as deep anesthesia before evacuation frequently produces more hypotension. The large-bore pericardiocentesis needle should be left in the pericardial space for continued evacuation during the preparation and initial surgical procedure to maintain decompression of the pericardial chamber. Once the pericardium is opened, there is usually an explosive evacuation of blood and clots with immediate improvement of the patient's cardiodynamic situation.

In three instances I have observed patients with some but not all of the indicative findings of pericardial tamponade, that is, without evidence of markedly elevated CVP and without extensive widening of the mediastinum but very labile CVP and mean arterial pressures. In these three cases the patients were returned to surgery, and localized clot obstruction of the left atrium was found. Immediately on evacuation of this large left atrium–compressing clot, there was dramatic improvement in the cardiac status. Others have reported similar instances of local chamber tamponade.

Cardiac arrhythmias

The arrhythmias occurring in the postoperative cardiac surgical patient are recognized by alarm tapes, reevaluated by replay systems, and generally diagnosed and treated similar to the arrhythmias occurring under other conditions; their diagnosis and specific care has been outlined in other chapters in this text. Today it is a constant effort for the family practitioner specializing in areas other than cardiology or internal medicine to keep up with the critical care staff with regard to knowledge of the interpretation, treatment, and consequences of the varying arrhythmias.

■ What arrhythmias occur in the postoperative cardiac surgical patient and how are they managed?

Sinus tachycardia is common in the immediate postoperative period and frequently is a response to hypovolemia, metabolic alterations, pain and apprehension, dehydration, myocardial irritability caused by anoxia, hypercapnia, or medications. It is most frequently treated by caring for the underlying causes: analgesia for pain, administration of adequate fluids for dehydration, decreasing or eliminating certain tachycardia-promoting drugs, appropriate respiratory control with arterial gas titration, and so forth. Occasionally sinus tachycardia requires digitalization, but before this is instituted digoxin levels are obtained to ensure that the tachycardia is not a sign of digitalis toxicity. In later postoperative periods if tachycardia persists, propranolol hydrochloride (Inderal) is often utilized but only in otherwise very stable patients.

Premature ventricular beats (PVB's) commonly occur at some phase in the postoperative period and should precipitate special attention, as they are frequently precursors of ventricular tachycardia and possibly ventricular fibrillation. Again, conditions such as anoxia, hypokalemia (especially when digitalis is being given), myocardial ischemia, and acid-base imbalances are frequently causative factors, but if PVB's continue once the suspected cause is corrected (such as administration of potassium in hypokalemia states) and occur more often than three to five times each minute, an IV bolus (25 to 100 mg) of lidocaine (Xylocaine) is given. At the same time a continuous lidocaine drip should be started and titrated to control the ectopic beats. Precaution is used to avoid lidocaine toxicity manifested by seizures and other CNS abnormalities and occasional suppression of myocardial contractility.

Patients with known preoperative ventricular ectopic beats can prophylactically be given 350 mg of procainamide (Pronestyl) orally every 4 hours at the time of admission and continued on this dosage by IV route postoperatively until oral medications can be reinstituted. The 350 mg is then given orally every 4 hours until it can be decreased to 500 mg every 6 hours.

Phenytoin (Dilantin) can be given by either IV or IM route in individuals sensitive to lidocaine and can be the drug of choice when the ectopic beats are associated with digitalis toxicity. Phenytoin is administered by the IV route in 100 mg increments for a total initial dose of 300 to 500 mg followed by 100 to 200 mg given by the IM or IV route every 6 hours for maintenance, with conversion to oral dosage when feasible.

Quinidine can be utilized in IM doses of 200 to 600 mg every 6 hours and 100 to 400 mg in slow titrated piggyback IV drips every 6 hours; however, there have been potential complications with the use of IV quinidine, and this drug is used only after exhaustion of other methods.

Propranolol (Inderal) has been more frequently recommended for control of both atrial and ventricular ectopic beats, but because of its hypotensive potentials, it use is usually limited to the more stable postoperative patient.

Atrial and occasionally ventricular pacing can be utilized to override ectopic beats by suppression if pacing wires were left in place at the time of surgery. This occasionally requires rates well over 100 beats/min, and the taxation of the myocardium must be considered.

Ventricular tachycardia is a frequent precursor of ventricular fibrillation and is treated in a manner similar to PVB's; however, when nonrelenting ventricular tachycardia persists, electrical conversion (cardioversion) is indicated.

Ventricular fibrillation, unless converted immediately or assisted by cardiopulmonary compression and ventilation, is associated with imminent death. The early treatment of the often preceding PVB's or ventricular tachycardia is hopefully a preventive measure against the development of ventricular fibrillation, but once it occurs, appropriate measures are instituted and when conversion is completed, preventive measures are reinstituted.

Supraventricular arrhythmias, such as atrial fibrillation and flutter, can be associated with very rapid ventricular response and are associated with poor atrial contractions, with ventricular filling and cardiac output often decreased. If the patient has not previously been treated with digitalis, this is the treatment of choice, but if conversion is unsuccessful in the face of adequate digitalization, electrical conversion may be indicated. When this arrhythmia develops in surgery with the heart exposed, electrical conversion is attempted at that time. Cardioversion requires relatively low voltage and can frequently be accomplished on the ward or in the emergency room with use of IV diazepam (Valium). The treatment of atrial flutter when associated with low cardiac output is similar to that of atrial fibrillation. Propranolol is occasionally used when vital signs are stable, but before using this drug surgeons usually prefer arrhythmia control to be fully in the hands of the cardiologist.

Paroxysmal atrial tachycardia (PAT), when diagnosed, is first treated with attempts at carotid sinus massage, eyeball pressure, and various Valsalva maneuvers. When not associated with heart block and in a nondigitalized patient, refractory PAT's are treated with rapid digitalization. If the PAT is associated with block and potassium depletion is present, potassium should be replaced; if still refractory, phenytoin (Dilantin) therapy should be instituted.

Premature atrial contractions (PAC's) are not uncommon in postoperative patients and are more frequent in association with valvular surgery; if not treated, atrial fibrillation or flutter will often develop. Recommended treatment is IM or oral (if the patient is able) quinidine, with 200 mg (300 mg orally) given every 6 hours.

Atrioventricular (AV) dissociation may be noted at the time of surgery in the repair of ostium primum, endocardial cushion, or ventricular septal defects. It can also occur during aortic and tricuspid valve replacement. If the block occurs at the time of surgery, it is more likely that permanent pacemaking modes will be required postoperatively. Temporary or permanent pacemaker wires can be inserted at surgery. AV dissociation and heart block not infrequently occur following mitral valve surgery. However, this is usually temporary and may be associated with digitalis toxicity and hypokalemia and may respond to potassium replacement and cessation of digitalis administration. Slow nodal rhythms (45 to 60 beats/min) may be managed by use of isoproterenol, atropine, or if temporary pacemaker wires are in place, atrial or ventricular pacing.

Cardiac arrest

The treatment of true cardiopulmonary arrest or ventricular fibrillation with apnea is a topic that could require volumes for complete discussion. However, certain basics will be mentioned. A marked contribution to the increased survival rate in cardiac surgical patients has resulted from prompt recognition of ventricular fibrillation and other life-endangering arrhythmias with appropriate conversion. The rapid institution of cardiopulmonary resuscitation in those individuals refractory to defibrillatory measures has also contributed to salvage rates. *All* practitioners, regardless of their specific areas of specialty, should be capable of appropriate cardiopulmonary resuscitation as a single rescuer or as a member of a full resuscitation team. The reader is referred to the American Heart Association reference material related to proper cardiopulmonary resuscitation techniques.

■ **What are some of the basic considerations with respect to cardiopulmonary resuscitation?**

The recognition of cardiac arrest is more easily expedited in the critical care unit where the patient is still connected to the monitoring and signaling devices. If the recognized condition is ventricular fibrillation, often simple defibrillation is adequate to restore appropriate cardiac function; however, if the heart is refractory to defibrillation, immediate cardiac compression and ventilation are instituted. Initially the patient should be ventilated, after clearing the airway, with 3 to 5 full breaths, cardiac compression should be instituted until a solid object can be placed under the chest, and the resuscitation team should be summoned. If the patient was not previously utilizing endotracheal or tracheal respiratory assistance, mouth-to-mouth or manual bag ventilation should be used with the appropriate airways until all the necessary equipment for endotracheal intubation, including an individual capable of performing the intubation, are present. A frequent mistake made by inexperienced personnel is to use critical resuscitation time in attempting intubation when the patient can be appropriately ventilated with a manual breathing bag and airway. Infusion lines are established as resuscitation is in progress.

All medications and equipment necessary for cardiopulmonary resuscitation and the potential minor complications that can occur should be present on the emergency cart. In addition to the usual items, this should include cutdown trays, large needles in case a tension pneumothorax must be decompressed, rib spreaders, material for simple tube thoracostomy, tracheostomy tray, suction apparatus, equipment for CVP line placement, materials for an arterial line, and monitoring equipment. The more commonly used medications such as epinephrine, sodium bicarbonate, lidocaine, calcium chloride, digitalis preparations, isoproterenol (Isuprel), metaraminol (Aramine), levarterenol (Levophed), phenytoin (Dilantin), morphine sulfate, and succinylcholine (Anectine) should be close at hand, preferably in prefilled syringes.

Extension of the neck to ensure a patent airway, 1½- to 2-inch compression of the sternum 60 to 80 times a minute, interposed with ventilation between the fifth and sixth compression, continual evaluation of the femoral and/or carotid pulses to check the effect of compression, blood gas measurements, and sodium bicarbonate administration should be carried out simultaneously.

When cardiac standstill is evident, intracardiac injection of 5 to 10 ml of a 1:10,000 concentration of epinephrine may be performed rapidly, with reinstitution of cardiac compression. If ventricular fibrillation occurs, defibrillation is utilized, and if unsuccessful and accompanied by a weak fibrillation pattern, 500 to 1000 mg of intracardiac calcium chloride (5 to 10 ml of a 10% solution) is given. These techniques are repeated until adequate cardiac output is established. Defibrillation is accomplished using 100 to 400 watt-seconds, usually starting at the lower levels. Electrode paste should be used to prevent burning and to ensure adequate contact. If the blood pressure is established but is too low for adequate perfusion, the various modes previously described for low cardiac output syndrome are instituted. Chest x-ray films should be obtained periodically to rule out pneumothorax resulting from intracardiac injections and forceful ventilation and to pursue evidence of possible aspiration or a misplaced endotracheal tube.

If external cardiac compression is unsuccessful as determined by the arterial monitor or lack of palpable carotid and femoral pulses, an incision is made in the fourth or fifth left intercostal space (if the previous operative incision is not as accommodating), and open cardiac massage is employed. If the pericardium for some reason has not previously been violated, it should be opened at a point located anterior to the phrenic nerve. A chest tray prepared for minor surgery with rib spreaders should be on the emergency cart or readily available. Open massage procedures are most often necessary in emphysema patients, patients with immobile chests, and when the pericardium has been widely opened for the cardiac surgery.

Once adequate circulation is restablished, it is necessary that a complete reevaluation be carried out; all laboratory studies—electrolyte evaluation, blood gas determination, digoxin level, hemoglobin concentration, hematocrit, ECG, chest x-ray films cardiac enzymes and isoenzymes—should be reevaluated. All appropriate measures should be taken to avoid recurrence of the cardiac arrest.

It is recommended that the use of analgesics and muscle relaxants be discontinued in the operating room so that the patient will be relatively alert on arrival in the unit. Sedation can be instituted once the status of the CNS is known.

Peripherovascular complications

Because of the usual generalized atherosclerosis in a large number of adult cardiac and especially coronary surgery patients, peripheral arterial occlusions in perfused and even nonperfused vessels can occur with relative frequency.

■ What are the signs and symptoms indicative of peripheral vessel obstruction?

Coldness, pallor, blotchy discoloration, loss of pulses with delayed venous and capillary refilling, and paresthesias and pain during activity or rest of an extremity are indicative of acute arterial obstruction. Evidence of these signs in one extremity and not in any others is even more conclusive of local arterial obstruction.

If signs of arterial obstruction appear in both lower extremities, this may indicate embolic or thrombotic blockage of the aortoiliac bifurcation or even a distal aortic dissection. Once this diagnosis is highly suspected or established, immediate surgical intervention is necessary, as the prognosis is frequently related to the efficacy and speed with which successful surgical intervention and correction are employed.

Occasionally a severely ischemic and swollen leg is indicative of the anterior tibial compartment syndrome resulting from anoxia and edema after femoral artery perfusion; this requires femoral artery embolectomy, reconstruction, or even multiple compartment fasciotomies for complete restoration of circulation and prevention of limb loss.

■ What venous problems can occur during the postoperative phase?

Phlebothrombosis or thrombophlebitis of the lower extremities is the most common venous complication occurring in the postoperative cardiac patient. It is usually well treated prophylactically with adequate hydration in the preoperative, operative, and postoperative phases, compressive wraps or antiembolic stockings placed in the operating room or on arrival in the intensive care unit, and the adequate use of a footboard for continual foot and leg activity. Frequent removal and reapplication of thromboembolic stockings or wraps periodically or as necessary combined with appropriate progressive activities and mobilization have previously been described. Phlebothrombosis and thrombophlebitis can occur in the upper extremities as a result of the use of irritating IV medications, and I have encountered three instances of total occlusion of the subclavian-axillary venous drainage of the upper extremity with typical phlegmasia cerulea dolens (severe purplish edematous and painful extremity) that required immediate surgical intervention and evacuation of clots by Fogarty catheter thromboembolectomy and irrigation with heparinized saline solution.

In cases of phlebothrombosis or thrombophlebitis of the lower extremities surgery is almost never indicated (unless phlegmasia cerulea dolens occurs), and as soon as it is safe, heparin therapy and/or low molecular weight dextran administration is started. Phenylbutazone (Butazolidin) is useful as an adjunctive drug in thrombophlebitis, but when used in combination with dextran or other anticoagulant-like drugs, bleeding complications can occur. Other side effects possible with this drug prevent its usage by many practitioners. If there are contraindications to the utilization of heparin and the patient has exhibited pulmonary emboli, if pulmonary emboli have occurred while the patient has been undergoing anticoagulation therapy, or if there is evidence of septic pulmonary embolization, surgical interruption of the inferior vena cava is imperative.

Pulmonary embolization

As in all postoperative cases, the threat of fatal or near fatal pulmonary embolization is always present and thus requires a high index of suspicion and acuity on the part of the critical care practitioner.

■ How is pulmonary embolization in the immediate postoperative period recognized?

In the responsive or conscious patient the rapid development of dyspnea associated with cyanosis, pleuritic-type chest pain, tachycardia, initial onset of mild hypotension followed by normal or elevated blood pressure, signs and symptoms of bronchospasm, hemoptysis, apprehension, and hypoxia (evidenced by arterial blood concentrations) either alone or in combination is highly indicative of pulmonary emboli. Later findings include signs of pulmonary hypertension as manifested by findings on auscultation, x-ray films, and ECG or in combination with pleural friction rub, x-ray evidence of peripheral infiltrates, or hypovascularity with or without pleural effusion.

■ How are pulmonary emboli treated?

If the diagnosis is fully established and it is safe to do so, heparin anticoagulation is instituted. Heparin is the only drug of choice for the first 7 to 10 days, and its administration by IV route is preferred. The therapeutic anticoagulation levels are evaluated by either activated clotting time, partial thromboplastin time, or Lee-White bleeding and clotting time studies.

As previously mentioned, surgical intervention is recommended only in cases where recurrent embolization occurs under anticoagulation, when anticoagulation is contraindicated, or if septic embolization is suspected. Pulmonary embolectomy is seldom indicated and reserved only for those patients exhibiting a course of continual deterioration despite nonsurgical treatment. Although this patient presents a poor surgical risk, utilization of the partial bypass instituted prior to diagnostic pulmonary arteriography and preceding anesthesia induction for removal of the pulmonary embolus increases the potential of survival.

PULMONARY COMPLICATIONS

Strict attention to preoperative, operative, and postoperative pulmonary care provides the greatest means for decreasing the increased respiratory morbidity and/or mortality seen among cardiac surgery patients in the postoperative period.

■ What prophylactic measures are taken to decrease pulmonary complications?

Depending on the history and physical examinations, inclusive of chest x-ray films and baseline pulmonary function, a patient may appropriately be assessed preoperatively as to total pulmonary function, including arterial gas concentrations. If there is any question of emphysema, bronchitis, asthma, bronchiectasis, airway obstruction, or pulmonary insufficiency with chronic or potential infection, the patient is preoperatively treated with an intensive prophylactic and therapeutic regimen, as previously mentioned.

These therapeutic modalities utilized preoperatively include preoperative education with respiratory assistance devices (intermittent positive pressure breathing and incentive spirometry), adequate utilization of mucolytic agents, humidification and bronchodilators as indicated, the use of postural and/or percussive postural drainage, and in cases where there is the suspicion of preoperative infection, appropriate therapy with antibiotics.

As previously mentioned, preoperative sputum cultures are obtained regardless of the history or findings so that appropriate therapy can be instituted in the immediate postoperative period if signs of pulmonary infection are present.

Abstinence from smoking and/or isolation from smoke-filled rooms at least in the immediate preoperative period (hopefully for weeks or months preoperatively) is urged.

The education of the patient is appropriate and productive postoperative deep breathing and coughing exercises are stressed.

■ What important measures are utilized during surgery to prevent postoperative pulmonary complications?

During pump perfusion and especially during long pump runs proteins are probably denatured and the physiologic characteristics of surfactant are altered, therefore making the cardiopulmonary bypass patient prone to atelectasis. When surfactant is altered or decreased, any partial or total collapse of the lung or alveoli can be associated with troublesome postoperative atelectasis. It is standard policy to apply varying intermittent pressures of inflation before, during, and after perfusion.

Antibiotics are added to the pump or given intravenously, and although their primary purpose is to prevent any mediastinal or cardiac infection from the skin or other sources, this probably adds prophylaxis to pulmonary infection.

In cases with extenuating circumstances that require longer than usual pump runs, excessive transfusion of blood, and maintenance of somewhat lower than optimum mean pressures on the pump, additional precautionary measures are taken, including the use of microfilters for blood (to prevent platelet aggregate pulmonary emboli) and the occasional use of IV or pump steroids to hopefully prevent perfusion ("pump") lung.

Every precaution should be taken to prevent regurgitation and aspiration of gastric contents. The high acid content of the gastric secretions, when brought in contact with the pulmonary mucosa, can predispose to overwhelming and diffuse aspiration pneumonia. If at any time during the operative or postoperative period aspiration is suspected, bronchoscopy and bronchial irrigation using a sodium bicarbonate and steroid solution is employed along with the administration of systemic corticosteroids and antibiotics. Today this complication occurs rarely because of the adequate use of nasogastric suctioning, appropriate inflations of the endotracheal tube cuffs, and decrease in overenthusiastic tendencies to feed or give the patient oral intake before the gastrointestinal tract has returned to normal function.

■ What specific complications can occur in the postoperative period and how are they prevented?

Atelectasis is a patchy, segmental lobar or total airless collapse of a lung, usually as a result of proximal bronchial obstruction from retained thick secretions, obstructing tubes, or aspirated material. It is usually accompanied by temperature elevations from 100° to 104° F, increases in pulse and respiratory rates, and evidence of AV shunting by the arterial gases, and it is confirmed by decreased breath sounds and excursions on the involved side and x-ray evidence of increased densities.

When major atelectasis occurs, mediastinal shift toward the affected side and frequently elevation of the diaphragm are evident on the chest x-ray film. Atelectasis appears to be one of the most common postoperative complications; by strict interpretation of the x-ray films, this appears in some form in at least 30% of the postoperative cases in which the pump was used. Frequently the only sign is visualization on the x-ray film of minimum infiltration or discoid atelectasis in the basilar segments. This is probably associated with the decreased surfactant, vascular congestion, and decreased ventilation of these areas during bypass.

The recommended therapy for this minimum or more involved atelectasis is frequent tracheobronchial suction, administration of adequate volume for ventilation, frequent use of the sigh mechanisms on the respirator, and when possible, constant positive end-expiratory pressure (PEEP) to maintain inflation of all areas and segments of the lung. Stimulation of deep breathing and coughing (using pillow supports over the incision for splinting) and appropriate use of humidification, mucolytic agents, and if not contra-

indicated, bronchodilators are also necessary adjuncts to both the treatment and the prevention of atelectasis.

Adequate use of pain medication prior to suctioning, pulmonary therapy, and coughing exercises enables the patient to obtain full respiratory excursions and produce better coughs. Postoperative complications are decreased with the use of the midsternotomy incision in contrast to the other chest incisions, because its solid bone-to-bond closure produces less pain in the postoperative period and use of this incision usually avoids entering either thoracic cavity. One of the most painful of all chest incisions is the posterolateral approach, with the anterolateral, the anterior inframammary, and the parasternal mediastinal incisions being progressively less painful.

Pneumothorax occurs in a small percentage of cases where pleural violation was not suspected and is usually recognized on the routine postoperative chest x-ray films. When first noticed, repeat x-ray films are obtained to ensure against progression, and if significant increase is present, immediate tube thoracostomy with underwater seal drainage is essential. Evaluation of chest excursion and auscultation combined with percussion lead to early recognition of this entity. Whenever ventilatory problems occur without other positive findings, pneumothorax should be suspected. A high index of suspicion should be maintained after any intracardiac injections following cardiopulmonary resuscitation procedures.

Pleural effusion associated with blood or serous accumulation in one chest cavity or the other occurs to some degree in a fair percentage of patients. If respiratory embarrassment develops with abnormal arterial blood gas concentrations or if the fluid increases, therapeutic aspiration and/or tube thoracostomy should be instituted.

Bronchial aspiration occurs infrequently today, but if moderate aspiration is visualized, it is recommended that the endotracheal tube be irrigated, while the patient is frequently turned, with a combination of saline solution, bicarbonate solution, and steroids. The mixture should contain sodium bicarbonate in a concentration of 2.3% to 2.5%. If irrigation is inadequate, bronchoscopy with therapeutic aspiration and irrigation with similar solution is indicated, followed by the use of steroids. The incidence of this complication can be lessened by the judicious use of the nasogastric tube and avoidance of the overzealous use of ice chips and other oral intake before gastrointestinal tract activity is established.

Inadequate ventilation is identified by visual and auscultation evaluation combined with frequent blood gas assessment. Causes of inadequate ventilation include inappropriately low volumes, decreased oxygen concentrations, lack of adequate humidification, poor use of end-expiratory pressures, improper placement of the endotracheal tube, and all previously mentioned factors such as atelectasis, pneumothorax, hemothorax, and hydrothorax, as well as endotracheal and airway resistance associated with a too-small tube or nonaspirated secretions. In patients whose ventilatory studies are not adequate after the third or fourth day using endotracheal intubation, a tracheostomy should be instituted for better toileting and prevention of ventilatory cuff and endotracheal tube problems.

Infection can also occur as the result of inadequate ventilation, inappropriate suctioning, and general inability to eliminate pulmonary secretions, as well as from aspiration and atelectasis occurring after using the pump. Once infection occurs, a very enthusiastic regimen must be employed, including sputum cultures and sensitivity tests, more vigorous pulmonary modalities, and appropriate antibiotic therapy. I have found a somewhat increased incidence of infection resulting from many of the gram-negative organisms, especially *Serratia marcescens,* after the prophylactic use of cephalosporins. Certain otherwise nonpathogenic bacteria can become opportunists when prophylactic antibiotics are used. When pulmonary infection occurs in a patient taking more than adequate doses of antibiotics, gentamicin sulfate and/or carbenicillin are frequently added to the antibiotic regimen. When marked atelectasis occurs on either the left or right side as a result of retained secretions and does not clear within a 6- to 8-hour period or respiratory efficiency is decreased, bronchoscopy with therapeutic aspiration and irrigation is rapidly instituted to prevent progressive pulmonary infection and/or abscess.

Perfusion ("pump") lung is a condition exhibited by progressive patchy atelectasis and worsening hypoxia and in late stages is associated with hypercapnia, acidosis, and severe hypoxemia. The characteristics of this entity closely parallel those of posttraumatic pulmonary insufficiency, and unless reversal is enacted in the early phases, death frequently ensues. It is often mandatory to treat this condition with continuous ventilatory support utilizing the mode of PEEP, corticosteroids, and all the previously mentioned pulmonary modalities.

RENAL COMPLICATIONS

Postoperative acute renal failure is a dreaded complication and is not infrequently encountered following cardiopulmonary bypass. The precipitating factors seem to be preexisting chronic renal disease or continual insult associated with the cardiac condition requiring surgery. This, in addition to possible decreased perfusion of the kidneys during bypass or associated hypotensive episodes or physiologic renal vasoconstriction from drugs, can precipitate the condition. The accumulation of serum and urine hemoglobin after moderate red blood cell destruction during bypass procedures in association with the previously mentioned factors predisposes to the development of renal failure. The shifting of body fluids with functional dehydration has also been suggested as a definite precursor to renal failure in bypass patients.

■ **What modes of therapy can be utilized in the prophylactic treatment of acute renal failure?**

When possible, maintenance of adequate hydration in the preoperative, operative, and postoperative periods with balanced electrolyte solutions is recommended. The hydration levels can be monitored by the amount of urinary output, the CVP, and the atrial pressure in the immediate postoperative period.

The use of high perfusion rates and flows during bypass with use of an osmotic diuretic such as mannitol is prophylactic, especially in cases where plasma and urine hemoglobin levels are elevated.

Preoperative microscopic evaluation of the

urine for casts and inflammatory cells with cultures and sensitivity tests for infections followed by appropriate urologic consultation when abnormal can help prevent the acute renal problem.

■ **What factors or signs suggest the development of acute renal failure?**

When urinary output is low in the postoperative period (below 20 ml/hr), it usually is a reflection of low cardiac output or dehydration, but it can be an early indication of renal failure. However, occasionally relatively static or high flows of urine can be present but with fixed low specific gravities; this can also be a manifestation of early renal failure.

The progressive elevation of the blood urea nitrogen (BUN) and serum creatinine and the continued decrease in urinary output despite adequate hydration with elevation in serum potassium levels and microscopic urinary pigments usually confirm the suspected diagnosis.

■ **What findings differentiate between renal failure, low cardiac output, and dehydration as the cause of decreased urine output?**

The rapid influx of 500 to 1000 ml of fluid (in a patient whose cardiodynamics can tolerate this) over a 2- to 3-hour period will usually establish whether or not a patient is dehydrated. If the urinary output increases with this measure, the patient is probably dehydrated or hypovolemic.

If overall cardiac output appears low and hypotension is present, the use of one of the inotropic agents that does not cause peripheral constriction in the renal capillary beds will usually elevate the blood pressure, and if urinary output increases, the decreased urinary flow was probably associated with low cardiac output.

When the preceding two measures fail along with increased doses of diuretics (in refractory cases doses as high as 200 mg of furosemide [Lasix] have been used in bolus form), the assumption of acute renal failure is probably confirmed.

■ **How is acute renal failure managed?**

When the diagnosis is highly likely and no response to the previously described measures has occurred, a nephrologist joins the team, takes over the management of fluids, and manages dosages of drugs excreted by or toxic to the kidney.

When the potassium and BUN levels cannot adequately be controlled by restriction of potassium and protein intake, exchange resins (administered through the rectum or nasogastric tube) are necessary, and if these are ineffective, peritoneal dialysis and/or preparation for hemodialysis can be instituted. Once a firm diagnosis of renal failure is established, the institution of each hemodialysis appears to result in a higher percentage of return of renal function.

It has been recommended by some that any urine volume below 30 ml/hr signals danger of impending renal failure. It is thought that a particularly useful test of impending tubular necrosis is a measurement of the urine-to-plasma ratio with regard to urea nitrogen. When the ratio is 10 or below, it is indicative of renal failure; however, when the ratio is 30 or above the patient is most likely suffering from dehydration alone. In the range between 10 and 30 the situation is considered to be impending or possibly incipient but still potentially reversible tubular necrosis.

With most individuals once the diagnosis of renal tubular damage has been ascertained, every effort should be made to restrict the intake of water, sodium chloride, and particularly potassium. Since patients subjected to open-heart surgery will not have a prolonged period of intestinal ileus, they will be taking oral fluids relatively soon, and excessive loading with fluids and potassium is possible. In renal failure any tendency for the serum sodium level to fall is usually indicative of excessive fluid intake.

POSTOPERATIVE FEVER AND INFECTION

Preoperative precautions such as antibacterial showers, clean linen, pulmonary prophylaxis, and preoperative antibiotic administration as well as intensive protective measures in the postoperative period have made major problems with infection relatively rare in the cardiac surgical patient.

■ **What are common causes for temperature elevations seen during the postoperative period?**

Fevers occurring in the first 24 to 48 hours postoperatively are usually associated with varying degrees of atelectasis and retained pulmonary secretions, as in most postoperative surgical patients. These temperatures are usually under 102° F orally and respond most often to continuation of the antibiotics, vigorous suctioning, deep breathing, coughing and other pulmonary modalities, and the simple administration of rectal acetaminophen (Tylenol) or salicylates. When the rectal temperatures persist at 101° to 102° F, simple cooling measures or use of a cooling blanket are helpful. Some of the temperature elevations immediately following use of the pump are also probably associated with increased red blood cell destruction, fluid shifts, and so forth.

Total refractoriness of fever to all therapeutic modes suggests CNS involvement, possibly from poor cerebral perfusion or embolic phenomenon.

High fevers occurring between the third and fifth days may indicate pulmonary infection as a result of nonresolved atelectasis, or possible urinary infection or septicemia. Any fevers that develop late or are refractory to active therapeutic regimens are evaluated with cultures of the wounds, sputum, blood, and urine. If the temperature elevations persist, antibiotics are withheld for 12 to 24 hours while blood cultures are reobtained, preferably during periods of temperature spikes.

Fevers that occur between the seventh and tenth days are more indicative of fluid accumulations or cavity infections, and careful scrutiny of all wound areas will not infrequently reveal serum or infected accumulations. Another cause, although rare, is pulmonary embolic phenomenon and is usually associated with dyspnea, slight tachycardia, mild hypertension, and pleural or pericardial friction rubs.

High fever on the seventh to tenth postoperative days can also indicate endocarditis and/or infection of a prosthetic graft or valve. When this is suspected, both venous and arterial blood samples are submitted for culture and sensitivity. Occasionally arterial blood samples have been responsible for establishing the diagnosis of mycotic infections of prosthetic valves.

It is relatively common to have low-grade temperature elevations persist despite antibiotics and appropriate hydration and in the face of normal white blood cell counts and sedimentation rates. On the recommendation of the cardiologist or epidemiologist all antibiotics and most nonessential drugs are often withheld, with frequent return of the temperature to normal.

Fever during the second postoperative week associated with pleuritic pain, pericardial friction rub, ECG evidence of pericarditis, and occasionally high lymphocyte and eosinophil counts may constitute a form of postcardiotomy syndrome that is treated initially with salicylates and/or acetaminophen (Tylenol) and occasionally with steroid medication (10 mg of prednisone four times a day for a period of 3 days), frequently with dramatic response.

The fever of bacterial endocarditis is often associated with chills and moderate to marked elevation of the white blood cell count and sedimentation rate. The signs and symptoms usually occur anywhere from the first week to multiple months after the surgical procedure. (More delayed onset of signs and symptoms is not uncommon in fungal endocarditis.) Dyspnea, peripheral embolic phenomenon (with peripheral petechiae or Quincke's pulse), splenomegaly, and/or the development of new murmurs are all significant signs in bacterial endocarditis.

Low grade fever (99° to 100.6° F) can occur from the first to the fourteenth postoperative day in patients with viral infections who not uncommonly are found to have normal white blood counts and even negative cold agglutinin titers. The possible explanation of the normal white blood counts and negative cold agglutinin titers could be explained by the amount of steroids used during bypass surgery.

Again, it is emphasized that the incidence of incisional, pulmonary, and sternal infections has been almost nil with diligent preoperative, postoperative, and operative precautions and with the use of antibiotics in *all* these phases.

GASTROINTESTINAL COMPLICATIONS

Complications of the gastrointestinal tract are usually quite rare and are kept to a minimum because of certain basic standards of care.

■ How are gastrointestinal complications prevented?

Whenever there is evidence by physical examination or on the postoperative chest x-ray films of gastric distention, nasogastric tubes are placed for decompression of the stomach.

Severe gastrointestinal distention with torsion and acute peptic ulceration with perforation are not unknown in the immediate postoperative period.

Liquids and ice chips are withheld until gastrointestinal activity is evident. Since sucking of ice chips is accompanied by moderate amounts of swallowed air for such a small fluid yield, I believe it is imperative that the patient be given nothing orally for a maximum of 12 and often 24 hours in the immediate postoperative period.

Individuals who have experienced problems with gastric hypersecretion, duodenal ulcer, peptic esophagitis, or acid indigestion will agree that coffee, tea, apple juice, and salty bouillons create epigastric distress and appear to produce moderate hyperacidity and distress. Therefore once bowel sounds are heard and abdominal distention is not present, a bland palatable diet is instituted. Once this is tolerated for 12 to 24 hours, the patient is allowed a more select or therapeutic diet (diabetic, low salt, and so forth). In no case in the immediate postoperative period is coffee, hot spicy soup, or bouillon allowed because of gastric acid secretion and fear of bronchial aspiration.

Gastrointestinal bleeding, particularly in patients with peptic esophagitis and duodenal ulcer, is not uncommon and is diagnosed in a manner similar to a routine workup.

INVOLVEMENT OF THE CENTRAL NERVOUS SYSTEM

Postoperative minor or major psychotic reactions, focal neurologic deficit, or total flaccid paralysis and coma can all occur during the postoperative phase.

■ **What frequent abnormalities of the CNS are manifested postoperatively and what is the cause and treatment?**

Major and minor personality disorders are not infrequently seen in postoperative patients. Occasionally specific causes are evident, such as a history of chronic alcoholic intake or preoperative personality problems treated with tranquilizing medications. However, frequently there is no history or specific etiology to explain postoperative signs and symptoms of paranoia, agitation, intermittent lack of coherence, disorientation, memory lapses, hallucinatory episodes, or bizarre motor actions during rest. The combination of the stress of the surgery, some degree of atherosclerotic cerebrovascular insufficiency, constant deprivation of sleep, some conscious or subconscious recollection of actual portions of the surgery, or possibly embolization of small amounts of air or other minute particulate matter during the pump run are all possible contributing factors.

These conditions usually require a magnitude of reassurance for the patient, relatives, and practitioners. Ignoring or antagonizing the irrational, confused patient usually only intensifies the problem. Appropriate sedation and establishment of sleep for the patient appears to be the single most important therapy, and this is frequently accomplished by withholding all activities if possible from midnight until 5 or 6 AM (with a respectively quiet unit during those hours) and utilization of a mild tranquilizing medication such as diazepam (Valium). In uncontrollable patients or those with a history of chronic ethanolism, chlorpromazine (Thorazine), chlordiazepoxide (Librium), or in dire necessities, IV alcohol is used. The majority of the confusion and bizarre activity episodes usually subside within 72 to 96 hours, but this period seems like weeks and months to the family and professional staff. With recovery, the patient can usually recall the episode in a very hazy postnightmarish manner, and this recall is often present for months or years.

■ **What are the less common but more serious CNS abnormalities that can occur?**

Total lack of consciousness without response to pain or other stimuli can occur in the immediate postoperative period from cerebral edema, continual embolization of air during the pump run, massive intracerebral embolization of clot or debris, or even intracerebral hemorrhage.

Generalized stupor and lack of response with focal signs are more often associated with small embolic phenomenon but nevertheless can herald postoperative neurologic defects or even death.

Progressive lightening of the coma with improvement is an encouraging sign, and when it occurs within the first 24 to 48 hours, carries a prognosis of minimum residual sequelae.

If no major response is obtained in the first 3 to 4 hours and there is no evidence to support analgesic dosage as the cause, neurologic consultation is obtained and a postoperative EEG and/or CT scan is immediately ordered and compared with the preoperative study. Caloric tests of the eardrums and evaluation for doll's eyes are performed by the neurologist or neurosurgeon. If there is any question of brain damage, methods to decrease cerebral edema are instituted. Corticosteroids given three or four times a day are administered over a 3- to 4-day period, the head and torso are maintained at approximately 30 degrees of elevation to decrease cerebral edema, overhydration is avoided with administration of adequately balanced salt solutions, and the judicial use of diuretics is instituted. Osmotic diuretics, such as mannitol and urea compounds (Urevert) are used less frequently today because of the associated rebound edema phenomena that can complicate recovery.

During this phase of CNS insult it is imperative that appropriate ventilation with normal or high concentrations of oxygen be maintained with normal or minimally elevated partial pressures of carbon dioxide.

Additional treatment includes hypothermia to decrease the metabolic needs of the CNS, phenytoin (Dilantin), or diazepam (Valium) to control seizures or convulsions, and when the suspected etiology is embolizing clot, utilization of heparin anticoagulation, when safe.

In cases where the specific etiology of the strokelike symptoms is not established, selective carotid arteriograms may be required. However, most symptomatic carotid artery stenosis or ulcerations have been discovered and evaluated preoperatively by auscultation and/or arteriography and surgically corrected before any cardiac surgical procedure is performed.

Occasionally patients will demonstrate delayed effects from analgesics and/or muscle relaxants used during surgery. These patients will frequently appear alert enough to be extubated, giving the surgeon a false sense of security. Then, as the patient is ready to leave the operating room or recovery facility, he will develop shallow respirations, become hypercapnic, and require emergency assisted ventilation and reintubation.

OTHER COMPLICATIONS
■ What other complications can occur in the postoperative cardiac surgical patient?

Fluid and electrolyte imbalances not infrequently occur; however, the administration of and reasons for appropriate electrolyte therapy have previously been described (Chapter 19).

Myocardial ischemia, infarction, or congestive failure can occur in these coronary occlusion–prone patients, but the management of these conditions is similar to that of any patient with these diagnoses. It is essential that these complications be recognized promptly so that the patient does not leave the unit or hospital with an existing infarction, impending arrhythmia, or congestive heart failure.

Psychologic dependency occurs in a fair number of cardiac surgical patients as a result of their having been in an atmosphere offering continuous expert attention. When transferred after 3 or 4 days to telemetry on the ward, it is important that the patient be assured that this transfer is an indication of excellent postoperative recovery.

BIBLIOGRAPHY FOR CHAPTERS 17-20

Adams, P. X., et al.: Clinical experience using potassium-induced cardioplegia with hypothermia in aortic valve replacement, J. Thorac. Cardiovasc. Surg. **75:**564, 1978.

Alexander, J. W.: Nosocomial infections, Curr. Probl. Surg. Aug., 1973.

Alpert, J. S., and Francis, G. S.: Manual of coronary care, Boston, 1977, Little, Brown & Co.

Aspinall, M. J.: Nursing the open heart surgery patient, New York, 1973, McGraw-Hill Book Co.

Austen, W. B., and Mundth, E. D.: Postoperative intensive care in the cardiac surgical patient, Prog. Cardiovasc. Dis. **11:**229, 1968.

Bachmann, F.: Disseminated intravascular coagulation, Disease-A-Month, Dec., 1969.

Bachmann, F., and Pichairut, O.: Surgical bleeding, Med. Clin. North Am. **56:**207, 1972.

Bartlett, R. H., Gazzaniga, A. B., and Geraghty, T. R.: Respiratory maneuvers to prevent pulmonary complications: a critical review, J.A.M.A. **244:**1017, 1973.

Bartlett, R. H., Gazzaniga, A. B., Brennan, M., and Hanson, E. L.: Studies in pathogenesis and prevention of postoperative pulmonary complications, Surg. Gynecol. Obstet. **137:** 925, 1973.

Beall, A. C., Jr., Fred, H. L., and Cooley, D. A.: Pulmonary embolism, Curr. Probl. Surg., Feb., 1964.

Behrendt, D. M., and Austen, G. W.: Patient care in cardiac surgery, Boston, 1972, Little, Brown & Co.

Berk, J. L., Sampliner, J. E., Artz, J. S., and Vincour, B.: Handbook of critical care, Boston, 1976, Little, Brown & Co.

Brandenberg, R. O.: Medical problems of aortic valve replacement, Prog. Cardiovasc. Dis. **7:**531, 1965.

Buchbinder, N. A., and Roberts, W. C.: Leftsided valvular acute infective endocarditis, Am. J. Med. **53:**20, 1972.

Buckberg, G. D., et al.: Studies of the effects of hypothermia on regional myocardial blood flow and metabolism during cardiopulmonary bypass, in the adequately perfused beating, fibrillating, and arrested heart, J. Thorac. Cardiovasc. Surg. **73:**87, 1977.

Burman, S. O.: Intra-aortic balloon pumping for low cardiac output syndromes, Surg. Clin. North Am. **55:**101, 1975.

Bushnell, S. S.: Respiratory intensive care nursing, Boston, 1973, Little, Brown & Co.

Calvin, J. W., Stemmer, E. A., Steedman, R. A., and Connolly, J. E.: Clinical application of parasternal mediastinotomy, Arch. Surg. **102:**322, 1971.

Clowes, G. H. A., Jr.: Surgery of the lung, esophagus and mediastinum. In Kinney, J. M., et al., editors: Manual of preoperative and postoperative care, Philadelphia, 1967, W. B. Saunders Co.

Cohn, H. E., and Capelli, J. P.: The diagnosis and management of oliguria in the postoperative period, Surg. Clin. North Am. **47:**1187, 1967.

Connolly, J. E., Wakabayashi, A., German, J. C., Stemmer, E. A., and Serres, E. J.: Clinical experience with pulsatile left heart bypass without anti-coagulation for thoracic aneurysms, J. Thorac. Cardiovasc. Surg. **62:**568, 1971.

Constant, J.: Bedside cardiology, Boston, 1969, Little, Brown & Co.

Cooley, D. A., and Hallman, G. L.: Surgical treatment of congenital heart disease, Philadelphia, 1966, Lea & Febiger.

Craver, M. C., Sams, A. B., and Hatcher, C. F.: Potassium-induced cardioplegia. Additive protection against ischemic myocardial injury during coronary revascularization, J. Thorac. Cardiovasc. Surg. **76:**24, 1978.

Damman, J. F., Jr., Thumg, N., Christlieb, I. I., Littlefield, J. B., and Muller, W., Jr.: The management of the severely ill patient after open-heart surgery, J. Thorac. Cardiovasc. Surg. **45:**80, 1963.

Danielson, G. K., and Ellis, F. H., Jr.: Low cardiac output and cardiac arrhythmias after open heart surgery. In Hardy, J. D.: Critical surgical illness, Philadelphia, 1971, W. B. Saunders Co.

Dismukes, W. E., et al.: Prosthetic valve endocarditis, Circulation **48:**365, 1973.

Ellis, F. H., Jr.: Surgery for acquired mitral valve disease, Philadelphia, 1967, W. B. Saunders Co.

Engleman, R. W., et al.: Cardiac tamponade following open-heart surgery, Circulation **41**(suppl. 11):165, 1970.

Finland, M.: Current problems in infective endocarditis, Mod. Concepts Cardiovasc. Dis. **41:**53, 1972.

Fraser, R. S., Rossall, R. E., and Dvorkin, J.: Bacterial endocarditis occurring after open heart surgery, Can. Med. Assoc. J. **96:**1551, 1967.

Friedman, B.: Cardiac surgery: dependency and apprehension complicate nursing care. Cardiac surgery: skilled nursing during the critical postoperative period, Nursing '74 **4:**33, 1974.

Goldin, M. D.: Intensive care of the surgical patient, Chicago, 1971, Year Book Medical Publishers, Inc.

Gott, V. L., Brawley, R. K., Donahoo, J. S., and Griffith, L. S. C.: Current surgical approach to ischemic heart disease, Curr. Probl. Surg., May, 1973.

Guntheroth, W. G., Morgan, B. C., and Mullins, B. S.: Effect of respiration and venous return and stroke volume in cardiac tamponade. Mechanism of pulsus paradoxus, Circ. Res. **20:**381, 1967.

Harrison, D. C., Kerber, R. E., and Alderman, E. L.: Pharmacodynamics and clinical use of cardiovascular drugs after cardiac surgery, Am. J. Cardiol. **26:**385, 1970.

Hegeman, C. O., Rappaport, I., and Berger, W. J.: Superficial temporal artery cannulation, Arch. Surg. **99:**619, 1969.

Holzer, J., et al.: Effectiveness of dopamine in patients with cardiogenic shock, Am. J. Cardiol. **32:**79, 1973.

Hudak, C. M., Gallo, B. M., and Cohn, T.: Critical care nursing, Philadelphia, 1973, J. B. Lippincott Co.

Javid, H., et al.: Neurological abnormalities following open-heart surgery, J. Thorac. Cardiovasc. Surg. **58:**502, 1969.

Juler, G. L., Stemmer, E. A., and Connolly, J. E.: Complications of prophylactic digitalization in thoracic surgery patients, J. Thorac. Cardiovasc. Surg. **58:**352, 1969.

Kantrowitz, A. R., Phillips, S. J., Butner, A., Tjønneland, S., and Haller, J. D.: Technique of femoral artery cannulation for phase-shift balloon pumping, J. Thorac. Cardiovasc. Surg. **56:**219, 1968.

Karliner, J. S.: Dopamine for cardiogenic shock, J.A.M.A. **226:**1217, 1973.

Kinney, J. M.: The recovery room and intensive care patient. In Kinney, J. M., et al., editors: Manual of preoperative and postoperative care, Philadelphia, 1967, W. B. Saunders Co.

Kirklin, J. W.: Advances in cardiovascular surgery, New York, 1973, Grune & Stratton, Inc.

Kirklin, J. W., and Nunn, S. L.: The cardiovascular system in care of the surgical patient. In Kinney, J. M., et al., editors: Manual of preoperative and postoperative care, Philadelphia, 1967, W. B. Saunders Co.

Kloster, F. L., Bristow, J. D., and Griswold, H. E.: Medical problems in mitral and multiple valve replacement, Prog. Cardiovasc. Dis. **7:**504, 1965.

Laufman, H.: Hematologic crises in surgery. In Hardy, J. D.: Critical surgical illness, Philadelphia, 1971, W. B. Saunders Co.

Levitsky, S.: New insights in cardiac trauma, Surg. Clin. North Am. **55:**43, 1975.

McGoon, D. W.: Techniques of open-heart surgery for congenital heart disease, Curr. Probl. Surg., Apr., 1968.

Melrose, D. G., Dreyer, B., Bentall, H. H., and Baker, J. B. E.: Elective cardiac arrest, Lancet **2:**21, 1955.

Meltzer, L. E., Pinneo, R., and Kitchell, J. R.: Intensive coronary care, Philadelphia, 1970, The Charles Press, Publisher.

Moffitt, E. A., Sessler, A. D., and Kirklin, J. W.: Postoperative care in open-heart surgery, J.A.M.A. **199:**129, 1967.

Nelson, R. M., Jenson, C. B., and Smoot, W. M., III: Pericardial tamponade following open-heart surgery, J. Thorac. Cardiovasc. Surg. **58:**510, 1969.

Neville, W. E.: Care of the surgical cardiopulmonary patient, Chicago, 1971, Year Book Medical Publishers, Inc.

New, H. C.: Antimicrobial agents—mechanisms of action and clinical usage, Curr. Probl. Surg., June, 1973.

Oaks, W. W., and Moyer, J. H.: Pre- and postoperative management of the cardiopulmonary patient, New York, 1970, Grune & Stratton, Inc.

Payne, D. D., De Weese, J. A., Mahoney, E. B., and Murphy, G. W.: Surgical treatment of traumatic rupture of the normal aortic valve, Ann. Thorac. Surg. **17:**223, 1974.

Quick, A. J.: Bleeding problems in clinical medicine, Philadelphia, 1970, W. B. Saunders Co.

Randall, H. T.: Fluid and electrolyte therapy. In Kinney, J. M., et al., editors: Manual of preoperative and postoperative care, Philadelphia, 1967, W. B. Saunders Co.

Roberts, W. C., Buchbinder, N. A.: Right-sided infective endocarditis, Am. J. Med. **53:**7, 1972.

Secor, J. S.: Coronary care—a nursing specialty, New York, 1971, Appleton-Century-Crofts.

Soroff, H. S., Birtwell, W. C., and Giron, F.: Assisted circulation. In Norman, J. C., editor: Cardiac surgery, New York, 1972, Appleton-Century-Crofts.

Spodick, D. H.: Acute cardiac tamponade, pathology, physiology, diagnosis and management, Prog. Cardiovasc. Dis. **10:** 64, 1967.

Standards for cardiopulmonary resuscitation (CPR) and emergency cardiac care (ECC), J.A.M.A. **227**(suppl.):834, 1974.

Tector, A. J., et al.: Coronary artery wounds treated with saphenous vein bypass grafts, J.A.M.A. **225:**282, 1973.

Van Meter, M.: Chest tubes—basic techniques for better care, Nursing '74 **4:**48, 1974.

Von Hippel, A.: Chest tubes and chest bottles, Springfield, Ill., 1970, Charles C Thomas, Publisher.

Wakabayashi, A., Connolly, J. E., Stemmer, E. A., and Nakamura, Y.: Clinical experience with heparinless, veno-arterial bypass without oxygenation for the treatment of acute cardiogenic shock, J. Thorac. Cardiovasc. Surg. **68:**687, 1974.

Walter, C. W.: Blood donors, blood transfusions. In Kinney, J. M., et al., editors: Manual of preoperative and postoperative care, Philadelphia, 1967, W. B. Saunders Co.

Wheat, M. W., et al.: Acute dissecting aneurysms of the aorta, J. Thorac. Cardiovasc. Surg. **58:**344, 1969.

Wilson, J. W.: The pulmonary cellular and subcellular alteration of extracorporeal circulation, Surg. Clin. North Am. **54:** 1203, 1974.

Yang, S. S., Bentivoglia, L. G., Maranhao, V., and Goldberg, H.: From cardiac catheterization data to hemodynamic parameters, Philadelphia, 1972, F. A. Davis Co.

CHAPTER 21

Human heart transplantation

Jack Copeland

HEART TRANSPLANTATION: HUMAN EXPERIMENTATION OR THERAPEUTIC MODALITY?

Since the first human heart transplant in December 1967, over 350 patients in the world have received transplanted hearts (Fig. 21-1). Initial enthusiasm led to a surge of heart transplants, with over 100 done in the year following the first operation. The early mortality rates were extremely high. Candidates chosen as recipients were generally moribund with far-advanced multisystem disease. Also, most heart surgeons were inexperienced in the treatment of cardiac rejection and the complications of immunosuppressive therapy.

By 1970 the number of transplants throughout the world had dropped to 20 per year, and since that time there has been a small increase, particularly in the last several years. At the present time approximately 30 to 40 heart transplants are performed each year with over half of these at Stanford University. Since 1967 human heart transplantation has been transformed from a theoretical concept to a clinical research experience and finally to a procedure that under the proper circumstances can be offered to patients in a number of centers throughout the United States and the world.

■ What experimental findings led to human heart transplantation?

Much of the fundamental research in heart transplantation research took place at Stanford University under the guidance of Dr. Norman Shumway. The initial impetus for laboratory experimentation with heart transplantation was brought about by an improved surgical technique for heart transplantation in dogs, described by Dr. Richard Lower and Dr. Shumway in 1961. This procedure, called "orthotopic transplantation," simplified what had previously been an extremely difficult surgical technique to a technique that could be completed with surgical precision within 45 minutes. This technique was similar to the method now used for human heart transplantation, which is shown in Fig. 21-2. The recipient's heart was removed, leaving over half of the posterior or atrial chambers of the heart for anastomosis to the donor heart. The atrial level of anastomosis obviated the need for making multiple smaller vascular connections for the superior and inferior venae cavae and the pulmonary veins. The current human transplantation technique involves running suture lines between the donor and the recipient atrial cuffs, followed by a running suture line connecting the donor with the recipient aorta, and finally, a running suture line that connects the donor with the recipient pulmonary artery.

Next there followed a number of laboratory experiments on dogs that were vital to the further development of heart transplantation. One initial finding was that in a period of 4 to 7 days after the heart transplant, dogs rejected the transplanted heart in much the same way as they rejected skin grafts or kidney transplants. When

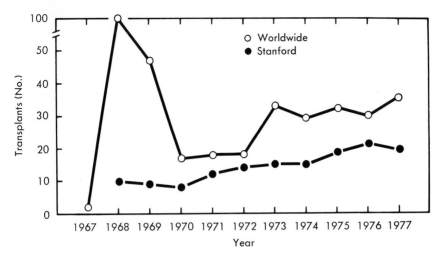

Fig. 21-1. Comparison of worldwide vs. Stanford University heart transplantation numbers, 1967-1977.

heart rejection became severe, the animals died. Drugs for treatment of rejection similar to those used in treating kidney transplants were administered to suppress the dog immune system. These consisted of steroids and azathioprine. Early detection of rejection based on the amplitude of the QRS complex on the dog's electrocardiogram was first reported. When the QRS voltage dropped by 10% to 20% on a given day, there was a high degree of correlation with early rejection changes in the transplanted heart. Use of the electrocardiogram as a guide for treatment of rejection by withholding steroids until a fall in QRS voltage was observed led to the first 1-year survival of dogs with transplanted hearts.

The rejection process was studied and found to be initiated by the appearance of small lymphocytes in the interstitium of the heart. This was generally accompanied by mild edema and followed shortly thereafter by further lymphocytic infiltration, then by polymorphonuclear leukocytes, and finally by hemorrhage into the myocardium, further edema, and necrosis or death of myocytes. Decreases in blood flow through the coronary arteries and in the cardiac output were dramatic; however, they did not occur until late in the rejection process and therefore could not serve as early indicators for treatment of rejec-

tion. On the other hand, it was clear that rejection begins before impairment of heart function occurs, and therefore rejection can be treated before the patient suffers the symptomatic consequences of congestive heart failure and low cardiac output.

Finally, a series of experiments was designed to examine the function of denervated hearts. In transplanting the heart all nerve supplies are cut and are not reestablished after the transplant procedure. Therefore the heart is without sensory nerves, or nerves from the parasympathetic and sympathetic nervous systems that govern heart rate. To study this problem, hearts were removed from and then reimplanted into the same dogs. Long-term survivors of this autotransplantation procedure were found to survive with no signs of heart failure and to be able to exercise at nearly the same level as dogs with normally innervated hearts.

With this basic information as a background, it was quite natural for further fundamental developments in heart transplantation to take place at Stanford. Since these experiments, a number of advances have been made in the treatment of patients with heart transplants. However, the primary problems confronted by the heart transplant surgeon and immunologist have not changed.

They still center around the rejection of foreign tissue by the immune system. The suppression of the immune system leads to opportunistic infection and therein lies the delicate balance between adequate immunosuppression and the prevention of infection that must be sought in transplantation patients.

HEART TRANSPLANTATION— THE STATE OF THE ART
■ What is the scope of the current heart transplantation effort?

Two to three human heart transplants each month are performed at Stanford University. The activity in other geographic areas is more spo-

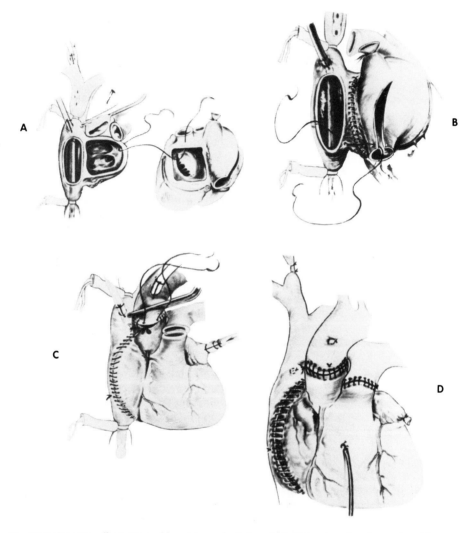

Fig. 21-2. Stepwise illustration of heart transplantation. **A,** Initial suture has been placed between cuffs of left atrium. Donor heart is then lowered into pericardial cavity and left atrial suture lines are completed. **B,** Beginning of right atrial suture line. **C,** Atrial suture lines have been completed and aortic suture line is nearly finished. **D,** All suture lines are completed and a temporary pacemaker wire is shown on right ventricular surface.

radic; however, the interest in heart transplantation has spread to a number of centers, and it appears that there will be an increase in the number of heart transplants in the near future.

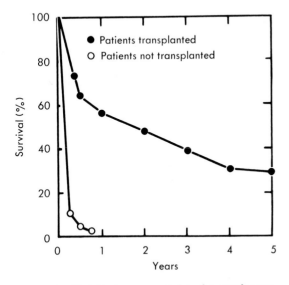

Fig. 21-3. All patients represented in this graph were chosen as potential recipients. Those represented by open circles (n = 35) died while awaiting donor heart. Those represented by closed circles (n = 136) received transplanted hearts.

■ How successful is heart transplantation?

The success of heart transplantation must be judged in a population of patients with terminal heart disease who have an extremely poor prognosis and in fact will probably die within 1 year (Fig. 21-3).

Fig. 21-3 depicts the status of the entire Stanford group of potential heart transplant recipients as of January 1978. The 35 patients represented by the open circles were chosen as potential heart transplant recipients but died before a suitable donor heart became available. The 136 patients represented by the black circles were chosen as potential recipients and did receive transplanted hearts. Those patients in the transplanted group had a markedly superior survival rate as compared to those who did not receive transplants. Thus a group of patients who can benefit from heart transplantation has been identified, and it has been shown that if they do not receive a transplanted heart, their prognosis is uniformly fatal. For those patients who do receive a transplanted heart, the outlook has improved since 1968. The 1-year survival rate at Stanford for heart transplantation grouped by years is shown in Fig. 21-4.

At present the chance of survival for 1 year following heart transplantation appears to be between 65% and 70%. Following the first year, the mortality rate for recent heart transplant recipi-

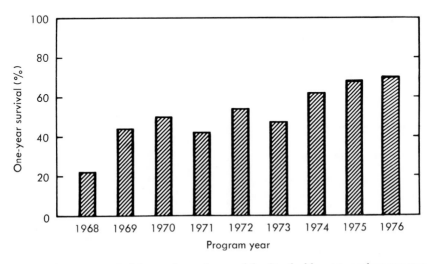

Fig. 21-4. One-year survival figures for each year of the Stanford heart transplant program.

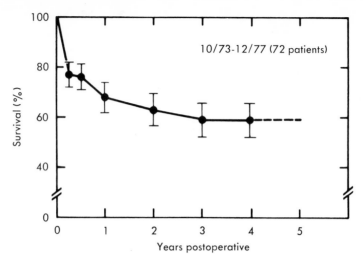

Fig. 21-5. Actuarial survival for heart transplant recipients at Stanford from 10/73 to 12/77.

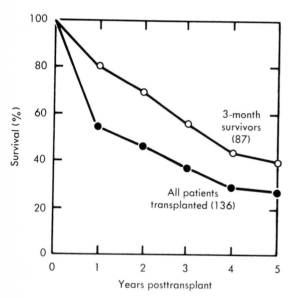

Fig. 21-6. Actuarial survival for all patients in Stanford heart transplant program as of 1/78. Patients who survive initial 3 months (open circles) have better long-term survival.

ents has been approximately 2% to 5% per year (Fig. 21-5). The summary for all patients receiving heart transplants at Stanford is shown in Fig. 21-6. This includes all patients from January 1968 to January 1978 and indicates a 5-year survival of approximately 30%. If the current trends indicated in Fig. 21-5 continue to hold, it is anticipated that the 5-year survival rate following heart transplantation will soon approach 50%.

■ **What causes death after heart transplantation?**

In the transplant group at Stanford there were 81 patient deaths as of January 1978. Over half of these were due to infection as shown below:

Cause of death	Number of patients
Infection	42
Acute rejection	17
Graft arteriosclerosis	
Proliferative	5
Atherosclerotic	6
Pulmonary hypertension	4
Malignancy	4
Cardiovascular accident	2
Suicide	1

Acute rejection was the second most common cause of death, followed by a smaller number of deaths caused by arteriosclerosis in the transplanted heart resulting in myocardial infarction.

■ Why have survival statistics in heart transplantation improved?

Recipient selection. During the first years of human heart transplantation only moribund patients were chosen as potential recipients. Many of these patients had multisystem disorders, including liver and kidney failure and severe chronic obstructive pulmonary disease. With this type of potential recipient, heart transplantation was successful in only rare and exceptional cases. Through a process of trial and error a set of criteria for the selection of potential recipients was established. While these criteria are not always binding, they serve as guidelines in choosing potential heart transplant recipients. Those guidelines are: (1) patient age of 50 or less, (2) no diabetes mellitus, (3) no active infectious process, (4) no evidence of current pulmonary infarction, (5) pulmonary vascular resistance of less than 10 Wood units, and (6) no multisystem disease (including kidney failure, liver failure, pulmonary failure, cardiovascular accident, or neoplasm). Each of these criteria was established on the basis of experience with human transplant patients. Patients over the age of 50 were generally found to be unable to tolerate the stress of the transplant and immunosuppressive therapy and had an increased mortality rate. Immunosuppressed patients with diabetes mellitus were found to have increased susceptibility to infection. Patients with active infections often developed fatal exacerbations of these infections after the implementation of immunosuppressive therapy. Patients with pulmonary infarctions before the transplant uniformly developed posttransplant abscesses in the areas of infarction unless the infarcted area was given an opportunity to heal completely into a scar. In the few transplant patients whose elevation in pulmonary vascular resistance was greater than 10 Wood units, acute right heart failure accompanied by arrhythmias occurred, and all of these patients died. The normal donor heart was unable to pump against the recipient's high pulmonary vascular resistance.

Increased availability of donor hearts and improved methods for donor heart procurement. Generally, patients with irreversible brain death below the age of 35 with no history of heart disease and no evidence of heart damage at the time they receive their fatal injury can be considered potential donors. In male donors 30 to 35 years of age it is prudent to obtain a coronary arteriogram to rule out the possibility of early coronary artery disease in the donor heart. In females the donor age range may be extended up to 40 years, if again the precaution of coronary arteriography is taken before accepting the donor heart. Other guidelines include the absence of systemic infection and malignancy in the donor.

In the past it has been most convenient to transport the donor, with respiratory support, to the hospital where the heart transplant is performed so that the donor heart can be removed immediately prior to removal of the recipient's heart, minimizing the period of myocardial ischemia. Recently, improvements in the preservation of hearts removed from donors have enabled cardiac transplant surgeons to remove the donor heart at a distant institution, cool it rapidly with a "cardioplegic" (high potassium) solution, and transport the heart maintaining a temperature of approximately of 4° C. Procurement of hearts in this manner has reduced the cost of donor transport and maintenance prior to the time of heart transplantation and in this way increased the general availability of donor hearts. Also, cooperative networks of tissue banks in large metropolitan areas have made more organs available for transplantation.

Treatment of rejection. Improved ability to diagnose and treat rejection of the heart is another major factor in improving patient survival after heart transplantation. Electrocardiographic QRS voltage amplitude in the heart transplant recipient is an extremely sensitive test for the diagnosis of early rejection. When the QRS voltage falls by approximately 20%, it is likely that rejection is occurring. Unfortunately, the electrocardiogram, while extremely sensitive, is not highly specific for rejection. The QRS voltage amplitude may fall because of falling hematocrit, change in body temperature, increased fluid in the pericardial or pleural spaces, systemic infection, and pneumothorax. Signs of heart failure such as a third heart sound (gallop rhythm), the occurrence of edema, paroxysmal nocturnal dyspnea, and pulmonary edema unfortunately occur after the heart rejection is well under way, and they are of little value in the early diagnosis of rejection episodes.

Currently the standard procedure for the diag-

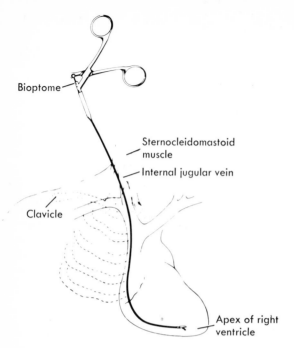

Bioptome

Sternocleidomastoid muscle

Internal jugular vein

Clavicle

Apex of right ventricle

Fig. 21-7. Drawing of heart biopsy procedure. This is done percutaneously via right internal jugular vein after administering local anesthetic.

nosis of rejection is the endomyocardial biopsy. As indicated in Fig. 21-7, this technique is performed by placing an endomyocardial bioptome into the right ventricle via the right internal jugular vein. A fluoroscope is used to view the bioptome tip.

Several biopsies are taken during the procedure and examined for histologic changes. If it is necessary to make an immediate diagnosis, frozen sections of the biopsies can be taken. More reliable information with regard to the presence or absence of rejection can be obtained from examining permanent sections stained with hematoxylin and eosin. Treatment for rejection is therefore based on microscopic examination of the myocardium.

Another indicator of rejection that may be helpful in the future is the level of T-lymphocytes or thymus-derived lymphocytes in the blood. This class of lymphocytes takes part in the rejection of grafted tissue rather than the B-lymphocytes,

which are derived from the bone marrow and do not invade the grafted organ. A simple way of estimating the level of these cells in the blood is called the "E-rosette" titer, which is based on the phenomenon of agglutination of sheep red blood cells around T-lymphocytes. When the level of T-lymphocytes rises, the likelihood of rejection is increased. The place of this technique in the diagnosis and treatment of rejection has not yet been defined.

Treatment of infection. Suppression of the immune system in heart transplant patients makes even the slightest infection a life-threatening occurrence, whether it is bacterial, viral, fungal, nocardial, or protozoan. In the Stanford experience 386 infections had occurred as of January 1978. They are listed by type as follows:

	Number of infections	Number of patients
Bacterial	235	94
Viral	66	54
Fungal	48	44
Protozoan	19	19
Nocardial	18	18

There were only 42 deaths from infection. It is likely that use of prophylactic broad-spectrum antibiotics at the time of transplantation, vigorous attempts at prompt diagnosis of infection, and treatment of infection with high doses of antibiotics for prolonged periods of time have reduced the death rate from infection. The most common location for infection in these patients has been the lungs. When a pulmonary infection is suspected, transtracheal needle aspiration of pulmonary secretions is performed using a percutaneous technique via the cricothyroid membrane. If an area of infiltrate or a coin lesion is seen on routine x-ray examination, full lung tomograms are taken. Infiltrates or coin lesions that cannot be diagnosed on the basis of transtracheal aspiration are diagnosed by transthoracic percutaneous needle aspiration. After obtaining all indicated culture specimens, when infection is strongly suspected, broad-spectrum antibiotic coverage is maintained until culture results become available. A constant vigilance for other sites of infection including the nasopharynx, kidney, bladder, and central nervous system has also proved worthwhile.

Prevention of graft arteriosclerosis. There has never been evidence of reinnervation of a transplanted human heart. In patients with transplanted hearts that develop coronary arteriosclerosis, there is no warning sign of myocardial ischemia since the patients have no nerve supply and therefore do not experience angina pectoris. It became apparent in 1970 that there was a great incidence of accelerated arteriosclerosis and painless myocardial infarction 2 to 4 years after heart transplantation. In fact, by the fourth postoperative year over 80% of patients were found to have significant coronary arteriosclerotic narrowing. For this reason, yearly coronary arteriography was instituted in 1971, and a trial regimen was begun that consisted of 100 mg dipyridamole orally four times per day, warfarin sodium to maintain the prothrombin time one and a half to two times above control level, a low fat diet, and an exercise program. While this regimen was instituted on an empirical basis, it seemed to be directed against factors that might contribute to the arteriosclerotic process. An hypothesis was made that immunologic damage occurred in coronary arteries, which led to platelet deposition and mural thrombosis followed by intimal proliferation and the deposition of lipids. Each part of the trial regimen was directed against one of these elements. Since the institution of that regimen, there has been a significant reduction in the incidence of coronary arterial lesions in heart transplant patients at Stanford.

Rabbit antithymocyte globulin (RATG) in the treatment of heart rejection. Beginning in 1973, rabbit antithymocyte globulin has been used in addition to corticosteroids and azathioprine in the treatment of rejection. This substance is produced by extracting thymocytes from human thymus glands, injecting these thymocytes into rabbits, and collecting their serum after several weeks. After purification, this antibody against T-lymphocytes is administered by intramuscular injection usually into the anterior thigh muscles. This substance has a specific action on the immune system, that is, a reduction in the number of T-lymphocytes, as opposed to the general immunosuppressive actions of steroids and azathioprine. Therefore there has been an increasing tendency to use RATG more liberally in the treatment and prevention of rejection episodes. Following intramuscular injection of this substance, there is an intense local reaction characterized by erythema, swelling, and pain. These injections often become the focus of a great deal of anxiety on the part of patients and constitute one of the great challenges to nursing care. It has been observed that a gentle, supportive, and kind nurse can make these injections much more tolerable to patients.

Retransplantation of the heart. Diagnosis of either irreversible rejection of the heart at any time after transplantation or the presence of severe coronary arteriosclerosis in a transplanted heart implies imminent death of the recipient. In those two situations it has been found worthwhile to attempt a second heart transplantation. Eight patients at Stanford have received a second heart transplant and one patient has received a third. Five of these patients are still alive, including three who have survived for 1 year or more following retransplantation. Of the four patients who died, three died of infections and one died of cerebral embolus. The problems that one might anticipate from retransplantation of the heart have not been prohibitive. There has been no change in surgical technique, and there have been no technical problems. The ever-present tendency for recipients to become infected has been no greater than in patients receiving one heart transplant, and thus far the results have been extremely encouraging and have given a further surgical alternative to patients with severe malfunction of their transplanted hearts.

HEART DONOR MANAGEMENT
■ **What are the criteria for brain death?**

The ability to diagnose brain death in patients with irreversible cerebral injury has made transplantation of the human heart possible. It has permitted maintenance of the function of healthy hearts in potential donors until the hearts can be removed for transplantation. The diagnosis of brain death generally consists of a battery of findings, including the following: The donor must be proven not to have blood levels of any sedative or narcotic drug that could result in severe central nervous system depression. He must be shown to have no spontaneous movement or respiration and no reflexes, either musculoskeletal or ocular as determined by cold caloric testing. He must have a flat electroencephalogram. Finally, if possible, it is most reassuring to have evidence of severe brain damage that is either grossly obvious or apparent on computed axial tomography or cerebral arteriograms. Once the diagnosis of brain death is made, it is truly an act of human kindness on the part of physicians and bereaved relatives to refer the potential donors to transplant surgeons. This requires both time and effort and can be a trying experience for all involved.

■ **What problems are encountered in supporting the heart donor?**

The donor with brain death generally has lost the homeostatic mechanisms that normally maintain blood pressure and temperature. Marked fluctuations in blood pressure may be seen including severe hypertension, but the general trend in blood pressure curves followed for 6 hours or more is downward, and support with an α-adrenergic agent such as metaraminol is usually necessary. The body temperature should be maintained in a normal physiologic range with a heating blanket. In addition, the donor may have diabetes insipidus caused by failure of the hypothalamus to secrete vasopressin. This condition is treated by replacing the urine output with an equal volume of intravenous fluid to prevent dehydration and by periodic administration of vasopressin (Pitressin).

Heart donors have the usual pulmonary problems of comatose patients, including inadequate clearing of secretions and atelectasis in dependent areas. These are complicated by the tendency for patients with intracranial damage to develop "neurogenic" pulmonary edema.

■ **What criteria determine a suitable donor?**

In addition to being pronounced dead on the basis of irreversible cerebral injury, there are several other important guidelines in determining which patient is a suitable heart donor. Males below the age of 30 and females below 40 without any history of heart disease, intrathoracic trauma or infection, or malignancy, and with an electrocardiogram that fails to demonstrate cur-

rent injury and a chest x-ray study that reveals a "normal" heart are generally acceptable. Older potential donors (males age 30 to 35 and females age 40 to 45) may be acceptable if coronary arteriography fails to disclose arteriosclerotic lesions.

The donor must be compatible with the recipient in the ABO blood typing system. A "negative" lymphocyte cytotoxicity test in which donor lymphocytes are not killed by recipient serum is helpful in predicting that preformed antibodies against donor tissue are not present. A size match, while not absolutely necessary, is desirable. If a large disparity in size exists between the donor and the recipient, it is usually acceptable to proceed if the donor is much larger than the recipient but not if he is much smaller.

■ **How is the donor managed after all criteria have been met?**

There are two ways of procuring donor hearts. As mentioned earlier, the donor may be supported and transported to the transplant hospital where the heart is removed at the time of the transplant procedure, or the heart may be removed, preserved by flushing cold (4° C) cardioplegic solution through the coronary arteries, and rapidly transported to the transplant hospital. Three to four hours of "ischemic" time may be encountered with the latter method.

HEART RECIPIENT MANAGEMENT
■ **What is appropriate preoperative care?**

In most cases heart recipients have undergone intensive diagnostic procedures prior to their referral for possible heart transplantation. The general guidelines for recipient selection noted previously apply. In addition intensive psychosocial screening for the patient and his family is done to seek out contraindications to performing transplantation and to obtain some estimate of the psychosocial impact of heart transplantation on the potential recipient. Heart failure is treated maximally during the waiting period prior to transplantation, and in the immediate preoperative period the heart recipient has blood drawn for type and cross match and is usually treated with a loading dose of azathioprine.

Intraoperatively, the heart recipient receives a large dose (generally 500 mg) of methylprednisolone intravenously after discontinuation of cardiopulmonary bypass and 125 mg intravenously every 8 hours thereafter for 3 to 4 doses. Postoperative care includes strict reverse isolation and intensive care of the intubated recipient with standard postcardiac surgical monitoring of electrocardiogram, arterial pressures, arterial blood gases, temperature, and urine output. The patient's heart rate and blood pressure are maintained generally with isoproteronol or dopamine. It has been noted that heart recipients have limited cardiac outputs during the first several postoperative days and that support of contractility and heart rate are necessary.

By the first postoperative day, removal of the endotracheal tube is often possible. Following this, the patient is treated with progressive ambulation and a salt-free and low fat diet. Prednisone, 100 mg/day orally is started. This dosage is reduced by 5 mg each day. Treatment with azathioprine is begun at a level of approximately 2 mg/kg/day and maintained at that level as long as there is no drop in white blood count or evidence of secondary liver disease. Treatment with rabbit antithymocyte globulin is given daily for the first 3 days following transplantation, then every other day for three more doses. The diagnosis of acute rejection episodes is made on the basis of ECG's twice daily, weekly heart biopsies, and clinical findings based on close follow-up of the patient.

Treatment of rejection episodes includes 1 g/day methylprednisolone intravenously for 3 days, a new cycle of rabbit antithymocyte globulin given daily for three doses and then every other day for three doses, an increase in the prednisone dose to 100 mg/day and tapering more gradually, heparinization, and treatment with furosemide (Lasix) as indicated. During intervals between rejection episodes when evidence suggestive of rejection is found such as T-cell elevation above baseline levels, treatment with increased dosages of prednisone and antithymocyte globulin may suffice. A number of other long-term medications are used in the treatment of these patients, including nystatin (Mycostatin) vaginal suppositories that are sucked and swallowed in order to decrease the growth of yeast in the patient's gastrointestinal tract. Antacids are taken to reduce gastric acidity. Special antibiotic mouthwashes are often used to reduce oral flora. Diuretics are used periodically. Electrocardiograms twice daily and weekly heart biopsies are done in an attempt to diagnose rejection early.

Physical and psychosocial rehabilitation efforts are made as soon as the patient is able to cooperate, which is usually within the first postoperative week. Plans for discharge are made as the patient progresses, and generally most patients can be discharged within 2 months following the transplant. Rehabilitation and close follow-up continue for the remainder of the patient's life, and it is of interest that a high degree of rehabilitation has been attained by 90% of patients who have survived for 1 year or longer.

CHAPTER 22

Replantation following traumatic amputation

Bruce M. Achauer, Arthur H. Salibian, and David W. Furnas

■ How long has replantation surgery been performed?

The patron saints of replantation are the twin brothers, Cosmos and Damian.[1] According to legend the saints appeared to a devout follower who was moribund from a cancer of the leg. The saints removed the diseased leg and replaced it with that of a Moor who had died earlier that day. Thus the black leg was attached to a white body. While replantation may be nothing new for saints, it has taken surgeons a long time to evolve the routine replantation of parts. Ambrose Paré made a breakthrough in surgery when arterial ligatures were developed in 1540. Alexis Carrell was awarded the Nobel Prize for developing a method of vascular anastomosis in 1902. However, vascular surgery came into its own during the Korean War.

The microscope was introduced to the operating room in the 1920's by an otolaryngologist, Nylen of Stockholm. The microscope has been used for middle ear surgery since that date. The next group of surgeons who adopted the microscope were the ophthalmologists in the 1940's. It was a neurosurgeon, Jacobson,[2] who introduced the term "microvascular surgery" in 1960. In 1962 an arm was successfully replanted by Malt.[3] Reports from China appeared at virtually the same time.[4] However, these did not represent microvascular cases. In 1967 Kamatsu and Tamai[5] reported a successful thumb replantation. Subsequently, series running into the hundreds have been reported, and the replantation of severed parts, even very small ones, is a routine occurrence in many centers throughout the world.

■ What were the technical hurdles?

The growth of microvascular surgery was slow for a number of technical reasons. Not only were the techniques tedious to develop and pass on, but the instrumentation and *suture* material were slow in evolving. Commercially available microvascular sutures were not produced until the 1970's. A great deal of time was spent trying to develop nonsuture-type repairs of arteries because suturing was thought to be too difficult. Today, however, 10-0 (22 μ) and 11-0 (18 μ) sutures are readily available. Special clamps had to be produced to avoid trauma to small vessels being repaired, and many modifications have been made in existing *microscopes* to allow two surgeons to see the same operative field and routinely repair vessels of 1 mm in diameter and smaller. The steps in performing a vascular anastomosis are illustrated in Fig. 22-1. Parallel to the development of microvascular surgery is the microscopic repair of nerves. Smith[6] in New York developed this for repair of divided facial nerves. Millesi[7] in Vienna has many years of experience in peripheral nerve repair and has shown the value of the accurate repair that only a microscopic approach can offer. During the last decade there has been an explosion in the applications of microvascular techniques to tissue

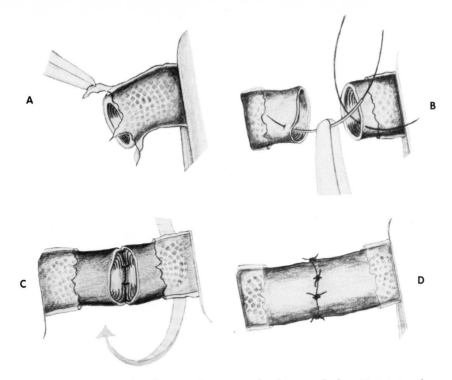

Fig. 22-1. A, Vessel ends are placed in special microvascular clamps and adventitia is stripped to prevent its falling into lumen. **B,** Interrupted sutures are placed anteriorly. **C,** Clamp is rotated 180 degrees to complete suturing posterior wall. **D,** No narrowing of lumen should be produced by repair.

transfer from one part of the body to another.[8] For example, the mouth and jaw area can be reconstructed in a one-stage operation, transferring groin skin with attached iliac crest bone to the mouth area.[9] Infertility problems, both the reversal of vasectomies and fallopian tube repair, have been corrected by microscopic procedures.[10] Even lymph vessels, in cases of lymphedema, have been reconstructed.[11]

■ What are the results of replantation?

Digital replantation has been very encouraging considering that the first replant was performed only a decade ago. The results in the future should be even more promising.

The primary concern in a replant is survival; however, the final outcome of the procedure depends on the useful *functional* and sensory recovery. With proper patient selection an 80% to 90% success rate can be achieved in replantation of digits. Patients in their 20's and 30's with clean-cut injuries have the best survival rates. Injuries through the metacarpal bone have a better chance of survival after replantation than distal amputations because of the larger vessel size. The results in revascularization and replantation are comparable.

The functional results following replantations have not been well documented. Weiland[12] reported 47% good to excellent results on 17 patients who underwent primary flexor and extensor tendon repairs. The patients were able to flex the tip of the finger to within 1.5 cm from the distal palmar crease with a loss of less than 30 degrees of extension. The best functional results are obtained in thumb amputations in which the important carpometacarpal joint is usually spared. Injuries through the digital sheath give the poorest results because of flexor tendon adhesions.

Sensibility determines the functional recovery of the hand, as recently assessed by Gelberman and co-workers.[13] Fifty percent of the patients studied had two-point discrimination less than 10 mm, and 70% were able to differentiate between heat and cold, and dull and sharp objects. All patients studied had protective sensation. Return of sensation was also found to be related to the blood flow in the digit. If the blood flow was less than 75% of that in the normal digit, the sensory recovery was poor.

The cosmetic appearance of replanted digits has been good in spite of bone shortening and atrophy. In distal injuries preservation of the esthetic unit of fingernail and pulp gives a more pleasing appearance than any prosthetic device.

In our series of 40 replantations at the University of California, Irvine, we have had seven failures, giving us a success rate of 82.5%. If avulsion injuries were excluded, our success rate would be 90%.[14]

■ What are the indications for replantation?

The most important step in replantation of amputated parts is making the correct initial decision to go ahead with the attempted replantation. It is possible to do greater harm than the initial trauma if an inappropriate decision is made. Once a part has been reattached, it is a very difficult emotional decision for a patient to agree to having it amputated even though it is totally useless. Thus in the case of hand injury *function* must be kept in mind throughout. The following are some of the factors that should influence the decision.

Part amputated. If half or more of the *thumb* is amputated, every attempt should be made to replant the part unless there is some absolute contraindication. A thumb, of course, constitutes a very important functional part of the hand and even if it is relatively immobile or does not have normal sensation, it is extremely useful as a post to oppose function in the remaining normal digits. Reconstruction of the thumb after it has been amputated is difficult and is almost never as good as a replanted thumb. Replantation of the

amputated thumb is one of the most worthwhile operations in surgery today.

Replantation of the single amputated finger should be done only under special circumstances. Loss of the *index* or *small* finger causes virtually no functional deficit, and the remaining three-fingered hand can be quite acceptable from the standpoint of appearance. Replanting the *long* or *ring* finger produces a stiff, relatively insensitive finger in the middle of an otherwise normal hand. Thus the function of the entire hand is diminished. Extenuating circumstances would include an extremely young patient in whom growth and development have yet to occur and a much better than average result can be expected. In addition, some people, for instance, a woman who is about to be married and loses the ring finger of the left hand, may have tremendous emotional investment in the amputated part. In this case appearance takes precedence over function, but this decision is not easily made. Amputated tips of fingers can be replanted, and to some people this is extremely important. Again, this is primarily for appearance, although there might be overriding occupational considerations. Of course, *multiple digit amputations* indicate replantation. If all four fingers are amputated, usually an attempt is made to replant as many fingers as possible. This is a good way to "hedge your bets" in case one or more digits is lost in the postoperative period.

Condition of amputated part. Ideally, one would like a clean-cut injury for consideration of replantation (Fig. 22-2). Unfortunately, this is not usually the case (Fig. 22-3). If there are multiple-level injuries, a replantation may not be possible. Also, if the amputated part is crushed, it may not be salvageable. Parts that are avulsed present a particular problem. The vessel may be destroyed for several centimeters proximal to the amputation and doom any replantation. One indication that this might have occurred is called "ribbon sign"[15] along the area of the digital vessels demonstrating a long area of tissue damage. In the thumb replant shown in Fig. 22-4 there was damage further down the thumb, but it was not severe enough to prevent replantation. Avulsion injuries are often impossible to replant. In cases of mul-

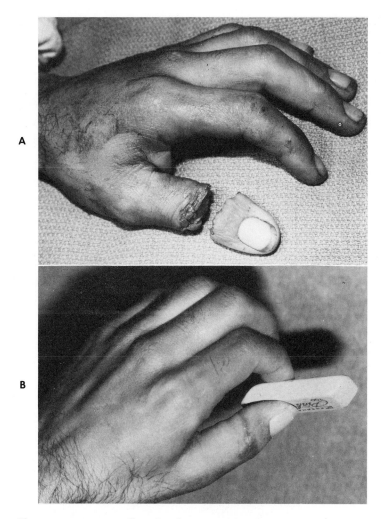

Fig. 22-2. Clean saw amputation allowed replantation of thumb of this carpenter who was able to return to work 8 weeks following injury.

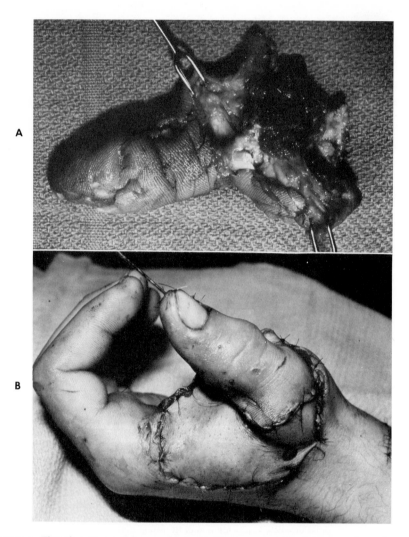

Fig. 22-3. A, Thumb amputated by saw blade. **B,** Despite extensive damage replantation was successful.

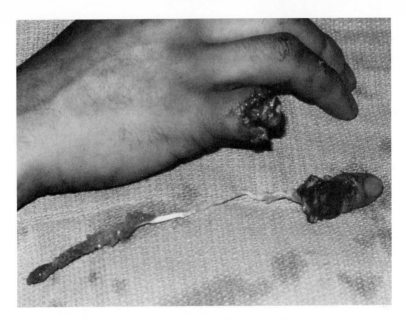

Fig. 22-4. Typical avulsion injury resulting in extensive tissue damage and not suitable for replantation.

tiple injuries substitutions can be made. In Fig. 22-5 the small finger was replanted at the thumb position. The *level of injury* is significant also. Injuries distal to the distal interphalangeal joint are extremely difficult to treat because there are virtually no veins at this point. Amputations at the wrist level are not uncommon, and a very useful result is usually obtained. Amputations around the elbow can be very complicated and it is difficult to preserve function. Amputations at more proximal levels pose special problems because of the muscles involved. Muscle tissue becomes necrotic very quickly, and if circulation is not established within a short time, the resulting muscle necrosis will doom the replantation to failure. However, amputated parts in which there is no muscle can be replanted several hours following amputation and success can be anticipated.

Status of patient. Age is of course very important. Older people who are prone to stiff joints must be selected carefully for replantation. All phases of recovery in older patients are poor. Nerve regeneration, joint mobility, bone healing, and tendon healing are delayed and make complications more likely. In children every effort

should be made to attempt replantation of almost any severed part because they have tremendous potential for recovering function. Psychologic trauma caused by growing up with missing parts can be severe. Despite the smaller vessels in children, replantations can be quite successful. The degloving ring avulsion injury shown in Fig. 22-6 is a good example. A degloving injury is rarely replantable, and a single digit, particularly a ring finger, is almost never replantable. However, in this child an excellent result was obtained.

The *mental status* of the patient is of some consideration. Often a part may be amputated during a suicide attempt; this greatly complicates the postoperative period of rehabilitation. If the injury occurred because the patient was intoxicated, be alert for delirium tremens in the postoperative period.

The occupation of the patient is important. Heavy laborers may well function better without a replantation, whereas people who meet the public may be very self-conscious if they are missing a part.

Patients with *multiple trauma* may not be candidates for replantation. For example, someone

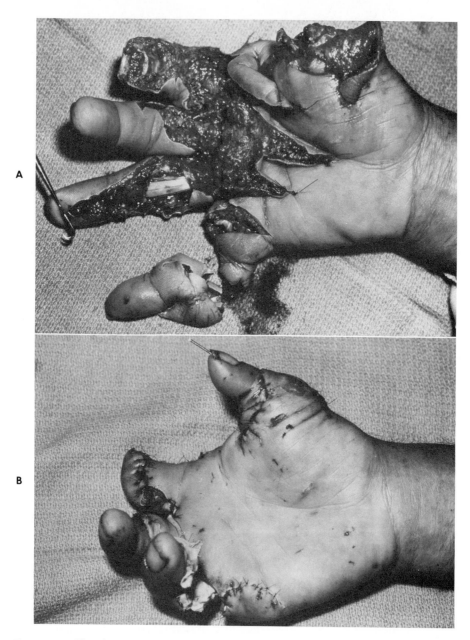

Fig. 22-5. A, Thumb is missing but there is an amputated small finger. **B,** Substituting finger for thumb restored hand function.

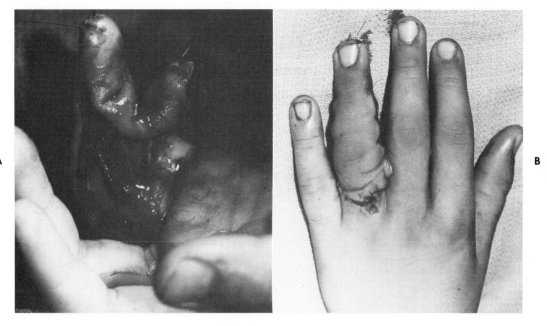

Fig. 22-6. A, Typical ring avulsion injury of skin and neurovascular structures. **B,** Circulation was restored using microvenous graft.

with a head injury and abdominal trauma or multiple other fractures may be too ill to undergo a multihour procedure, and anticoagulants may be contraindicated.

Replantation up to 36 hours after amputation has been reported if the amputated part is kept cold.[16] In the future, if storage techniques are improved, replantation may be possible several days after injury, allowing recovery from life-threatening injuries.

■ What are the steps in replantation?

Replantation surgery is unique in many aspects, one of which is that there is not only the patient, but the amputated part to consider. It is hoped that they both arrive at the same hospital at about the same time. This is certainly not always the case. The amputated part must be handled properly initially or the procedure cannot be carried out. The amputated part should be placed in a moist gauze (Fig. 22-7, *A*). Hypotonic solutions such as plain or sterile water must not come in contact with exposed tissue. The amputated

part should then be placed in a plastic bag (Fig. 22-7, *B*) so that moisture does not escape and the part does not become waterlogged from surrounding solutions. This bag should then be placed in ice (Fig. 22-7, *C*) and covered on all sides. Dry ice should not be used as this will cause freezing, which produces tissue necrosis. Parts should then be x-rayed and taken to the operating room while the patient is being prepared. If practical, the operation can begin on the amputated part while the patient is being readied for surgery. A great deal of time must be spent in properly *identifying* the vessels, nerves, and tendons that are to be repaired and also to debride and clean the wound and shape the bone. Once all of the structures have been identified, they are tagged with different colored sutures so that they do not have to be relocated. After this has been completed, the same procedure is carried out on the amputation stump. If there is a great deal of tissue damage, severe shortening may be necessary. If there is a clean cut, shortening may be minimized to preserve function. Lately, the use of

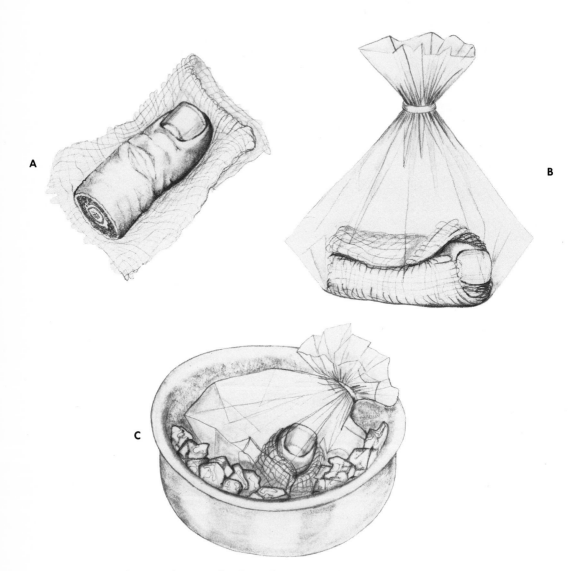

Fig. 22-7. A, Amputated part is placed in saline-moistened gauze. **B,** Digit placed in plastic bag. **C,** Immersed in ice.

interposition microvenous grafts[15,17] has decreased the necessity for extreme shortening. The first step in the actual replantation is securing a solid *bony fixation*. This is usually done with longitudinal or crossed Kirschner wires. The larger structures are repaired first. In the finger this would include the flexor and extensor tendons. At this point the arterial reconstruction is done. The parts are usually identified using loupe *magnification* (4.5× to 6× magnification). The microscope is then brought into position for the arterial repair. The technique of *arterial repair* is illustrated in Fig. 22-1. When the arterial clamps have been removed and circulation is established, the venous drainage can be inspected directly. An attempt is made to *anastomose the veins* that bleed the most profusely after releasing the arterial clamp. If possible, several venous anastomoses are done, usually two for each artery repaired. After successful completion of the arterial and venous anastomoses, the *nerves* are repaired. In past years the major interest was to establish circulation, and surgeons would do the tendon and nerve repairs at a later date. It was soon discovered, however, that reoperating in the area of microvascular anastomosis was very difficult and that better functional results could be obtained if all structures were repaired initially. *Skin closure* can produce complications if it is too constrictive. A very loose closure, a skin graft, or possibly a flap may be necessary. There will usually be some bleeding from the site of anastomosis and if the blood does not have ready access through the incision, a hematoma will develop and the ensuing pressure will occlude the anastomoses.

■ How is the circulation monitored?

An experienced microvascular surgeon can usually tell at a glance the status of a replantation. If there is difficulty with an arterial anastomosis, the replanted part will be quite *pale* and the part will feel empty and cold. If the arterial anastomosis has some function but the venous anastomosis has difficulties, there will be a *blue* congested appearance. Capillary refilling is one of the most common forms of circulation check. It is certainly useful but it can be misleading. Positive capillary refill can be seen on totally amputated segments of tissue. Also manipulation of replanted parts by many observers is not a good idea. A more reliable clinical test is to stick a small needle into the replanted part and observe any bleeding. If a drop of bright red blood appears fairly promptly, this is excellent evidence of intact circulation. Again, this method should not be repeated too often. Small temperature probes have been used to monitor replanted digits. This clinical tool is very useful when performed under strictly controlled conditions. Photoplethysmography has been used and may become more useful in the future.[18] Transcutaneous or percutaneous oxygen measurements are being investigated.[19] The surgeon can locate an area over the vascular anastomosis for checks with a *Doppler* probe. This is a useful way for the nursing staff to monitor the circulation.

■ What parts other than hands can be replanted?

Scalp. It is not uncommon for someone with long hair who works around machinery to sustain a scalping injury. This has classically been treated by skin grafting over which a wig must be placed. Often there was not stable wound healing of the scalp. The first scalp replantation was done in 1975[20] and several successes have followed (Fig. 22-8). It is an extremely rewarding procedure because the scalp has many suitable vessels and usually heals very well. Often the ear, eyebrow, or forehead may be included in the amputated part.[21] All of these can be replanted and the results are usually superb.

Facial parts. A replanted upper lip and nose are illustrated in Fig. 22-9.[22] Ears have been replanted when attached to an avulsed scalp segment. We have performed one ear replantation, which eventually failed. An incomplete ear amputation was revascularized by Hayhurst, resulting in complete success.[23]

Penis. Penile amputations are rare, but this extremity can be replanted as well as any other. The urethra is repaired for stabilization and two arteries are repaired from one vein because of the relatively large size of the veins. Anticoagulation must be kept at a minimum because of the large vascular spaces, which may tend to bleed. An ex-

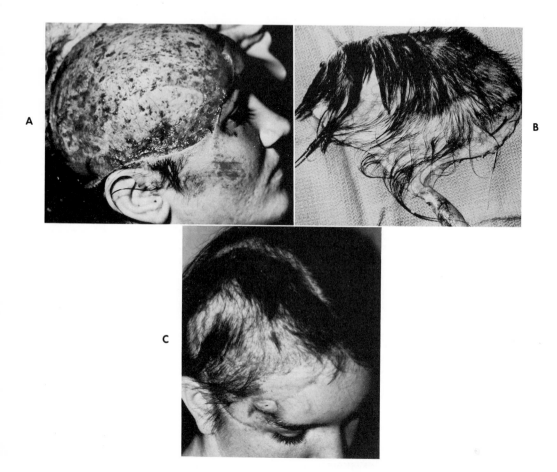

Fig. 22-8. A, An 18-year-old female car wash employee whose long hair became tangled in the rotating shaft of one of the brushes. **B,** Amputated specimen. **C,** Postoperative view at 1 month showing complete survival of the replanted scalp. (From Buncke, H. J.: Plast. Reconstr. Surg. **61**:666, 1978. With permission of the American Society of Plastic and Reconstructive Surgeons, Inc.)

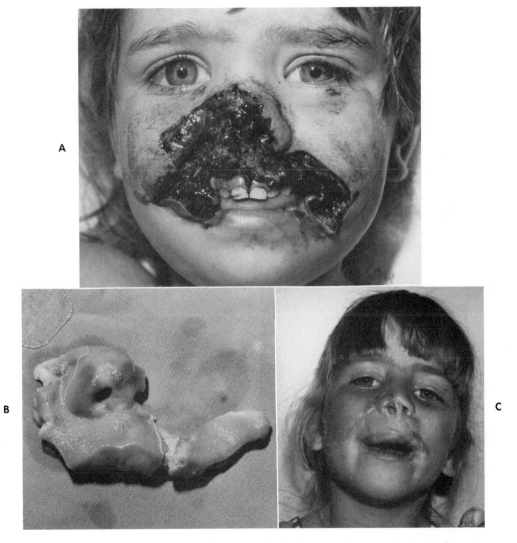

Fig. 22-9. A, Missing facial tissue secondary to dog bite. **B,** Amputated part found after family sent to search for it. **C,** Replanted tissue. (From James, N. J.: Plast. Reconstr. Surg. **58:**623, 1976. With permission of the American Society of Plastic and Reconstructive Surgeons, Inc.)

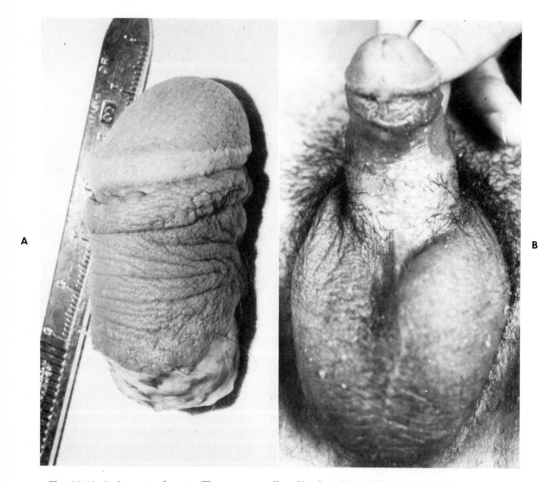

Fig. 22-10. A, Amputated penis. These are usually self-inflicted. **B,** Following replantation, normal urinary function was restored and some sensation returned. (From Cohen, B. E., et al.: Plast. Reconstr. Surg. **59**:276, 1977. With permission of the American Society of Plastic and Reconstructive Surgeons, Inc.)

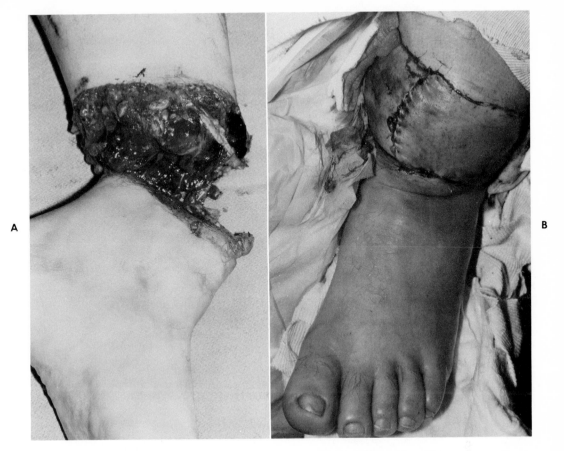

Fig. 22-11. A, Amputated foot secondary to industrial accident. **B,** Replanted foot. This was eventually amputated because of persistent osteomyelitis.

ample of this is illustrated in Fig. 22-10. The reported cases had good urinary flow postoperatively and some are even capable of erection.[24]

Lower limb. Although finger and hand replantations have become common, lower limb replantation is still quite rare. There are several reasons for this. First, a prosthetic replacement for a foot or lower leg offers a much better substitute than those for a thumb or hand. Second, because the force required to amputate a foot is so great, there is usually a great deal of crush injury, making considerable shortening necessary and thus greatly reducing the functional result. The patient pictured in Fig. 22-11 obtained a success-

ful revascularization; however, the foot was amputated because of chronic osteomyelitis before any ambulation occurred. Forefoot and heel[25] replantations in children have been reported. Toes have been replanted. Although toes are certainly not necessary for gait, open-toed shoe styles make a strong case for this in women. One of the most dramatic pictures to be presented from the Chinese cases is of a lower limb replantation to the opposite stump. In this situation, both legs were amputated and the most replantable part was placed on the most suitable stump, producing a very functional result and a very unusual photograph![16]

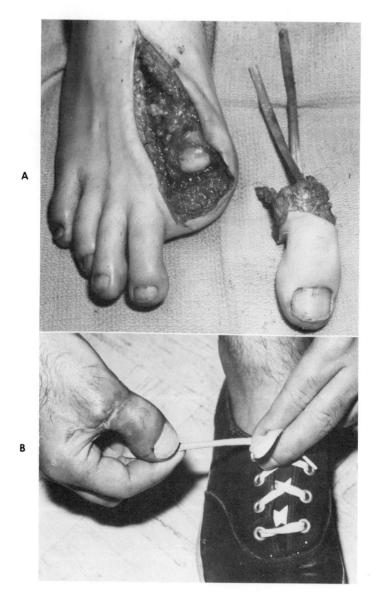

Fig. 22-12. A, Great toe removed in preparation for transfer to hand. **B,** Function of great toe transplant.

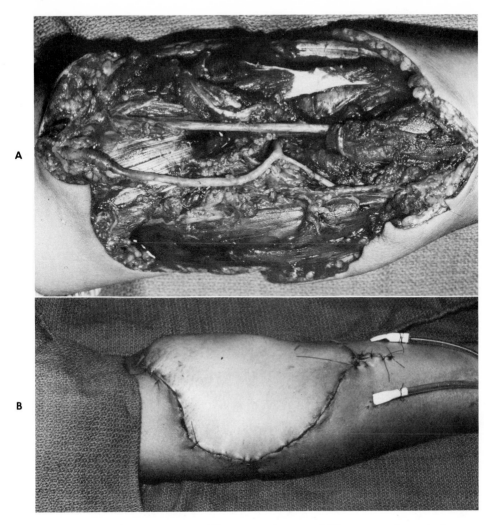

Fig. 22-13. A, Vascular reconstruction following gunshot wound. Flap coverage is required to protect vein grafts. **B,** Free flap taken from groin. Microvascular anastomoses of groin vessels to vein graft in area providing circulation for flap.

■ What are other uses of microvascular surgical techniques?

Flap transfer. In hand reconstruction the first or second toe can be transferred to the hand in a in a one-stage operation, bringing in all of the same elements that were present in the missing digit.[26] This is particularly useful in thumb reconstruction, as illustrated in Fig. 22-12. Flap tissue can be transferred in one stage using these techniques. The most common example is a flap of skin and subcutaneous tissue taken from a groin based on the superficial circumflex iliac artery and vein. These can then be anastomosed to arteries in the recipient bed. In the patient shown in Fig. 22-13 a gunshot wound of the forearm required revascularization of the hand by a vein graft. This then required coverage with a flap.

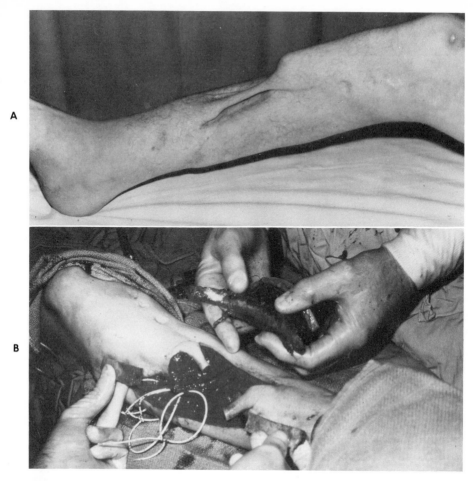

Fig. 22-14. A, There is long defect in tibia with intact fibula and inadequate skin coverage for standard bone graft. **B,** Section of rib is held with intercostal vessels overlying surgeon's index finger. Attached to rib is subcutaneous tissue, muscle, and skin overlying rib. Hands on inferior aspect hold iliac crest bone grafts that were wedged between intact fibula and tibia. **C,** Postoperative appearance showing healed skin flap. There is solid bony union, and there has been marked hypertrophy of vascularized bone graft. Patient is now able to ambulate quite satisfactorily on this leg.

Instead of the multistaged traditional method, this was done in a one-stage operation.

Composite flap transfer. Extending the concept of tissue transfer one stage further, several types of tissue such as skin and bone can be transferred. An example is shown in Fig. 22-14 in which a rib and overlying skin were transferred to a lower limb to reconstruct a traumatic defect of both skin and tibia.

■ **What drugs are used in microvascular surgery?**[27]

Anticoagulants

Heparin. Heparinization was used routinely in the early days of replantation. It has several shortcomings that discourage its use. There is almost always profuse bleeding from the anastomosed vessels, usually requiring multiple transfusions. Additionally, the patency rate of vessels repaired

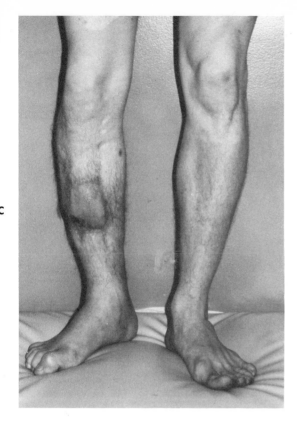

C

Fig. 22-14, cont'd. For legend see opposite page.

using heparin is no greater than those of untreated controls. Often heparin will be given in one dose intraoperatively when there is some technical difficulty or possibly in a low dose treatment of 5000 units twice daily. Heparin solution (100 U/ml) is used routinely for irrigating vessels at surgery.

Dipyridamole (Persantin). Dipyridamole is an anti-inflammatory agent with an action similar to aspirin, but it is also a vasodilator. It was developed originally for use in angina patients. It has proved useful in the postoperative care of replantation patients and is a recommended drug. The dosage is 100 mg every 6 to 8 hours.

Aspirin. Aspirin is extremely effective in preventing platelet aggregation. Also, the use of aspirin usually does not result in excessive bleeding. Aspirin is generally given intraoperatively,

then continued for several weeks postoperatively. Interestingly, the effects of aspirin are detectable after a dose of 3 mg/kg and they persist for 5 to 7 days.

Dextran. Dextran also helps prevent platelet adhesion. It is given in a 6% solution; the low molecular weight variety is usually used. The infusion is started intraoperatively and the concentration reaches its maximum immediately after the end of the infusion. However, the maximum antithrombotic effect occurs 4 hours after the end of an infusion. Dextran 70 has been shown to be more effective than dextran 40. One unit is usually given on each of the first few postoperative days.

Reserpine. Reserpine also produces platelet adhesiveness. It can be administered intra-arterially and results in a prolonged depletion of vessel wall catecholamine content. The maximum dose is 1 mg intra-arterially daily and it should not be used for more than 3 to 4 days.

Antispasmodics

Vessel spasm is one of the greatest enemies of the microvascular surgeon. Warm solutions of 2% lidocaine (Xylocaine) (without epinephrine), papaverine, chlorpromazine, or magnesium sulfate have been used. A recent study by Swartz[28] has shown these to be of benefit in preventing thrombosis. Vasodilatation can also be obtained by long-acting axillary block or epidural infusion. Some workers have even left catheters in the axillary sheath for continuous infusion of anesthetic agents. We have successfully used a vein graft at the site of the anastomosis as a conduit for local administration of topical lidocaine (Xylocaine) in the postoperative period.[29] Postoperative administration of chlorpromazine is also useful because it is known to inhibit the second phase of platelet aggregation and it reduces anxiety because of its tranquilizing effect. This reduction in anxiety can help produce vasospasm. Recommended dosage is 10 mg orally every 8 hours for about a week. Isoxsuprine may play an important role in the future. Laboratory studies and early clinical trials show promise.[30]

REFERENCES

1. Danilevicius, Z.: Cosmos and Damian, the patron saints of medicine in art, J.A.M.A. **201:**1021, 1967.

2. Jacobson, J. H., and Suarez, E. L.: Microsurgery in anastomosis of small vessels, Surg. Forum **11**:243, 1960.
3. Malt, R. A., and McKhann, C.: Replantation of severed arms, J.A.M.A. **189**:716, 1964.
4. Ch'en, C. W., Ch'ien, Y. C., and Pav, Y. S.: Salvage of the forearm following complete traumatic amputation; report of a case, Chin. Med. J. **82**:623, 1963.
5. Komatsu, S., and Tamai, S.: Successful replantation of a completely cut-off thumb, Plast. Reconstr. Surg. **42**:374, 1968.
6. Smith, J. W.: Microsurgery of peripheral nerves, Plast. Reconstr. Surg. **33**:317, 1964.
7. Millesi, H.: Nerve grafting. In Converse, J. M., editor: Reconstructive plastic surgery: principles and procedures in correction, reconstruction, and transplantation, ed. 2, Philadelphia, 1977, W. B. Saunders Co., p. 3227.
8. Buncke, H. J., Furnas, D. W., Gordon, L., and Achauer, B. M.: Free osteocutaneous flap from a rib to the tibia, Plast. Reconstr. Surg. **59**:799, 1977.
9. Daniel, R. K.: Mandibular reconstruction with free tissue transfers, Ann. Plast. Surg. **1**:346, 1978.
10. Cerruti, R. A., Jepson, P., Furnas, D. W., and Silber, I.: Vasovasostomy, Urology **3**:209, 1974.
11. O'Brien, B. M., Sykes, P. J., and Threlfall, G. N.: Microlymphaticovenous anastomoses for obstructive lymphedema, Plast. Reconstr. Surg. **60**:197, 1977.
12. Weiland, A. J., et al.: Replantation of digits and hands: analysis of surgical techniques and functional results in 71 patients with 86 replantations, J. Hand Surg. **2**:1, 1977.
13. Gelberman, R. H., Urbaniak, J. R., Bright, D. S., and Levin, L. S.: Digital sensibility following replantation, J. Hand Surg. **3**:313, 1978.
14. Furnas, D. W., Salibian, A. H., and Achauer, B. M.: Genesis of a replantation program, Am. J. Surg. **136**:21, 1978.
15. Van Beck, A. L., Kutz, J. E., and Zook, E. G.: Importance of the ribbon sign, indicating unsuitability of the vessel in replanting a finger, Plast. Reconstr. Surg. **61**:32, 1978.
16. Buncke, H. J., et al.: Replantation surgery in China: report of the American replantation mission to China, Plast. Reconstr. Surg. **52**:477, 1973.
17. Biemer, E.: Vein grafts in microvascular surgery, Br. J. Plast. Surg. **30**:197, 1977.
18. Jobsis, F. F., Barwick, W. J., and Boyd, J. B.: Optical monitoring as a research and clinical method to assess tissue metabolism and blood flow. In Serafin, D., and Buncke, H. J., Jr.: Microsurgical composite tissue transplantation, St. Louis, 1978, The C. V. Mosby Co., p. 191.
19. Achauer, B. M., Black, K. W., Beran, A. V., and Huxtable, R. F.: Transcutaneous Po_2 monitoring of flap circulation following surgery. In Lucey, J. F., editor: Blood gas monitoring, New York, 1979, Alan R. Liss, Inc., p. 517.
20. Miller, G. P., Anstee, E. J., and Snell, J. A.: Successful replantation of an avulsed scalp by microvascular anastomoses, Plast. Reconstr. Surg. **58**:133, 1976.
21. Buncke, H. J., Rose, E. H., Brownstein, M. J., and Chater, N. L.: Successful replantation of two avulsed scalps by microvascular anastomoses, Plast. Reconstr. Surg. **61**:666, 1978.
22. James, N. J.: Survival of large replanted segment of upper lip and nose, Plast. Reconstr. Surg. **58**:623, 1976.
23. Nahai, F., Hayhurst, J. W., and Salibian, A. H.: Microvascular surgery in avulsive trauma to the external ear, Clin. Plast. Surg. **5**:423, 1978.
24. Cohen, B. J., May, J. W., Daly, J. S., and Young, H. H.: Successful clinical replantation of an amputated penis by microneurovascular repair: case report, Plast. Reconstr. Surg. **59**:276, 1977.
25. Zook, E., VanBeek, A. L., and Wavak, P. W.: Replantation of the heel in a child, Ann. Plast. Surg. **2**:154, 1979.
26. Cobbett, J. R.: Free digital transfer: report of a case of transfer of a great toe to replace an amputated thumb, J. Bone Joint Surg. **51**:677, 1969.
27. Ketchum, L. D.: Pharmacological alterations in the clotting mechanism: use in microvascular surgery, J. Hand Surg. **3**:407, 1978.
28. Swartz, W. M., Brink, R. R., and Buncke, H. J.: Prevention of thrombosis in arterial and venous microanastomoses by using topical agents, Plast. Reconstr. Surg. **58**:478, 1976.
29. Furnas, D. W., and Salibian, A. H.: Vein graft conduit for delivery of topical drugs to a microvascular anastomosis, Plast. Reconstr. Surg. **63**:129, 1979.
30. Finseth, F., and Adeberg, M. G.: Experimental work with Isoxsuprine for prevention of skin flap necrosis and for treatment of the failing flap, Plast. Reconstr. Surg. **63**:94, 1979.

CHAPTER 23

Endocrine and metabolic disorders

Bernhard G. Anderson

The endocrine system consists of glands that secrete hormones directly into the bloodstream. As customarily defined, the endocrine glands include the pituitary, thyroid, parathyroids, adrenals, ovaries, testes, and the islet cells of the pancreas. The hypothalamus, part of the brain, secretes "releasing" factors or hormones that release or inhibit the secretion of the hormones of the anterior pituitary gland. In pregnancy the placenta has important endocrine functions.

A wide variety of organs and cells secrete hormones directly into the blood but are not usually classified as endocrine glands. The kidneys secrete erythropoietin, which stimulates red blood cell production, and renin, which raises the blood pressure through the angiotensin system and affects aldosterone secretion by the adrenal cortex. Gastrointestinal hormones include secretin and gastrin. Prostaglandins, kinins, and serotonin are chemical compounds found in blood that are of diverse or uncertain origin and have important physiologic effects. They are sometimes classified as hormones, although they are not customarily included as part of the endocrine system. The endocrine status of the pineal gland and the thymus is uncertain.

Metabolism refers to a complex variety of biochemical processes that occur in organs, tissues, and cells of the body and are concerned with the utilization of oxygen and food for energy and growth. Metabolic disorders are closely related to various endocrine functions, and hormones serve as regulators of many metabolic processes.

The action of hormones depends on a specific interaction between the hormone and a receptor that is usually located in a cell or in the cell membrane. The regulation of hormone activity is complex. Most endocrine disorders are associated with excessive or deficient secretion of hormones.

This chapter is concerned with the major endocrine and metabolic disorders that may be encountered in the management of critically ill patients. The frequency of occurrence of these disorders will depend in part on the type of patients seen in a particular hospital or critical care facility. Although adrenal disease as a cause of adrenal insufficiency is rare, adrenocortical insufficiency secondary to suppression of adrenocortical function by treatment with adrenal steroids is common. Diabetic ketoacidosis and hypercalcemia are relatively common. Some of these disorders are encountered infrequently.

The following topics will be discussed in this chapter: adrenocortical hormones, adrenocortical insufficiency, calcium disorders (hypercalcemia and hypocalcemia), diabetic ketoacidosis, hyperglycemia nonketotic hyperosmolar coma, hypoglycemia, pheochromocytoma, thyroid disorders (hyperthyroid crisis and myxedema coma), and water metabolism and antidiuretic hormone (deficiency and excess).

ADRENOCORTICAL HORMONES

The adrenal cortex secretes various steroid hormones—the most important are cortisol and aldosterone. Androgens, estrogens, and progestins are also secreted but are functionally less important. Cortisol, the major glucocorticoid, contributes to the maintenance of the blood glucose level mainly by promoting gluconeogenesis from amino acids; thus it is protein catabolic. Cortisol increases the glomerular filtration rate and thus enhances water diuresis. Glucocorticoids also have lympholytic and eosinopenic effects and tend to increase the number of erythrocytes in the blood. Various other glucocorticoid effects include stimulation of the central nervous system, increased gastric acidity, and fat mobilization. Of great importance are the anti-inflammatory and the immunosuppressive actions of glucocorticoids. These actions are the basis for the therapeutic use of cortisol and related glucocorticoids in a wide variety of diseases. Aldosterone, the major mineralocorticoid, promotes the retention of sodium and the excretion of potassium by the kidneys. Cortisol, although primarily a glucocorticoid, also has mineralocorticoid effects when given in large amounts.

■ **What interrelations govern the hypothalamus, anterior pituitary gland, and adrenal cortex?**

Corticotropin (ACTH), secreted by the anterior pituitary gland, stimulates the adrenal cortex to produce cortisol. Diurnal variation in the release of corticotropin normally occurs so that it is released in the greatest amounts about 4 AM to 6 AM and in the least amounts about 12 hours later. The secretion of cortisol closely follows the release of corticotropin. A servoregulatory mechanism operates to stimulate the release of corticotropin when the plasma cortisol level falls and to suppress corticotropin when the plasma cortisol level rises. Stress—including trauma, infections, psychic factors, and a wide variety of illnesses—stimulates the release of corticotropin and consequently the secretion of cortisol. Stressful stimuli apparently induce the hypothalamus to secrete corticotropin-releasing factor.

■ **What governs aldosterone secretion?**

Aldosterone is not under direct corticotropin control but is regulated mainly by the renin-angiotensin system. Aldosterone secretion increases in response to a reduction in intravascular volume such as occurs with sodium depletion, acute hemorrhage, or severe fluid losses.

■ **What are synthetic steroids?**

Hydrocortisone is the pharmacologic name for synthetic cortisol. Synthetic adrenocortical steroids have been produced that have potent glucocorticoid effects with little or no mineralocorticoid effects. These agents include prednisone, prednisolone, triamcinolone, betamethasone, and dexamethasone. They are widely used for their anti-inflammatory effects and other glucocorticoid effects. Fludrocortisone is a synthetic mineralocorticoid that resembles aldosterone.

ADRENOCORTICAL INSUFFICIENCY

Acute adrenocortical insufficiency is precipitated by stress in patients with chronic adrenocortical insufficiency, anterior pituitary insufficiency, or adrenocortical suppression from glucocorticoid therapy. In patients without previous adrenal disorders adrenocortical failure is rare but may result from adrenal hemorrhage or infarction.

■ **How is it recognized?**

Manifestations of adrenocortical insufficiency include weakness, hypotension, shock, fever, and reduced consciousness. Hyperpigmentation of the skin and mucous membranes is seen in patients with chronic primary adrenocortical insufficiency. The serum sodium concentration is usually low and the potassium level high in primary adrenocortical failure but not in cases secondary to pituitary insufficiency or suppression by previous corticosteroid treatment. The blood glucose level tends to be low and the blood urea nitrogen level elevated. The diagnosis is confirmed by finding a low value for plasma cortisol or 17-hydroxycorticosteroids, but treatment must be started immediately when there is reasonable suspicion without awaiting laboratory confirmation.

■ **What is the treatment?**

1. Hydrocortisone, 100 mg, should be given intravenously at once. A water-soluble preparation of hydrocortisone such as the sodium succinate or phosphate form is used. Additional hydrocortisone in 5% dextrose and 0.9% saline (sodium chloride) is infused intravenously at a rate of 10 mg of hydrocortisone per hour for 24 hours; alternatively, 50 mg of hydrocortisone can be given intramuscularly every 6 hours.

2. An intravenous infusion of 5% dextrose in 0.9% saline, 1 L, should be started immediately. The total fluid replacement in the first 24 hours is about 3 L, usually 5% dextrose in 0.9% saline. Thereafter 1 L of 5% dextrose in 0.9% saline daily is usually adequate, with 5% to 10% dextrose in water making up the remainder of the fluid requirements.

3. No potassium is given in the first 24 to 48 hours because the serum potassium level is already elevated. Later, maintenance amounts of potassium will be needed, usually 40 to 60 mEq daily given as potassium chloride.

4. Vasopressors such as norepinephrine or metaraminol may be needed if the hypotension does not respond to hydrocortisone, fluid, and sodium replacement.

5. The hydrocortisone dose is reduced to 25 mg every 6 hours on the second or third day and progressively reduced to reach maintenance amounts of 20 to 30 mg daily in divided doses within 1 week. This can usually be given orally after the acute crisis has subsided.

6. A mineralocorticoid is usually needed to promote sodium retention when the hydrocortisone dose is less than 60 mg/day. Fludrocortisone is given orally; the average dose is 0.1 mg daily.

7. Fluids can be given orally as soon as tolerated, followed by a regular diet that usually obviates the need for sodium and potassium supplements.

8. Precipitating causes and concurrent diseases should be identified and treated appropriately.

■ What is secondary adrenocortical insufficiency?

Secondary adrenocortical insufficiency is due to deficiency or suppression of corticotropin. Cortisol is deficient, but aldosterone secretion is not greatly decreased. Therefore sodium depletion is uncommon, and mineralocorticoids are seldom needed. The treatment is otherwise the same as for primary adrenocortical insufficiency.

■ How should stress be managed?

Management of stress in patients with adrenocortical insufficiency is concerned with providing optimal support for patients with chronic ad-

renal insufficiency, hypopituitarism, or recent adrenal corticosteroid therapy (within 6 months) who have major acute illnesses or trauma or are undergoing surgery. Similar management is appropriate for patients undergoing elective bilateral adrenalectomy. Hydrocortisone is given intravenously at a rate of 10 mg/hour beginning ½ to 1 hour before the induction of anesthesia. Alternatively hydrocortisone can be given intramuscularly in doses of 50 mg every 6 hours. Some physicians prefer to give cortisone acetate intramuscularly in doses of 50 to 100 mg beginning 12 hours before surgery. The other details of management are similar to those described in the preceding section.

CALCIUM DISORDERS

Calcium is important in various membrane transport systems, which accounts for its effects on nerve, muscle, and heart function. About one half of the calcium in the blood plasma is bound to plasma proteins or complexed with other ions; the other half is ionized and physiologically available. Although *total* calcium concentration in the serum is usually measured, the *ionized* calcium is the important fraction that determines its physiologic activity. Thus total calcium concentration may be low in patients with low plasma protein levels, but the ionized calcium fraction may be normal. Alkalosis decreases and acidosis increases the ionized fraction of calcium. Hypercalcemia depresses neuromuscular excitability and causes bradycardia, cardiac arrhythmias, and impaired renal function. Hypocalcemia increases neuromuscular excitability and causes tetany.

■ What factors regulate calcium metabolism?

Calcium metabolism is regulated by parathyroid hormone, thyrocalcitonin, and vitamin D. A deficiency of parathyroid hormone leads to hypocalcemia, whereas an excess of parathyroid hormone produces hypercalcemia. This hormone has two major effects: (1) it maintains the plasma concentration of calcium at its normal level, about 9 to 11 mg/dl (values differ among laboratories), and (2) it promotes the renal excretion of phosphate. Thyrocalcitonin, which is secreted by the thyroid gland, lowers the plasma calcium level. Vitamin D promotes calcium absorption from the gut, contributes to the maintenance of a normal plasma calcium level, induces the calcification of new bone, and increases the renal excretion of calcium.

Hypercalcemia

■ What causes hypercalcemia?

Hypercalcemia may be caused by tumors metastatic to bone and occasionally by neoplasms that secrete a parathyroid hormone–like substance. Hyperparathyroidism is a classic cause of hypercalcemia. Less common causes of hypercalcemia include hypervitaminosis D, the milk-alkali syndrome, multiple myeloma, sarcoidosis, Paget's disease in immobilized patients, thiazide diuretics, hyperthyroidism, and adrenal insufficiency.

■ What is the treatment of hypercalcemia?

The urgency and vigor with which treatment must be pursued depends on the severity of the hypercalcemia. A patient with a serum calcium concentration in excess of 15 mg/dl is usually in critical condition and requires intensive care. It is important to monitor the fluid intake and output, body weight, serum electrolyte concentrations, electrocardiogram, and central venous pressure. Fluid overload must be prevented. Adverse changes in the serum concentrations of sodium, potassium, calcium, and magnesium may occur. Agents that lower the serum calcium level include: (1) drugs that increase the urinary excretion of calcium, such as saline and furosemide; (2) drugs that increase calcium precipitation or retard bone dissolution, such as phosphates and mithramycin; and (3) measures that decrease the gastrointestinal absorption of calcium.

■ Specifically what measures are indicated?

1. Hydration is accomplished with isotonic sodium chloride solution 3 to 5 L given over 24 hours.

2. Furosemide is administered in doses of 40 to 120 mg every 4 to 6 hours to induce sodium and calcium excretion. Potassium losses from diuresis will need to be replaced.

3. Phosphates may be given, provided that renal function is adequate and the patient is not hyperphosphatemic. Preparations containing monobasic and dibasic sodium and potassium phosphate may be given orally; the equivalent of 2 to 3 g of phosphorus is given daily in divided doses. Neutra-Phos contains 250 mg of phosphorus per capsule (which should be dissolved in 75 ml of water). Phospho-Soda contains 1 g of phosphorus per 8 ml; 4 ml diluted in 200 ml of water can be given 3 or 4 times daily. Preparations of neutral phosphate can be infused intravenously slowly, 50 mmoles over 6 to 8 hours, but the use of these preparations is hazardous.

4. Mithramycin may be effective in patients with hyperphosphatemia or impaired renal function. A single dose of 25 μg/kg of body weight is administered in 0.9% sodium chloride solution slowly over 3 to 4 hours. This may be adequate to lower the serum calcium level to normal within 48 to 72 hours. This drug is potentially toxic.

5. Prednisone, 60 to 80 mg daily, may be helpful, but its effects are too slow (several days) in an acute situation. It is usually not effective in patients with hyperparathyroidism.

Not all of these measures are needed in all patients with hypercalcemia. Hydration and diuresis may be sufficient to restore the serum calcium level to normal in the milder cases of hypercalcemia.

Hypocalcemia

■ What are the causes and signs of hypocalcemia?

Acute hypocalcemia may develop within a few hours postoperatively if the parathyroid glands have been damaged or removed in patients undergoing thyroidectomy. Chronic hypocalcemia occurs in hypoparathyroidism, rickets, and osteomalacia; occasionally it may be a manifestation of magnesium deficiency.

Acute hypocalcemia increases neuromuscular irritability and tetany may occur. Chvostek's sign (twitching of the side of the face in response to tapping over the facial nerve in front of the ear) is usually positive. The serum calcium level is low. Neuromuscular irritability and tetany may occur in patients with alkalosis, although the total serum calcium level is normal. In patients with chronic hypocalcemia, tetany may be induced by alkalosis.

■ How should hypocalcemia be treated?

Effective measures in treating hypocalcemia include calcium, vitamin D, and possibly magnesium as follows.

1. In an urgent situation calcium gluconate, 10 ml of a 10% solution, should be given intravenously over several minutes. Great caution is mandatory if the patient is receiving digitalis or its glycosides because of the synergistic effects of calcium and digitalis on the heart. In less acute situations calcium salts can be given orally; 10 to 25 g of calcium lactate or calcium gluconate may be needed daily. Dietary calcium should be increased but dietary phosphates decreased. Milk products should be avoided because they are rich in phosphates as well as calcium. Sedation may be helpful.

2. Hypocalcemia after thyroid or parathyroid surgery may be temporary, lasting only a few days or a few weeks. If the condition appears to be permanent or cannot be controlled by calcium given orally, vitamin D is prescribed. Calciferol in doses of 200,000 units daily is given, with reduction of the dose as the serum calcium concentration is restored to normal. Dihydrotachysterol may be preferable because of its quicker onset and shorter duration of action; the dosage range is 0.2 to 1 mg/day. The serum calcium concentration should be monitored frequently (initially every week, then less often) to maintain the serum calcium level at about 9 to 10 mg/dl. Hypercalcemia from overtreatment must be avoided.

3. Magnesium deficiency sometimes accompanies hypocalcemia, and the hypocalcemia may not respond to treatment unless the magnesium deficiency is corrected. Magnesium sulfate, 2 ml of a 50% solution, may be given intramuscularly in an acute situation. In patients with severe magnesium depletion, 2 mEq of magnesium per kilogram of body weight may be given intravenously over 4 to 6 hours.

Chronic hypocalcemia may not require treatment. Patients with hypocalcemia secondary to low plasma protein levels may have a normal ionized fraction of calcium in the blood and need no treatment for hypocalcemia.

DIABETIC KETOACIDOSIS

Diabetic ketoacidosis is a metabolic emergency caused by a deficiency of insulin or resistance to its action. The failure to metabolize glucose leads to overproduction of glucose by the liver and hyperglycemia. The metabolism of fat is accelerated but is incomplete; this produces an accumulation of ketones, acetoacetic acid, and beta-hydroxybutyric acid. A severe degree of metabolic acidosis results, together with excessive amounts of acetone and ketones in the blood and urine. The osmotic diuresis induced by the hyperglycemia produces severe dehydration with depletion of sodium and potassium.

The clinical manifestations include weakness, polyuria, and polydipsia with dehydration, hyperpnea, and coma in severe cases. Ketoacidosis is precipitated in patients with diabetes mellitus by intercurrent diseases, especially infections or failure to take insulin. Ketoacidosis sometimes is the presenting problem in patients with previously unrecognized diabetes mellitus.

■ What are the laboratory data?

The blood glucose level is high, usually in the range of 400 to 800 mg/dl. The serum pH is low (a pH of 7.1 indicates a doubling of the hydrogen ion concentration). The serum bicarbonate concentration is low—in severe cases less than 10 mEq/L. Tests for acetone and glucose in the serum and urine are strongly positive. Leukocytosis is common. The serum sodium concentration may be low, normal, or high, depending on the severity of dehydration and degree of sodium depletion. The serum potassium concentration may be normal in the presence of a severe body potassium deficit because the acidosis causes an intracellular-to-extracellular shift of potassium. The severity of the patient's condition is more closely related to the degree of acidosis than to the degree of hyperglycemia.

■ How should diabetic ketoacidosis be treated?

Insulin, fluids, and potassium are the most important requirements. Prompt initiation of treatment and meticulous attention to patient care are essential for a successful therapeutic outcome.

■ How much insulin is needed?

For many years large amounts of insulin were thought to be necessary to overcome insulin resistance and reestablish the metabolism of glucose. Therapeutic failure was often attributed to the use of inadequate amounts of insulin. Since 1972, the efficacy of small doses of insulin has been recognized and the use of "low-dose" regimens has attained widespread acceptance.

■ **What is low-dose insulin therapy?**

Insulin in amounts as little as 2 to 10 units per hour given by constant intravenous infusion can be effective in the treatment of diabetic ketoacidosis. Similarly small doses of insulin can be effective when given by the intravenous or intramuscular route at hourly intervals.

■ **What are the advantages of low-dose insulin therapy?**

Hypoglycemia and hypokalemia are less likely to occur as complications of treatment. The low-dose protocols are simple to implement and seldom require hourly adjustments in the dose of insulin.

■ **What are the disadvantages of low-dose insulin therapy?**

Some patients may not respond to low doses of insulin. Rarely, patients with excessive resistance to insulin may be encountered, and these patients may require several hundred units of insulin for successful treatment. Little is gained by attempting to use the minimum effective dose of insulin and much may be lost.

■ **Which method of insulin therapy is recommended?**

1. Promptly give 10 to 25 units of regular insulin intravenously as the initial dose. In milder cases this priming dose may be omitted.

2. Give 10 units of insulin per hour by continuous intravenous infusion.

3. If the blood glucose level does not decrease substantially within 2 hours, increase the dose of insulin to 20 units per hour. In more severe cases, increase the dose to 100 units per hour.

4. When the blood glucose level declines to 250 mg/dl or less, decrease the rate of insulin infusion to 2 to 5 units per hour. Alternatively, insulin may be given intramuscularly or subcutaneously at intervals of 1 to 2 hours. The dose should be adjusted in accordance with the blood glucose level.

■ **Is insulin adsorbed to containers and tubing?**

Some loss of insulin may occur from adsorption to glass or plastic bottles and tubing, but the amount lost is small. This problem can be avoided by diluting the insulin in a 1% solution of serum albumin or by running 100 ml of a solution of 5 units of insulin per deciliter through the tubing before using the tubing to administer insulin to the patient.

■ **What fluids and electrolytes are indicated?**

Several liters of fluid are usually needed in the first 24 hours.

1. Sodium chloride, 0.9% solution, 1 L, should be given intravenously in the first hour. Additional amounts of isotonic sodium chloride solution are given subsequently at slower rates of infusion.

2. Potassium replacement should be instituted within 1 hour of starting insulin therapy unless the patient is oliguric or hyperkalemic. Potassium chloride is given intravenously at a rate of 20 mEq/hr. The total potassium deficit may be 200 to 500 mEq; 100 to 200 mEq of potassium should be replaced in the first 12 hours.

3. Phosphorus depletion probably occurs in most patients with diabetic ketoacidosis, but the optimal dose of phosphorus for replacement is unknown. Some of the potassium replenishment can be given as potassium phosphate solution.

4. Dextrose solution, 5% in water, should be started when blood glucose level falls below 300 mg/dl. This is given to furnish fuel for energy, prevent hypoglycemia, and inhibit ketoacidosis.

5. Sodium bicarbonate is recommended if the serum pH is less than 7.0 or if the serum bicarbonate concentration is less than 5 mEq/L. Bicarbonate, 50 to 100 mEq, is given as sodium bicarbonate solution intravenously. The use of excessive amounts of bicarbonate may be hazardous; cardiac arrhythmias, alkalosis, and aggravation of phosphorus and potassium deficiencies may occur.

■ **What other measures are indicated?**

1. A urethral catheter may be needed in anuric or comatose patients, but catheters should be avoided because of the danger of infection.

2. Gastric lavage with warm isotonic saline solution may be advisable if gastric dilatation or persistent vomiting occurs.

3. An adequate airway must be established if the patient is comatose.

4. The search for and treatment of precipitating causes of the ketoacidosis should be initiated promptly.

■ **What monitoring procedures are useful?**

Frequent determinations of the blood glucose level, serum pH, and serum electrolyte concentrations are essential. Tests for glucose and ketones in the urine at hourly intervals are helpful. The ECG may provide evidence of hypokalemia. Accurate records of fluid intake and output, amounts of insulin and electrolytes given, and results of laboratory tests are indispensable. A "flow sheet" that shows the essential data in readily comprehensible form is highly desirable.

■ **When can intermediate or long-acting insulin preparations be used?**

As soon as the patient recovers from the acute episode of ketoacidosis, an appropriate diet and intermediate or long-acting insulin preparations such as NPH or the lente insulins can be prescribed.

■ **How are diabetic patients managed during surgery?**

Surgical procedures require special management in diabetic patients. For patients taking insulin, one half of the usual daily dose of lente or NPH insulin is given on the morning of surgery, together with a slow infusion of 5% dextrose in water. This may be supplemented with additional doses of short-acting insulin, depending on the blood glucose level. Usually the urine should be tested for glucose and acetone every 2 to 4 hours postoperatively, and insulin should be administered depending on the urine glucose concentration and the response to previously administered doses of insulin. As the patient improves and is able to tolerate food, the previously established insulin regimen can be implemented. Hypoglycemia must be carefully watched for and promptly treated.

■ **What adjustments in insulin dosage should be made during acute illness?**

Diabetic patients with acute illness, especially infections or gastrointestinal disturbances, may require increased or unpredictable amounts of insulin. In these situations it may be advsiable to use short-acting insulin preparations. This facilitates frequent modifications of the dosage of insulin as may be required during rapidly changing circumstances.

■ **What types of metabolic acidosis may be associated with diabetic ketoacidosis?**

Lactic acidosis and alcoholic ketoacidosis are forms of metabolic acidosis that should be considered in the differential diagnosis.

■ **What is lactic acidosis?**

Lactic acidosis is an uncommon but extremely severe disorder that may occur in diabetic as well as nondiabetic patients. It is usually precipitated by anoxia. The serum lactate:pyruvate ratio usually exceeds 10:1. An unexplained "anion gap" in the concentration of electrolytes in the serum occurs. Sodium bicarbonate should be given to counteract the acidosis. Fluid deficits should be replaced. Insulin may be needed in diabetic patients.

■ **What is alcoholic ketoacidosis?**

Alcoholic ketoacidosis refers to a severe form of metabolic acidosis that occurs in chronic users of excess amounts of alcohol (ethanol). After prolonged bouts of drinking alcoholic beverages with inadequate food intake, gastrointestinal distress and vomiting occur. The ketone levels in the blood, especially beta-hydroxybutyrate, are increased. The blood glucose concentration seldom exceeds 300 mg/dl. Hypoglycemia sometimes occurs. The condition usually responds to the intravenous administration of dextrose solutions. Fluid and electrolyte deficits should be replaced. Insulin is not usually needed unless the blood glucose level exceeds 300 mg/dl. These patients may be excessively sensitive to the effects of insulin.

HYPERGLYCEMIC NONKETOTIC HYPEROSMOLAR COMA

This syndrome characteristically occurs in patients with maturity-onset diabetes mellitus, although it can occur at any age. The characteristic features of this disorder are severe dehydration and hyperglycemia without ketoacidosis—

hence the term "hyperglycemic nonketotic hyper-osmolar coma." The syndrome is precipitated by concurrent disease. Relative insulin deficiency leads to hyperglycemia and osmotic diuresis. In the absence of adequate fluid replacement, extremely severe dehydration occurs. Mental obtundation is profound, with or without coma. Mild ketosis may be found. The blood glucose level may be extremely elevated. The condition is fatal if untreated.

■ **What is the treatment?**

Hydration is essential in the treatment of hyperglycemic nonketotic hyperosmolar coma. An isotonic solution of sodium chloride, 1 or 2 L, is given initially, intravenously. Hypotonic saline, 0.45% solution of sodium chloride, is given subsequently. Dextrose solutions are contraindicated until the blood glucose concentration has decreased below 300 mg/dl; then dextrose solutions are given to provide water without excess sodium. Water deficits of 8 to 10 L or more are common. Potassium replacement will almost always be needed, and larger amounts will usually be required earlier than in patients with diabetic ketoacidosis.

■ **How much insulin is needed?**

There is some evidence that the insulin requirements in hyperglycemic nonketotic coma are less than in diabetic ketoacidosis. However, excessive insulin resistance as well as insulin sensitivity does occur in this syndrome, and the insulin requirements usually approximate those in diabetic ketoacidosis. Regular insulin should be given promptly: 10 to 25 units initially intravenously, followed by 10 units per hour by continuous intravenous infusion. The dose should be increased if the response is inadequate. For the first 24 hours the blood glucose level should be maintained above 250 mg/dl.

Lactic acidosis occasionally occurs as a complication and requires bicarbonate therapy. Concurrent diseases must be searched for and treated appropriately.

HYPOGLYCEMIA

The brain is dependent almost entirely on glucose for its metabolism. Therefore it is extremely important that hypoglycemia be recognized and treated promptly. In critically ill patients hypoglycemia is probably most commonly encountered in diabetics receiving insulin. Other causes include impaired liver function with inadequate food intake, adrenal insufficiency, insulinomas and other insulin-producing tumors, and a variety of drugs but mainly the sulfonylureas and phenformin (oral antidiabetic agents). Neuromuscular irritability, tremor, excess sweating, and tachycardia occur in response to epinephrine release by the adrenal medulla. With more severe degrees of hypoglycemia convulsions or coma may occur. The blood glucose concentration is usually less than 50 mg/dl. Treatment should be started on reasonable suspicion without awaiting the results of the blood glucose determination.

■ **What is the treatment of hypoglycemia?**

Dextrose (d—glucose) is the specific treatment for hypoglycemia. Dextrose should be given intravenously in severe situations; 10 to 25 g are usually adequate, but more may be needed. Because of its high viscosity, 50% dextrose solution is difficult to inject: 20% solutions are easier. Alternatively, glucagon can be given subcutaneously, intramuscularly, or intravenously in doses of 1 to 5 mg; it is effective in patients with excess insulin but not in patients with impaired liver function.

For the milder hypoglycemic reactions to insulin in diabetic patients orange juice administered orally in amounts of 120 to 180 ml may be sufficient. Frequent feedings, especially bedtime feedings, are helpful in preventing hypoglycemia in patients treated with long-acting insulin.

For severe cases of hypoglycemia in patients with insulin-producing tumors, diazoxide may be helpful as well as cortisone acetate or other glucocorticoids.

PHEOCHROMOCYTOMA

Paroxysmal or sustained hypertension occurs in patients with pheochromocytoma, a tumor of the adrenal medulla or sympathetic nerve endings. These tumors secrete norepinephrine and epinephrine, are uncommon, and are curable by surgery. Labile hypertension associated with palpitation, headache, and excessive sweating are characteristic manifestations. The diagnosis is established by finding excessive urinary excretion of catecholamines or their metabolites. Hypertensive crises may occur. Preoperative and postoperative care requires special pharmacologic management.

■ **What drugs are indicated for treatment?**

Phentolamine (Regitine) and phenoxybenzamine (Dibenzyline) are useful to control blood pressure. Both are α-adrenergic blocking agents; they inhibit the effects of catecholamines but do not alter their synthesis or degradation. Phentolamine is short acting; repeated doses of 1 to 5 mg intravenously may be needed to control paroxysmal hypertension. Phenoxybenzamine is longer acting; doses of 40 to 100 mg orally every 12 hours are given for more sustained control of the hypertension. Propranolol (Inderal), a β-adrenergic blocker, is useful in controlling catecholamine-induced arrhythmias, tachycardia, angina, and sweating. Doses of 40 mg or more every 4 to 6 hours may be needed. When possible, it is probably wise to establish α-adrenergic blockade before giving β-adrenergic blockers so as to avoid unopposed α-adrenergic stimulation.

■ **What precautions should be observed?**

Drugs to be avoided—because they release catecholamines—include metaraminol (Aramine), methyldopa, guanethedine, and the tricyclic antidepressants. Organic iodine dyes used in arteriography are potent releasers of catecholamines; therefore arteriography should not be performed until the patient is adequately treated with phenoxybenzamine.

■ **What preoperative and surgical management is advisable?**

In preparation for surgical removal of a pheochromocytoma, patients are usually treated with phenoxybenzamine for 2 weeks or longer to stabilize the blood pressure. Opinions differ concerning the advisability of continuing the drug up to the time of surgery or stopping it 2 or 3 days before surgery. Hypotension may follow the removal of a pheochromocytoma. Norepinephrine is given intravenously under careful monitoring to raise the blood pressure. Blood volume restoration is important to control postoperative hypotension; these patients tend to have decreased plasma volume.

THYROID DISORDERS

Thyroid function is not acutely altered during the course of nonthyroidal diseases, but two thyroid disorders that require intensive treatment may be encountered—*hyperthyroid crisis* and *myxedema coma.*

Hyperthyroid crisis
■ **What is meant by hyperthyroid crisis?**

Hyperthyroid crisis, known also as "thyroid storm," refers to an acute severe exacerbation of hyperthyroidism. Although rare, it is fatal if untreated and has a significant mortality even if treated. The crisis may be precipitated by trauma, surgery, or intercurrent diseases in patients with uncontrolled hyperthyroidism. In hyperthyroid patients given iodides exacerbation of the hyperthyroidism may occur after withdrawal of iodides because of accelerated release of thyroid hormones from the unblocked thyroid gland. Severe hyperthyroidism can be unmasked after abrupt withdrawal of propranolol in patients with unrecognized or untreated hyperthyroidism.

■ **How is thyroid storm recognized?**

Extreme tachycardia or atrial fibrillation, fever, and profound weakness occur. The common manifestations of hyperthyroidism are usually observed including goiter, warm moist skin, tremor, and muscle weakness. Ophthalmopathy may or may not be present. The diagnosis of thyroid storm is arbitrary—customary criteria include a heart rate in excess of 140 per minute and fever without other cause in a critically ill hyperthyroid patient. Laboratory tests to confirm the diagnosis include abnormally high concentrations of free and total thyroxine (T_4) and triiodothyronine (T_3) in the serum. The thyroidal uptake of radioactive iodine is usually elevated but cannot be determined promptly.

The urgency of the situation demands that treatment be started before laboratory confirmation of the diagnosis can be obtained.

■ **What is the treatment?**

Specific treatment is directed at inhibiting the secretion and release of excess thyroid hormones (T_4 and T_3) and counteracting their effects.

1. Antithyroid drugs should be given in large doses—propylthiouracil, 200 mg, or methimazole

(Tapazole), 20 mg every 6 hours orally or by gastric intubation (no preparations for parenteral use are available). These drugs block the synthesis of new thyroid hormone. Propylthiouracil is preferable because it also inhibits the peripheral conversion of thyroxine to triiodothyronine.

2. Iodine in the form of sodium or potassium iodide, 0.5 to 1.0 g, is given orally or intravenously every 12 to 24 hours, but not until the patient has received a blocking dose of propylthiouracil or methimazole. Iodides inhibit the synthesis and release of thyroxine from the thyroid.

3. Adrenergic blocking agents are helpful because thyroxine and triiodothyronine potentiate the effects of catecholamines. Guanethedine orally and reserpine intramuscularly have been used. The most effective drug currently available is propranolol; doses of 20 to 40 mg or more are given orally every 4 to 6 hours. In an urgent situation propranolol should be given intravenously— 0.5 mg initially and 1 to 2 mg every 4 to 6 hours slowly and cautiously. The oral route is safer.

■ **What supportive measures are indicated?**

1. Fluids to correct dehydration and replace losses of sodium and potassium are given intravenously.

2. Dextrose with large amounts of vitamin B complex is needed. The hypermetabolism associated with hyperthyroidism requires increased amounts of vitamin B.

3. Hydrocortisone, 200 to 300 mg daily, is recommended during the acute phase (although adrenal insufficiency is ordinarily not present).

4. Hypothermia may be needed if cool wet packs or ice packs are ineffective.

5. Digoxin or shorter acting glycosides may be needed, as well as quinidine or other antiarrhythmic agents. The dose of digoxin may be higher than usual because of the accelerated metabolism.

6. Diuretics may be needed if congestive heart failure or pulmonary edema occurs.

7. Sedation with phenobarbital or diazepam may be helpful.

8. Appropriate treatment of precipitating or concurrent diseases should be initiated.

Improvement should occur in 24 to 48 hours with recovery from the acute phase within a few days. Treatment of the hyperthyroidism with anti-thyroid drugs and propranolol, with appropriate modifications in dosage, is then continued until the patient is euthyroid. Definitive therapy with radioactive iodine or thyroidectomy or long-term antithyroid drug therapy can then be selected.

Myxedema coma
■ **What is myxedema coma?**

Myxedema coma is a severe degree of thyroid hormone deficiency that occurs in patients with untreated hypothyroidism of long duration. Although uncommon, it is extremely important to recognize the disorder and treat it effectively. It is fatal if untreated and has a high mortality rate even with treatment. The characteristic signs of myxedema (severe hypothyroidism) are usually present: typical facies, nonpitting edema, cold dry skin, myoedema and delayed relaxation of tendon reflexes (unless the patient is areflexic), bradycardia, and usually hypotension. Mental obtundation is severe. Hypothermia is common (several degrees below normal) but may not be recognized with the usual clinical thermometer.

■ **What induces myxedema coma?**

The precipitating factors in myxedema coma include infection, trauma, cerebrovascular thrombosis, myocardial infarction, and drugs that depress the central nervous system. Carbon dioxide retention may occur in association with alveolar hypoventilation.

■ **What laboratory tests are helpful in diagnosis?**

Abnormally low values for total thyroxine (T_4) concentration in the serum are characteristic. The T_3 concentration is low but may also be low in various nonthyroidal diseases. The serum TSH (thyroid stimulating hormone) concentration is elevated in primary hypothyroidism but not in cases of hypopituitarism. The cerebrospinal fluid protein may be elevated. Hyponatremia may occur in association with inappropriate secretion of antidiuretic hormone. Hypercholesterolemia is common in myxedema, but the serum cholesterol concentration may not be elevated in chronically ill and undernourished patients. The electrocardiogram usually shows sinus bradycardia, low voltage of the QRS complexes, and low or flat T waves.

How should myxedema coma be managed?

Treatment may have to be started on the basis of reasonable suspicion without waiting for the results of confirmatory laboratory tests despite the hazard in patients with heart disease. Replacement of the deficiency of thyroid hormone is specific. Levothyroxine sodium is given intravenously. The usual dose is 0.5 mg. Some physicians prefer to give 0.25 mg initially and 0.25 mg again in 24 hours. As an alternative, liothyronine (triiodothyronine) may be given in doses of 25 μg every 6 to 12 hours for 24 to 48 hours. This is given orally because parenteral preparations may be unavailable. After initial replacement, levothyroxine, 50 μg daily, is given. As the patient improves, maintenance therapy with levothyroxine can be given orally. The average maintenance dose is 0.15 mg daily but varies from 0.1 to 0.3 mg daily.

What supportive measures are indicated?

1. Ventilation is important, if necessary assisted ventilation, with the judicious use of oxygen.

2. Prevention of further heat loss is important, and gentle external warming may be used cautiously. Rapid warming should be avoided.

3. Fluid replacement should be accomplished slowly; excess sodium should be avoided. Dilutional hyponatremia may be encountered, requiring water restriction. Potassium deficiency may need replenishment. Dextrose is given intravenously if hypoglycemia occurs.

4. Hydrocortisone, 200 mg daily, in divided doses is recommended because of the possibility of adrenocortical insufficiency.

5. Digoxin may be needed if congestive heart failure is present. The dose may be lower than usual because of the hypometabolism.

6. Vasopressors may be needed if the hypotension does not respond to levothyroxine.

7. Appropriate treatment for precipitating and concurrent diseases should be initiated.

WATER METABOLISM AND ANTIDIURETIC HORMONE

The antidiuretic hormone (ADH), vasopressin, controls the reabsorption of water by the kidneys. ADH is secreted by specialized cells in the hypothalamus and stored in the posterior lobe of the pituitary gland. The secretion of ADH is regulated by osmoreceptors located in the anterior hypothalamus. These receptors are sensitive to changes in the osmolality of the plasma. The plasma osmolality increases with a rise in solute concentration in the plasma, caused either by an increase in solutes or a loss of water. The osmolality decreases with a fall in solute concentration, caused either by a decrease in solutes or a gain of water. An increase in plasma osmolality stimulates the secretion of ADH, which promotes the renal tubular reabsorption of water. A decrease in plasma osmolality inhibits the secretion of ADH and thus promotes the renal excretion of water.

Although many factors affect water metabolism, this discussion is concerned with primary disturbances in ADH secretion.

What is diabetes insipidus?

Diabetes insipidus is characterized by severe polyuria and polydipsia caused by inadequate antidiuretic hormone activity. The cause of the disorder is a lesion of the hypothalamic nuclei that secrete ADH or of the posterior lobe of the pituitary gland. Brain tumor or trauma is a common cause, but some cases are without known cause. These patients excrete large amounts of dilute urine, 4 to 10 L/day. This is accompanied by intense thirst so that the patients consume large amounts of water. Provided that the patient has free access to water, osmotic equilibrium can be maintained. But unconscious patients and those who for any reason cannot drink freely are subject to severe dehydration that can be fatal.

How is the diagnosis made?

The possibility of diabetes insipidus is suggested in patients with head trauma or recent pituitary surgery who excrete excessive amounts of urine with low specific gravity (less than 1.010). This must be distinguished from impaired renal concentration ability and a response from diuretic agents or fluid overload.

What is the treatment of diabetes insipidus?

Vasopressin (Pitressin) is effective in treating diabetes insipidus. For acute or temporary situations an aqueous vasopressin solution is used because of its short duration of action. The usual dose is 5 to 10 units given subcutaneously every 4 to 6 hours. (Because of its vasoconstrictive effects, it should be used with caution in patients with coronary artery disease.) For more sustained effect vasopressin tannate (Pitressin tannate in oil) is used. Each ampule contains 5 units/ml. The dose range is 0.2 to 1 ml given intramuscularly. The duration of action varies from 24 to 72 hours. The dose and frequency of administration should be adjusted to the individual patient's need, so as to maintain a urine volume of 1 to 3 L/24 hr. The ampule should be warmed to body temperature and shaken thoroughly to ensure that the active drug is suspended evenly in the oil. Fluid intake and output should be carefully monitored. The patient's daily weight and determination of urinary specific gravity or osmolality are helpful guides. For maintenance therapy, synthetic lysine vasopressin (lypressin) nasal spray is available.

■ **What is nephrogenic diabetes insipidus?**

Nephrogenic diabetes insipidus is a renal tubular defect characterized by inability of the kidneys to respond to ADH. There is no deficiency of ADH in this condition; therefore the administration of vasopressin is not effective treatment. Restriction of fluids and the administration of thiazide diuretics may be helpful. The mechanism of action of thiazides in this condition is incompletely understood; probably they are effective by inducing a sodium deficit.

■ **What is the syndrome of inappropriate ADH secretion?**

The syndrome of inappropriate ADH secretion is characterized by the inability to secrete a dilute urine in the presence of decreased plasma osmolality and normal renal function. The physiologic events resemble those that occur following the administration of excess amounts of ADH; the plasma osmolality and serum sodium concentrations are low, while the urine contains sodium and is relatively concentrated. Edema is not usually present. Excess ADH activity has been postulated to be the cause of this disorder, but the cause is obscure.

This syndrome has been described in a variety of clinical situations including central nervous system disorders, myxedema, and various malignant neoplasms.

■ **Is treatment indicated?**

Treatment is strict limitation of fluid intake to correct the hyponatremia. The condition is resistant to the administration of sodium, particularly isotonic sodium chloride solution.

SUMMARY

Endocrine and metabolic disturbances occur in a variety of conditions in critically ill patients. Stress initiates an adrenal response, mediated by the hypothalamus and anterior pituitary gland, that provides increased amounts of adrenocortical hormones, which are important in many metabolic processes. Although adrenal insufficiency is uncommon, adrenocortical steroids are frequently used in pharmacologic doses for their anti-inflammatory and supportive effects. Diabetes mellitus is relatively common and diabetic ketoacidosis is often precipitated by acute illness in diabetic patients. Hyperglycemic nonketotic hyperosmolar coma is a serious complication of acute diseases associated with dehydration in diabetic patients. Hypercalcemia occurs in a variety of disorders that disturb calcium homeostasis. Thyroid function is not usually disturbed in patients with nonthyroidal diseases, but hyperthyroid crisis and myxedema coma, although rare, require prompt intensive treatment. Derangements of water and electrolyte metabolism are common in critically ill patients and are closely related to various endocrine functions.

Specific plans for treatment are presented for the major endocrine and metabolic disorders that occur in critically ill patients. Alternative therapeutic regimens may be effective. Meticulous attention to patient care is essential.

BIBLIOGRAPHY

Alberti, K. G. M. M.: Low-dose insulin in the treatment of diabetic ketoacidosis, Arch. Intern. Med. **137:**1367, 1977.

Cohen, A. S., Freiden, R. B., and Samuels, M. A., editors: Medical emergencies. Diagnostic and management procedures from Boston City Hospital, Boston, 1977, Little, Brown & Co.

Kreisberg, R. A.: Diabetic ketoacidosis: new concepts and trends in pathogenesis and treatment, Ann. Intern. Med. **88:**681, 1978.

Myers, W. P. L.: Differential diagnosis of hypercalcemia and cancer, CA **27:**258, 1977.

Williams, R. H., editor: Textbook of endocrinology, ed. 5, Philadelphia, 1974, W. B. Saunders Co.

Wilmore, D. W.: The metabolic management of the critically ill, New York, 1977, Plenum Publishing Corp.

CHAPTER 24

Management of renal failure

D. E. Gentile

■ What is the functional role of the kidneys?

In man, kidneys are paired organs, each weighing about 140 g, located retroperitoneally in the dorsal part of the abdomen, partially above and below the twelfth ribs. Although small in size, they receive approximately 20% to 25% of the cardiac output each minute. Microscopically each kidney contains 1 to 1.25 million functional units, the nephrons, one of which is illustrated in Fig. 24-1. Filtration of the plasma takes place at the glomerulus, and the filtrate thus formed is altered on its course through the nephron by tubular reabsorption and secretion until an appropriate (for the body's needs) quantity and quality of urine is produced at the terminal portion of the nephron. The calyces, pelves, ureters, and bladder are simply conduits and do not further alter the composition of the urine.

Renal function is complex and not limited to the elimination of urea and other waste products of metabolism from the body via the urine. Normally functioning kidneys allow man a considerable amount of freedom in the type and amount of food and liquid ingested and the environmental conditions that are endurable. By producing urine that is hypertonic (concentrated) or hypotonic (dilute), relative to the "tonicity" of plasma water, and by varying the excretion of electrolytes, the kidneys contribute greatly to the maintenance of the normal composition of body fluids, a state necessary for the proper function of all body cells and organs. Because the urinary excretion of acids or alkali can be altered to help maintain

body fluid pH within narrow limits, the kidneys together with the lungs and the body buffer system protect man from major swings in pH that may result from the ingestion of excessive acids or alkali, from the production of acid from neutral dietary precursors, or from clinical conditions leading to excessive losses of acids or alkali from

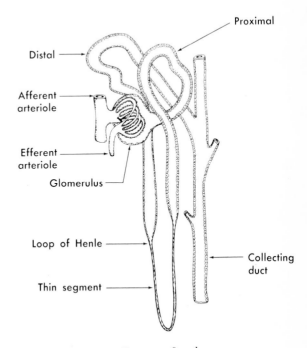

Fig. 24-1. Diagram of nephron.

441

the body, as may be seen in severe vomiting or diarrhea.

Apart from these "regulatory" functions, the kidneys play a role as endocrine organs by producing hormones that affect red blood cell formation (erythropoietin), blood pressure control (renin and prostaglandins), and the secretion of aldosterone by the adrenal glands (renin-angiotensin system). An additional aspect of kidney function includes metabolic processes, for example, the conversion of vitamin D to an active metabolic form and the degradation of insulin, parathormone, and gastrin.

Since the kidneys are involved in numerous and fundamental processes, it is easy to see why there are far-reaching, complex, and serious manifestations of renal functional impairment. Fortunately the large number of nephrons present in each kidney comprise a "reserve force," so that although subtle biochemical changes may be present with mild to moderate degrees of kidney disease, relatively normal homeostasis may be maintained, and the patient may feel quite well until 70% to 80% of the nephron mass has been destroyed.

■ **How does examination of the urine help in the evaluation of kidney function? What are the components of routine urinalysis?**

Simple *observation* of the urine can provide evidence of disease of the urinary tract or kidneys. For instance, if the urine is cloudy, the presence of pyuria (pus cells in the urine) and thus urinary tract infection may be suspected. Red urine will usually indicate the presence of blood but may be caused by hemoglobin or myoglobin in the urine and may be seen in certain types of porphyria or in some persons after the ingestion of beets. Other colors may be seen after the ingestion of certain dyes (methylene blue plus medications containing various dyes).

Milky urine may be seen when pus, phosphate crystals, and, in rare cases, lymphatic fluid are present in the urine. Foamy, sticky urine is characteristic of marked proteinuria.

The *specific gravity* is a measurement of the density of the urine and is affected by the number as well as the molecular weight of the solids present. Specific gravity should always be inter-

preted in the context of the patient's state of hydration. Normal kidneys can vary in urinary specific gravity over a wide range (1.001 to 1.040), producing high specific gravity (concentrated) urine when the patient has been without fluids for some time and is relatively dehydrated. Low specific gravity (dilute) urine is present normally when the patient has taken in (or has been administered) more fluids than are absolutely required. The specific gravity can be misleading when large amounts of glucose are present, giving falsely high readings. The specific gravity may be inappropriately high in clinical states where a positive water balance exists, such as congestive heart failure and hypoalbuminemia. In these situations, although intrinsic renal damage is not present, diminished renal blood flow leads to inappropriate urinary concentration.

Although not performed as part of the routine urinalysis, measurement of the urine *osmolality* gives more precise information than specific gravity about urinary concentration and dilution and is often used in cases where such information is needed.

Measurement of the urinary *pH* may provide information relating to the patient's acid-base balance and will also indicate abnormal renal responses to an existing acid-base problem. Inherited or acquired defects in the acidification process of the urine (renal tubular acidosis) are frequently associated with alkaline urine in the presence of metabolic acidosis. A clue to the diagnosis is the inappropriate pH of the urine in a situation where normal kidneys would be elaborating maximally acidified urine. Inappropriate acidification of the urine can be seen in cases where marked body potassium depletion exists, as in prolonged vomiting caused by duodenal ulcer with obstruction.

Urine is routinely tested for the presence or absence of *glucose*. A positive test is usually caused by the presence of an elevated serum glucose level. In normal situations glucose is filtered at the glomerulus and completely reabsorbed by the proximal tubules when serum glucose concentration is normal or slightly elevated. In abnormalities of glucose reabsorption (renal glycosuria) glucose is present in the urine despite a normal serum concentration.

Qualitative tests for *protein* are part of the routine urinalysis. A commonly used test is the addition of sulfosalicylic acid to the clear supernatant of centrifuged urine with observation of the degree of precipitation present. This gives semiquantitative information on the amount of protein present. When abnormal amounts of protein are present qualitatively, quantitative tests are performed on timed (12- or 24-hour) collections. Up to 150 mg of protein may be present normally in 24 hours. In a variety of kidney diseases abnormal amounts of protein are present, and qualitative tests will be positive for protein. In general the largest amounts of protein are seen in patients with primary glomerular diseases, especially those producing the nephrotic syndrome.

Microscopic examination of the centrifuged urinary sediment is a critical test. Whenever possible, it should be performed carefully on the first morning specimen (usually the most concentrated). The sediment is, in a sense, a biopsy without surgery or needle aspiration of the kidney and can provide specific information when performed by an experienced observer. The presence of an excessive number of casts and the type of cells or crystals contained in them may give positive identification of the disease process present. The presence of red blood cells in casts, for instance, strongly suggests glomerulonephritis; white blood cell casts indicate pyuria as originating from one or both kidneys. Other formed elements such as *oval fat bodies* (lipid-laden tubular epithelium), *doubly refractile fat bodies* (cholesterol esters), and *crystal casts* give specific information indicating the disease state producing renal functional impairment.

■ **What is the significance of serum creatinine, creatinine clearance, and blood urea nitrogen?**

The most common quantitative estimate of kidney function used clinically is *creatinine clearance. Creatinine* is an inert substance that is formed from the dehydration of creatine in muscle, is not metabolized further (significantly), and is excreted, for practical purposes, simply by the process of filtration at the renal glomerulus. Its production (and thus excretion) is a function of the muscle mass of the individual. Males have greater creatinine production and excretion than females, the difference between the two being proportional to muscle mass. Despite the facts that (1) measurement of the serum creatinine is not exact because of the presence of an interfering noncreatinine chromogen in the serum and (2) small amounts of creatinine are added to the urine by tubular secretion, as well as glomerular filtration in man, for clinical purposes the creatinine clearance is equivalent to the *glomerular filtration rate* (GFR), as shown in the following formula:

$$GFR = \frac{U_{cr} \times V}{P_{cr}}$$

where U_{cr} = urinary creatinine concentration, V = urinary flow rate (usually milliliters per minute), and P_{cr} = plasma creatinine concentration. Average GFR values for normal young men is 125 ± 15 ml/min/1.73 m^2 of body surface area. For normal young women the average is 110 ± 15 ml/min/1.73 m^2 of body surface area.

Since urine flow rate is used in the calculation of GFR, accurately timed collections of urine are necessary for valid results. The serum creatinine level is inversely proportional to the creatinine clearance, but because normal serum creatinine concentrations can vary according to the size and muscle mass of the patient, a single serum creatinine determination may not provide precise information regarding the absolute level of renal function. For example, a serum creatinine concentration of 3.0 mg/100 ml in a 90-pound woman may indicate renal functional impairment comparable to that seen in a 200-pound muscular man whose serum creatinine concentration is considerably higher.

Blood urea nitrogen (BUN) is a measure of the major end product of protein metabolism in man (urea). The BUN is normally below 20 mg/100 ml and rises when renal functional impairment is present. Since urea is reabsorbed by the tubules, its clearance may be affected by the urine flow rate. The level of BUN is affected not only by changes in glomerular filtration and urine flow rate but also by the rate of urea production. BUN may be elevated in the presence of stable renal function following the ingestion of large protein loads and also in situations where rapid protein breakdown is taking place, such as in patients who have suffered extensive trauma, those who have infection, and in others following major surgery. These factors must be considered before drawing conclusions about renal functional status simply from the level of BUN. For example, in a patient who has extensive gastrointestinal bleeding (protein load) or is extremely catabolic the BUN may rise significantly with only a small increment in the serum creatinine level. This situation is called *prerenal azotemia* and means that nonrenal factors are accountable for a demonstrated rise in BUN.

Many of the routinely measured electrolytes and blood chemistries are affected by renal abnormalities and will be discussed, where pertinent, subsequently. X-ray and isotope studies provide much information about the structure and function of the urinary tract. These tests provide data of diagnostic and therapeutic significance but are not, in the strictest sense, studies of renal function.

■ **Of what use is renal biopsy in the diagnosis and management of kidney disease?**

Evaluation of kidney tissue by routine microscopy, by special immunofluorescent techniques, and by electron microscopy has provided help in the diagnosis of specific renal and systemic disorders and serves as a guide to the therapy and prognosis in many renal (especially glomerular) disorders. Whereas renal biopsy may be performed as an open surgical procedure, the technique of percutaneous renal biopsy is most commonly used.

■ **What precautions are taken before performing renal biopsy?**

The following checks should be made:
1. The presence and location of two kidneys should be demonstrated.
2. Coagulation studies should be normal.
3. Urinary tract infection should be ruled out.
4. The patient should be cooperative and understand the reason for the biopsy as well as the potential benefits and risks involved.

■ **What are some potential complications of renal biopsy?**

Bleeding may take place. This may occur into the renal collecting system, producing gross hematuria, sometimes with clot formation and renal colic, or it may be perinephric (retroperitoneal); in addition, significant bleeding can be hidden and only become evident when a blood pressure or hematocrit drop is noted.

Minimal bleeding is routine. On rare occasions (less than 1%) bleeding is sufficient to require transfusion. Bleeding massive enough to require nephrectomy is even less common.

The close monitoring of vital signs and the observation of the urine after biopsy is required to detect early signs of significant bleeding. Grossly bloody urine is not uncommon and is more likely to occur in severely uremic patients or patients with uncontrolled hypertension. Bright red urine may be present when relatively small amounts of blood are present, and it is useful to quantitate the amount of bleeding by centrifugation of the urine in a hematocrit centrifuge.

Injury, or sampling of other structures, although uncommon, may occur. Infection is also rare. The exact frequency of the occurrence of arteriovenous fistula is unknown, but rarely is it of clinical significance.

ACUTE RENAL FAILURE
■ **What is acute renal failure?**

Acute renal failure is the sudden onset of diminished renal function usually, but not always, accompanied by oliguria. (Oliguria is customarily defined as a urine output of less than 400 ml/24 hr.) There are occasional cases of true acute renal failure wherein normal or large amounts of urine are formed. In these instances the condition is called *nonoliguric acute renal failure*. Sudden failure of kidney function may occur in patients with previously normal kidneys or in those who have preexisting kidney disease. The designation of acute signifies not only the nature of onset but also suggests the possibility of reversible renal failure.

■ **How can acute renal failure be distinguished from chronic renal failure?**

Chronic renal failure is the result of a parenchymal disease process of both kidneys that has been present for months or years with gradual, irreversible deterioration of renal function. Urine output is often normal until the latest stages of the disease. In rare situations chronic renal failure may have an "acute" course, as in certain cases of *rapidly progressive glomerulonephritis, bilateral renal cortical necrosis,* and *multiple myeloma.* At times it is difficult to distinguish acute from chronic renal failure or to quantitate the effects of an acute insult on renal function in a patient with underlying kidney disease. It is critical to make the distinction, since specific treatment for remediable causes of acute deterioration of renal function will have a favorable impact on the patient's long-term course.

In the evaluation of any patient with renal failure it is important to review completely the patient's medical history for information concerning previous kidney disease or hypertension. A review of past medical records, if available, will provide useful information whether there is positive evidence of renal involvement or not.

Evaluation of kidney size and the absence or presence and severity of anemia may also provide differential information. With chronic parenchymal renal disease and renal failure of a severe degree there is usually a reduction in the size of the kidneys. Evaluation of renal size can be accomplished by kidney-ureter-bladder (KUB) testing, tomography, or infusion intravenous pyelogram (IVP) with tomography.

Although visualization of the kidneys using contrast material and x-ray films may not be ideal, sufficient information can be obtained by utilizing large doses of contrast material. This rule of diminished renal size in chronic disease is not absolute, however, since there are certain chronic disease processes that may be associated with normal or large kidneys even though significant renal failure is present. Examples of these include *polycystic kidney disease, diabetic glomerulosclerosis,* and *renal amyloidosis.*

Anemia of chronic renal failure will be discussed later in greater detail, but in general chronic renal failure is accompanied by anemia that becomes more severe as the level of renal function diminishes. The presence of normal or near-normal hemoglobin concentration and hematocrit level in a patient with significant renal functional impairment who is not dehydrated suggests the presence of a relatively recent deterioration of renal function.

■ What are the causes of acute renal failure?
Renal ischemia

Renal ischemia may result from hypotension following traumatic, surgical, or obstetric hemorrhage; *disseminated intravascular coagulation;* severe dehydration from gastrointestinal or other fluid losses, for example, exposure to excessive environmental heat; "third spacing," as may be seen following extensive third-degree burns or following bowel surgery; and after vascular surgery, especially of the aorta and/or renal arteries.

Toxins

Certain drugs and chemicals exert specific nephrotoxicity. A partial list of these includes the following:

Agents that may cause acute renal failure
Antibiotics: gentamicin, kanamycin, colistin, neomycin, amphotericin, sulfonamides
Metals: mercury, lead, arsenic
Carbon tetrachloride
Ethylene glycol
Radiographic contrast materials
Anesthetic agents: methoxyflurane, halothane
DDT and other insecticides

Agents that may cause interstitial nephritis
Analgesics: phenacetin
Methicillin

Agents that may cause nephrotic syndrome
Penicillamine
Trimethadione, paramethadione
Gold

With both "ischemic" and "toxic" acute renal failure the pathologic lesion often seen is necrosis of the renal tubules. Thus a common synonym for acute renal failure associated with these causes is *acute tubular necrosis.* It is of interest, however, that tubular necrosis may not be seen on renal biopsy or at autopsy in a significant number of cases of acute oliguric renal failure following an ischemic episode. The renal histology may appear normal, suggesting that a purely functional abnormality may be present, perhaps related to the abnormal distribution of renal blood flow.

Parenchymal renal disease

Severe acute glomerulonephritis of any type may lead to acute oliguric renal failure. Diffuse interstitial nephritis of acute onset and unknown origin as well as interstitial nephritis related to drugs and infection has been noted to produce acute renal failure. In patients with underlying vascular disorders, such as diabetes mellitus, *necrotizing papillitis* may result from infarction of the renal papillae caused by a combination of medullary interstitial infection and vascular insufficiency. Papillary necrosis may also occur as the result of prolonged, excessive ingestion of phenacetin and perhaps other analgesics, but leads to gradual chronic renal functional impairment rather than acute renal failure.

Nephron obstruction

Intrarenal (nephron) obstruction may occur as the result of deposition of a number of materials, including uric acid crystals, oxalate crystals, the precipitation of sulfonamides, and the precipitation of abnormal globulins such as those found in the urine of patients with multiple myeloma. In each of these cases the presence of large amounts of a relatively insoluble substance and dehydration of the patient combine to produce precipitation of the substance in nephrons.

■ What is prerenal failure?

Normal renal blood flow is approximately 1200 ml/min and comprises approximately 20% of the cardiac output. In situations where vascular volume depletion exists, defense mechanisms to maintain circulation to other vital organs result in decreased blood flow to the kidneys. As a result, renal function tests may be abnormal and urine flow rate may diminish, although parenchymal renal damage has not occurred. When this happens, it is important to detect the problem early and take measures to correct it rapidly before full-blown true acute renal failure develops. Close clinical surveillance alone may give sufficient clues to establish the presence of volume depletion. If the patient develops oliguria while under clinical observation, a review of the recent trend in body weight may demonstrate inordinate weight loss over several days, suggesting negative water balance. Measurements of the central venous pressure or the pulmonary wedge pressure, if low, provide evidence for volume depletion. If the patient is not absolutely confined to bed, the simple observation of a postural (standing) drop in blood pressure may give added weight to the possibility that volume depletion exists.

A trial of IV fluids, including normal saline solution, mannitol, or a solution containing albumin may lead to correction of vascular volume deficit, increased rates of urine formation, and restoration of the BUN and serum creatinine concentration toward normal. The amount of the solutions given and the rates at which they are given depend on the degree of volume depletion that is suspected clinically, the age and cardiovascular status of the patient, and the response of arterial pressure and central venous pressure or pulmonary wedge pressure to the fluid administration. An important point to keep in mind is the fact that concentrated albumin solutions increase vascular volume to a greater degree than would be expected from the volume of solution administered, since the colloid osmotic pressure of protein infused leads to a shift of water from "compartments" outside of the blood vessels to the vascular compartment. When these diagnostic or therapeutic fluid administration maneuvers are made, the most serious potential complication is circulatory overload with congestive heart failure and pulmonary edema. This danger is increased when acute renal failure is present.

At times when the circulatory state and the state of hydration of the patient are equivocal or the patient has known or suspected borderline cardiac function, it is safer to attempt to stimulate renal perfusion and urine formation by the administration of potent diuretics such as furosemide or ethacrynic acid. It is frequently necessary to give relatively large IV doses of these agents in order to determine if a response will take place. Doses in the range of 200 to 600 mg of furosemide are generally safe but should not be given rapidly or directly into a central venous pressure catheter. In the latter instance the potential for causing cardiac arrhythmias exists. Larger doses of these drugs have been reported to produce transient or permanent deafness on rare occasions. Care should be taken not to administer large doses to patients who are receiving potentially ototoxic antibiotics such as aminoglycosides (for example, gentamicin), since the combined effects of the diuretic and antibiotic are more likely, although not proved, to cause eighth nerve damage.

■ **What measures should be taken to exclude urinary obstruction as a cause for acute oliguria?**

Obstruction to the flow of urine must always be considered when evaluating a patient with acute oliguria. Obstruction of the ureters, bilaterally, is unusual but can occur.

If bilateral ureteral obstruction is the cause of oliguria, its detection and relief can be lifesaving. Increasing experience with renal ultrasound has shown this procedure to be particularly well suited for investigation of the critically ill patient. Ultrasound provides a safe, noninvasive, portable, and reasonably accurate method for demonstrating the presence of hydronephrosis and/or ureteral dilatation and the presence or absence of retroperitoneal or pelvic masses, which may cause ureteral obstruction.

When the clinical situation strongly suggests obstruction, bilateral retrograde catheterization of the ureters may become necessary to rule out obstruction. Isotope scanning techniques may also safely help to rule out obstruction in certain cases.

■ **What are the causes of bilateral ureteral obstruction?**

The causes of bilateral ureteral obstruction are as follows:
1. Pelvic tumor with local invasion
2. Retroperitoneal lymphadenopathy, as seen with lymphomas and leukemia
3. Idiopathic retroperitoneal fibrosis
4. Deposition of urate crystals in the ureters (This may be seen in patients with extreme hyperuricemia following treatment of neoplasms with cytotoxic agents or following the injection of radiologic contrast materials in hyperuricemic, dehydrated patients.)
5. Accidental ligation of both ureters during pelvic surgery
6. Bilateral ureteral calculi (rare)

■ **What specific problems are seen in patients with acute renal failure?**

The specific problems seen in these patients may be summarized as:

1. Nutritional complications
2. Water balance difficulties
3. Electrolyte disturbances
4. Uremic manifestations
5. Infection
6. Gastrointestinal bleeding

This list may oversimplify the problems encountered in the management of patients with acute renal failure. More commonly than not the patient is desperately ill as a result of recent severe trauma or burns or extensive surgery, with or without infection. Thus the problems caused by the patient's underlying disease state are compounded by a second, critical clinical problem. Treatment with drugs is made more complicated and recovery from the primary problem that led to the development of acute renal failure is made more tenuous.

■ **What are the nutritional requirements of patients with acute renal failure?**

Patients who have acute renal failure following trauma, burns, or surgery are extremely catabolic, breaking down their own tissue stores to meet their massively increased energy requirements. Over a relatively short time period severe nutritional deficits can occur and, perhaps more important, excessive breakdown of protein stores leads to a rapid rise in BUN. This in turn leads to the early development of uremia. For many years it has been recognized that the provision of nonprotein calories may decrease the rate of protein breakdown, and the usual treatment was the administration of hypertonic glucose solutions or, if the patient could take food orally, carbohydrate and fat calories were given. Quantitative limits were placed on this form of treatment because fluid intake was limited by the presence of oliguria and because of difficulties encountered in administering IV hypertonic solutions. In addition, the necessary level of conservation of protein breakdown could not be effectively accomplished. Similar problems were encountered in attempting to achieve oral nutritional replacement therapy because patients were frequently anorexic and had nausea and vomiting. In the case of a patient who does not require hemodialysis therapy, supportive dietary measures can be utilized but usually at the expense of nutritional needs. If the patient is not ill enough to need dialysis, a temporary state of malnutrition may be tolerated until recovery occurs.

It has been shown that *total parenteral nutrition* utilizing a mixture of essential amino acids and hypertonic glucose solutions administered via a caval catheter may be used to satisfy the nutritional needs of some patients, especially those who are not oliguric. This form of therapy is based on the observation that the administration of essential amino acids may produce better utilization of protein nitrogen.

The absolute caloric needs vary according to the underlying disease states. Severely burned or posttraumatic patients may initially have a caloric requirement of 4000 to 5000 calories/day.

Patients who require dialysis (the majority of patients with acute renal failure) can have more effective alimentation and/or caloric intake than those treated conservatively, since frequent dialysis allows restoration of fluid balance and removal of potentially toxic protein metabolites, as well as the maintenance of normal serum electrolyte concentrations. Special aspects of nutrition in dialysis patients will be discussed in Chapter 27.

Anabolic steroids have been used to minimize negative nitrogen balance in acute renal failure, but their effects have not been dramatic.

■ How is rational fluid therapy achieved in the conservative management of acute renal failure?

Since oliguria is present in most patients with acute renal failure, overhydration and circulatory overload are a constant threat. It is virtually impossible to give a patient no fluid because of the need for medications and calories. The general goals in management are to produce negative water balance when the patient is overhydrated at the onset, or to maintain a zero water balance if the patient is normally hydrated. (In the situation where the patient is underhydrated to begin with, trials at restoration of normal hydration in an effort to reestablish urine flow will, ideally, have led to a state of normal hydration.) Estimation of the state of hydration must be made from day to day by physical examination, looking for the presence or absence of edema, hypertension, postural hypotension, abnormal skin turgor, and pulmonary congestion.

Accurate daily weight of the patient is of critical importance in assessing water balance, since sharp swings in body weight over short time periods are attributable to changes in water balance rather than to changes in dry body mass. Since a gradual fall in dry mass can be expected to occur because of the catabolic state of the patient and inadequate nutrition, a fall in body weight of about ½ pound/day is expected if water balance is achieved.

A number of formulas have been devised for calculating fluid requirements, for example, an intake of 500 ml plus the measured output for 24 hours. These formulas are useful for initiating therapy but must be altered according to the patient's specific needs as determined by weight changes and physical findings. Patients who are febrile or exposed to high ambient environmental temperatures will require more fluid administration than those who are not, since insensible water loss and perspiration will be greater at higher temperatures.

■ What are the manifestations of hyperkalemia and what measures are taken to prevent them?

The clinical environment in which acute renal failure develops sets the stage for dramatic increases in the level of serum potassium. Trauma, surgery, and infection all lead to cellular breakdown with the release of intracellular potassium to the circulation. When coupled with the inability to excrete potassium, concomitant extracellular acidosis secondary to renal failure, and tissue ischemia secondary to hypotension and poor perfusion, rapid rises in serum potassium levels can take place. Although flaccid paralysis and anxiety may occur as a result of hyperkalemia, the most serious adverse effects are on cardiac conduction. Characteristic changes are seen in the ECG, generally when the serum potassium concentration reaches and exceeds 6.5 mEq/L (Fig. 24-2). As the serum potassium levels increase in the toxic range, there is progressive evidence of cardiac depression, and death can occur from cardiac standstill or ventricular fibrillation in a matter of minutes. Unfortunately there is no direct correlation between the absolute serum level of potassium and the changes seen

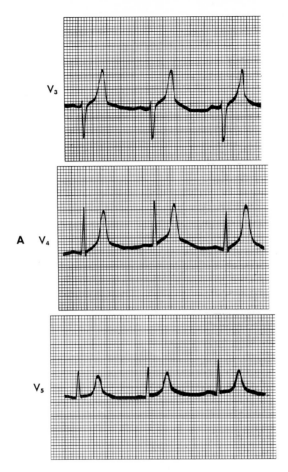

Fig. 24-2. A, Peaked T wave with narrow base from a patient with a serum potassium concentration of 6.6 mEq/L. *Continued.*

in the ECG; cardiac monitoring and serial ECG's are necessary for observation of the effects of potassium toxicity. This lack of correlation exists because the ratio of the extracellular to intracellular concentrations of potassium, rather than the serum level per se, is responsible for the deleterious electrical effects.

A rising serum potassium concentration in the toxic range comprises a *medical emergency that requires immediate measures for control.* Removal of potassium from the body is specifically desired and is most effectively achieved by dialysis (most efficiently by hemodialysis). Fatal levels of hyperkalemia may develop before the prepara-

tion for dialysis can be made, and one or all of the following measures may be used definitively or as interim therapy:

1. *Infusion of sodium bicarbonate.* Sodium ion antagonizes the effect of potassium on the myocardial cell membrane, and the rise in extracellular pH caused by the bicarbonate leads to a movement of potassium into the cells.

2. *Calcium solutions* (calcium gluconate or calcium chloride). Calcium ion antagonizes the effect of potassium at the myocardial cell membrane.

3. *Glucose and insulin infusion.* This combination causes the movement of potassium into the

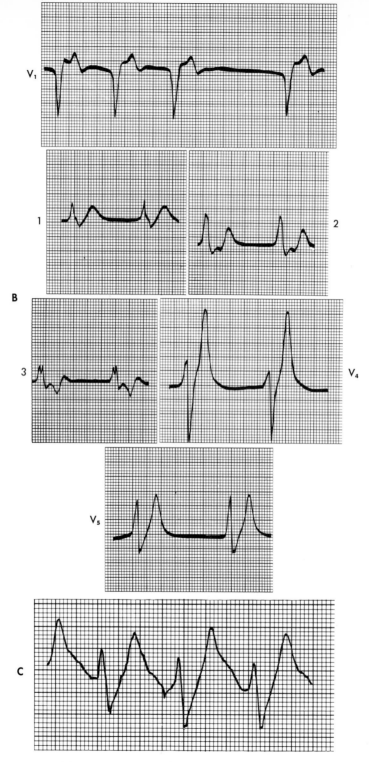

Fig. 24-2, cont'd. B, Wide QRS complex with loss of P waves and peaked T waves from a patient with a serum potassium concentration of 7.5 mEq/L. **C,** Very wide QRS complex, AV dissociation, and "sine" wave pattern from a patient with a serum potassium concentration of 8.3 mEq/L.

cells temporarily. One unit of regular insulin is given for every 3 to 4 g of glucose. Thus 50 ml of 50% dextrose in water can be given with 8 units of regular IV insulin.

4. *Cation-exchange resins* (specifically sodium polystyrene sulfonate [Kayexalate]). These selectively exchange sodium (to the patient) from potassium (from the patient) and can be given either orally or by retention enema. When given orally or by enema with 70% sorbitol or 20% dextrose in water, the resultant loss of water via the gastrointestinal tract may enhance the removal of potassium. When given by retention enema, it is imperative that the enema be retained for a period of 30 to 60 minutes in order to allow efficient exchange to take place. A theoretical exchange of 3 mEq of potassium/g of resin used is predicted but somewhat less occurs in clinical use.

These measures may be sufficient treatment in themselves but more often than not peritoneal dialysis or hemodialysis must be instituted to maintain safer serum potassium levels. Control of potassium intake is mandatory in the subsequent management of the patient.

■ What consideration must be given to other ions in the management of acute renal failure?

In oliguric acute renal failure sodium restriction is necessary to avoid hypertension and congestive heart failure. In the nondialyzed oliguric patient absolute avoidance of sodium is necessary. Low concentrations of serum sodium may sometimes be observed but are more often caused by dilution of the extracellular fluid by excessive water administration prior to the recognition of oliguria rather than to true sodium depletion. In nonoliguric patients measurement of the sodium excretion will be necessary to arrive at a rational prescription for appropriate sodium intake.

Low serum levels of calcium may be observed in some patients and are related to phosphate retention. No clinical symptoms are usually observed unless the rapid correction of acidosis is achieved by the administration of alkali. Frank tetany may develop under these circumstances and will require the administration of calcium.

Antacid therapy is usually given to minimize the occurrence of gastrointestinal ulceration. Aluminum hydroxide gels should be used for this purpose, since other antacids contain magnesium that may be absorbed in sufficient quantities by the gastrointestinal tract, further increasing the level of serum magnesium, which is already elevated by the presence of renal failure. Specific therapy for acidosis is not usually given, but protein restriction instituted to minimize azotemia will diminish acid production from metabolism. In modern medical practice calcium, phosphate, magnesium, and acid-base metabolism are more effectively managed with dialysis therapy.

■ What factors affect survival in acute renal failure?

As already pointed out, acute renal failure does not usually occur as an isolated condition but as a complication of serious medical problems. Thus the nature and severity of the underlying problem are the ultimate factors in survival. A patient with third-degree burns over 90% of the body surface, for example, has a poor prognosis whether or not renal failure develops. Dialysis therapy has resulted in an improvement in the mortality statistics for posttraumatic acute renal failure from a World War II death rate of greater than 90% to one of approximately 67% among Korean War casualties.

Although the survival rate did not improve during the Vietnam war, the *incidence* of acute renal failure in severely traumatized military men was decreased by two thirds. Refinement of surgical, cardiovascular, and fluid and electrolyte resuscitative techniques very likely have played a major role in this reduced morbidity. Most of the worldwide experience shows little improvement in survival during recent years, owing in part to the fact that patients in older age groups and those undergoing bold modern surgical procedures present more serious and complicated medical problems than were seen before.

The chief cause of death among patients with acute renal failure is infection. This is especially true in patients who have had abdominal injuries and/or abdominal surgical procedures. Whether the presence of renal failure makes these patients more susceptible to infection or longer survival allows infectious complications to develop is not definite, but both factors are probably significant.

The presence of an indwelling urethral catheter is a potential source of urinary tract infection and sepsis. This form of instrumentation is unnecessary in most patients with acute renal failure and should be avoided.

Another relatively common complication in some reports is gastrointestinal bleeding. The combination of stress and the effects of uremia in producing defects in coagulation plays a role in producing this complication.

■ Does renal function return to normal following recovery from acute renal failure?

In cases of acute renal failure associated with renal hypoperfusion or tubular necrosis virtually complete recovery of renal function can be expected. Measurements of glomerular filtration rate usually approach normal after several weeks or months. Occasionally abnormalities in concentrating ability and other discrete tubular functions have been seen for a number of months after recovery. There is no known increased susceptibility to the development of a second episode of acute renal failure. If acute renal failure is associated with glomerulonephritis, interstitial nephritis, papillary necrosis, or bilateral cortical necrosis, residual renal functional impairment and hypertension are more likely to develop.

CHRONIC RENAL FAILURE

Diffuse parenchymal renal disease, regardless of etiology, ultimately leads to the development of *end-stage renal failure* with the symptom complex of uremia. Although specific diseases may impart particular characteristics to the clinical picture, patients who have far-advanced kidney failure can effectively be considered as a single group. The specific cause of the uremic syndrome is unknown, but its development is related to the retention of toxic products of protein metabolism, as well as to general derangement of the body's content and concentration of normal constituents such as sodium, potassium, bicarbonate, hydrogen ions, calcium, phosphorus, and magnesium. The following discussion will consider the manifestations or consequences of chronic renal failure and the general principles involved in conservative management.

■ What diseases cause chronic renal failure?

There is considerable overlapping in any classification of renal disease. The partial list given here serves to indicate the variety of disease processes that lead to renal failure:

1. Glomerular disease (*acute* and *chronic glomerulonephritis* of diverse etiologies). *Systemic lupus erythematosus* and other collagen vascular diseases can be included in this category even though they produce significant vascular and interstitial lesions.

2. Primary interstitial lesions. This includes *chronic pyelonephritis* and *nephritis of analgesic abuse.*

3. Congenital renal anomalies. *Polycystic kidney disease, medullary cystic disease,* and *hypoplastic kidneys* are the most common causative agents in this category.

4. Obstructive uropathy. Obstruction may occur at any point in the urinary tract and may be intrinsic or extrinsic. Thus obstruction may be caused by urethral stricture or posterior urethral valves with vesicoureteral reflux, or there may be obstruction of the ureters, either congenital or caused by involvement by neoplasm or urinary stones.

5. Other. Other categories of renal disease include metabolic disorders such as gout and nephrocalcinosis secondary to hyperparathyroidism, vascular disease such as nephrosclerosis related to hypertension, and tubular disorders such as the Fanconi syndrome.

■ Is there a difference between chronic renal failure and uremia?

In the strictest sense there is a difference. As renal function deteriorates, abnormalities in the blood and body chemistries are present and will become more abnormal as the destruction of the nephron population takes place. Anemia and hypertension may be present as well, but the patient may continue daily activities with no awareness of the chronic illness present. At some point in time a variety of symptoms will develop, including fatigability, somnolence, nausea and vomiting, pruritus, muscle cramps, paresthesias, easy bruisability, and symptoms of circulatory overload. These symptoms, some or all of which may be present in a single patient, signify the presence of symptomatic uremia.

■ What hematologic abnormalities are present in uremia, and how are they managed?

Normocytic normochromic anemia is a common concomitant of renal failure. The more severe the renal failure, the more severe is the anemia. Both decreased red blood cell production and shortened survival of red blood cells contribute to the anemia. Decreased production of erythropoietic factor from diseased kidneys (the chief source of this substance in the body) is the major cause of decreased red blood cell production, whereas unknown factors in uremic serum and changes in small blood vessels as a result of hypertension lead to a shortened life span of red blood cells. Other factors contributing to anemia are the propensity of uremic patients to bleed from the gastrointestinal tract and possibly diminished iron absorption from the intestines.

The treatment of anemia is generally not effective unless uremic factors are removed. Occasionally transfusions are necessary because of symptoms directly attributable to anemia, especially in patients with significant coronary vascular disease. Because of hypertension and chronic circulatory overload, packed red blood cells should be used. It was formerly thought that previous blood transfusions jeopardized the success of a kidney transplant. This was felt to be due to the formation of antibodies by the patient, which when stimulated at the time of transplantation, lead to a higher incidence of rejection. This has not been found to be the case. Indeed, it has been shown that those patients receiving cadaveric donor kidney transplants, who have received several transfusions with packed red blood cells before the transplant, have a better record of graft survival than patients who have received no transfusions. Treatment with vitamins and iron does not lead to an improvement in anemia in patients not receiving maintenance hemodialysis.

Bleeding, especially from the gastrointestinal tract and mucous membranes of the nose and mouth, is a common consequence of uremia. While the primary cause of bleeding may be disturbances in these tissues themselves, a qualitative defect in platelet function plays an important contributing role. This abnormality can be corrected by dialysis.

Decreased leukocyte counts are seen in uremic patients and may be associated with increased susceptibility to infections. Multiple factors in a debilitating illness, however, probably contribute to this decreased resistance to infection.

■ Is hypertension inevitable in uremia?

Most patients with advanced renal failure have hypertension. However, those that do not have hypertension exhibit relatively large urinary volumes and rates of sodium excretion. These patients are likely to have primary interstitial rather than glomerular disease and frequently have a background of obstructive uropathy.

Hypertension, when present, is related to salt and water excess and/or the effect of increased renin production by diseased kidneys. The principles of treatment include the achievement of optimum salt and water balance by diet manipulation and the use of diuretics and various antihypertensive agents suited to the specific needs of the patient. As with other causes of hypertension, optimum control of blood pressure is required to decrease the likelihood of coronary and cerebrovascular complications and also to prevent additional damage to already severely compromised kidneys. Drugs commonly used in the treatment of hypertension include diuretics (thiazides, furosemide, and ethacrynic acid), methyldopa, hydralazine, propranolol, guanethidine, and diazoxide.

■ Pericarditis is a common manifestation of uremia. How is it recognized and treated?

Prior to the availability of hemodialysis and transplantation, pericarditis was usually present shortly before the death of a patient with uremia. More recently it has been recognized that pericarditis may occur prior to the terminal phase of renal disease and may occur in patients whose uremia is relatively well controlled by hemodialysis. Pericardial inflammation may be present with or without chest pain and can be detected by careful frequent examination of the heart, listening closely for a pericardial friction rub.

In uremia there is a tendency for the formation of hemorrhagic pericardial fluid that may rapidly increase in quantity and produce *cardiac tamponade,* that is, interference with blood return to the heart and thus decreased cardiac output as a result of "constriction" of the heart by fluid under considerable pressure in the pericardial cavity. When tamponade is developing, the pericardial friction rub may disappear, but there are increasing signs of elevated jugular venous pressure. Arterial blood pressure will fall, a narrow pulse pressure will be noted, and paradoxical pulse (systolic pressure decreased more than 10 mm Hg in inspiration as compared to expiration) will be present.

The patient who is at risk for developing uremic pericarditis must be closely monitored with regard to these clinical signs. Emergency measures will be required to reverse the serious hemodynamic complications of cardiac tamponade. Pericardiocentesis setup should be immediately available and used when clinically indicated. The removal of fluid from the pericardial sac by needle aspiration may result in dramatic improvement, but this may be only temporary, because rapid reaccumulation of fluid can occur and because the pericardial fluid may be "loculated" and thus not adequately removed by one or two needle aspirations. In these cases open (surgical) pericardiotomy may be required with the creation of a pericardial "window" to allow continuous drainage of newly formed pericardial fluid into the mediastinum. At times it is necessary to excise the visceral pericardial membrane in order to reduce the surface producing the inflammatory fluid, to allow free drainage of the mediastinum, and to prevent development of adherent, constrictive pericarditis. The infusion of steroids into the pericardial cavity has been used following either pericardiocentesis or open pericardiotomy with apparent reduction in the inflammatory response that produces pericardial effusion.

■ **What are the gastrointestinal manifestations of uremia?**

Anorexia, nausea and vomiting, and gastrointestinal bleeding caused by "uremic enterocolitis" are commonly seen. These add to the discomfort and disability of the patient and require supportive therapy. The bleeding that occurs, while usually not massive, may lead to sufficient blood loss to make transfusion necessary. Conservative treatment with diet, as discussed subsequently, in addition to antiemetic drugs will lead to relief of some of these symptoms if sufficient residual renal function is present.

■ **What are the neurologic manifestations of uremia?**

The most marked neurologic symptoms are as follows:

1. Somnolence and lethargy, loss of deductive ability, delusions, hallucinations, progressive obtundation, and finally coma when an advanced degree of azotemia is present
2. Peripheral neuropathy, both sensory (paresthesias and loss of vibratory position and sense) and motor, with variable degrees of weakness
3. Possibly seizures (frequently associated with hypertension)
4. Neuromuscular irritability with cramping, muscle twitching, shooting pains, gross myoclonic jerks, and asterixis (flapping tremor similar to that seen in severe liver disease and with respiratory acidosis)

■ **Why does bone disease occur in association with uremia?**

Marked disorders of calcium and phosphorus metabolism occur in renal failure. These are caused by several metabolic abnormalities, including the following:

1. *Disordered vitamin D metabolism.* This leads to reduced responsiveness to the administration of normal or very large doses of vitamin D. The liver and the kidneys are responsible for the conversion of vitamin D to its (presently known) most active form, 1,25-dihydroxycholecalciferol. A deficiency of this metabolite leads to the decreased absorption of ingested calcium from the intestine. Over a period of time this contributes to diminished mineralization of bone. In children growth is affected and ricketslike lesions develop. In adults bone pain and pathologic fractures may occur. Vitamin D affects bone metabolism directly, but the significance of this action is presently not well understood.

2. *Secondary hyperparathyroidism.* This occurs as a result of retention of phosphate with consequent lowering of serum calcium levels as renal failure progresses. Again, there is demineralization of bone and the characteristic bone lesion of hyperparathyroidism, that is, *osteitis fibrosa cystica,* develops. Mobilization of calcium from bone in the presence of high serum phosphate levels may lead to deposition of calcium

phosphate in many tissues of the body (*metastatic calcification*). When deposition is in critical areas, significant symptomatology may occur, such as heart block from deposition in the cardiac conduction system and painful arthritis from deposition in the synovium and bursa of joints. Pruritus is associated with increased calcium deposition in the skin, and "uremic red eyes" occur with conjunctival deposits.

3. *Chronic metabolic acidosis.* This probably contributes to bone demineralization but is not the major factor in producing this complication.

■ Are measures taken to prevent or minimize skeletal complications?

Efforts are made to maintain normal concentrations of calcium and phosphorus in the serum, although this by no means guarantees the desired result. Therapeutic efforts include the following:

1. The provision of adequate dietary calcium, in the range of 1.2 g/24 hr for adults, should be undertaken.

2. The reduction and maintenance of serum phosphate at normal levels should be accomplished with the use of aluminum hydroxide gels. (Magnesium-containing gels are contraindicated because magnesium absorption may take place and contribute further to the already increased levels of serum magnesium seen in renal failure.) *Aluminum hydroxide should be given immediately following a meal.*

3. Vitamin D may be given, but large doses are required. Because of abnormal rates of metabolism, there is the distinct possibility of "overshooting" the desired effect, with the result being that increased metastatic calcification may take place. Safer and more effective prevention and treatment of some forms of bone disorders in uremia may be made possible with the use of 1,25 dihydroxy vitamin D (calcitriol), which is clinically available.

4. Correction of metabolic acidosis, when severe, should be achieved.

5. Partial or complete parathyroidectomy may be necessary, depending on the long-range therapeutic plans for the patient and the severity of the disorder.

Additional measures are taken in patients whose renal functions have deteriorated sufficiently to require maintenance hemodialysis.

■ What is uremic pneumonitis?

X-ray and pathologic findings similar to those seen in pulmonary edema are found in patients with uremia. Since hypertension and circulatory overload are commonly present, it is difficult to separate purely cardiovascular factors from metabolic factors that may be causing these findings. It is entirely possible that exudate formed from uremic capillary abnormalities is the cause for the x-ray appearance of the "uremic lung," but the evidence is not conclusive. This finding usually accompanies far-advanced uremia, and control is achieved by eliminating uremia by conservative means or by dialysis and also by relieving circulatory congestion.

Another finding related to the lungs in uremia is pleuritis with friction rub and pleural effusion. Again, this is usually seen with advanced renal failure.

■ What are the dermatologic manifestations of uremia?

Pruritis is a common and sometimes persistent complaint of uremic patients. The cause for this is not known but has been related to calcium deposition in the skin.

Uremic patients have a distinctive yellowish pallor that may be related to the retention of "urochrome" pigment plus the effects of anemia.

Purpura and ecchymosis are commonly seen and are related to abnormal platelet function, perhaps increased capillary fragility, and other unknown factors.

Rashes are commonly seen. The fact that uremic patients receive multiple medications probably contributes to this manifestation.

■ What is the role of diet in the treatment of uremia?

Although a specific uremic "toxin" has not been identified, it is clear that the end products of protein metabolism play a major part in producing uremic symptoms. The symptoms are usually not evident until marked impairment of renal function exists, and restriction of protein intake is not necessary until symptomatic uremia is present. Diets high in essential amino acids (high biologic value protein) have been found to have a greater effect on reducing azotemia (and also uremic symptomatology) than diets low in protein but not high in essential amino acids. When protein-restricted diets containing high biologic value protein are given with sufficient carbohydrate and fat calories (approximately 30 calories/kg), reduction in BUN and improvement in symptoms occur in patients with marked renal functional impairment, that is, creatinine clearance less than 5 ml/ min. As a result, dialysis therapy may be deferred for several months. Adequate nutritional and social (and emotional) requirements of the patient rarely allow reduction of protein intake below 0.5 to 0.7 g of protein/kg of body weight. Lack of patient acceptance of the diet is the main obstacle to "successful" dietary management.

Sufficient intake of vitamins is necessary. Other factors in dietary management include the close supervision of calcium, sodium, potassium, and water balance of uremic patients. Considerable individualization of diet is required for each patient, depending on the peculiarities of mineral balance observed.

■ What renal and extrarenal factors can be controlled to produce optimum renal function in patients with advanced renal failure?

The appropriate measures to take include the following:
1. Ideal control of hypertension
2. Elimination of urinary infection
3. Control of congestive heart failure
4. Prevention of volume depletion (dehydration)
5. Removal of urinary obstruction
6. Elimination of protein loads that may be produced by gastrointestinal bleeding or by tissue catabolism secondary to infection or to the use of drugs that lead to protein breakdown, such as adrenocorticosteroids and tetracyclines
7. Correction of electrolyte imbalances, especially sodium depletion

■ What problems related to drug therapy exist in patients with renal failure?

The metabolism of many drugs requires excretion by the kidney or conversion to inactive forms

by the kidney. It is evident that the dosage of many drugs must be altered in patients with renal failure in order to avoid dangerous side-effects and complications. The following list shows several drugs commonly used in uremic patients, the dose of which may be unchanged in some cases or reduced in others as renal functional impairment progresses:

Drugs that should be avoided in renal failure
Antibiotics: tetracycline, chlortetracycline, demethylchlortetracycline, cephaloridine, nitrofurantoin, nalidixic acid, neomycin
Other agents: triamterene, spironolactone, azathioprine, chlorpropamide, phenformin, gold

Drugs that should be significantly reduced in dose in renal failure
Antibiotics: gentamicin, kanamycin, streptomycin, amphotericin, polymyxin B, colistin, vancomycin, pentamidine(?)
Other agents: phenobarbital, procainamide, quinidine, allopurinol, digoxin, tolbutamide(?)

Drugs that require little or no change in dose in renal failure
Antibiotics: cephalothin, chloramphenicol (decreased dose with associated hepatic disease), erythromycin, clindamycin, ampicillin, carbenicillin, cloxacillin, methicillin, penicillin G, doxycycline
Other agents: acetylsalicylic acid, secobarbital, codeine, diazepam, glutethimide, morphine, lidocaine, atropine, propranolol, diazoxide, hydralazine, methyldopa, furosemide, phenytoin

For a complete discussion of this subject, refer to the monograph on drugs in renal failure by Bennett and co-workers.

BIBLIOGRAPHY

Bennett, W. M., Singer, I., and Coggins, C.: A practical guide to drug usage in adult patients with impaired renal function—a supplement, J.A.M.A. **223:**991, 1973.

Bennett, W. M., et al.: Drugs and renal disease, London, 1978, Churchill Livingstone.

Brenner, B. M., and Rector, F. C., Jr.: The kidney, Philadelphia, 1976, W. B. Saunders Co.

Earley, L. E., and Gottschalk, C. W.: Strauss and Welt's diseases of the kidney, ed. 3, Boston, 1979, Little, Brown & Co.

Lewis, E. J., and Magill, J. W., editors: Proceedings of the Conference on Nutritional Aspects of Uremia, Oct. 23, 1967, Am. J. Clin. Nutr. **21:**349, 1968.

Papper, S.: Clinical nephrology, Boston, 1971, Little, Brown & Co.

Pitts, R. F.: Physiology of the kidney and body fluids, Chicago, 1974, Year Book Medical Publishers, Inc.

CHAPTER 25

Renal transplantation

Donald C. Martin

The past decade has seen renal transplantation pass from an experimental, clinical procedure to an established method for rehabilitation of patients crippled by chronic renal failure. Important contributions by urologists have played a role in making this possible. Today, transplantation remains in the hands of a few surgeons and urologists who have taken extra training in order to prepare themselves for their role in this treatment. This is necessary since the clinical problems encompass many unique characteristics, and there are too few patients to require expertise by all surgeons and urologists. This chapter is intended to provide the reader with a basic background of knowledge in renal transplantation.

■ **Which patients are selected for renal transplantation?**

The criteria for selection of recipients have evolved over the past 10 years. Advanced, irreversible renal failure remains the most important criterion. The presence of certain systemic diseases, such as lupus erythematosus, diabetes mellitus, Fabry's disease, amyloidosis, and others, no longer constitutes an absolute contraindication. Clearly the extent of extrarenal disease must be evaluated on an individual basis. Although renal grafts have functioned in recipients with cystinosis and oxalosis, the demonstrated precipitation of crystals in the graft suggests the utilization of renal transplantation for these patients is of questionable merit.[1]

Renal transplantation in Fabry's disease remains of uncertain benefit. The expectation that the grafted kidney would supply the deficient enzyme—α-galactosidase and prevent or inhibit the deposition of ceramide trihexoside in tissues—has not been proved.[2]

A normal functioning lower urinary tract is desirable for renal transplantation, but grafts can be successfully implanted with drainage via an isolated ileal conduit. Long-term success has been achieved in such patients.[3]

The American College of Surgeons–N.I.H. Registry of Transplants has published data that show that renal transplantation in the very young (less than 3 years of age) and the elderly (greater than 50 years of age) is associated with a lower percentage of success.[4] Transplant surgeons will usually evaluate such candidates on an individual basis.

The renal diseases that lead to transplantation in more than 15,000 patients are listed below:

Disease	Percent of total
Glomerulonephritis	56.0
Pyelonephritis	13.1
Polycystic disease	5.4
Nephrosclerosis	4.9
Congenital obstructive disease	1.4
Nephritis secondary to drugs	1.3
Diabetic glomerulosclerosis	1.2
Familial nephropathy	1.2
All others	15.5

It is anticipated that diabetic renal disease will make up a larger percent of recipients in the future as many more of these patients are being treated with chronic renal dialysis. Patients with malignancy, active infection, active peptic ulcer disease, diverticulitis, severe vascular disease, or serious psychiatric illness are excluded from transplantation.

■ When is the recipient subjected to a preliminary bilateral nephrectomy?

The preparation of all renal transplant recipients with preliminary bilateral nephrectomy, once a common practice, is no longer wisely utilized. Nephrectomy in recipients is indicated only for very specific indications. The most important indication is the presence of chronic infection. The urinary tract of the recipient must be sterile at the time of transplantation. This will require bilateral nephroureterectomy for some patients.

Persistent hypertension while on dialysis was once a frequent indication for pretransplant nephrectomy. This is less frequently necessary today. The control of fluid balance, ultrafiltration on dialysis, and potent antihypertensive drugs together often allow satisfactory control of blood pressure.

■ How are kidney donors selected?

Renal transplantation has advanced because one of the paired organs in a living donor can be employed with no functional impairment to the donor.

Living donors. The criteria for the use of familial donors have evolved with our knowledge of histocompatibility testing. The donor should be a willing volunteer under no duress. Since the establishment of 18 years as the age of legal majority, the donor should be 18 years of age or older in order to give legally acceptable consent. Identical twin transplantation poses no immunologic barrier and is, therefore, the ideal combination. Compatible siblings are preferred next followed by parental donors.

The use of nonrelated living donors has largely been abandoned as they offer little, if any, advantage over cadaveric donor renal transplantation.

The evaluation of a donor will include the histocompatibility tests to be described later and the following tests: (1) history and physical examination; (2) complete blood count; (3) urinalysis; (4) urine culture; (5) 24-hour urine for protein and creatinine clearance; (6) serum electrolytes,

blood urea nitrogen, creatinine, uric acid, calcium, and phosphorus; (7) fasting and 2-hour postprandial blood sugars; (8) tests for hepatitis-associated antigen; (9) chest x-ray film; (10) electrocardiogram; (11) excretory urogram; and (12) renal arteriogram.

Cadaveric donors. Much of the increase in the number of renal transplants of recent years is attributable to the increasing availability of cadaveric organs. Seventy percent of all transplants are now from cadaveric donors. In certain instances, a cadaveric organ transplant will be selected in preference to a living donor.

Most cadaveric donors today fit the criteria of brain death, so the organs may be salvaged while the circulation remains intact. This provides better kidneys, facilitates postoperative care, and makes the procedure safer for the recipient. Many states have initiated statutes that clarify the legal basis of cerebral death.

Cadaver donors must have no history of renal disease, hypertension, or processes that could be transmitted to the recipient. Patients with malignancy and infection are obviously excluded.[5]

In brain-injured patients fluids may be restricted in order to reduce brain swelling. Because of these considerations, many donors are identified who are dehydrated with poorly perfused kidneys.

When brain death has been established in the donor, it is desirable to maintain perfusion and function of the kidneys prior to nephrectomy. This may be accomplished by expanding the blood volume with saline, colloid, mannitol, or all three. If the blood pressure in the prospective donor has to be maintained by means other than fluids, the use of dopamine is preferred. Immediately prior to cadaver donor nephrectomy, large volumes of fluids and mannitol may improve renal blood flow so that dopamine or vasoconstrictor drugs may be discontinued. A rapid infusion of mannitol is useful in achieving this end.

Donor nephrectomy is performed in the operating room under careful sterile conditions.

■ What is the role of tissue typing in kidney transplantation?

A number of compatibility tests are now routine in renal transplantation. The first consideration is ABO blood type. The donor and recipient must be compatible in the same manner as for blood transfusions. Generally, donor and recipient are of the same ABO blood group, but type "O" may be considered the universal donor and type AB the universal recipient. Therefore a transplant can be made from a type O donor to a type A recipient but not the reverse. The Rh factor does not appear important in renal transplantation and need not be identical.

HLA. The HLA antigens are transplantation antigens on the cell surface of nucleated cells. They can be detected on peripheral lymphocytes, renal tubular cells, and skin fibroblasts with a simple in vitro cytotoxicity test employing specific sera and complement. They are detected clinically on lymphocytes as these cells are readily available and give good reactions.

The HLA antigens are more than 40 in number, segregating as four allelic pairs. They are inherited as allelic pairs on subloci close to one another on the sixth chromosomes. The new nomenclature for each sublocus is to designate the first series as HLA-A 1, HLA-A 2, HLA-A 3, HLA-A 9, HLA-A 10, and HLA-A 11. Those antigens of the second series are now designated HLA-B 5, HLA-B 7, HLA-B 8, HLA-B 12, and HLA-B 13. In addition there are HLA-CW 1, HLA-CW 2, and so forth and HLA-DW 1, HLA-DW 2, and so forth for the C and D loci.

Those antigens evaluated at international workshops but not yet clearly defined are given the designation HLA-AW 28, HLA-BW 14, HLA-CW 1, or HLA-DW 1, depending on the locus.

Each individual may be expected to have four HLA specificities of the A and B series: two of each as an allelic pair, as one specificity of each series is inherited on the chromosome from each parent. An example of the inheritance of HLA antigens is given in the following:

	Father	
Haplotype	A	B
HLA antigens	1-8	3-7
Children	A and C	A and D
	1, 8, 2, 12	1, 8, 9, 13

	Mother	
Haplotype	C	D
HLA antigens	2-12	9-13
Children	B and C	B and D
	3, 7, 2, 12	3, 7, 9, 13

In the preceding the capital letters are used to represent the chromosome, and the numbers are the HLA specificities. Each chromosome has a specificity from the first series (HLA-A) and one from the second series (HLA-B). Each pair of specificities on a chromosome is termed a haplotype. It can be seen that the simple laws of genetics determine that each child will share one haplotype with the mother and one with the father. This means that renal transplantation from parents to offspring will always be associated with one haplotype compatibility but also with one haplotype incompatibility.

We have illustrated the genetics of HLA with only the A and B locus antigens, as most clinical tissue typing has been done with these loci. In familial tissue typing compatibility for A and B will mean compatibility at C and D because these are on the same chromosome. In tissue typing outside of family members, no such compatibility will exist, as the C and D locus antigens segregate independent of A and B.

It can be seen that there are only four possible combinations of haplotypes (chromosomes) so that there is a one in four likelihood that siblings will share both haplotypes. When two siblings have both haplotypes in common, they are termed "HLA identical." This is most important in clinical renal transplantation, as grafts between HLA identical siblings have an excellent prognosis. Approximately 90% of such transplants will be functioning at 1 and 2 years. Furthermore these recipients require smaller doses of immunosuppressive drugs and are usually free from graft rejection crises. These recipients do require some form of immunosuppression despite the favorable prognosis.

Transplantation from parent to child and between siblings who share only one haplotype is not as successful. A larger percentage will fail because of immunologic rejection. It is obvious that when a sibling is available or when more than one sibling may be considered a prospective donor, HLA typing should be done in search for an HLA identical donor.

Testing individuals for HLA may not always reveal four specificities. In some individuals one, two, or three specificities may be found. This may be explained either by a homozygous allel; that is, both parents have the same HLA specificity or there is an as yet unidentified HLA antigen present.

It was hoped that typing for HLA and selecting donor recipient pairs for transplantation from cadaver donors would greatly improve clinical results. This has not been the case. With more than 30 HLA specificities in the A and the B series segregating in random fashion in the population, it is extremely difficult to identify an HLA identical cadaver kidney donor for a given recipient. Even more disheartening are the results. In transplantation from four antigen-compatible donors to recipients in cadaveric transplantation, there is only a 9% better result in comparison with four antigen-incompatible transplants. These facts suggest that while HLA antigens are now readily detectable by a simple in vitro cytotoxic method, they are not strong antigens with regard to the ultimate fate of renal transplants.

MLC. When lymphocytes of two different individuals are placed in cell culture, they are able to detect antigens on one another and respond by proliferation to blast formation. This is the basis of the mixed lymphocyte culture test of compatibility (MLC). It appears the MLC test detects a separate set of antigens distinct from HLA-A and B segregating independently in the general population. These are termed HLA-DW 1, HLA-DW 2, and so on. To identify an HLA-D antigen the investigator must have a cell of known antigenic makeup in contrast to a known serum used for detection of HLA-A and HLA-B. The HLA-D antigens are, therefore, termed cell-determined antigens (CD), while the HLA-A and HLA-B are termed serum-determined antigens (SD). The mixed lymphocyte culture test is made a one-way reaction by alternately blocking proliferation of one of the cells in culture with mitomycin C or another similar inhibitor. In this way the investigator can determine which cell in culture is responding to the antigen with blast formation. Cells are incubated in culture for several days for this test and blast formation is quantitated by incorporation of tritiated thymidine. It can be seen that this test requires much more time, equipment, and cells than sera. All these factors make it difficult or impossible to utilize the MLC test for clinical cadaver renal transplantation. One of the difficulties in working with the MLC

test is that almost all reactions are positive with cell proliferation. Investigators are currently attempting to quantitate the degree of reaction by calculating a stimulation index.

The stimulation index may be utilized in clinical transplantation to select a parent or one haplotype-matched sibling donor in a family. While most different individuals react positively in MLC, HLA identical siblings usually do not stimulate. The MLC reaction between HLA identical but nonrelated individuals is usually positive. This suggests MLC reactions are more important than HLA, as the results of clinical renal transplants in these two circumstances clearly show a more favorable result with a negative MLC (that is, between HLA identical siblings).

A number of centers are energetically employed in the identification of MLC antigens with the goal of characterizing a given individual's MLC determinants in a manner comparable to our present ability to characterize HLA.

■ **What is the cross match test for transplantation?**

Cytotoxins. The sera used in the development of our understanding of the HLA antigen system are those that contain naturally occurring cytotoxic antibodies. These antibodies are capable of killing lymphocytes in vitro in the presence of complement. The antibodies occur as a consequence of immunization through pregnancy and whole blood transfusions. They may also develop following tissue or organ allografts.

If these naturally occurring cytotoxins are present in a renal graft recipient and have a cytotoxic effect on the antigens of the donor, one may see a rapid immunologic destruction of the graft. To prevent this occurrence, a cross match test is always made, testing recipient serum against donor lymphocytes. This is a routine compatibility test to be done immediately prior to all renal transplants.

The presence of cytotoxins in an individual or in a group of prospective candidates to receive a renal graft may be determined by testing the serum of each individual against the lymphocytes from a large number of random donors.

At UCLA in the laboratory of Dr. Paul Terasaki, individual sera may be tested against 50 to

100 different donor cells.[6] Only when a large number are tested can we determine with reasonable confidence whether or not an individual has been sensitized by exposure to HLA antigens.

When renal transplant recipients develop cytotoxins from exposure to HLA antigens of leukocytes in whole blood transfusions, it is more difficult to find a kidney donor to which they do not exhibit a positive cross match reaction. This observation has led to the widespread use of frozen red cells that are devoid of leukocytes and have little if any HLA antigens present.

The study of development of cytotoxins following transfusions has led to some very interesting observations with regard to immunity. If one looks at a large population of patients receiving whole blood transfusions and plots the percent with cytotoxins against the number of transfusions, it will be apparent that the percent positive will increase with the number of transfusions. However, after more than 20 transfusions, approximately 50% of the population will not develop cytotoxins.

When cadaver renal transplants are made into patients who have received multiple transfusions and have never developed cytotoxins, the prognosis for function at 1 year is 80%. This is in contrast to approximately 30% success with cadaver renal transplantation into patients with cytotoxins.

It would thus appear that the response to HLA antigens in whole blood identifies a segment of the population with a more active immune response, one more likely to reject a kidney graft. This group is termed "responders" in contrast to those who have multiple transfusions, do not develop cytotoxins, and are less likely to reject a kidney and who are termed "nonresponders." Not all transplant surgeons agree with the difference in graft results of "responders" and "nonresponders" to HLA antigens. A group in Minnesota has published results that they interpret to show no difference in transplants comparing responders to nonresponders.

Some have postulated that the individuals who receive leukocytes in transfusions but do not develop cytotoxins are instead producing a blocking or enhancing antibody that favors subsequent renal transplantation.

Transplantation centers all over the world are now reporting improved graft survival in recipients who have received blood transfusions prior to renal transplantation.

The patients who have never had a transfusion have the poorest percent success and those with more than 20 transfusions the best. Patients who receive intermediate numbers of transfusions lie between these limits.

■ What are the special considerations for nephrectomy in transplantation?
Living related

The donor nephrectomy for renal transplantation is a unique surgical procedure in that it is surgery performed on one individual for the benefit of another. It entails risk with no personal physical benefit. The psychologic benefits are self-evident.

The surgeon performing donor nephrectomy must understand the needs of the transplant surgeon with regard to the length of artery and vein, length of ureter, and blood supply to the ureter.

To provide a kidney that will be in optimum condition for 30 to 40 minutes of ischemia and yet function promptly in the recipient, we make every effort to ensure good renal perfusion. This begins with intravenous fluids for the donor, overnight, prior to nephrectomy; 1500 ml of 5% dextrose and half-normal saline is a good quantity of fluid. After the induction of anesthesia, we pass a urethral catheter in the donor so that a diuresis may be induced during surgery without distending the bladder. The donor is well hydrated throughout the procedure. Vasopressors are not used should relative hypotension occur with anesthesia and positioning of the patient, but rather adequate expansion of the blood volume is used to maintain blood pressure and renal perfusion. The use of 50 g of mannitol will often enhance renal perfusion and ensure a good diuresis during nephrectomy.

Cadaver donor nephrectomy

The cadaver donor nephrectomy is carried out in the operating room with all sterile precautions. In California statutes clarify the position of cerebral death so that kidneys may be removed with an intact circulation.

The donor is frequently the victim of a severe head injury, in which circumstance he or she may be kept dehydrated. After brain death has been certified, the perfusion and function of the kidneys is improved by rapid infusion of electrolyte solutions and mannitol. The donor is given 10,000 units heparin and phentolamine (Regitine), 15 mg, prior to nephrectomy. The kidneys are removed transperitoneally with an effort to obtain the full length of the renal arteries and veins and a long segment of ureter. A transverse upper abdominal or a long midline incision provides good exposure.

■ **How may kidneys be preserved for subsequent use in transplantation?**

The kidney to be transplanted may be kept ex vivo for many hours or several days. Two methods of preservation are currently in widespread use. They may be looked on as complementary. The washout method of renal preservation employs a cold electrolyte solution of a composition to approximate the concentrations within cells. The sodium is low and potassium high. These solutions were developed at UCLA first by Dr. Geoff Collins[7] and later modified by Dr. Stephen Sacks.[8] Human kidneys have been preserved 24 to 38 hours by simple washout cooling, stored in a cold container, and transplanted with immediate function after revascularization. The upper limit of safe preservation by this method has not been established, but it is apparent that 24 hours of preservation is readily accomplished.

For renal preservation of 2 to 3 days, a perfusion system of the type developed by Belzer is necessary.[9] These machines use a cryoprecipitated plasma or an albumin solution of electrolyte composition comparable to the blood. The principal factor in all forms of renal preservation is cooling. Kidneys are kept at 2° to 8° C for optimal results.

■ **How is the kidney implanted into the recipient?**

The technique of placing the renal transplant in the iliac fossa using the iliac vessels for revascularization was first employed by Küss[10] and was used successfully by Murray in the first transplant between identical twins.[11] It has taken its place as the standard operation for renal transplantation. The procedure is performed extraperitoneally by means of an incision lateral to the rectus muscle in the lower abdomen.

The renal vein is anastomosed end to side to the external iliac vein. The renal artery is anastomosed end to end with the internal iliac artery. The kidney should be allowed to take a position in the iliac fossa that seems natural. No attempt is made to place the graft in one position. The ureter of the graft is anastomosed mucosa to mucosa in the floor of the bladder.

In transplantation into small children, particularly with adult size kidneys, the iliac fossa and the iliac vessels may not accommodate the graft. In these circumstances the transplant is placed intra-abdominally in the lower lumbar area with venous anastomosis to the inferior vena cava and arterial anastomosis to the aorta or to the common iliac artery.

Drainage of the wound is not employed by many transplant surgeons. We have used the closed drainage of the Hemovac system for many years and regularly obtain 200 to 400 ml of fluid over 24 to 48 hours. This is mainly lymph. We have rarely observed a primary lymphocele in our series, whereas others report them in a significant percentage of cases.

The urethral catheter is used to drain the bladder in those patients exhibiting a brisk diuresis as in transplantation from living donors. The catheter is removed in 24 to 48 hours. When the graft does not function immediately, as in transplantation from cadaveric donors, we do not employ urethral catheter drainage and have observed no adverse effects. Our patients may void the small volumes of urine produced by such grafts.

■ **What are the important considerations in the ICU immediately after renal transplantation?**

The early postoperative management of the recipient of a renal transplant is concerned with fluid and electrolyte balance. A careful record of intake and output is necessary. Daily body weights are an important method of assessing fluid balance. The recipient of a kidney from a living donor may experience a profound diuresis caused by fluid and osmotic particles. This patient will need precise replacement of fluid volume and electrolytes. Determination of urinary sodium and potassium is helpful in guiding electrolyte replacement. During osmotic diuresis, the urine will contain 75 to 100 mEq of sodium. This is replaced by administering one-half normal saline with added sodium bicarbonate. The urinary potassium is extremely variable and may need replacement in some patients. Serum electrolytes will be determined at 4-hour intervals the first 24 hours following transplantation and daily thereafter. The complete blood count including platelet count is obtained daily. Leukopenia and thrombocytopenia are important indicators of bone marrow depression by azathioprine (Imuran). This is an undesirable consequence of immunosuppressive therapy.

■ Which drugs are used to achieve immunosuppression and prevent graft rejection?

The immunosuppressive drugs are employed in variable doses according to the experience and idiosyncracies of the individual transplant surgeon. I employ azathioprine in a dose of 4 mg/kg body weight per day for the first 2 days of therapy and generally give 1.5 mg/kg body weight thereafter unless a fall in leukocytes or platelets indicates bone marrow depression. This calls for drastically reduced doses or even temporary cessation of azathioprine. It is undesirable to withhold azathioprine, as graft rejection as been observed even with severe leukopenia. For this reason, the goal of azathioprine administration is to achieve immunosuppression without bone marrow depression.

Corticosteroids in the form of prednisone or methylprednisolone (Solu-Medrol) are the next mainstay of immunosuppression. We give Solu-Medrol, 1 g, intravenously daily for 1 to 2 weeks and then switch to oral prednisone. The large doses of Solu-Medrol are appropriate in recipients of cadaver kidneys when the graft is not functioning because of ischemic injury. In this circumstance one cannot detect the development of a rejection crisis so we treat the patient with the full doses of Solu-Medrol we would give to a patient experiencing graft rejection. When renal function is good, alterations in function become the hallmark of the rejection crisis. To detect alterations in graft function, we determine the serum creatinine and BUN daily for the first 2 or 3 weeks and three times per week thereafter for 1 to 2 months. Failing renal function calls for increased doses of corticosteroids.

Antilymphocyte globulin is given intramuscularly or intravenously in some centers for 2 to 8 weeks. This is an adjunct to the use of azathioprine and prednisone.

■ What are the signs and symptoms of an allograft rejection crisis?

The diagnosis of an acute allograft rejection crisis may manifest by one or all of the following physical symptoms and signs:

1. Fever
2. Pain at the site of the graft
3. Swelling of the graft
4. Change in bruit audible over the graft
5. Hypertension
6. Oliguria
7. Reduction in urinary sodium
8. Lymphocytes in the urinary sediment
9. Fibrin split products in the urine
10. Leukocytosis
11. Thrombocytopenia
12. Rising BUN and serum creatinine
13. Reduced renal blood flow by isotopic measurements
14. Circulating cytotoxins
15. Accumulation of radioactive fibrin in the graft

The occurrence of allograft rejection is extremely variable. It is more likely to be accompanied by several of the above shortly after transplantation, but will often be silent with only a rise in serum BUN and creatinine later. Treatment of the rejection crisis is by administration of Solu-Medrol, 1 g, intravenously daily for 3 to 5 days. We also give local irradiation to the graft, 150 R, on alternate days for three doses.

Renal biopsy is rarely necessary to establish the diagnosis of a graft rejection. The wide spectrum of histologic changes seen in transplanted kidneys, even those with good function, makes interpretation of renal biopsy difficult. We have found the blood clearance of hippuran to be a valuable method of evaluating renal function following transplantation.[12,13]

When renal function has stabilized at an optimum level, it is desirable to have an excretory urogram to serve as a baseline study and to detect any unsuspected obstructive uropathy.

■ What is the role of renal isotope scans after transplantation?

In transplantation from cadaver donors, the ischemic injury to the graft may result in markedly impaired function for 1 to 4 weeks. During this time, the patient is supported by frequent hemodialysis. The integrity of this poorly functioning graft is determined by the gamma camera and radionuclide imaging with technetium 99 and I^{131} radiohippuran. Serial determinations are made during the period of oliguria. Hippuran excretion can be detected with minimal volumes of urine per 24 hours. These observations support the continued use of immune suppression until graft function ensues with recovery from ischemic injury. Quantitative estimations of hippuran clearance by the kidney can be made when renal function is poor.[13]

■ What are the important urologic complications after renal transplantation?

The medical and surgical complications following renal transplantation are the major factors that mandate the need for specialized training for transplant surgeons and restrict performance to major medical centers. The performance of surgery in the chronically ill patient then subjected to immunosuppression opens the host to a variety of unusual infections and other complications.

The urologic complications of transplantation are similar to those seen in other patients undergoing ureteral surgery. Added dimensions are a compromised blood supply to the ureter and immunosuppression.

Ureteral obstruction may occur at the uretrovesical junction at any time after transplantation but is most likely early. Obstruction can be identified by an excretory urogram or by hippuran scan. Tension on the anastomosis, edema, and misplaced sutures may play a role. Extrinsic obstruction of the graft ureter by the spermatic cord or extravesical fibrosis have been described. Obstruction can be relieved by a temporary ureteral intubation with passage of a catheter cytoscopically or by reanastomosis of the graft ureter to the bladder. When open surgical intervention

is necessary, we favor reanastomosis to the bladder whenever feasible. Utilization of the recipient ipsilateral ureter is a good second choice.

Ureterocutaneous fistula is the most dangerous urologic complication. Persistence of urinary leakage with associated infection in an immune suppressed patient has led to many fatalities in the past. Through experience, we have learned to obtain early correction of the fistula or to sacrifice the transplanted kidney and save the patient. Fistula will develop if the initial ureterocystostomy is not performed carefully. Ureteral necrosis can occur if the transplanted ureter is not provided with an adequate blood supply. The graft rejection process may compromise ureteral blood supply and lead to necrosis with a ureterocutaneous fistula. When the fistula is the result of compromised blood supply, we favor correction using the recipient ipsilateral ureter with a ureteropyelostomy so that only the renal pelvic blood supply of the graft is needed for a successful outcome. We favor prompt surgical intervention in patients with urinary fistula as the risk of persistent fistula with infection is great.

Vesicocutaneous fistula will occur if the original cystotomy is not closed carefully or if infection erodes the suture line. If this is a partial leak, it can be managed by urethral catheter drainage.[14-17]

■ What are the important surgical complications?

Lymphocele. The division of large lymphatic vessels about the iliac artery and vein may lead to an accumulation of lymphatic fluid in the wound. As mentioned earlier, careful ligation of these lymphatics and temporary wound drainage will usually prevent this occurrence. Some patients have been reported to develop a large collection of lymph adjacent to the graft kidney. This can be recognized as an expanding mass in the lower abdomen, displacing the bladder and graft ureter. Treatment may be aspiration or, more definitively, marsupialization of the wall of the lymphocele with the peritoneal cavity.[18]

Gastrointestinal

Peptic ulcer disease. The increased gastric acid secretion induced by corticosteroid therapy may lead to peptic ulcer disease. The prophylactic application of antacids will protect most patients. When high-dose steroids are used, we give ant-acids every 2 hours. All patients are kept on antacids following transplantation. Rarely will ulcer surgery be necessary to control gastrointestinal bleeding or relieve persistent pain. The indications in transplant patients are the same as those for other patients.

Pancreatitis. Corticosteroid therapy may also result in pancreatitis. This may be acute or chronic. It can be a life-threatening illness. Conventional medical management is indicated.[19,20]

Diverticulitis. Transplantation into the older age group will increase the likelihood of treating patients with diverticulosis. Patients on immuno-suppression may be more prone to develop acute diverticulitis. This has proved fatal in some cases. Preoperative assessment of the colon may be indicated before transplantation in older patients, particularly those with a history of diverticulosis or bowel problems.[21,22]

Spontaneous rupture of the graft. The transplanted kidney may develop edema from ischemic injury or the rejection process. Marked graft swelling has led to spontaneous rupture of the kidney.[23] The patients frequently have abrupt onset of pain and swelling in the graft site. There may be significant hemorrhage manifest by a fall in hematocrit. The ruptured kidney is usually badly damaged, and most often nephrectomy is indicated. We have successfully repaired one graft. Lord collected 26 cases of graft rupture in Australia and New Zealand.[24] Graft nephrectomy was necessary in 20.

■ Which complications are attributable to the corticosteroid therapy?

In addition to the complications of the immunosuppressive regimen, there are those complications that occur in any group of patients on corticosteroids. These are the most frequent in a group of transplant patients.

Aseptic necrosis of the femoral head. Aseptic necrosis of the femoral head is seen in approximately 5% to 10% of patients. It is a cause of pain and disability. The pain may occur weeks or months before radiographic changes are seen. This complication can be anticipated in patients

who require larger doses of prednisone in order to maintain the function of the graft, but in our experience it appears to occur as an individual idiosyncratic event, as it will be seen shortly after the initiation of therapy in one patient and not after many years in another. Reconstruction of the total hip has successfully rehabilitated many patients.

Premature development of cataracts. The premature development of cataracts is another relatively frequent and unpleasant complication of the use of corticosteroids. While this might be anticipated more frequently in the older recipient, it is seen at all ages. Surgical intervention is indicated along the same guidelines used for other patients.

The catabolic effect of corticosteroids is seen very obviously in the skin and subcutaneous tissues of patients on long-term therapy. This will manifest by easy bruising and marked intracutaneous hemorrhage.

■ What are the important infections after transplantation?

Opportunistic infections. The immunosuppressed patient does not appear more vulnerable to the common upper respiratory infections. The serious infections are those that rarely affect individuals with an intact immune system. Pulmonary infections caused by the fungi *Aspergillus, Nocardia,* and so on are life-threatening in all and fatal in some patients. The protozan pulmonary infection due to *Pneumocystis carinii* is an example of infection caused by altered host resistance. This organism must be identified by lung biopsy and the use of a silver methenamine tissue stain. Specific therapy in the form of pentamidine isethionate is available and may salvage some patients. Antifungal agents have been used successfully in transplant patients, even those with less than optimal renal function.[25]

The ubiquitous virus of cytomegalic disease is frequently found in the urine or lungs of transplant recipients with severe infections. Whether this represents a primary infection or a secondary state is not certain. Unless cytomegalic titers are determined serially in individual patients, it is difficult to interpret this test. The efficacy of cytosine arabinoside therapy is open to question.

Table 25-1. Results of renal transplantation by donor source

Donor source	Graft function 1 year (%)	Graft function 2 years (%)
HLA identical	85.0	79
Other siblings	79.9	73.7
Parent	71.7	61.1
Cadaver donor	50.6	42.6

Table 25-2. Results of renal transplantation by age

Recipient's age at transplant	Graft function (%)				
	1 year	2 years	3 years	4 years	5 years
0-5	37	21	20	20	20
6-50	52	44	39	35	34
51-60	42	31	26	25	25

■ **What are the results of transplantation?**

The results of renal transplantation are of great interest to all. There has been only a slight improvement over the past 5 years. The mortality rate for recipients has declined so that surgeons are learning to be more skillful, both technically and with immunosuppressive regimens. Results must be viewed with regard to donor source (Table 25-1).[26]

The results may be further evaluated with regard to the age of the recipient (Table 25-2). This reveals results are not as good in the very young and in the elderly with kidneys from cadaver donors.[4]

■ **What are the special considerations for children?**

The prospect of long-term renal dialysis is unpleasant for both the patient and the family. Transplant surgeons have, therefore, treated children with chronic renal failure with optimism and enthusiasm. Children tolerate the surgical procedures and immunosuppressive regimens well. There is one major additional consideration for the pediatric age group and this regards growth. The administration of prednisone is attended with variable growth patterns both in transplant recipients and other pediatric patients. For this reason, results will often be better if the pediatric patient has already passed successfully through the major growth cycle. Patients with retarded growth because of long-standing chronic renal disease may resume growth but rarely is "catch-up" growth observed. Except for the very young, the results of renal transplantation in children are generally good.[27-29]

REFERENCES

1. Barnes, B. A., et al.: The 12th report of the human renal transplant registry, J.A.M.A. **233**:787, 1975.
2. Philippart, M.: Kidney transplantation in Fabry's disease, N. Engl. J. Med. **289**:270, 1972.
3. Kelly, W. D., Merkel, F. K., and Markland, C.: Ilial urinary diversion in conjunction with renal homotransplantation, Lancet **1**:222, 1966.
4. Barnes, B. A., et al.: The 11th report of the human renal transplant registry, J.A.M.A. **226**:1197, 1973.
5. Martin, D. C., Rubini, M., and Rosen, V. J.: Cadaveric renal homotransplantation with inadvertent transplantation of carcinoma, J.A.M.A. **192**:752, 1965.
6. Terasaki, P. I., Mickey, M. R., and Kreisler, M.: Presensitization and kidney transplant failures, Postgrad. Med. J. **47**:89, 1971.
7. Collins, G. M., Bravo-Shugarman, M., and Terasaki, P. I.: Kidney preservation for transportation, Lancet **2**:1219, 1969.
8. Sacks, S. A., Petritsch, P. H., Linder, R., and Kaufman, J. J.: Renal autotransplantation, Am. J. Surg. **128**:402, 1974.
9. Belzer, F. O., and Kountz, S. L.: Preservation and transplantation of human cadaver kidney, Ann. Surg. **173**:394, 1970.
10. Küss, R., Teinturier, J., and Milliez, P.: Quelques essais de graffe de rein chez l'homme, Me. Acad. Chir. **77**:755, 1951.
11. Merrill, J. P., Murray, J. E., Harrison, J. H., and Guild, W. R.: Successful homotransplantation of the human kidney between identical twins, J.A.M.A. **160**:227, 1956.
12. Awad, W., Bennett, L., and Martin, D. C.: Detection of renal homograft rejection reaction with a single dose of radiohippuran, J. Urol. **100**:223, 1968.
13. Martin, D. C., Hunter, J. L., Lawton, M. B., Berke, R. A., and Morton, M. E.: Serial radionuclide quantitative function studies for evaluation of renal transplants, J. Urol. **112**:2, 1974.
14. MacKinnon, K. J., et al.: Cadaver renal transplantation: emphasis on urological aspects, J. Urol. **99**:486, 1968.
15. Martin, D. C., Mims, M. M., Kaufman, J. J., and Goodwin, W. E.: The ureter in renal transplantation, J. Urol. **101**:680, 1969.
16. Starzl, T. E., et al.: Urological complications in 216 human recipients of renal transplants, Ann. Surg. **172**:1, 1970.
17. Belzer, F. O., et al.: Prevention of urologic complications after renal allotransplantation, Arch. Surg. **101**:449, 1970.

18. Schweizer, R. T., Cho, S., Kountz, S. L., and Belzer, F. O.: Lymphoceles following renal transplantation, Arch. Surg. **104**:42, 1972.

19. Johnson, W. C., and Nabseth, D. C.: Pancreatitis in renal transplantation, Ann. Surg. **171**:309, 1970.

20. Penn, I., et al.: Acute pancreatitis and hyperamylasemia in renal homograft recipients, Arch. Surg. **105**:167, 1972.

21. Penn, I., Brettschneider, L., Simpson, K., Martin, A., and Starzl, T. E.: Major colonic problems in human homotransplant recipients, Arch. Surg. **100**:61, 1970.

22. Demling, R. H., Salvatierra, O., and Belzer, F. O.: Intestinal necrosis and perforation after renal transplantation, Arch. Surg. **110**:251, 1975.

23. Koostra, G., Meyer, S., and Elema, J. D.: "Spontaneous" rupture of homografted kidneys, Arch. Surg. **108**:107, 1974.

24. Lord, R. S. A., Effeney, M. B., Hayes, J. M., and Tracy, G. D.: Renal allograft rupture, Ann. Surg. **177**:268, 1973.

25. Koppel, M. H., Coburn, J. W., Rosen, V. J., Davis, A., and Rubini, M. E.: Transplantation pneumonia: the importance of early open lung biopsy for etiologic diagnosis, Clin. Res. **17**:120, 1969.

26. Barnes, B. A., et al.: Renal transplantation in congenital and metabolic diseases, J.A.M.A. **232**:148, 1975.

27. Fine, R. N., et al.: Renal transplantation in young children, Am. J. Surg. **125**:559, 1973.

28. De Shazo, C. V., et al.: Results of renal transplantation in 100 children, Surgery **76**:461, 1974.

29. Talwalkar, Y. B., Harner, M. H., Musgrave, J. E., Lawson, R. K., and Campbell, R. A.: Pediatric renal transplantation, West. J. Med. **123**:1, 1975.

BIBLIOGRAPHY

Amos, D. B.: Transplantation antigens. In Saliston, D., Jr., editor: Textbook of surgery, Philadelphia, 1972, W. B. Saunders Co., p. 438.

Bach, F. H., and Kisken, W. A.: Predictive value of mixed leukocyte cultures for skin allograft survival in man, Transplantation **5**:1046, 1967.

Callender, C. O., et al.: Anti-HLA antibodies: failure to correlate with renal allograft rejection, Surgery **76**:573, 1974.

Calne, R. Y., and Murray, J. E.: Inhibition of the rejection of renal homografts in dogs by Burroughs-Wellcome 57-322, Surg. Forum **12**:118, 1961.

Carrel, A.: The ultimate result of a double nephrectomy and replantation of one kidney, J. Exp. Med. **14**:124, 1911.

Cochrum, K., Perkins, H., Payne, R. D., Kountz, S. L., and Belzer, F. O.: The correlation of MLC with graft survival, Transplantation Proc. **5**:391, 1973.

Goodwin, W. E., et al.: Human renal transplantation, I. Clinical experiences with six cases of renal homotransplantation, J. Urol., **89**:13, 1963.

Hamburger, J., et al.: Renal transplantation, Baltimore, 1972, The Williams & Wilkins Co., p. 80.

Hardy, J. D.: High ureteral injuries: management by autotransplantation of the kidney, J.A.M.A. **184**:97, 1963.

Hume, D. M., Merrill, J. P., Miller, B. F., and Thorn, G. W.: Experiences with renal homotransplantation in the human: report of nine cases, J. Clin. Invest. **34**:327, 1955.

Ibels, L. S., Stewart, J. H., Mahoney, J. F., and Shiel, A. G. R.: Deaths from occlusive arterial disease in renal allograft recipients, Br. Med. J. **3**:552, 1974.

Kaufman, J. J., Alferez, C., and Nararrete, R. V.: Autotransplantation of a solitary functioning kidney for renovascular hypertension, J. Urol. **102**:146, 1969.

Kissmeyer-Nielsen, F., Olsen, S., Petersen, V. P., and Fjeldborg, O.: Hyperacute rejection of kidney allografts, associated with pre-existing humoral antibodies against donor cells, Lancet **2**:662, 1966.

Leiter, E., Kim, K. H., and Glabman, S.: Urinary reconstruction by pyeloureteral anastomosis in human renal transplants, J. Urol. **109**:28, 1973.

Marshall, V. F., Whitsell, J., McGovern, J. H., and Miscall, B. G.: The practicality of renal autotransplantation in humans, J.A.M.A. **196**:1154, 1966.

Opelz, G., and Terasaki, P. I.: Histocompatibility matching utilizing responsiveness as a new dimension, Transplant Proc. **4**:433, 1972.

Opelz, G., Sengar, D. P. S., Mickey, M. R., and Terasaki, P. I.: Effect of blood transfusions on subsequent kidney transplants, Transplant Proc. **5**:253, 1973.

Penn, I., and Starzl, T. E.: Malignant tumors arising de nova in immunosuppressed organ transplant recipients, Transplantation **14**:407, 1972.

Pierce, J. C., Madge, G. E., Lee, H. M., and Hume, D. M.: Lymphoma, a complication of renal allotransplantation in man, J.A.M.A. **219**:1593, 1972.

Sacks, S. A., Petritsch, P. H., and Kaufman, J. J.: Canine kidney preservation using a new perfusate, Lancet **1**:1024, 1973.

Salvatierra, O., Jr., Kountz, S. L., and Belzer, F. O.: Polycystic renal disease treated by renal transplantation, Surg. Gynecol. Obstet. **137**:431, 1973.

Sheil, A. G. R., et al.: A controlled clinical trial of machine perfusion of cadaveric donor renal allografts, Lancet **2**:287, 1975.

Starzl, T. E., Marchiora, T. L., Porter, K. A., Iwasaki, Y., and Cerilli, G. J.: The use of heterologous antilymphoid agents in canine renal and liver homotransplantation and in human renal homotransplantation, Surg. Gynecol. Obstet. **124**:301, 1967.

Starzl, T. E., et al.: Cyclophosphamide and human organ transplantation, Lancet **1**:70, 1971.

Ting, A., and Terasaki, P. I.: Influence of lymphocyte-dependent antibodies on human kidney transplants, Transplantation **18**:371, 1974.

CHAPTER 26

Management of the renal transplant patient

Joyce R. Hostetler

The patient with irreversible renal failure faces three possible alternatives: no treatment and death, chronic dialysis (either peritoneal dialysis or hemodialysis), or transplantation. The renal failure patient is burdened with many decisions, perhaps one of the most significant being the choice of requesting transplantation. Renal transplantation is, as a rule, given some consideration by the renal failure patient following many traumatic changes in his life-style. Patients sometimes choose transplantation at the time they are notified of their renal failure and presented with the various modalities of treatment. Thus transplantation may occur during the predialysis stage of renal failure. Others may select transplantation months or years after beginning dialysis. The many restrictions associated with dialysis create numerous psychologic stresses. Some changes affecting the renal failure patient include:

1. Diet
2. Ability to work
3. Freedom and activity
4. Economic deprivation
5. Decreased sexual function
6. Altered body image
7. Change of role within family structure
8. Increased dependency

The inability of the patient to cope with one or more of these areas may lead to a request for transplantation. The end-stage renal disease patient encounters a complex world of medical and surgical decision making associated with numerous psychosocial problems.

Patient management requires a team effort including:

Nephrologists
Transplant surgeons
Psychiatrists
Psychologists
Nurses
Social workers
Dieticians
Many other skilled health personnel

By necessity the patient becomes an individual dependent on members of the medical community for lifesaving decisions and intervention. Very few find this an easy transition.

The renal failure patient comes to transplantation in need of information, sometimes with unrealistic expectations, and always with a great deal of hope for an improved quality of life. Successful transplantation offers greater rehabilitation and a better quality of life than dialysis. Patients who remain on chronic dialysis long enough to acquire numerous medical complications may no longer be able to tolerate the additional risks attendant with transplantation. Clearly, it is in the best interests of the dialysis patient to have early and periodic opportunities to discuss renal transplantation.

The transplant recipient is never free from medical supervision because of: (1) the possibility of graft rejection, which may occur weeks, months, or even years after surgery, and (2) the complications of immunosuppressive drugs. Patient management is an ongoing process requiring long-term monitoring of graft function. Included in the care of the transplant recipient is frequent interaction with the family. Organ procurement or the clinical management of the end-stage renal disease patient involved in the transplant process is the responsibility of the transplant coordinator.

The objective of this chapter is to present an overview of transplantation to the nursing community focusing on the nurse-patient relationship. The nursing staff devotes a great deal of time interacting with the patient and his family in their attempt to cope during this crisis period, thus portions are devoted to the psychosocial aspects of transplantation.

Although the protocols for management of the transplant patient may vary in different centers throughout the United States, they are basically the same. The procedures described in this chapter relate to the functions of a transplant team at the University of California at Irvine.

■ How are patients referred for transplantation?

Referral may occur in one of several ways. The patient may initiate the evaluation process by personally contacting the transplant center and requesting an interview. However, the majority of patients are referred by their attending physician who contacts the transplant center and requests an interview with the patient. On occasion the dialysis nurse will, at the request of the physician, make the necessary arrangements to have a patient interviewed and evaluated.

■ What is involved in an evaluation interview with a potential transplant recipient?

The initial interview focuses on three areas: (1) patient education, (2) patient assessment, and (3) data collection including medical history. Great care must be taken to give the patient unbiased information, including both the positive and negative aspects of transplantation. The patient may request the presence of a spouse or entire family at the initial interview, particularly if the possibility of a living related donor exists within the nuclear family.

Topics discussed during the interview include:
1. Medical history including family members

2. Acquisition of past medical records, x-ray films, and renal biopsy slides
3. Pretransplant laboratory tests required for matching donors with recipients, including ABO, histocompatibility tests, cytotoxic antibodies, cross matching, and MLC
4. Statistical success rates of kidney grafts as related to donor source
5. Identification of possible donors within the nuclear family
6. Diagnostic studies required for workup, which may include voiding cystourethrogram, barium enema, pulmonary function studies, or stress electrocardiogram
7. Skin tests for tuberculosis, mumps, histoplasmosis, and coccidioidomycosis
8. Pretransplant interview with social worker including donor and recipient
9. Interview and evaluation by transplant surgeon
10. Placement on cadaver waiting list and uncertain length of time before kidney becomes available
11. Preoperative procedures such as dialysis and transfusion
12. Surgical risks, incision site, anesthesia, length of stay in ICU, undetermined length of hospitalization, signs and symptoms of rejection
13. Postoperative monitoring of kidney function by laboratory tests and renal scans
14. Immunosuppressive drug therapy and related complications
15. Need for patient cooperation in long-term monitoring of graft function

A candidate form is then completed with all pertinent information regarding the patient, family members, occupation, financial status, hemodialysis data and medical history. An evaluation workup may require weeks or months to complete.

■ How is a living related donor evaluated and prepared for nephrectomy?

At the time of the initial interview with the potential kidney recipient, the possibility of obtaining a kidney from a family member is discussed. Selecting a donor can be a crisis for the entire family. Many times a patient will declare the willingness of a family member to donate, and on inquiry the prospective donor emphatically declines. Another approach is to have the potential recipient refer the donor to the transplant center for information. A reluctant donor will fail to follow through with the referral. Perhaps the most difficult and time-consuming aspect of living related transplants is the identification of a willing donor within the nuclear family. A screening period and decision-making process may take months or even years. The spouse of a potential related donor may exert pressure against the donation. The family system of donor selection is clearly at its most efficient very early in the selection process and works primarily in the direction of excluding some family members from participation. Because of subtle family pressures, the person selected by the family may be the one that would be least missed if problems arose. When a child is the recipient, the search for a donor is easier and the crisis of decision making is less acute than for an adult. Mothers generally view donation of a kidney as an obligation to their children and are motivated by guilt. A spouse may offer to donate, but is not considered as there is no biologic relationship. Some motives for donation are strong altruistic drives, religious beliefs, or guilt in past relationships.

When a donor or donors have been identified, an interview is conducted, preferably with the spouse or significant other present. Information is given to all concerned regarding the necessary laboratory tests, which include an IVP and renal arteriogram. These studies are not without risk, but are necessary to establish normal function and anatomy of the kidneys. The potential donor needs to be informed as to the surgical risks, possible rib resection, site of incision, anesthesia, influence of nephrectomy on life-style, expected length of convalescence, financial burden, and the advantages of transplanting living related donor kidneys as compared to cadaver organs. An opportunity is given to the donor to talk to an individual who has experienced organ donation for a family member. The donor has an evaluation by the social worker for the purpose of exploring his relationship with the recipient, ventilating any reservations he might have regarding the donation, discussing the pos-

sibility of graft rejection, and verbalizing his fears and anxieties surrounding major surgery and resultant altered body image. This nonthreatening interview presents an opportunity to the potential donor to withdraw his offer. The spouse or significant other is encouraged to attend the interview.

Much tension and apprehension are associated with an elective nephrectomy. If a donor demonstrates behavior indicating a reluctance to donate, the physician may offer an opportunity to the patient to terminate the evaluation and supply a plausible medical excuse to the recipient and family. Because of the crisis nature of living related transplantation, the medical and nursing staff, including the social worker, provide emotional support and medical information to the donor, recipient, and families on a continuing basis in an effort to allay fear and anxiety. A pretransplant psychosocial evaluation of donor and recipient enables the medical and nursing staff to understand the individuals' coping mechanisms with previous stress situations so that they may be sustained during this totally new, unique crisis period.

On completion of the basic laboratory tests and IVP, the potential donor is presented to the transplant team, composed of surgeons and nephrologists, for evaluation. If accepted, the donor is hospitalized for a renal arteriogram. Following this procedure, the transplant may be scheduled at the convenience of the surgeon, donor, and recipient.

Preoperative teaching of the living related donor begins with the initial interview. Reinforcement of information and reassurance is necessary throughout the donation process. Statistics reveal that nephrectomy with a healthy donor is a relatively safe surgical procedure. Mortality risk has been calculated as 0.05%. The living related donor is admitted on the day prior to transplantation. Routine preoperative laboratory studies are performed and the transplant surgeon may request another cross match between donor and recipient. IV fluids are started on the evening prior to surgery. The patient is then given information related to the activities of the following day such as preoperative medication, approximate time of departure for surgery, time spent in the recovery room, and subsequent return to the surgical ward. The patient is also taught the importance of turning frequently, coughing, deep breathing, and methods for minimizing discomfort during these procedures. The donor is informed of the availability of medication postoperatively for discomfort as ordered by the physician. Deep breathing exercises using various techniques begin on the first postoperative day to prevent pulmonary complications. Early ambulation is encouraged by the medical staff. Lenient visiting hours exist on the day of surgery as family support is much needed by the donor. It is not uncommon for a family donor to experience depression during the postoperative period. This may be caused by: (1) loss of a vital organ, (2) the altered body image, and (3) feelings of neglect resulting from the focus of attention postoperatively shifting from the donor to the recipient.

Discharge from the hospital occurs, as a rule, on the seventh postoperative day. The donor will require medical checkups for several months. Normal activity is resumed after the sixth week of convalescence.

■ What preoperative care is given the transplant recipient?

The patient awaiting transplantation must be maintained in optimal condition for surgery. At the time of admission the patient must be free of infection, particularly in the urinary tract and dialysis access site. Careful physical examination must be performed to detect any condition that would jeopardize a patient once immunosuppressive drug therapy is initiated. Pretransplant dialysis is performed and transfusion of packed cells is indicated if the hematocrit is less than 28. The patient is generally euphoric with a totally optimistic outlook prior to surgery. Despite the uncertainty of the procedure, the majority of patients are eager for the surgery, with a focus on graft acceptance rather than the possibility of graft rejection. The patients readily share their feelings regarding transplantation with the nursing staff. Because of the emergency nature of cadaveric transplantation and the need to hurry the patient through the various preoperative procedures, it is essential that the nursing staff exhibit a calm, confident approach to the patient to prevent adding to his feelings of anxiety. Continuous patient education is practiced by the transplant nursing staff, and the patient's involvement in his care is encouraged. Frequently, the recipient expresses curiosity regarding the cadaver donor, and the usual policy is to reveal the donor's age and sex but withhold information regarding actual identification. Information related to the postoperative period is reviewed with the patient: the need for a urinary catheter for 1 or 2 days and hematuria for several days following surgery, Hemovac drainage from the incision, frequent testing of blood, early ambulation, 24-hour stay in ICU, IV drug therapy for approximately 3 days, and monitoring of renal function with isotope scans.

■ What postoperative care is given the transplant recipient?

Immediately after surgery, the transplant recipient arrives in the intensive care unit from the postanesthesia room for a stay of approximately 24 hours. As the patient arrives, an assessment can be made of:

1. The patient's level of consciousness and degree of pain
2. The intravenous lines, noting site, type of solution, and flow rate
3. The abdominal dressing, noting drainage and presence of Hemovac, and recording site of incision
4. The Foley catheter, noting patency and drainage
5. The location of vascular access site and presence of bruit
6. The vital signs, avoiding extremity with shunt or fistula
7. The patient's weight
8. The patient's most recent electrolytes

Nursing responsibilities focus on observation of kidney function by accurately monitoring hourly intake and output, weight, serum BUN and creatinine, and maintaining critical fluid and electrolyte balance. Patient education revolves around helping the patient avoid sources of infection, verbalizing symptoms, and detecting early signs of complications. Vital signs, output, and electrolytes are frequently reported to the surgical staff. In this crucial postoperative period the nurse caring for the transplant recipient must accurately observe and report any changes, subtle or obvious, in the patient's status. Immunosuppressive drug therapy is administered as ordered by the physician. Progressive ambulation is started on the first postoperative day. Ice chips may be tolerated on the first postoperative day with dietary increase dependent on the patient's overall status. On the second postoperative day the patient is returned to the surgical ward and assigned a private room. The recipient then faces an unknown period of hospitalization filled with uncertainty. His length of stay may vary from 2 weeks to 2 months, depending on renal function and complications. Azathioprine and methylprednisolone (Solu-Medrol) are administered intravenously for 2 or 3 days; thereafter oral dosages are prescribed. The patient must, once again, be prepared for the undesirable side-effects of the immunosuppressive drugs. Patient education revolves around drug therapy, dosages and identification, monitoring of graft function, subjective symptoms of infection, interpretation of laboratory values, and the necessity of various tests such as renal scans, chest x-ray examinations, and the use of dialysis support while waiting for adequate renal function. Ambulation is encouraged to improve circulation and bowel function and to prevent pulmonary complications.

Just prior to discharge the patient's medications are reviewed, as well as signs and symptoms of rejection or infection. Instructions are given regarding recording of daily weight, temperature, and urine output. The patient is instructed to contact the transplant team if he notes a temperature greater than 100° F, pain over the grafted kidney, marked decrease in urine output, rapid weight gain, and any signs of possible infection either at the site of the incision or in the upper respiratory tract.

Daily telephone contact is made between the patient and the transplant nurse coordinator for the first few weeks as this is the critical period for infections and rejection crises. Blood samples are taken every other day and clinic visits are made weekly for approximately 1 or 2 months depending on the patient's status. As the recipient's renal function becomes more stable, laboratory tests and clinic visits are less frequent.

A wide range of emotional behavior may be observed in the transplant recipient during the first few critical months following surgery. Complications and rejection crises may cause the patient to become angry, depressed, frightened, suicidal, demanding, critical of the medical and nursing staff, and at times openly hostile.

The social worker and nursing staff provide emotional support for the patient by permitting him to ventilate his feelings of anxiety. During the uncertain few weeks following a transplant, kidney function may fluctuate and patients erroneously feel the surgery has been a failure. They may be sustained during this period by merely offering encouragement and hope for a successful outcome of the transplant. Particularly during crucial periods, the patient needs to turn to people in whom he has the most trust. He fears abandonment by the medical and nursing team as he may already have experienced abandonment by significant others in his personal life. In the event of graft failure the patient has to cope with a grief period manifested by depression, a sense of loss, and mourning. Some patients in this situation are reluctant to return to their dialysis unit and will request a transfer to another facility.

■ **What complications may occur in the long-term management of the transplant recipient?**

The transplant recipient requires medical supervision for as long as he keeps the grafted kidney. Complications occurring in the early postoperative period frequently relate to technical problems associated either with the procurement of the organ or transplantation. The rejection phenomenon is a major problem that may occur at any time after surgery. Complications related to immunosuppressive drug therapy may arise during the early postoperative period or months and even years following transplantation. Sepsis and pulmonary infections during the first year are two dreaded complications that contribute greatly to the mortality rate of renal transplantation.

The responsibility of the nurse is to observe and assess the patient for early signs and symptoms of infections and rejection. The importance of reporting health problems to the transplant team is encouraged as many complications require immediate attention and can be better managed in the early stages. Frequently the transplant recipient merely needs an explanation of various symptoms and reassurance that the problems he is experiencing are normal for individuals on immunosuppressive drug therapy. Because of the anxiety related to possible loss of the grafted kidney, recipients require a great deal of emotional support, particularly for the initial 3 months following transplantation.

Some physical problems the recipient may experience include (1) steroid acne, (2) fatigue, (3) loss of hair or, conversely, hirsutism, (4) weight gain, (5) cushinoid or moon facies, and (6) enlarged abdomen. Purple-red striae may appear on the legs, abdomen, and breasts; joint pains may accompany a rapid reduction in prednisone dosage; upper respiratory or viral infections such as herpes are quite common occurrences; and hypertension may continue to be a problem following transplantation. Many patients welcome the assistance of a dietician who will offer guidelines for caloric intake and subsequent weight reduction. Changes in body image are distressing to many patients and they need to ventilate their feelings regarding alterations in physical appearance. Physical changes may have a profound effect on the emotional and social facets of an individual's life.

The nurse monitoring long-term graft function may never become lax regarding the observation and recording of laboratory test results, for deviations may occur years after transplantation even in the most stable recipient. A rise in BUN and creatinine may herald a rejection crisis; a reduction in hematocrit may accompany the early stages of a failing kidney or gastrointestinal bleeding. Leukopenia or thrombocytopenia may indicate the need to alter azathioprine dosage. Observation of an abnormal laboratory value requires a repeat of the test before initiating medical action.

The patient experiencing a rejection crisis becomes frightened and may become angry or depressed. Many patients will try to blame the rejection phenomenon on their drug therapy, diet, activities, physicians, God, or numerous external factors. Rejection crises are treated with either intravenous methylprednisolone or an increase of oral prednisone dosage. The nurse must provide continuous information regarding the rejection process and the medical treatment. Tests, drugs, and side-effects may have to be explained many times because of the patient's use of defense mechanisms such as denial and rationalization. The transplant recipient must constantly be offered encouragement and hope, for the threatened loss of the grafted kidney is accompanied by fear and depression. Long-term use of immunosuppressive drugs may result in: (1) drug-induced diabetes, (2) aseptic necrosis of the femoral head, (3) fragility of blood vessels resulting in bruising, (4) thinning of the skin, (5) gastric ulcers, (6) cataracts requiring surgery, and (7) malignancy. Nurses offer valuable assistance by instructing the patient and his family about the changes in health status and by providing emotional support and counseling during the periods requiring medical or surgical intervention.

■ What is the role of the emergency room and intensive care unit nurse involved in cadaveric organ donation?

Perhaps one of the most important functions the emergency room and ICU nurse can perform in organ donation is to identify a potential donor. Much credit must be given to critical care nurses in assuming responsibility for the initiation of procedures leading to the eventual removal of organs for transplantation. A nurse familiar with the criteria for defining brain death developed by the Ad Hoc Committee of the Harvard Medical School may well be the key factor responsible for an increased availability of cadaveric kidneys. The criteria are as follows:

1. *Unreceptivity and unresponsivity*—There is a total unawareness to externally applied stimuli and inner need and complete unresponsiveness.
2. *No movements or breathing*—Observations by physicians over a period of at least 1 hour are adequate to assure that there are no spontaneous movements or response to stimuli.
3. *No reflexes*—The pupils will be fixed and dilated. Head turning or caloric irrigation of the ear elicits no eye movement. There is no evidence of postural activity (decerebrate or other). As a rule, the tendon reflexes cannot be elicited.

4. *Flat electroencephalogram*—Of great confirmatory value is the flat or isoelectric EEG. We must assume that the electrodes have been properly applied, that the apparatus is functioning normally, and that personnel in charge are competent.
5. *Findings consistent for 24 hours*—All of the above tests shall be repeated at least 24 hours later with no change.
6. *Absence of intoxication or hypothermia*—The above criteria have validity only if hypothermia (temperature below 90° F) or CNS depressants are excluded.

The criteria outlined have been quite generally accepted since 1968.

Legislation to clarify the legal acceptance of brain death and facilitate the procurement of cadaveric organs for transplantation has been enacted in a number of states.

The California brain death statute (Health and Safety Code, Section 7180) effective September 27, 1974, defines the determination of death, and The Uniform Anatomical Gift Act (Section 7150) provides for the donation of human tissue for transplantation at the time of death, either by the decedent or the next of kin.

Another California legislative milestone was the approval of Senate Bill No. 542 on August 23, 1975, which enables each individual possessing a driver's license in the State of California to make an anatomical gift, effective on death, by merely completing a sticker affixed to the back of the license.

Cadaver kidney donors are individuals who have suffered total and irreversible cessation of brain function. The most frequently seen and accepted cadaver donors are those individuals who fall into one of the following categories:

1. Vehicular trauma with resultant head injury
2. Homicide or suicide gunshot wound to the head
3. Drowning
4. Intracranial hemorrhage as a result of ruptured vascular malformations

The most suitable donors are young persons who have suffered head injury without concomitant intra-abdominal injury. They should have no history of renal disease, hypertension, malignancy, or infection that could be transmitted to the recipient. Generally, donors over the age of 55 are rejected because of the possibility of vascular disease in the kidneys. Trauma victims dead on arrival are not acceptable donors because of nonviable kidneys.

The nurse interested in participating in organ donation may initiate the process by communicating with the patient's attending physician to learn if there is a possibility of survival. If the patient is a candidate for life-support systems and irreversible brain death is established, the physician may, or may not, be willing to participate in organ donation. The responsibility of the physician to approach the grieving family with a medical explanation of the patient's status and request a consent form signature for the removal of kidneys and possibly eyes, heart, and liver is indeed a matter of great concern. Many physicians are, understandably, reluctant to perform this most unpleasant task. In determination of brain death, legal protection is provided the attending physician by requiring independent confirmation of the death by another physician. It is mandatory that neither physician be a member of the transplant team.

Assuming that the physician is willing to obtain consent of next of kin, the nurse may then contact the coroner for consent of removal of organs and provide pertinent patient information. The next of kin, in order of priority, according to the Uniform Anatomical Gift Act are:

1. The spouse
2. An adult son or daughter
3. Either parent
4. A guardian of the decedent at the time of death
5. Any other person authorized or under the obligation to dispose of the body

When both consents have been obtained, it is generally the nurse's responsibility to contact the nearest Regional Organ Procurement Agency (ROPA) transplant center for the purpose of reporting the prospective donor and receiving instructions related to sending of blood samples for tissue typing, cross matching, and maintenance of the donor. The nurse may act as liaison between the transplant team and the attending physician. Notifying a ROPA or transplant center does not constitute a commitment on the part of the hospital or the patient's family. On occasion, a family may, while maintaining a vigil, reverse their decision to donate organs. Emotional support must be provided by the nursing staff for the grieving family and spiritual support should be obtained if requested.

The nurse reporting a prospective donor should have the patient's chart on hand. She may be asked to provide the following information:

1. Name, age, sex, race
2. Attending physician and confirming physician
3. ABO group
4. Admitting date and diagnosis
5. Neurologic evaluation
6. Establishment of brain death
7. Date and time of declaration of death
8. Cause of death
9. Consent from next-of-kin
10. Coroner's consent
11. Has the patient been given vasopressors? Which ones? How much?
12. What other drugs have been given to the patient?
13. What are the last known hourly output, BUN, creatinine, blood pressure, temperature, urine analysis?
14. Any indication of cancer, infection, or history of renal disease or hypertension

If it is determined that the patient is a suitable potential donor, the nurse will be asked to draw and send to the laboratory 70 ml heparinized blood for tissue typing and cross matching prior to the nephrectomy.

Participation in organ donation can be a rewarding experience for the critical care nurse, particularly if the transplant center informs the unit of the disposition of the donated organs.

■ **What is the role of the operating room nurse in the removal of cadaveric organs?**

The operating room receives notification of a potential cadaver donor from the intensive care unit. A tentative time of nephrectomy will be established, depending on the availability of the operating room and staff. The operating room should be set up for a standard, sterile laparotomy including vascular instruments. A minimum of four liters of lactated Ringer's solution or nor-

mal saline solution that has been packed in ice or refrigerated for at least 2 hours prior to surgery is required. It is recommended that a respiratory therapist be present in the operating room to maintain oxygenation of the donor throughout the procedure. The nephrectomy is performed by the transplant team, accompanied by procurement technicians and nurses who are specially trained to assist in the procedure, particularly following the removal of the organs from the donor. Preservation supplies and drugs are brought to the surgical suite by these personnel.

The donor is prepared for laparotomy under careful sterile procedures with the maintenance of mechanical support. The nurse must obtain a coroner's case number and document it on the chart. Following the removal of consented organs, the body is released to the mortician.

Participation in cadaver organ donation is not without profound emotional impact on the nursing staff. Many aspects of neurologic nursing may be depressing; however, the operating room staff is unique in that they willingly contribute their efforts to the final act of the donor. This is contrary to daily efforts and emphasis on prolonging life. Although some individuals experience negative feelings, these are generally outweighed by the positive aspects of the procedure, which is related to the number of lives benefited by the gift of a healthy organ.

BIBLIOGRAPHY

Abram, H. S., and Buchanan, D. C.: Organ transplantation: psychological effects on donors and recipients, Surg. Rounds, **1**(2):22, 1978.

Bernstein, D. M.: The organ donor, J.A.M.A. **237**(24):2643, 1977.

Blount, M., and Kinney, A. B.: Chronic steroid therapy, Am. J. Nurs. **74**(9):1626, 1974.

Chatterjee, S. N., and Payne, J. E.: Difficulties in obtaining kidneys from potential postmortem donors, J.A.M.A. **232**(8):822, 1975.

Felix, K. S.: Total patient care, the team approach to transplantation, Nurs. Clin. North Am. **4**(3):451, 1969.

Hayes, C. P., Jr., and Gunnells, J. C., Jr.: Selection of recipients and donors for renal transplantation, Arch. Intern. Med. **123**:521, 1969.

Kobrzycki, P.: Renal transplant complications, Am. J. Nurs. **77**(4):641, 1977.

Light, J. A., Perloff, L. J., and Spees, E. K., Jr.: Medical legal, and ethical aspects of organ transplantation, Milit. Med. **140**(9):632, 1975.

Masland, R. L.: When is a person dead? Res. Staff Phys. **21:**48, 1975.

Milne, J. F.: Psychosocial aspects of renal transplantation, Urology **IX**(6):82, 1977.

Muslin, H. L.: Psychiatric aspects of renal failure, Am. J. Psychiatry **127**(9):105, 1971.

Ringden, O., Friman, L., Lundgren, G., and Magnusson, G.: Living related kidney donors: complications and long-term renal function, Transplantation **25**(4):221, 1978.

Robbins, K. C., and Powers, A. M.: Renal transplantation. In Gaelo, B., Hudak, C., and Lohr, T., editors: Critical care nursing, ed. 2, Philadelphia, 1977, J. B. Lippincott Co., p. 363.

Sachs, B. L.: Renal transplantation: a nursing perspective, Garden City, N.Y., 1977, Medical Examination Publishing Co., Inc.

Schumann, D.: The renal donor, Am. J. Nurs. **74**(1):105, 1974.

Simmons, R. G., Hickey, K., Kjellstrand, C. M., and Simmons, R. L.: Family tension in the search for a kidney donor, J.A.M.A. **215**(6):909, 1971.

Spanos, P. K., et al.: Complications of related kidney donation, Surgery **76**(5):741, 1974.

Stuart, F. P.: Selection, preparation and management of kidney transplant recipients, Med. Clin. North Am. **62**(6):1381, 1978.

Veith, F. J., et al.: Brain death, J.A.M.A. **238**(15):1651, 1977.

Wolf, Z.: What patients awaiting kidney transplant want to know, Am. J. Nurs. **76**(1):92, 1976.

CHAPTER 27

Principles of hemodialysis

N. D. Vaziri

In the predialysis era potentially reversible acute renal failure was associated with a high mortality rate. Return to the normal state for surviving groups involved prolonged periods of convalescence and disability. Management of such patients at that time consisted of rigid dietary restriction of fluids, proteins, sodium, and potassium. The consequence of this dietary restriction was a catabolic state with loss of muscle mass and other tissues that prolonged the recovery time and delayed the assumption of normal activities following the improvement of renal function.

Because of their uremic environment, malnutrition, and underlying disorders, patients were decidedly prone to develop systemic infections. Sepsis was the most common cause of death in patients with acute renal failure. Among those who survived, additional catabolic effects of systemic infection further prolonged the convalescent period. Uremic pericarditis with its serious consequences, that is, pericardial tamponade and constrictive pericarditis, was very common. Uremic neuropathy was frequently seen. Sensory and motor neuropathies were quite disabling and could last for many months after recovery from acute renal failure.

Anemia was invariably present and often very profound. Severe fluid overload and resultant congestive heart failure and pulmonary edema were extremely prevalent. These could occur even in the face of the most severe restriction of sodium and fluid intake with total body weight loss. It was the endogenous water from tissue breakdown that overloaded patients' damaged hearts, not the ingested or parenterally infused fluids.

End-stage chronic renal failure was a hopeless and terminal condition. With the advent of dialysis techniques and their proper use the high mortality and morbidity associated with acute renal failure has improved significantly, and patients with acute renal failure are allowed adequate dietary protein intake and are dialyzed early before uremic symptoms and complications supervene. Therefore positive nitrogen balance is maintained and wasting and uremic complications are prevented while the acute renal failure follows a course toward complete recovery. When the kidney function improves, the patient is in a good physical and mental condition and is able to resume normal life.

End-stage renal failure is no longer synonymous with death. Patients with nonfunctioning kidneys can be maintained on long-term dialysis for many years with relative comfort and productivity. It should be mentioned, however, that even though the development and perfection of dialysis technology has been one of the greatest breakthroughs in the field of medicine, it is far from being a perfect substitute for a normal kidney.

The kidney can be envisioned as a gland with both endocrine and exocrine functions. The result of its exocrine function is the formation of urine, which is the end product of glomerular filtration, tubular secretion, and tubular reabsorption. The kidney is responsible for elimination of metabolic waste products, excretion of exogenous toxins, maintenance of acid-base balance, and fluid and electrolyte homeostasis. Excretory function of the kidney is a smooth, sensitive, and continuous process and responds to physiologic needs of the body so properly that the composition and volume of body fluids are kept within normal limits despite wide variability of dietary content and fluid intake.

In addition to their excretory role, kidneys serve the following important endocrine functions:

1. Kidneys are responsible for the production of *erythropoietin*, a polypeptide hormone that regulates erythrocyte formation in the bone marrow. Lack of erythropoietin in patients with end-stage renal failure is one of the causes of the anemia that is always associated with renal failure.

2. Conversion of *vitamin D* to its active metabolite (1,25-dihydroxycholecalciferol) occurs in the kidney. In the absence of a functional kidney, dietary vitamin D or its endogenous counterpart remains inactive. Therefore a state of vitamin D resistance supervenes, resulting in the development of rickets or osteomalacic bone disease.

3. Kidneys secrete *renin*, which, by generating angiotensin II, regulates extracellular fluid volume and arterial blood pressure. Angiotensin II is one of the most potent vasoactive agents and causes severe vasoconstriction and raises the blood pressure. It is also capable of stimulating the secretion of aldosterone, which is a sodium-conserving hormone. By virtue of its sodium-conserving properties, aldosterone can expand extracellular fluid volume.

4. A variety of prostaglandins with diverse physiologic roles is produced by the kidneys.

5. Kidneys are target organs for parathyroid hormone, aldosterone, and antidiuretic hormone (ADH).

6. Kidneys are responsible for partial degradation of the insulin secreted by the pancreas, as well as parathyroid and antidiuretic hormones.

From the preceding discussion it becomes obvious that the kidney is an important member of the endocrine system. It directly secretes hormones, regulates secretion of some hormones by other glands, responds as a target organ to hormones produced elsewhere in the body, and par-

ticipates in the deactivation of some hormones. Needless to say, dialysis does not replace the endocrine function of the kidneys. It is not even an adequate substitute for their excretory function, since it lacks the smoothness and continuity of normal renal operation.

Dialysis treatments are given intermittently, which result in rapid changes in the composition and volume of the internal milieu. They permit the accumulation of waste products, hydrogen ion, sodium, potassium, other substances, and frequently excess water during the interdialytic intervals. Therefore dialysis patients undergo recurrent fluctuation of the composition and volume of body fluids, which is contrary to the normal physiologic state and has adverse short- and long-term consequences.

By expressing these negative views, I do not intend to be pessimistic, but rather to present a realistic view. In fact, during the past two decades with the development and evolution of dialysis technology, a great deal of progress has been made in the management of end-stage renal failure.

■ **What are the basic elements in hemodialysis?**

The basic elements involved in the process of hemodialysis are the patient, the dialyzing membrane (artificial kidney), and the dialysis machine, the source of dialysis fluid. Accessory devices, that is, connecting tubes, various pumps, and so on, are obviously necessary to bring these elements together and make the process mechanically feasible.

Patient

The patient serves as the source of blood; therefore it is necessary to have access to the bloodstream. This is accomplished through surgically created arteriovenous communications referred to as vascular access. Various forms of vascular access and their proper care will be discussed later in this chapter.

Dialyzer

Dialyzers consist of permeable membranes across which exchange processes between blood and dialysis fluid take place. They are usually

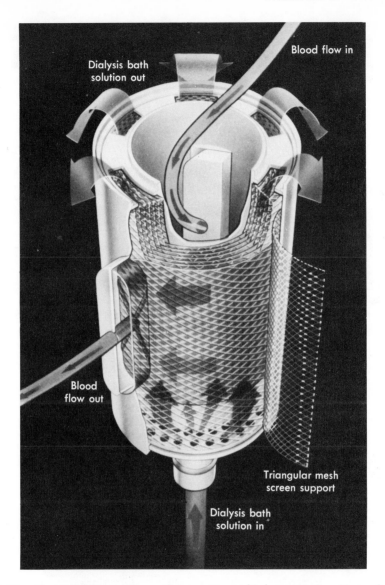

Fig. 27-1. Ultra-Flow II Coil Hemodialyzer. (Courtesy Travenol Laboratories, Inc., Morton Grove, Ill.)

made of cellophane or Cuprophan, which are cellulose derivatives. The basic difference between various dialyzers is in their physical arrangement. Several sizes of each kind are usually available. In the following paragraphs we will try briefly to describe the basic structure of the various commercially available dialyzers.

Coil hemodialyzers. In coil hemodialyzers the dialyzing membrane is made into a tubelike structure that is wound around a central core and supported by woven screens or unwoven lattices. Dialysate reaches the membranes through the perforations in the supporting structure, while the blood is continuously pumped into the tubelike membrane (Fig. 27-1). Depending on the number of coils (1, 2, or 4), total surface area

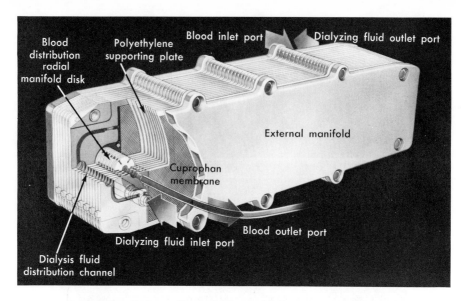

Fig. 27-2. Parallel Plate Dialyzer. (Courtesy Travenol Laboratories, Inc., Morton Grove, Ill.)

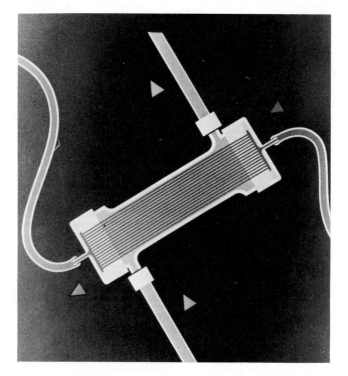

Fig. 27-3. Hollow Fiber Artificial Kidney. (Courtesy Cordis-Dow Corporation, Miami, Fla.)

(0.7 to 2.5 m²), kind of cellulose used (cellophane, Cuprophan), width of the blood channels, and supportive structure, a multitude of coil hemodialyzers have been manufactured.

Parallel flow hemodialyzers (Kiil). The parallel flow dialyzers consist of two dialyzing membranes placed between two supportive surfaces in parallel fashion. Blood flows between the two membranes and dialysate flows on the outside (Fig. 27-2). These dialyzers are characterized by small priming volumes and low internal resistance.

Hollow fiber or capillary dialyzers. The hollow fiber hemodialyzers consist of a large number of microtubules made of deacetylated cellulose acetate. The capillaries are jacketed in a plastic cylinder and sealed on each end into a tube sheet (Fig. 27-3). Blood passes through the capillaries continuously, while dialysate flows in and out of the plastic case, bathing blood-containing microcapillaries. Capillary dialyzers are characterized by their small size, easy storage, and very small priming volumes; however, because of their higher thrombogenicity, larger doses of heparin are required when these dialyzers are used.

Dialysis machine (dialysate source)

The dialysis machine is responsible for the production and delivery of dialysate. Many brands of dialysis machines are available. Depending on the mechanics of dialysate production, these machines can be categorized into four groups.

Central delivery system. In the central delivery system large volumes of dialysate are made by mixing appropriate amounts of concentrated solution with treated water. Dialysate is then delivered through pipelines to each individual patient treated in the dialysis unit. This system has several advantages: the size of the individual machines is quite small, the risk of mistakes in making individual baths is nonexistent, the problem of malfunction of the proportioning system is avoided, and the patient care area remains clean.

There are some disadvantages: the large size of initial investment and the inability to make adjustments according to individual patient needs.

Batch system. In a batch system each machine has its own tank with an average capacity of 120 L of dialysate. The tank is filled with treated water, and the proper amount of concentrate is then added to provide ideal concentration. The advantage of this system is the possibility of making individual adjustments in dialysate composition depending on biochemical abnormalities. The disadvantages include the large size of each machine, the spillage of water and dialysate on the floor during mixing and draining processes, and the possibility of making mistakes by adding too much, too little, or no dialysate to the tank with its serious consequences.

Proportionating machines. In the proportionating system treated water enters the machine from a central reservoir and is mixed with the concentrated solution on a continuous basis. Fresh dialysate is produced in this manner and delivered to the dialyzer. The advantage of these machines is their small size. Their disadvantage is the risk of malfunction of the proportionating pump, which can have serious consequences.

Dialysate regenerating system. The dialysate regenerating machines have been in use for several years and have practically eliminated the need for large volumes of dialysate. Only 1 to 2 L of dialysate is needed for the operation of these machines. In contrast to all the other systems, the dialysis fluid is not discarded after passage through the dialyzer; instead it is passed through two cartridges containing various adsorbents. The adsorbents remove various metabolic waste products as well as potassium, phosphorus, calcium, magnesium, and so on, and refresh the dialysate, which can be recirculated. To avoid hypocalcemia, calcium is constantly added to the dialysate.

As a result, portable dialysis machines no bigger than a suitcase have become a reality. A stable, well-trained dialysis patient will no longer be imprisoned by the giant kidney machine and can travel with more freedom.

■ What are the indications for short-term hemodialysis?

The indications for short-term hemodialysis can be divided into two major categories: renal and nonrenal. The renal indications include acute renal failure and reversible deterioration of stable chronic renal disease. The nonrenal indications to be considered are intoxication with dialyzable drugs; severe fluid overload refractory to other modalities of treatment; metabolic acid-base disturbances, for example, lactic acidosis or severe metabolic alkalosis; severe electrolyte abnormalities, for example, hyperkalemia, hypercalcemia, hypermagnesemia, or hyponatremia; and marked hyperuremia.

During the past two years several groups have reported on successful hemodialytic treatment of chronic schizophrenia and protracted psoriasis. Further investigations are required to confirm these preliminary observations.

■ **When is the right time to start hemodialysis treatment in acute renal failure?**

With the increasing availability and improvement of dialysis techniques, the approach to the management of acute renal failure has changed considerably. Dietary protein restriction as a means of uremia control is no longer justifiable. Dialysis treatment should be started early rather than late. Most nephrologists believe that dialysis should be started before the patient becomes symptomatic. The following findings call for the initiation of dialysis without delay:

1. Hypercatabolic states as suggested by the rapid rise of creatinine and urea such as is seen in patients with systemic infection and crushing injuries
2. Marked azotemia (BUN more than 100 mg)
3. Hyperkalemia
4. Marked metabolic acidosis
5. Any of the following uremic symptoms: Gastrointestinal manifestations—anorexia, nausea, or vomiting; central nervous system (CNS) symptoms—reversal of sleep patterns, changes of mental status, asterixis, or convulsions; cardiovascular manifestations—pericarditis, congestive heart failure, or pulmonary congestion; or hematopoietic system symptoms—bleeding diathesis (platelet dysfunction resulting from uremia) or anemia

■ **Are there any contraindications to the use of hemodialysis?**

There are no absolute contraindications to the use of hemodialysis; however, under the following conditions hemodialysis may be difficult or somewhat dangerous:

1. Hemodialysis is not recommended when systemic heparinization is contraindicated, for example, in the presence of actively bleeding peptic ulcers, fresh intracranial hemorrhage or head trauma, or hypersensitivity to heparin preparations. Under most circumstances the use of regional heparinization or miniheparinization (administration of very small amounts of heparin) allows hemodialysis to be used with a minimum of difficulty. If major problems are anticipated, peritoneal dialysis should be considered. In the presence of pericarditis regional or miniheparinization should be used to avoid hemopericardium and tamponade.

2. Patients with severe cardiovascular disease and instability may present problems with hemodialysis. These patients may not tolerate the relatively rapid changes of internal milieu and intravascular volumes imposed by hemodialysis. They should undergo peritoneal dialysis.

3. Young children and elderly patients in whom the creation and maintenance of functioning vascular access is difficult should not undergo hemodialysis. These patients may be better treated with peritoneal dialysis.

4. Patients suffering overdoses of drugs that have high tissue- and protein-binding properties respond to peritoneal dialysis better than hemodialysis, for example, those patients with phenytoin (Dilantin) and glutethimide poisoning.

■ **What are the criteria for starting maintenance dialysis in patients with chronic renal failure?**

Patients with chronic renal failure should be monitored closely. It is often possible to predict the course of the disease with some certainty when the patient has been studied for some time. It is ideal to create an arteriovenous fistula or one of the other means of internal vascular access a few months prior to the expected date when dialysis will be needed. The availability of a reliable vascular access for use when it is needed gives a sense of security to both patient and physician. In general when creatinine clearance falls below 10 ml/min or when the first symptoms of uremia develop, dialysis should be started; patients who start later respond less favorably to dialysis. The indications for the immediate initiation of dialysis in patients with chronic renal failure are the same as those for patients with acute renal failure.

■ **What are the requirements for admission to a long-term dialysis program?**

With the wide availability of federal funds for the care of patients with end-stage renal failure, the acceptance standards for a long-term dialysis program set by dialysis committees have become quite liberal. Factors such as age and underlying systemic disorder are no longer used as reasons for denying a patient the right to live in most centers. In other words, the patient is the main decision-maker. Patients with terminal metastatic cancer who do not wish to continue the agony are not treated with dialysis. The acceptance of patients with profound psychiatric disorders is frequently a difficult decision. These patients can cause severe disturbances in the dialysis units, terminate their lives by opening the vascular access, project their paranoid ideas on dialysis personnel, and become a source of threat to the others. Nevertheless, in the opinion of most practitioners psychiatric disorder does not justify denial of a person's right to live.

■ **What are the objectives of home dialysis programs, and what criteria are required?**

Because of the tremendous financial impact of in-center maintenance dialysis, home dialysis programs have been strongly supported and encouraged by the federal government and private agencies. In addition to its much lower cost, home dialysis provides a more complete and natural rehabilitation.

The following lists some of the criteria required for a home hemodialysis program:

1. The physical structure of the patient's residence should be suitable for installation of water deionizer, reservoir, plumbing system, dialysis machine, and drainage system.

2. The patient should be eager to participate and assume the major role in self-dialysis with minimum assistance at home.

3. The patient should be trainable and reliable.

4. The availability of a willing and interested related dialysis assistant, for example, spouse, parent, or child, is an absolute requirement, since even when the patient is perfectly self-sufficient, there are emergency situations where the aid of a second person is vitally important. However, since severe psychologic problems such as role reversal, emotional blackmailing, sense of dependency for life on the other person, and severe guilt feelings in cases of real or potential mistakes can be and have been encountered, the tendency is to assign the patient the major role in self-dialysis and use the assistant for minor tasks and emergency situations.

■ **Should dialysis patients be given any special diet?**

Restriction of dietary sodium, potassium, and fluid intake is frequently necessary in dialysis patients. A day-to-day weight change in dialysis patients reflects the balance of their fluid intake and output rather than a real alteration of body mass. Patients with good urine output may be allowed more or less liberal fluid intake. In general a weight gain of 0.5 kg/day is permitted between dialyses. A "no-added" salt (4 g/day), low potassium, and liberal protein diet is usually prescribed.

These statements hold true in both acute and chronic renal failure patients treated with hemodialysis. It is worthwhile to mention that salt substitutes contain large amounts of potassium and should not be used in patients with renal failure.

■ **What drugs are routinely prescribed for dialysis patients, and what is the reason behind their use?**

Since intermittent dialysis does not completely remove all the dietary phosphorus, the plasma phosphorus concentration is frequently elevated. Prolonged elevation of serum phosphorus levels results in soft tissue and vascular calcifications and progressive bone damage. For this reason hyperphosphatemia should be controlled. This is achieved by the use of phosphate-binding antacids (aluminum hydroxide) that bind dietary phosphate and prevent its absorption from the intestines. The dose of aluminum hydroxide should be adjusted by careful monitoring of the plasma phosphorus level. In order to achieve its maximum phosphate-lowering effect, aluminum hydroxide should be given with or after each meal.

Because of its abundance in various foods, a low phosphate diet is not practical.

Since water-soluble vitamins are removed by dialysis, supplementation with therapeutic multi-vitamins is necessary. Folic acid loss is particularly significant and, if not replaced, results in severe anemia. The daily use of 1 to 2 mg of folic acid is mandatory to prevent folate deficiency anemia.

A small amount of iron is lost with each dialysis, and iron absorption may be impaired in patients with renal failure. As a result, some of these patients are iron deficient. When iron deposits in the patient's bone marrow are reduced or lacking, the administration of oral or parenteral iron will be helpful.

Patients who have excess iron stores because of repeated transfusions or excessive iron administration should not be given additional iron, since it can cause hemosiderosis and organ damage.

Patients with chronic renal failure are frequently in a negative calcium balance. Their fecal calcium content is often more than their dietary intake. A variety of therapeutic approaches have been taken to overcome this problem, including the use of high calcium dialysates (3.5 mEq/L), therapeutic doses of vitamin D, and oral administration of calcium carbonate. Variable results have been reported with each of these modalities. It is mandatory that hyperphosphatemia is controlled before attempts are made to improve calcium balance. If the serum calcium level is raised while the serum phosphorus level is elevated, calcium phosphate will precipitate in vascular walls and soft tissues, causing vascular and tissue damage.

■ **What are the major criteria by which adequacy of dialysis is judged?**

Several parameters are used to judge adequacy of dialysis treatment:

1. Patient's general condition and sense of well-being
2. Degree of anemia and its progression or improvement
3. Nerve conduction velocity (NCV) and electromyographic (EMG) abnormalities (NVC and EMG studies are most commonly used to assess the adequacy of dialysis. These studies can be done serially twice a year.)
4. Degree of azotemia as judged by average plasma urea and creatinine levels
5. Fluid balance, blood pressure control, and cardiac status
6. Muscle mass and dry body weight
7. Presence or absence of uremic symptoms

The deterioration of these parameters calls for more intensive dialytic treatment.

■ **What is the minimum dialysis requirement per week?**

No single minimum dialysis requirement suits all dialysis patients. Depending on the patient's residual renal function, size, and dietary and metabolic load, the dialysis requirements vary. In other words, a special dialysis program in terms of length and frequency should be tailored for each individual patient. However, the average patient requires a minimum of 18 hr/m² of dialysis per week.

The hour–square meter concept refers to the product of dialysis time in hours multiplied by the surface area of the dialyzing membrane. For instance, when a patient is dialyzed three times a week, 6 hours each time with a dialyzer with a 1 m² surface, the weekly dialysis will be 18 hr/m², as calculated below:

$$3.0 \times 6.0 = 18 \text{ hr/week}$$
$$T \times S = 18.0 \times 1.0 = 18 \text{ hr/m}^2$$

in which T = time on dialysis in hours per week and S = surface area of dialysis membrane in square meters.

According to this concept, the dialysis time can be shortened if the dialysis surface is increased. By utilizing large surface area dialyzers or two dialyzers in parallel or in series, a significant reduction of dialysis time has become possible.

Although the clearance of small molecules, for example, urea and creatinine, with the large surface area, fast dialysis technique is satisfactory, its efficiency in removing midsized molecules, which are thought to be responsible for uremic neuropathy, may be suboptimal. The technique is still new, and more experience is required to answer this and many other questions that may be raised in the future. With the advent of highly permeable membranes, adequate dialysis may be accomplished with shorter dialysis treatments.

■ What is the extent of rehabilitation?

The degree of rehabilitation is quite variable. Approximately 28% of these patients are capable of doing all usual activities, 34% are unable to perform strenuous work, 24% are unable to do ordinary activities, and 14% need assistance for primary self-care. The results are generally much worse in patients with advanced diabetes.

Table 27-1. Survival statistics of patients on maintenance hemodialysis*

Source	Type of program	1-year survival (%)	2-year survival (%)
European Dialysis and Transplantation Association	In-center	84	72
	Home	92	85
Peter Bent Brigham Hospital	In-center	93	86
	Home	88	78
1972 National Dialysis Registry		90	80

*In comparison with renal transplantation, dialysis is superior to cadaver and inferior to live related renal transplantation as far as mortality rates are concerned.

■ What is the long-term survival rate of patients on maintenance hemodialysis treatment, and how does it compare with the data for renal transplant recipients?

The mortality rate in the long-term dialysis population is approximately 10% per year. According to some statistics, home dialysis is slightly superior to in-center dialysis with respect to survival. This has not been a consistent finding, however, and it may reflect a greater physical and psychologic stability among home dialysis patients as compared to the in-center dialysis group. Table 27-1 shows the 1- and 2-year survival statistics obtained from three different sources.

■ What is the significance of the dialyzability of various drugs?

It is quite important to know if a drug is dialyzable or not, and if it is, to what extent. Dialysis can be used to enhance the elimination of dialyzable drugs from the body in case of drug overdose. Patients with renal failure frequently have multiorgan disorders requiring multiple drug therapy. Furthermore, because of their increased susceptibility, the incidence of infections requir-

Table 27-2. Drug dialyzability

Drug	Significant removal by dialysis Hemo-	Significant removal by dialysis Peritoneal	Drug	Significant removal by dialysis Hemo-	Significant removal by dialysis Peritoneal
Antibacterial agents			Isoxazolyl penicillins	No	No
Ampicillin	Yes	No	Kanamycin	Yes	Yes
Carbenicillin	Yes	Yes	Lincomycin	No	No
Cephalexin	Yes	Yes	Methenamine mandelate	?	?
Cephaloridine	Yes	Yes	Methicillin	No	No
Cephalothin	Yes	Yes	Metronidazole	?	?
Cephapirin	Yes	Yes	Nalidixic acid	?	?
Cephazolin	Yes	Yes	Neomycin	Yes	?
Chloramphenicol	Yes	?	Nitrofurantoin	Yes	?
Chloroquine	?	?	Penicillin G	Yes	?
Clindamycin	No	No	Pentamidine	?	?
Dapsone	?	?	Pyrimethamine	?	?
Dia-mer-sulfonamides	Yes	?	Quinine	?	?
Erythromycin	?	?	Sodium colistimethate	No	No
Gentamicin	Yes	Yes	Streptomycin	Yes	?
Griseofulvin	?	?	Tetracycline	Yes	No

Continued.

Table 27-2. Drug dialyzability—cont'd

Drug	Significant removal by dialysis		Drug	Significant removal by dialysis	
	Hemo-	Peritoneal		Hemo-	Peritoneal
Antibacterial agents—cont'd			Levodopa	?	?
Tobramycin	Yes	?	Lithium	Yes	Yes
Trimethoprim	Yes	?	Phenothiazines	No	No
Vancomycin	No	No	Tricyclic antidepressants	No	No
Antituberculous and anti-			Trimethadione	?	?
fungal agents			Succinimides	?	?
Amphotericin B	No	No	Immunosuppressant and		
Cycloserine	?	?	antineoplastic drugs		
Ethionamide	?	?	Bleomycin	?	?
Ethambutol	Yes	?	Busulfan	?	?
5-Fluorocytosine	Yes	?	Cyclophosphamide	Yes	Yes
Isoniazid	Yes	?	Cytosine arabinoside	?	?
P.A.S.	?	?	Doxorubicin	?	?
Pyrazinamide	?	?	5-Fluorouracil	Yes	Yes
Rifampin	No	No	6-Mercaptopurine and	?	?
Viomycin	?	?	azathioprine		
Drugs used in the treatment			Methotrexate	?	?
of arthritides and inflam-			Vinca alkaloids	?	?
matory disorders			Anticoagulants and		
Allopurinol	?	?	cardiac glycosides		
Colchicine	No	No	Digitoxin	No	No
Glucocorticoids	?	?	Digoxin	No	No
Gold	No	?	Heparin	No	No
Indomethacin	?	?	Warfarin	?	?
Phenylbutazone	Limited		Diuretics		
Probenecid	?	?	Acetazolamide	Yes	?
Hypoglycemic drugs			Aminophylline	Yes	?
Acetohexamide	?	?	Ethacrynic acid	?	?
Chlorpropamide	?	?	Furosemide	No	No
Insulin	?	?	Mercurials	?	?
Phenformin	?	?	Metolazone	?	?
Tolbutamide	No	No	Spironolactone	?	?
Analgesics and soporific			Thiazides	?	?
drugs			Triamterene	?	?
Acetaminophen	Yes	?	Antihypertensive drugs		
Acetylsalicylic acid	Yes	Yes	Diazoxide	Yes	?
(aspirin)			Guanethidine	?	?
Barbiturates			Hydralazine	?	?
Long acting	Yes	Yes	Methyldopa	Yes	?
Short acting	No	No	Minoxidil	?	?
Chloralhydrate	Yes	?	Reserpine	No	No
Diazepam	No	No	Antiarrhythmic agents		
Diphenhydramine	?	?	Lidocaine	No	?
Ethchlorvynol	No	?	Phenytoin	No	No
Meprobamate	No	No	Procainamide	Yes	?
Opiates	?	?	Propranolol	No	No
Pentazocine	?	?	Quinidine	?	?
Propoxyphene	No	?	Miscellaneous drugs		
Drugs used in neuropsy-			Cimetidine	Yes	Yes
chiatry			Clofibrate	?	?
Anticholinesterases	?	?	Methimazole	?	?
Haloperidol	?	?	Propylthiouracil	?	?

ing antibiotic therapy is quite high in these patients. Sufficient blood levels of antibiotics or other drugs are quite vital to obtain the pharmacologic effects. If the drug is dialyzable, its plasma concentration may fall below therapeutic levels following dialysis. As a result, the underlying disorders will cease to be under control. By proper adjustment of the dose and administration of dialyzable drugs at the end of dialysis, this problem can be avoided. Table 27-2 provides information as to the dialyzability of some of the more commonly used drugs.

BIBLIOGRAPHY

Arthur, G., et al.: Clinical maintenance hemodialysis with a sorbent-based low-volume dialysate regeneration system, Trans. Am. Soc. Artif. Intern. Organs **17**:253, 1971.

Bailey, G. L., editor: Hemodialysis principles and practice, New York, 1972, Academic Press, Inc.

Bennett, W. M., Singer, I., and Coggins, C. J.: A guide to drug therapy in renal failure, J.A.M.A. **230**:1544, 1974.

Bremmer, B. M., and Rector, F. C., editors: The kidney, Philadelphia, 1976, W. B. Saunders Co.

Earley, L. E., and Gottschalk, C. W., editors: Strauss and Welt's diseases of the kidney, ed. 3, Boston, 1979, Little, Brown & Co.

Massry, S. G., and Sellers, A. L., editors: Clinical aspects of uremia and dialysis, Springfield, Ill., 1976, Charles C Thomas, Publisher.

Pendras, J. P., and Stinson, G. W., editors: The hemodialysis manual, Seattle, 1970, Edmark Corporation.

Shaldon, S.: Haemodialysis in chronic renal failure, Postgrad. Med. J. suppl., p. 3, November 1966.

Shimizu, A., et al.: Straight arteriovenous shunt for long-term hemodialysis, J.A.M.A. **216**:645, 1971.

Winchester, T. F., et al.: Dialysis and hemoperfusion of poisons and drugs—update, Trans. Am. Soc. Artif. Int. Organs **23**:762, 1977.

CHAPTER 28

Hemoperfusion and vascular access

N. D. Vaziri, K. S. Mirahmadi, and Mary Anne Robinson

HEMOPERFUSION

Activated charcoal has a great affinity to bind and adsorb various substances. For this reason it has been used orally to remove toxins from the gastrointestinal tract for many years.

In 1964 Yatzidis[1] reported that by passing blood through a bed of activated charcoal one can remove various substances from the blood. Since then many investigators have used activated charcoal to remove uremic toxins in patients with renal failure, hepatic toxins in patients with liver failure, and exogenous toxins in patients with drug overdose. Rosenbaum[2] has reported that similar results can be achieved by using different types of resin instead of activated charcoal.

■ **What are the different types of hemoperfusion cartridges?**
Cartridges containing activated charcoal

B-D Hemodetoxifier (Becton, Dickinson & Co.) The B-D Hemodetoxifier contains 100 g of uncoated activated carbon particles deposited on a polyester film and wound into a coil with a fine mesh filter to prevent embolization of charcoal particles. The carbon particles used in these cartridges are made of coconut shell charcoal. Since the charcoal particles are not coated in this cartridge, its clearances are quite high. Unfortunately the risk of thrombocytopenia is greater with this cartridge than with those containing coated particles.

Homocol (Sandev Ltd.). The Homocol cartridge contains 300 g of activated charcoal coated with acrylic hydrogel. Since the activated carbon particles are coated, use of this cartridge is associated with a lower incidence of thrombocytopenia. Its clearance of various toxins has been maintained in an acceptable range by its greater charcoal particle content.

Adsorba 300C (Gambro). The Adsorba 300C cartridge contains 300 g of cellulose-coated activated charcoal. This cartridge is highly effective in removing various toxins, and the related incidence of thrombocytopenia is very low.

ACAC hemoperfusion system. Since 1956 Chang and his group[3] have been involved in the development of artificial cells with microencapsulated enzymes and other biologically active materials. Recently they introduced albumin-coated activated charcoal (ACAC) for treatment of uremic patients. The cartridge, which contains 300 g of ACAC, has a very good clearance for various substances and is associated with a low incidence of thrombocytopenia.

Cartridges containing resins

Various forms of resins have been used to develop biocompatible hemoperfusion cartridges, including the DX-60 cartridge (Extracorporeal Inc.) and the Amberlite XAD-4. The Amberlite XAD-4 cartridge contains 650 g of an uncoated uncharged resin with a special adsorptive property for lipid-soluble substances. Thrombocytopenia has been reported in patients treated with resin cartridges.

■ **How do you connect the patient to the hemoperfusion cartridge?**

As in hemodialysis, the patient should have a blood access for hemoperfusion. An arteriovenous

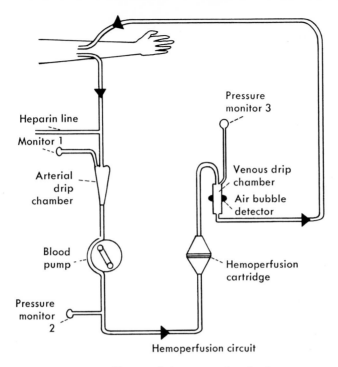

Fig. 28-1. Hemoperfusion connection circuit.

shunt is commonly used in patients who need few hemoperfusion treatments. Percutaneous femoral vein catheters can be used to perform one or two hemoperfusion treatments, especially in patients with drug overdose. Fig. 28-1 shows the hemoperfusion connection circuit. Monitor 1 indicates the pressure between the patient's arterial blood supply and the blood pump; in case of hypotension this monitor will register a low pressure. Monitor 2 is helpful in calculating the pressure drop across the cartridge; if there is clot formation inside the cartridge, this monitor will show high pressure. Monitor 3 indicates the patient's venous resistance.

■ **What are the complications of hemoperfusion?**

Thrombocytopenia

The platelet count may decrease markedly during hemoperfusion; this is more common in cartridges containing uncoated charcoal particles.

Hemoperfusion is relatively contraindicated in patients with thrombocytopenia. Some centers use routine platelet transfusion after hemoperfusion, especially in patients with liver failure. In patients with drug overdose, hemoperfusion does not cause profound thrombocytopenia and replacement is not necessary.

Leukopenia

White blood cells may decrease with hemoperfusion, but this is transient and does not cause serious clinical problems.

Hemolysis

Lysis of red blood cells can occur with hemoperfusion, but it is not common.

Clotting factor deficiencies

The hemoperfusion cartridge may remove various clotting factors from the circulation, possibly resulting in bleeding diathesis in patients undergoing hemoperfusion. Fresh frozen plasma can replace the missing clotting factors and correct the problem.

Clot formation

Occasionally, owing to inadequate heparinization or other reasons, blood may clot inside the hemoperfusion cartridge. This situation is signified by a very high pressure reading on the pre-cartridge monitor (monitor no. 2) and necessitates replacement of the clotted cartridge.

Hypotension

Hypotension has been reported during hemoperfusion, and this may be related to the removal of pressor amines by the cartridge. Administration of intravenous fluids and pressor agents is sometimes necessary to correct this problem.

Embolization

Embolization of charcoal particles has been reported in animal studies, but in the currently available hemoperfusion cartridges the use of very fine mesh filters has minimized this complication.

Air emboli

High negative pressure on the arterial side or faulty blood lines may cause air embolization in the hemoperfused patient. Air bubble detector devices are generally used to detect and prevent air embolization.

■ What is the clearance of various substances by hemoperfusion?

Activated charcoal does not adsorb urea, phosphate, or electrolytes, but it removes creatinine, uric acid, and middle molecular uremic toxins satisfactorily. When the blood flow is maintained at 300 ml/min, the clearances of creatinine and uric acid may be as high as 250 ml/min. Similar clearances can be achieved for phenobarbital, salicylates, and glutethimide. Unlike hemodialysis, in hemoperfusion the charcoal cartridge may become saturated after a few hours, and the clearance may drop very rapidly. Hemoperfusion is the treatment of choice in cases of poisoning with fat-soluble toxins such as glutethimide, highly protein-bound substances, and large molecular

size compounds. Unlike hemodialysis, one cannot remove fluid from the blood by hemoperfusion; therefore its use in the treatment of renal failure is limited.

■ What are the advantages of using a cell separator in hemoperfusion?

To minimize the problems of thrombocytopenia and loss of white and red cells, some centers use a cell separator device in conjunction with hemoperfusion. In this system the cell separator separates the plasma from the cells. After the plasma fraction passes through the cartridge, it is mixed with the blood cells before it is returned to the patient.

■ What are the indications for hemoperfusion?

Drug overdose

Hemoperfusion has been used very successfully in the treatment of various forms of acute poisoning. Commonly known toxins such as barbiturates, glutethimide, salicylate, and paraquat can be removed by hemoperfusion. Hemoperfusion is used only in those patients with drug overdose who are critically ill; therefore most overdose patients do not need hemoperfusion. Overdose patients with deep hypotension, hypoventilation, or progressive clinical deterioration should be considered for hemoperfusion if the drug is one that can be removed by hemoperfusion.

Hemoperfusion may be indicated when the following plasma concentrations are found: phenobarbitone, >10 mg%; other barbiturates, >5 mg%; glutethimide, >4 mg%; methaqualone, >4 mg%; salicylate, >80 mg%; meprobamate, >10 mg%. Since the plasma concentration is very low in patients with tricyclic antidepressant overdose, hemoperfusion is not very effective. In acetaminophen (Tylenol) overdose, hemoperfusion has little to offer because of the short half-life of the drug and the early occurrence of toxic injury in the course of the disease.

Renal failure

Hemoperfusion has been used in conjunction with hemodialysis for the treatment of patients with chronic renal failure. Chang,[4] who has worked in this area since 1956, recently reported his experience with ACAC hemoperfusion. He used a cartridge containing 300 g of albumin-coated activated charcoal (ACAC) with a surface area of 2.5 m^2. Charcoal granules were 2 to 5 mm in diameter and the priming volume of the cartridge was 200 ml. He found that with a blood flow of 300 ml/min, the urea clearance was negligible, but the clearances for creatinine, uric acid, and middle molecules were 230, 235, and 100 ml/min, respectively. Charcoal hemoperfusion is not capable of removing urea, phosphate, electrolytes, and water from the blood; therefore it must be used in conjunction with hemodialysis in uremic patients. For these reasons, hemoperfusion has not yet gained widespread clinical use in the treatment of renal failure.

Liver failure

The mortality of acute hepatic failure with Grade III or IV hepatic encephalopathy may be as high as 80% to 90%. In contrast to the kidney, heart, or brain, the liver has a great capacity for regeneration following injury. Therefore supportive measures to sustain life in a patient with acute hepatic failure might allow sufficient time for hepatocellular regeneration and eventual survival.

Various supportive measures including exchange transfusion, cross-circulation with a human volunteer, pig liver perfusion, peritoneal dialysis, and hemodialysis with Cuprophan membrane have failed to improve survival. Recently Gazzard and co-workers[5] published their experience in 22 patients with acute fulminant hepatic failure treated with charcoal hemoperfusion. They reported 50% survival in their series, which represents a considerable improvement over the 17% survival obtained in nonhemoperfused patients with hepatic failure. Since then, a few other centers have reported improvement of coma after hemoperfusion in patients with hepatic encephalopathy.[6] Unfortunately, owing to the high risk of thrombocytopenia and bleeding diathesis in these patients, the widespread use of hemoperfusion in hepatic coma is not yet practical.

VASCULAR ACCESS

The vascular access is the "lifeline" of the patient with end-stage renal disease on long-term hemodialysis treatment. It consists of a high blood flow circuit surgically created to provide easy access to the patient's circulation in order to perform hemodialysis. Hemodialysis cannot be performed without an adequate blood access; therefore proper care and maintenance of the vascular access is extremely important.

There are two major classes of vascular access: external arteriovenous shunts and internal arteriovenous fistulas.

External arteriovenous shunts

An external arteriovenous (AV) shunt is created by the surgical insertion of a Teflon-Silastic cannula into an artery and another into the corresponding vein. The two cannulas are joined externally when not in use. The primary advantage of an AV shunt is its immediate usability for short-term dialysis or hemoperfusion. However, they are not very durable and frequent repairs and/or revisions are often necessary to maintain adequate patency. There are several types of AV shunts, described as follows.

Quinton-Schribner shunt

The Quinton-Schribner shunt is created by inserting the Teflon tips of the Silastic cannulas directly into the artery and the corresponding vein. End-to-end anastomosis is used to secure the vessel to the cannula. The Quinton-Schribner shunt is primarily placed in the distal portions of the extremities, utilizing relatively small vessels such as the radial artery and cephalic vein or the posterior tibial artery and saphenous vein.

Allen-Brown shunt

The Allen-Brown shunt is often utilized to create an access for hemodialysis. The cannula used in this type of AV shunt has a Dacron sleeve at the proximal tip, which is fused to the Silastic cannula. The Dacron sleeve is anastomosed end to end or end to side to large vessels such as the brachial artery and cephalic vein.

Thomas shunt

The Thomas shunt uses a Dacron patch, which is fused to the proximal end of the Silastic cannula. The Dacron patch is sutured to the vessel

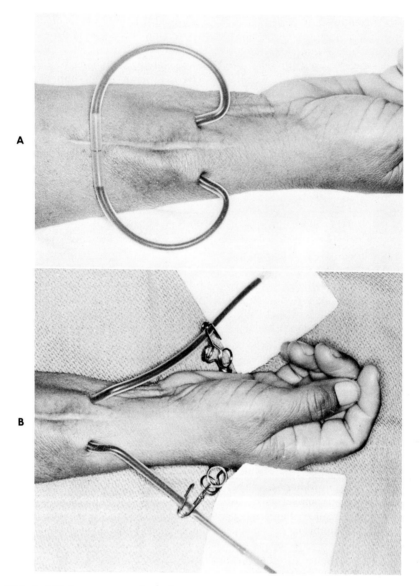

Fig. 28-2. A, A-V shunt connected together with Teflon adapter. **B,** Shunt shown with arterial and venous sides disconnected. Note bulldog clamps on each side of shunt.

by an end-to-side anastomosis. These shunts are primarily placed on very large vessels such as the femoral artery and saphenous or femoral vein.

Buselmier shunt

The Buselmier shunt is a compact, U-shaped, somewhat rigid Silastic prosthesis. This type of shunt is placed in vessels that are in close proximity to each other. The U-shaped portion of the external part contains protruding inlets for easy access to the circulation.

■ What are the major complications of the external AV shunts, and how are these treated?

External AV shunts are prone to many complications because of their exposure to the external environment. Possible disconnection and subsequent blood loss is a major risk with these shunts. The constant exposure to the outside increases the risk of infection. Furthermore, the external AV shunts clot quite frequently.

Infections

Although local infections in the area of the AV shunts are common, they are relatively easy to control. Systemic infections are usually caused by extension of local infections. Therefore meticulous shunt care is highly recommended to prevent the occurrence of these infections. Unexplained fever in a dialysis patient should suggest a possible shunt infection. Shunt infection may cause tenderness, redness, and edema around the cannula sites. The patient may complain of burning pain. Blood and site cultures should be obtained and local and systemic treatments instituted. Since *Staphylococcus aureus* is usually responsible for shunt infection, appropriate antibiotics such as vancomycin and cloxacillin are commonly used in treating these infections. Meticulous aseptic techniques should be used in handling the AV shunt. Daily cleaning with antibacterial agents and solutions should be performed as well as regular changing of sterile dressings.

Bleeding

Bleeding caused by the dislodgment or disconnection of the AV shunt is a major risk. This may

result from accidental or suicidal pulling or cutting of the shunt. All patients with AV shunts should carry bulldog clamps, which can provide immediate hemostatis when cannulas are disconnected.

Clotting

Thrombosis is a common complication of the AV shunts. Loss of audible bruit and palpable thrill, darkening of the blood content of the cannula, and reduced shunt temperature are indications of clotting. Predisposing conditions include (1) insufficient blood flow through the shunt caused by its mechanical malposition such as kinking of the Silastic tract; (2) reduced blood flow through the shunt owing to a low cardiac output, as seen in shock, dehydration, and hypotension; (3) hypercoagulability states, as seen after surgery; and (4) local infections of the shunt.

■ What is the procedure for declotting a shunt?

Commercial disposable declotting trays are available for the declotting procedure. They usually contain all the necessary equipment, such as a 12-inch polyethylene catheter with leur lock connector, Teflon adaptors, and 20-ml syringes. The following steps are recommended for declotting:

1. Prepare the shunt and the surrounding area with an antibacterial agent such as Betadine solution after removing all dressings.
2. Prepare a sterile field with sterile towels. The person declotting the shunt must use aseptic techniques when performing this procedure.
3. Prepare warm heparinized saline using 1000 units of heparin for each 100 ml of normal saline.
4. Prepare syringes, adaptors, and catheters.
5. Use sterile bulldog clamps to clamp both sides of the clotted shunt.
6. Separate the shunt with a sterile shunt spreader.
7. Release the bulldog clamp; reclamp if bleeding occurs.
8. Remove the clot by gently pulling on it, if

possible. Use the syringe with heparinized saline to gently aspirate the clot from the shunt.

9. If aspiration is unsuccessful, insert the polyethylene catheter and attempt to aspirate the clot.
10. Repeat this procedure if necessary.
11. When the shunt is declotted, irrigate the cannula with the heparinized solution and reconnect the shunt. Never inject more than 1 to 2 ml of solution into the arterial line since this may result in serious embolic complications.
12. If this procedure is unsuccessful, the use of an embolectomy (Fogarty) catheter may be necessary. The catheter is inserted into the cannula past the clot or obstruction, the balloon tip is inflated, and the clot is gently pulled out.

To prevent repeated clotting, continuous infusion of heparinized solution into the shunt via a T-tube adaptor may be necessary. Sometimes the attempts to declot the shunt are unsuccessful, and surgical revision may be required.

■ Can fibrinolytic agents be used to declot shunts?

Streptokinase and urokinase have been used to declot shunts, and several studies have shown their efficacy in this situation. Fibrinolytic agents convert plasminogen into plasmin, which in turn reverses the clotting process by its active fibrinolytic effect. In the case of streptokinase, 250,000 IU of this product is dissolved in 2 ml of 5% dextrose in water. This is infused slowly into the clotted cannula. The cannula is then clamped, and the fibrinolytic agent is left in the cannula for 2 hours. After this the cannula is unclamped, aspirated, and flushed with normal saline. Heparin infusion may be used to prevent recurrence of clotting. Oral administration of warfarin (Coumadin) may be prescribed as well.

Internal arteriovenous fistulas

An internal arteriovenous (AV) fistula is created by subcutaneous surgical anastomosis of an artery and a neighboring vein. Internal AV fistulas can provide a high flow circuit needed to perform hemodialysis. Percutaneous needle cannulation provides access to the internal AV fistulas. The internal AV fistulas are best suited for the patient on long-term hemodialysis treatment. The internal AV fistulas last longer than the external AV shunts. They provide freedom of motion for the bearing limb and are esthetically superior to the external AV shunts. Furthermore, the infectious complications are less common. The internal AV fistulas usually require some time to develop and mature before they can be used. Several types of AV fistulas are used to provide access to the circulation, including the following.

Cimino fistula

The Cimino fistula is a common type of internal fistula that is usually placed in the arm. The side of the radial artery is surgically opened and anastomosed to the end of the cephalic vein. The vein and its branches become dilated and arterialized, thus providing a high flow circuit capable of supplying adequate blood flow to the artificial kidney for hemodialysis (Fig. 28-3).

Saphenous graft

The saphenous graft is not used as commonly as the Cimino fistula. It is usually placed when attempts to create other fistulas fail. There are two methods of creating a saphenous fistula. One procedure is by surgically anastomosing a branch of the saphenous vein to the femoral artery. As a result, the saphenous vein becomes dilated and arterialized and converts to an internal fistula. Because the anatomic location of the fistula in the groin area increases the risk of infection, this type of fistula is used infrequently. Another method of creating a saphenous fistula is by grafting a piece of the saphenous vein to the arm vessels; the saphenous graft in the arm is used for cannulation.

Bovine graft

The bovine fistula utilizes the denatured carotid artery of a calf. This heterograft is surgically connected to an artery and a vein, producing a subcutaneous conduit that is quite easy to cannulate.

Synthetic conduits

In recent years synthetic materials have been successfully used to create internal accesses. By anastomosing polytetrafluoroethylene (PFTE)

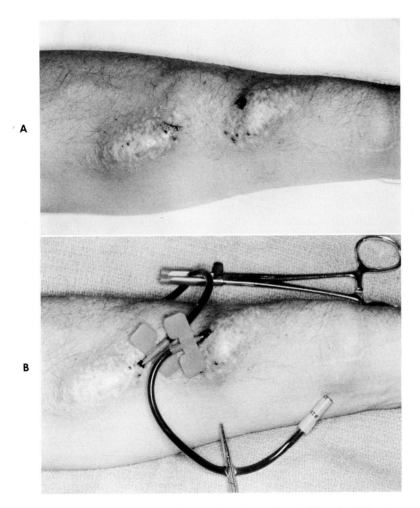

Fig. 28-3. A, Cimino A-V fistula (internal) created in September, 1970, and still functioning. **B,** Cimino fistula with 14-gauge needles inserted. Needle on right is directed toward radial artery and uses arterial blood flow. Needle on left is for venous return.

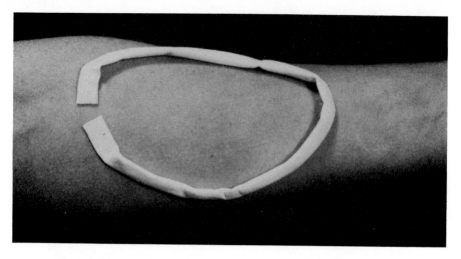

Fig. 28-4. Photograph of a PFTE conduit used to create an internal access.

conduits to various vessels, durable and efficient internal fistulas can be created. The diameter and the length of these grafts can be determined prior to implantation. Synthetic and bovine grafts lack the myoelastic contraction of the normal vessels, resulting in the prolonged puncture site bleeding seen in some patients after dialysis. These grafts can be used as early as 1 to 4 weeks after their placement (Fig. 28-4).

■ **What are the common complications of internal arteriovenous fistulas, and how are these treated?**

In comparison to the external AV shunts, the internal AV fistulas have a lower incidence of complications. However, these complications are usually more difficult to treat. They include infections, clotting, and prolonged puncture site bleeding following cannula withdrawal.

Fistula infections can be local or systemic. It is usually more difficult to treat an infected AV fistula than an AV shunt. The extremity that bears the infected fistula may be edematous and painful. Redness and tenderness may be present, and the patient may have fever. Blood and site cultures should be taken and antibiotic therapy initiated. If possible, the infected fistula should not be utilized for dialysis to prevent possible systemic dissemination. Infection may pre-

dispose to clotting; therefore monitoring and assessment of bruit and thrill are important for early detection of thrombosis. It may be necessary to remove the infected AV fistula or graft when infection cannot be irradicated with conservative therapy.

Local trauma, multiple punctures, and infections can predispose the AV fistula to clotting. The usual signs of clotting include diminished bruit and thrill, poor blood flow, hardening of the fistula tract, pain, and discoloration. Surgical revision or construction of a new fistula is necessary in this situation.

Prolonged bleeding from the puncture sites after dialysis can be due to a variety of reasons, including (1) large size of the needles and the corresponding defect in the vascular wall; (2) high blood flow and pressure; (3) presence of circulating heparin and resultant enhanced thrombin inhibition and delayed clot formation; and (4) lack of myoelastic contraction, which is important for normal hemostatic mechanism in case of synthetic conduits. Other possible causes of prolonged bleeding may be intrinsic in nature, such as platelet dysfunction associated with uremia. Usually, digital compression is used to stop bleeding from the sites; however, it may take as long as 15 to 30 minutes before the bleeding stops. Topical thrombin has proved effective in reducing puncture site bleeding time by 50%. Topical thrombin (5000 units in 5 ml of diluent) can be applied to the puncture sites during needle withdrawal. This should be followed by digital compression applied to the bleeding sites. Exogenous thrombin provides rapid fibrin clot formation at or near the surface of the skin; its subsequent propagation through the bleeding tract results in rapid hemostasis.

REFERENCES

1. Yatzidis, H.: Recherches sur l'epuuration extra renale a L'aide du charbon actif, Nephron **1**:310, 1964.
2. Rosenbaum, J. L., Kramer, M. S., Raja, R., Winstens, S., and Dalal, F.: Hemoperfusion for acute drug intoxication, Kidney Int. (Suppl.) **10**:341, 1966.
3. Chang, T. M. S.: Microcapsule artificial kidney, Kidney Int. (Suppl.) **10**:218, 1976.
4. Chang, T. M. S.: Microcapsule artificial kidney: including updated preparative procedures and properties, Kidney Int. (Suppl.) **10**:218, 1976.
5. Gazzard, B. G., et al.: Charcoal hemoperfusion in the treatment of fulminant hepatic failure, Lancet **I**:1301, 1974.
6. Gelfand, M. C., Knepshield, J. H., Cohan, S., Ramirez, B., and Schreiner, G.: Treatment of hepatic coma with hemoperfusion through coated charcoal, Kidney Int. **10**:239, 1976.

BIBLIOGRAPHY

Bahuth, J.: Expanded polytetrafluorethylene as an arteriovenous conduit for hemodialysis, dialysis, and transplantation, November, 1977.

Barbour, B. H., Lasette, A. M., and Koffler, A.: Fixed-bed charcoal hermoperfusion for the treatment of drug overdose, Kidney Int. (Suppl.) **10**:333, 1976.

Gelfland, M. C., Knepshield, J. H., Cohen, S., Ramirez, B., and Schreiner, G.: Treatment of hepatic coma with hemoperfusion through polyacrylamide hydrogel-coated charcoal, Kidney Int. (Suppl.) **10**:239, 1976.

Goulding, R.: Experience with hemoperfusion in drug abuse, Kidney Int. (Suppl.) **10**:338, 1976.

Hampers, C. L.: Long-term hemodialysis, ed. 2, New York, 1974, Grune & Stratton, Inc., p. 243

Mindich, B., et al.: Human umbilical cord vein for vascular replacement, Surgery **81**:152, 1977.

Porter, J. M., and Goodnight, S. H., Jr.: The clinical use of fibrinolytic agents, Am. J. Surg. **134**:217, 1977.

Rosenbaum, J. L., Kramer, M. S., and Raja, R.: Resin hemoperfusion for acute drug intoxication, Arch. Intern. Med. **136**:263, 1976.

Shane, G.: Vascular access for hemodialysis. In Massry, S. G., and Sellers, A. L., editors: Clinical aspects of uremia and dialysis, Springfield, Ill., 1976, Charles C Thomas, Publisher, vol. III, ch. 17, p. 504.

Vaziri, N. D., and Robinson, M. A.: Topical thrombin and control of bleeding from cannulation sites in dialyzed patients, J. Dialysis **2**:393, 1978.

CHAPTER 29

Complications of hemodialysis and their management

N. D. Vaziri

End-stage renal disease, once a terminal event, is now being converted by dialysis technology to a chronic debilitating condition. Life itself may be prolonged for many years, but its quality is widely variable because of medical and nonmedical problems. Long-term dialysis patients, in addition to being susceptible to the diseases contracted by other persons, are prime targets for many other disorders that are more or less peculiar to them. This chapter is intended to briefly review these complications and discuss their prevention and management.

The complications may be related to vascular access difficulties, defective dialysis apparatus, improper fluid composition, anticoagulation, dialysis of essential nutrients, infections, consequences of shunt declotting procedure, rapid alterations of extracellular fluid volume and composition, failure to adhere to the dietary and drug regimen, socioeconomic and psychologic problems, hyperlipidemia and accelerated atherosclerosis, chronic anemia, renal osteodystrophy, secondary hyperparathyroidism, hypertension, dialysis-associated pericarditis, or other cardiac complications.

■ **What are the complications caused by the rapid changes of extracellular fluid volume and composition imposed by dialysis?**
Hypotension

Hypotension is a common occurrence during dialysis. It is usually caused by rapid volume depletion and/or production of vasodepressor sub-stances during dialysis. It responds to the reduction of blood flow rate and IV infusion of saline or colloid solutions.

Transient dyspnea at end of dialysis

Occasionally patients develop a transient tachypnea and mild shortness of breath immediately after completion of dialysis. This seems to be related to a mild but sudden increase of intravascular volume resulting from the rapid return of blood content from the artificial kidney and tubing system to the patient. In a short period of time the excess fluid is sequestered throughout the extracellular compartment and symptoms improve.

Disequilibrium syndrome

Disequilibrium syndrome is a clinical disorder that occurs during or immediately after dialysis. It may be mild, manifesting with headaches, nausea, vomiting, and drowsiness. When severe, there may be involuntary jerking movements, disorientation, psychosis, convulsions, coma, and markedly elevated cerebrospinal fluid (CSF) pressure. It is accompanied by EEG changes that point to the central nervous system (CNS) origin of these clinical manifestations. The EEG changes consist of diffuse slowing of the basal rhythm and occasional paroxysms of high voltage spikes. Pathologically, swelling of nerve cells and cerebral edema characterize this syndrome. The syndrome is most likely to occur with the first few dialyses in the following situations:

1. In severely azotemic patients
2. When prolonged and overly efficient dialysis is given
3. In the presence of a preexisting neurologic disorder

The disorder occurs paradoxically while biochemical abnormalities of the patient's extracellular fluid are being corrected.

The pathogenesis of the syndrome is not well understood. However, it seems to be caused by a disequilibrium between intracellular and extracellular fluids. The following factors have been incriminated in the pathogenesis of disequilibrium syndrome:

1. Reduction of extracellular fluid osmolality resulting from the removal of urea by dialysis and more importantly, a drop in its sodium concentration.* Lower extracellular fluid osmolality relative to intracellular fluid causes a shift of water into the cell and resultant cell swelling.

2. Increased intracellular and cerebrospinal fluid acidosis. Dialysis can rapidly correct the extracellular fluid acidosis by increasing its bicarbonate concentration. With correction of renal acidosis, pulmonary compensation will disappear. As a result, the partial pressure of carbon dioxide (Pco_2) rises. In contrast to bicarbonate ions, CO_2 equilibrates across the cell membrane quite rapidly. Therefore Pco_2 inside the cell rises while bicarbonate is still low; as a result intracellular pH falls. The same mechanism is operative across the blood-brain barrier, causing cerebrospinal fluid acidosis.

3. Reduction of oxygen delivery to the tissues. This relates to the effect of blood pH on the oxygen-hemoglobin dissociation curve. In the presence of acidosis the affinity of hemoglobin for oxygen is reduced. As a result, a more complete unloading of oxygen is expected at the tissue level. Rapid correction of acidosis with dialysis reverses this effect and may transiently impair tissue oxygen delivery in these anemic patients.

4. Hypoglycemia. This may be caused by reversal of insulin resistance and removal of glucose by dialysis.

5. Idiogenic osmoles. A marked increase in the osmolality of the brain has recently been shown in uremic animals after rapid dialysis. This is not due to an increased sodium, potassium, chloride, calcium, magnesium, or urea content of the brain. Since the nature of the osmotically active substances that are responsible for the observed rise in brain osmolality is not known, they have been termed idiogenic osmoles. Increased osmolality of brain cells results in a shift of water from the extracellular fluid to the intracellular space and causes brain edema and intracranial hypertension.

Treatment and prevention. Several modalities of treatment and prevention have been used with variable results. By slow IV infusion of mannitol or hypertonic sodium chloride solutions during dialysis, the symptoms may be minimized or eliminated. This is accomplished through maintaining extracellular fluid osmolality. The administration of phenytoin (Dilantin) prior to dialysis can reduce the symptoms.

In my experience the best way of preventing disequilibrium syndrome is to reduce the duration and flow rates of the first few dialysis treatments and increase their frequency. This results in the gradual rather than sudden correction of extracellular fluid abnormalities, allowing parallel correction of intracellular fluid with time.

Postdialysis syndrome

Postdialysis syndrome is a very common problem among the long-term dialysis population. It manifests as weakness, fatigue, and dizziness, and occasionally headaches, nausea, and muscle cramps. Symptoms start after dialysis and last 12 to 24 hours. The problem reappears with each dialysis and is very annoying. I believe this syndrome is a mild recurrent form of disequilibrium syndrome.

Paradoxical hypertension

Severe hypertension can occur when the patient undergoes drastic ultrafiltration. This is called paradoxical because the usual response is hypotension rather than hypertension. It is caused by the increased release of vasoactive

---

*The sodium concentration in all conventional dialysates is around 130 mEq/L. It is about 155 mEq/L in the water fraction of plasma and extracellular fluid. Therefore most dialysates are hypotonic with respect to sodium and are capable of reducing the extracellular fluid sodium concentration.

agents, that is, renin-angiotensin and catecholamines, in response to volume depletion. Treatment consists of the IV infusion of saline solution to replete intravascular volume and relieve vascular hyperreactivity.

■ **What complications can arise from the dysfunction of dialysis apparatus and inappropriate dialysate formulation?**
Mechanical blood loss

Blood losses caused by rupture of the dialysis membrane or disconnection of the tubing system are discussed elsewhere.

Clotting of artificial kidney

Clotting occurs when the patient is not adequately heparinized and/or the blood flow through the dialyzer is slow. In microcapillary kidneys many of the microfibers may be occluded by blood clots without being noticed. This can markedly reduce the efficiency of dialysis. With coil dialyzers clotting is readily suspected by a rapid increase of the venous resistance and visual detection of the clot in the tubing system. Because of their relatively large priming volume, clotting in coil dialyzers is associated with significant blood loss.

Adequate anticoagulation with careful monitoring of clotting time and provision of good blood flow are essential for the prevention of this problem.

Hemolysis

Hemolysis is occasionally seen in dialysis patients under the following circumstances:

1. Dialysis against hypotonic bath. This is occasionally encountered when the person who is responsible for dialysis forgets or fails to add adequate amounts of concentrate to the tank before dialysis is started. Malfunction of the proportionating machines can also create a similar problem. Exposure to hypotonic medium results in the swelling and rupture of red blood cells as they pass through the dialyzer.

Patients often complain of shortness of breath, chills, back pain, feeling ill, nausea, and vomiting. Because of the release of hemoglobin into plasma, blood content of the venous line appears glossy and simulates cherry syrup. Dialysis should be discontinued immediately. Serial hematocrit and electrolyte determinations should be performed. The patient's blood should be typed and cross matched and transfusion started if a significant drop in hematocrit is observed or if the patient becomes symptomatic from the acute exacerbation of anemia. Because of the release of intracellular potassium, serum potassium levels may rise to dangerous concentrations and should be carefully watched. In order to avoid this serious complication, the routine measurement of dialysate conductivity before starting dialysis should be mandatory.

2. Tight occlusion of the blood pump. This results in traumatic breakdown of the red blood cells as they pass through the pump. Finding many red blood cell fragments (schistocytes) on a smear taken from the blood leaving the pump suggests the diagnosis and calls for correction of the problem.

3. Copper-induced acute hemolysis. A few cases of acute hemolysis resulting from dialysis with copper-contaminated dialysates have been reported in the literature. Contamination was caused by the release of copper from copper tubing in dialysate-making machines. In all cases water deionizer was exhausted, allowing delivery of acid water capable of dissolving copper to the dialysate-making machine. Greenish discoloration of the dialysate should indicate the possibility of copper contamination.

4. High dialysate temperature. Excess heating of dialysis fluid is another cause of hemolysis during the dialysis procedure.

5. Increased chloramine content of the tap water subsequent to chlorination. This may result in production of methemoglobin and hemolysis. Addition of ascorbic acid to the dialysate prevents this.

Air embolism

Air embolism is one of the most serious complications of hemodialysis. The following conditions can predispose to the development of air embolism:

1. Use of a blood pump
2. High negative pressure that sucks the air from around the needle and releases the dissolved gas as free bubbles in the blood

3. Empty bottles connected to the blood line
4. Defective and broken lines, providing an entrance for air into the blood line

I have seen fatal cases of air embolism subsequent to starting the machine with an *unprimed* kidney and tubing system! The severity of the disorder depends on the volume and rapidity of air entering the circulation, as well as on the patient's position at the time of the incident. A small amount of air slowly infused into the circulation is dissolved in the plasma and usually causes no significant problems. When a sizable bolus of air rapidly enters the venous circulation, it finds its way along the bloodstream toward the right atrium and ventricle. Subsequent contractions of the heart against the air-blood mixture create tremendous amounts of foam, filling the right ventricle and pulmonary vascular bed and impeding blood return to the left ventricle and systemic circulation. Some air bubbles find their way through the naturally occurring central pulmonary arteriovenous shunts or cardiac septal defects to various organs, including brain and retinal vessels.

Clinical findings consist of sudden onset of dyspnea, cough, cyanosis, respiratory arrest, and loss of consciousness. Churning of the foam may be audible on auscultation of the heart, and air bubbles may be seen in retinal vessels on careful funduscopic examination. Examination of the tubing system frequently reveals the presence of residual air in the tubing system, helping to establish the diagnosis.

As for every other disorder, the best treatment for air embolism is its prevention. This is achieved by avoiding high negative pressures, checking for defective and leaky tubing systems, using collapsible plastic instead of rigid glass IV fluid containers, and clamping the IV line before the container is completely empty. Electronic air-detecting devices are also helpful.

In the case of suspected air embolism, *dialysis should be stopped* and the source of air eliminated immediately. The patient should be placed *on the left side* with the feet higher than the head, in order to trap the air bolus in the right ventricle and allow enough time (20 to 30 minutes) for its resolution in the blood. Oxygen should be administered in high concentration.

In the case of respiratory arrest or severe distress, *assisted respiration is necessary. A needle or catheter aspiration* of the right side of the heart to remove the trapped air and foam may be necessary to make resuscitative measures successful.

If available, the patient should be placed in a hyperbaric chamber. Under high barometric pressures the solubility of nitrogen in the plasma increases; air bubbles disappear and clinical improvement ensues. Decompression of the chamber should be performed very slowly, since sudden decompression results in the appearance of air bubbles in the blood and diffuse fatal air embolization.

Leukopenia

The number of circulating white blood cells drops significantly during the first 30 minutes of dialysis. It returns to normal in about 1 hour. Margination and aggregation of the white blood cells within the pulmonary capillaries seem to be responsible for the phenomenon. It should be mentioned that this phenomenon occurs invariably with each dialysis in all patients and is mediated by activation of the complement system. Although it is not usually associated with any significant clinical problems, it can cause acute cardiorespiratory difficulties in susceptible individuals.

Hypernatremia

Hypernatremia is another complication caused by the inappropriate formulation of dialysate. Severe hypernatremia with a hyperosmolar state has occurred as a consequence of ion-exchange water softener malfunction, allowing delivery of water with a high sodium concentration to the dialysate-making machine. Headaches, excess thirst, blurry vision, and disorientation characterize this syndrome.

Water intoxication

Water intoxication is also caused by the inappropriate formulation of dialysis fluid when its sodium concentration is below 120 mEq/L. It is characterized by signs of increased intracranial pressure, that is, headaches, nausea, vomiting, confusion, convulsion, and coma.

Hypokalemia

Most dialysis patients are dialyzed against zero or very low potassium baths. Although this is often necessary for the removal of excess potassium, at times a profound hypokalemia is encountered. Clinical symptoms of hypokalemia are muscular weakness, ileus, and cardiac arrhythmias that could be life threatening in digitalized patients. Therefore serum potassium concentrations should be checked periodically to avoid this complication.

Hard water syndrome

The calcium content of tap water can be quite high. Ion-exchange water softeners are used to remove the calcium content of tap water. Malfunction of the water softener can release excess calcium into the water. When this water is mixed with ordinary concentrate, the resultant dialysate will have a very high calcium concentration. Dialysis against such dialysate will result in the influx of calcium from the bath to the patient and cause hypercalcemia. Clinical symptoms include weakness, lethargy, anorexia, vomiting, hypertension, and burning of the skin. The diagnosis is confirmed by measurement of the calcium content of the bath and the patient's plasma.

Treatment and prevention are obvious, that is, correction of the malfunctioning apparatus and calcium concentration of dialysate.

Fluoride excess

The fluoride content of dialysates is quite high in cities where water supplies are artificially fluoridated or areas where the content of fluoride in the water is naturally high. Fluoride can cause osteosclerosis and some other bony and dental changes, but it has generally been thought to be harmless. Recently, however, the possibility of its role in the pathogenesis of progressive renal osteodystrophy has been raised. Therefore the safety of high fluoride dialysate is quite uncertain at the present time.

Hyper- and hypoglycemia

At the present time most conventional hemodialysis fluids are either glucose free or contain no more than 200 mg of glucose. Therefore hyperglycemia and reactive hypoglycemia associated with hemodialysis are no longer observed.

However, in the past when baths containing high concentrations of glucose were used for ultrafiltration purposes, these complications were commonly seen. With peritoneal dialysis, in which the dialysates have a high glucose content, hyper- and hypoglycemia remain among the consequences of this procedure. For further information, refer to Chapters 30 and 31.

■ **What are the complications caused by failure to adhere to the dietary and drug regimen?**

Despite the wide variability of dietary intake, the volume and composition of the body fluids remain relatively unchanged. Kidneys play a major role in maintaining the homeostasis of the internal milieu, which is vital to the proper function of all the cells and organ systems.

Dialysis patients who are functionally or anatomically without kidneys lack these regulatory mechanisms. Therefore the volume and composition of their body fluids are altered every time they eat or drink.

Although dialysis treatment is intended to replace the excretory function of the kidney, because of its intermittent nature, it does not simulate the function of normal kidneys, which have the minute-to-minute control of homeostasis of the internal milieu. The purpose of dietary and drug regimens prescribed for these patients is to minimize these fluctuations, which have immediate and long-term adverse effects on various organs. The dietary and drug regimens recommended for dialysis patients were discussed earlier in detail. Here I will discuss various problems that can result from failure to adhere to these recommendations.

Fluid overload

The ingestion of excess fluid by these patients results in expansion of their body fluids, including the intravascular and interstitial compartments. This in turn elevates the blood pressure and increases the load on the heart, resulting in congestive heart failure and pulmonary edema.

In catabolic patients endogenously produced water from the breakdown of tissues can produce congestive heart failure and pulmonary edema in the absence of excess exogenous fluid intake and weight gain.

The ingestion of excess salt can cause expansion of the extracellular fluid by shifting water from the intracellular to the extracellular compartment. Therefore fluid and sodium ion intakes should be restricted to prevent these catastrophic events. When they happen, emergency dialysis with ultrafiltration should be performed. If this is not possible, phlebotomy with plasmaphoresis and the return of packed red blood cells should be considered.

Hyperkalemia

Renal failure patients cannot handle large loads of potassium. The ingestion of potassium-rich foods, for example, fruits and milk, results in a rapid rise of their serum potassium. Severe hyperkalemia causes muscle weakness and even paralysis of various muscle groups, including the respiratory muscles. It has serious cardiac toxicity. As plasma potassium increases above 6 to 7 mEq/L, the T waves become tall and peaked, the P-R interval is prolonged, P waves disappear, QRS complexes are prolonged, and idioventricular rhythm and cardiac arrest follow sequentially with gradual increments of plasma potassium.

Emergency treatment is necessary if fatal cardiac complications are to be avoided. Potassium ion can be driven into the cells by IV infusion of sodium bicarbonate or insulin and glucose mixtures. IV calcium gluconate counteracts the cardiac effects of hyperkalemia, but it is dangerous in digitalized patients.

A sodium-polystyrene sulfonate (Kayexalate)–sorbitol mixture (ion-exchange resin) given orally or by enema can lower plasma potassium ion by removing it through the gastrointestinal tract. Emergency dialysis against zero or, if not available, a low potassium ion bath is the most direct answer.

It should be noted that hyperkalemia may occur in postsurgical catabolic patients (sepsis or crush syndrome), or patients with hemolysis or gastrointestinal bleeding in the absence of exogenous potassium ion intake. This is caused by the release of potassium ion associated with the breakdown of tissues or red blood cells. Frequent dialysis treatments and administration of Kayexalate are helpful in bringing this hyperkalemia under control.

Hyperphosphatemia

Intermittent dialysis is not adequate to remove all the phosphorus that enters the body fluids from dietary sources and bone resorption. Hyperphosphatemia is therefore a common finding in dialysis patients. Aluminum hydroxide administered with meals binds dietary phosphate and prevents its absorption. It is routinely prescribed for dialysis patients to control hyperphosphatemia. Failure to administer aluminum hydroxide results in lowering of the serum calcium level, increased vascular and soft tissue calcification, and progression of renal osteodystrophy. To adjust the dose of aluminum hydroxide and determine the reliability of the patient in taking the drug, the serum phosphorus level should be checked at regular intervals.

Hypermagnesemia

The kidney is the main route of magnesium ion (Mg^{++}) excretion. Use of Mg^{++}-containing antacids or laxatives by renal failure patients can result in marked elevation of plasma Mg^{++}. Hypermagnesemia results in development of the following:

1. Depression of neuromuscular conductivity and thereby weakness of skeletal muscles, hypo- and areflexia, and paralysis of respiratory muscles
2. Suppression of the CNS, resulting in confusion, lethargy, and coma
3. Cardiac conduction and contractility defects, resulting in various blocks and cardiac arrest

To prevent these complications, the use of Mg^{++}-containing antacids and laxatives should be prohibited in renal failure patients. Treatment includes dialysis using a low Mg^{++} bath.

Megaloblastic anemia

Failure to take folic acid supplements results in the deterioration of preexisting anemia in these patients. This is discussed in some detail with respect to the drug regimen (Chapter 27).

■ What problems can arise in association with the vascular access?

A multitude of local and systemic complications can arise from vascular access, whether it is one of the internal or external arteriovenous shunts.

Clotting

Thrombosis is the most common complication of arteriovenous shunts. Disappearance of the thrill and bruit and, in the case of external shunts, visual detection of clot in the cannulas confirm the diagnosis. Predisposing factors include the following:

1. Reduced blood flow through the shunt caused by hypotension, pericardial tamponade, tight bandage, or sleeping on the extremity bearing the shunt may contribute to the development of thrombosis.

2. There is a high incidence of clotting of the blood access following major surgical procedures, regardless of their nature. This has been attributed to the so-called hypercoagulable state associated with surgically induced tissue damage (release of tissue thromboplastin, and so on).

3. Local trauma and multiple punctures can induce thrombosis by damaging the endothelium.

4. Local infections predispose to thrombosis.

External shunts can be declotted, as discussed elsewhere. In the case of internal shunts, surgical thrombectomy has been tried with variable success.

Heparin infusion through a T tube intermittently every 4 hours or continuously by a Harvard pump can be given on a short-term basis to prevent recurrent clotting. Small doses of coumadin, dipyridamole (Persantine), or aspirin have been used successfully on a long-term basis.

Embolization

The injection of heparinized saline solution into the arterial cannula during the declotting procedure can dislodge the clot and push it upward against the blood flow. The clot can then be carried to various organs by the bloodstream. When the injected volume is high enough to move the clot to the aortic arch, cerebral embolization can occur. With lower volumes embolization and ischemic necrosis of the extremity may develop.

Pulmonary embolism following declotting of the venous cannulas has also been reported. Arterial embolization can be prevented by avoiding the injection of more than 1 to 2 ml of declot-ting solution into the arterial line. Treatment consists of emergency embolectomy whenever possible following angiography.

Infection

Blood access infections can be local or become systemic. In general, infections are more common but easier to control in external arteriovenous shunts. They are less common but more difficult to eradicate in internal shunts. Local infections consist of cellulitis, abscess formation, or infection around the cannula. These infections have at times caused separation of the cannula and life-threatening blood loss. They are usually caused by *Staphylococcus aureus*, but other organisms such as *Streptococcus* and *Pseudomonas* are also seen. Meticulous shunt care and systemic antibiotics may eradicate the infection; however, at times removal of the cannula or closure of the internal shunt is necessary.

Systemic infections include septicemia, septic pulmonary embolism with resultant lung abscess, and endocarditis. One of the problems that is occasionally encountered is persistent fever in a patient with internal or external shunt who has no evidence of local infection. The question that arises is whether the shunt should be dismantled or not. In my experience infection without local manifestation is quite uncommon. Nevertheless, endovasculitis of arteriovenous fistula can occur with minimum local signs and yet behave like endocarditis. Endovasculitis should be treated just like endocarditis, with 4 weeks of treatment using appropriate antibiotics. If antibiotics fail to improve the symptoms of infection, the shunt should be dismantled.

Vancomycin, which is effective against *Staphylococcus*, is a favorite antibiotic in the treatment of blood access infections. Because of its long half-life in patients without kidney function, injection of 1000 mg of vancomycin every 10 days provides adequate coverage.

Pseudoaneurysm

Pseudoaneurysm is an uncommon complication of external arteriovenous shunts. It is usually seen in shunts that have survived an episode of local infection and occurs as a pulsatile mass.

Phlebitis

Phlebitis can be seen with both external and internal shunts. It is characterized by severe pain, since blood with arterial pressure flows through the inflamed vein. A cord may be palpable along the vein. It usually results in clotting of the shunt. Anticoagulation therapy with elevation and heat application are used to treat this condition.

Skin erosion

Skin erosion consists of ulceration of the skin overlying the subcutaneous segment of cannula. The development of erosion is often followed by local infection and subsequent clotting of the shunt. Prevention includes leaving some subcutaneous soft tissue between the cannula and overlying skin at the time of shunt placement. Padding with sterile cotton at pressure points is helpful after the shunt is inserted.

Dermatitis

Dermatitis is a common complication. It is usually caused by hypersensitivity to adhesive tapes, antibiotic ointments, or pHisoHex. It responds to the discontinuation of the allergen and the use of corticosteroid-containing ointments.

Joint separation

Joint separation results from separation of the external ends of the arterial and venous cannulas. When occurring at night or remaining unnoticed, this can result in life-threatening blood loss. This is more likely to happen when the shunt is old and the external ends are worn out. For this reason old shunts should be trimmed for a tight connector fit.

Cannula avulsion

The most common cause of cannula avulsion is local shunt infection resulting in weakening or necrosis of the vessel wall. Suicidal or accidental pulling of the shunt has also been reported. Cannula avulsion is associated with significant blood loss.

High output cardiac failure

External arteriovenous shunts usually do not cause high output cardiac failure, since their flow rate is about 200 to 350 ml/min, which is only a small fraction of the cardiac output. However, arteriovenous fistulas, saphenous vein grafts, and bovine grafts that have very high blood flows can impose a significant load on the heart and cause cardiac enlargement and failure. Measurement of cardiac output before and after temporary obstruction of the arteriovenous shunt demonstrates its hemodynamic significance. Determination of pulse rate before and after temporary manual occlusion of the shunt is a simple bedside examination to demonstrate significant arteriovenous shunting. If the pulse rate drops by 10 or more counts per minute or cardiac output increases significantly following temporary occlusion of the shunt, the patient's cardiac failure is likely to improve by surgical correction of the shunt directed toward reducing its flow.

Steal syndrome

In the presence of an external or internal arteriovenous shunt, which is a low resistance circuit, more blood preferentially flows through the arteriovenous shunt. If the patient also has peripheral vascular disease, shunting of the blood away from the extremity will cause ischemia. Ischemia may be characterized by intermittent claudication, pain on elevation of the involved extremity, cooler temperature compared to the contralateral side, decreased arterial pulses, and prolonged blanching time. At times ischemic gangrene results. Treatment consists of reduction of the blood flow through the shunt or its surgical removal.

■ What are the complications of anticoagulation in dialysis patients?

Anticoagulation is necessary to prevent clotting of the blood during its extracorporeal circulation. Systemic or regional heparinization is used for this purpose. *Bleeding* from various sources, for example, intracranial, gastrointestinal, wound, or intrapericardial areas, can occur subsequent to heparinization. Uremic patients, because of their underlying platelet dysfunction, are even more prone to serious bleeding disorders following heparinization than are other patients. Patients in whom systemic anticoagulation is contraindicated may be dialyzed with *regional heparinization*. This involves the continuous infusion of heparin into the arterial line of the dialyzer to prevent clotting outside the body. Equivalent amounts of protamine sulfate are simultaneously infused into the venous line to neutralize the effect of heparin when the blood returns to the circulation. Accordingly, by this pharmacologic maneuver adequate anticoagulation is achieved in the extracorporeal circuit without affecting the systemic coagulation profile.

One of the problems frequently encountered following regional heparinization is *heparin rebound*. This is characterized by depression of the coagulation parameters and occasionally bleeding a couple of hours after termination of the procedure. It is caused by faster metabolism of protamine sulfate as compared to heparin, which results in the appearance of heparin effect after the protamine sulfate is completely metabolized. Administration of additional protamine sulfate at this time reverses the rebound phenomenon.

The development of *allergic reaction* to the animal protein content of heparin occasionally creates a major problem. Heparin allergy usually appears as severe pruritus following the administration of heparin. The solution to this problem is to switch from pork mucosa heparin to beef lung heparin.

■ What are the infectious complications of hemodialysis?

It is a well-known fact that uremia lowers the resistance to infection. The repeated transfusions required by some hemodialysis patients expose them to blood-borne infections. Furthermore, the use of external shunts or repeated cannulations of internal fistulas with each dialysis provide a convenient port of entry for various organisms. The infections that are more commonly seen in this population include blood access infections, viral hepatitis, cytomegalovirus infections, and pyrogenic reaction. Bacterial endocarditis, osteomyelitis, and various other infections have also been reported with increased frequency in these patients.

Blood access infections

Local and systemic infections originating from the blood access were discussed earlier.

Viral hepatitis

Viral hepatitis is one of the most serious problems associated with chronic dialysis. Dialysis patients and staff are frequently exposed to blood and its derivatives. Many outbreaks of hepatitis among the patients and staff have occurred in dialysis units, resulting in tremendous morbidity and significant mortality.

Hepatitis can be caused by a multitude of viruses and other microorganisms as well as the toxic or immunologic injuries resulting from various drugs and toxins. There are two major forms of viral hepatitis: hepatitis B (long-incubation, Au_1-positive, HAA-positive, or serum hepatitis) and hepatitis A (short-incubation, Au_1-negative, or HAA-negative hepatitis). In contrast with the old concept, hepatitis A can be transmitted not only by the oral route but also through parenteral means. Similarly, hepatitis B can be transmitted not only parenterally, but also through oral, respiratory, sexual, and personal contact.

Although the use of blood and its derivatives is the major cause of hepatitis, HAA-positive hepatitis may occur in untransfused persons. This probably results from the transmission of the virus from one patient to the other by contaminated dialysis equipment, personnel, toilet facilities, dining utensils, personal contacts, and so on. The incidence of anicteric asymptomatic disease with chronic antigenemia is quite high among dialysis patients. It is frequently severe and symptomatic among the dialysis personnel with transient antigenemia. Because of the prevalence of asymptomatic disease in patients, it is necessary to perform monthly screening tests, liver function tests, and hepatitis-associated antigen (HAA) determinations. There are no false positive results for HAA, but depending on the sensitivity of the testing method and the time of sampling in relation to the time of exposure, there is a 20% to 50% chance of registering a false negative result. Therefore a negative HAA test does not rule out hepatitis B.

Abnormal liver function does not always indicate viral hepatitis. The differential diagnosis list is long and includes infectious and noninfectious causes.

Noninfectious causes of hepatitis

Drugs: methyldopa (Aldomet), methyltestosterone chlorpromazine, phenytoin (Dilantin), indomethacin (Indocin), griseofulvin, synthetic estrogens and progestins, and so on

Toxins: alcohol, plasticizers used in manufacturing dialysis tubing, inorganic phosphorus, carbon tetrachloride, and so on

Anesthetics: halothane and methoxyflurane

Postsurgical: probably caused by morphine, produces benign and self-limited hepatic dysfunction

Infections

Cytomegalovirus and various other viruses, miliary tuberculosis, leptospirosis, tularemia, brucellosis, amebiasis, mononucleosis, hepatitis associated with pneumonia and sepsis, and so on

Miscellaneous

Hemosiderosis secondary to repeated transfusions and parenteral iron, cirrhosis, neoplasm, biliary obstruction, and so on

Since hepatitis A and B are both transmitted by oral and parenteral routes, the prevention and control methods are the same and are aimed at two fronts:

1. Prevent the introduction of the virus to the unit.
   a. Restrict transfusions and use frozen packed red blood cells when necessary. Hepatitis viruses are destroyed as a result of the procedures necessary to prepare frozen packed red blood cells; therefore the use of this preparation minimizes the risk of hepatitis.
   b. Screen dialysis candidates and prospective personnel for liver function and the presence of HAA.
2. Take measures to prevent the spreading of the disease when hepatitis has occurred.
   a. Exercise meticulous nursing techniques of aseptic and contagion precautions.
   b. Screen patients and personnel monthly for liver function and the presence of HAA.
   c. Personnel contracting hepatitis should be excused from work until such time when the HAA test is negative.
   d. Limit blood transfusions to very symptomatic patients or in preparation for surgery. The advantage of using frozen packed red blood cells over the use of other products was discussed earlier.
   e. Serve meals with disposable utensils and prohibit eating and smoking by the personnel in the unit.
   f. Separate the patients' toilet facilities from those of the personnel. Install knee-operated faucets and pedal-operated soap dispensers.

g. Enforce personal hygiene.
h. Vigorously cleanse the dialysis machine following rupture of the coil.
i. Avoid spilling blood and other fluids on the floor.

This list of precautionary measures is by no means complete, and the reader is referred to specific sources for additional information.

Cytomegalovirus infection

Cytomegalovirus infection is seen in immunosuppressed hosts. It can cause hepatitis, pericarditis, nephritis, enteritis, pneumonitis, and mononucleosis-like syndromes.

Pyrogenic reaction

Pyrogenic reaction results from the passage of some bacterial endotoxins from the bath into the circulation. It is characterized by fever and shaking chills during or shortly after dialysis. It is caused by bacterial growth in the tap water used for making dialysate. Pyrogenic reaction is not a true infection, since the bacteria do not enter the body.

■ What complications can arise from chronic renal failure in dialysis patients?

With the advent of the dialysis technique, the natural course of end-stage renal failure has changed. With partial substitution of the excretory function of the kidney by long-term dialysis, patients can live for many years despite a lack of functioning kidneys. As a result, many metabolic defects that would not have become manifest fully had the patient died of uremia will do so with prolongation of life. These include renal osteodystrophy, peripheral neuropathy, nerve deafness, dialysis dementia, muscle cramps, anemia, pericarditis, accelerated atherosclerosis and hyperlipidemia, and sexual problems.

Renal osteodystrophy

Renal osteodystrophy consists of one or a combination of several of the following disorders:

1. Renal dwarfism, which refers to growth retardation caused by the onset of renal failure early in life.
2. Rickettsia or osteomalacic bone disease, which is caused by the impaired metabolic activation of vitamin D by the kidney. Vitamin D in

its original form is biologically inert and needs metabolic activation in the liver and kidney in order to become biologically active. In the absence of a functioning kidney vitamin D remains inactive, resulting in the development of osteomalacic bone disease and the impairment of calcium absorption from the intestines.

3. Bone disease related to increased parathormone secretion. The impairment of phosphate excretion in chronic renal failure results in the elevation of plasma phosphate. Since the product of calcium and phosphate is constant ($Ca \times PO_4 = K$), an elevation of serum phosphate results in a lowering of serum calcium. Furthermore, as discussed earlier, the impairment of vitamin D metabolism in renal failure interferes with calcium absorption from the intestines and bones and further depresses the plasma calcium level. A reduction of the plasma calcium level stimulates the parathyroid gland to secrete large amounts of parathyroid hormone. Parathyroid hormone causes bone resorption to normalize serum calcium level. Prolonged elevation of parathyroid hormone results in development of osteitis fibrosa cystica. Bone pain, fragility, x-ray abnormalities, and severe pruritus are among the clinical findings of secondary hyperparathyroidism.

4. Soft tissue and vascular calcifications. This is caused by high phosphate levels enhancing the precipitation of calcium phosphate in soft tissues and vessel walls. Vascular calcifications probably contribute to these patients' ischemic heart disease and peripheral vascular insufficiency.

5. Osteosclerosis. Osteosclerosis is apparent on x-ray films as a relative increase in radiopacity of some areas of the skeleton. This increased density does not mean stronger bony structure; rather, it has been shown to be abnormal and fragile. Osteosclerosis is caused by the abnormal deposition of calcium and phosphate in immature matrix and/or is a reflection of fluoride toxicity, as discussed earlier.

A variety of therapeutic modalities have been advocated for the treatment and prevention of renal osteodystrophy. These include control of hyperphosphatemia by dialysis and phosphate-binding agents, such as aluminum hydroxide, by far the most important and effective therapy; dialysis

against high calcium baths, that is, 3.5 to 4 mEq/L, to suppress parathyroid hormone and improve negative calcium balance; administration of oral calcium carbonate; use of therapeutic doses of vitamin D; or performance of subtotal parathyroidectomy, which frequently alleviates pruritus and improves bone disease.

Dialysis against high calcium baths and the administration of oral calcium carbonate or therapeutic doses of vitamin D can be quite dangerous if carried out without controlling hyperphosphatemia, since by elevating the level of plasma calcium while the serum phosphate level is high, soft tissue and vascular deposition of calcium can be enhanced, which is quite damaging.

Peripheral neuropathy

Peripheral neuropathy is one of the known complications of uremia. Dialysis treatment can slowly improve the patient's peripheral neuropathy. However, nerve conduction studies and electromyography frequently show residual abnormalities. There is indirect evidence to suggest that the accumulation of some as yet unidentified middle molecules normally cleared by the kidney is responsible for the development of peripheral neuropathy. The clearance of these molecules by dialysis is reduced when the dialysis time is short and flow rates of blood and dialysate are high. Such inadequate dialysis treatments can result in the development of progressive disabling neuropathy, although the patient's urea and creatinine levels are adequately reduced.

Nerve deafness

Nerve deafness of varying severity is very common among long-term dialysis patients. The pathogenesis of this deafness is not clearly understood. It may be part of the uremic neuropathy, but the possibility of exposure to ototoxic drugs cannot be ruled out. Recently preparations used for the sterilization and preservation of dialysis membranes and tubing systems have been incriminated.

Dialysis dementia

Dialysis dementia was first described by Alfrey and his associates in 1972. Subsequently several other groups reported similar observations in their dialyzed patients. The disorder begins with speech abnormalities such as stuttering and slowing. This is followed by the development of dizziness and dyspraxia of the speech, tremulousness, asterixis, seizures, myoclonus, dyspraxia of movement, loss of ability to concentrate, impairment of memory, personality changes, depression, paranoia, hallucinations, ataxia, and inability to speak and perform self-care. The disorder is progressive with a fatal outcome and fails to respond to more adequate dialysis treatments and various pharmacologic agents.

The cerebrospinal fluid usually shows normal cell count and chemistries. Electroencephalogram (EEG) reveals generalized slowing, delta bursts, and spike activity. These changes are more pronounced after dialysis than before dialysis. Histologic examination of brain on autopsy shows normal tissue except for occasional areas of edema and gliosis. Use of tap water for preparation of dialysate was implicated in several reports. Elevated tin and aluminum levels have been found on histochemical analysis of the brain tissue and have been implicated in the genesis of dialysis dementia by some investigators. However, the pathogenesis and effective treatment of this syndrome remain poorly understood.

Muscle cramps

Muscle cramps during and after dialysis are quite common among patients undergoing hemodialysis treatment. The pathogenesis of this annoying problem is not clearly known. Rapid fall of extracellular fluid osmolality owing to sodium and chloride removal with subsequent water shift into the cells and cell swelling has been implicated. The beneficial effect of high dialysate sodium concentration and mannitol administration supports this contention. Reduced oxygen unloading to the tissues owing to increased blood pH and reduced red blood cell level of 2,3-diphosphoglycerate induced by dialysis has also been suggested as a possible mechanism.

Anemia

Anemia is an almost universal finding among the dialysis population. It is disabling and very difficult to control. Multiple factors are involved in the pathogenesis of this anemia:

1. Lack of *erythropoietin,* a polypeptide hormone secreted by the kidneys that is responsible for the formation of red blood cells by the bone marrow.

2. Defective iron utilization by erythroid precursors. The amount of iron stored in the reticuloendothelial cells of these patients is usually increased, but it cannot be utilized for hemoglobin synthesis. This abnormality is commonly seen in most of the chronic diseases.

3. Blood loss. Because of uremic platelet dysfunction, gastrointestinal and other sources of occult blood loss are common in these patients. Furthermore, with each dialysis, some blood, although a small amount, is lost.

4. Short red blood cell life span. The uremic environment has adverse effects on erythrocytes and results in the premature destruction of red blood cells. When red blood cells from normal persons are transfused into a uremic patient, the life span of these cells shortens. Transfusion of a uremic patient's red blood cells to a normal person normalizes the cells' life span. These data indicate that the early destruction of red blood cells in uremic patients is caused by the abnormal environment, not an intrinsic defect in the red blood cells. Increased splenic destruction of red blood cells has recently been shown to contribute to the anemia of some dialysis patients. Such patients may benefit from splenectomy.

5. Decreased iron absorption from the gastrointestinal tract has been implicated by some investigators. However, more recent investigations have shown that intestinal absorption of iron is often normal in these patients.

6. Folic acid, which is essential for red blood cell production, is washed out of the circulation during dialysis.

7. Bone marrow depression, caused by the uremic environment, deficiency of erythropoietin, and the lack of various essential nutrients, plays a major role in the pathogenesis of anemia in dialysis patients.

8. Drug-induced anemia, for example, by methyldopa (Aldomet), should always be suspected.

The treatment of the anemia of chronic renal failure presents an extremely difficult problem. *Folic acid* in doses of 1 to 2 mg/day should be given to all dialysis patients to make up for losses with dialysis. Oral or parenteral *iron* should be given only to those patients in whom the saturation of iron-binding proteins and serum ferritin level are low and the bone marrow iron stores are depleted.

Testosterone derivatives stimulate erythrogenesis in the bone marrow in the presence of some erythropoietin. They are used orally as methyltestosterone on a daily basis or in IM injectable depot forms given every 1 to 4 weeks. These derivatives are almost always effective in raising the patient's hematocrit by a few points. Their drawbacks, however, include androgenic effects on female patients (increased hair growth and voice changes), possible atherogenic effect, and cholestatic jaundice caused by methyl derivatives.

Cobalt compounds can raise the hematocrit through stimulating an impairment of oxygen utilization by the cells, which signals the bone marrow to produce more red blood cells. Improvement of tissue oxygenation, which is the goal in the treatment of anemia, is not achieved by the use of cobalt compounds.

Blood transfusions, although resulting in the dramatic improvement of anemic symptoms and providing a sense of strength and well-being, produce only transient effects and are associated with great risks. The adverse consequences of repeated transfusions are as follows:

1. There is a high risk of viral hepatitis and transmission of other infectious agents such as cytomegalovirus and various bacteria that contaminate blood during its preparation.

2. The patient's own erythrogenic mechanism is suppressed because of the availability of exogenous red blood cells.

3. Hemosiderosis—with each transfusion a significant amount of iron enters the body and must be stored in reticuloendothelial cells following the destruction of red blood cells. The accumulation of enormous amounts of iron in the liver, pancreas, heart, skin, and other tissues damages these organs.

4. The development of antibodies against white blood cell and platelet antigens results in febrile reactions during future transfusions.

5. The formation of antibodies against various

minor blood group antigens with multiple transfusions makes it difficult to find compatible blood for emergency or elective purposes in the future.

Therefore it is recommended that transfusions be restricted for the treatment of highly symptomatic patients or in preparation for surgery.

Pericarditis

Two distinct forms of pericarditis can be recognized in these patients:

1. Uremic pericarditis. This is a fibrinous and hemorrhagic pericarditis that is found in untreated or underdialyzed patients. It improves and gradually clears with adequate dialysis treatments.

2. Dialysis-associated pericarditis. This occurs in the face of adequate dialysis treatment. It is also fibrinous and hemorrhagic and is characterized by fever, leukocytosis, chest pain, pericardial friction rub, and effusion. It usually does not respond to more adequate dialysis treatment. Its etiology is as yet obscure. Viral, bacterial, and fungal cultures and serologic tests have been unrevealing. Improvement may follow the use of indomethacin (Indocin) or corticosteroids.

At times pericardial effusion increases and pericardial tamponade results. This requires emergency pericardiocentesis and decompression of the heart chambers to improve the cardiac output and reduce venous pressure. Occasionally surgical pericardiectomy or creation of a pericardial window should be performed.

Patients with pericarditis should be closely monitored for the development of cardiac tamponade. Rapid distention of the jugular veins, arterial hypotension, marked paradoxical pulse pressure (more than 10 mm Hg), dyspnea, hepatomegaly, and hepatojugular reflux suggest significant pericardial effusion and cardiac tamponade.

These patients should undergo dialysis with regional or miniheparinizations to avoid hemopericardium.

Accelerated atherosclerosis and hyperlipidemia

Coronary artery disease is the most common cause of death among long-term dialysis patients. The incidence of myocardial infarction in these patients is several times higher than that of patients with type II hyperlipidemia. It takes only a few years to develop a severe atherosclerosis that would have otherwise taken many decades. Although the pathogenesis of accelerated atherosclerosis in dialysis patients is not clearly understood, several factors seem to be responsible:

1. Hypertension. The majority of dialysis patients are hypertensive. This hypertension is usually but not always volume dependent. It drops following dialysis with ultrafiltration and gradually rises again with reexpansion of the extracellular volume between dialyses. It is often difficult to use antihypertensive drugs to control this hypertension. With the use of these drugs the patient's blood pressure drops to subnormal levels during and after dialysis, which interferes with the dialysis procedure and with the patient's activity afterward.

2. Fluctuations of intravascular volume impose an excess load on the heart and cause cardiomegaly and recurrent episodes of cardiac failure.

3. Anemia and the presence of arteriovenous shunts produce a high output state that further increases the load on the heart.

4. Vascular calcification, discussed with renal osteodystrophy, enhances the development of coronary artery disease.

5. Type IV hyperlipidemia with marked elevation of plasma triglyceride levels is extremely prevalent among dialysis patients. The pathogenesis of this hyperlipidemia is not well understood yet. Whatever the causes of hyperlipidemia, it contributes to accelerated atherosclerosis.

6. The level of uric acid in these patients is frequently above normal.

7. A diabetic glucose tolerance curve is usually exhibited. Abnormal carbohydrate metabolism is a well-known phenomenon in these patients.

8. Testosterone preparations commonly used for the treatment of anemia are known atherogenic substances.

All these factors and perhaps other as yet unrecognized conditions predispose these patients to accelerated atherosclerosis and death from ischemic heart disease and cerebrovascular accidents. There is no definite treatment or prevention for this complication. Nevertheless, at the present state of knowledge the following steps appear to be advisable in reducing the risk and severity of the disorder:

1. Low carbohydrate and saturated fat diet
2. Adequate hypertension control
3. Use of lipid-lowering drugs when necessary
4. Avoidance of androgenic steroids when possible
5. Control of hyperphosphatemia and hyperparathyroidism

Sexual problems

Impotency, sterility, and amenorrhea are extremely common among dialysis patients. Androgenic steroids sometimes improve impotence in male patients, but the effect is transient. Psychotherapy may be helpful.

■ What are the socioeconomic and psychologic impacts of long-term dialysis?

Maintenance dialysis is a very expensive treatment. It can easily drain all the financial resources of an average family in a short period of time. Although the various governmental agencies will cover the expenses involved in the care of end-stage renal disease, this usually does not begin until all the family resources are exhausted. The poor state of health and the disruption of the patient's time schedule caused by the time spent for dialysis itself and the traveling to and from the dialysis center frequently interfere with the patient's work and productivity.

Depending on dialysis for living, fear of sudden death from disruption of vascular access, hyperkalemia or pulmonary edema, severe dietary restrictions, impaired sexual activity, changes of self- and body images because of disfiguring external and internal shunts and multiple surgical scars, sense of being rejected from society, and many other social, personal, financial, and psychologic problems are faced by these patients every day. Each patient's reaction to the stress is somewhat different. Depression and denial are commonly encountered, whereas suicide by opening the shunt or ingestion of large quantities of potassium-containing foods and other self-destructive means are rarely seen.

Psychotherapy, especially the help and support of social workers and dialysis personnel, is extremely important in improving the patient's psychologic attitude.

BIBLIOGRAPHY

Abram, H. S., Moore, G. L., and Westervelt, F. B.: Suicidal behavior in chronic dialysis patients, paper presented at the one hundred twenty-third annual meeting of the American Psychology Association, May, 1970.

Alfrey, A. G., et al. Syndrome of dyspraxia and multifocal seizures associated with chronic hemodialysis, Trans. Am. Soc. Artif. Intern. Organs **18:**257, 1972.

Bailey, G. L., editor: Hemodialysis principles and practice, New York, 1972, Academic Press, Inc.

Bennett, W. M., Singer, I., and Coggins, C. J.: A guide to drug therapy in renal failure, J.A.M.A. **230:**1544, 1974.

Bussell, J. A., Abbott, J. A., and Lim, R. C.: A radial steal syndrome with arteriovenous fistula for hemodialysis, Ann. Intern. Med. **75:**387, 1971.

Editorial: Air embolism, Dialysis & Transplantation J., p. 13, April/May 1972.

Arthur, G., et al.: Clinical maintenance hemodialysis with a sorbent-based low-volume dialysis regeneration system, Trans. Am. Soc. Artif. Intern. Organs **17:**253, 1971.

Halper, I. S.: Psychiatric observations in chronic dialysis program, Med. Clin. North Am. **55:**177, 1971.

Kaegi, A., et al.: Arteriovenous-shunt thrombosis, N. Engl. J. Med. **290:**304, 1974.

Kennedy, A. C., et al.: The pathogenesis and prevention of cerebral dysfunction during dialysis, Lancet **1:**790, 1964.

Kjellstrand, C. M., et al.: Considerations of the middle molecule hypothesis 11—neuropathy in nephrectomized patients, Trans. Am. Soc. Artif. Intern. Organs **19:**325, 1973.

Knight, A. H., et al.: Hepatitis-associated antigen and antibody in haemodialysis patients and staff, Br. Med. J. **3:**603, 1970.

Manzler, A. D., and Schreiner, A. W.: Copper-induced acute hemolytic anemia, Ann. Intern. Med. **73:**409, 1970.

Massry, S. G., and Sellers, A. L., editors: Clinical aspects of uremia and dialysis, Springfield, Ill., 1976, Charles C Thomas, Publisher.

Port, F. K., Johnson, W. J., and Klass, D. W.: Prevention of dialysis disequilibrium syndrome by use of high sodium concentration in the dialysate, Kidney Int. **3:**327, 1973.

Siddiqui, J. Y., et al.: Causes of death in patients receiving long-term hemodialysis, J.A.M.A. **212:**1350, 1970.

Thomas, P. K., et al.: The polyneuropathy of chronic renal failure, Brain **94:**761, 1971.

Tyler, H. R.: Neurologic disorders in renal failure, Am. J. Med. **44:**734, 1968.

CHAPTER 30

Principles of peritoneal dialysis

N. D. Vaziri

The term "dialysis" refers to the diffusion of water and solutes across a permeable membrane separating two fluid compartments. Factors governing this process are the permeability characteristics of the membrane, the osmotic and hydrostatic pressures on each side, and the differential concentration of individual solutes in each compartment. *Water* molecules move freely across the membrane. Although this movement is bidirectional, the net transport of water occurs from the hypotonic to the hypertonic compartment. The rate and the direction of *solute* transport depends on the size of the molecules, the differential concentrations in each compartment, and the mass flow. The smaller the molecule, the higher is its permeability. However, if a highly diffusible substance binds with high molecular weight substances, such as proteins, the molecule will lose its diffusibility.

Hydrostatic forces are also important in the mass transport of water and solutes. The direction of movement is from the high pressure to the low pressure compartment. The result of these various interactions is the achievement of a state of *equilibrium* in which the algebraic sum of osmotic and hydrostatic forces becomes equal on both sides of the membrane. Therefore no *net* water and solute transport can occur, since the rate of transport in one direction is equal to the other. Diffusion and mass transport processes are quite rapid in the beginning but slow down in time as pressure and concentration gradients gradually dissipate. These principles form the basis for the use of *dialysis treatment* in clinical medicine. This treatment is aimed at the elimina-

tion of endogenous or exogenous toxins, the correction of electrolyte and acid-base abnormalities, and/or the removal of excess fluids. This requires a mechanism that brings the patient's circulating blood in contact with a physiologic solution through a permeable membrane. In such a system undesirable compounds present in the patient's blood can be washed out by diffusion into the dialysate. Furthermore, equilibration of the patient's plasma with dialysate that has desirable electrolyte concentrations helps to normalize the patient's electrolyte and acid-base abnormalities.

Dialysis involves three major elements:
1. Blood
2. Dialyzing membrane
3. Dialysis fluid (dialysate)

Accessory devices are obviously necessary to bring these elements together and to make the process mechanically feasible. In peritoneal dialysis, the mesenteric and peritoneal capillary circulation provides the blood supply. The peritoneal membrane, consisting of the capillary wall, a thin layer of connective tissue, and the mesothelial lining, makes up the dialyzing membrane.

With this brief introduction, the basic concepts and techniques involved in peritoneal dialysis will be presented and an attempt made to answer some of the questions that are important in understanding these concepts and in managing patients undergoing peritoneal dialysis.

■ How is the peritoneal catheter inserted?

It should be ascertained that the bladder is empty and there are no masses in the way before attempting to insert the catheter. This is done by careful examination of the abdomen and straight catheterization of the bladder when necessary. Failure to do so may result in catastrophic entry to a distended bladder, an abdominal aortic aneurysm, a tumor mass, or a polycystic kidney instead of the peritoneal cavity.

To reduce the patient's anxiety, premedication may be given with diazepam (Valium) or other preferred medications. The patient should be in the supine or semisupine position. The skin under the umbilicus is shaved properly, cleansed with iodine or other preferred solutions, and draped as for a laparotomy. The skin and underlying tissue are deeply infiltrated with a local anesthetic agent, for example, 1% procaine. An extremely small midline incision is made about one third of the way from the umbilicus to the pubic bone. The scalpel blade is inserted into the anterior wall of the abdomen until it is felt to grate on the linea alba. A small incision is ex-

tended in the linea alba. The reason for selecting the midline for introducing the catheter is its relative avascularity, which reduces the risk of significant bleeding. Through this incision the catheter with the stylet in place is inserted. With a short thrust the peritoneum is penetrated. The patient may experience some pain as the parietal peritoneum is stretched and should be made aware ahead of time that this pain will occur in order to prevent uncontrolled movements that may interfere with proper catheter placement.

It may be advisable to ask the patient to contract the abdominal wall muscles while the catheter is being pushed through the incision. As soon as the peritoneum is pierced, the stylet should be removed and the catheter advanced. It should be aimed posteriorly and inferiorly toward the small pelvis through right or left paravertebral gutter. Usually about 50 cm of the catheter enters the abdomen. Some of the older catheter sets in-

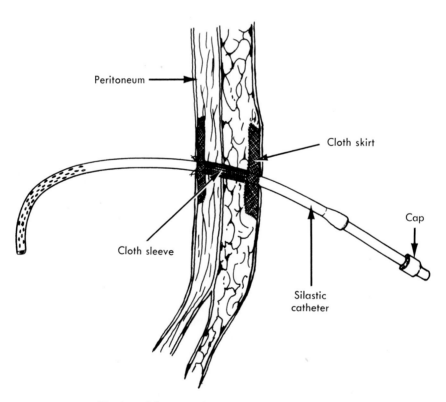

Fig. 30-1. Schematic of Tenckhoff's catheter in place.

clude a trocar through which the peritoneal catheter is advanced, and the trocar is removed after the catheter is properly placed. The position of the catheter is important in ensuring an adequate flow of irrigation fluid. The catheter is usually advanced with ease. Difficulty in passing the catheter is usually caused by the presence of the omentum in the way and rarely by its extra- or retroperitoneal localization. The difficulty is usually overcome by manipulating the catheter or infusing 1 or 2 L of dialysis fluid through the catheter and subsequently readjusting and advancing it.

Needless to say, the team performing the procedure should wear masks, gloves, hats, and sterile gowns and should exercise extreme aseptic measures. To prevent the inadvertent displacement of the catheter, a couple of stitches are placed along the incision and the catheter is tied to the skin. The catheter is then connected to the inflow system (Figs. 30-1 and 30-2).

■ What is the dwell time?

Dwell time refers to the period of time between the beginning of inflow and the end of drainage.

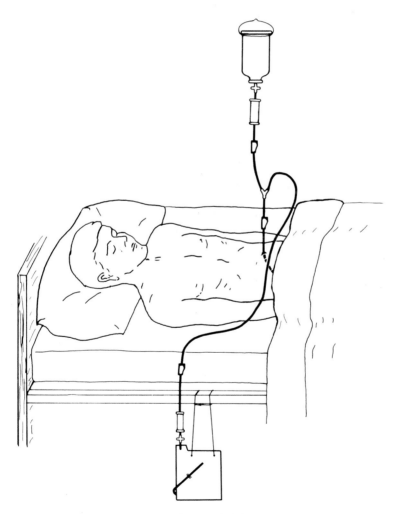

Fig. 30-2. Peritoneal dialysis.

■ **What about the volume, duration, and number of exchanges?**

It is important to remember that the *dialysis fluid should be warmed to body temperature* before it is used. Introduction to the peritoneal cavity of the fluid at a subnormal temperature not only causes discomfort to the patient, but also reduces the efficacy of dialysis by constricting the peritoneal vascular bed and reducing its blood flow. With regard to volume, up to 2 L of fluid is allowed to flow into the peritoneal cavity by gravity as rapidly as possible with each exchange. This should take no longer than 5 to 10 minutes. If the flow is slow, the catheter should be repositioned, since its tip may be buried in the omentum. The volume of administered fluid on each run should be tailored according to the patient's size, age, and pulmonary status. The introduction of large amounts of fluid into the abdomen of a patient with respiratory failure may adversely affect pulmonary ventilation by restricting the diaphragmatic excursion, particularly in the supine position. This is mostly a hypothetical consideration, however, and with proper positioning of the patient and slight adjustment of fluid volumes such problems are readily avoided.

Fluid is allowed to remain in the peritoneal cavity for 15 to 30 minutes. During this time the necessary exchanges between fluid and circulating blood in the peritoneal capillaries take place. The abdomen is drained by a siphon effect through the closed system. When the system is patent, the gravity drainage should occur quite rapidly and should take no longer than 10 minutes. When the flow slows down, manual compression of the abdomen toward the catheter may result in a temporary increase of flow into the drainage container. This procedure is repeated continuously for 12 to 48 hours and occasionally for 72 hours, depending on the clinical response and the nature of the disease for which peritoneal dialysis is being used. It should be kept in mind that the *longer the duration of the procedure the higher is the risk of peritoneal infection. Specimens of drainage fluid should be sent for bacterial culture and sensitivity tests periodically.* Careful records should be kept of the exact time of starting and ending each exchange, the drugs added, the vital signs, and the fluid balance. When dialysis is completed, the catheter is removed and the wound closed with additional stitches or clamps and covered with sterile gauze.

■ **What is the clearance, and what is the role of the dwell time?**

The effectiveness of dialysis is determined by the peritoneal clearance. Clearance can be simply defined as the volume of plasma that is completely cleared of the substance under consideration in 1 minute by peritoneal dialysis. It is calculated using the following formula:

$$C = \frac{C_D \times Q_D}{C_P}$$

in which C = clearance in milliliters per minute, C_D = concentration in outflow fluid, C_P = concentration in blood or plasma, and Q_D = rate of dialysate flow in milliliters per minute as determined by dividing the outflow volume by the length of the dwell time.

Clinical and experimental investigations have shown that urea and potassium have the highest peritoneal clearances. The clearances of creatinine, uric acid, phosphate, and sulfate are almost equal, at a level lower than urea and potassium and higher than calcium and magnesium.

Serial measurements of urea concentration in dialysis fluid have shown that the concentration rises quite rapidly during the first 20 to 30 minutes. Thereafter urea enters the peritoneal fluid at a much slower rate. This is caused by a reduction of the concentration gradient with time; in fact, in 2 hours a state of equilibrium is achieved. Urea and other clearance studies have been done using various dialysate flow rates. Urea clearance improves as the dialyzing rate is increased. A maximum clearance of 28.5 ml/min is achieved with a dialyzed volume of 3.5 L/hr. Further increase in dialyzed volume may result in a reduction of urea clearance. Therefore *a dialysis volume of 2.5 to 3.5 L/hr provides the most efficient and economical condition.*

■ **What is meant by continuous as opposed to intermittent flow?**

Two basic ways of irrigating the peritoneum exist—continuous flow and intermittent flow.

In the continuous method two catheters are placed. Dialysate enters through one and drains through the other on a continuous basis.

The popular method is intermittent flow, in which a predetermined volume of dialysate is rapidly infused into the peritoneal cavity. Some time is allowed for equilibration and the exchange processes between fluid and blood, following which the old fluid is drained and fresh fluid introduced.

The risk of infection, leakage, and traumatic complications is highest using the continuous method, for obvious reasons, and the urea clearance may be lower as a result of the shortcut taken between the inflow and outflow channels, shorter equilibration time, and lower concentration gradients.

■ **What is the ideal composition of irrigating fluid?**

There is no single ideal dialysis fluid. The ideal fluid for one patient with a particular problem may be unsuitable for another person with a different problem. In general the dialysis fluid should have the following properties:

1. It must permit the maximum diffusion of metabolic waste products or exogenous toxins.
2. It must be capable of correcting the patient's volume abnormalities, for example, volume overload.
3. It should be able to normalize the patient's electrolyte and acid-base abnormalities.

When the purpose of dialysis is merely the elimination of uremic toxins or dialyzable exogenous poisons, dialysis fluid should contain physiologic concentrations of electrolytes and 1.5% glucose. When hyperkalemia is present, a potassium-free dialysate should be used to enhance the elimination of excess potassium. In cases of hypercalcemia or hypermagnesemia, calcium and magnesium ions should be reduced or preferably removed from the dialysate, respectively.

When fluid overload is the major problem, a hypertonic solution containing 4% to 5% glucose should be used. Frequently multiple problems coexist, requiring complex considerations. In fact, as the patient's clinical and biochemical status changes during and/or as a result of dialysis, the composition of fluid may need to be changed and proper adjustments made to meet new physiologic requirements; therefore close follow-up and the frequent clinical and laboratory evaluation of patients undergoing short-term peritoneal dialysis is quite important. Many of the necessary alterations can be made by using different commercially available dialysates of various composition and by the addition of necessary substances to them. However, there have been occasions when a homemade peritoneal dialysate specifically designed for certain patients has been necessary. For instance, almost all the commercial preparations contain lactate and a few of them acetate as the base substance. These organic anions are readily converted to bicarbonate under ordinary circumstances. However, patients with lactic acidosis are not capable of converting lactate. Therefore the use of lactate-base dialysates not only fails to correct the patient's acid-base disturbance, but will even exaggerate it. In such situations I have ordered bicarbonate base dialysate to be made. Because of the pharmacologic incompatibility of calcium and magnesium with bicarbonate (precipitation of calcium and magnesium carbonate), the solution must be free of calcium and magnesium ions. Use of this dialysate has been very successful in improving the patient's acid-base balance, and by careful monitoring of the patient's serum calcium and magnesium levels and the IV infusion as needed of calcium compounds, the development of significant hypocalcemia or hypomagnesemia in these patients has been prevented.

Fructose and sorbitol have been used in place of glucose to generate osmotic forces for the removal of excess fluids. Peritoneal dialysis with solutions containing sorbitol has occasionally caused reversible alterations of mental status, mild liver function test abnormalities, nausea, and vomiting. For this reason the Food and Drug Administration has recently removed these products from U.S. markets; however, 1.4 to 1.8 g sorbitol solutions are still used in other countries. Table 30-1 provides the list and composition of most of the commercially available peritoneal dialysis fluids.

■ **What drugs, if any, are added to dialysis fluid?**

To prevent clotting of the catheter, it is customary to add 500 to 1000 units of *sodium lipoheparin* to each 2 L of dialysis fluid for the first two to four runs. If the drainage fluid remains or turns clear, no more heparin is used in subse-

Table 30-1. Commercially available peritoneal dialysis solutions

Manufacturer	Product	Available sizes (ml)	pH	Components (mEq/L)						
				Na+	K+	Ca++	Mg++	Cl−	Lactate	Acetate
Abbott Laboratories	Inpersol D-1.5-W	1000, 2000	5.2	140.5	0	3.5	1.5	101	44.5	0
	Inpersol D-4.25-W	200		140.5	0	3.5	1.5	101	44.5	0
Cutter Laboratories, Inc.	Peridial 1.5D	1000, 2000	5.4	132	0	3.5	1.5	102	35	0
	Peridial 4.25D	2000	5.4	132	0	3.5	1.5	102	35	0
McGaw Laboratories	Peritoneal dialysis solution with 1.5% dextrose	1000, 2000		140	0	4.0	1.5	100.5	0	45
	Peritoneal dialysis solution with 1.5% dextrose and low sodium	1000, 2000		132	0	3.5	1.5	102	35	0
	Peritoneal dialysis solution with 4.25% dextrose	2000		140	0	4.0	1.5	100.5	0	45
	Peritoneal dialysis solution with 4.25% dextrose and low sodium	2000		132	0	3.5	1.5	102	35	0
Travenol Laboratories	Dianeal with 1.5% dextrose	1000, 2000	5.5	141	0	3.5	1.5	101	45	0
	Dianeal K with 1.5% dextrose	1000	5.5	141	4	3.5	1.5	101	45	0
	Dianeal 137 with 1.5% dextrose	2000	5.5	132	0	3.5	1.5	102	35	0
	Dianeal K-141 with 1.5% dextrose	2000	5.5	132	4	3.5	1.5	106	35	0
	Dianeal with 4.25% dextrose	2000	5.0	141	0	3.5	1.5	101	45	0
	Dianeal 137 with 4.25% dextrose	2000	5.5	132	0	3.5	1.5	102	35	0
	Dianeal K-141 with 4.25% dextrose	2000	5.5	132	4	3.5	1.5	106	35	0

Table 30-2. Intraperitoneal antibiotics

Antibiotic	Dose (mg/L)	Safe blood level ($\mu g/ml$)	Half-life
Ampicillin	50	50-100	Short
Cephalothin (Keflin)	50	50-100	Short
Carbenicillin	200	200	Short
Methicillin	100	100-200	Short
Gentamicin	10	10-12	Long
Kanamycin	10	10-15	Long
Vancomycin	15	15-25	Long
Amphotericin	2.5	2.5	Long

quent passages. However, if the return is blood tinged, heparin use should be continued until the drainage fluid clears.

When the patient has peritonitis or contamination has occurred during the procedure, antibiotics can be mixed with the fluid. Highly effective local and systemic levels of antibiotics are usually achieved by the addition of antibiotics to peritoneal dialysis fluid (Table 30-2).

Most of the peritoneal dialysates are potassium free. To avoid hypokalemia, the patient's plasma potassium levels should be carefully monitored. When the plasma potassium level is normal or subnormal, 2 to 4 mEq of potassium chloride can be added to each liter of dialysate to maintain a normal potassium balance.

Isoproterenol (Isuprel) can be added to the dialysis fluid to improve the efficiency of dialysis. This improvement is the result of increased peritoneal blood flow and vasodilatation induced by the drug. Sodium nitroprusside has been recently tried successfully to increase peritoneal dialysis.

Albumin has been added to dialysates in order to enhance the removal of protein-bound substances such as salicylates. This is quite costly and should be used only in cases of severe intoxication.

Dialysis with cottonseed oil has been used in the treatment of patients with glutethimide overdose and intoxication with other lipid-soluble agents. This procedure carries with it the risk of fat embolism and is quite messy.

Peritoneal dialysis with fluids containing tromethamine (THAM) has been used in the treatment of patients with barbiturate overdose.

THAM is an organic base that can bind weak acids and their salts. Therefore its addition to peritoneal dialysis fluids enhances the elimination of barbiturates from the circulation. Because of its affinity for weak acids, it can lower the Pco_2 in the blood, which is transient and clinically unimportant. Its absorption from the peritoneum is quite slow, which is a point in favor of its use.

■ **What are the causes of poor drainage and dialysis fluid retention, and what can be done to correct them?**

A mild to moderate positive balance is commonly seen with the first few exchanges of peritoneal dialysis. This is caused by pooling of small amounts of fluid in parts of the peritoneal cavity that are not readily drained by the catheter when the catheter tip is not located in the most dependent part of the small pelvis. This should not cause any undue anxiety, since with subsequent passes the balance becomes progressively negative. However, if the drainage stops or slows down while significant amounts of fluid are still in the abdomen, this may indicate that the catheter tip is buried in the omentum. By applying mild pressure to the lower abdomen on both sides, elevating the head of the bed, rotating the patient or carefully repositioning the catheter, the drainage can usually be improved and the retention eliminated. If all these measures fail, the catheter should be removed and examined for clots in the lumen. Sometimes catheter malfunction is caused by peritonitis, ileus, or constipation. The other cause of drainage problems is malplacement of the catheter outside the peritoneum, that is, within the adipose tissue of the abdominal wall or retroperitoneal space. This is occasionally encountered when the procedure is performed by an inexperienced person on an obese patient and calls for the removal of the catheter and its proper replacement.

■ **Does the body absorb the glucose content of the peritoneal dialysate?**

The concentration of glucose in peritoneal dialysis fluids is much higher than in plasma. This concentration gradient results in the diffusion of glucose from the peritoneal cavity to circulating blood. At a dialyzed volume of 2.5 L/hr a total of 300 to 750 g of glucose may be absorbed per day, which provides a large quantity of calories. In nondiabetic patients the blood sugar level can rise to as high as 300 mg/100 ml. Although this may not create any major problems in nondiabetic patients, it can produce significant difficulties in diabetic patients. Therefore blood sugar levels should be carefully monitored and the insulin dose adjusted in diabetic patients.

■ **Is ultrafiltration possible using peritoneal dialysis, and if so, how?**

In contrast to hemodialysis, the control of hydrostatic forces for the purpose of ultrafiltration is not possible in peritoneal dialysis. However, *osmotic forces can be used very effectively*. By adding high concentrations of glucose, fructose, or sorbitol to the dialysate, it can be made hypertonic (2.5% to 4% glucose or 1.5% to 1.8% sorbitol). This hypertonicity results in the movement of water from intravascular to peritoneal spaces and in the removal of large quantities of water. For the purpose of effective ultrafiltration *shorter transit times* (10 to 20 minutes) are desirable. With prolonged dwell times increasing amounts of osmotic agent are absorbed into the circulation, which not only limits the effective ultrafiltration but can also create serious complications.

■ **What are the indications for short-term peritoneal dialysis?**

Under most circumstances peritoneal and hemodialysis can be utilized interchangeably. The choice between the two is usually made on medical grounds. However, simplicity of the technique, possibility of rapid initiation, independence from the surgical team to provide vascular access, freedom from complicated space-occupying machinery, and lack of the need for specially trained personnel tend to favor the choice of peritoneal dialysis over hemodialysis.

In some patients peritoneal dialysis is superior to hemodialysis. Patients who need only one or two dialyses may be better managed by peritoneal dialysis. For example, when dialysis is needed to treat severe intractable congestive heart failure, significant amounts of fluid can be removed by peritoneal dialysis over 1 to 2 days. Furthermore,

acute hemodynamic changes that may occur with hemodialysis and can cause cardiovascular complications are avoided.

Intoxication with drugs that have low circulating levels and high tissue- and protein-binding capacities will respond to peritoneal dialysis, which is a slow and prolonged process, more readily than to hemodialysis. Drugs such as phenytoin (Dilantin) and glutethimide fall into this category.

In situations where anticoagulation is contraindicated, for instance, in patients with internal bleeding, cerebral trauma, or hemorrhage and following neurosurgical procedures or hemorrhagic pericarditis, peritoneal dialysis is safer than hemodialysis.

In very young children, elderly patients, and those with severe cardiovascular diseases or shock, peritoneal dialysis is preferable.

Because of its lower risk of intermittent bacteremia, hypotension, and bleeding caused by heparinization, peritoneal dialysis is probably superior to hemodialysis following open-heart surgery, particularly prosthetic valve replacement.

Patients with acute renal failure after various major abdominal or transabdominal retroperitoneal surgeries have undergone peritoneal dialysis with satisfactory results. Therefore recent abdominal surgery does not seem to be a contraindication to peritoneal dialysis. However, in the presence of fresh wounds and multiple drains it may be quite a messy procedure. It should be noted that many postoperative patients have ileus, which renders catheter insertion somewhat difficult, and also atelectasis, which predisposes to pulmonary infections. These patients should be treated with intermittent positive pressure breathing (IPPB) and pulmonary toilet. In addition, the volume of their peritoneal dialysis exchanges should be reduced to avoid further compression and atelectasis of the lung tissue. The general indications for short-term peritoneal dialysis are as follows:

1. Acute renal failure
2. Reversible deterioration of chronic renal failure
3. Various intoxications
4. Severe fluid overload refractory to other therapeutic means

5. Acid-base disturbances

6. Major electrolyte and some metabolic disturbances

7. In awaiting the maturation of arteriovenous fistula and the initiation of chronic hemodialysis

8. In treatment of peritonitis by adding antibiotics to dialysis fluids

Beneficial results have been reported with peritoneal dialysis in acute hemorrhagic pancreatitis. The improvement has been attributed to the removal of vasoactive substances released from necrotic pancreatic and other tissues.

■ Are there any contraindications to the use of peritoneal dialysis?

There are no absolute contraindications to peritoneal dialysis, especially if the risk of hemodialysis is higher than that associated with peritoneal dialysis. The following list enumerates those conditions in which peritoneal dialysis may be associated with a high incidence of various complications:

1. In the presence of diffuse skin infection or cellulitis of the abdominal wall the catheter can transport the pathogenic organisms to the peritoneal cavity and cause peritonitis.

2. Diffuse intra-abdominal malignancy and previous peritonitis are associated with a higher risk of viscus perforation. This is also true in cases involving small children and cachectic individuals. Under these circumstances prior infusion of some dialysate into the peritoneal cavity through a 15-gauge, 10 cm long needle to distend the abdomen followed by aspiration of fluid from the projected site of catheter insertion ensures free access to the peritoneal cavity and reduces the risk. Surgical insertion of the catheter under direct vision is the other alternative.

3. With severe bleeding diathesis, the correction of the hemostatic abnormality, if possible, prior to catheter placement is ideal. If it is not possible, surgical placement of the catheter under direct vision may be the procedure of choice.

4. Peritoneal catheter insertion in patients with ileus is associated with an increased risk of viscus perforation, drainage difficulty, and poor clearance. Furthermore, severe bowel distention may preclude the use of adequate exchange volumes.

5. The presence of abdominal drains may result in a leakage of the fluids and peritoneal infection.

6. In the presence of diaphragmatic gaps the dialysate may find its way up to the thoracic cavity and embarrass pulmonary function. By placing the patient in a sitting or semisitting position, the difficulty may be eliminated.

7. Preexisting asymptomatic hernias may enlarge or become symptomatic as a result of peritoneal dialysis. This is caused by the increased intraperitoneal tension generated by large volumes of fluid. It can be prevented by avoiding abdominal overdistention and by the use of local supportive devices.

8. The inability to maintain adequate dietary intake is a definite contraindication to long-term peritoneal dialysis. This is because of the significant obligatory protein loss with peritoneal dialysis that results in a depletion syndrome if the dietary intake is insufficient.

■ Can peritoneal dialysis be performed in the presence of acute peritonitis?

The answer is definitely yes. In fact, by combining the systemic and local antibiotic therapy, faster and more complete recovery of peritonitis can be accomplished. It is important to mention that the degree of protein loss with peritoneal dialysis is much greater in patients with peritonitis than those without peritonitis. It could be as much as 60 g or more daily.

■ How does peritoneal dialysis compare with hemodialysis, and what are the major differences, advantages, and disadvantages?

1. The surface area of the artificial kidney is variable, depending on the choice of dialyzer. The surface area of the adult peritoneum is fixed at about 1.8 m² (almost equal to skin surface).

2. The permeability characteristics of the membranes are different. The peritoneal membrane is much more permeable, allowing the passage of larger molecules, in contrast to artificial kidney membranes that have limited permeabilities.

3. Blood flow, hydrostatic pressure, and dialysate flow rate can be easily regulated in hemodialysis by means of the various pumps and

clamps, whereas only dialysate flow can be altered in peritoneal dialysis.

4. Hemodialysis baths are always isosmolar, and ultrafiltration is achieved by manipulation of the hydrostatic forces. In the case of peritoneal dialysis, hydrostatic forces are almost constant, but osmotic forces are variable.

5. With hemodialysis the clearance of small molecules is several times higher than in peritoneal dialysis. This results in a rapid correction of extracellular fluid biochemical abnormalities, which may cause disequilibrium syndrome. Because of the slowness of biochemical changes in peritoneal dialysis, disequilibrium syndrome is practically nonexistent.

6. In hemodialysis abrupt changes of blood volume caused by extracorporeal circulation may result in hypotension at the onset of the treatment or during ultrafiltration, and mild congestive heart failure at the end on return of the blood, which suddenly increases the load on a borderline compensated heart.

7. With peritoneal dialysis it is easy to change the composition of dialysate as the patient's laboratory findings and state of hydration change. This is more difficult in the case of hemodialysis because of the rapidity of the patient's biochemical changes and the large volume of dialysis fluids.

8. Because of its relatively low clearance rates, peritoneal dialysis may not be an adequate treatment for hypercatabolic patients in whom tremendous amounts of waste products are generated. Under these circumstances the use of long and frequent hemodialysis treatments with or without peritoneal dialysis is advisable.

9. Hemodialysis is more efficient in the rapid correction of severe fluid overload and pulmonary edema. The same is true in the case of severe hyperkalemia and other electrolyte abnormalities.

10. Peritoneal dialysis is associated with a loss of 20 to 80 g of protein daily.

11. The longer duration of peritoneal dialysis and the maintenance of the same position in bed is frequently tiresome.

12. The consequences of the absorption of large amounts of glucose with peritoneal dialysis has been discussed.

13. Peritoneal dialysate should be sterile. This is not a requirement for hemodialysis fluids, since bacteria cannot pass through hemodialysis membranes.

14. There is no need for systemic or regional heparinization during peritoneal dialysis. This is an absolute necessity in the case of hemodialysis; therefore peritoneal dialysis may be the procedure of choice in patients who should not be treated with anticoagulants.

15. There is no need for a vascular access in peritoneal dialysis and no risk of air embolism, clotting, rupture of the dialyzer, or many other complications that are associated with hemodialysis.

BIBLIOGRAPHY

Andersson, G., et al.: Glucose absorption from the dialysis fluid during peritoneal dialysis, Scand. J. Urol. Nephrol. **5:**77, 1971.

Baran, H., et al.: Kinetics of protein loss during peritoneal dialyses, Pol. Med. J. **11:**277, 1972.

Boen, S. T.: Kinetics of peritoneal dialysis, Medicine **40:**243, 1961.

Brewer, T. E., et al.: Indwelling peritoneal (Tenckhoff) dialysis catheter. Experience with 24 patients, J.A.M.A. **219:**1011, 1972.

Deger, G. E., and Wagoner, R. D.: Peritoneal dialysis in acute uric acid nephropathy, Mayo Clin. Proc. **47:**189, 1972.

De Santo, N. G., et al.: Haematoma of rectus abdominis associated with dialysis, Br. Med. J. **3:**281, 1972.

Edwards, D. H., Gardner, R. D., and Williams, D. G.: Rupture of a hernial sac: a complication of peritoneal dialysis, J. Urol. **108:**255, 1972.

Gault, M. H.: Peritoneal solutions, Can. Med. Assoc. J. **108:**325, 1973.

Greenblatt, D. J.: Fatal hypoglycaemia occurring after peritoneal dialysis, Br. Med. J. **2:**270, 1972.

Henderson, L. W.: Peritoneal ultrafiltration dialysis: enhances urea transfer using hypertonic peritoneal dialysis fluid, J. Clin. Invest. **45:**950, 1966.

Holm, J., Lied En, B., and Lindqvist, B.: Unilateral pleural effusion—a rare complication of peritoneal dialysis, Scand. J. Urol. Nephrol. **5:**84, 1971.

Kahn, S. I., Garella, S., and Chazan, J. A.: Nonsurgical treatment of intestinal perforation due to peritoneal dialysis, Surg. Gynecol. Obstet. **136:**40, 1973.

Kessler, J.: Peritoneal dialysis and dialysate volumes, N. Engl. J. Med. **286:**110, 1972.

Mattocks, A. M., and El-Bassiouni, E. A.: Peritoneal dialysis: a review, J. Pharm. Sci. **60:**1767, 1971.

Maxwell, M. H., et al.: Peritoneal dialysis. I. Technique and applications, J.A.M.A. **170:**916, 1959.

Pirpasopoulos, M., et al.: A cost-effectiveness study of dwell times in peritoneal dialysis, Lancet **2:**1135, 1972.

Rae, A., and Pendray, M.: The advantages of peritoneal dialysis in chronic renal failure, J.A.M.A. **225:**937, 1973.

Raja, R. M., et al.: Hyperosmotic coma complicating peritoneal dialysis with sorbitol dialysate, Ann. Intern. Med. **73:**993, 1970.

Rosato, E. E., et al.: Peritoneal lavage treatment of experimental pancreatitis, J. Surg. Res. **12:**138, 1972.

Scurrell, A. M.: Peritoneal dialysis—a five-year evaluation, Nurs. Times **69:**929, 1973.

Sharma, B. K., et al.: Peritoneal dialysis in resistant congestive heart failure and pulmonary oedema, J. Indian Med. Assoc. **58:**159, 1972.

Sheppard, J. M., et al.: Lactic acidosis: recovery associated with use of peritoneal dialysis, Aust. N.Z. J. Med. **2:**389, 1972.

Stoltz, M. L., Nolph, K. D., and Maher, J. F.: Factors affecting calcium removal with calcium-free peritoneal dialysis, J. Lab. Clin. Med. **78:**389, 1971.

Vaziri, N. D., et al.: Bicarbonate-buffered peritoneal dialysis—an effective adjunct in the treatment of lactic acidosis, Am. J. Med. **67:**392, 1979.

Vidt, D. G.: Recommendations on choice of peritoneal dialysis solutions, Ann. Intern. Med. **78:**144, 1973.

Wardle, E. N.: Simple method for detection of infection of peritoneum during dialysis, Br. Med. J. **2:**518, 1973.

CHAPTER 31

Maintenance peritoneal dialysis

N. D. Vaziri

During recent years long-term peritoneal dialysis has become a valuable alternative to maintenance hemodialysis in the management of patients with end-stage renal failure. The high risk of peritonitis, the need for repeated painful insertions of peritoneal catheters, and the high cost of dialysis fluids were among the factors limiting the utilization of peritoneal dialysis on a long-term basis in the past.

With the advent of implantable peritoneal catheters, automated dialysis machines, and improved aseptic techniques, home and in-center long-term peritoneal dialysis procedures are gaining increased popularity among physicians and patients. The implanted catheter provides a long-term access to the peritoneal cavity, thereby eliminating the need for the painful reinsertion of the catheter with each dialysis and reducing the risk of infection.

The catheters (Tenckhoff catheters) are made of Silastic, which is soft, pliable, quite compatible with peritoneal membrane, and therefore nonirritating. The part of the catheter that lies in the wall of the abdomen is equipped with one or two Teflon cuffs. Fibroblasts grow into the Teflon cuffs providing satisfactory fixation of the catheter to the abdominal wall and a reliable barrier against bacterial penetration of the peritoneal space.

Automated machines provide unlimited amounts of sterile pyrogen-free dialysate by mixing a sugar-electrolyte concentrate with water. Pure pyrogen-free sterile water is produced in the machine from tap water by several processes, including reverse osmosis, heating, and filtration through several membranes and cartridges. Therefore the problem of handling large volumes of expensive premade dialysates and its tremendous financial impact has been resolved.

A predetermined volume of dialysate is delivered and drainage disposed of intermittently through a closed system. The dialysate temperature, inflow, outflow, and dwell times are automatically regulated.

In contrast to hemodialysis, peritoneal dialysis is a slow and smooth process, and sudden hemodynamic changes requiring close attention and immediate action are not expected.

The procedure can be started by an unattended, trained patient at home, proceed during sleep, and be terminated in the morning. As a result, daytime activity will not be compromised, since all the required 30 to 40 hours of dialysis per week can be done at night.

The number of institutions providing maintenance in-center and home peritoneal dialysis programs is rapidly growing, and the cost of operation is becoming competitive with hemodialysis. In the near future we will undoubtedly witness the universal expansion of this technique with a lower cost of operation.

■ **What are the causes of failure of the indwelling catheter to drain properly, and how may they be diagnosed and managed?**

Failure of the indwelling catheter to drain properly may be caused by one of the following problems:

1. Malposition of the catheter. This usually results from omental entanglement during implan-

tation of the catheter. It should be suspected when the catheter malfunction occurs during the early postimplantation period. Upper or midabdominal pains are frequently observed when suctioning is applied. The pain is caused by traction of the omentum with suctioning. The diagnosis is confirmed by abdominal x-ray studies following injection of 3 to 5 ml of contrast medium (Renografin). It is corrected by repositioning of the catheter.

2. Internal obstruction. This is usually caused by tissues sucked into the catheter lumen through its side perforations. It is more commonly seen in children and is more likely to occur when the side perforations are large. The diagnosis is confirmed by injection of radiopaque dye into the catheter under an image intensifier. An attempt should be made to remove the incarcerated tissue fragments and reposition the catheter. If this fails to solve the problem, a new catheter should be placed.

3. Obstruction caused by peritoneal infections. This is usually associated with asymptomatic or mild or recurrent infections and may be a sequela of a healed infection. The development of pain with rapid infusion of dialysate suggests the diagnosis. Anatomic confirmation can be achieved by x-ray study of the abdomen following injection of 10 to 20 ml of radiopaque dye into the catheter. The study will show poor diffusion of the dye throughout the abdomen and perhaps encasement of the catheter by surrounding tissues. Catheter replacement followed by 3 to 4 weeks of intraperitoneal and systemic antibiotic therapy will solve the problem.

4. Constipation. Constipation is one of the causes of functional and reversible catheter obstruction. A history of constipation, negative x-ray studies, and improvement following the use of purgatives suggest the diagnosis. Measures that improve bowel function will correct catheter malfunction.

■ What are the primary indications for maintenance peritoneal dialysis?

There are certain groups of patients who do not tolerate hemodialysis treatment well and may be better treated with long-term peritoneal dialysis. These include the following:

1. Young children. Although providing vascular access and performing hemodialysis is possible even in infants, the procedure is difficult and the access is hard to maintain. Furthermore, hemodialysis is psychologically much more traumatic than painless peritoneal irrigation through an implanted catheter during sleeping hours at home, which allows full-time school attendance and liberal activities. Early renal transplantation is the other alternative. However, because of the accompanying long-term steroid therapy, children undergoing transplantation usually grow and mature very poorly. For this reason it is advisable to defer transplantation to a later time when reasonable growth and maturation have occurred. This classic concept has been recently challenged. In the interim these patients should be maintained on dialysis and a high protein calorie diet.

2. Elderly patients. The elderly, particularly those persons over 60 years of age with major cardiovascular disorders, are good candidates for maintenance peritoneal dialysis. Providing and maintaining functional vascular access is frequently difficult in these patients because of prevalent atherosclerotic peripheral vascular disease. In addition, these patients are frequently sensitive to the sudden hemodynamic changes and rapid alterations of the biochemical composition of internal milieu imposed by hemodialysis. For these reason they react more favorably to maintenance peritoneal dialysis.

3. Patients with severe cardiovascular disease and instability. These persons are better candidates for peritoneal dialysis regardless of age.

4. Patients with contraindications to systemic or regional heparinization. These patients may have to use peritoneal dialysis. Recurrent bleeding peptic ulcer disease, dissecting aneurysms, or hypersensitivity to various heparin preparations are a few examples of the disorders affecting these persons.

5. Patients who lack reliable vascular access routes for hemodialysis. The number of suitable vessels for creation of vascular access and the survival of each vascular access route are limited. Consequently, with passage of time hemodialysis patients, particularly *diabetic* patients, run out of reliable vascular access routes. This

has always been a frustrating experience for those practitioners who deal with patients on long-term hemodialysis. However, with the advent and perfection of the maintenance peritoneal dialysis technique, lack of vascular access is no longer a hopeless situation.

6. Patients who require home dialysis but who live alone. For reasons of safety and simplicity unattended persons are quite capable of performing peritoneal dialysis with automated machines. This is not true with hemodialysis, in which life-threatening complications can occur at any minute during the procedure.

7. Patients who exhibit an inability to learn hemodialysis techniques. Self-hemodialysis techniques are more complicated than peritoneal dialysis techniques. In addition, the cannulation of arteriovenous fistulas and various grafts is quite painful. Home dialysis candidates who cannot or refuse to learn hemodialysis techniques should be considered for a maintenance home peritoneal dialysis program.

8. Patients who refuse transfusions because of ethnic beliefs. These persons should not undergo hemodialysis, since major blood loss or hemolysis necessitating transfusion is among the more common complications of hemodialysis. Peritoneal dialysis is the proper choice in these patients.

9. Hemodialysis and renal transplant candidates awaiting fistula maturation or transplantation surgery. These patients can be treated with peritoneal dialysis in the interim period.

■ **How are fluid retention and hypertension controlled in patients on maintenance peritoneal dialysis?**

Fluid and sodium intakes should be restricted in these patients. In addition, the osmolality of the dialysate should be adjusted by changing the dialysate glucose concentration so that fluids retained between dialyses can be removed. A 1.5% glucose dialysate usually does not remove any fluids; 2% to 2.5% solutions are suitable for most patients.

Hypertension may remain a problem despite control of extracellular fluid volume, requiring antihypertensive drugs or even bilateral nephrectomy.

■ **What are the complications of peritoneal dialysis?**

The complications of peritoneal dialysis can be divided into four categories: those related to insertion of the catheter, those caused by infection, metabolic complications, and miscellaneous complications.

Complications directly related to insertion of catheter

Intestinal perforation. Intestinal perforation is likely to occur when too much force is exerted to penetrate the peritoneum. Patients with ileus, diffuse intra-abdominal carcinomas, adhesions, previous peritonitis, and large uteruses are more prone to this complication. Surgical intervention may be necessary in such circumstances. However, according to a recent report, several patients with intestinal perforation subsequent to peritoneal catheter insertion have been treated conservatively with antibiotics and supportive measures with good results.

Bladder perforation. Perforation of the bladder has been reported in patients with urinary retention and distended bladder. For this reason it is mandatory to empty the bladder before attempting to insert the peritoneal catheter.

Intraperitoneal bleeding. Rupture of small abdominal wall vessels is not an uncommon complication. It is characterized by bloody fluid return that should clear readily. The addition of 5 mg heparin to each liter of dialysate is helpful to prevent obstruction of the catheter by blood clots. Heparin can be discontinued after the fluid turns clear. Large vessel injury is very unlikely; however, rapid development of shock and heavy bloody return should suggest this possibility or, alternatively, rupture of one of the solid organs. A mild bloody return may be indicative of peritoneal infection or neoplasm. It is occasionally seen during the first few days of the menstrual period even in the absence of endometriosis.

Hematoma of the abdominal rectus muscle and retroperitoneal penetrations are occasionally encountered.

Complications caused by infections

Peritonitis. Peritonitis is one of the major complications of peritoneal dialysis. Although it is frequently caused by infection, aseptic peritonitis is encountered with some frequency.

STERILE PERITONITIS. Sterile peritonitis is an aseptic inflammation caused by low dialysate pH, its marked hypertonicity and chemical impurities, and the presence of blood or pyrogens in the fluid. It is associated with symptoms of peritoneal irritation and an increased number of white cells in the drainage fluid. White cell counts in the fluid may be as high as 50 cells/mm³ or more, and this makes the fluid turbid. Sterile peritonitis can result in adhesion formation and peritoneal fibrosis.

INFECTIOUS PERITONITIS. Although some investigators have speculated that the infectious organisms originate from the bowel as a result of catheterization-induced lacerations, the most likely possibility is that the organisms are carried through the skin to the peritoneum by the catheter. It is important to realize that symptoms of peritonitis in these patients are frequently very mild or nonexisting. A high index of suspicion is necessary to make the diagnosis in early stages.

Late obstruction of the catheter that fails to correct with the irrigation may be the first sign of peritonitis. A low-grade fever, reduced appetite, weakness, or malaise are sometimes present. Mild abdominal discomfort and slight rebound tenderness or a blood-tinged fluid return may be the presenting signs.

Infected catheter exit or *subcutaneous catheter tract* should raise suspicion. With gram-negative infections a full-blown sepsis may develop. *By far the most common finding is turbidity of the drainage fluid. White blood cell count in the fluid frequently exceeds 300 to 500 cells/mm³.*

The Gram stain may confirm the presence of bacteria in the peritoneal fluid. Cultures and sensitivity tests should be done and treatment started immediately. The choice of antibiotic is dependent on the findings of a Gram-stained smear. Appropriate changes can be made later when the results of the culture and sensitivity testing become available, or if peritonitis fails to respond in 24 to 48 hours.

Treatment includes the addition of appropriate antibiotics and heparin to the irrigation fluid, which provides effective local and systemic antibiotic concentrations and prevents obstruction of

the catheter by fibrin clots. Unless the patient is markedly septic, there is no need for the administration of antibiotics through other routes. Small exchange volumes are used to reduce discomfort, and irrigation is carried on continuously for 3 to 4 days, by which time the infection should have cleared. Every-other-day dialysis with heparin and antibiotic-containing fluid is then carried on for 3 weeks more. If the biologic half-life of the antibiotic used is short (for example, cephalosporins), oral or parenteral administration will be indicated to maintain optimum plasma and tissue levels on the days off dialysis. Failure to respond to therapy or recurrence of infection may call for removal of the old catheter and placement of a new one in a different site.

Daily fluid culture and sensitivity tests are mandatory during treatment, since resistant organisms may emerge and new organisms superimpose, requiring a change in strategy. Delayed or inadequate treatment of peritonitis results in adhesion formation and peritoneal fibrosis that will complicate future catheterizations and markedly reduce the peritoneal dialysis clearances to the extent that peritoneal dialysis may have to be abandoned. Furthermore, protein losses with peritoneal dialysis increase tremendously in the presence of peritonitis, reaching levels as high as 60 to 80 g/day. Recommended intraperitoneal antibiotics and their doses are given in Table 30-2 (p. 519).

Since *Staphylococcus aureus* is one of the major causes of peritonitis in these patients, cephalothin may be a good starting drug while awaiting the results of the culture and sensitivity tests.

Loading doses of gentamicin, vancomycin, and kanamycin should be given parenterally prior to the initiation of their peritoneal administration.

Metabolic complications

Protein amino acid and vitamin losses. As discussed earlier, protein loss with dialysis fluid is a problem in long-term peritoneal dialysis patients. Under ordinary circumstances the loss is 10 to 20 g/dialysis, which amounts to 30 to 60 g/week. When peritonitis is present, losses can increase five to ten times. Although amino acid and vitamin losses have not been investigated thoroughly yet, their losses should be similarly significant.

Even calorie malnutrition may occur despite the absorption of large quantities of glucose from the bath. To avoid protein and vitamin depletion, a high protein diet with multiple vitamins and 2 to 4 mg/day of folic acid should be prescribed. If the patient is catabolic, parenteral hyperalimentation may be necessary. Patients who cannot maintain a good protein intake should not be treated with peritoneal dialysis; hemodialysis may be a better choice.

Consequences of glucose absorption. For obvious reasons a high glucose concentration in the peritoneal dialysate results in the absorption of large quantities of glucose into the circulation. This may be beneficial to patients with calorie malnutrition. In other patients it can cause obesity, hyperlipidemia (type IV), and hyperglycemia that may even require small doses of regular insulin (blood sugar levels more than 400 mg/L) for its control. In diabetic patients the insulin dose should be adjusted before their discharge to a home dialysis program.

Hyperosmolar coma caused by the preferential movement of water across the peritoneal membrane against a high osmotic gradient was discussed earlier. It is not uncommon with acute peritoneal dialysis, but because of the stability of the patients and the interrupted nature of the treatment (every other day), hyperosmolar coma is very rare in patients on long-term peritoneal dialysis, since the resultant mild hyperosmolar states are corrected by ingestion of free water and endogenous water production.

Electrolyte disturbances

HYPOKALEMIA. Patients dialyzed against zero or very low potassium dialysates may develop hypokalemia, which can cause weakness, ileus, and cardiac arrhythmias. This could be quite dangerous in patients receiving digitalis preparations.

HYPOCALCEMIA. Hypocalcemia may develop when a low calcium bath is used.

HYPERNATREMIA. Because of the excess loss of free water, hypernatremia may occur. This was discussed earlier.

Hypoglycemia. A hypoglycemia attack can occur following the termination of peritoneal dialysis. This is frequently seen when dialysates with high glucose concentrations are used. The pathogenesis of this hypoglycemia is as follows: Because of its high concentration in dialysis fluid, glucose is absorbed in large quantities during dialysis. This raises the levels of plasma glucose, which, in turn, stimulates insulin secretion by the pancreas. With the termination of dialysis, the influx of glucose to the circulation ceases immediately, but because of its long half-life, the insulin level remains elevated for several hours. During this period of time recurrent endogenous insulin reactions can occur. This reaction is self-limited and is treated with IV infusion of glucose and oral carbohydrates, just as reactions caused by exogenous insulin are treated. The development of palpitation, diaphoresis, agitation, confusion, coma, convulsion, and so on after peritoneal dialysis should suggest the diagnosis, and prompt treatment of hypoglycemia should be started. Failure to treat hypoglycemia may result in permanent brain damage.

Miscellaneous complications

Ascites formation. Some patients develop progressive and recurrent ascites during the interdialysis intervals, following the discontinuation of peritoneal dialysis, after renal transplantation, or when switching to hemodialysis programs. The reason for this phenomenon is not clear. However, it seems to be related to the prolonged use of low pH and hypertonic dialysates, which is believed to cause aseptic inflammation of the peritoneal membranes. The fluid is quite rich in protein and relatively cell free. At times the rate of its accumulation is such that unless it is regularly drained, it can cause respiratory embarrassment. In these cases, if the catheter is not infected, it should be left in place for some time to drain the fluid, hoping that it will clear spontaneously.

Pleural effusion. Pleural effusion in patients with chronic renal failure may be caused by fluid retention and congestive heart failure. Acute massive effusion following peritoneal dialysis, however, is probably caused by a shift of the intra-abdominal fluid to the thoracic cage through a preexisting or evolving diaphragmatic defect.

Abdominal pain. Peritoneal dialysis through the indwelling Silastic catheter should be painless. The presence of pain may be caused by one or a combination of the followed conditions:

1. Peritonitis (as previously discussed)
2. Adhesions around catheter
3. Low dialysate pH (less than 5.5)
4. Free air within the peritoneal cavity as a result of inadequate deaeration of fluid by the machine or inadvertent infusion of air into the peritoneal cavity and characterized by pain in the shoulders and interscapular area following assumption of an upright position; can be corrected by assuming Trendelenburg or knee-chest position to let the air out through the catheter
5. Unrelated disorders such as appendicitis, peptic ulcer disease, and gaseous distention of intestines

CONTINUOUS AMBULATORY PERITONEAL DIALYSIS

Continuous ambulatory peritoneal dialysis (CAPD) was first introduced by Popovich and his associates[1,2] in 1976 as a modality in the treatment of chronic renal failure. Since that time, several other reports have been published by the same group as well as other investigators. In this system, peritoneal dialysis fluid is continuously present in the peritoneal cavity except for brief periods of drainage of the old fluid and instillation of the fresh solution five times a day. Indwelling peritoneal catheters similar to those used in maintenance peritoneal dialysis are used to provide access to the peritoneal space. After each drainage and instillation of fresh fluid, the patient is disconnected from the tubing and the indwelling catheter is capped. The patient is then free to resume his or her normal daily activities while internal dialysis is in progress. The procedure is carried out every day and represents a continuous portable dialysis system. In contrast to conventional intermittent dialytic treatments, the long periods of confinement and relative immobility and marked fluctuations of body fluid volumes and composition are totally avoided with CAPD.

■ How is CAPD performed?

Indwelling Tenckhoff peritoneal catheters should be placed in all patients. Between the periods of fluid drainage and instillation, the external end of the catheter is capped and held close to the skin by a dressing and supportive gauze belt.

The drainage and instillation are performed five times a day between 7 AM and 11 PM, 3 to 4 hours apart, using conventional potassium-free peritoneal dialysis fluids. After drainage of the old fluid, 2 L of fresh fluid (in adults) are instilled into the peritoneal cavity. Needless to say, the fluid should be warmed to 37° C before instillation; however, some patients have used fluids at ambient temperature without difficulty. The instillation and drainage occur by gravity and on the average take 10 to 20 minutes, respectively. Aseptic measures should be observed meticulously throughout the procedure to avoid peritonitis. An accurate account of inflow and outflow volumes should be kept, and daily body weight should be recorded by the patient. In case of significant weight gain (fluid retention) and development of edema, dialysate containing 4.5% glucose could be used once or twice a day to remove excess fluids. The remaining exchanges should be carried out using 1.5% dextrose solution.

■ Does CAPD provide acceptable control of biochemical and clinical abnormalities?

CAPD represents an effective ambulatory internal dialysis since it provides acceptable control of azotemia and salt and water balance in patients with end-stage renal failure. The clearance of small molecules by CAPD approaches the dialysate flow rate and compares well with other dialytic techniques on a weekly basis. The weekly clearance of larger solutes in this system is six times greater than with hemodialysis.

Limited experience has shown more satisfactory control of hypertension in patients undergoing CAPD as compared to other dialytic modalities. This is probably due to better control of fluid overload. Improvement in the sense of well-being, energy, and appetite, as well as in daily activities and overall productivity, has been reported following institution of CAPD.

■ What are the desirable features of CAPD?

CAPD has several advantages including the following:

1. Achievement of continuous steady state chemistries

2. Requires short home training period
3. Can be done by the patient alone and practically anywhere
4. Provides internal dialysis, compatible with unlimited mobility
5. Requires no electricity, running water, or complicated equipment
6. Is performed without anticoagulation or blood access
7. Does not cause blood loss or significant hemodynamic stress
8. Requires minimal dietary restriction and is potentially less expensive than other dialytic modalities; no major initial investment necessary
9. Provides better clearance for larger molecules per week as compared to hemodialysis
10. Prolongs catheter life because of the daily use

■ **What are the disadvantages of CAPD?**

Undesirable features of CAPD include:
1. High incidence of peritonitis (has occurred every 10 weeks in a series of patients undergoing CAPD); usually responds to therapy promptly
2. Significant protein loss ranging from 10 to 20 g/day
3. Lower weekly urea clearance (60% of the hemodialysis clearance rate)
4. High cost of premade dialysate and difficulty with the shipments and storage of monthly supply of dialysates
5. Possible depletion of important large molecular substances

■ **Is there any way to reduce the incidence of peritonitis with CAPD?**

Subsequent to the original reports by Popovich and co-workers[1,2] in which glass containers were used, Oreopoulos and associates[3] introduced a new technique that made CAPD much easier and safer. Instead of 2 L bottles, they used 2 L collapsible plastic bags with short connecting tubes that are readily attached to the peritoneal catheter. Following inflow, the bag is left attached to the connection tube and is carried while rolled up in a cloth waist purse under the clothing. At the end of the exchange the same bag is used to drain the old fluid, after which it is removed and replaced by a new one. This technique has resulted in a dramatic reduction of the incidence of peritonitis to one episode every 10.5 patient months. This is still higher than the incidence of peritonitis with maintenance intermittent peritoneal dialysis using an automated delivery system at home (one episode every 18 patient months). Therefore further improvement is needed to make the procedure as safe as maintenance intermittent peritoneal dialysis with automated systems.

REFERENCES

1. Popovich, R. P., et al.: The definition of a novel portable wearable equilibrium peritoneal dialysis technique, Trans. Am. Soc. Artif. Intern. Organs **5**:64, 1976.
2. Popovich, R. P., et al.: Continuous ambulatory peritoneal dialysis, Ann. Intern. Med. **88**:449, 1978.
3. Oreopoulos, D. G., and Robson, M.: Ambulatory dialysis, Ann. Intern. Med. **89**:147, 1978.

BIBLIOGRAPHY

Baillod, R. A., et al.: Home dialysis in children and adolescents, Proc. Eur. Dialysis Transplant. Assoc. **9**:335, 1972.
Berlyne, G. M., et al.: Amino acid loss in peritoneal dialysis, Lancet **1**:1339, 1967.
Blumenkrantz, M.: Maintenance peritoneal dialysis as an alternative for the patient with end-stage renal failure, Clin. Dig. **6**:1, 1977.
Boen, S. T.: Kinetics of peritoneal dialysis, Medicine **40**:243, 1961.
Boyer, J., et al.: Hyperglycemia and hyperosmolality complicating peritoneal dialysis, Ann. Intern. Med. **67**:568, 1967.
Crossley, K., et al.: Intraperitoneal insulin for control of blood sugar in diabetic patients during peritoneal dialysis, Br. Med. J. **1**:269, 1971.
Edwards, S. R., and Unger, A. M.: Acute hydrothorax, a new complication of peritoneal dialysis, J.A.M.A. **199**:853, 1967.
Henderson, L. W.: Peritoneal ultrafiltration dialysis: enhances urea transfer using hypertonic peritoneal dialysis fluid, J. Clin. Invest. **45**:950, 1966.
Johnson, P. J.: Bidirectional permeability of human peritoneum to substances of widely varying molecular weight, Master's thesis, University of Washington, 1973.
Lindner, A., and Tenckhoff, H.: Nitrogen balance in patients on peritoneal dialysis, Trans. Am. Soc. Artif. Intern. Organs **16**:255, 1970.
Mallette, W. G., et al.: A chemically successful subcutaneous peritoneal access button for repeated peritoneal dialysis, Trans. Am. Soc. Artif. Intern. Organs **10**:396, 1964.
Maxwell, M. H., et al.: Peritoneal dialysis. I. Technique and applications, J.A.M.A. **170**:916, 1959.
Rae, A., and Pendray, M.: The advantages of peritoneal dialysis in chronic renal failure, J.A.M.A. **225**:937, 1973.

Simmons, J. M., et al.: Relation of calorie deficiency to growth failure in children on hemodialysis and growth response to calorie supplementation, N. Engl. J. Med. **285:**653, 1971.

Stauch, M., et al.: Factors influencing protein loss during peritoneal dialysis, Trans. Am. Soc. Artif. Intern. Organs **13:** 172, 1967.

Tenckhoff, H.: Peritoneal dialysis today: a new look, Nephron **12:**420, 1974.

Tenckhoff, H., et al.: One year's experience with home peritoneal dialysis, Trans. Am. Soc. Artif. Intern. Organs **11:** 11, 1965.

CHAPTER 32

Accelerated or malignant hypertension

N. D. Vaziri

Malignant hypertension is defined by the presence of extreme acute elevation of diastolic blood pressure usually in excess of 120 to 140 mm Hg and one or more of the following disorders:

1. Hypertensive retinopathy with papilledema
2. Hypertensive encephalopathy
3. Renal involvement
4. Acute deterioration of left ventricular function with left ventricular failure and even florid pulmonary edema, and angina or myocardial infarction

In addition to these major manifestations, microangiopathic hemolysis and some as yet unexplained constitutional manifestations such as weight loss, anorexia, malaise, debility, and fever are commonly present in this syndrome. Because of a multitude of pathophysiologic conditions that could predispose to malignant hypertension, it should be considered as a syndrome rather than a single disease entity.

Before the advent of effective therapy, early death from uremia, cerebrovascular accident, and heart failure was inevitable, and the life expectancy after the diagnosis of malignant hypertension was less than 2 years. The prognosis has improved significantly with early administration of potent antihypertensive agents and supportive measures. Five-year survival now exceeds 33%. The term "accelerated hypertension" is sometimes used interchangeably with "malignant hypertension," but accelerated hypertension frequently refers to a recent significant increase over previous hypertensive levels or symptoms and signs of malignant hypertension without papilledema.

532

■ **What is the incidence and prognosis of malignant hypertension?**

Since malignant hypertension can occur in the course of any hypertensive disease, the successful control of the various forms of hypertension may significantly reduce the incidence of the malignant phase. Before the advent of effective antihypertensive therapy, as many as 6% to 8% of hypertensive conditions would progress to the malignant or accelerated phase. Subsequently an incidence of about 1% has been reported by several investigators. The peak incidence of the syndrome is observed in the middle-aged population. It is more prevalent in males than in females and more common in American blacks than in whites.

With regard to prognosis in untreated patients, the mortality rate is 90% in 2 years; however, with early and vigorous treatment, malignant hypertension seems to be reversible.

■ **What are the underlying conditions associated with malignant hypertension?**

Malignant hypertension can occur during the course of practically any hypertensive disorder. In the majority of cases (40%) malignant hypertension develops in patients having a history of *essential hypertension,* particularly when untreated or inadequately controlled. *Chronic interstitial nephropathy* and *chronic glomerulonephritis* constitute the underlying predisposing conditions in about 20% and 15% of the cases of malignant hypertension, respectively. Other, less prevalent, predisposing conditions include: polyarteritis nodosa, unilateral renal artery stenosis, postpartum hypertension, eclampsia, radiation nephritis, congenital renal disorders, hydronephrosis, pheochromocytoma, renal thromboembolic phenomena, scleroderma, Cushing's syndrome, primary aldosteronism, renal tuberculosis, and use of estrogen and oral contraceptive agents.

Malignant hypertension with no preexisting hypertension or other known disorders also occurs with some frequency. Most of the patients in this category are young black males.

■ What is known about pathogenesis of malignant hypertension?

The pathogenesis of vascular lesions in malignant hypertension is controversial. Some investigators feel that a high level of blood pressure in itself is responsible for the observed pathologic changes. When severe hypertension is produced by a marked constriction of the renal artery in experimental animals, intimal proliferation and necrotizing arteriolitis develop in most vascular beds, but vessels of the kidneys with stenosed arteries, which are protected against high arterial pressure, are spared. This and several other experiments suggest the direct role of high intraarterial pressure in the pathogenesis of vascular lesions in malignant hypertension.

However, several clinical and experimental observations suggest that severe hypertension may not account completely for the pathogenesis of malignant nephrosclerosis. There is evidence to suggest that in the malignant phase of hypertension, some vasopressor substance or substances are released by the kidneys owing to vasospasm. This, in turn, increases the degree of vascular reactivity and histologic lesions, thus leading to further narrowing of the vessels with release of increasing amounts of the vasopressor substance. A vicious circle is therefore established. Common findings of very high levels of renin, angiotensin, and aldosterone in the malignant phase of hypertension, dramatic improvement of hypertension with reduction of peripheral vascular resistance, and increased cardiac output after bilateral nephrectomy support the role of the kidney in the pathogenesis of malignant hypertension.

The common association of microangiopathic hemolysis and intravascular coagulation with malignant hypertension has been noted for over a decade. To date, it is not known whether malignant hypertension is the cause or the effect of microangiopathic hemolysis and coagulation.

■ What renal lesions can result from malignant hypertension?

The great majority of patients with malignant hypertension develop a rapidly progressive renal lesion called malignant nephrosclerosis. Occasionally the kidneys are spared, but this is the exception rather than the rule. With prompt and adequate antihypertensive therapy, one can modify the course and diminish or prevent the development and progression of renal lesions.

The gross appearance and size of the kidney depend on the underlying renal disease; for instance, small contracted kidneys are seen with preexisting benign nephrosclerosis, large scars with chronic pyelonephritis, and normal-size kidneys in de novo malignant nephrosclerosis. Petechial hemorrhages on the surface of the kidneys are due to rupture or arterioles.

Histologic findings consist of three major changes:

1. Proliferative endarteritis. This involves the afferent and interlobular arteries and gives rise to a so-called "onion peel" appearance. It is thought to be due to fibroblastic proliferation of subendothelial connective tissue and results in severe narrowing or obliteration of arteriolar lumina. This marked arteriolar narrowing or obliteration in turn causes renal parenchymal ischemia and damage. This lesion can develop with great rapidity. Some investigators regard it as highly specific for malignant hypertension.

2. Necrotizing arteriolitis. This lesion is characterized by fibrinoid necrosis of the afferent arteriolar walls and their infiltration with polymorphonuclear cells. Intratubular and parenchymal hemorrhages with vascular rupture are the consequence of this lesion. Many authors consider necrotizing arteriolitis as characteristic of malignant hypertension.

3. Necrotizing glomerulitis. This is characterized by precipitation of fibrinoid material and polymorphonuclear infiltration in the tufts of glomeruli whose afferent arterioles have necrotizing

arteriolitis. These glomerular changes may progress to cellular proliferation, mimicking chronic glomerulonephritis. The irregular and focal glomerular involvement in malignant nephrosclerosis (rarely more than one third glomeruli) differentiates it from chronic glomerulonephritis, which shows a widespread distribution. Pathologic changes associated with underlying disorders, when present, are also seen. Proliferation endarteritis and necrotizing arteriolitis may occur in organs other than the kidneys, for example, the gastrointestinal tract, pancreas, liver, adrenal glands, and so on. Clinical and laboratory manifestations of malignant nephrosclerosis consist of marked proteinuria, microscopic or gross hematuria, cylindruria, oliguria, and progressive azotemia.

■ What is hypertensive encephalopathy?

Hypertensive encephalopathy is one of the manifestations of malignant or accelerated hypertension. Its clinical picture consists of a wide spectrum of diverse neurologic aberrations that develop acutely as a result of severe blood pressure elevation. The symptoms and signs vary from severe headache, nausea, vomiting, blurring of vision, and confusion to transient blindness, paralysis, seizures, stupor, and deep coma. Findings suggest that focal neurologic deficits can also develop; however, they are quite rare and should suggest other CNS pathology. As a result of marked cerebral edema, fatal cerebellar herniation may occur. This event may be associated with performance of a lumbar puncture. In most cases the cerebrospinal fluid (CSF) pressure and protein concentration are elevated. Neurologic manifestations sometimes reverse themselves in a few days following effective control of hypertension, but at times recovery is prolonged or incomplete. Pathologic findings include arteriolar wall thickening and necrosis, brain edema, and areas of hemorrhage.

■ Is malignant hypertension preventable?

According to the result of a Veterans Administration Hospital cooperative study[1] on essential hypertension, medical management of subjects reduced the incidence of congestive heart failure, hypertensive retinopathy, and kidney failure. In this study no treated patient developed malignant hypertension. Although no such controlled studies have been done to examine the effect of antihypertensive therapy in prevention of the malignant phase in patients with renal hypertension, it seems reasonable to assume that a similar result could be achieved.

■ How is a patient with malignant hypertension managed?

The diagnosis of malignant hypertension calls for immediate emergency hospitalization and institution of effective antihypertensive therapy. Bedrest and sedation usually help in lowering the blood pressure in most hypertensive patients. The mechanism of this response is not clear, but it may have to do with reduction of the circulating blood volume and/or removal from a stressful environment. Close monitoring and observation of the patient's condition and adherence to dietary and drug programs are more possible in the hospital environment. Patient education with regard to the severity of his condition and its future management should be accomplished at this time.

A low sodium diet is mandatory and is a useful adjunct in the treatment of this condition, as well as in the treatment of all the other hypertensive disorders. Remarkable reductions in blood pressure levels and significant improvement in the prognosis of patients with both benign and malignant hypertension have been demonstrated by various investigators with the use of the "rice-fruit" diet or other low sodium diets.

Use of antihypertensive drugs is the mainstay in the treatment of malignant hypertension. A variety of effective agents are now available. In the absence of severe renal insufficiency, administration of these drugs, along with the general measures mentioned previously, will usually result in a favorable response. A brief discussion of the mechanisms of action, indications, contraindications, routes of administration, and side-effects of these drugs follows.

Diazoxide (Hyperstat)

Diazoxide, when rapidly injected intravenously, is very effective in lowering arterial blood pressure. It is usually given in a dose of 5 mg/kg body weight in children and 300 mg in adults. The antihypertensive effect of diazoxide appears in 30 seconds and lasts for 3 to 8 hours. If the desirable effect is not achieved with the first bolus, the dose can be repeated in half an hour. The patient's blood pressure should be monitored regularly every 30 minutes to 1 hour. Although severe hypotension may develop as a result of this drug, it is relatively uncommon. Because of its rapid and dramatic effect, low incidence of hypotension, and ease of administration and subsequent monitoring, diazoxide has become the most popular drug in the management of malignant hypertension. Some of its side-effects are fluid retention, hyperglycemia, reflex tachycardia, and increased myocardial ischemia in patients with coronary artery insufficiency.

Sodium nitroprusside

Sodium nitroprusside (NTP) is one of the most effective antihypertensive agents manufactured. Its only route of administration is intravenous. It is a direct vasodilator like hydralazine and diazoxide. The drug is available in the form of sterile powder, which is usually dissolved in 5% dextrose in water (60 mg nitroprusside/1000 ml of 5% DW) and slowly infused intravenously. The rate of infusion is determined and adjusted by careful and frequent monitoring of the patient's blood pressure. The onset and duration of the action of nitroprusside is within a few seconds. It consistently lowers the blood pressure in most patients, including those who are resistant to all the other drugs, does not result in tachyphylaxis (resistance to the drug), and has a low toxicity. When in solution, it becomes deactivated on exposure to light; therefore the bottle should be covered by a dark bag to prevent this phenomenon. The blood thiocyanate level should be measured periodically in patients receiving nitroprusside, since thiocyanate toxicity has been reported in such patients. A reversible hypothyroidism can occur with prolonged nitroprusside treatment. Following withdrawal of nitroprusside, the thyroid function returns to normal spontaneously.

Hydralazine (Apresoline)

Hydralazine is a potent antihypertensive drug. It has a direct effect on the smooth muscles of the arterioles and causes vasodilatation. Reflex tachy-cardia, throbbing headaches, and development of a lupuslike syndrome are among its major side-effects. Because of reflex tachycardia, myocardial oxygen consumption increases with the use of this drug. Angina and myocardial infarction may develop in patients with ischemic heart disease if tachycardia is not controlled. Simultaneous use of propranolol not only counteracts this effect, but also potentiates the antihypertensive action of hydralazine. This combination is quite effective and very popular. Intramuscular or intravenous injections of hydralazine in doses of 5 to 30 mg every 4 to 6 hours is frequently adequate for control of malignant hypertension in most patients. In large doses hydralazine can cause agitation and anxiety, which may be confused with symptoms of hypertensive encephalopathy. If after 2 hours blood pressure cannot be controlled with parenteral hydralazine, another agent should be used.

Trimethaphan camphorsulfonate (Arfonad)

Trimethaphan camphorsulfonate and other ganglionic blocking agents exert their antihypertensive action by competitive inhibition of acetylcholine in sympathetic ganglia, thus preventing postsynaptic depolarization. With slow, intravenous infusion, trimethaphan camphorsulfonate exerts a potent blood pressure–lowering effect that is potentiated by postural effects. Need for constant monitoring of blood pressure, parasympatholytic side-effects (for example, urinary retention, constipation, ileus), and development of resistance to the drug are among its major disadvantages.

Reserpine

By depleting the catecholamine stores of postganglionic fibers, reserpine and other rauwolfia preparations interfere with adrenergic neurotransmission and thereby reduce peripheral vascular resistance. Reserpine can be administered intramuscularly in doses of 1 to 2.5 mg in a hypertensive crisis. There is usually a delay of 1½ to 2½ hours in onset of its antihypertensive response, and its duration of action is about 7½ to 8 hours. Delayed response and different individual sensitivity to reserpine and its side-effects (mainly, nasal congestion, peptic disorders, and central nervous system depression) are among the disadvantages of this drug.

• • •

With parenteral use of one of these preparations, blood pressure should be promptly lowered to a safe level, particularly when hypertensive encephalopathy is present. In order to achieve satisfactory blood pressure control without parenteral drugs, an oral antihypertensive program should be initiated simultaneously or shortly afterwards in conjunction with a tapering off and final discontinuance of the parenteral drugs.

A close association between microangiopathic hemolysis and malignant hypertension has been recognized for over a decade; however, a definite cause and effect relationship between the two has not been established. Heparin and dipyridamole (Persantin) have been used by some investigators to prevent intravascular coagulation in these patients with the assumption that malignant hypertension is associated with intravascular coagulation. The results have not been favorable, and the use of anticoagulants is not recommended in such patients at the present time.

■ **What is the role of dialysis in patients with malignant nephrosclerosis?**

Renal failure with uremia is a common complication of malignant hypertension. In the predialysis era 95% of the mortality related to malignant hypertension was caused by uremia. In addition to its lifesaving value in uremic subjects through correction of azotemia, electrolyte, and acid-base disturbances, dialysis can differentiate and separate the metabolic from the hypertensive component of encephalopathy. Furthermore in the face of renal insufficiency, fluid retention becomes a problem and contributes to the elevation of blood pressure. Dialysis (hemo- or peritoneal) with ultrafiltration and removal of the excess fluids contributes to the control of the patient's hypertension.

■ **Is there any role for surgery in the management of malignant hypertension?**

A minority of patients in whom malignant hypertension is associated with a surgically cor-rectable lesion (for example, pheochromocytoma, renal artery stenosis, primary aldosteronism, or coarctation of the aorta) will benefit from the surgical removal or correction of the lesion and should undergo the proper surgical procedure.

Bilateral nephrectomy in patients with malignant hypertension results in the dramatic improvement of their hypertension. When kidneys are functional or potentially functional (acute reversible renal failure), bilateral nephrectomy for the purpose of blood pressure control is inappropriate and should not be considered. Even in the presence of irreversible renal damage and maintenance hemodialysis, this procedure should be avoided as much as possible, since anephric patients present a difficult problem with regard to the degree of anemia, bone disease, and volume and electrolyte disorders. There is a subgroup of patients with malignant nephrosclerosis on maintenance hemodialysis in whom severe hyper-reninemia, volume-independent hypertension anorexia, loss of lean body mass, and progressive deterioration of the general condition constitute the clinical picture. This subgroup should undergo bilateral nephrectomy. The procedure may also be beneficial in patients who are undergoing renal transplantation.

REFERENCE

1. Veterans Administration Cooperative Study Group on Anti-hypertensive Agents: II. Results in patients with diastolic blood pressure averaging 90 through 114 mm Hg, J.A.M.A. **213:**1143, 1970.

BIBLIOGRAPHY

Brain, M. C., et al.: Microangiopathic hemolytic anemia: the possible role of vascular lesions in pathogenesis, Br. J. Haematol. **8:**358, 1962.

Brain, M. C., et al.: Treatment of patients with microangiopathic hemolytic anemia with heparin, Br. J. Haematol. **15:**603, 1968.

Brest, A. N., et al.: Mechanisms of antihypertensive drug therapy, J.A.M.A. **211:**480, 1970.

Del Greco, F., et al.: Association of accelerated (malignant) hypertension in a patient with primary aldosteronism, J. Clin. Endocrinol. Metab. **26:**808, 1966.

Dolliery, C. T., et al.: Clinical pharmacology of beta-receptor–blocking drugs, Clin. Pharmacol. Ther. **10:**765, 1969.

Drano, J., et al.: Malignant hypertension, Arch. Intern. Med. **133:**791.

Feingold, L. N., et al.: Control of cachexia and ascites during chronic hemodialysis by bilateral nephrectomy, Ann. Intern. Med. **78:**829, 1973.

Finnerty, F. A., et al.: Clinical evaluation of diazoxide, a new treatment for acute hypertension, Circulation **28**:203, 1963.

Finnerty, F. A., et al.: Influence of extracellular fluid volume on response to antihypertensive drugs, Cir. Res. **26 & 27** (suppl 1): 72, 1970.

Gifford, R. W., and Richards, N. G.: Hypertensive encephalopathy: Part 1. Etiology, pathology and clinical findings, Curr. Concepts Cerebrovas. Dis. **5**:43, 1970.

Gunnells, J. C., et al.: Peripheral and renal venous plasma renin activity in hypertension, Ann. Intern. Med. **71**:555, 1969.

Harrison, T. S., et al.: Malignant hypertension in pheochromocytoma: correlation with plasma renin activity, John Hopkins Med. J. **130**:329, 1972.

Heptinstall, R. H.: Malignant hypertension: a study of 51 cases, J. Pathol. **65**:423, 1953.

Kincaid-Smith, P., McMichael, J., and Murphy, E. A.: The clinical course and pathology of hypertension with papilledema (malignant hypertension), Q. J. Med. **27**:117, 1958.

Kincaid-Smith, P., et al.: Dipyridamole and anticoagulants in renal disease due to glomerular and vascular lesions: a new approach to therapy, Med. J. Aust. **1**:145, 1970.

Linton, A. T., et al.: Microangiopathic hemolytic anemia and the pathogenesis of malignant hypertension, Lancet **1**:1277, 1969.

McCormack, L. J., et al.: Effects of antihypertensive treatment in the evolution of renal lesions in malignant nephrosclerosis, Am. J. Pathol. **34**:1011, 1958.

Mroczek, W. J., et al.: The importance of the rapid administration of diazoxide in accelerated hypertension, N. Engl. J. Med. **285**:603, 1971.

Mroczek, W. J., et al.: Malignant hypertension: kidney too good to be extirpated, Ann. Intern. Med. **80**:754, 1974.

Nickerson, M.: Antihypertensive agents and the drug therapy of hypertension. In Goodman, L. S., and Gilman, A., editors: The pharmacologic basis of therapeutics, ed. 4, New York, 1970, Macmillan Inc., p. 728.

Nickerson, M.: Drugs inhibiting adrenergic nerves and structures innervated by them: III. Adrenergic neuron blocking agents. In Goodman, L. S., and Gilman, A., editors: The pharmacologic basis of therapeutics, ed. 4, New York, 1970, Macmillan Inc., p. 570.

Page, I. H., et al.: Cardiovascular actions of sodium nitroprusside in animals and hypertensive patients, Circulation **11**:188, 1955.

Papper, S., and Vaamonde, C. A.: Nephrosclerosis. In Strauss, M. B., and Welt, L. G., editors: Diseases of the kidney, Boston, 1971, Little Brown & Co., p. 735.

Perera, G. A.: The accelerated form of hypertension: a unique entity? Trans. Assoc. Am. Physicians. **71**:62, 1958.

Pickering, G.: Reversibility of malignant hypertension, Lancet **1**:413, 1971.

Pohl, J. E., and Thurston, H.: Use of diazoxide in hypertension with renal failure, Br. Med. J. **4**:142, 1971.

Prichard, N. C.: Propranolol as an antihypertensive agent, Am. Heart J. **79**:128, 1970.

Schottstaedt, W. F., and Sokolow, M.: The natural history and course of malignant hypertension with papilledema, Am. Heart J. **45**:331, 1953.

Smirk, F. H., and McQueen, E. G.: Use of mecamylamine in the management of hypertension, Br. Med. J. **1**:422, 1957.

Stunkard, A., et al.: Studies on hydralazine: evidence for a peripheral site of action, J. Clin. Invest. **33**:1047, 1954.

Tcherdaroff, P., et al.: The present status of symptomatic surgical treatment for arterial hypertension. In Gross, F., editor: Antihypertensive therapy: principles and practice, an international symposium, New York, 1966, Springer-Verlag, p. 394.

Volle, R. L., and Koelle, G. B.: Ganglionic stimulating and blocking agents. In Goodman, L. S., and Gilman, A., editors: The pharmacologic basis of therapeutics, ed. 4, New York, 1970, Macmillan Inc., p. 585.

CHAPTER 33

Pediatric hypertension

N. D. Vaziri and G. Madani

■ How is hypertension in children defined?

Because of wide variation of blood pressure values among the general population, accurate definition of hypertension (HTN) in both children and adults has been difficult. However, based on the recent recommendation of the task force on blood pressure control in children, HTN should be diagnosed when blood pressure measurements obtained on two separate occasions exceed the 95th percentile or 140 and 90 mm Hg for systolic and diastolic pressures, respectively. Standard charts have been developed through multicenter collaborative studies supported by the National Institutes of Health in 1977. In these nomograms the distribution of systolic and diastolic pressures among children age 2 to 18 years is shown for each age group. The patient's percentile point can be determined by referring to these charts (Fig. 33-1).

■ When and how should we investigate hypertension in children?

Medical evaluation is indicated in all patients with moderate to severe hypertension as well as those asymptomatic patients whose blood pressure has been above the 95th percentile point on two separate occasions. The workup should include the following points:

1. Accurate family history with special reference to hypertension
2. Complete physical examination with emphasis on target organs, that is, eyes, brain, heart, and kidneys
3. Attempts to exclude secondary hypertension

4. Adjustment of blood pressure according to age, weight, and height
5. Determination of blood pressure in child's parents and siblings
6. Laboratory investigations as indicated

In children with severe hypertension, immediate evaluation and treatment are necessary since uncontrolled accelerated hypertension can result in serious target organ damage. Patients with isolated systolic hypertension should be observed closely as target organ damage may occur in such patients without diastolic hypertension.

■ How should we measure blood pressure in children and infants?

The width of the blood pressure cuff should be sufficient to cover the upper two thirds of the child's arm. The ultrasound technique for blood pressure measurement has replaced the conventional flush method in premature and full-term infants. Either technique can be used in older infants and children. A number of factors and conditions affect the blood pressure measurement in children. These include the child's size and position, unfamiliar surroundings, anxiety, and difficulty in detecting Korotkoff sounds.

■ What is the role of inheritance in pediatric hypertension?

A familial tendency seems to exist for systolic and diastolic hypertension in children of all ages, virtually extending to the first weeks of life. Elevated blood pressure has been reported in 28% of children with one hypertensive parent and 41%

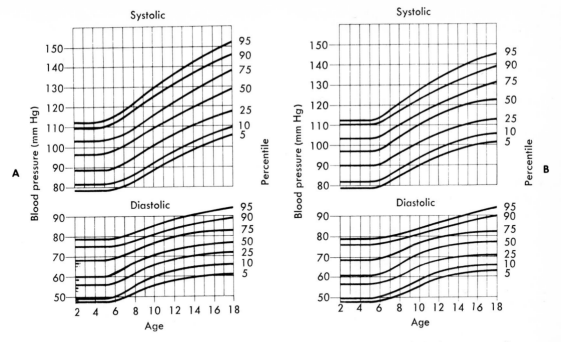

Fig. 33-1. Percentiles of blood pressure measurement in **A,** boys and **B,** girls (right arm, seated). (From Report of the Task Force on Blood Pressure Control in Children: Pediatrics **59**[Suppl.]:803, 1977.)

of children whose parents are both hypertensive. The role of heredity in the pathogenesis of hypertension has been suggested by the study of hypertension in twins and the lack of correlation between the blood pressure in nonbiologic parents and their adopted children.

Besides the familial tendencies, several other factors appear to contribute to the development of hypertension. These include sodium intake, obesity, stress, and physical activity.

■ What are the causes of hypertension in children?

As with the adult variety, hypertension in children may be idiopathic (*essential hypertension*) or caused by an underlying pathologic condition (*secondary hypertension*). Secondary HTN is much more prevalent in children than adults. The major causes of secondary hypertension are:

1. Unilateral and bilateral renal parenchymal or vascular abnormalities, such as various nephritides, renal artery stenosis, tumors, and so on
2. Vascular abnormalities, such as coarctation of aorta
3. Endocrine disorders, including Cushing's disease, pheochromocytoma, aldosteronomas, congenital adrenal hyperplasia, and so on
4. Neurologic disorders including bulbar poliomyelitis, increased intracranial pressure, and so on
5. Metabolic causes, for example, hypercalcemia, gouty or diabetic nephropathy
6. Drug-related hypertension, such as that induced by sympathomimetic agents, corticosteroids, amphetamines, licorice, and so on

HYPERTENSIVE CRISIS IN CHILDREN

Severe uncontrolled hypertension constitutes a major threat to life and various vital organs and should be regarded as a medical emergency. It is referred to as accelerated hypertension when it complicates the course of a preexisting hypertension, or malignant hypertension when it occurs as an acute event. It can cause severe hypertensive encephalopathy, retinopathy, and nephropathy, as well as acute left ventricular failure. The most common manifestation of hypertensive crisis in children is encephalopathy. This may be characterized by headaches, visual abnormalities, seizures, coma, and many other diverse neurologic abnormalities.

■ What are the most common causes of hypertensive crisis in children?

As with adults, hypertensive crisis can occur in the course of any hypertensive disorder and represents a syndrome with diverse etiologies. The most common causes, however, are acute postinfectious glomerulonephritis, hemolytic uremic syndrome, Henoch-Schönlein purpura, lupus erythematosus nephritis, membranoproliferative glomerulonephritis, chronic interstitial nephritis, chronic renal failure, renal vascular hypertension, renal transplant rejection, pheochromocytoma, various drugs, and untreated or poorly treated essential hypertension.

■ What are the symptoms and signs of hypertensive crisis?

The patient may complain of severe headaches, vomiting, visual disturbances, and shortness of breath. Convulsions or alteration of mental status may be the presenting symptoms. Physical examination may reveal exudates, hemorrhages, papilledema, and arteriolar constriction on funduscopic examination. Gallop rhythm with pulmonary congestion and rales may signify left ventricular failure owing to tremendous increase in the left ventricular afterload. Renal involvement may be characterized by hematuria, proteinuria, oliguria, and rising blood urea nitrogen and creatinine concentrations. Microangiopathic hemolytic anemia with fragmentation of red blood cells, hypokalemia, and secondary hyperaldosteronism are often present.

■ What should we remember about neonatal hypertensive crisis?

Hypertensive crisis is quite uncommon in neonates. When it occurs, it is hard to diagnose because measurement of blood pressure is often difficult and the clinical manifestations of hypertensive crisis are easily misinterpreted in these babies. The systolic pressure can be easily measured with a Doppler device or an oscillometer even when the baby is quite small. Congestive heart failure is the most common manifestation of hypertensive crisis in neonates.

The finding of an abdominal mass should suggest intra-abdominal hemorrhage or renal etiology for the baby's hypertension; absent or diminished femoral pulses suggest coarctation of aorta; and umbilical artery catheterization can result in thrombus formation and, when placed very high, can produce renal artery thrombosis and thereby severe hypertension. Medical treatment is often effective in controlling neonatal hypertensive crisis; however, surgical approaches such as thrombectomy, nephrectomy, or other procedures may be necessary.

■ How should we manage hypertensive crisis?

As with adults, children with hypertensive crisis should be hospitalized and treated immediately. Investigations to determine the etiology of severe hypertension should be postponed or conducted simultaneously with the efforts to control the hypertensive crisis. Convulsions can be treated with diazepam (Valium). Diuretics can be used in patients with evidence of marked fluid overload, congestive heart failure, and pulmonary edema. Potent antihypertensive drugs should be used parenterally to control the intense vasoconstrictions that are usually associated with severe hypertension. Aggressive antihypertensive treatment is indicated in children with diastolic pressures exceeding 110 to 130 mm Hg with or without encephalopathy, cardiac, renal, or retinal changes. The most popular drug currently used in the treatment of hypertensive crisis in children is diazoxide, which is relatively safe and quiet effective in this setting. Sodium nitroprusside, hydralazine, and reserpine can be used as well. The mode of action, side-effects, and various other properties of these agents have been briefly presented previously. Various drugs used in this condition and their pediatric dosages are listed in Table 33-1. Oral antihypertensive agents should be started as soon as possible so that parenteral agents can be tapered and discontinued.

Table 33-1. Drugs used in the treatment of hypertensive crisis and their pediatric dosage

Agent	Dose	Mode of action
Agents with very rapid onset		
Trimethaphan	0-1 mg/kg/min (IV)	Ganglionic blockade
Sodium nitroprusside	0.5-8 μg/kg/min (IV)	Direct vasodilator
Agents acting within minutes		
Diazoxide	5 mg/kg (IV rapid)	Direct vasodilator
Hydralazine	0.1-0.2 mg/kg (IV)	Direct vasodilator
Agents acting within hours		
Reserpine	0.7 mg/kg (IM)	Catecholamine depletion
Methyldopa	5-10 mg/kg (IV infused over 30-60 min)	Adrenergic blockade
Agents used in catecholamine-mediated hypertension		
Phentolamine	0.05-0.1 mg/kg (IV)	α-Adrenergic blockade
Phenoxybenzamine	0.5-1 mg/kg (oral or IV)	α-Adrenergic blockade

When hypertensive crisis is due to pheochromocytoma, intravenous phentolamine is administered for prompt control of hypertension. Thereafter, phenoxybenzamine is given orally to sustain an adequate α-adrenergic blockade. β-adrenergic blockade with propranolol or other such preparations is often necessary as well.

BIBLIOGRAPHY

Bauer, S. B., et al.: A complication of umbilical-artery catheterization, N. Engl. J. Med. **293**:1032, 1975.

Dinsdale, H. B., Robertson, D. M., and Haas, R. A.: Cerebral blood flow in acute hypertension, Arch. Neurol. **31**:80, 1974.

Lassen, N. A., and Agnoli, A.: The upper limit of autoregulation of cerebral blood flow on the pathogenesis of hypertensive encephalopathy, Scand. J. Clin. Lab. Invest. **30**:113, 1972.

Plumer, L. B., Kaplan, G. W., and Mendoza, S. A.: Hypertension in infants—a complication of umbilical arterial catheterization, J. Pediatr. **89**:802, 1976.

Report of the Task Force on Blood-Pressure Control in Children. Prepared by National Heart, Lung, and Blood Institutes. Pediatrics **59**(suppl. 5), Part 2, 1977.

Skinhöj, E., and Strandgaard, S.: Pathogenesis of hypertension encephalopathy, Lancet **1**:461, 1973.

CHAPTER 34

Management of the burn patient

Patricia Allyn and Robert Bartlett

The skin is a remarkable organ, protecting the body from the environment and keeping fluids in and infection out. Burn damage to the skin of any magnitude is a serious injury. Nowhere in medicine is the coordination of a team of doctors, nurses, therapists, technicians, and laboratory and operating room personnel so important. The seriously burned patient is the ultimate challenge in critical care because of the complexity of medical and nursing management. Even though the magnitude of injury may be massive and prolonged, survival and rehabilitation can be expected as soon as the burn surface is covered with healthy skin.

■ What is the pathophysiology of burns?

Thermal injury to the skin causes cellular necrosis, capillary damage, capillary thrombosis, and denaturation of collagen and other proteins in the skin and subcutaneous layers. The depth of the burn is proportional to the amount of heat and length of time it is applied (Table 34-1).

A first-degree burn causes erythema of the skin and only slight damage to the uppermost layers, occasionally causing blistering. Second-degree burn encompasses all the range between this and the extreme of third-degree burn but by definition implies that some of the layer of epithelial cells that generates new skin is intact. Second-degree burns can therefore be expected to heal by the generation of new skin and reepithelialization. A third-degree burn is that in which the skin and all its appendages (sweat glands, hair follicles, and sebaceous glands) are completely destroyed by the injury, so that the patient has a

thick layer of coagulated necrotic skin (eschar) on top of viable subcutaneous fat. Third-degree burns will always require skin grafting or some other method of closure for healing to be complete. Fourth-degree burns extend into muscle and bone.

Immediately after the injury, it is often difficult to judge the depth of the burn, but some general characteristics can usually be recognized. The capillary injury of second- and third-degree burns results in leakage of plasma from blood into the interstitial space of the subcutaneous fat and damaged skin. In addition, large amounts of water are lost from the surface of the burn by evaporation. This is most obvious in second-degree burns where the surface is moist and oozing plasma, but the charred eschar of third-degree burns is also very permeable to water vapor. The evaporation of water from the surface causes cooling of the patient. The loss of plasma into the burned area and loss of water from the burned area to the atmosphere results in a rapid diminution of blood volume, specifically plasma volume, causing a concentration of red blood cells or a rise in hematocrit. As the blood volume falls and the hematocrit rises, viscosity increases, making it harder for the heart to pump the small amount of blood remaining. Cardiac output falls, perfusion of other vital organs falls, and unless the fluid is replaced, the patient with a major burn will die very promptly from plasma loss. Consequently, most of the effort in the first 2 days after an extensive burn is directed at replacing plasma that has been lost into the tissues and dealing with the later resorption of this plasma back

Table 34-1. Characteristics of various depths of burns

Depth of burn	Cause	Surface	Color	Pain sensation
First degree	Sun or minor flash	Dry, no blisters	Erythematous	Painful, hyperesthetic
Second degree	Flash or hot liquids	Blisters, moist	Mottled red	Painful, hyperesthetic
Third degree	Flame	Dry	Pearly white or charred	Little pain, anesthetic
Fourth degree	Sustained flame or electrical	Charred, cracked	Charred, black	Little

into the vascular space. Plasma loss begins immediately after the burn and continues at a high rate for 12 to 15 hours, after which it gradually diminishes; the edema phase is generally finished within 48 hours.

All of these phenomena become more severe with increasing depth and extent of the burn. The extent is expressed as the percentage of body surface involved with second-, third-, and fourth-degree burns. This is estimated by mapping the burn on a chart and calculating the percent of body involved (Fig. 34-1).

The second largest problem confronting the patient with major burns is infection. Once the edema phase has been passed and the patient is taking nourishment orally and normal hemodynamics have been reestablished, a large amount of necrotic skin exposed to the atmosphere on one side and covered by subcutaneous fat on the other side is left. This necrotic skin is an excellent culture medium and becomes colonized with bacteria quite rapidly. The principal effort of burn care between the fourth day and the fourth week is devoted to preventing infection in this necrotic skin while waiting until the surface is healed or ready for grafting.

The subcutaneous fat will generally not accept a skin graft until it has formed a significant layer of granulation tissue with its rich capillary bed that will vascularize and maintain a split-thickness skin graft in a viable condition. Granulation tissue begins to form at the interface between healthy and damaged tissue within days of the burn, but the complete formation of granulation tissue requires 3 to 6 weeks. The time from burn to grafting can be shortened by debriding eschar and assuring good nutrition.

Preventing infection in the eschar is accomplished with topical surface antibiotic agents that keep the eschar free of invasive infection with bacteria. Associated with this, daily cleansing and antiseptic washing of the surface with removal of dead tissue decreases the exposure of the surface to bacteria and minimizes the chance for infection. Most of the drugs used to destroy bacteria on the surface of the eschar also inhibit granulation tissue and epithelialization and therefore prolong the time for healing somewhat.

Other organs besides the heart and skin are vulnerable in the burn patient. Pulmonary complications are the most common cause of death after burn injury. This may be because of smoke inhalation, fluid overload, pulmonary capillary damage, or a combination of these. Renal failure may occur, particularly in fourth-degree burns associated with myoglobin or hemoglobin urea. Paralytic ileus is common if septicemia occurs. Stress ulcers with upper gastrointestinal bleeding are also associated with sepsis. CNS symptoms are common and reversible, ranging from confusion or depression to seizures and coma.

During the weeks before surface healing or grafting, careful attention must be paid to joints, muscles, and ligaments under the area of the burn. Immobilization may result in contractures and loss of function very rapidly, so that exercise of the full range of motion of all joints in the area of the burn and night splinting to prevent deformity are essential parts of burn management. Proper nutrition is also essential, as grossly excessive amounts of calories are required to run the metabolic machinery after a severe burn. After discharge these patients should be observed for several months to assist with their complete rehabilitation and return to normal life.

INSTRUCTIONS FOR COMPLETING THIS FORM

1 COLOR IN THE BURN

Shade or color in the body diagrams to represent as closely as possible how the burn looks to you when viewing the patient from a directly anterior and/or directly posterior direction. Ignore the dashed lines on the diagrams while doing this.

2 CIRCLE AGE FACTOR

Since body proportions change from infancy to adulthood and since these changes mainly affect relative head and lower extremity proportions, this table allows you to choose the most appropriate body proportions for the age of the patient. Ages 0, 1, 5, 10, and 15 years and adult are given. Choose the age closest to that of the patient and use the H (head), T (thigh), and L(leg) percentage factors in the column below the age selected. To avoid mistakes, circle these numbers

3 CALCULATE EXTENT OF BURN

Each body part listed in the calculation table is indicated on the anterior and posterior body diagrams by dashed lines. The percentage of total body surface area for each body part is printed either on the diagram or in the age factor table (step 2). If the shaded or colored area in the body diagram covers an entire body part, the whole percentage figure for that part is entered into the calculation table. If the shaded area covers only a fraction of a body part, then that fraction of the percentage figure is entered. For example, if an anterior chest burn covered about one third of the trunk, then one third of 13, or 4%, would be entered in the space for "trunk" in the anterior column. When all body parts have been considered, subtotals are made for anterior and posterior burned areas. The grand total then represents an estimate of the percent of total body area burned. This number is most frequently referred to as the "size of the burn."

■ **How is the determination made as to the degree of emphasis to be placed on the physiologic, surface, and functional management of the burn patient?**

The physiologic, surface, and functional management processes involved in treating the burn patient are equally important in assuring good results but require different emphasis at different times. This changing emphasis is diagrammed in Fig. 34-2. Physiologic management is of primary importance during the resuscitation phase and remains important until the time the surface is covered. Direct surface management is of minimum importance for the first few days following the burn injury but becomes progressively more important until the time of grafting, when surface management is paramount. Functional management must be stressed within the first 24 hours of burn injury to prevent tissue damage that may lead to irreversible structural loss. This is particularly true in severe burns of the hands and the eyes. As long as joint motion is maintained during emergency management, little attention need be paid to functional management until the time the surface is covered with skin. Then functional management becomes the most important aspect of care and continues to be of major importance for 6 to 12 months.

Although the individual aspects of care can be described in this fashion, the team approach to the patient requires that each individual who approaches the burn patient must be well versed in all aspects of management and their interrelationships. This is particularly important with regard to psychologic management and rehabilitation. All burn patients should be treated as any other ill patient in the hospital. Cosmetic appearance and function should be discussed freely but minimized in the acute phase and throughout the patient's course. If the patient leaves the hospital with a healthy mental status, social adjustment will be much easier.

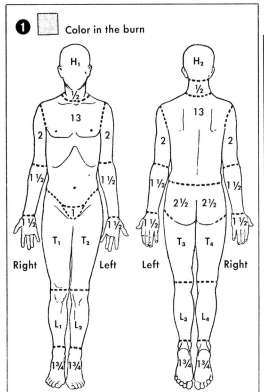

❶ Color in the burn

Right   Left   Left   Right

❸ Calculate extent of burn

	Anterior	Posterior
Head	H_1	H_2
Neck		
Right arm		
Right forearm		
Right hand		
Left arm		
Left forearm		
Left hand		
Trunk		
Buttock		
Perineum		
Right thigh	T_1	T_4
Right leg	L_1	L_4
Right foot		
Left thigh	T_2	T_3
Left leg	L_2	L_3
Left foot		
Subtotal		
% Total area burned		%

❷ Circle age factor

	Percent of areas affected by growth Age					
	0	1	5	10	15	Adult
$H_{(1\ or\ 2)} = \frac{1}{2}$ of the head	9½	8½	6½	5½	4½	3½
$T_{(1,2,3\ or\ 4)} = \frac{1}{2}$ of a thigh	2¾	3¼	4	4¼	4½	4¾
$L_{(1,2,3\ or\ 4)} = \frac{1}{2}$ of a leg	2½	2½	2¾	3	3¼	3½

Fig. 34-1. Estimation of size of burn by percent.

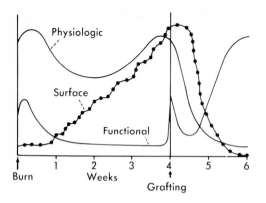

Fig. 34-2. Emphasis in burn management.

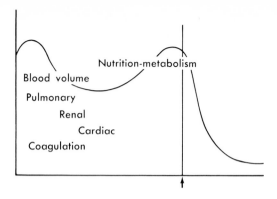

Fig. 34-3. Physiologic management.

■ **What survival rates are anticipated in the care of burn patients?**

Survival is expected for patients less than 60 years of age with uncomplicated burns covering up to 60% of the body surface. Death in these patients is usually related to smoke inhalation or other concomitant injury. Among young patients with burns over 60% to 80% of the body surface 50% survive, but survivors with burns of over 80% are rare. Death is usually caused by pulmonary insufficiency. At Orange County Medical Center 93% of the patients who survived major disfiguring or deforming burns underwent successful rehabilitation and resumed normal life.

This chapter outlines a plan for the critical care of the burn patient. Although there are several alternative methods of physiologic and surface care, these methods have produced the best results in burn care today based on survival, hospital stay, and rehabilitation. Other management approaches will be mentioned where appropriate. The interested reader is referred to the bibliography for further details.

PHYSIOLOGIC MANAGEMENT

Major emphasis is placed on physiologic management from the time of admission until the time that the surface is ready for skin grafting. During this time all major organ systems are vulnerable to failure in the burn patient, and organ function must be carefully monitored and failure prevented or vigorously treated when it occurs.

Specific areas of concentration in physiologic management are outlined in Fig. 34-3.

■ **What initial measures should be considered in the care of the critically burned patient?**

All patients with second- or third-degree burns over greater than 20% of the body surface area should be admitted to the hospital. All children and infants with second- or third-degree burns over 15% or more of the body surface area should also be admitted. The full management protocol outlined here should be instituted for all patients who are admitted to the hospital and then modified according to physiologic response.

Emergency care

Rapid cooling of a thermal injury will minimize the depth of tissue damage and is the only appropriate first aid that should be carried out at the scene. If the patient is seen during or immediately after the burn or if the surface is no longer warm, topical cooling is not necessary; in fact, it may be detrimental. Beyond that time the surface should be simply covered with a sheet or towel (which need not be sterile) and the patient should be prepared for transfer to a burn center. A third- or fourth-degree burn will not be painful, and although the patient will be apprehensive and worried, medication for pain will not be required. Second-degree burns are quite painful on exposure to air. This pain may be alleviated by wet dressings applied to the surface. Tepid water on a towel or sheet will suffice during transfer. No other topical agents should be applied; no débridement should be done. A large IV line should be attached and colloid infusion begun if 30 minutes or more will elapse before the patient arrives in the burn unit.

Emergency room care

All clothing should be completely removed to facilitate examination, and the patient should be covered with a clean sheet. Vital signs should be measured and blood drawn to evaluate complete blood count (CBC), blood urea nitrogen (BUN), blood sugar, type and cross match, and carboxyhemoglobin. If the patient is hypotensive or appears to have any signs of respiratory distress or facial burns, arterial blood gases should be measured. Simultaneously, one large plastic catheter should be inserted into a peripheral vein for fluid administration and a central venous catheter of the largest possible diameter should be inserted by direct puncture or cutdown. Venipuncture and cutdown procedures may be performed through burned tissue with impunity. The position of the central venous catheter must be verified by chest x-ray film, usually taken in the emergency room. Fluid infusion may be begun in the peripheral venous catheter and dextrose and water infusion in the central venous catheter. A bladder catheter should be placed to measure urine output and a nasogastric tube should be passed. Chest x-ray films should be taken, and the patient readied for transfer to the critical care area. Diazepam (Valium) may be given by IV route for sedation. Rarely narcotics may be required for pain. All of this should be accomplished in 15 minutes or less.

If the patient has obvious respiratory distress, severe deep burns around the head and neck, or burn injury extending into the palate or pharynx on direct examination, tracheal intubation will be necessary. A nasotracheal tube should be passed when feasible, but prolonged and repeated attempts at intubation may exacerbate the edema; this job should be performed by the most experienced member of the team. If intubation is impossible, tracheostomy may be done, but only on extremely rare occasions.

Concomitant injuries may be cared for after an adequate airway is established. If the patient has a condition requiring immediate operation (compound fractures, intracranial bleeding, intra-abdominal bleeding), he should be taken to the operating room and treatment for the burn surface becomes of low priority. Closed fractures are splinted. Skeletal traction, if necessary, may be carried out through burned tissue without concern.

Burn unit admission

If the patient is significantly hypotensive, is suffering severe respiratory insufficiency, or has an initial blood pH below 7.30, he should be taken directly from the emergency room to the burn unit. If these findings are not present, the patient should be taken to a hydrotherapy room, preferably adjacent to the burn unit, where he should be weighed and bathed in a large tub with warm water, sodium hypochlorite, and Betadine solution. All loose tissue should be debrided at this time without anesthesia. Blisters should be opened and debrided, and all hair-bearing areas near or in the burn area shaved. If foreign material such as dirt and tar is present, more extensive cleaning may be required. Pain medication may be given by IV route for the first time during this phase of management. It is not necessary to shave the entire head in burns of the face or scalp. If the patient's condition is unstable, débridement, washing, and dressing should be carried out as quickly as possible in bed in the burn unit while more intensive monitoring and therapy is taking place.

After the initial cleaning of the surface, topical antibiotic dressings should be quickly applied and the patient placed in bed in the burn unit in a semisitting position. Hands and feet should be elevated if burned. ECG monitoring is initiated at this time, along with hourly measurement of blood pressure, pulse, central venous pressure, urinary output, respiratory rate, tidal volume, and fluid intake. Temperature should be monitored continuously; an over-the-bed radiant heater may be added to prevent hypothermia (Fig. 34-4).

This phase of management should take no longer than 1 hour. Consideration should then be given to placement of an intra-arterial catheter, a pulmonary artery catheter, and Kirschner wire

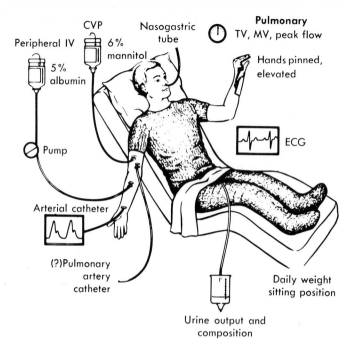

Fig. 34-4. Initial management and monitors.

pins in fingers for severely burned hands; escharotomies should be performed on any area that appears to be constricting. Arterial catheters should be placed for any patient with severe smoke inhalation injury, any patient who requires intubation, or any patient with unstable blood pressure. Pulmonary artery catheters should be floated into patients with preexisting myocardial disease, massive burns, or preexisting pulmonary disease. Metal pins should be placed to maintain the proximal interphalangeal joints in full extension for patients with third-degree burns of the hands. Hand management is discussed extensively later. The hands should be placed in anticlaw splints and elevated.

Escharotomies should be carried out early in the course of management for all patients who have extensive circumferential burns of extremities, neck, or chest. When in doubt, the escharotomy should not be done, and the blood supply or chest expansion carefully monitored at hourly intervals, escharotomy being performed within

the first 6 to 12 hours if significant constriction occurs. Escharotomy usually can be done without anesthesia using a knife blade or cautery, and bleeding from the skin edges is minimal. If bleeding does occur, it must be controlled by electrocautery. If the patient requires escharotomy, an extensive procedure should be done, extending down to and including fingers, on both sides of the wrist or ankle, and proximal to normal tissue, which may include the chest wall. Escharotomies over the chest wall to facilitate chest expansion should be done in grid fashion, including both vertical and horizontal incisions. IV morphine or similar narcotics should be used for pain. IV diazepam (Valium) or similar drugs should be used to calm agitated patients. Ketamine anesthesia is useful when pin placement is required, but this should not be used to anesthetize the patient simply because of agitation.

Once the initial management is instituted as outlined in Fig. 34-4, attention should be turned to hemodynamic and fluid resuscitation.

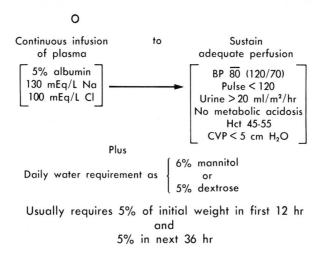

O

Continuous infusion   to   Sustain
of plasma   adequate perfusion

$$\begin{bmatrix} 5\% \text{ albumin} \\ 130 \text{ mEq/L Na} \\ 100 \text{ mEq/L Cl} \end{bmatrix} \longrightarrow \begin{bmatrix} \text{BP } \overline{80} \text{ (120/70)} \\ \text{Pulse} < 120 \\ \text{Urine} > 20 \text{ ml/m}^2/\text{hr} \\ \text{No metabolic acidosis} \\ \text{Hct 45-55} \\ \text{CVP} < 5 \text{ cm H}_2\text{O} \end{bmatrix}$$

Plus

Daily water requirement as $\begin{cases} 6\% \text{ mannitol} \\ \text{or} \\ 5\% \text{ dextrose} \end{cases}$

Usually requires 5% of initial weight in first 12 hr
and
5% in next 36 hr

Fig. 34-5. University of California Irvine Medical Center burn "formula."

■ What should be known about hemodynamics and blood volume in the care of the burn patient?

Fluid management is the most important part of the early care of the burn patient. The goals of successful fluid management are to maintain adequate perfusion and supply metabolic demands while maintaining pace with the rate of plasma loss into and water evaporation through the burned surface; this should not result in an overload of the extracellular space in the lungs with large amounts of salt and water. Studies by Moore[1] showed that a large burn can sequester approximately 10% of the body weight in the extracellular space, and the fluid that is sequestered is essentially plasma. This fluid is reabsorbed after 48 hours and excreted over the ensuing 7- to 10-day period. These studies are incorporated into the "Brigham Burn Budget," which we follow.

Although a 5% albumin colloid solution is preferred for further resuscitation, many centers achieve good results by infusing crystalloid solutions such as lactated Ringer's solution only. Studies by Monafo and co-workers[2] and Moylan and associates[3] suggest that the total amount of sodium ion is the critical factor in successful burn resuscitation. This has led some investigators to infuse hypertonic saline solution or lactated Ringer's solution to provide the required amount of sodium ion with less fluid volume. Several formulas have been devised to calculate the fluid requirements of the burn patient. The Baxter formula dictates the use of 4 ml of Ringer's lactate solution per kilogram per percent burn.[4] We recommend that crystalloid solutions be avoided during resuscitation because they may preferentially collect in the interstitial space in the lung, leading to pulmonary complications hours or days later. Burn formulas for fluid management are loose approximations to provide a general idea of the amount of fluid to have on hand during the acute management stage.

The fluid plan followed in the University of California Irvine Medical Center burn unit is outlined in Fig. 34-5. Simply stated, a plasma substitute is infused at a rate sufficient to maintain adequate arterial perfusion. This will require approximately 10% of the body weight in colloid solution during the first 48 hours, half of that during the first 12 hours. Blood pressure, central venous pressure, urine output, and hematocrit are measured every hour initially, and every 2 to 4 hours thereafter until the patient's condition becomes stable. Urinary output should remain between 20 and 50 ml/hr in adults, and mean arterial pressure should remain above 80 mm Hg. If the mean arterial pressure is below 80 mm Hg or if the urine output is less than 20 ml/m²/hr, the infusion rate is increased until these parameters are improved, or until the central venous pressure is 10 cm H_2O or the pulmonary artery diastolic pressure is 20 cm H_2O. The hematocrit is a valuable index of plasma loss in the burn patient. The hematocrit should be carefully followed and maintained between 40% and 50% with plasma infusion. A rapidly dropping hematocrit during resuscitation is usually a sign of excessive plasma infusion and is treated by slowing the infusion, not by transfusion of blood. Some red blood cells are lost in the presence of burn injury but generally not enough to require a transfusion.

The relationship between the blood volume and cardiac function is monitored by estimating perfusion by the criteria just mentioned and measuring central venous or right atrial pressure. The patient should be in normal acid-base status without metabolic acidosis. Usually the severely burned patient will have a moderate respiratory alkalosis. If metabolic acidosis exists, it should be treated with sodium bicarbonate or tromethamine (THAM) buffer, followed promptly by a more rapid infusion of plasma substitute.

Pulmonary artery pressure monitoring[5] provides a much more sensitive index of blood volume and cardiac function relationships than central venous pressure monitoring. Pulmonary artery pressure monitoring should be instituted in any patient who remains hypotensive or acidotic while on an appropriate fluid replacement regimen or in any patient who has signs of myocardial depression with central venous pressure above 10 cm H_2O. The relationships between pulmonary artery and central venous pressure monitoring are shown in Fig. 34-6, and interpretation of the pulmonary artery pulse contour as a guide to fluid management is shown in Fig. 34-7. It is suggested that correct fluid resuscitation is usually associated with a central venous pressure of 0 to 5 cm H_2O; central venous pressure over 10 cm H_2O is usually associated with left ventricular failure and pulmonary edema accumulation.

Water with 5% dextrose in solution should be infused to replace insensible water losses, which will usually be excessive if the burn surface is wet and exudative. Occlusive dressings minimize surface evaporation to some extent. The water re-

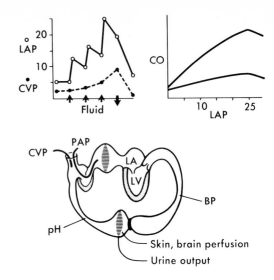

Fig. 34-6. Central venous and pulmonary artery pressure monitoring.

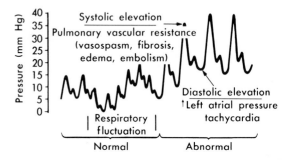

Fig. 34-7. Pulmonary artery pressure interpretation. (From German, J. C., Allyn, P. A., and Bartlett, R. H.: Arch. Surg. **106:**788, 1973.)

quirement for an adult will be approximately 2000 ml/day. The water requirement for a child or infant can be calculated as 1000 ml/m^2 of body surface area or as three fourths of the estimated blood volume. Electrolytes should be infused if electrolyte solution is lost through vomiting, diarrhea, or nasogastric tube suction. Initially there may be hemoglobin or myoglobin in the plasma from hemolysis and muscle destruction. In this case, infusion of a diuretic drug is instituted to attempt to prevent acute renal failure secondary to pigment casts. In general the insensible water loss is replaced with 5% mannitol solution during the first 24 hours if pigment is present in the serum or urine. Mannitol, ethacrynic acid, or furosemide may also be used. There is no need for additional diuretic drugs. The urine output is such a valuable monitor of fluid replacement and perfusion that artificially changing the volume or composition of the urine with potent diuretics is not a wise practice. Fluid management continues with the previously mentioned parameters in mind until capillary integrity is reestablished and spontaneous diuresis occurs, usually 48 to 72 hours after the burn. If the fluid is reabsorbed from the burn area, renal function must be excellent to prevent hypervolemia.

■ How is renal damage in the burn patient detected and managed?

Although cardiac output may fall early after burn injury, properly managed fluid resuscitation will avoid classic acute tubular necrosis in virtually every case. If fluid resuscitation is inadequate for any reason and acute tubular necrosis does occur, it may be seen as anuric or polyuric renal failure. In either case, renal damage is best detected by abnormalities of urinary electrolytes, so that all urine is saved in 24-hour intervals for the first 3 days after the burn has occurred. In this way urinary electrolytes and urea can be present with the stress of the burn. Urinary sodium levels will be less than 10 mEq/L and urinary potassium levels higher than 60 mEq/L. Urine area levels should be 10 to 20 times the blood urea. If the urinary sodium concentration is over 50 mEq/L, and the potassium concentration is under 20 mEq/L, renal tubular damage is present.

When renal failure does occur following burn injury, it is usually associated with hemolysis or muscle destruction. When fourth-degree burns are suspected, induced diuresis with mannitol or furosemide should be instituted.

When renal failure occurs in burn patients secondary to pigment load, acute tubular necrosis, or relative renal insufficiency with normal urine volume, renal function should be replaced or augmented with dialysis. Peritoneal dialysis can be carried out, but hemodialysis is preferred. As soon as the diagnosis of renal failure is made, an arteriovenous shunt should be placed, preferably through nonburned tissue to permit securing of the shunt. Daily dialysis may be instituted and carried out for 6 to 8 hours prior to tubbing and debriding daily. The use of vigorous hemodialysis in the five massively burned patients at Orange County Medical Center prolonged life in three patients to the point where grafting was possible. Only 22 cases of dialysis treatment of renal failure in burned patients have been reported in the literature (including the five cases just cited) with four survivors.[6]

Technical considerations in dialysis

Aggressive hemodialysis in the massively burned patient requires the assemblage and coordination of a team of medical, nursing, and allied critical care personnel. Hemodialysis is definitely preferable to peritoneal dialysis, except in small children. A standard silicone rubber shunt may be placed in any available extremity, usually in an area of burn eschar. Because of the quality of the tissue, great care must be taken to avoid dislodging the shunt during dialysis, hydrotherapy, and dressing changes. Burn patients exhibit definitely hypercoagulable signs during the second and third week following the burn injury, and clotting of the venous limb of the shunt is a common complication, resulting in many revisions. The shunt is commonly used to infuse hypertonic glucose solutions during hyperalimentation. Infection around the shunt or septicemia from the shunt has not been a problem. The treatment protocol may include daily tubbing in a Hubbard tank containing water and chlorine bleach and cleaning the burn surfaces with Betadine solution. The surface should be dressed with antibiotics (mafenide acetate [Sulfamylon Cream] or silver sulfadiazine). The shunt area should be thoroughly washed and redressed daily, along with the rest of the burn area.

On the few occasions where arteriovenous hemodialysis has resulted in sustained hypotension in a patient with precarious hemodynamic status, venovenous dialysis has been achieved by the passage of a large catheter into the inferior vena cava for outflow with a peripheral vein used as a return route. It is easy to achieve flows of

200 to 300 ml/min with this technique and hypotension does not result, but the large caval catheter cannot be left in position and must be replaced with each dialysis.

Hemodialysis flows of 200 to 300 ml/min may be used, usually with ultrafiltration and regional heparinization. The patient should be weighed daily after dialysis, with all dressings off, and prior to hydrotherapy. Weight loss during dialysis should be monitored by the use of a bed scale. It is easiest to begin dialysis early in the morning and continue until 1 or 2 PM. The patient is usually mentally and physiologically most stable immediately after dialysis, at which time all dressings should be removed and the patient tubbed, debrided, redressed, and returned to bed. Bleeding with dressing and débridement has been less following dialysis than when dialysis is done after débridement. As in any high mortality group of patients, one of the most important aspects of

patient care is the maintenance of enthusiasm and optimism among the treatment team.

■ **What pulmonary complications may be anticipated in the burn patient?**

Pulmonary complications are the most common cause of death in burn patients. For example, in a series of 100 patients reviewed in the Orange County Medical Center burn unit in 1971 and 1972, 22 had pulmonary complications, and 19 of these patients died.[7] This 20% incidence and 86% mortality associated with pulmonary complications is typical of results from other units. The factors in the pathogenesis of pulmonary complications are outlined in Fig. 34-8. Exogenous factors (primarily smoke inhalation) and endogenous factors (circulating myocardial depressants and other humoral factors) combine to produce alveolar collapse and increased interstitial water in the lung. This results

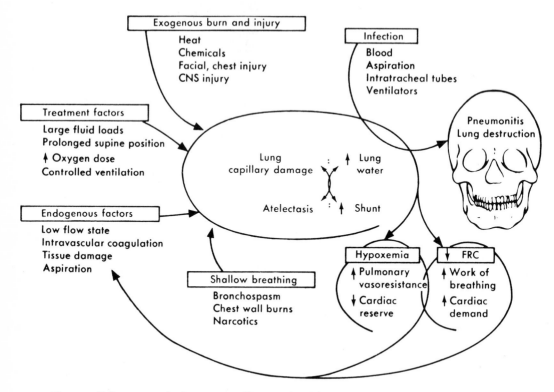

Fig. 34-8. Pathogenesis of pulmonary insufficiency. (Modified from Achauer, B. M., et al.: Ann. Surg. **177:**311, 1973.)

in hypoxemia and decreased functional residual capacity and further complicates peripheral perfusion. The edematous lung is susceptible to infection, and bacterial pneumonitis is a common fatal complication.

Lung damage from smoke inhalation is caused by the toxic effects of volatile vapors from completely burned materials on the respiratory epithelium and alveoli.[8] These vapors, which include formaldehyde and other aldehydes and ketones, are formed when wood, upholstery, paint, and so forth burn. Lung damage occurs when the fumes are inhaled over a prolonged period of time. Consequently, pulmonary damage from smoke inhalation occurs in patients who have been in fires in enclosed spaces. The best indicator of smoke inhalation is the presence of soot in the sputum, and this may persist for several days. Carboxyhemoglobin may indicate the severity of smoke inhalation if measured soon after the injury.

Smoke inhalation alone carries a high mortality from brain death secondary to hypoxia or overwhelming pulmonary insufficiency in the first few hours. The patient who survives a smoke inhalation injury more than 12 hours has a good prognosis. Smoke inhalation in association with any surface burn creates more serious pulmonary problems than smoke inhalation or burn alone.

Endogenous pulmonary damage from inadvertent fluid overload may be minimized by using colloid solution for resuscitation and by using pulmonary artery pressure as a guide to fluid replacement as previously outlined. Avoiding endotoxin in the bloodstream by debriding eschar and keeping the surface clean and avoiding low-flow states with potential intravascular coagulation and lysosomal enzyme release are also important in preventing pulmonary capillary damage and myocardial depression. Circulating myocardial depressants have been identified in burned skin, and this may add to interstitial pulmonary edema.

Pulmonary complications secondary to upper airway obstruction from burn edema itself are managed by intubation of the trachea through the nose or the mouth for the 4 or 5 days during the edematous phase. Tracheostomy is usually not necessary to relieve upper airway obstruction.

Management with a mechanical ventilator is also unnecessary for the patient with upper airway obstruction.

The best guide to pulmonary parenchymal damage is arterial Po_2 at a known concentration of oxygen in inspired air (FIO_2). Hypoxemia during air breathing may be the only sign of impending pulmonary damage early after the burn. Chest x-ray films are usually normal during the first 24 hours. Progressive hypoxemia is one of the indications for mechanical ventilation with lung parenchymal damage. An indwelling arterial catheter should be placed in all patients whose history or blood gas concentrations suggest impending pulmonary complications, and intubation with mechanical ventilation is instituted when indicated. The use of intentional dehydration with diuretics and positive end-expiratory pressure is helpful in smoke inhalation syndrome. Large doses of corticosteroids may be given to the smoke inhalation patient to minimize edema and humoral damage to lung capillaries, although the value of this medication has not been definitely proved.

Using the principles of recognition, prevention, and management, the incidence of pulmonary complications in the University of California Irvine Medical Center burn unit has decreased to 15%, with an overall mortality of 50%.

■ What nutritional and metabolic management modalities should be considered?

Burn injury imposes a hypermetabolic catabolic state with increased caloric expenditure and rapid wasting of fat and lean body mass. The patient with a moderate burn can lose 10% of body weight in a period of 2 to 3 weeks. Patients who rapidly lose 15% to 20% of body weight reach a state of energy crisis characterized by hypothermia, bradycardia, coma, and hyponatremia that has a high mortality rate if not promptly treated with calories. The hypermetabolic state has been related to heat loss as a result of water evaporation from the surface.[9] Water loss through burn or eschar reaches a level two to three times the amount of water loss through intact skin. This is minimized by the occlusive dressings that are used in our unit. The complications of desiccation evaporation (hypernatremia, rising hematocrit, and intense thirst) are not seen in our patients. Studies by Zawacki[10] and other investigators have shown that when water loss is totally eliminated by occlusive plastic dressings, the hypermetabolic state persists. The hypermetabolic state seems to be related to the extent and the depth of the burn and is associated with high catecholamine levels and high steroid levels. In patients who are not septic this hypermetabolism reaches an extreme two times the baseline level.

Although some have considered that the hypermetabolic state always occurred and was attended with lean tissue loss, this is not necessarily the case. In a recent study measuring caloric expenditure by indirect calorimetry, it was found that weight loss could be prevented and could, in fact, be promoted during the healing phase of burn injury by meeting the caloric expenditure on a day-to-day basis. Normal caloric expenditure is 40 to 55 calories/m²/hr. In burn patients a caloric intake of at least 100 calories/m²/hr should be assured by oral intake, tube feeding, or occasionally by IV nutrition. This should be accompanied with careful measurement of body weight daily. If the patient loses weight on this regimen, indirect calorimetry should be carried out and actual caloric expenditure calculated.

Higher metabolic rates are associated with a larger percentage of burn and with the amount of third-degree burn. Caloric intake is calculated daily, and if the intake falls behind caloric expenditure on oral intake, a nasogastric feeding tube should be passed and tube feedings added. The tube feeding may be formulated by a hospital dietary department and should have a milk and meat base. The caloric strength can be varied from ¾ to 1½ calories/ml. If caloric requirements cannot be met by oral intake and gastric tube feeding, IV nutrition may be instituted using 10% Intralipid by a peripheral vein or 25% glucose by a central venous catheter. Both of these IV caloric substrates should be supplemented with 5% amino acid solution as a nitrogen source. The average caloric expenditure between the first and third weeks of burn management from this study is illustrated in Fig. 34-9. These charts can be used to estimate caloric expenditure based on total body surface burn or, better, on percent of full-thickness burn.[11]

Maintaining good nutrition, particularly positive caloric and nitrogen balance, is essential in achieving survival and satisfactory healing in all extensively burned patients. Appetite is poor in burn patients, and almost every patient with

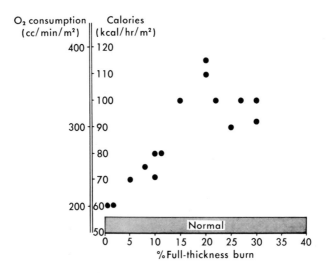

Fig. 34-9. Caloric expenditure vs full-thickness burn.

burn covering 50% or more of total body surface will require tube feedings.

■ What changes in coagulation and platelet mechanisms may be anticipated in the burn patient?

Extensive changes in coagulation and platelet mechanisms occur in burn patients. These changes were not widely recognized and were incompletely studied until recently. In a recent report[12] detailed studies of coagulation, platelet count and function, and fibrinolysis were made in 11 extensively burned patients.

Hemostasis is normally accomplished by a series of enzyme reactions involving the soluble protein clotting factors and ending in the formation of fibrin, as well as the adhesion and aggregation of platelets, forming a platelet plug. Fibrin clots contain plasminogen, which becomes activated to plasmin, a fibrinolytic enzyme, and destroys fibrin, resulting in fibrin degradation products (FDP). Partial thromboplastin time, prothrombin time, and thrombin time are screening tests that cover clotting factors I to XII. The changes that occur in clotting factors after burn injury with colloid resuscitation include a drop in clotting factor level (manifested as a rise in screening test time) occurring during the first 24 to 48 hours following burn injury. This is primarily caused by dilution with the fluid used for resuscitation. Factor VIII is manufactured by the liver in response to stress, and its level rises during this period. The clotting factors gradually increase thereafter, reaching normal or supernormal levels associated with shorter screening test times, so that the burn patient exhibits hypercoagulable signs between the second and fourth weeks following burn. The drop in clotting factors does not reach clinically significant levels in these patients. Fibrinolysin (plasminogen-plasmin) activity is not elevated in burn patients, and FDP levels remain normal (essentially absent) throughout the course of burn injury.

The most significant changes occur in platelet count and function, as shown in Fig. 34-10. Platelet count drops following burn injury, partly as a result of dilution and partly from other mechanisms that remain to be determined. The platelet count reaches the lowest level on the second or third day following burn and is associated with platelet malfunction (thrombocytopathia) at the same time. Any surgical procedure carried out during this time may encounter severe bleeding typical of thrombocytopenia and thrombocyto-

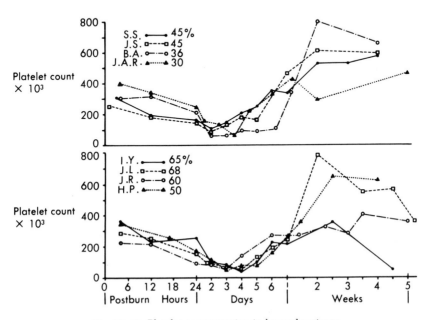

Fig. 34-10. Platelet concentration in burned patients.

pathia, that is, gradual continued oozing that stops with cautery or direct pressure and starts again within an hour and is unresponsive to further mechanical efforts at control. This type of bleeding can cause exsanguinating hemorrhage but is misleading because of the slow continuous oozing nature of the bleeding. When this type of bleeding occurs, it must be treated with platelet concentrates or fresh blood with active platelets. Platelet count returns to normal by the end of the first week and is above normal from the second to the fifth week following burn injury.

Hence if surgical procedures are required early in the course of management, they should be done within the first 24 hours, if possible, or delayed until the platelet count has begun to rise. Rising platelet count is associated with a return of normal platelet function. The use of fresh-frozen plasma, vitamin K, or other efforts aimed at supporting clotting factors are unnecessary maneuvers. Since there is no evidence of consumption coagulopathy as such, heparin therapy is contraindicated. During the late healing phase and at the time of grafting the patient's blood is truly hypercoagulable; granulating beds that are debrided are commonly seen to clot very promptly. Thromboembolic phenomena, however, are exceedingly rare in burn patients. The mechanism of thrombocytopenia and the role of platelet-active drugs in the prevention of thrombocytopenia are under investigation. If gram-negative septicemia occurs in a burn patient, thrombocytopenia will result, and this is a good guide to sepsis. One patient in the series mentioned previously developed thrombocytopenia associated with *Klebsiella* septicemia from a septic thrombophlebitis. This is also the only patient (I. Y.) who showed a delayed drop in platelet count in Fig. 34-10.

Thrombocytopenia per se should not be treated unless associated with significant bleeding. The prophylactic administration of platelets simply because the count is low is not indicated and is in fact contraindicated, as platelet antibodies may develop.

Blood transfusion is required frequently in the management of burn patients, particularly when active surface eschar excision is carried out. The average requirement of a patient burned over 50% of the body is 10 to 20 units of blood during hospitalization.

■ **What should be known about immunology and reticuloendothelial function in the burn patient?**

Host defense mechanisms against bacteria, fungus, or viral infection must be maintained in the burn patient. Reticuloendothelial function, including phagocytosis, bacterial clearance, and bacterial killing by circulating white cells and tissue histiocytes, has been extensively studied in burn patients. Severe leukocytosis in the range of 20,000 to 50,000/mm^3 (primarily with polymorphonuclear leukocytes and monocytes) is common in extensively burned patients.

Serum immunologic factors follow patterns similar to serum clotting factors, with initial depression followed by return to normal and maintenance of normal or slightly elevated levels throughout the course of treatment. This includes the study of immunoglobulins, complement, and antibody responses. Cellular immunologic responses in the form of lymphocyte physiology have been studied by Munster and associates[14] and others. They show a predominance of β-lymphocytes following burn injury with significant alteration in cellular immunity.

The supplementation of immune responses by bacterial vaccines or passive immunization with hyperimmune serum has been extensively investigated in burn patients, particularly with regard to *Pseudomonas aeruginosa.*[15] This line of investigation has not been pursued in the Orange County Medical Center burn unit, as septicemia is exceedingly rare (three to four instances per year) and is usually associated with diverse organisms among which no particular endemic strain predominates. In fact, studies related to sepsis in general, rare new opportunistic organisms, methods of surface bacterial counting, wound biopsy, and control of surface sepsis with biologic dressings have all been unnecessary, because surface infection and systemic infection simply do not occur. This is primarily the result of maintaining adequate nutrition, as mentioned previously, and maintaining a clean burn surface, as mentioned subsequently.

■ **What gastrointestinal management modalities should be considered?**

Patients with extensive burns develop ileus for the first day or two following burn injury, and a nasogastric tube should be utilized with all burn patients for gastric suction during this time. One or two hourly instillations of antacid may be carried out during the acute period, followed by the placement of antacid or food in the stomach at least every hour during the remainder of the course of extensively burned patients. As soon as peristalsis returns, as evidenced by active bowel sounds and passage of stool of flatus, feeding is begun, preferably directly by mouth or by nasogastric tube if the patient cannot eat. Occasionally ileus may complicate later phases of burn management, and this is managed by nasogastric suction. Rarely bleeding may occur from the gastric mucosa, which is evidenced by occult blood–positive gastric aspirate. Extensive bleeding should be unusual, and gastric bleeding requiring transfusion or operation is rare. In many adult burn units stress ulcer with burn injury (Curling's ulcer) is a common occurrence.[16] Lack of Curling's ulcer in some burn units may be associated with the frequent instillation of antacid or food into the stomach and the lack of sepsis. The best treatment for massively bleeding stress ulcers in other patients may be extensive subtotal or total gastrectomy.

Pancreatitis has complicated burn management in four patients at the Orange County Medical Center, all of whom were extensively burned patients with very deep burns. Pancreatitis has occurred late in the course of management and has been associated with deep muscle necrosis, ileus, and peritonitis. This complication was lethal in two of the four patients involved. The etiology is unknown. Pancreatitis should be considered in patients with extensive burn injury, ileus, and peritoneal findings.

■ What CNS and neuropsychiatric management modalities should be considered?

"Burn encephalopathy" has been described and is usually associated with sepsis, hypoxia, smoke inhalation, shock, or hyponatremia. A toxin in burned skin has been described that may alter brain capillary permeability.[17] Abnormal CNS function is common in major burn patients and ranges from confusion and disorientation to stupor, seizures, and coma. This encephalopathy is usually not associated with septicemia and the exact cause is unknown. This metabolic enceph-

alopathy is totally reversible and essentially never leaves organic sequelae.

Reversible peripheral neuropathies have been reported following burn injury, and muscle weakness is a common complaint. Weakness usually occurs in directly burned and grafted areas; the exact cause is difficult to delineate.

Psychiatric and psychologic management plays a major part in burn patient care. Many burn patients have psychologic disorders before burn injury, in fact, causing burn injury. These include senility, chronic brain syndrome, alcoholism and its sequelae, drug abuse and its sequelae, and a variety of personality disorders. If the patient was not psychologically disturbed before burn injury, he may become so, particularly if the burn will be disabling or severely disfiguring. Every effort should be made to treat the burn patient as capable of total rehabilitation. Burn scars should be freely discussed but minimized, and the patient should be assured that reconstructive procedures will make the appearance acceptable. At the same time every patient should be cautioned that every burned area will result in scarring; his adjustment to this fact must begin early in the course of management. All the staff involved with the care of burn patients should be encouraged to participate in the psychologic care from the time of admission, primarily by this type of prophylaxis. The help of a psychiatrist is rarely necessary but extremely valuable on occasion.

SURFACE MANAGEMENT
■ What surface management is recommended?

During the first week of hospitalization the wound itself is of secondary importance to physiologic considerations. However, the essence of burn care revolves around burn wound management. An interest in topical antibiotics and the use of total exposure treatment in the last two decades has diverted attention from aggressive mechanical care of the burn wound. It is recommended that appropriate burn unit protocol include the following: vigorous daily cleaning of the burn surface in a hydrotherapy tank, direct débridement, and tangential excision of eschar at frequent intervals followed by semiocclusive dressings. Use of this type of surface management virtually eliminates burn wound sepsis so that patient isolation, precautionary procedures, and efforts at quantitating surface flora are unnecessary. As long as the surface is kept clean, the type of surface antibiotic used is relatively unimportant. The vehicle and ease of application become the major considerations. This type of surface management is continued until the entire burn surface is covered with healthy granulation tissue, at which time split-thickness skin grafting is done. This usually occurs 20 to 25 days after burn injury. Grafting may be done with a combination of postage stamp, mesh graft, and sheet graft techniques, and a 95% to 100% take may be expected with every grafting procedure.

The only satisfactory alternative method of surface care is immediate or early (first 5 days) excision of eschar down to viable tissue or fascia and immediate surface coverage either with autograft or skin substitute followed by autograft.[18] This approach has been evaluated from time to time, and it has been found to be a favorable one for only small burns (15% of body surface or less). Inadequate graft take (40% to 60%) in most early excisions merely results in a fresh wound that requires formation of granulation tissue before regrafting can be done. This results in no ultimate saving of time and the possible risks associated with a major operative procedure early in the patient's course. Satisfactory temporary skin coverage would make this surface management technique preferable to current methods. This method of surface care will become preferable when satisfactory skin substitutes are developed. Silicone membrane, homograft, and pigskin in this connection have all been found to be lacking.[19,20] The use of true skin transplantation (homograft associated with pharmacologic immune suppression) after early excision has been satisfactorily carried out by Burke[21] in a few massively burned pediatric patients. Further evaluation of this radical procedure and continued evaluation of skin substitutes will eventually lead to early excision and coverage as a method of choice. Specific details in surface management protocol are outlined in Fig. 34-11.

Recommended protocol involves open wards without isolation precautions, cleaning and tubbing in water and hypochlorite solution carried

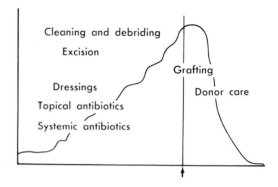

Fig. 34-11. Surface management.

out every day and pursued to the point of documented sterility after tubbing each day, excision of eschar beginning as soon as the platelet count is adequate and continued until a satisfactory granulating wound is obtained, and closed wounds with occlusive dressing using topical antibiotic cream, permitting the total mobility of patients.

Open wards

The philosophy of open wards is possible because of adequate surface management and is very important in the physiologic and psychologic care of the patient. The only precautions are covering of street clothes with a gown when entering the burn unit and washing of hands between caring for each patient when the patients or bedside accoutrements are handled.

Cleaning

Cleaning of the surface must be carried out at 24-hour intervals to be effective. Bacteria multiply in a logarithmic fashion and may reach levels capable of invasive infection if the surface is allowed to go more than 24 hours without vigorous cleaning and antiseptics. The burn surface is cleaned by immersion in water containing sodium hypochlorite solution (Clorox, in a ratio of 1:300 units of water). This amount of hypochlorite corresponds to 1 gallon per Hubbard tank, ½ gallon per small tank, or one glass per bathtub or large bucket. The hypochlorite destroys the bacteria it contacts and also coagulates proteins on the surface to facilitate cleaning and removal. After immersion in the warm hypochlorite tub for 10 to 20 minutes, the surface should be actively cleaned by scrubbing with a soft cloth using Betadine solution. The surface should be cleaned until all protein exudate has been removed from the surface, and eschar, debrided deep dermal or fat tissue, or granulation tissue is exposed. This is commonly associated with a small amount of bleeding. Loose necrotic tissue, if present, should be removed by sharp débridement; this may be done without anesthesia but does require heavy narcotic dosage on a daily basis. Every patient should be cleaned in this fashion every day, regardless of the extent of the burn. Rarely, a massively burned patient or smoke inhalation patient with unstable pulmonary or hemodynamic status may be cleaned in bed, but this is difficult. Patients should be submerged in the hypochlorite tub with central venous catheters, fresh incision, all manner of open wounds, fractures, chest tubes, arterial catheters, tracheostomy wounds, and so on. It is interesting that osteomyelitis associated with the presence of skeletal pins and wound infection in fresh operative sites are virtually absent with this surface cleaning protocol.

Excision of eschar

The excision of eschar should be begun as soon as adequate platelet count and function is assured (beginning on the fifth or sixth day following the burn) and carried out every 3 to 4 days until a satisfactory granulation surface is present. Excision may be carried out tangentially using hand-held dermatomes of the Weck, Goulian, or Campbell grafting knife variety. The first excision may be done without anesthesia and carried to the point of pain or bleeding. This is partly therapeutic but primarily diagnostic to identify areas of second- and third-degree burn. Major débridement is associated with bleeding and is never begun until a solid IV line is in place and blood is available.

Following this initial débridement, subsequent excisions may be carried out utilizing IM ketamine anesthesia in a dose of 3 to 4 mg/kg. *Ketamine* has greatly facilitated burn management and is used extensively. Gag and cough reflexes are preserved with ketamine anesthesia, the patient is semiresponsive, excessive muscle tone and posturing result, maintaining normal body temperature, and the drug can be administered to patients in the tub in any position. Over 1000 doses of ketamine anesthetic have been administered in this fashion to burn patients at University of California Irvine Medical Center with no significant physiologic complications. Psychologic complications in the form of "bad trips" or frightening nightmares occurred in 16% of patients initially. This has decreased to approximately 5% with the extensive use of diazepam (Valium) during induction and during emergence from ketamine anesthesia.

The tangential excision may be carried out in vigorous fashion down to fat or fascia where necessary, limited by the appearance of viability and bleeding. Major bleeding may be controlled with electrocautery carried out simultaneously with the débridement. Total hemostasis with cautery must be achieved before surface dressings are applied. The only significant complications that have followed this type of management have been those related to the underestimation of bleeding, causing hypovolemia with shock requiring fluid and blood transfusion for resuscitation.

Closed wounds

Closed wounds may be achieved by the application of topical antibiotic cream dressings after tubbing. Dressing may be carried out by burn unit critical care staff. Antibiotic cream impregnated into fine-mesh gauze rolls should be applied to the surface. Supplemental antibiotic cream may be added to the surface lightly and the entire dressing held in place with an elastic netting (Surgifix) dressing. Care must be taken to avoid circumferential wrapping, particularly in the early phase, when edema is present. These techniques are illustrated in Fig. 34-12.

After dressings are applied patients should be encouraged to be up and around. Any patient who is satisfactorily ambulatory may be discharged home to return at 24-hour intervals for cleaning, tubbing, débridement, and redressing until the time of grafting. Burns covering up to 40% of the body may be primarily managed on an outpatient basis unless significant pulmonary,

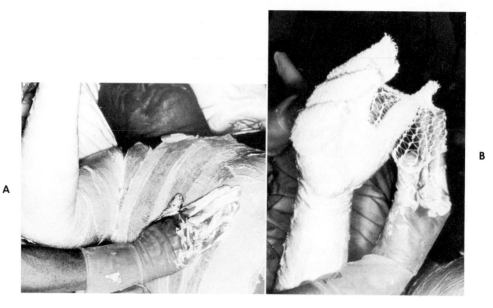

Fig. 34-12. Dressing technique.

nutritional, metabolic, or social complications do not permit this management.

The type of topical antibiotic is not particularly important from a bacteriologic point of view as long as the surface is vigorously cleaned daily. Consequently, the material that has the best application characteristics without pain and is the most economical is the favored material. At present this is *silver sulfadiazine* (Silvadene), a hydrophilic cream containing 1% silver sulfadiazine that has good bactericidal properties and is not painful on application. Mafenide acetate (Sulfamylon Cream) has equal bactericidal properties and ease of applicability, but it is associated with a burning pain on application and may cause mild metabolic acidosis by carbonic anhydrase inhibition. The 1% *sodium sulfadiazine* solution may be prepared in the pharmacy and has good working characteristics and an adequate bactericidal activity, although it is not as good as silver sulfadiazine in this regard. Consequently, sodium sulfadiazine is recommended for use in small burns, on an outpatient basis, or in the treatment of major burns with open areas after grafting. Silver sulfadiazine and sodium sulfadiazine are virtually free of complications. Although skin sen-

sitivity and rash have been reported, this has been observed in only three cases. *Candida albicans* and *Staphylococcus aureus* are commonly cultured from the surface in small amounts in patients treated with silver sulfadiazine. Gramnegative organisms are also found in patients treated with sodium sulfadiazine. This topical colonizing flora is insignificant, does not cause invasive infection, and is not specifically treated until the time of grafting.

Betadine ointment has good bactericidal properties and causes mild burning on application but is in a gel base that is difficult to manage. It becomes liquid at body temperature and runs freely from the surface, staining linen and personnel. *Neosporin* has caused deafness in some patients and should not be used for topical burn care. *Furacin* is readily available, painless on application, and moderately inexpensive. It is associated with a 10% to 30% skin sensitivity and is not recommended for use for that reason. The use of *0.5% silver nitrate solution,* reapplied frequently to gauze dressings, has been practiced in many institutions. This is an excellent bactericidal agent but forms a black silver chloride precipitate on virtually all surfaces with which it comes in

Table 34-2. Topical antibiotic preparations

Preparation	Cost*
Mafenide (Sulfamylon Cream)—4 oz tube	$ 4.84
Silver sulfadiazine (Silvadene) in 400 g jar	$17.44
Betadine ointment in 454 g jar	$13.32
Furacin ointment—5 pounds	$40.20
Neosporin in 15 g tube†	$ 1.20
Neosporin G in 15 g tube†	$ 1.70

*1980 prices.
†Not used for large burns.

contact. Consequently, it is unpopular as a topical agent. Use of this material may be associated with marked electrolyte abnormalities. A comparison of various antibiotic preparations is shown in Table 34-2.

■ How is a granulating wound managed?

After eschar is removed granulation tissue begins to form on the surface. Commonly a period of several days exists wherein healthy granulation tissue is present, associated with remnants of eschar, coagulated dermis, exposed muscle, bone, tendon, or fat. During this time the granulation tissue may be managed with a topical antibiotic dressing along with the rest of the surface, as described previously. This keeps the granulation area clean and free from invasive infection. The surface will remain healthy if nutrition is good. Skin grafting may be carried out when the entire surface is ready. The use of human homograft skin,[22] banked frozen homograft skin,[23] fresh xenograft (pig) skin, and frozen radiated banked xenograft skin[24] is advocated in many other centers. All these techniques of management of the granulating wound have been evaluated and found to be equal or inferior to the dressings previously outlined. Skin prostheses such as silicone rubber membrane and collagen membrane have been extensively evaluated and are not significantly better than gauze dressings alone. Eventually a skin prosthesis will be available that has good adherence and bactericidal properties. At that time this material will be the preferred management for granulating wounds.

The granulation tissue can be managed in this fashion for as long as 3 or 4 weeks if necessary. This is required only when a burn cannot be completely covered at the time of the initial grafting (burns greater than 40% of body surface area). Granulation tissue dressed in conventional fashion for longer than 1 month becomes progressively fibrotic associated with poor blood supply, a pale firm appearance, and a fascialike appearance when scraped and debrided. This "hypermature" granulation tissue can be avoided by periodic débridement of the granulation tissue by mechanical means or the use of topical 1% silver nitrate.

After skin grafting the areas of granulation tissue are commonly left between postage stamp grafts or interstices in mesh grafts. These areas may be managed by the techniques just outlined with daily vigorous removal of protein transudate from the surface.

■ What factors should be considered when grafting is required?

The philosophy of grafting techniques should be to achieve total autogenous skin coverage at the earliest possible time. This should be done in the interest of patient survival and may sometimes be done at the expense of late cosmetic results but never at the expense of functional result. For example, in a patient with third-degree burns of hands, face, and all of both legs, the legs would be grafted first to achieve surface coverage and survival, with hands and face taking second priority. With surface management as just outlined, grafting would usually be carried out between 20 and 25 days after the burn, permitting grafting of hands and face 1 to 2 weeks later. This policy does not result in severe disfigurement or disability problems. The postage stamp method used for most grafting results in a checkerboard appearance. In general, however, the cosmetic late results of stamp grafting compare favorably with sheet or mesh grafting and the advantages of the technique as outlined subsequently warrant its use.

After considering the priority of surface to be covered, the next consideration is to achieve the surface coverage rapidly. It is recommended that no more than 2 hours be spent in the operating room performing a grafting procedure (except for the hands or face, which may require longer). Approximately 30% to 40% of the body surface area may be covered with graft at a single sitting in 2 hours with an expectation that 95% to 100% will take in every patient.

■ How should donor sites be managed?

It is recommended that split-thickness skin graft ranging from 0.008 inch in small children to 0.012 inch in adults be used. These thin grafts promote good surface takes. Over hands and face thicker grafts may be used (up to 0.014). After skin is taken from the donor site the surface should be allowed to clot by exposure to air. Material to be applied to the donor site should be saturated with blood to allow fibrin to mesh into its surface. Clots should be gently wiped off and the donor site material (thin silicone membrane at present) applied to the surface. This may be held in place with tape if extensive turning is required. Donor site covers should be rolled where necessary to eliminate transudate. They should be left in place until the donor site heals and the material falls off spontaneously. If donor site coverages are rubbed off in the process of extensive turning and grafting, silicone membrane may be replaced or dressing with silver sulfadiazine instituted. Donor sites provide excellent models of partial skin damage and are commonly used for studies of topical agents or skin substitutes. Although infection in donor sites is extremely unusual, these sites should be treated with topical cleaning when it does occur. Donor sites heal well in 7 to 10 days regardless of the method of management. The major consideration in selecting a dressing for donor sites is to leave the patient mobile and free of pain. Silicone membrane has the best characteristics in this regard.

■ What operating room policies should be considered?

Every patient undergoing skin grafting should be tubbed in hypochlorite solution prior to going to the operating room. All hair-bearing skin in areas of potential donor sites should be shaved in the tub at the same time. The burns should be topically washed with Betadine and wrapped in moist towels.

In the operating room the following equipment is necessary for all burn grafting: heating blanket on the bed, temperature sensor in the patient, at least one good IV line for major grafting, and ECG monitoring. Ketamine anesthesia associated with diazepam (Valium) is recommended, and narcotics and nitrous oxide may be given at the discretion of the anesthesiologist. Endotracheal intubation is never necessary despite extensive turning and revision of position. Temperature must be followed carefully. Blood loss should be followed primarily by pulse rate or blood pressure where appropriate, although in many patients the blood pressure cannot be measured because of the lack of an available site. Often the task of an extensive grafting appears to be so massive that the novice surgeon is frozen into immobility. All members of the grafting team must be exhorted to continue to participate rapidly in the various procedures in order to achieve a short time for the patient to be under anesthesia.

After grafting is completed and the grafts are held in place with nylon netting or sutures, the patient may be returned directly to the burn unit. Grafts and/or donor sites on extremities should have topical pressure applied by firm Kerlix gauze wrapping immediately after grafting; this should be left in place overnight and carefully removed the next day. Wrapping should never be placed over unprotected graft or over hands or face, and wrapping is not practical on the trunk.

Extra donor skin that is removed in the operating room and not required for grafting should be placed in saline solution with antibiotics and refrigerated for possible future use. This skin may be used up to 1 week following grafting for application to granulating areas. In general the preservative solution is prepared with 1 g of cephalothin (Keflin)/L of saline solution.

■ How is late surface care managed?

After grafting, the mesh and sheet grafts should be cared for by frequent (every 4 hours) pressure with cotton-tipped applicators to eliminate any transudate or exudate. Grafts should be left exposed to the air during this period. Collections under grafts should be aspirated or removed through small incisions. Sheet grafts and mesh grafts should be left exposed at all times except on those rare occasions when stents are used, in which case the grafts should be left exposed beginning 48 hours after grafting. Rolling and cleaning of the surface by the critical care unit staff should be carried out until the grafts are firmly adherent (3 to 5 days). On the third or fourth day the patient may be gently dipped in the hypochlorite tub without vigorous cleaning. On the fifth day all netting and rubber covers may be gently removed. On the sixth or seventh day the use of closed dressings with silver or sodium sulfadiazine may be reinstituted if there are any open areas on the surface.

As soon as the surface is completely covered with skin, light gauze and elastic wraps may be applied to all grafts on extremities and mobility encouraged. When total surface coverage has been achieved, the patient should be measured for elastic pressure garments over grafted or healed second-degree burn areas. Elastic wraps should be continued until that time to maintain pressure on the burns, to mold collagen into a flat pattern, and to protect the delicate new epithelium.

The healed second-degree or grafted third-degree surface always itches and has varying degrees of pain. Itching may be treated with antihistamines (diphenhydramine [Benadryl] or hydroxyzine [Atarax]), and pain may usually be adequately treated by topical pressure. The healed surface always proceeds through a period of hypertrophy of scar with rapidly proliferating collagen and fibroblasts below the epithelium, resulting in a raised, erythematous, itchy, and hyperesthetic surface. This process continues for 4 to 6 months following the burn, then gradually regresses over the ensuing year as fibrosis eliminates the capillary bed in hypertrophic scar. Hypertrophic scarring can be minimized by topical application of pressure as outlined subsequently. All patients should be cautioned that hypertrophic scarring will inevitably occur. Resurfacing or reconstructive procedures are contraindicated until prompted by joint deformity or psychologic disability. The surface becomes dry very easily, and the patient should be advised to use lanolin ointment on the surface to maintain lubrication.

FUNCTIONAL MANAGEMENT
- **What functional management modalities should be considered?**

Cases in which the patient survives a major burn but becomes a physical or social cripple

should not occur. Proper functional management, as outlined in Fig. 34-13, will prevent this situation. Functional management in the acute phase is as essential a part of critical care as physiologic monitoring or surface cleaning.

Prophylaxis

Joint function. The prevention of contracture deformity requires meticulous attention to detail. Characteristically the burn patient attempts to maintain a fetal-like position, one of flexion and adduction. This position must be assiduously avoided, as it leads to contracture. The major concern is with those patients who have burns that cross the flexor surface of the joint or that are lateral to this surface. Efforts toward preventing disabling contractures should begin on admission to the burn unit with proper positioning and splinting.

Hand. Splints should be fabricated and applied, even if the patient's fingers have been pinned.

Elbows. Elbows should be placed in full extension and supination. If this position is difficult to maintain, extension splints may be necessary.

Neck. Deformities of the neck are severely disabling and great care should be taken to prevent such contractures. The neck should be positioned in hyperextension. *No pillows should be used!* A crib mattress placed on top of a regular mattress with the head over the edge of the crib mattress is a good method for positioning. An isoprene neck conformer may be fabricated and applied as soon as the edema decreases. This device should be worn essentially 24 hours each day.

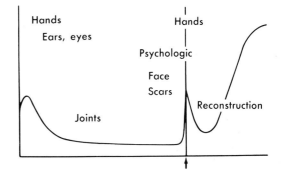

Fig. 34-13. Functional management.

Axilla. The patient should be positioned with the arms in 90 degrees of abduction. If this position is difficult to maintain, elbow splints will assist.

Hips. The lower extremities should be placed in full extension with the legs abducted approximately 15 degrees to prevent dislocation at the hip and flexion contractures. The prone position is excellent if the patient can tolerate it.

Feet. The feet should be held in 90 degrees of flexion to prevent heel cord shortening. This position may be maintained by using a footboard or posterior splints.

■ **How often should exercise of the range of motion be employed?**

Maintaining joint range of motion in the burn patient is a prime concern, as any limitation will affect the patient's ultimate functional level. Each joint should be taken through the complete range of motion at least once daily. If the patient is responsive, he should be taught self-ranging. If any loss of range is observed, the occupational therapist should be notified so that corrective measures can be taken before the contracture becomes established. The hand is an exception to this procedure. If the burn is second-degree or less, full range of motion is encouraged. If the patient has third-degree burns crossing the dorsum of the hand, extreme flexion may damage the extensor hood mechanisms and should be used with caution.

On healing of second-degree burns the patient should be encouraged to move as much as possible. Early attention to self-care needs such as feeding and hygiene should be encouraged. Splinting devices should be applied mainly at night to maintain the proper functional position, and the patient should be involved in active exercise during the day.

■ **How are grafting and skeletal traction managed?**

If pins are used in the wrist for positioning after grafting, wrist flexion should be avoided, as this results in mechanical hyperextension of the metacarpophalangeal joints and flexion of the proximal interphalangeal joints. The patient (while in traction) should be taught isotonic exer-

cises to prevent loss of muscle bulk and weakness.

■ **What techniques may be employed in post-grafting functional management?**

The goal of the entire burn team should be to assist the patient in reaching the highest possible functional level.

Pressure and collagen molding

Collagen molding in the healing burn by the application of continuous pressure can improve the ultimate appearance of healed or grafted burns. Two weeks after healing or grafting, the occupational therapist should measure the patient for pressure garments to cover all major burn areas. Once fitted, the patient should be instructed to wear the garment 24 hours each day. If additional pressure is indicated for specific areas of scarring, individually fitted isoprene inserts may be fabricated for placement under the garment. The patient should be encouraged to wear the pressure garments until the grafts have matured, approximately 1 year after the burn.

Prophylactic splints

Prophylactic splints may be used primarily as a precaution against contracture or to prevent recurrence of a contracture. These splints are usually worn at night for a length of time determined by the practitioner or therapist.

Active splints

Progressive splinting. Progressive splinting is a useful tool for improving range of motion when established contractures occur. The splints may be fabricated from isoprene and applied directly to the flexor surface of the extremity. The progressive splinting process calls for continuous wearing of the splint from one therapy session to the next. The range of the splint is gradually increased on a daily basis until full range of motion is achieved.

Dynamic splints. Dynamic splints are splints that allow the patient to perform active motion. These splints are particularly helpful in reducing edema in the newly (after 5 days or more) grafted hand.

Exercise. After healing of second-degree burns

or grafting of third-degree burns, a vigorous exercise program should be initiated. The patient should be treated at least once daily with passive stretching and active and resistive exercise. Passive exercise must begin early after healing or grafting if functional use of the extremity is to be accomplished. Active exercise should be stressed, particularly in the activities of daily living. Resistive exercise should be given to prevent imbalance of muscle power and generalized weakness and as an assist for overcoming contractures. The patient should be encouraged to take an active role in the rehabilitative process. Each patient should be instructed in a home program and given written directions for exercise and splinting. By the time the patient is discharged from occupational therapy, he should be wearing the pressure garment as prescribed and should be reliably doing passive stretching and exercise as outlined by the therapist.

■ **What vocational rehabilitation assistance is available?**

Vocational rehabilitation should be available for those patients having difficulty returning to their former employment. The patient may be referred directly to the state department of vocational rehabilitation or may be referred to the occupational therapy department, who will contact a vocational counselor.

■ **What protocol for hand management should be employed?**

Prompt and early management of burned hands is required for a satisfactory functional result. As soon as the immediate physiologic needs have been met and stabilized, a hand management plan should be initiated. Usually the hand burn victim has an extensive total body burn. The dorsum of the hand is almost always involved, and this thin skin is easily destroyed, exposing and damaging extensor tendons and the dorsal hood. Palmar burns are unusual, and deformity from palmar burns is rare. Because of edema and extensive tendon exposure, the patient tends to keep the hands in metacarpophalangeal hyperextension, proximal interphalangeal flexion, and distal interphalangeal flexion. This position is most comfortable and is naturally assumed. It will lead to severe disability associated with extensor tendon rupture and boutonnière deformity if not quickly managed.

Principles of management require *proximal interphalangeal and distal interphalangeal joint fixation in extension* to prevent extensor tendon rupture with *metacarpophalangeal joint motion*, including a full 90 degrees of flexion to stretch the metacarpophalangeal collateral ligaments. This is usually accomplished by simple elevation, active and passive motion, and anti-claw splints. The patient with obvious third-degree burns of the hand and arm is treated according to the protocol outlined by Achauer et al.[25]

SUMMARY

The physiologic management principles in the acute burn patient are the same principles that apply to any generalized or localized capillary leak syndrome (pancreatitis, peritonitis, anaphylaxis, portal vein thrombosis, and so on). Careful cardiac and pulmonary monitoring and therapy are essential. Equally important are surface management and functional management. These modalities are often not considered part of critical care or the duty of the burn practitioner. These *are* responsibilities of the critical care physicians, nurses, and allied team members and are of the most critical nature and must not be neglected.

REFERENCES

1. Moore, F. D.: The body weight burn budget—basic fluid therapy for the early burn, Surg. Clin. North Am. **50:**1249, 1970.
2. Monafo, W. W., Chuntrasakul, C., and Ayvazian, V. H.: Hypertonic sodium solutions in the treatment of burn shock, Am. J. Surg. **126:**778, 1973.
3. Moylan, J. A., Jr., Reckler, J. M., and Mason, A. D., Jr.: Hypertonic lactate saline resuscitation in thermal injury, Surg. Forum **22:**49, 1971.
4. Baxter, C. R.: Fluid therapy of burns, sixth national burn seminar, J. Trauma **7:**69, 1967.
5. German, J. C., Allyn, P. A., and Bartlett, R. H.: Pulmonary artery pressure monitoring in acute burn management, Arch. Surg. **106:**788, 1973.
6. Bartlett, R. H., Gentle, D. E., Allyn, P. A., Nitta, D. E., and Quasha, A.: Hemodialysis in the management of massive burns, Trans. Am. Soc. Artif. Intern. Organs **19:**269, 1973.
7. Achauer, B. M., et al.: Pulmonary complications of burns: the major threat to the burn patient, Ann. Surg. **177:**311, 1973.
8. Zikria, B. A., Ferrer, J. M., and Floch, H. F.: The chemical factors contributing to pulmonary damage in smoke poisoning, Surgery **71:**704, 1972.

9. Gump, F., and Kinney, J. M.: Caloric and fluid losses through the burn wound, Surg. Clin. North Am. **50:**1235, 1970.
10. Zawacki, B. E.: The microcirculation of skin after burning: its relation to tissue edema and viability, sixth annual meeting of the American Burn Association, Cincinnati, Ohio, 1974.
11. Bartlett, R. H., Allyn, P. A., Geraghty, T., and Wetmore, N.: Nutritional management based on oxygen consumption and caloric balance measurements, sixth annual meeting of the American Burn Association, Cincinnati, Ohio, 1974.
12. Bartlett, R. H., et al.: Changes in coagulation and platelet function following burn injury, sixth annual meeting of the American Burn Association, Cincinnati, Ohio, 1974.
13. Bartlett, R. H., and Allyn, P. A.: Pulmonary management of the burned patient, Heart Lung **2:**714, 1973.
14. Munster, A., et al.: Cell-mediated immunity after thermal injury, Ann. Surg. **177:**139, 1973.
15. Alexander, J. W., et al.: Prevention of invasive *Pseudomonas* infection in burns with a new vaccine, Arch. Surg. **99:**249, 1969.
16. Artz, C. P.: Curling ulcer, annual report, Ft. Sam Houston, Texas, 1954, Brooke Army Medical Center, Surgical Research Unit.
17. Allgower, M., et al.: Study of burn toxins, Ann. N.Y. Acad. Sci. **150:**807, 1968.
18. Haynes, B. W., Jr.: Early excision and grafting in third degree burns, Ann. Surg. **169:**736, 1969.
19. German, J. C., Wooley, T. E., Achauer, B., Furnas, D. W., and Bartlett, R. H.: Porcine xenograft burn dressings—a critical reappraisal, Arch. Surg. **104:**806, 1972.
20. Tavis, M., Harney, J., Thornton, J., Woodruff, A., and Bartlett, R. H.: Modified collagen membrane as a skin substitute: preliminary studies, sixth annual meeting of the American Burn Association, Cincinnati, Ohio, 1974.
21. Burke, J. F.: The use of skin transplantation and immunosuppression in the treatment of extensive full thickness thermal burns, fifth annual meeting of the American Burn Association, Dallas, Texas, 1973.
22. Shuck, J. M., Pruitt, B. A., Jr., and Moncrief, J. A.: Homograft skin for wound coverage, Arch. Surg. **98:**472, 1969.
23. Berggren, R. B., and Lehr, H. B.: Viability of frozen human skin, Mod. Med. **34:**134, 1966.
24. Rappaport, I., Pepino, A. T., and Dietrick, W.: Early use of xenografts as a biological dressing in burn trauma, Am. J. Surg. **120:**144, 1970.
25. Achauer, B. B., Bartlett, R. H., Furnas, D. W., Allyn, P. A., and Wingerson, E.: Internal fixation in the management of the burned hand, Arch. Surg. **108:**814, 1974.

BIBLIOGRAPHY

Artz, C. P., and Moncrief, J. A.: The treatment of burns, ed. 2, Philadelphia, 1969, W. B. Saunders Co.

Boswick, J. A., editor: The surgery of burns, Surg. Clin. North Am. **50:**entire issue, 1970.

Feller, I.: International bibliography on burns, Ann Arbor, Mich., 1969, American Burn Research Corporation.

Feller, I., and Archambeault, C.: Nursing the burned patient, Ann Arbor, Mich., 1973, Institute for Burn Medicine.

Furnas, D. W.: A bedside outline for the treatment of burns, Springfield, Ill., 1969, Charles C Thomas, Publisher.

Lynch, J. B., and Lewis, S. R.: Symposium on the treatment of burns, vol. 5, St. Louis, 1973, The C. V. Mosby Co.

Monafo, W. W.: The treatment of burns, St. Louis, 1971, Warren H. Green, Inc.

Moyer, C. A., and Butcher, H. R., Jr.: Burns, shock, and plasma volume regulation, St. Louis, 1967, The C. V. Mosby Co.

Polk, H. C., Jr., and Stone, H. H.: Contemporary burn management, Boston, 1971, Little, Brown & Co.

CHAPTER 35

Care of the neurologic patient

Harry Friedman

Many neurologic syndromes encountered in clinic or hospital practice do not reach the level of critical care requirements such that minute-to-minute observation is mandatory. Although many of these conditions progress inexorably to death, such as progressive degenerative processes, these disorders require little more than good custodial care. It is primarily in the areas of trauma to the brain, spinal cord, and contiguous structures, neoplasia, certain infectious-inflammatory processes, toxic states, and vascular disease that emergency situations arise that require decisive and aggressive approaches at all echelons of management. The purpose of this chapter is to point out those entities in neurologic-neurosurgical practice that may be encountered in the foregoing categories wherein the application of high standards of diagnostic skill and management, as well as quality critical care, must be exercised. The usual and some unusual complications will be mentioned. Diagnostic studies, including biochemical, neurophysiologic, and neuroradiologic studies, will be considered. The limitations as well as the usefulness of the lumbar puncture will be stressed. Diagnostic and therapeutic neuropharmacology will be mentioned.

Recognizing the importance of critical care, there will be sections dealing with general treatment measures as well as bedside critical care management in specific or unusual situations.

In enumerating those neurologic or neurosurgical conditions that could be classified as "true emergencies," the list would include acute bacterial meningitis, cerebral hemorrhage in its various forms, acute cerebrovascular occlusion, decompensation of the CNS in the presence of neoplasms, pituitary apoplexy, some forms of cerebral trauma such as depressed skull fractures, cerebral contusion, the various traumatic cerebral hemorrhages, spinal cord injury, status epilepticus, and certain intoxications. The cardinal signs of deterioration and usual means of management will be discussed.

TRAUMA
■ What are the general principles of treating the severely head-injured patient?

The focus of primary care should be on prevention of secondary CNS damage, since complications that follow such trauma can be more detrimental than the initial injury itself. The effect of injury to the brain consists of two parts: the initial injury with its direct effect on the brain and the subsequent metabolic and structural changes. The former includes the force of injury imparted directly to the brain with torsional or stretch effects. The latter consists of alterations in acid-base balance, changes in circulation, edema, and impairment of oxygen and glucose utilization through damage to enzyme systems. Current treatment methods can do little for the injury itself once it has occurred, but several treatment methods may ameliorate some of the aftereffects.

A thorough history and complete physical examination are of vital importance in predicting the patient's subsequent course. For example, different kinds of automobile accidents can produce different injuries depending on the direc-

Table 35-1. Signs associated with head injury and observations or treatment

Sign	Observation/treatment
Oculomotor or third cranial nerve paralysis resulting from direct injury; compression of nerve between the temporal lobe uncus and tentorium caused by hematoma or edema or kinking around posterior cerebral artery; most significant cranial nerve in indication of rising intracranial pressure	Observe briskness of reaction of pupil to light by checking each pupil individually with flashlight to measure direct, not consensual, reaction; darken room; approach laterally; check every 15 min at first. Observe changes in speed of reaction. Observe difference in size of pupils (ipsilateral dilation with third nerve compression). Report change in equality *immediately;* dilation with fixation is a late sign with a poor prognosis. Observe for other eye signs. While checking eyes, look for foreign bodies, including contact lenses, and remove, if possible.
Increased systolic pressure and/or widened pulse pressure and slow pulse caused by increased systole from attempt to transport sufficient oxygenation in face of rising intracranial pressure, pulse eventually slowing reflexly as blood pressure rises	Check blood pressure and pulse every 15 min at first. Lood for other injuries if blood pressure falls and pulse increases. Be sure airway is adequate for oxygenation, especially in presence of facial, neck, and chest injuries
Decreased movement, strength, and sensation in extremities resulting from lesion and/or increased pressure in cerebral hemisphere or brain stem, compression of motor fibers from midbrain to spinal cord against the tentorium, or spinal cord injury	Check every 15 min for spontaneous equal movement of all extremities. If an extremity does not move spontaneously, record type of stimuli, if any, that causes movement. Check for purposefulness of movements. Check strength and equality of handgrips; check for drift of outstretched arms. Observe for decorticate and decerebrate posture. (Decorticate posture involves abducted and rigidly flexed arms. Decerebrate posture is characterized by rigidly extended extremities, arched back, and toes turned inward.
Seizures resulting from direct trauma to cerebral tissues, cerebral edema, foreign bodies in brain, or hypoxia	Note beginning point, progression, and duration. Suction excessive saliva; stay with patient; protect the airway. Try to differentiate drowsiness and confusion of postictal state from progressive irritability and lethargy associated with increasing intracranial pressure.
Vomiting caused by increased intracranial pressure or swallowing blood, especially if food or alcohol was ingested just prior to accident	Observe vomiting, which may be projectile. Suction promptly; remove suction catheter from tubing and put tubing directly in mouth to remove large, undigested food particles that obstruct catheter. Turn patient to side to prevent aspiration; keep entire spine in straight alignment when turning. Pass nasogastric tube as ordered. Remove foreign bodies from mouth, including dentures. Look for sources of bleeding in mouth.
Restlessness resulting from rising intracranial pressure, pain, hypoxia, or urinary retention	Elevate head of bed 30 degrees unless contraindicated by shock; never put in Trendelenburg position. Avoid having bright lights on face continuously. Maintain a relatively quiet environment with few distractions. Make instructions to patient simple and understandable; avoid speaking in loud tones even if patient is loud and abusive. Check for distended bladder and catheterize, especially if abdominal trauma is suspected.

Table 35-1. Signs associated with head injury and observations or treatment—cont'd

Sign	Observation/treatment
	Restrain as needed; patient may require leather restraints. Improperly applied or excessive restraint can increase restlessness further. Only protective covering to keep patient from removing tubes and dressings may be needed and can be made by placing a folded washcloth in the palm of hand with finger surfaces separated and then wrapping a 3-inch elastic bandage around entire hand and up the arm about 6 inches. Tape securely; remove at least every 8 hours to check circulation to hands.
Cerebrospinal fluid leakage usually caused by disruption of mucous membranes in basilar skull fracture, primarily risking infection	Observe for clear drainage from nose and ears; bloody drainage that produces a relatively colorless halo around a spot of blood usually indicates the presence of cerebrospinal fluid leak (bull's eye sign).
	If drainage is excessive, use only a loose, dry sterile dressing.
	Use good hand washing technique.
	Do not suction nasally in presence of this drainage.
	Discourage nose blowing or sneezing. Cerebrospinal fluid produces a positive reaction on dextrose testing.

tion of impact to the head. Motorcycle and bicycle accidents may produce depressed skull fractures, whereas falls and diving accidents and those associated with a moving vehicle often result in spinal injuries.

Preexisting medical problems such as those seen in diabetes, cardiac disturbances, and epilepsy as well as alcoholic or drug ingestion frequently precipitate a fall, leading to serious head injuries. The seriousness of these injuries may be compounded by the chronic use of drugs such as anticoagulants. In these instances treatment of the preexisting problem should be undertaken simultaneously with the CNS injury evaluation.

The level of consciousness can be altered by other factors also, such as concurrent abdominal injury (ruptured spleen, contused kidney, lacerated liver, or perforated urinary bladder), causing a rapid or insidious blood loss that can seriously compromise the body's total circulating blood volume and the large amount of oxygenated blood required by the brain. *"Head injury alone does not cause shock."* Hypovolemia may cause hypoxia of the neuronal and support cells, further edema of the cerebral tissue, and loss of consciousness. Hypovolemia and hypoxia from chest injuries (pneumothorax, hemo-

thorax, or flail chest) can result in the same problem. In addition to causing a reduced level of consciousness, hypoxia causes restlessness that can contribute to a rise in intracranial pressure. One should also be alert to the possible development of adult respiratory distress syndrome ("shock lung"), which may accompany cerebral insults—especially trauma—either primarily or secondarily.

Head injuries are commonly accompanied by neck injuries, which should always be suspected until proved to be absent. High cervical cord, laryngeal, or tracheal damage may alter the level of consciousness. Since consciousness, or the patient's awareness of self and surroundings, is a result of total body function, the practitioner must always suspect and observe for associated conditions that may alter the patient's consciousness. It is important to assess the patient's orientation to time, place, and person. The head-injured patient should be aroused during normal sleeping hours and questioned regarding these three aspects as part of routine patient care and observation.

The neurologic signs listed in Table 35-1 are usually associated with changes in the patient's sensorium, and appropriate intervention is rec-

Table 35-2. Common drugs, dosages, and routes of administration used in the care of the head-injured patient

Drug	Dose	Route	Comments
Methylprednisolone	20-40 mg q 6 hr	IV, then IM	Dose tapered gradually as discontinued, or depot injection given day before termination of steroid if given for more than 3 days; antacid given with each dose to prevent gastrointestinal bleeding from stress or steroid; steroid used to decrease cerebral edema
Mannitol, 20%	30-50 ml/hr	IV	Diuretic to reduce extracellular fluid volume and decrease cerebral edema if hematoma is absent
Furosemide	40-80 mg 1 4-6 hr	IV	Cerebral diuretic
Phenobarbital	30-60 mg q 4 hr	IV, IM, or PO	Anticonvulsant; more rapid acting than phenytoin.
Diazepam	5-10 mg initially, then repeated every 30 min as needed	IV	Anticonvulsant for persistent unrelieved seizures; may be necessary initially until phenytoin level effective; patient observed for respiratory depression and depression of level of consciousness
Propoxyphene	32-65 mg q 3-4 hr as needed	PO	Analgesic
Acetaminophen	325-650 mg q 3-4 hr as needed	PO or PR	Analgesic, antipyretic
Acetylsalicylic acid	300-600 mg q 3-4 hr as needed	PO or PR	Analgesic, antipyretic
Codeine	30 mg q 3-4 hr as needed	IM or PO	Narcotic analgesic
Tetanus toxid	0.5 ml	IM	For active immunity
Human tetanus immune globulin (Hyper-Tet)	250-500 units	IM	For passive immunity

ommended. The usual pharmacologic preparations and dosages used in the care of the head-injured patient are outlined in Table 35-2.

Whether surgery is needed or not, several treatment modalities can be followed. The patient should be on the side or back with nasogastric drainage to prevent aspiration. The head of the bed should be elevated 30 degrees to enhance venous drainage from the brain. Oxygenation should be accomplished with a mask or binasal cannula. Intravenous fluid should be kept below 2 L every 24 hours. Steroid solutions using either methylprednisolone or dexamethasone may be given every 6 hours together with antacids either by nasogastric tube or in the form of IM injection of anticholinergic medication, for example glycopyrrolate or cimetidine IV. Because of the danger of adrenal suppression, tapering dosages of corti-

costeroids should be given, starting on the fourth or fifth day. Caution should be exercised in giving cerebral diuretics until the presence of an intracranial clot is ascertained, since pharmacologic decompression may precipitate further bleeding.

Currently being evaluated in the management of severe increased intracranial pressure is the use of high dose steroids, for example 500 mg to 1 g of methylprednisolone every 6 hours. It is too early to state if this will become a standard treatment but it appears promising.

The following factors related to nursing care should be considered: frequent turning and use of sheepskin, footboards, antiembolic stockings, and cardiac monitoring. In addition, periodic testing of electrolyte concentrations, arterial blood gas levels, glucose concentration, and blood urea nitrogen (BUN) should be performed. In-

Table 35-3. Classification of various types of acute head injuries and treatment

Anatomic location	Type of injury	Usual CNS signs or symptoms	Treatment
Skull	Linear fracture	Those of underlying brain injury	Observation if uncomplicated
	Depressed fracture	Same as linear fracture	Surgical decompression with brain débridement or hemorrhage evacuation as indicated
	Frontal basilar fracture	Cerebrospinal fluid rhinorrhea, periorbital ecchymoses, pneumocephalus	Elevation of head, antibiotics, surgical closure if rhinorrhea persists for more than 1 week or if recurrent episodes of meningitis occur
	Petrobasilar fracture	May be associated with CN VII and CN VIII dysfunction, otorhinorrhea, Battle's sign	Observation, possibly antibiotics
Meninges and their spaces	Epidural hemorrhage	"Lucid interval," progressive deterioration, ipsilateral dilated pupil, skull fractures crossing meningeal artery groove	Urgent decompression
	Dural laceration	Those of underlying brain injury, venous oozing (if compound injury) from lacerated dural sinus	Elevation of head and packing of wound, surgical débridement and closure
	Subdural hemorrhage	Those of underlying brain injury, progressive deterioration, may be acute or chronic	Evacuation of hemorrhage
	Subarachnoid hemorrhage	May be mild or severe depending on brain injury and presence or absence of associated arterial spasm	Observation if uncomplicated by collection of blood or other surgical CNS lesion
Brain	Concussion	Mild headache, nausea, vomiting, dizziness; no focal signs or unconsciousness	Observation
	Contusion	History of unconsciousness, transient focal signs, prolonged elevated intracranial pressure, possibly signs of severe focal damage with cerebral edema	Observation if mild or transient; steroids, hyperventilation, intracranial pressure monitoring, internal decompression if severe
	Laceration	As with contusion	Exploration and débridement if suspected; often an incidental finding during decompression
	Intracerebral hemorrhage	Usually associated with deepened consciousness and focal signs of damage	Evacuation of clot; if in frontal, occipital, or temporal lobe, subtotal lobectomy

dwelling bladder catheters should be avoided, if possible, to prevent cystitis and proximal urethral damage. Since fever is often present in head injuries, this should be treated with appropriate antipyretics. The indiscriminate use of antibiotics should be discouraged and should be reserved for use when clear indications of infection are present or imminent. A bowel regimen, including use of stool softeners and periodic enemas, should be instituted early. Early and frequent mobilization of joints and extremities will help prevent pressure sores, contractures, calcium loss, and negative nitrogen balance. In addition, this will help promote venous drainage and maintain muscle tone.

The onset of shock in the head-injured patient

demands that a search be made in other body cavities for its cause, since head injuries do not cause shock, as emphasized previously.

Table 35-3 summarizes the various head injuries and indicates appropriate treatment.

■ What ancillary diagnostic tests may be performed in the workup of the head-injured patient?

Skull x-ray films, including anteroposterior Towne and horizontal beam brow-up lateral views, should be obtained. The horizontal beam brow-up lateral view should be obtained rather than the often performed vertical beam lateral view with the patient's head rotated in the supine position, since a cervical spine fracture may be present associated with the head injury. Also, pneumocephalus sphenoid sinus fluids levels are easier to observe if the head is in the brow-up position. Stereoscopic lateral views help delineate the location and extent of fractures and/or foreign bodies such as indriven bone fragments and bullet paths.

Cervical spine x-ray films to show C7-T1 should be routinely performed in the head-injured patient for the reasons alluded to previously.

Computed axial tomography of the head is a radiologic technique that can very accurately locate lesions and may give a clue as to the nature of the lesion. Because location of hematomas and degree of brain shift can be so accurately determined by this study, it has supplanted arteriography as the study of choice in most neurosurgical centers when studying trauma.

In the absence of computerized tomographic equipment, assessment can still be performed by arteriography. Both sides of the head should be studied, either with bilateral injections of contrast material or by the cross-compression technique utilizing a single site injection. The patient who has not shown focal signs, who has not had asymmetric pupils (in the absence of orbital injury), and who is reasonably alert can usually be safely observed without having arteriography. The patient suffering a head injury who has asymmetric pupils should undergo exploratory surgery immediately without expending valuable time in performing diagnostic studies. The co-existence of orbital trauma should not deter immediate exploration, since severe intracranial trauma capable of producing a dilated pupil may be present.

Caloric irrigation of the external ear canals coupled with determination of doll's eye responses (oculocephalic reflex) may be helpful in determining the extent of brain stem injury.

Rating scales are coming into general use in an attempt to standardize treatment. These enable different groups to compare data more meaningfully. In addition they have some prognostic value. Two such scales are the Glasgow Coma Scale and the Ransohoff Scale.

■ What is the general plan for treating the comatose patient in the emergency room when no history is available?

1. Rapidly check airway, ventilation, and pulse; examine pupils, response to pain, and presence of focal neurologic signs; determine vital signs and external signs of trauma to head and the rest of the body including spine.
2. Provide airway and oxygen; endotracheal tube is preferred.
3. Draw blood for electrolyte, glucose, BUN, toxicology screening, arterial blood gas tests, and complete blood count.
4. Give by IV 50 ml of 50% glucose solution.
5. Obtain ECG.
6. Obtain x-ray films and CT scan.
7. Perform lumbar puncture after ascertaining that no mass effect is present on CT scan or arteriography.
8. Insert nasogastric tube.

■ What are some conditions that may cause increased intracranial pressure?

1. Cellular and/or vascular disease or injury, producing cerebral edema or bleeding
2. Space-occupying lesions
3. Obstruction of ventricular and cerebrospinal fluid pathways
4. Interference with venous drainage from intracranial cavity
5. Meningitis
6. Hypoxia, acute or chronic
7. Chronic obstructive pulmonary disease

■ **What are the signs and symptoms of increased intracranial pressure?**

1. Increasing headache with or without vomiting
2. Restlessness
3. Diminishing alertness and noticeable changes in the level of consciousness
4. Irregular pupils that may be dilated on the side of a hemorrhage
5. Decreased pulse rate
6. Decreased respirations (Periods of apnea may eventually occur.)
7. A gradual increase in blood pressure as extremes in pressure are reached
8. Possible weakness or paralysis on one side of the body
9. Convulsions
10. Increased cerebrospinal fluid pressure

■ **How is intracranial pressure monitored?**

There are two general methods of monitoring intracranial pressure: those using extracerebral techniques and those using intraventricular catheters. The extracerebral methods require placement of either a direct-reading subarachnoid screw or a transducer. The method of intraventricular cannulation not only permits direct reading but affords the opportunity of rapidly reducing pressure by simply draining off cerebrospinal fluid.

The critical care practitioner caring for the neurosurgical patient must make continuous, astute, intelligent observations and must also have the ability to interpret and record his or her observations in order that lifesaving measures may be instituted at the appropriate moment. Special charts for "neuro checks" for use by the nurse are in use in many intensive care units. Organ swelling (the result of fluid or mass) elsewhere in the body presents only modest implications; however, brain edema, hematoma formation, and progressive hydrocephalus threaten life itself. Irreversible damage may occur when nerve cells are rendered hypoxic, as when increased pressure is developing and impairing CNS circulation, since nerve cells cease functioning under such conditions.

Experience has shown that, despite all the space-age monitoring devices now available for use in critical care, close observation by the bedside practitioner of specific *body functions* serves as the best guide for assessing intracranial pressure. Some important areas of observation to be considered in the care of the seriously ill neurologic patient are consciousness, blood pressure and pulse, ocular signs, vomiting, weakness or paralysis, temperature, respiration, pain, and convulsion.

Consciousness

The practitioner should be aware that actual *squeezing of the brain* may occur as pressure builds up in the cranial cavity, especially if caused by a space-occupying lesion. As the intracranial pressure begins to increase, the patient may appear asymptomatic.

Diffuse compression may affect numerous brain regions, including the reticular formation. The result is that confusion, disorientation, and delerium are often observed during the early stages of increased intracranial pressure. Deep coma and other complications may follow unless early corrective measures are taken to decrease the pressure.

Blood pressure and pulse

One of the most reliable indications of rising intracranial pressure is pulse slowing, which reflexly occurs as extracranial carotid circulation encounters an abnormally elevated head of pressure in the intracranial circulation as a result of alterations in autoregulatory mechanisms. Blood pressure may rise, but this is usually a terminal event as autoregulation fails and the full head of blood pressure is transmitted into the arteriolar circulation.

Ocular signs

Normally the pupils are equal in size and react on response to light. The neurologically injured patient should be observed closely for changes in the pupils' size, equality, and reaction to light. Should an intracranial hemorrhage occur, a dilated, fixed pupil may be observed on the affected side; that is, it will not react on exposure to a light directed on the pupil. A fixed dilated pupil demands immediate determination of cause.

Funduscopic examination may reveal the

presence of subhyaloid or splinter hemorrhages, the former suggesting intracranial hemorrhage and the latter suggesting increasing intracranial pressure. Papilledema is rarely seen before 18 to 24 hours. If present, vision is usually unaffected.

Medial deviation of an eye may result from increased intracranial pressure causing traction on the sixth cranial nerve with resultant paresis of the lateral rectus muscle. Skew deviation of the eyes may be the result of cerebellar or brain stem compression.

Vomiting

Vomiting, sometimes projectile, is a common symptom of increased intracranial pressure; characteristics and frequency of all vomiting should be reported to the principal practitioner.

Since vomiting or strain of any kind, for example, while using the bedpan, should be avoided to prevent further increase in the pressure, the bedside practitioner should do everything possible to control vomiting, strain in defecation, or undue patient activity.

Weakness or paralysis

Progressive hemiparesis, spasms, and hypertonicity may be the result of compression of a hemisphere or of the brain stem. The first indication that progressive hemiparesis is impending may be a positive Babinski response (a fanning and dorsiflexion of the toes when the sole of the foot is stroked). This should be reported immediately to the principal practitioner.

Temperature

A hyperthermic condition will increase the patient's metabolic needs; therefore it is important that every measure be employed to avoid an increase in body temperature.

Respiration

The most important task that the bedside practitioner must carry out religiously is to maintain a clear airway. Increased intracranial pressure and hypoxia in the respiratory center of the medulla will result in respiratory changes. The hypoxia itself increases cerebral edema. The early signs of respiratory failure are irritability, anxiety,

and restlessness. The respiratory rate begins to rise and becomes shallow, the nares flare in and out, there is a decrease in the tidal volume and vital capacity (the use of bedside spirometric measurements is helpful), the pulse rate and blood pressure rise, sweating and cyanosis occur, and consciousness is lost. Again, the body's compensatory mechanisms come into play, and the accessory muscles of respiration work at an early stage; then the chest wall and abdomen cease to move. Snoring and stertorous respirations may be noted initially, followed by Cheyne-Stokes type respiration as progress toward death occurs. Altered respiratory states are extremely serious in the neurologic patient and immediate corrective action must be initiated if possible. The patient may require mouth-to-mouth respiration or intubation and mechanical ventilatory support until the increased intracranial pressure has been brought under control.

Pain

Since headache is a significant symptom of increasing intracranial pressure, it is important to record its location, duration, and severity.

Convulsion

Accurate observation and recording may provide vital information that will be useful in the treatment of the patient, since the type of seizures may indicate the area of the brain being focally irritated. The bedside practitioner should protect the patient (use of padded tongue blades, plastic airways, and *firm* padding of some kind to prevent the patient from self-harm as a result of falling against bed rails, and so on) and observe the seizure, noting kind; movements (clonic or tonic); duration; level of consciousness *preceding, during,* and *after* the seizure; when the seizure began to progress; and the direction of head and eye movement.

■ How is the patient with spinal injury handled?

Although opinion varies as to the definitive treatment of spinal fractures as far as time and type of surgery, certain points need to be stressed regarding early care. The patient should be immobilized in a supine position on a sheepskin or alternating pressure mattress. Stabilization of the head (with sandbags and a towel roll placed under the neck) should be instituted until definitive treatment is performed. The two-mattress bed technique or one of the turning type beds should be used for the patient with cervical spine injury in traction as well as other spinal fractures. Early tracheostomy may be necessary.

Patients with residual function in extremities can be managed on a regular bed with a trapeze bar attached. Constant catheterization is becoming less popular. Instead, intermittent catheterization to reduce infection and enhance bladder training is being recommended by urologists. Vital signs should be observed, especially in high spinal injuries because of the possible occurrence of vasomotor instability. In addition temperature-regulating mechanisms may be disturbed, resulting especially in the preservation of heat, for example, the lightest bedclothes may produce high rises in temperature. A bowel regimen should be instituted early, consisting of the administration of stool softeners, laxatives, and enemas, all on a regular schedule, to prevent impaction.

■ How are patients with malingering or hysterical brain or spinal cord injury detected?

All patients, regardless of the initial impression or the patient's past history, should be treated as if certain injury exists. In two areas, however, suspicion may be aroused; these are the apparently unconscious patient and the apparently paralyzed patient.

False unconsciousness may be suspected in an individual suffering an injury too minor to have produced unconsciousness and exhibiting fluttering or opening and closing of the eyelids. Catatonic posturing may be possible; for example, an extremity may maintain itself in a raised position. The patient may resist verbal commands or application of painful stimuli but may awaken quickly when ammonia is applied to the nostrils.

The state of hysterical spinal injury may be suspected when a nonanatomic sensory pattern is present, and no lesion may be localized on x-ray films. Caution must be used here, since a myelop-

athy may be produced in the absence of fracture. The application of painful stimuli will aid in exposing the hysterical or malingering state.

■ How is status epilepticus handled?

Phenytoin in the usual dosages for seizure disorder is generally ineffective because of its slow metabolism in the liver. However, 300 to 500 mg intravenously with careful observation of cardiac function may be helpful. Currently IV or IM phenobarbital, diazepam, or IV sodium amobarbital may be given according to the following schedule:

PHENOBARBITAL: Adult, 30 to 60 mg given by IM route every 4 to 6 hours, with 20 to 30 mg given by IV route slowly for the initial therapy

SODIUM AMOBARBITAL: Adult, 250 to 500 mg given by IV route every 4 hours, with drip of 1 g in 1 L of fluids to run 24 hours, then stop to allow patient to awaken; constant monitoring of vital signs is imperative

DIAZEPAM: Adult 5 to 10 mg given by IV route slowly or 5 to 10 mg given by IM route every 6 hours

PHENYTOIN: Adult, 100 mg given by IM or IV route to institute chronic treatment

CEREBROVASCULAR ACCIDENTS
■ How is the diagnosis of stroke made?

Stroke, or cerebrovascular accident (CVA), is manifest by the sudden appearance of symptoms referable to a particular vascular distribution after other cerebral catastrophes such as trauma, tumor, or abscess have been eliminated as possibilities. The latter is important, since mass lesions may be silent until they suddenly deteriorate; this is unusual, however, since a careful history will usually reveal that subtle symptoms have been present over a period of time. The cardinal sign of CVA is its suddenness in onset in the absence of prior deterioration. It may be manifest by either interruption of blood flow to an area by thrombosis or embolization or by hemorrhage, either intracerebral or subarachnoid.

Occlusion of the common carotid artery may produce a picture of total contralateral hemiparesis or hemiplegia; dysphasia or aphasia, if involving the dominant hemisphere; and contralateral visual field involvement. Cortical and deep sensory involvement may be present. A lesion in the area of the anterior cerebral artery may produce contralateral leg weakness and may include the contralateral face by involving the artery of Heubner proceeding to the face area of the internal capsule. Middle cerebral artery occlusion produces contralateral hemiparesis or hemiplegia involving mainly face and arm, speech difficulty if in the dominant hemisphere, and right-sided field deficits.

■ How is the patient with uncomplicated subarachnoid hemorrhage treated?

Early arteriography and lumbar puncture should verify the diagnosis of subarachnoid hemorrhage (SAH) and the location of the aneurysm, as well as the hemodynamic characteristics of the cerebral circulation around the aneurysm. For the patient who is to have a direct surgical approach to the aneurysm, it is best to delay surgery until the risk of spasm has passed. Meanwhile the patient is to maintain strict bedrest and quiet environment, lying flat in bed with nothing given rectally. Stool softeners should be given. Antihypertensive medication should be given for severe rises in blood pressure.

For an aneurysm of the internal carotid artery that is to be treated by common carotid artery gradual ligation, surgery can be carried out early using the same principles of care just outlined, which will continue to apply until complete occlusion is accomplished.

■ What are the usual causes of embolization to cerebral arteries?

Cerebral embolization arises from cardiac causes such as chronic atrial fibrillation, cardioversion-initiated or spontaneous fragmentation of mural thrombi (as from old myocardial infarction), fragmentation of valvular vegetations, parodoxical embolization through patent foramen ovale, and as a complication of cardiac surgery. Septic emboli may occur in cases of subacute bacterial endocarditis. Marantic emboli may occur when neoplastic cells pass a patent foramen ovale.

■ What is the medical treatment of stroke?

Adequate nutrition, oxygenation, and early rehabilitation of such patients are indicated. In acute stroke an adequate airway must be provided, and aspiration should be prevented. Nasal oxygenation to maintain a high Po_2 to the marginal areas of ischemia (too high a Po_2 may produce cerebral vasoconstriction) should be provided. A mixture of oxygen and carbon dioxide at about 6 L/min will provide the high Po_2 required plus a measure of vasodilatation to enhance flow. If the patient cannot swallow, IV nutrition may be given, but nasogastric feedings are more desirable, since the tube serves as a means of emptying the stomach between feedings, it necessary, to reduce the possibility of aspiration while providing a route of nutritional support not possible with conventional means of IV feeding. Anticoagulation should be considered for the patient with transient ischemic attacks, especially if an ulcerative plaque is observed on arteriogram. Also, the patient with brain stem ischemia should be considered for anticoagulation. Aqueous heparin in a dose of 4000 to 5000 units given by IV administration every 6 hours should be adequate. It should not be used if blood pressure is high (above 170 to 180 mm Hg systolic and/or above 110 mm Hg diastolic).

■ When is surgery indicated for stroke?

Surgical intervention in stroke depends on the manifestations of the stroke. There are three general areas for surgical intervention: carotid artery stenosis or occlusion, intracerebral hematoma, and cerebral aneurysm. These are discussed here in general terms. Acute occlusion of the extracranial portion of the carotid artery, if discovered within the first 6 to 8 hours, should be considered a possible indication for exploration. Waiting too long may predispose the patient to develop a hemorrhagic infarct in the area of ischemia. Also, the patient with transient ischemic attacks referable to a specific carotid stenosis should be considered for endarterectomy. Cerebral revascularization techniques are coming into use in some situations.

The patient who has suffered an intracerebral hematoma, especially of the nondominant hemisphere or the cerebellum, should be considered for early surgical removal of the clot. The same is true for the patient suffering an intracerebral hematoma from rupture of an intracranial aneurysm. Otherwise the subarachnoid hemorrhage patient should have a period of waiting before definitive surgery on the aneurysm should be considered, as noted previously.

■ How is cerebellar hemorrhage best managed?

Cerebellar hemorrhage is best handled by early surgical decompression. The diagnosis is made in a patient usually with a hypertensive history who develops sudden, severe headache with vomiting, unsteady gait, and other specific signs of cerebellar dysfunction. Ventriculography, arteriography, or computed axial tomography may support the diagnosis, but little time should be lost in performing decompression, since progression to the comatose and decerebrate state can occur quite rapidly. With a history and physical examination suggesting this picture, it is justifiable to operate without performing contrast studies, since the course may be rapid and irreversible and valuable time lost.

■ What are some of the neurologic complications of cardiovascular surgery?

The embolization of cholesterol plaques is the usual cause of neurologic dysfunction. Air and fibrin clot embolization from valves can occur. Also a hypercoagulable state may occur. There is recent evidence that fat embolization can occur after median sternotomy. Focal neurologic deficits may occur after carotid artery surgery because of the embolization of fibrin clots, incomplete plaque removal, improper shunt positioning, and intimal dissection with arterial occlusion. Paraplegia caused by intercostal artery interruption, especially of the great radicular artery of Adamkiewicz, may occur after aortic surgery.

■ What are the potential complications of common carotid artery ligation for aneurysm?

There are three potential sources of complications: ischemia, embolization, and carotid artery erosion. Ischemic symptoms, that is, focal deficits, may arise during the turning down of the clamp. This is treated by reopening the clamp. Embolization may occur near the completion of occlusion when a bruit appears, signaling tur-

bulence at the clamp site, or if the clamp has been placed too far distal from the carotid bifurcation. If embolization is suspected, immediate arteriotomy with evacuation of the clot is necessary.

Rarely a clamp erodes the artery. This may be signaled by slow swelling at the surgical site or a slow ooze of blood from the incision, or it may be catastrophic with a large gush of blood and rapid swelling. Direct pressure should be applied until the artery can be exposed and repaired. If rapid deterioration of the patient is imminent, then reopening the operative wound before reaching surgery to control bleeding may be necessary.

CNS INFECTIONS

■ What are the most common meningeal infecting agents in descending order of frequency, and what is the most effective antibiotic treatment of each?

1. Viral agents (enterovirus, mumps). Treatment is supportive in most cases, although cytosine arabinoside may be given in papovavirus infections.
2. *Neisseria meningitidis.* Pencillin G (adult, 20 million units/day), ampicillin (400 mg/ kg/day given by IV route in children 2 months of age or older), chloromycetin, or a sulfonamide may be given.
3. *Haemophilus influenzae* (in children 7 years of age or younger). Ampicillin (100 to 200 mg/kg/day) or chloramphenicol (50 to 100 mg/kg/day) is recommended.
4. *Diplococcus pneumoniae.* Penicillin G (20 million units/day) or erythromycin (1 to 4 g/day) may be administered.
5. *Streptococcus pyogenes* (groups A and B). Penicillin G or erythromycin is recommended.
6. *Escherichia coli* (or other gram-negative bacilli, especially in neonates and after neurosurgical procedures). A combination of ampicillin with gentamicin (6 mg/kg/ day) or kanamycin may be given. Cephalosporins are also useful. Gram-negative ventriculitis may be treated by a combination of intraventricular gentamicin and carbenicillin.
7. Coagulase-positive *Staphylococcus* (brain abscess, surgical infection). Penicillin G,

ampicillin, or methicillin (100 to 300 mg/kg/day) may be used.

8. *Mycobacterium tuberculosis.* Isoniazid (adult, 30 mg/kg/day), ethambutol (15 mg/kg/day), or streptomycin (adult, 1 g/day; children, 20 mg/kg/day) is effective. Pyridoxine should be given to patients taking isoniazid.

9. *Cryptococcus neoformans* and other fungi. Amphotericin B (adult, 1 to 2 g/day) is recommended.

10. *Listeria monocytogenes.* Ampicillin, streptomycin, or chloramphenicol may be given.

11. *Enterococcus* (in neonates). Penicillin G or ampicillin may be given.

12. *Treponema pallidum.* Penicillin G or tetracycline (20 mg/kg/day) is useful.

13. *Leptospira.* Penicillin G or tetracycline is the preferred treatment.

■ **What are the usual causes of brain abscess?**

Retained foreign bodies introduced by trauma such as depressed bone fragments, hair, clothing, and dirt form one group causing brain abscess. Another cause, although less likely, is abscess complicating meningitis associated with frontobasilar or petrobasilar skull fractures. Chronic purulent otitis media is associated with brain abscess. Metastatic abscess from another source of infection such as the pulmonary or cardiac system accounts for some brain abscesses.

Cerebral aneurysms may result from mycotic cardiac emboli and may lodge in the walls of cerebral arteries. They usually cause episodes of subarachnoid hemorrhage. Characteristically they are multiple and located in areas considered unusual for congenital aneurysms; that is, they are located along the smaller, more distal branches of the major cerebral circulations. Frequently subarachnoid hemorrhage is the first clinical manifestation of subacute bacterial endocarditis. Furthermore the patient who demonstrates low-grade fever with the appearance of a diastolic murmur, or splinter, or petechial hemorrhage with neurologic deterioration may have either cerebral abscess or cerebral mycotic aneurysm.

■ **How may the patient who has focal neurologic deficits and purulent discharge from the ear be best managed?**

A careful neurologic history and examination should be performed to determine the duration of the suspected cerebral lesion and whether it is located in the cerebellum or temporal lobe, the two most likely locations of focal cerebritis or abscess resulting from chronic purulent otitis. Temporal lobe abscess usually produces contralateral hemiparesis, dysphasia if in the dominant hemisphere, and occasionally visual field impairment along with papilledema. Cerebellar abscess usually produces ipsilateral dystaxia, dysmetria, and nystagmus on the side of the lesion. One must be careful not to confuse unsteadiness with hemiparesis.

Following this drainage, material is sampled for culture and sensitivity, and the patient is given large doses of antibiotics, following which cerebral arteriography or computed tomography is performed to help delineate the location of the lesion. The otolaryngologist will then perform a mastoidectomy to institute drainage. Immediately after this the neurosurgeon should carry out the appropriate procedure, either excision of the abscess or aspiration and drainage. If it is determined that the cerebral lesion is focal cerebritis rather than abscess, the administration of large doses of IV antibiotics is the treatment of choice until the cerebritis resolves or an abscess finally walls off. If the latter occurs, the appropriate neurosurgical procedure should be instituted.

Early drainage of the otitis is required to prevent sepsis and to enhance recovery from the subsequent craniotomy, particularly if only a drainage procedure is performed, since continuing bacterial contamination will probably produce continuing infection. Furthermore, sudden rapid neurologic deterioration can occur as a result of cerebral edema, increased intracranial pressure, or subdural or intraventricular rupture of the abscess.

■ **What are some of the acute and chronic complications of meningitis?**

Focal or generalized convulsive seizures are commonly seen and may actually be the initial symptoms. Generalized sepsis may occur and, particularly in meningococcal meningitis, the Waterhouse-Friderichsen syndrome (WFS) with adrenal and circulatory collapse can occur. WFS may actually be a manifestation of disseminated intravascular coagulopathy with the adrenal dysfunction being a secondary, not a primary, phenomenon. It is thought that the adrenal gland may suffer ischemic changes as a result of platelet aggregations and thus, in part at least, produce the systemic deterioration characteristic of WFS.

Chronic complications include cerebral or subdural abscess, usually from late or incomplete therapy. Normal pressure hydrocephalus is occasionally seen as a late effect caused either by blockage of the cerebrospinal fluid outflow at the aqueduct or absorption over the vertebral convexity at the pacchionian granulations.

■ **What are some important facets of infectious polyneuritis?**

Infectious polyneuritis is best known as the Guillain-Barré syndrome and is often considered to be a true medical emergency.

If the course of the disease indicates a rapidly ascending paralysis, mechanical ventilation may be indicated, and preparation for a possible tracheostomy should be carried out. Special bedside care may be required to observe and record the patient's progress properly. Bulbar signs such as hoarseness, choking, or respiration by accessory muscles indicate that mechanical ventilation may be imminently necessary.

The prominent sign is a bilateral facial palsy. Other symptoms besides paralysis include painful tactile and thermal hyperesthesia, usually aural in distribution, or hypoesthesias and tenderness of muscles. Extraocular muscle function may be impaired. Cerebrospinal fluid shows an elevated protein content that will rise on subsequent determinations without a corresponding increase in cells. By contrast, poliomyelitis produces a cerebrospinal fluid leukocytosis. A recent history of possible viral exposure may strengthen the suspicion that this disease is present.

CNS TUMORS

■ **Why might patients with a cerebral tumor undergo sudden deterioration?**

The two primary causes of sudden change are hemorrhage and edema. Hemorrhage within the tumor produces an intracerebral hematoma with sudden increase in intracranial pressure. Edema in the area of the brain around a tumor may increase as the tumor size increases. During hypoxic or ischemic episodes or during sudden pH changes or other as yet unknown occurrences, cerebral compensation fails, with subsequent sudden increase in cerebral edema and thus increased intracranial pressure.

In general the more malignant types of tumor hemorrhage, probably because they may have abnormal vessels within the tumor or may erode normal cerebral vessels. Glioblastoma multiforme, metastatic malignant melanoma, and other malignant metastatic tumors produce hemorrhage.

Sudden deterioration caused by edema or hemorrhage requires immediate oxygenation, ventilatory support, large IV and IM doses of steroids, and immediate surgical decompression. Mannitol or urea may be given but should be reserved for the period immediately preceding and during craniotomy. Postoperative monitoring of intracranial pressure is a useful adjunct to detect those changes that may indicate impending deterioration.

■ **When should a spinal cord tumor be handled as an emergency?**

Whether the patient has a history of previous malignancy or not, if progressive signs and symptoms referable to a particular level of the spinal cord are present and especially if these findings are less than 1 week in duration, early surgical decompression should be accomplished. If there are no x-ray findings coincident with the level of neurologic deficit, a myelogram to confirm the level should be performed prior to surgery and a marker placed over the spine at the proper level. The time spent waiting for surgery should be kept to a minimum, since recovery of lost neurologic function or prevention of further deterioration is enhanced by early decompression.

COMPLICATIONS THAT MAY FOLLOW DIAGNOSTIC NEUROLOGIC PROCEDURES

■ What is the usefulness of the lumbar puncture?

In clinical practice the lumbar puncture (LP) is most helpful in determining the presence of absence of subarachnoid hemorrhage and the presence or absence of an infection or inflammatory process. Regarding the former, uniform color in three tubes indicates the presence of subarachnoid hemorrhage, and a yellow supernatant indicates that it is at least 12 hours old. A traumatic LP may be indicated by variations in the amount of blood in the collecting tube and a clear, colorless supernatant, especially if the clinical history suggests a course lasting more than 12 hours. The presence of clear, colorless cerebrospinal fluid with a lymphocytic response is usually suggestive of aseptic (viral) meningitis or tuberculous or fungal meningitis. The clinical picture and appropriate smears will help differentiate between these. A cloudy cerebrospinal fluid is usually present with acute bacterial meningitis.

■ What are the contraindications to LP?

The presence of papilledema until the mass effect in the head is excluded, a pineal shift on the Towne projection of skull x-ray films, and focal neurologic signs before a mass effect is excluded usually contraindicate LP. There is rarely a need to perform LP in a case of head injury or suspected tumor, since other studies will be more definitive, and LP may produce a rapid deterioration.

■ What are some complications of neuroradiologic procedures and their treatment?

Carotid arteriography may be associated with the production or aggravation of focal neurologic signs by means of intra-arterial thrombosis or occlusion requiring exploration for the reestablishment of flow, sheath injections, accidental air injection, or embolization from the needle or adjacent atheromatous plaques. Hemorrhage into adjacent tissues can cause pain, swelling, and tracheal compression. This may require endotracheal intubation or tracheotomy. Allergic reactions to the contrast material may occur and are treated as any allergic reaction.

Retrograde brachial arteriography may cause catheter embolization (if one is used), arterial spasm, or embolization distally with varying degrees of ischemia to the forearm and hand. Spasm may be treated with local injections of lidocaine or simple warm packs. Occlusion by embolus requires immediate arteriotomy and evacuation of thrombus. The median nerve may be injured by too medial a needle passage. Dissecting hematoma in the neurovascular compartment may cause compression of the median and ulnar nerves and of the brachial artery. This requires instant fasciotomy and hematoma evacuation.

Pneumoencephalography may be associated with severe headache, nausea, and vomiting. These are best treated by placing the patient in a flat position and administering appropriate medication. Seizures or a sudden increase in intracranial pressure may occur, especially if an irritating lesion is already present. Anticonvulsant medication, antiedema agents, and definitive treatment of the offending lesion will usually handle these complications. One must always observe for temporal lobe or cerebellar herniation in the presence of mass lesions.

Ventriculography may be attended by the same complications, except that herniation is less likely to occur.

Myelography is sometimes accompanied by headache, unsteadiness, nausea, and vomiting. An additional hazard is the production of increased neurologic deficits when the needle is placed below the level of the block. Early decompression of the lesion causing the block is necessary to avoid this occurrence.

■ How do various drugs affect pupillar size (acute intoxication)?

Morphine, heroin, narcotics in general, and nerve gases produce meiosis. Dilated pupils may be produced by the following (pupillary response is spared): glutethimide, atropine, cocaine, amphetamines, ganglionic blockers, botulism, alcohol (may produce unequal pupils), and LSD-type drugs.

Table 35-4. Endocrine-metabolic states ascociated with CNS disease

Metabolic disturbance	Associated neurologic state	Clinical diagnosis	Laboratory diagnosis	Treatment
Panhypopituitarism	Pituitary adenoma; may be sudden as in pituitary apoplexy	Headaches, visual field deficit, endocrine disturbance	Low thyroid-stimulating hormone levels, low 17-hydroxycorticoid and 17-ketogenic steroid levels, low gonadotropin levels	Removal of tumor, hormonal replacement
Inappropriate secretion of antidiuretic hormone	Several, including SAH, subdural hematoma, tumor	Hyponatremia	Low serum sodium level, high urine sodium level; low serum osmolality, high urine osmolality; high urine specific gravity; normal renal and adrenal function	Treatment of underlying CNS condition; restriction of fluids; administration of concentrated saline solution (for example, 300 ml of 3% sodium chloride) if total body sodium depletion is suspected
Hyperosmolar nonketotic	Head injury, usually	Stupor, hyperglycemia	High serum glucose, acidosis, no acetone in serum	IV insulin
Diabetes insipidus	Pituitary tumor; usually postoperative complication of pituitary surgery; blunt head trauma	Marked diuresis of a dilute urine (several hundred milliliters per hour)	Low urine specific gravity	Aqueous vasopressin for first 3 days; vasopressin tannate in oil after first 3-4 days; fluids to match urine output plus approximately 500 ml/24 hr; electrolyte levels monitored

■ What conditions and/or drugs may bring about papilledema (not caused by intracranial mass lesions)?

The conditions and/or drugs producing papilledema are as follows:

Addison's disease
Bilateral ischemic optic neuropathy (giant cell arteritis)
Birth control pills
Chronic steroid administration
Diabetes mellitus
Guillain-Barré syndrome or other conditions causing an increase in cerebrospinal fluid protein
Hurler's syndrome
Hypertension
Hyperthyroidism
Hypervitaminosis A
Hypoparathyroidism
Lead poisoning
Nalidixic acid
Polycythemia vera
Rocky Mountain spotted fever
Sarcoidosis
Sickle cell anemia
Steroid withdrawal
Systemic lupus erythematosus
Tetracycline
Thrombotic thrombocytopenia purpura
Tuberculous meningitis
Upper cervical spine masses

Table 35-4 identifies several endocrine and/or metabolic states associated with CNS disease and indicates the appropriate treatment for each.

BIBLIOGRAPHY

Aaron, H., editor: Handbook of antimicrobial therapy, New Rochelle, N.Y., 1974, Medical Letter, Inc.
Advisory Council for the National Institute of Neurological Disease and Blindness: A classification and outline of cerebrovascular disease, Neurology **8:**1, 1958.

Bartter, F. C., and Schwartz, W. B.: The syndrome of inappropriate secretion of antidiuretic hormone, Am. J. Med. **42:** 790, 1967.

Bruce, D. A., et al.: Regional cerebral blood flow, intracranial pressure and brain metabolism in comatose patients, J. Neurosurg. **38:**131, 1973.

Caveness, W. F., and Walker, A. E.: Head injury, Philadelphia, 1966, J. B. Lippincott Co.

Coates, J. B., and Meirowsky, R. M.: The Neurosurgery of trauma, Office of the Surgeon General, Washington, D.C., 1965, United States Army.

DeBakey, M. E., et al.: Cerebral arterial insufficiency: one to eleven year results following arterial reconstructive operation, Am. Surg. **161:**921, 1965.

Dennis, L. H., Cohen, R. J., Schachner, S. H., and Conrad, M. E.: Consumptive coagulopathy in fulminant meningococcemia, J.A.M.A. **205:**183, 1968.

Fisher, C. M., Picard, E. H., Polack, A., Dalal, P., and Ojemann, R. G.: Acute hypertensive cerebellar hemorrhage: symptoms and surgical treatment, J. Nerv. Ment. Dis. **140:** 38, 1965.

Friedman, H., and Odom, G. C.: Expanding intracranial lesions in geriatric patients, Geriatrics **27:**105-115, 1972.

Jennett, B., and Teasdale, G.: Aspect of coma after severe head injury, Lancet **1:**878, 1977.

Lundberg, N. I., Troupp, H., and Loren, H.: Continuous recording of the ventricular fluid pressure in patients with severe, acute traumatic brain injury, J. Neurosurg. **22:**581, 1965.

Merritt, H. H.: A testbook of neurology, ed. 5, Philadelphia, 1973, Lea & Febiger.

Murphy, F., and Maccubbin, D. A.: Carotid endarterectomy: a long term follow-up study, J. Neurosurg. **23:**156, 1965.

Odom, G. L., Tindall, G. T., Cupp, H. B., and Woodhall, B.: Neurosurgical approach to intracerebral hemorrhage in cerebrovascular disease, J. Nerv. Ment. Dis. **41:**145, 1966.

Plum, F., and Posner, J. B.: The diagnosis of stupor and coma, ed. 2, contemporary neurology series, Philadelphia, 1972, F. A. Davis Co.

Salmon, J. H.: Ventriculitis complicating meningitis, Am. J. Dis. Child. **124:**35, 1972.

Toole, J. F., and Patel, A. N.: Cerebrovascular disorders, New York, 1967, McGraw-Hill Book Co.

Whisnant, J. P., Matsumoto, N., and Eleveback, L. R.: The effect of anticoagulant therapy on prognosis of patients with transient cerebral ischemic attack in a community, Mayo Clin. Proc. **48:**844, 1973.

Youmans, J. R.: Neurologic surgery, Philadelphia, 1973, W. B. Saunders Co.

CHAPTER 36

Nursing care of the neurologically injured patient

Ellen Beam Rudy

The neurologically injured patients encountered in a critical care unit are there primarily for three reasons, (1) astute and accurate assessments of physiologic parameters, (2) monitoring of diagnostic and treatment measures used in the management of care, and (3) skilled nursing care. Evaluation of clinical symptoms and the measures necessary to prevent secondary neurologic damage may well determine the degree of recovery the patient experiences. For these reasons it is important for nurses responsible for the neurologically injured patient to base their clinical judgment on scientific knowledge and accurate assessments.

CRANIAL TRAUMA OR PATHOLOGY

One of the events most feared by man is his loss of mental capacity. For this reason, any injury or disease that involves damage to the brain threatens what, in fact, makes man human. Man's brain is his uniquely human organ. The brain cannot be regenerated, repaired, or homotransplanted. It accumulates no metabolic debts, and unless supplied continuously by an effective circulation carrying large amounts of oxygen and glucose it suffers irreparable damage. Thus the integrity of the intact nervous system must be the first goal in therapeutics to prevent additional or secondary neurologic damage to the patient with cranial trauma or pathology.[1]

■ What is the first objective in bedside care of the neurologically injured patient?

The first area of responsibility is to establish and maintain a patent airway and to maintain adequate ventilation. Head-injured patients with an obstructed airway will often die from the respiratory obstruction before the brain trauma. When necessary, an oral or nasal airway should be inserted, and frequent aseptic suctioning with proper oxygenation may be necessary to control secretions and prevent obstruction. If the patient has had head trauma, suctioning should be done through the mouth until it has been determined that no damage has been done to the dura causing leakage of spinal fluid into the nasal cavity.

When possible, the patient should be placed on his side so that the tongue will not occlude the airway. In patients with head trauma the oral cavity is often injured causing the swallowing of blood and subsequent vomiting. This side positioning will facilitate the drainage of vomitus from the oral cavity and lessen the likelihood of aspiration pneumonia as a complication to the neurologic problems.

Side positioning is also recommended following cranial surgery to facilitate oral drainage and airway patency. Drainage of secretions and respiratory toilet may further be facilitated in postcraniotomy patients by placing patients flat in bed on their abdomen in the swimmers position

583

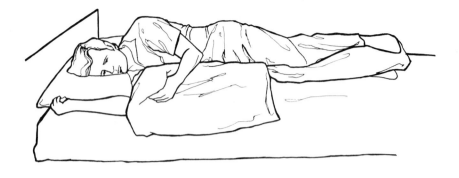

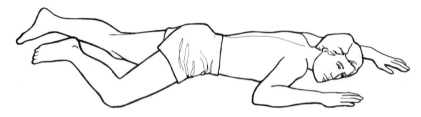

Fig. 36-1. Side position and swimmer's position.

(Fig. 36-1). Care should be taken in any positioning to avoid neck and hip flexion, which contribute to increasing the intracranial pressure.

If airway patency or adequate ventilation cannot be maintained by use of an oral or nasal airway, the patient may require the insertion of an endotracheal tube and subsequently a tracheostomy may be necessary. The institution of ventilatory support from a respirator should be based on the evaluation of arterial blood gases. Respiratory patterns indicating neurologic damage will be discussed in more detail under the section on the neurologic assessment.

Too often not enough emphasis has been placed on the importance of adequate ventilation and respiratory toilet in the case of the patient with a neurologic problem. Proper positioning, adequate suctioning, and knowledgeable assessment of blood gases can contribute immeasurably to the prevention of brain hypoxia and respiratory infections, which may delay and impede recovery.

■ **What are the nursing responsibilities in monitoring and assessing the patient's condition?**

Good clinical judgment by the critical care nurse in care of the neurologically injured patient is based on astute, accurate assessment of the patient. There are generally two major categories of assessment, the initial or baseline assessment and the continuous or ongoing assessment performed at the bedside. Both are important and will be discussed in detail.

NEUROLOGIC ASSESSMENT

One important point should be made about the term "assessment." The data collection, which includes the determination of level of consciousness, vital signs, and sensory and motor deficits, is prerequisite to the assessment on which clinical judgment is based. The assessment activity by the nurse is what she decides based on the synthesis of all the data collected. The following questions should be addressed with each assessment:

What is the neurologic status of the patient?
Is his condition improving or deteriorating?
Are the changes expected or should a physician be notified?
Based on the assessment, what nursing measures should be instituted, and which ones should be avoided?

Baseline neurologic assessment

A complete history and physical examination are vitally important for planning care of a neurologically injured patient. The initial history and physical are usually done by the medical staff, and the medical management is initiated. However, since ongoing neurologic evaluations will be the responsibility of the critical care nurse, a detailed neurologic assessment is required as a baseline for further evaluations. An example of an initial assessment is given in Fig. 36-2, with the major parts of the examination being cerebral function, cranial nerve function, cerebellar function, and motor and sensory function.

Ongoing bedside assessment

Frequent neurologic assessments performed at the bedside are designed to give information that indicates improved neurologic status or deteriorating status, suggesting an increase in intracranial pressure. The major areas to be evaluated are level or state of consciousness, vital signs, cranial nerve function, and motor function, and sensory system function.

Level of consciousness

Changes in levels of consciousness are considered the most important external indication of changes in intracranial pressure. The nursing staff in constant contact with the patient are better equipped than any other health team members to recognize changes in behavior that may indicate a change in the level of consciousness.

Consciousness may be thought of as having two components, one being its crude "off-on" quality, which research now shows to be a relationship between the reticular activating system of the brain stem, thalamus, and cerebral cortex, and the content area that is dependent completely on the functions of the cerebral hemisphere.

According to Plum:

The present physiologic concept of consciousness is that it depends upon close interaction between the intact cerebral hemispheres and the central gray matter of the upper brainstem. The (cerebral) hemispheres contribute most of the specific components of consciousness, including language, memory, intellect, and learned responses to sensory stimuli. But in order for the cerebrum to function, the organism must be aroused or activated by more caudally placed mechanisms that reside in the thalamus, hypothalamus, midbrain and upper pons. An important component of this arousal mechanism is located within the ascending reticular activating system; other brainstem systems also influence cerebral cortical activity and the state of consciousness.[1]

The reticular activating system is not one structure in the brain but instead is composed of neurons that start in the upper end of the spinal cord, are throughout the brain stem, and extend upward throughout the central portion of the thalamus into the hypothalamus, and into areas adjacent to the thalamus. Collectively these areas of diffuse neurons are known as the *reticular activating system* (RAS). This system controls the overall degree of central nervous system activity, including control of wakefulness and sleep and control of at least part of our ability to direct attention toward specific areas of our conscious minds.

Stimulation to the RAS can come from several sources and is helpful in understanding wakefulness in normal individuals as well as patients with head injuries. One source of stimulation is sensory stimuli such as pain, visual, and auditory signals. This explains why a painful stimulus is frequently used to determine the level of consciousness in a comatose patient. A decrease in response to painful stimuli indicates a higher degree of brain stem damage. It also helps explain the lack of sleep (increase in wakefulness) experienced by some patients in an ICU setting with the sensory overload that they experience from constant visual and auditory stimuli.

A second source of stimulation to the RAS and

Assessment criteria

Name: _____

Date: _____

Admission diagnosis: _____
BP _____ T _____ P _____ R _____

Cerebral function
I. Level of consciousness
   Wakefulness
      Alert
      Lethargic—drowsiness, inaction, and indifference in which responses are delayed and incomplete, an increased stimulus may be required to evoke a response.
      Obtundurate—duller indifference in which little more than wakefulness is maintained.
      Stupor—the state from which the subject can only be aroused by vigorous and continuous external stimulation.
      Coma—psychologic and motor responses to stimulation are either semiappropriate movements in response to noxious stimuli or with only primitive reflexes (sucking, corneal) or completely lost with no response at all.
   Content
      Oriented completely
      Automatism
      Confused, to what degree
      Delirium
      Unresponsive
II. Calculations
      Perform simple calculations
III. Memory
      Short term—repeats back number series, repeats recent events

Data

Comments:

Comments:

Comments:

Comments:

Comments:

Comments:

Assessment criteria

IV. Affect—mood
      Labile
      Hostile
      Abusive
      Flat
      Appropriate
      Inappropriate
V. Abstract reasoning
      Relates meaning of proverbs
VI. Thought content
      Delusional
      Paranoid
      Obsession with one idea
      Appropriate and intact
VII. Speech
      Clear
      Slurred
      Rambling
      Aphasic (describe)
Cortical-sensory
   I. Visual
      Looks at objects and identifies
   II. Auditory
      Interprets sounds
   III. Tactile
      Identifies objects in hand with closed eyes (stereognosis)
      Opens-closes safety pin
Cranial nerves
   I. Olfactory
      Smell
   II. Optic
      Fields of vision
      Visual acuity
      Structures
      External—red reflex, optic disc, vessels, retina, macula
      Internal—red reflex, optic disc, vessels, retina, macula
   III. Oculomotor
      Eyelids
      PERRLA
      EOM (extraocular movement)
   IV. Abducens
      EOM

Data

Comments:

Comments:
Comments:

Comments:

Comments:
Comments:
Comments:

Comments:

Fig. 36-2. Initial neurologic assessment tool.

Assessment criteria	Data
V. Trigeminal	Comments:
Facial sensation	
Clench jaws	
Corneal reflex	
VI. Trochlear	Comments:
EOM	
VII. Facial	Comments:
Frown, smile, close eyes	
Taste	
VIII. Acoustic	Comments:
Weber test	
Caloric ice water test	
IX. Glossopharyngeal } test together	Comments:
X. Vagus	
Gag reflex	
Swallowing	
Uvula symmetry	
Phonation	
Taste	
XI. Spinal accessory	Comments:
Neck and shoulder movement	
XII. Hypoglossal	Comments:
Protrudes tongue in midline	
Cerebellar function	
Coordination	Comments:
Rapid alternating movements	
Gait	
Toe-to-heel	
Romberg	Comments:
Involuntary movements	
Tremors—intension, resting	
Fasciculations	
Choreatic	
Athetoid	
Spasm	
Convulsions	

Assessment criteria	Data
Motor functions	Comments:
Size of muscles	
Symmetric	
Atrophy	
Muscle tone	
Normal	
Flaccid	
Rigid	
Spastic	
Decerebrate	
Decorticate	
Muscle strength	
Normal	Right
Weakness	Left
Absent	
Sensory	Comments:
Tactile	
Superficial pain	
Deep pain	
Vibratory sense	
Temperature	
Position and motion sense	
Two-point localization	
Extinction	
Deep tendon reflexes	Comments:
Achilles—0 absent	
Patellar—1 diminished	
Biceps— 2 normal	
Triceps— 3 brisk	
Plantar— 4 hyperactive	

Summary of significant findings:

Assessment:

Fig. 36-2, cont'd. For legend see opposite page.

wakefulness is the cerebral cortex itself. This is experienced by people who cannot "turn their brain off" and go to sleep. Overstimulation of the cerebral cortex through excitement, anxiety, or worry are examples that produce wakefulness.

Finally the RAS can be stimulated by motor activity. This is because an exceedingly large number of nerve fibers that pass from the motor regions of the cerebral cortex also go to the RAS. Therefore motor activity that is produced through activity of the motor cortex also stimulates the RAS to produce wakefulness. This helps explain the need to "move around to wake up" and also the increase in response by some comatose patients during the period of bathing and bedmaking by the nurse. The stimulation of the motor system through passive body movements produces some stimulation to the RAS and wakefulness. Unfortunately this point is often missed by nurses in reporting patient responses. Following bathing, turning, back care, and other motor stimuli, patients will often respond to less noxious stimuli (lower levels of pain) that will be needed at a later, more restful period. This does not usually indicate a change in the level of consciousness, but rather a decrease in motor stimulation compounded with the sensory stimulus that produces a response.

The "content" part of consciousness—the thinking, feeling, controlling part—is directed by the cerebral cortex. As just discussed, the "conscious-unconscious" part of wakefulness is directed by the reticular activating system located in the brain stem (midbrain, pons, and medulla) and in the diencephalon, which stimulates the cerebral cortex. Based on this knowledge, it becomes clearer why patients can show a profound decline in content but retain full wakefulness, or why patients may remain oriented to person, place, and time (the old standby questions) and be slowly becoming less and less wakeful. The symptoms and brain involvement then are different and purport different concerns. *Both evaluations are important, but it seems reasonable to assess them separately.*

Vital signs

Blood pressure and pulse. A change in vital signs without a change in level of consciousness suggests the presence of other medical problems. The nurse should be alert to other signs of blood loss or circulatory problems. Changes in vital signs are usually a late effect of increasing intracranial pressure.

The classic symptoms of an increasing systolic blood pressure, widening pulse pressure, and decreasing pulse rate, which have for years been taught as signals of increasing intracranial pressure, have *not* been found to correlate well with changes in intracranial pressure documented through cranial ventricular monitoring. When these classic vital sign changes are seen transiently, they probably reflect hypoxia of the brain stem secondary to decreased perfusion pressure. As pressure within the skull increases because of edema, hemorrhage, blocked cerebrospinal fluid (CSF), or lesion growth (remember the three factors: cells, blood, CSF), there is pressure on the blood vessels within the brain causing a decrease in the blood supply to the brain tissue. The central nervous system response to this ischemia is one of the most powerful of all the activators of the sympathetic vasoconstrictor system. It is a compensatory mechanism whereby the blood pumped to the brain is under increased pressure so that it can reach the ischemic areas of the brain to provide both oxygen and glucose. This CNS ischemic response operates as an emergency arterial pressure control system that acts rapidly and extremely powerfully to prevent further decrease in arterial pressure whenever blood flow to the brain decreases dangerously close to the lethal level. This otherwise unwarranted rise in blood pressure is an attempt by the body to maintain nutrition in the neurons. At the same time that the systemic hypertension is occurring, a progressive bradycardia owing to vagal slowing of the heart may be noted. Baroreceptors in the aorta and carotid arteries sense the increase in pressure and thus stimulate the vagus nerve, which causes the pulse to slow. When these vital signs are progressive and sustained, the vital sign changes may well represent decompensation within the brain and the time for intervention is past and death is usually the result.[2,3]

Respirations. Respiratory patterns may be very significant in patients with head injury or pathology. Respiration serves several purposes, including metabolic gas exchange, communication, and heat regulation. In addition, the respiratory system is endowed with a number of protective reflexes, some of which influence the respiratory rate and depth; others induce coughing, sneezing, and yawning. The principal integration and regulation of these several functions are achieved by respiratory neurons located in the medulla oblongata and lower pons. This "respiratory center" is, in turn, influenced by structures at higher levels of the nervous system as well as by changes in its local chemical environment. In general a low blood pH indicating an acid condition causes increased deep respirations, while a high blood pH indicating an alkaline condition will decrease the rate and depth of respirations. Neurologic disorders frequently produce breathing abnormalities. Diseases or increasing pressure on the cerebrum or upper brain stem commonly induces disturbances in the respiratory rate and rhythm that do not interfere with gas exchange. A word of caution is in order. Metabolic and neurogenic influences on the respiratory act often overlap and interact so that one must interpret respiratory changes cautiously. The alert nurse will recognize respiratory rhythm and rate changes and report them. Blood gas evaluations are usually called for to help distinguish metabolic from neurogenic influences. Any degree of CO_2 retention will further increase intracranial pressure because of its cerebrovasodilator effects, and therefore adequate ventilation with maintenance of a clear airway is essential for the patient with increased intracranial pressure.

CNS respiratory failure results when the respiratory-integrating neurons in the medulla oblongata become damaged or diseased. The original insult could be from a subdural hematoma causing increasing intracranial pressure with resulting herniation of the medulla and respiratory arrest. An alert nurse can assess impending signs of respiratory failure. Central respiratory failure produces defects in the respiratory rate and rhythm, and symptoms usually evolve through progressive stages.

Severe bilateral hemisphere dysfunction impairs the nonchemical influences on the act of breathing even more, and in addition in many

such patients there is an increased respiratory responsiveness to chemical stimuli. As a result, many of them develop a breathing pattern with regular oscillations between hyperpnea and apea. This is Cheyne-Stokes respiration. The regular waxing and waning, being dependent on stimuli reaching the respiratory system, has a period length equal to twice the lung-to-brain circulation period.

Involvement of anatomic centers in the posterior hypothalamus and midbrain produces moderate pulmonary edema in many patients, and a pattern of hyperpnea (rapid respiration) with a low Pco_2 combined with a below-normal Po_2 is the result.

A less common manifestation of midbrain-upper pontine lesions is a true central hyperventilation. It is marked by respiratory rates of as high as 25 to 40/min, low Pco_2 and above normal Po_2.

Damage at or below the pons produces irregular breathing patterns. These may take various forms from cluster breathing and gasping to ataxic patterns where the depth and timing of the next breath cannot be predicted.

All of these latter patterns are associated with abnormal blood gas values and underventilation, which tend to accentuate whatever neurologic injury is already present.

Extensive damage or depression of the medullary reticular formation generally destroys the central control of respiration and produces severe hypoventilation or apnea.

In most intensive care centers the patients are placed on artificial ventilation before many of these severely deteriorated patterns are manifested. The problem of weaning these patients from artificial support is almost impossible if brain stem damage has occurred.[4]

Temperature. Temperature changes are rarely used as indications of increasing intracranial pressure. There are, however, several important points the critical care nurse needs to remember about temperature changes. In most instances of an elevated temperature the possibility of an infection should be evaluated. Pulmonary infections are very common in immobile patients or in patients with tracheostomy or endotracheal tubes. Indwelling catheters and arterial and intravenous lines are also possible sources of infection to the patient. If an infection is suspected, treatment should be initiated immediately. Patients with head injuries or following cranial surgery will often be on a cortisone preparation to decrease cranial edema. One side-effect of these medications is the inhibition of the body's normal response to infection. An elevated temperature may be the first indication of such a problem.

The body's temperature control mechanism is in the hypothalamus of the brain. A lesion or increased pressure in this area could interfere with the body's ability to regulate its temperature. For this reason, with all comatose patients the use of a hypothermia blanket to reduce temperature should be closely monitored. Damage to the temperature-regulating area of the brain can result in abnormal responses to the hypothermia treatment resulting in subnormal temperatures in the patient. When symptoms of intracranial pressure are present, it is suggested that temperatures be lowered very slowly to prevent overcompensation.

Cranial nerve functions

Continuing neurologic assessments in intensive care units should be expanded from measur-

Table 36-1. Assessment of cranial nerve function

Cranial nerve	Name	Type	Function
I	Olfactory	Sensory	Smell
II	Optic	Sensory	Visual fields, visual acuity
III	Oculomotor	Motor	Pupil constriction, accommodation, EOM*—doll's eyes (superior rectus, inferior oblique, inferior rectus, medial rectus)
IV	Trochlear	Motor	EOM* (superior oblique)
V	Trigeminal	Motor	Opens and closes jaw, muscles of mastication
		Sensory	Sensations from three branches: ophthalmic—forehead, cornea; maxillary—cheek; mandibular—jaw, mucous membrane of mouth
VI	Abducens	Motor	EOM*—doll's eyes (lateral rectus)
VII	Facial	Motor	Muscles of face and scalp, frown, smile, puff cheeks, close eyes
		Sensory	Taste anterior two-thirds of tongue
VIII	Acoustic	Sensory	Auditory—hearing, vestibular—equilibrium
IX	Glossopharyngeal	Motor	Swallow, gag, phonation
		Sensory	Taste posterior one-third of tongue
X	Vagus	Motor	Swallow, gag, phonation; slows heart, contracts bronchial muscles
		Sensory	Sensation in larynx, trachea, lungs, esophagus, posterior ear
XI	Spinal accessory	Motor	Moves head, shrugs shoulder
XII	Hypoglossal	Motor	Tongue movement

*EOM—extraocular movement.

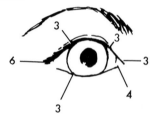 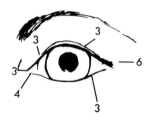

ing only the third cranial nerve function (pupil size and response to light) to an evaluation of several of the cranial nerves. Listed in Table 36-1 are the 12 cranial nerves and their functions.

The cranial nerves of primary importance to the critical care nurse are those generally associated with eye function (II, III, IV, VI). However, because the origin of the cranial nerves is in the area of the brain stem, an evaluation of other cranial nerve functions is important in determining the level of the cranial lesion or involvement. For example, the corneal reflex tests the trigeminal nerve (V), and the gag reflex tests the glossopharyngeal (IX) and vagus (X) nerves. Absence of these reflexes indicates brain stem involvement. Loss of the corneal reflex most frequently encountered in comatose patients may lead to inflammation and ulceration of the cornea owing to loss of blinking and excess dryness of the corneal area. This condition can cause permanent eye damage and loss of vision. Nursing care should include an evaluation of the corneal reflex and dryness of the cornea. The eyes should be lubricated with artificial tears or an ophthalmic ointment and covered with an eye shield or taped shut to prevent dryness. Regular cleansing and assessment of the eye should be part of the routine physical care of these patients.

Assessment of eye function as part of the ongoing neurologic assessment is done to determine lesions at the level of the third cranial nerve. Eyes should be assessed for equality of pupils, response to light, and abnormal movements. It should be noted that many people with no neurologic deficiency have unequal pupils. Unless the difference between the pupils is great, this point should be kept in mind and other signs of third nerve involvement such as sluggish pupil constriction or diminished ability to move the eye toward the nose (medial rectus function) are found. It is also worth noting that a direct blow to an eye such as often accompanies a head injury may result in lack of normal pupillary changes and this may confuse a neurologic assessment.

The best way to assess pupil size is to ask the patient to look straight ahead focusing on something across a semidarkened room. In this way the pupils will remain dilated enough to measure

them with a millimeter ruler and assess their size. The nurse should then bring a flashlight up the side of the eye until the pupil constricts and then to the opposite eye to check its constriction. One eye is examined at a time, while the other eye is covered to prevent consensual constriction.

Testing pupillary response to light involves testing both the optic (II) and oculomotor (III) nerves. The optic nerve must be intact for the light to cause stimulation to the eye. The perception of light by the optic nerve then stimulates the oculomotor nerve to cause constriction of the pupil. The iris of the eye is influenced by two parts of the brain, the third cranial nerve or oculomotor nerve and the brain stem. The oculomotor nerve contains parasympathetic nerve fibers and when stimulated by light will constrict the pupil. The brain stem contains sympathetic nerve fibers and when stimulated will cause dilation of the pupil. This is a normal response. However, overstimulation of the oculomotor nerve from medication such as morphine or prostigmine or intracranial pressure compressing the sympathetic fibers in the hypothalamus and brain stem can cause very constricted or "pinpoint" pupils. Atropine acts in the opposite way causing dilation of pupils. For this reason a good understanding of pharmacology is important in recognizing exactly what can be attributed to increased intracranial pressure (IIP) and what to drug action. It is important to remember that the action of the oculomotor nerve is parasympathetic. It is also important to know that the oculomotor nerve goes from the ciliary body behind the iris of the eye directly along the floor of the brain above the tentorial membrane to its origin in the brain stem. It does not cross paths; pressure on the right oculomotor nerve will affect the right pupil, and pressure on the left oculomotor nerve will affect the left pupil. Enough pressure on this nerve will cause it to cease functioning and the sympathetic influence of the brain stem will result in a dilated pupil.

Major injury to the midbrain, as in central infarction or hemorrhage or in the compression and distortion wrought by transtentorial herniation, nearly always interrupts both sympathetic and parasympathetic pathways. The resulting pupils are in midposition (4 to 5 mm) fixed to light and sometimes irregular and slightly asymmetric.

In stuporous or comatose patients reflex eye movements may be elicited to test the integrity of the brain's pathways to the muscles of the eyes. The most common of these reflexes include the following.

1. The *oculocephalic reflex* or *"doll's eyes"* phenomenon is demonstrated if the head is rotated to the right and the eyes deviate left. The nerves controlling lateral gaze are the abducens (VI) cranial nerve from the pons and the oculomotor (III) cranial nerve from the midbrain. The vestibular apparatus at the acoustic (VIII) cranial nerve transmits information about head position to the pons; that information enters the lower pons, ascends to the upper pons and midbrain, and exits the appropriate cranial nerves causing the eyes to deviate to the side opposite the turning. This positive response indicates an intact brain stem. Loss of the doll's eye response indicates brain stem impairment. An exception is the negative "doll's eye" response seen in sedative drug intoxication. This is the only metabolic encephalopathy in which negative doll's eye response is seen. This is an important point because drug-induced coma is very common.[5]

2. The *oculovestibular reflex* refers to reflex conjugate eye movements, or nystagmus, or both. After examining the ear for intactness at the tympanic membrane, the patient's head is elevated 30 degrees, and ice water is slowly syringed into the ear canal. In patients with an intact brain stem the stimulation to the vestibular portion of the acoustic nerve transmits this stimulus to the pons and the sixth cranial nerve and up to the midbrain and the third cranial nerve. The sixth nerve causes the eye closest to the irrigated ear to move laterally, while the third nerve causes the opposite eye to move medially followed by rapid rotation in the opposite direction by both eyes. This results in horizontal nystagmus with slow movement toward the irrigated ear and rapid movement away. In the comatose patient you may see the eyes move slowly toward the irrigated ear and remain there 2 to 3 minutes; the rapid movement away has disappeared. This response indicates the lesion is supratentorial or metabolic and the brain stem is intact. If, however, the response is extremely abnormal such as downward deviation and rotary jerking of one eye, the lesion is in the brain stem or cerebellum.[4-6]

3. The *ciliospinal reflex* is initiated by pinching the neck of the patient and watching the eye pupil on the same side (ipsilateral) dilate. Absence of this reflex in the comatose patient indicates brain stem impairment.

With coma from brain stem lesions, reflex eye movements are depressed or abnormal. With midbrain or pontine lesions on the medial side, the eye on the side of the lesion fails to adduct on reflex movements. Lateral pontine lesions cause eyes to deviate away from the side of the lesion, and reflex movements on that side are often blocked.

Papilledema. Nurses who want to become proficient in the use of the ophthalmoscope should certainly attempt to perfect these skills in an intensive care setting. Proper use of the ophthalmoscope can be taught in a few sessions with a nurse practitioner or physician, and including it in a neurologic assessment will perfect the nurse's skills if adequate supervision is provided. Adequate skilled supervision is necessary for nurses to gain skill and confidence in their findings. However, papilledema may require 18 to 24 hours to develop, so it may not be as helpful in assessing acutely developing intracranial pressure as the tools of observation already being used.

Motor and sensory system function

To evaluate the motor and sensory component of the body it is important to know what you are measuring, and if there is a deviation from normal, exactly what this could mean. The cerebral hemispheres of the brain are divided into lobes. These lobes are the frontal, parietal, temporal, and occipital. The portion of the brain primarily concerned with motor activity is located at the posterior portion of the frontal lobe, and the sensory component is adjacent to the motor area in the anterior portion of the parietal lobe.

If the patient is awake and alert, it is best to evaluate the sensory and motor functions of the extremities separately. For the sensory component, the patient is asked to close his eyes and identify the sharp or dull feeling of a safety pin on the face, arms, abdomen, thighs, and legs.

The sharp point of the pin should be felt without even breaking the skin. If an absence of this discrimination is found, further evaluation should be done to identify the boundaries of the deficit and the type and amount of stimulus needed to elicit sensation.

For the motor component, all extremities should be tested for voluntary movement and strength. The patient should be asked to move his hands, flex his arms, flex his legs, pull his arms up against resistance, and pull his legs up against resistance. It is often difficult to detect beginning muscle weakness from these maneuvers. For this reason, a better test of voluntary motor function at the upper extremities is to have the patient close his eyes and hold his arms straight in front of him for about 30 seconds. With motor weakness, the affected limb will begin to "drift" downward without apparent awareness of the patient.

For the lower extremities, muscle weakness may be more easily detected if the patient is allowed out of bed. His gait and ability to bear weight and lift his legs can be observed and evaluated at this time. If this is not possible, the bed maneuvers mentioned are sufficient.

If the patient is unable to follow verbal commands owing to a stuporous or comatose condition, the motor and sensory responses will need to be evaluated in another manner. Most abnormalities at the early or diencephalic stage of intracranial pressure signal damage to the pyramidal tract (corticospinal tract) somewhere between the cortex and the midbrain. The pyramidal tract serves as the major "thruway" for the nervous system signals that control voluntary muscles. Since the tract decussates (crosses) below the midbrain, any weakness, paralysis, or abnormal motor response on one side of the body indicates a brain lesion or pressure on the opposite side. For this reason it is important to evaluate motor and sensory activity with the difference of upper and lower extremities in mind but also comparison of left side to right side.

The nurse should observe any spontaneous movement of the extremities during periods of no stimulations, during periods of bathing and turning the patient, and during periods of noxious stimulation such as suctioning or injections.

From these observations she can determine the stimulus necessary to initiate motor activity and a description of the motor response. A purposeful motor response would be an attempt to turn away from the noxious stimulus or a movement to stop the stimulus. A nonpurposeful response might simply be the movement of extremities with no direction. An inappropriate or pathologic response includes decorticate and decerebrate responses.

It is usually necessary for the nurse to perform a neurologic evaluation at times other than during bathing or suctioning. For this reason, the level of sensory stimulation necessary to elicit a motor response may necessitate the use of painful stimuli. Light pressure by stroking an extremity should be tried first; if there is no response, deep pressure should be applied on the Achilles tendon or supraorbital ridge of the eye. If a more painful stimulus is needed, it should be remembered that pinching soft tissue such as squeezing the arm, leg, thigh, or chest will leave the patient with multiple bruises contributing to his already traumatized state. For this reason, it is suggested that when painful stimuli are applied, large muscle masses such as the trapezius (neck) or the gastrocnemius (calf) be used.

Again, a team approach and good communication between nursing staff and physicians is imperative. A physician is usually willing to discuss a patient's condition and exactly how important the evaluation of response to pain is to a particular patient. If response to deep pain or noxious stimuli must be elicited every time a neurologic assessment is done, then the nurse may have no alternative. A patient in a deep coma who has not responded to painful stimulus for some time would certainly warrant an evaluation by the nurse as to the necessity for continual repetition of measures to elicit such a response.

Pathologic motor responses. There are several motor responses that are pathologic and indicate extensive CNS damage. These include decorticate and decerebrate motor responses.

DECORTICATE AND DECEREBRATE MOTOR RESPONSES. The motor cortex gives rise to tracts that descend the spinal cord through both the pyramidal tract and the extrapyramidal tract. These two tracts have opposing effects on the tone of the body muscles. The pyramidal tract (corticospinal tract) causes continuous facilitation and therefore a tendency to increase muscle tone throughout the body. On the other hand, the extrapyramidal system transmits inhibitory signals through the basal ganglia and the bulboreticular system of the brain stem, with resultant inhibition of muscle action. When the motor cortex is destroyed, the balance between these two opposing effects may be altered. If the lesion is located discretely in the primary motor cortex where the large Betz cells lie, both pyramidal and extrapyramidal elements are affected equally and the patient loses essentially all purposeful or voluntary motor function, resulting in paralysis of the muscles. This does not mean that the muscles themselves cannot contract, but that the person's ability to control the movements is gone.

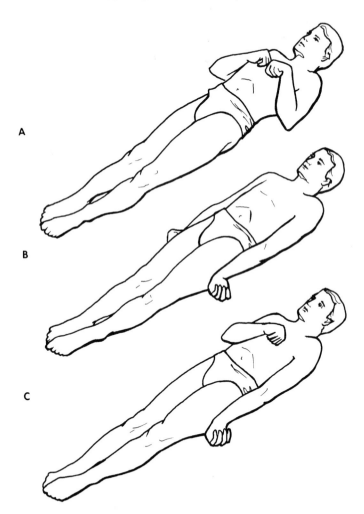

Fig. 36-3. Decorticate and decerebrate responses. **A,** Decorticate response. Flexion of arms, wrists, and fingers with adduction in upper extremities. Extension, internal rotation, and plantar flexion in lower extremities. **B,** Decerebrate response. All four extremities in rigid extension with hyperpronation of forearms and plantar extension of feet. **C,** Decorticate response on right side of body and decerebrate response on left side of body.

On the other hand, if the lesion is large enough to involve large portions of the sensorimotor cortex, both anterior and posterior to the primary motor area, these regions that normally transmit inhibitory signals through the extrapyramidal tracts will be injured. Therefore loss of extrapyramidal inhibition will lead to muscle spasm. If the lesion involves the basal ganglia as well as the motor cortex itself, the spasm is even more intense because the basal ganglia normally provide very strong inhibition of the bulboreticular system, and loss of this inhibition further exacerbates the excitation of muscles. This intense muscle spasm is frequently called a *"decorticate"* response and is characterized by flexion of the arms, wrists, and fingers with adduction in the upper extremities and extension, internal rotation, and plantar flexion in the lower extremities. In other words arms, wrists, and hands are folded inward and curled together across the chest, while the legs and feet straighten and turn outward (Fig. 36-3).

In *"decerebrate"* rigidity, the muscle spasm is of the antigravity muscles and is called extensor spasm. In this response all four extremities are in rigid extension with hyperpronation of the forearms and plantar extension of the feet. This response also indicates a loss of the inhibitory effect of the extrapyramidal tract, only this time the extensor muscles are primarily stimulated instead of the flexor muscles. This response indicates a lesion at the level of the brain stem. When a patient digressed to the point of only a decerebrate response, the prognosis is very grave. These pathologic motor responses will frequently be accompanied by deep coma, rapid breathing, and perhaps dilation of both pupils (Fig. 36-3).

IPSILATERAL MOTOR INVOLVEMENT. As mentioned earlier, a deficit in motor functioning on one side of the body generally indicates a brain lesion or pressure on the opposite side of the brain because the nerve fibers carrying motor function cross below the midbrain. There are instances, however, when pressure from brain tissue edema or a hematoma may push the brain toward the tentorial notch at an angle causing compression on the far side of the midbrain (uncal herniation)—the side opposite the lesion or hematoma. And in those few cases the signs of motor function deficit

will be on the same side (ipsilateral) as the lesion. However, with any pressure on the midbrain the deterioration is rapid and weakness or paralysis soon becomes bilateral.

Most motor abnormalities will occur because of pressure on the motor cortex above the midbrain. The example of ipsilateral involvement was given to cover other possibilities.

REFLEX MOTOR ACTIVITY. Reflexes most frequently evaluated by the critical care nurse are those already mentioned in the evaluation of the cranial nerves and include pupillary (III), corneal (V), gag (IX), and swallow (X) reflexes. Deep tendon reflexes may also be evaluated by the nurse who has become skillful in this maneuver. An intact tendon reflex requires a healthy peripheral sensory nerve, spinal nerve, dorsal root, cord synapse, motor root, motor nerve, neuromuscular junction and muscle.

The deep tendon reflexes most frequently tested and the spinal nerves they evaluate include:

Reflex	Spinal nerve
Achilles	S1, S2
Patellar	L2-4
Biceps and brachioradialis	C5, C6
Triceps	C6-8

The scale on which these reflexes are graded is:
0+   No response
1+   Diminished or weak reflex
2+   Normal reflex
3+   Brisk or stronger than normal reflex
4+   Hyperactive reflex

Superficial reflexes may also be tested. They are initiated by stroking the skin with a blunt object. Examples of superficial reflexes, the spinal nerve tested, and the normal response are listed in Table 36-2.

An abnormal response to the plantar reflex is called the *Babinski sign* (Fig. 36-4). As noted in Table 36-2, a normal response is a plantar flexion of all the toes. An abnormal response, or positive Babinski sign is dorsiflexion of the big toe with or without fanning of the other toes. This response is caused by injury to the pyramidal tract (corticospinal tract), which goes to the foot region. This positive Babinski response does not occur when the neurologic damage is only in the extrapyramidal system. Therefore the sign is often used clinically to detect damage specifically in the pyramidal portion of the motor cortex.[3]

■ **What are the major points in making the neurologic assessment or evaluation?**

The ongoing neurologic examination provides the critical care nurse with data about the major components of the neurologic system. From this data, the critical care nurse must determine the following.

Present neurologic status

All neurologic deficits such as decreased levels of consciousness, sensory, and motor impairments must be evaluated in terms of the baseline data. *Establish a trend* from the total assessment. A synthesis of the data should indicate if

the overall condition is improving or deteriorating.

Need for medical intervention

Based on the present neurologic status, the nurse must determine if the physician should be notified. There is *no substitute for prompt, accurate reporting of neurologic changes.* While medical management varies with the cause, from this assessment the physician can determine the medical or surgical treatment necessary to prevent further neurologic damage and even death. While it is always important to report signs of deteriorating neurologic functions, in some cases it is equally important to report improvement. An example of this would be increasing restlessness and increasing spontaneous movements from a patient who earlier had been comatose and re-

Table 36-2. Testing of superficial reflexes and their normal responses

Reflex	Maneuver	Spinal nerve	Normal response
Upper abdominal reflex	Stroke up from umbilicus	T7-9	Umbilicus moves up
Lower abdominal reflex	Stroke down from umbilicus	T10, T11	Umbilicus moves down
Cremasteric reflex	Stroke inner thigh	T12, L1	Scrotum moves up on that side
Plantar reflex	Stroke up outer side of sole of foot and across ball of foot	S1, S2	Plantar flexion of all toes
Gluteal reflex	Stroke skin of gluteal muscle	L4 through S3	Skin tenses at gluteal area

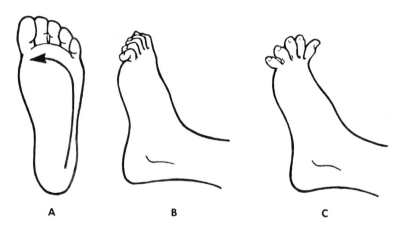

Fig. 36-4. Babinski's sign. **A,** Test maneuver; **B,** normal response; **C,** abnormal response.

sponded only to painful stimuli. This could be followed by increasing levels of awareness such as opening eyes to verbal stimuli and responding voluntarily to touch. While the overall picture indicates an improving neurologic condition, if restlessness becomes extreme, the safety of the patient may be endangered. The physician should be notified of the condition and medications to control restlessness may need to be ordered.

Need for nursing interventions

There are several nursing measures that should be routine for all patients with head trauma or cranial pathology. These measures are designed to decrease or avoid increasing intracranial pressure.

Measures that prevent hypercapnia (Pco$_2$ greater than 42 mm Hg) and hypoxia (Po$_2$ less than 50 mm Hg). Blood gas results must be closely monitored to prevent hypercapnia and hypoxia; airway patency must be maintained through proper positioning and adequate suctioning; and mechanical ventilator settings must be checked properly.

Limiting fluid intake. All IV fluid should be administered with a minidripper to prevent too rapid infusion of fluids. Accurate intake and output records must be kept to help judge hydration.

Positioning patients properly. All patients with head trauma should be positioned to prevent flexion of the neck or hips. There is evidence that head, neck, and extreme hip flexion increase intracranial pressure.[2] If there is evidence of increasing intracranial pressure, the head of the bed should be elevated to 30 degrees to improve venous drainage from the brain.

Avoiding Valsalva maneuvers. Any straining such as turning in bed, sitting up, or straining at stools can contribute to increasing pressure in the brain. Mauss and Mitchell[2] point out that these activities plus many other everyday activities cause spikes of intracranial pressure far above normal and are often well tolerated by patients. However, in some cases an acute increase in pressure can be neurologically damaging. For this reason, clinical judgments must be made as to which activities should be avoided or reduced and in which individual situation it is more important to avoid these activities than in others. Rou-

tinely all patients with a head injury or with cranial pathology should be taught to exhale when moving their bowels, fecal contents should be kept soft through diet, fluids, and stool softeners, and the patient should be assisted in turning and sitting up until the neurologic condition has stabilized. A Valsalva maneuver alone will probably not be sufficient to cause a sustained increase in intracranial pressure; however, its combination with other pressure-producing conditions may accelerate a deteriorating condition.

Avoiding excess talking about the patient's condition. Most nurses have been taught that in an unconscious patient hearing is one of the last senses to be diminished. However, in the daily stress of caring for unconscious patients, nurses too often forget this fact and may talk about the patient and his condition within hearing range of the patient. Recent research suggests that conversations with alert patients about their condition or conversations "over" unconscious patients increased the intracranial pressure of these patients. The degree to which this was damaging was not evaluated, but it does suggest another way in which nursing care can be directed to avoid adversely affecting the patient.[7]

■ What other physical assessment in addition to the neurologic assessment should be performed?

For the neurologically injured patient the neurologic assessment is the most detailed, but several other areas of physical assessment are also important.

Respiratory system

The importance of airway patency, proper ventilation to prevent hypercapnia and hypoxemia, and the respiratory patterns have already been presented. The critical care nurse should evaluate lung sounds frequently to determine areas of congestion and the need for suctioning. The nurse should be aware that in positioning the patient the dependent lung fields can become more congested. This is another reason for frequent repositioning of the patient and good respiratory toilet. If respiratory congestion does become a major problem, the use of postural drainage and respiratory physical therapy should be evaluated.

Both of the maneuvers of postural drainage and "cupping and clapping" can increase intracranial pressure and should be evaluated from the patient's neurologic tolerance to such therapies.

Cardiovascular system

Nearly all patients in a critical care unit have cardiac monitoring. For the patient with a head injury, it is important to recognize that the heart rhythm is influenced by the vasomotor center in the lower pons and upper medulla. The lateral portions send excitatory impulses through the sympathetic nerves to the heart, thus increasing the pulse rate. The medial portion sends inhibitory impulses to the heart through the parasympathetic (vagus) nerve, thus slowing the heart. Cardiac arrhythmias may occur because of pressure on the vasomotor center or, more commonly, because of metabolic alterations from respiratory disturbances that accompany brain disorders. Because of the immobility of comatose patients, peripheral pulses should be monitored to detect phlebitis owing to blood stagnation.

Renal system

Accurate measurement of intake and output is important to the patient with a head injury or cranial pathology. Disoriented and unconscious patients will need to have an indwelling Foley catheter. Daily catheter care, most commonly with povidone-iodine complex (Betadine) is important to prevent urinary infections. Careful monitoring of urinary output is important for the early recognition of diabetes insipidus.

Diabetes insipidus occurs when there is injury (trauma, edema) to the hypothalamic area of the brain with subsequent suppression of the production of antidiuretic hormone (ADH). With the loss of ADH the kidney excretes large amounts of dilute urine (specific gravity 1.001 to 1.005). While this condition is usually a temporary one, extreme dehydration and hypernatremia can occur if adequate fluid replacement is not met. In the unconscious patient the inability to demand water may be fatal without nursing observation and interventions.

Gastrointestinal system

For the patient who is able to move to ambulate or even move around in bed, assessment of bowel sounds may not be of major importance. However, through adequate fluids, nutrition, and stool softeners, straining during stools should be avoided as discussed earlier. Too often bowel elimination is ignored in the unconscious patient and the bowel may become impacted with stool. This situation can be avoided through adequate hydration, stool softeners, and the use of Fleet enemas to stimulate evacuation. Accurate elimination records should be kept on these patients, including stool elimination as well as urine. Frequent, small liquid stools should signal the possibility of impacted bowel with stool leakage around it. A digital examination can determine if this is the case.

■ What are the factors that contribute to intracranial pressure?

The intracranial contents consist primarily of tissue, blood vessels, and cerebrospinal fluid. Increases in any of these can result in an increase in intracranial pressure. The brain in encased in an unyielding skull. Normally the skull's rigidity affords a welcome protection to the vulnerable brain tissue. However, through direct injury or with the growth of a lesion inside the skull, the contents may expand and the skull than becomes a liability, essentially acting as a vise. This subsequent crowding of the brain tissue results in neurologic symptoms expressed through a decreased level of consciousness, increasing systolic blood pressure, widening pulse pressure, decreasing pulse rate, and various sensory and motor deficits.

If these symptoms go untreated, the brain tissue may suffer irreversible damage or even death if vital brain centers are destroyed through this crowding. The point to remember is that critical care nurses are in attendance 24 hours a day. It is through their knowledge and clinical judgment that signs of increasing intracranial pressure can be discerned and treated.[8]

■ What is the clinical picture of acutely increasing intracranial pressure?

From an anatomic standpoint, the brain is divided into the right and left hemispheres by an extension of the dura mater called the falx cerebri. From the posterior part of the falx cerebri, the dura flares out laterally forming the tentorium cerebelli. This supports the temporal and occipital lobes of the brain and separates the occipital lobes from the cerebellum. It also serves as a line of demarcation for description when referring to sites of cranial lesions, that is, supratentorial or subtentorial.

The clinical picture of a supratentorial lesion or injury-producing coma or stupor has several distinctive features. If a history is available, localizing symptoms such as frontal headaches, focal seizures, or other changes consistent with hemispheric disease will usually precede unconsciousness. Physically, most patients demonstrate a combination of focal hemispheric signs, for example, sensorimotor defect, aphasia, and visual field defect, reflecting the site of the original pathologic process plus diffuse signs of supratentorial dysfunction, indicating that the lesion is exerting remote effects on the opposite hemisphere and the deep encephalon. Unless the patient is in the terminal stages of brain involvement, no evidence of direct subtentorial brain stem dysfunction can be found. That is, pupillary and oculovestibular reflexes remain intact.

As brain contents are progressively pushed downward, the neurologic signs and symptoms evolve in a characteristic manner, beginning with impairment in the diencephalon functions on down to the brain stem. Acutely increasing intracranial pressure results in a characteristic constellation of symptoms as the forebrain is herniated downward into the tentorial notch.[1]

Supratentorial central syndrome

As diencephalic function becomes involved by downward herniation of this structure, a change in alertness or behavior will become apparent: The patient will gradually become more somnolent (lower consciousness, more sleepy). Respirations may be interrupted by deep sighs and occasional pauses (Cheyne-Stokes). Pupils may be small and equal and react to light briskly. The doll's eyes phenomenon may be present.

As herniation progresses, the clinical signs of midbrain failure develop: Respirations may change from Cheyne-Stokes to sustained central hyperventilation. Pupils dilate moderately and become fixed at midposition. Doll's eyes phenomenon becomes difficult to elicit. Coma has progressed beyond purposeful response and is replaced by bilateral decerebrate rigidity in response to noxious stimuli.

As the ischemia produced by the downward herniation of the brain stem through the incisura progresses, signs of lower pons and medulla failure develop: Hyperventilation is replaced by a more or less regular pattern of respiration, often rapid and shallow. Pupils are dilated and fixed. Doll's eyes movements are gone. Response to noxious stimulus is flaccid. Babinski response is evidenced bilaterally. Decompensation occurs now with respirations slow and irregular in rate and depth. The pulse rate will vary widely. Blood pressure falls.[9]

Uncal herniation and lateral brain stem compression

Expanding lesions developing in the lateral portion of the middle fossa or in the temporal lobe may be expected to shift the medial edge of the uncus and hippocampal gyrus toward the midline and through the incisural notch. The earliest sign is the unilaterally dilated pupil (on side of injury). Impaired consciousness may not be seen consistently in the early stage, but deterioration may proceed rapidly. Soon after pupil dilation, an external third nerve paralysis appears and the involved eye turns outward. The patient becomes stuporous and then deeply comatose. Motor function may be initially impaired ipsilaterally (owing to pressure displacing the brain medially, thus pressing the contralateral cerebral peduncle against its incisural border). It quickly becomes bilateral motor paresis or paralysis. Early doll's eyes movements indicate third nerve impairment, then disappear as the midbrain is compressed. Continued progression at this point is similar to central diencephalic midbrain syndrome[9].

Subtentorial syndrome

In compression or destruction from subtentorial lesions or injury the characteristic clinical feature is the presence of restricted and usually asymmetric signs of focal brain stem dysfunction (for example, specific cranial nerve dysfunction). This discrete localization is unlike metabolic lesions causing coma in which the signs commonly indicate incomplete dysfunction at several different levels of the brain, and it is also unlike supratentorial herniation, in which *all* function of any given level tends to be lost as the process progresses. Continued progression of intracranial pressure results in brain stem compression with subsequent death, usually respiratory arrest.[1]

■ **What are the common treatments when there is evidence of increasing intracranial pressure?**

There are both medical and surgical treatments for alleviating increasing intracranial pressure. The more commonly used treatments will be described.

Medical management

Corticosteroids. In most cases of head trauma and with postcraniotomy patients, corticosteroids will be used to reduce inflammation and thus reduce the cerebral edema. After a few days at a maintenance dose, the dosage will be reduced daily until it is discontinued. While corticosteroid drugs do help control cerebral edema, they are not fast acting and would not be useful where there is evidence of rapidly increasing intracranial pressure. Patients receiving corticosteroids should be watched for evidence of gastrointestinal bleeding and masked infectious processes.

Osmotic diuretics. By administering a hypertonic solution, it is possible to establish an osmotic gradient across the blood-brain barrier that removes water from the brain and reduces cerebral edema. The drugs most commonly used are a 30% solution of urea or a 20% solution of mannitol given intravenously. The reaction to these diuretics is fairly rapid and can offer short-term relief from cerebral edema. More aggressive treatment such as emergency burr holes may be necessary for longer lasting relief. In cases where cerebral bleeding is suspected, such as in a subdural hematoma, osmotic diuretics are contraindicated. In these cases a decrease in brain tissue size from the diuresis provides more room for the expansion of the hematoma.

Hyperventilation. Through the reduction of carbon dioxide in the blood, cerebral vasoconstriction will occur, thus decreasing the blood volume to the brain tissue. This reduction in blood volume results in a decrease in intracranial pressure. Hyperventilation can be sustained most

successfully in patients receiving ventilatory support from respirators. The lowering of the arterial Pco_2 through hyperventilation should be carefully monitored by frequent evaluation of arterial blood gases.

Fluid limit and patient positioning. Limiting fluid intake to 50 to 100 ml/hr and elevation of the patient's head to 30 degrees to facilitate venous drainage have been discussed. While both of these measures may help control cerebral edema to some degree, neither is very effective in patients with evidence of rapidly increasing intracranial pressure.

Surgical management

Burr holes. The removal of small circular portions of the skull (trephination), called burr holes, can be used to diagnose and treat subdural and epidural hematomas. The advantages of this procedure lie in low risk and speedy evacuation of the clot if the patient's condition is rapidly deteriorating. However, a subdural hematoma in an unusual place can escape detection.[10]

Craniotomy. The removal of large areas of the skull and opening the dura to allow room for brain swelling are aggressive measures occasionally employed to cope with cerebral edema. These measures are employed only in a life-and-death situation and cannot be considered very successful.

Ventricular catheter or subarachnoid screw. Both the ventricular catheter and the subarachnoid screw can be used to monitor intracranial pressure and to drain cerebrospinal fluid to help decrease intracranial pressure.

■ **What are the major nursing responsibilities related to intracranial monitoring?**

Each critical care unit that uses intracranial monitoring will have its own procedure for the insertion of the ventricular cannula or the subarachnoid screw. There are several points that should be remembered regardless of the procedure used for monitoring.

Be consistent in taking pressure readings. For each pressure reading the patient's head should be in the same position relative to the transducer. This may necessitate using a carpenter's level to line up the catheter with the transducer, or if the patient's head cannot be lowered, the level of the head should be consistent with each reading.

Establish a trend with the pressure readings. While there are reported normal ranges for intracranial pressure, 50 to 200 mm H_2O or 4 to 15 mm Hg, the "normal" will vary somewhat for each patient. Therefore an isolated reading is less meaningful than repeated readings that can be compared for changes over time. Pressure readings will be elevated if the patient is moving, coughing, sneezing, or is contracting abdominal muscles. These elevated pressures are temporary and readings should be repeated.

It should be stressed that a transient rise in intracranial pressure (ICP) is rarely damaging and, in fact, occurs in normal individuals during straining at stool, isometric exercises, and sexual intercourse. An elevated ICP is most damaging when the brain is no longer able to compensate for this increased pressure. Brain tissue, cerebrospinal fluid, and blood comprise the three major components of the intracranial volume. When there is a slight increase in one volume, compensation occurs by a slight decrease in another component. In the early states of cerebral edema, ICP remains normal as cerebrospinal fluid and blood volume are reduced. However, once the margin of compensation is exhausted, a further increase in volume creates a major rise in ICP and decompensation (tentorial herniation or herniation through foramen magnum) and death results.[11]

Recognize and avoid complications of intracranial monitoring. One of the major problems with any type of invasive monitoring procedure is the chance of *infection.* Rigid aseptic procedures must be maintained to prevent contamination and subsequent cranial infections.

The tube and oscilloscope must be observed for signs of *obstruction* of the intracranial catheter. If the waveform appears dampened, indicating obstruction of the catheter, the tubing should be checked for kinks or other obstructions.

All connections and stopcocks must be checked frequently for two further complications, leaks and overinfusion. If CSF is allowed to *leak* out of the intracranial monitoring system, the system is open for infection, and the intracranial pressure may become lowered allowing brain tissue to be sucked into the catheter or against the subarachnoid screw. If the monitoring system has an IV fluid bag for flushing the catheter, it must be checked to see that fluid does not accidentally infuse into the ventricle or subarachnoid space causing an increase in ICP with possible permanent neurologic damage or death.[5]

Future trends indicate that work is being done on a transducer that can be inserted into the intracranial space through a small twist drill hole, thus avoiding surgery in the operating room. Also a transducer has already been developed that does not require external leads. The problem is still one of artifact interference. Newer diagnostic procedures will allow better visualization of cerebral blood flow and will permit measurement of displacement and distortion of the brain. The ultimate measure of brain function is metabolism, and techniques for measuring it are under study.

■ **What is the nursing role in control of pain and restlessness in postcraniotomy patients or patients with head injury?**

Opiates and sedatives are avoided for patients with head injuries. These drugs further depress an already damaged nervous system, impair respirations, and increase stupor. For control of pain mild analgesics are used. Codeine is the drug of choice and should be used judiciously. While some degree of pain can be expected with head trauma and postcraniotomy, the nurse should be alerted to signs of increasing intracranial pressure if headaches persist or become worse even after medication. Headaches and periorbital edema may be early signs of increasing intracranial pressure in the alert patient.

Urinary retention may account for restlessness in lethargic or drowsy patients and is readily treated by catheterization. In the unconscious patient hyperactivity or extreme restlessness may be treated with short-acting barbiturates or mild tranquilizers. The nurse should provide an environment in which the patient cannot further traumatize himself by his thrashing and moving about in bed. This involves padding the side rails and covering elbows and heels with padding to prevent sheet burns. If possible, arm and leg restraints should be avoided as pulling against them increases intracranial pressure. A Posey belt, however, can help to keep the patient in bed without completely hampering movement.

An important point to remember is that patients who have been restless and become lethargic or stuporous without medication are, in fact, becoming less wakeful—a decreased level of consciousness. While the nurse may be relieved that the restlessness has ceased, the importance of the decrease in level of consciousness should not go unnoticed. A thorough neurologic assessment should be done to more completely evaluate the neurologic status and determine other signs that may indicate increasing intracranial pressure.

■ **In what way can the critical care nurse provide emotional and psychologic support for the family of the head-injured patient?**

The most important means available to the nurse for providing support to family members is through frequent, empathetic communication. The family who does not understand what is happening to the patient and why is faced not only with concern for the patient but also fear of the hospital care he is receiving. Many nurses feel that they will be asked a question they cannot answer or be asked for an outcome that they do not wish to predict. Questions like these can easily and rightfully be referred to the physician, but questions such as : Is he resting? Is the respirator still on? Does he talk much? and so on can be answered in a straightforward manner. There are no stock answers about how to give support to a family or family member, but concern and recognition of family needs are indeed a nursing responsibility. The major points to be conveyed to family members are that care and comfort are being provided for their loved one, that the family is not a bother, and questions they have are important and every attempt will be made to answer them.

The importance of communication between the nursing staff and the physician can again be a great asset in establishing what and how much should be said to the family about the patient's condition and prognosis. However, no one needs to give the nurse information before she can be a good listener or before she can express assurance of the care the patient is receiving from the nursing staff.

An experienced nurse will also recognize that family members are often the first to notice changes in consciousness, both signs of improvement and signs of deterioration. Any comment from a family member that indicates a change should be heeded and evaluated carefully. Of course, always be cautious of family members who want so badly for improvement that they see it when it is not there. Do not degrade or make light of it, try to understand and try not to support what is not there.

■ **What are the ethical issues involved in patients with a head injury or trauma?**

Nurses caring for patients with severe brain injuries will eventually become aware of the ethical and legal questions surrounding brain death and the use and misuse of technology to prolong life. In most cases the patient will have been placed on a respirator for ventilatory support and the question then becomes, "When do you stop the respirator?" The criteria most frequently used by the medical profession in determining when to discontinue ventilatory support is when the patient has:

1. Absence of all cerebral responsiveness
2. Absence of all cranial nerve reflexes
3. Absence of any spontaneous movement
4. No response to deep pain
5. Absence of spontaneous respirations when disconnected from the respirator for 3 minutes (some use Pco_2 >55 mm Hg and no spontaneous respirations)
6. Isoelectric EEG (not required in some states)

In spite of these criteria the question of who should decide—the physician? the family? a hospital committee?—has no easy answers. The critical care nurse, while having no direct power over these decisions, must develop an awareness of the ethical and legal issues surrounding such decisions. Nurses should become involved in institutional policy making and review committees that address such issues. Further, the nurse must become aware of the legal parameters surrounding her role in the care of these patients.

No one needs to remind the nursing staff of the physical and emotional drain as they care for severely brain-damaged patients and have contact with their families over a long period of time.

Recognizing this, nurses need to provide a support system among themselves and good communication with the medical staff so that nursing input into decisions for care of brain-damaged patients will be considered.

REFERENCES

1. Plum, F.: Disorders of the nervous system and behavior. In Beeson, P., and McDermott, W., editors: Textbook of medicine, Philadelphia, 1975, W. B. Saunders Co., p. 540.
2. Mauss, N. K., and Mitchell, P. H.: Increased intracranial pressure. An update, Heart Lung 5(6):919, 1976.
3. Guyton, A. C.: Textbook of medical physiology, Philadelphia, 1976, W. B. Saunders, Co.
4. Plum, F., and Brennan, R. W.: Differential diagnosis of altered states of consciousness. In Youmans, J. R., editor: Neurological surgery, vol. 1, Philadelphia, 1973, W. B. Saunders Co., p. 44.
5. Holloway, N. M.: Nursing the critically ill adult, Menlo Park, Calif., 1979, Addison-Wesley Publishing Co.
6. Plum, F., and Posnar, J.: Diagnosis of stupor and coma, Philadelphia, 1972, F. A. Davis Co.
7. Mitchell, P. H., and Mauss, N. K.: Relationship of patient-nurse activity to intracranial pressure variations: a pilot study, Nurs. Res. 27(1):4, 1978.
8. Rudy, E.: Early omens of cerebral disaster, Nursing '77 58, February, 1977.
9. Thomas, L. M.: Acute increased intracranial pressure and the pathophysiology of mass lesions. In Youmans, J. R., editor: Neurological surgery, vol. 2, Philadelphia, 1973, W. B. Saunders Co., p. 953.
10. Patterson, R. H., Jr.: Injuries of the head and spine. In Beeson, P., and McDermott, W., editors: Textbook of medicine, Philadelphia, 1975, W. B. Saunders Co., p. 753.
11. Halon, K.: Description and uses of intracranial pressure monitoring, Heart Lung 5(2):277, 1976.

BIBLIOGRAPHY

Beeson, P., and McDermott, W.: Textbook of medicine, Philadelphia, 1975, W. B. Saunders Co.
Conway, B. L.: Carini and Owens' neurological and neurosurgical nursing, ed. 7, St. Louis, 1978, The C. V. Mosby Co.
Langfitt, T. W.: Increased intracranial pressure. In Youmans, J. R., editor: Neurological surgery, vol. 1, Philadelphia, 1973, W. B. Saunders Co., p. 443.
Loughead, W. M., and Barnett, J. J. M.: Lesions producing spontaneous hemorrhage. In Youmans, J. R., editor: Neurological surgery, vol. 2, Philadelphia, 1973, W. B. Saunders Co., p. 709.
Neurological assessment in cranial trauma or pathology. Cranial trauma, National Critical Care Institute Library Series, Orange, California, 1978.
Ojemann, R. G.: Intracerebral and intracerebellar hemorrhage. In Youmans, J. R., editor: Neurological surgery, vol. 2, Philadelphia, 1973, W. B. Saunders Co., p. 844.
Thomas, L. M., and Gurdjian, E. S.: Intracranial hematomas of traumatic origin. In Youmans, J. R., editor: Neurological surgery, vol. 2, Philadelphia, 1973, W. B. Saunders Co., p. 960.
Walker, A. E.: Mechanisms of cerebral trauma and the impairment of consciousness. In Youmans, J. R., editor: Neurological surgery, vol. 2, Philadelphia, 1973, W. B. Saunders Co., p. 936.

CHAPTER 37

Clinical management of the obstetric patient

Irene Matousek and Chester B. Martin

There are sound reasons for the different management of women who are critically ill at any point in pregnancy from conception until the physiologic puerperal recovery approximately 6 weeks after delivery. First, there are alterations in maternal physiology and anatomy that may change or obscure physical findings or responses to stressful circumstances or medications. Second, there is the presence of the fetus, dependent for life support on a relatively intact maternal physiology.

In very early pregnancy the embryo is undergoing rapid proliferation of cells and differentiation of body systems. At this time pharmacologic insults from the administration of drugs are likely to occur. Hazards from radiation are also well documented, and there is serious cause to believe that an unfavorable maternal environment with altered body chemistry and a deficient supply of oxygen may have equally grave consequences.

■ **When does pregnancy become a concern in the management of a critical care patient?**

Pregnancy should be a concern from conception onward. It may be worthwhile to consider every woman during the reproductive years, from approximately age 12 to age 50, as a likely candidate for pregnancy unless proved otherwise. A rapid pregnancy screening test of urine and/or serum may be helpful in verifying an early pregnancy when history or clinical examination findings are equivocal.

When the patient is known to be pregnant, the inclusion of pregnancy on the patient's problem list ensures consideration of pregnancy in selecting clinical diagnostic techniques, therapeutic plans, and management. A critical illness of almost any sort may cause the pregnancy to terminate spontaneously. The termination of pregnancy in a critically ill woman may often result in the birth of a compromised infant.

It may be well to consider the advantages to the fetus of transportation, in utero, to a site where *both* mother and infant may have intensive care immediately available.

PHYSIOLOGIC CHANGES IN PREGNANCY

■ **What are some of the important changes in maternal physiology during pregnancy?**

The pregnant patient has an increase in blood volume, heart rate, and cardiac output (the amount of blood pumped each minute by the heart). Her blood pressure tends to be lower than in the nonpregnant state, especially during the middle period of pregnancy. The energy cost and increased cardiac work required by exercise is greater during pregnancy than at other times. This is of particular significance in the pregnant woman with cardiac or pulmonary disease and may reduce the tolerance for exercise or stress in such patients.

Kidney blood flow and urine filtration are normally increased by 30% to 50% during pregnancy. In addition, there is normally a dilatation of the ureters and slowing of urine flow during pregnancy. These changes predispose the pregnant patient to urinary tract infections, which, if severe, can be a threat to both maternal and fetal health.

■ What is the role of nutrition in pregnancy?

Although good nutrition is important at any time, it is especially so during pregnancy. Inadequate nutrition may contribute to many of the complications of pregnancy, including impaired fetal growth and preeclampsia-eclampsia (see subsequent discussions).

■ What are the important changes produced by the enlarging uterus?

As it grows, the uterus progressively displaces the other abdominal contents of the abdomen. In most normal women the displacement produces no symptoms or at most contributes slightly to unpleasant symptoms such as heartburn and epigastric fullness after meals. In women with deformities of the thoracic spine and rib cage, however, the upward displacement of abdominal contents may displace the diaphragm and restrict its movements sufficiently to produce respiratory embarrassment.

The displacement of many abdominal organs from their normal position, and the forward displacement of the abdominal wall by the enlarging uterus may alter the physical signs accompanying many acute intra-abdominal diseases and trauma. For example, in appendicitis the abdominal tenderness and localized signs of peritoneal irritation may appear much later in the course of the disease during pregnancy than in the nonpregnant state, and the tenderness when it appears may be located at or above the level of the umbilicus rather than in the usual right lower quadrant position. Similarly, with intra-abdominal bleeding or gastrointestinal perforation, signs of peritoneal irritation may appear only quite late in the course of the disease, and the early absence of these signs may lead to an initial misdiagnosis and mismanagement.

In the last third of pregnancy the weight of the uterus and its contents is carried anterior to the normal axis of weight bearing. This plus the hormone-induced softening of the connective tissue supports of joints predisposes the pregnant patient to postural back pain and, indeed, acute back injury.

Also during the last third of pregnancy the enlarging uterus compresses the pelvic veins and inferior vena cava. This in turn leads to slowing of the blood circulation in the pelvic and leg veins and predisposes the pregnant patient to the development of thrombophlebitis and thromboembolism, especially if she is immobilized because of illness or injury. Even ambulatory women have an increased risk of developing venous thrombosis, especially if there is any preexisting venous disease. Such measures as elastic support stockings, avoidance of long standing, and elevation of the legs when at rest are thus indicated in pregnant women with a history of thrombophlebitis or with existing varicose veins; leg elevation, elastic stockings, and regular examination for evidence of thrombophlebitis are indicated whenever a pregnant patient is immobilized or confined to bed because of illness or injury. It is important that the stockings be removed at least every 4 hours and reapplied to prevent constriction and impairment of blood flow. At the time of removal passive movement of the lower extremities may assist blood flow.

■ What are the goals for fetal management during critical care of the obstetric patient?

The primary goal is to provide the best possible maternal environment for the growing fetus. The developing fetus is dependent on its mother for an uninterrupted supply of oxygen. This in turn requires an intact supply of maternal red blood cells, adequate maternal blood pressure to ensure perfusion of the placenta, and sufficient arterial oxygen tension to promote diffusion across the placenta. Accordingly, transfusion should be considered for correction of severe anemia. Hypotension should be corrected by the restoration of effective blood volume (avoiding vasoconstrictive drugs, if possible, since these may impede uterine blood flow). Oxygen should be administered when there is maternal hypoxemia, hypotension, or severe anemia.

The fetus must be protected from pharmacologic and biochemical insults. The fetus very rapidly reflects altered maternal biochemical states. Almost all drugs cross the placenta, and many affect the fetus or newborn adversely.

The fetus is dependent on the mother for an adequate heat-losing mechanism. The high metabolic rate of the fetus creates heat, which must be transported to the mother for dissipation. This mechanism is essential to avoid stressing the fetal organism, both through the increased consumption of oxygen during hyperthermia and exhaustion of the cardiovascular system, which increases heart rate and cardiac output in an attempt to lose heat. The safe heat tolerance level for the human fetus is unknown, but it may be lower than that of the child or adult. Serious consideration should be given to treating the sustained elevation of temperature in critically ill pregnant women directly through the use of evaporation, cold packs, or other means. Aspirin and similar drugs of the prostaglandin synthetase-inhibitor group should be used with caution, if at all, for these drugs are potentially capable of altering the fetal circulation by causing premature closure of the ductus arteriosus.

The fetus is also dependent on the mother for nutrition. The essential substrates appear to be glucose and amino acids. Although the fetus apparently can tolerate short periods of deprivation, there is evidence that its neurologic development may be impaired by maternal ketoacidosis. For this reason the critically ill pregnant woman should receive sufficient calories to prevent the development of starvation, ketosis, and acidosis.

OBSTETRIC PROBLEMS IN THE FIRST HALF OF PREGNANCY

The most commonly encountered pregnancy-related problems requiring critical care during the first half of pregnancy are abortion, ectopic pregnancy, and pernicious vomiting.

Abortion

Abortion legally denotes the termination of pregnancy prior to the stage of fetal viability, that is, prior to 20 weeks after the last menstrual period (LMP), in most jurisdictions in the United States. Abortions may be spontaneous or induced; induced abortions further may be either therapeutic (performed through legitimate medical care channels) or illegal (criminal).

■ What are the symptoms and findings in spontaneous abortion?

The first clinical signs of spontaneous abortion are usually the appearance of vaginal bleeding accompanied by lower abdominal cramping pain. The bleeding results from separation of the placenta, whereas the cramps represent intense uterine contractions. The stage of abortion marked only by uterine bleeding with or without accompanying cramps but before dilatation of the cervix has begun is called "threatened abortion."

With further evolution of the abortion process the cervix begins to efface and dilate as a result of the uterine contractions. When the cervical dilatation and effacement can be detected on clinical examination, the abortion is said to be "inevitable." Considerable placental separation has usually occurred by this stage, and the bleeding may become quite heavy.

Dilatation of the cervix is usually followed shortly by expulsion of the products of conception (embryo or fetus, fetal membranes, and placenta). The expulsion phase is frequently accompanied by a further increase in the amount of vaginal bleeding. An incomplete abortion is one in which the conceptus has been partially expelled, but additional fragments of the placenta and fetal membranes remain within the uterus. A complete abortion is one in which all of the products of conception have been expelled. The stage of complete abortion is usually followed by a reduction in the severity of the cramps and in the amount of vaginal bleeding. During the latter half of the first trimester and in the first half of the second trimester the expulsion of the products of conception may occur piecemeal over several hours, and it is not unusual for fragments of placenta and fetal membranes to remain within the uterus following expulsion of the major portion of the products of conception. Retention of these placental fragments in utero may cause continued bleeding, and the degenerating placental material provides a rich growth medium for bacteria, which enter the uterine cavity through the dilated cervix. For this reason and in order to minimize the duration of pain and the amount of blood loss, incomplete abortion is usually terminated by curettage, and curettage is frequently performed even though the abortion may seem to have proceeded spontaneously to completion.

■ What are the chief critical care problems in spontaneous abortion?

The major problems of spontaneous abortion relate to blood loss, infection, and operative injury during completion of the abortion.

Any patient undergoing abortion is at risk for a major hemorrhage. Assessment of the amount of blood loss already sustained, establishment of a route for the rapid IV administration of fluids or blood, and arranging for the availability of crossmatched blood for replacement should be done very early in the care of these patients. These steps should be performed even if the patient is only experiencing minor bleeding when she is first seen, because the amount of hemorrhage may increase dramatically at any time.

When the patient is seen with threatened abortion signaled only by mild cramps and scanty vaginal bleeding, adequate treatment may consist of starting an IV infusion, restricting oral intake (in case later operative intervention is required), and observing her while at bed rest for a time. In a large proportion of these early cases the symptoms will subside, and the pregnancy will continue uneventfully. From 8 weeks' amenorrhea onward, the use of real-time ultrasound scanning to detect the presence or absence of embryonic heart action has proved very useful in differentiating those cases of threatened abortion with a high probability of continuation (positive heart action) from those in which eventual abortion is inevitable because of absence or death of the embryo (negative heart action). In other patients the pain and bleeding will increase and require evacuation of the uterus by curettage. When the patient is initially seen at the stage of inevitable or incomplete abortion, preparations should be set in motion for early curettage in order to minimize the amount of pain, the amount of blood lost, and the likelihood of ascending uterine infection. The oral administration of liquids, food, or medication should be avoided in anticipation of the use of anesthesia.

Serious intrauterine infection is not frequent in patients with spontaneous abortion unless the patient has delayed for a considerable time before seeking medical care. All patients should be examined for evidence of infection, however, because of the potential gravity of this complication. Suggestive findings include fever, uterine tenderness, and foul-smelling vaginal discharge or placental fragments. Hypotension and tachycardia disproportionate to the estimated amount of blood lost are potentially very serious clinical signs. Infected abortion can become a life-threatening complication because of the possibility of septicemia, septic shock, and invasive pelvic infections with virulent strains of *Streptococcus, Escherichia coli,* or *Clostridium,* which may inhibit the vagina and cervix.

In order to minimize the likelihood of introducing additional pathogenic organisms into the vaginal tract of patients undergoing abortion, pelvic examination should be carried out only following antiseptic cleansing of the vulva, and only sterile gloves and instruments should be employed. The number of pelvic examinations should be kept to the minimum required for diagnosis and treatment.

Operative injury to the uterus, cervix, and, in rare instances, even the bowel or pelvic supporting tissues may occur during the course of curettage and completion of an abortion despite the exercise of careful judgment and the employment of skillful technique. Simple uterine perforation usually requires only observation to exclude intraabdominal bleeding from the perforation site. More serious injuries may require active intervention. Since an injury may go unrecognized at the time by even an experienced surgeon, all patients should be observed carefully for evidence of blood loss or peritoneal irritation for several hours following curettage.

■ What critical complications may occur with therapeutic abortion?

The complications of the therapeutic termination of pregnancy depend on the means employed to empty the uterus. In the first trimester this is usually evacuation of the products of conception by means of a suction curette. The chief hazards of this route are laceration of the cervix during dilatation and perforation of the uterus during curettage. Either of these accidents may be followed by serious hemorrhage. In addition, perforation of the uterus may result in inadvertent injury to the bowel, with resulting peritonitis. Uterine infection may occur, even though the dilatation and curettage were carried out under surgical asepsis. The infection may become apparent early during the postoperative period or may appear several days later (especially if a few placental fragments have been left in the uterus). Patients should be observed for several hours under recovery room conditions following suction curettage in order to detect hemorrhage or peritonitis from unrecognized injuries. The patient should also be instructed on discharge to be alert for symptoms and signs of delayed postoperative infection and to return immediately should symptoms appear.

■ What are the problems associated with therapeutic abortion during the second trimester?

In the second trimester the uterus is larger, its contents are bulkier and more substantial, and the techniques for terminating pregnancy are less satisfactory than in the first trimester. All the methods presently in use carry the risk of potentially serious complications; patients undergoing midtrimester pregnancy termination must be observed carefully, both during and for several hours after the abortion, to detect problems at an early stage when treatment can be more effective and the likelihood of a life-threatening situation can be minimized. The methods for second trimester abortion most frequently employed at present are dilatation of the cervix and extraction of the uterine contents (D and E), induction of immature delivery by means of prostaglandins or by intrauterine injection of hypertonic solutions (saline, urea, or glucose), and abdominal hysterotomy. The serious hazards present with all these techniques are hemorrhage, injury to the uterus or cervix, and infection.

D and E is similar to the dilatation and curettage (suction) method employed for first trimester terminations except that, since the fetus is larger, both the degree of cervical dilatation required and the size of the instruments used for the extraction of uterine contents are larger than in the first trimester. Therefore the risk of cervical laceration and uterine perforation is also increased. Operative blood loss is usually greater, and placental fragments may be left behind in the uterus, leading to the risk of postoperative bleeding and infection up to several days after the procedure. These hazards notwithstanding, D and E remains the preferred technique in many clinics for pregnancy terminations up to 16 weeks' menstrual age.

The use of *prostaglandins* (PG's) to induce midtrimester abortion has increased greatly in recent years. These substances act directly on the myometrium to induce uterine contractions. In addition, PG's (especially PG-E_2) act on the cervix to induce softening and "ripening," thus favoring more rapid cervical dilatation. Intra-amniotic injection of PG-$F_2\alpha$ and intravaginal suppositories of PG-E_2 are methods presently approved for clinical use, and several other routes of administration and synthetic analogues of these compounds are undergoing clinical testing or are already approved for use in other countries. In some clinics, PG-E_2 suppositories are used to soften the cervix in preparation for D and E, and in others the administration of PG's is combined with the intravenous infusion of oxytocin or intra-amniotic instillation of hypertonic urea to increase the success rate and decrease the time required for the abortion. The PG's are very potent stimulators of uterine contractions and may occasionally cause uterine rupture or cervical laceration even when used alone. The incidence of these complications is increased when PG's are combined with oxytocin or other uterine stimulants. Another not infrequent problem with PG-induced midtrimester abortion is retention of the placenta, sometimes requiring curettage for completion of the abortion. Uterine or cervical lacerations, or incomplete expulsion of the placenta, can be causes for copious bleeding. With uterine rupture a large part of this bleeding may be intra-abdominal and thus not immediately apparent. Retention of placental fragments can also lead to bleeding and/or infection some days after the abortion itself. Thus during the induction of midtrimester abortion with PG's, the patient must be observed both for unusual vaginal blood loss and evidence of uterine rupture (abdominal pain, indications from pulse and blood pressure of concealed bleeding). The patient should be warned to return promptly for treatment should she develop fever, pain, or increased bleeding in the days following the abortion.

The PG's have many other actions besides those on the uterus and cervix. These frequently show up as distressing (although usually not dangerous) side-effects during their use to induce abortion. These side-effects include nausea and vomiting (often occurring quite suddenly and with little warning), increased intestinal motility leading to abdominal cramps and diarrhea, fever (which may complicate the ability to detect infection), and bronchospasm. Nursing personnel should be prepared for the occurrence of these side-effects and also be prepared to provide sympathetic and reassuring support to the patient experiencing these distressing symptoms.

Two other infrequent but serious complications of PG's should be noted. The first of these may occur when PG's are used to induce delivery in cases of missed abortion and intrauterine fetal death. The strong uterine contractions provoked by the PG's may force amniotic fluid and clot-promoting substances resulting from autolysis of the fetus and placenta into the maternal circulation. This can lead in turn to an extensive disseminated intravascular coagulation (DIC) syndrome with bleeding, circulatory collapse, and renal failure. A second problem may occur when PG's are combined with intravenous infusions, especially infusions containing oxytocin. PG's affect the distribution of blood flow within the kidney and may impair the ability to excrete an excessive water load. The antidiuretic effect of oxytocin accentuates this problem. Under these circumstances, the patient can develop water intoxication with convulsions or coma. Both the amount of IV fluids and urine production should be noted carefully during PG use, and an increasingly positive fluid balance should be promptly called to the attention of medical personnel.

Hypertonic solutions of sodium chloride, urea, or glucose, injected intra-amniotically, kill the fetus and damage the placenta and decidua, resulting in the production of endogenous PG's, labor, and expulsion of the uterine contents. The hazards associated with the use of hypertonic solutions include the following:

1. Rapid movement of fluid into the amniotic space, causing hypotension
2. Inadvertent IV injection, resulting in shock
3. Accidental injection into the myometrium, causing uterine necrosis and peritonitis
4. Release of clot-promoting substances from the degenerating placenta and decidua into the circulation, producing disseminated intravascular coagulation with consumption of clotting factors and a secondary bleeding disorder
5. In patients with cardiac and renal disease, retention of the excessive sodium within the vascular system and vessel walls, resulting in edema, hypertension, and even cardiac failure
6. With hypertonic glucose solutions, serious intrauterine infection

Although these complications are relatively infrequent, their occasional occurrence makes it advisable that patients undergoing midtrimester abortion be observed carefully for evidence of one or another of these problems for several hours following the intra-amniotic instillation of the hypertonic solution. Many authorities believe that these patients should be kept in the hospital until abortion has been completed.

The use of hypertonic injections into the amniotic cavity has been combined with the IV administration of oxytocin in order to shorten the injection-delivery time. This combination has also been found to result in an increased incidence of some of the complications mentioned previously. The addition of uterine stimulation with oxytocin to that resulting from the hypertonic solutions may also result in uterine rupture.

Abdominal hysterotomy is essentially a mini-cesarean section. This procedure has the obvious disadvantages of a major abdominal operation requiring a general anesthetic. Blood loss is often relatively high. In addition, the uterine incision is usually a vertical one in the body of the uterus, a location that carries the risk of rupture with major bleeding in a subsequent pregnancy. In a recent survey, abdominal hysterotomy was found to have the highest morbidity and mortality rates of all of the midtrimester abortion techniques in common use.

One further technique of midtrimester abortion should be mentioned, although its use seems to be declining. That is the use of Laminaria (dried seaweed that swells on absorption of water) or a bougie (such as a Foley catheter with a large volume bag) to effect gradual dilation of the cervix. This is then followed by D and E or by induction of uterine contractions with oxytocin to empty the uterus. The introduction and retention of foreign bodies for a period within the cervix carries the risk of infection, although in practice the incidence of this complication has been rather low. Cervical laceration, uterine perforation, and uterine rupture are further potential complications of abortion by this method.

■ **What are the serious complications that may occur following illegal abortion?**

The most frequent complications following illegal abortion are the same ones that occur after spontaneous or therapeutically induced abortion: hemorrhage, infection, and trauma. The frequency of these complications is probably increased, because the criminal abortionist is likely to be relatively uneducated, unskilled, and in some cases flagrantly careless and dirty. In addition, the patient is likely to delay seeking medical care, in the hope that her problem will go away and that she may remain undetected. When these patients do seek medical attention, they are likely to be suffering from severe and protracted hemorrhage or advanced pelvic or systemic infection. There may be intraperitoneal bleeding or peritonitis as a result of uterine perforation, and occasionally foreign bodies such as catheters and other objects are found within the abdominal cavity as a testimony to the abortionists's lack of skill. The patient known or suspected to have had a criminal abortion should have abdominal x-ray films taken to detect intraperitoneal air resulting from uterine perforation, intra-abdominal foreign bodies, and evidence of infection with gas-forming organisms in the pelvis. Many criminal abortion patients are critically ill when they are brought to the hospital and may require immediate, vigorous therapy of hypovolemic shock and advanced sepsis.

In some cases criminal abortion has been attempted by the injection of necrotizing solutions or pastes into the uterus. In these patients there may be extensive necrosis of pelvic tissue and advanced infection. Tetanus or gas gangrene infections may be present. Some of these substances may be nephrotoxic, moreover, adding the problems of renal shutdown to those of shock and sepsis.

Ectopic pregnancy
■ **What is ectopic pregnancy?**

Ectopic pregnancy refers to the implantation of the conceptus outside the main portion of the uterine cavity. This ectopic implantation most frequently occurs in the fallopian tube, but may also occur on the pelvic peritoneum and surface of other intra-abdominal organs (abdominal pregnancy), on the ovary (ovarian pregnancy), in the intramyometrial portion of the uterine tube (cornual pregnancy), or in the cervical canal (cervical pregnancy). Ectopic pregnancies rarely survive beyond the first trimester. Rupture of the implantation site (tube or uterine cornu) or placental separation are the usual events that terminate the pregnancy, and either can cause profuse intra-abdominal hemorrhage. Some abdominal pregnancies survive into the second or third trimester; however, the incidence of placental insufficiency and maternal complications (for example, bowel obstruction) is high and delivery of a live, mature fetus is unusual.

■ **What are the symptoms of ectopic pregnancy?**

The most frequent symptoms of ectopic pregnancy, especially tubal pregnancy, is abdominal pain. Other very common symptoms include vaginal bleeding and a history of delayed or missed menstrual period. Symptoms of shock may also be present.

Important physical findings suggesting ectopic tubal pregnancy include a pelvic mass—usually unilateral or posterior to the uterus—and the aspiration of nonclotting blood on culdocentesis. The uterus may be normal in size or enlarged one and one-half to two times. Hypotension, tachycardia, and pallor may be present if the intraperitoneal bleeding is severe.

■ What are the initial critical steps in the management of ectopic pregnancy?

The initial management steps in cases of suspected ruptured or bleeding ectopic pregnancy consist of establishing a large caliber IV line, assessing adequacy of circulation, and sending a blood sample for type and cross match. The patient should be observed carefully and frequently for evidence of actual or impending shock during the time when diagnostic procedures and preparations for definitive therapy are being carried out.

Pernicious vomiting
■ What is pernicious vomiting (hyperemesis gravidarum)?

Many pregnant patients experience some nausea and vomiting during the first trimester. These symptoms probably result from hormonal stimulation of the "vomiting center" in the brain stem. Usually the nausea and vomiting are mild and disappear toward the end of the first trimester. In a small minority of women, however, the nausea and vomiting are severe and protracted and may result in dehydration and ketoacidosis. Repeated episodes of nausea and vomiting can interfere markedly with maternal nutrition.

■ What is the danger of pernicious vomiting to the pregnancy?

In one large study of women with hyperemesis gravidarum there was a high incidence of abortion in patients suffering repeated episodes of severe nausea and vomiting. In addition, more recent studies have shown that there is an increased incidence of neurologic abnormalities in the infants of women who experienced ketonemia and ketonuria from any cause during their pregnancies.

■ Which patients with nausea and vomiting of pregnancy require urgent care?

The pregnant woman who has clinically apparent dehydration clearly needs hospitalization for correction of her fluid and electrolyte abnormalities. In addition, the urine of any pregnant woman with a history of more than occasional vomiting should be tested for the presence of acetone. Any pregnant woman exhibiting acetonuria is a candidate for hospitalization and IV fluid therapy. In many patients with hyperemesis gravidarum, the nausea and vomiting will subside when the patient is admitted to the hospital and her fluid and electrolyte abnormalities are corrected. Other patients will require antinauseant medications for relief of the nausea and vomiting. These medications should be selected carefully, especially during the first trimester, because some of them have been suspected of causing congenital anomalies.

OBSTETRIC PROBLEMS IN THE SECOND HALF OF PREGNANCY
■ What are the obstetric and other pregnancy-related problems requiring critical care during the second half of pregnancy?

The most important disorders—from the standpoint of severity or frequency—requiring critical care during the second half of pregnancy include bleeding complications (such as placenta previa and abruptio placentae), hypertensive disorders, premature rupture of the fetal membranes and premature labor. Urinary tract infections may occur at any time during pregnancy, but these can become life-threatening complications, especially for the fetus, during the latter months.

All pregnant patients become critical care patients during labor, delivery, and the early postpartum hours. Although most women go through the peripartum time without incident, the potential for damaging or life-threatening complications for both fetus and mother is at its greatest during this time.

Although many intercurrent medical diseases may complicate the management of pregnancy, certain maternal diseases such as diabetes, heart disease (especially obstructive valvular disease), chronic renal disease, and acute febrile illnesses are particularly noteworthy because of their relative frequency and because of the urgent maternal or fetal complications sometimes associated with them.

▪ What are the important bleeding complications during the second half of pregnancy?

The most important obstetric complications associated with vaginal bleeding during late pregnancy are placenta previa and premature separation of the placenta (abruptio placentae). Trauma to the vagina and cervix and lesions such as cervical erosions and cervical cancers may also cause bleeding during pregnancy, as at other times. Bleeding during the early or late postpartum period may result from lacerations of the uterus, cervix, or vagina; failure of the uterine muscle to contract following separation of the placenta; or the presence of fetal membrane or placental remnants within the uterus.

▪ What is the clinical situation characteristic of placenta previa?

Placenta previa refers to implantation of the placenta in the lower portion of the uterine cavity, adjacent to or even covering the cervical opening. Bleeding occurs when a portion of the placenta separates as a result of the normal thinning of the lower uterine segment and dilatation of the upper cervix, which takes place prior to labor in late pregnancy. Placental separation and consequent bleeding may also occur as a result of mechanical disturbance of the upper cervix or lower uterine segment that may occur during intercourse or vaginal examination.

The bleeding in placenta previa is typically painless and unassociated with regular uterine contractions. The uterus is soft and not tender. Because the placenta occupies the lower portion of the uterus, the fetal presenting part (breech or vertex) is usually displaced upward and may be palpated as "floating" relatively high above the pelvic inlet. In many cases the long body axis of the fetus may be oriented transversely or obliquely (transverse or oblique lie) instead of the usual position parallel to the maternal body axis. The fetal heart tones are usually normal and without the irregularity suggesting fetal distress, unless the amount of maternal blood lost has been great enough to produce (maternal) hemorrhagic shock.

Episodes of bleeding from placenta previa usually subside spontaneously unless interference causes additional placental separation or progres-sive labor has begun. Expectant management with bedrest under close medical supervision will usually permit the pregnancy to continue until the stage of fetal maturity (usually 37 weeks) if the bleeding occurs before this time. Since even gentle manipulation of the cervix may dislodge additional portions of the placenta and produce further bleeding, it is of utmost importance to avoid this possibility. For this reason vaginal examination should not be performed on any patient suspected of having placenta previa until this possibility has been excluded—usually by ultrasonographic scanning. The recent development of compact, relatively easy-to-operate real-time ultrasonic scanners with good picture quality has greatly increased the applicability of the technique in even urgent situations. The ability to determine placental location accurately by ultrasonography has virtually eliminated the need for the "double setup" examination in cases of late pregnancy bleeding. This latter procedure, so called because it was carried out in the operating room with anesthesia and surgical personnel in attendance and a "double setup" of instruments for either cesarean section or vaginal delivery, depending on the findings, in readiness, was formerly employed when (1) the duration of pregnancy at the time of the bleeding was 37 weeks' or more or (2) intervention was forced because of continuing blood loss or the onset of clinical labor. It is infrequently indicated today in an adequately equipped hospital.

▪ What are the clinical characteristics of premature separation of the placenta?

The symptoms and findings resulting from premature separation of the normally implanted placenta vary according to the degree of placental separation and, to a lesser extent, according to the mechanism responsible for the separation. The degree of premature separation can range from detachment of all or a major part of the placenta (abruptio placentae) to separation of only a small portion of the placental edge. The mechanism involved in the major placental separations appears to be most often disruption of the wall of one or more of the arteries supplying maternal blood to the placenta, permitting the escape of maternal blood under high pressure into the decidua (endometrium of pregnancy). The extravasated blood may dissect extensively in the decidual layer, leading to the separation of increasing amounts of the placental area. The most frequent cause of these arterial ruptures is thought to be focal degeneration and necrosis in the arterial wall and adjacent decidua. Such lesions occur with increased frequency in pregnancies complicated by chronic hypertensive disease or maternal cigarette smoking, and abruptio placentae occurs more often in hypertensive than in normotensive pregnant women and in smokers than in nonsmokers.

Less extensive and less dramatic placental separations result from local disruption of the placental attachments, especially at the placental margin. Such local separations may result from stresses imposed by unequal growth of the placenta and uterine wall and perhaps also tensions on the placental attachments occurring during uterine contractions. The maternal blood escaping into the decidua in these local separations is not under high arterial pressure, and the separation is less likely to extend.

Although only a small proportion of placental separations result from external trauma, trauma can indeed produce either local or extensive placental separation. Placental separation is more likely to occur in cases of abdominal trauma; however, severe accelerations or decelerations, as during automobile accidents, may stress the placental attachment to the point of separation even though there is no direct injury to the abdomen. The possibility of premature separation of the placenta should thus be kept in mind in the assessment of women who experience trauma during pregnancy.

The pregnant woman who has experienced a major degree of placental separation presents a fairly characteristic clinical picture. Vaginal bleeding is usually present, and this can be copious. In a small portion of cases the bleeding from placental separation is retained behind the placenta (concealed abruptions), and in these patients vaginal bleeding will be absent. Continuous abdominal and/or low back pain is likely to be present, and this may be severe. The uterus is frequently tender to palpation, especially if the area of abruption involves the anterior uterine wall.

Uterine contractions are usually present, and in some patients with severe abruptions very frequent uterine contractions combined with an increase in the resting tension (hypertonus) gives the impression of a continuous uterine contraction that does not relax. The fetal heart tones may be absent, or a slow or irregular fetal heart rate may give evidence of fetal distress. Major degrees of placental separation may be recognized easily from the history and physical findings.

The smaller degrees of premature separation of the placenta are more difficult to diagnose with certainty from the clinical findings alone. In particular it may be difficult to distinguish between a marginal separation of the placenta and bleeding from placenta previa without the aid of specialized techniques such as ultrasound scanning to demonstrate the placental location. Uterine pain, tenderness, and contractions may be minimal or absent with small placental separations. One important clue may often be obtained on abdominal examination, that is, the finding that the fetal presenting part (vertex or breech) is dipping deeply into the pelvis, and this suggests that a major degree of placenta previa is unlikely to be present. On the other hand, this finding does not exclude a marginal or low-lying placenta; thus digital vaginal examination should only be performed after placental localization studies have excluded placenta previa.

■ What are the management principles in premature separation of the placenta?

When the clinical symptoms and findings indicate a major degree of placental separation, prompt termination of the pregnancy by induction of labor or cesarean section is indicated if the fetus is still alive. The fetal heart rate should be monitored continuously and the fetus delivered by cesarean section if distress occurs. Induction of labor with fetal monitoring is usually also indicated for lesser degrees of premature placental separation when the complication occurs during the last 3 or 4 weeks of pregnancy, after the fetus has reached adequate maturity. Earlier than this time, the pregnancy may be managed expectantly under close observation if the bleeding subsides and there is no evidence of fetal distress.

■ **What other major maternal complications may occur with abruptio placentae?**

Hemorrhagic shock is a frequent complication of major placental abruptions because of the extensive maternal blood loss that may occur. In many patients, however, the blood pressure is maintained at normal or even elevated levels for a time even though major hemorrhage has occurred. If this possibility is not recognized, one may be lulled into a false sense of security in managing patients with placental abruption, only to be rudely surprised when circulatory collapse occurs abruptly. The patient with severe abruptio placentae, that is, the patient with abdominal pain and a tense, tender uterus, has probably lost 1000 to 1500 ml of circulating blood volume within a relatively short time after the onset of the abruption. In these patients it is a good practice to begin replacement with electrolyte solutions immediately after the complication is diagnosed. The urine output is usually a good indicator of the adequacy of the blood volume, and a low or falling output (below 50 to 75 ml/hr) suggests inadequate replacement. If the urine volume does not begin to increase following infusion of 1000 to 1500 ml of fluid, however, one should be wary of the possibility that acute renal failure has occurred. A central venous pressure catheter should be inserted at this point, if this has not already been done, and used as a guide to further fluid therapy in order to avoid volume overload and pulmonary edema.

Another major complication that may accompany abruptio placentae is the occurrence of a coagulation disorder. The most frequent coagulopathy encountered with abruptio placentae is disseminated intravascular coagulation with consumption of multiple clotting factors. In a very much smaller proportion of patients a fibrinolytic state may dominate. A blood sample for observation of clot formation and possible lysis should be drawn periodically throughout the management of patients with abruptio placentae. Even when a coagulopathy develops, however, specific replacement of fibrinogen and other clotting factors is usually necessary only if cesarean section delivery is required.

The third major complication that may accompany abruptio placentae is acute renal failure.

This occurs primarily because of renal ischemia resulting from severe blood loss. In patients with disseminated intravascular coagulation, fibrin thrombi in the renal glomerular capillaries may add to the impairment of kidney function.

■ **What other problems cause vaginal bleeding in late pregnancy?**

Lacerations of the vagina or cervix may produce copious bleeding because of the increased vascularity of these tissues during pregnancy. These lacerations may result from sexual activity or attempts to terminate the pregnancy. Caustic chemicals such as potassium permanganate are occasionally used for douching, and these may cause vaginal or cervical ulcerations with heavy bleeding. Cervical cancers may also be responsible for heavy bleeding during pregnancy. Vaginitis, cervicitis, or cervical erosions tend to produce only scanty bleeding, spotting, or blood-tinged discharge. Bloody mucus may be expelled at the onset of labor ("bloody show"). Any vaginal bleeding during late pregnancy must be assessed with caution, however, for the initial bleeding from placenta previa or premature placental separation may be very scanty in amount.

Rarely an abnormal insertion of the umbilical cord into the placenta or an atypical path of umbilical vessel branches will bring these fetal vessels close to the internal cervical opening, where they may be torn during cervical dilatation or vaginal examinations in labor. Fetal hemorrhage from these vessels can rapidly bring about fetal distress. For this reason the fetal heart rate should always be monitored for evidence of fetal distress when vaginal bleeding occurs in late pregnancy, even when there is no evidence of abruptio placentae or placenta previa.

■ **What are the initial measures in the management of the patient with vaginal bleeding in late pregnancy?**

Patients with vaginal bleeding in late pregnancy should immediately have the following procedures done:

1. A rapid assessment of the amount of blood lost
2. Provision made for blood replacement
3. An IV line placed for fluid therapy

4. Other indicated physiologic support such as oxygen administration

The first step is a rapid assessment of the amount of bleeding that has occurred or is occurring. When the patient describes bleeding greater than the peak of menstrual flow of if there is blood on the legs or clothing, it is wise to proceed as if a major bleeding complication is present. When abdominal pain and uterine tenderness are present, the possibility of abruptio placentae with concealed hemorrhage should be considered, even though external bleeding is minimal or absent. A large caliber IV line should be established immediately and kept open with a balanced electrolyte or normal saline solution. Tachycardia, hypotension, and pallor usually indicate that a major degree of blood loss has already occurred, and fluids should be administered rapidly. In any case blood should be tested for type and cross match.

After these steps have been accomplished, additional history may be obtained and physical examination carried out in order to determine further the cause of the bleeding. A gentle, careful speculum examination may be carried out in order to inspect the vagina and cervix for local lesions; however, pelvic examination may easily provoke an immediate massive hemorrhage if the bleeding results from placenta previa. Therefore, unless this cause of bleeding has been excluded, digital palpation of the upper vagina and cervix *should not* be performed except in the operating room under double setup conditions and even then only if the decision has been made to terminate the pregnancy. The fetal heart tones should be checked as part of the initial assessment, and continuous monitoring of the fetal heart rate (using external techniques) should be begun if the presumptive diagnosis is abruptio placentae or placenta previa or if the mother appears to be hypovolemic. When fetal distress is present, the administration of oxygen to the mother by means of a face mask may benefit the fetus while preparations are being made for definitive treatment.

The data base should be completed as soon as the patient's condition permits. This will include a well-defined history either from the patient or her family, a review of available records, comple-

tion of the physical examination, ultrasonographic examination (if not already done), and steps to obtain information from other pertinent sources such as the physician's office, clinic, or hospital.

■ **What are abnormally elevated levels of blood pressure during pregnancy?**

The expected blood pressure in young women during the childbearing years tends to be lower than the "normal" 120/80 mm Hg. The blood pressure tends to fall slightly during pregnancy in normal women, averaging about 5 mm Hg below nonpregnant levels during the latter part of the first trimester, the second trimester, and the early part of the third trimester. The midpregnancy fall in blood pressure may be exaggerated in patients with chronic hypertension. For this reason blood pressures greater than about 125/80 mm Hg should be regarded with suspicion during pregnancy.

■ **What are the hypertensive disorders that may complicate pregnancy?**

Blood pressures greater than 140 mm Hg systolic and 90 mm Hg diastolic are definitely abnormal during pregnancy. Lower readings are abnormal when they represent a rise of 30 mm Hg systolic or 15 mm Hg diastolic over nonpregnant or early pregnancy blood pressure.

The group of hypertensive diseases that may complicate pregnancy includes the following four categories:

1. *Preeclampsia-eclampsia.* This is a syndrome of unknown cause that occurs only during pregnancy or the early postpartum period. Preeclampsia is characterized by hypertension, generalized edema, and proteinuria. In eclampsia convulsions and/or coma are also present.

2. *Chronic hypertension.* This category includes women known or suspected to have chronic hypertensive disease. The elevated blood pressure may be the result of essential vascular hypertension, or it may be secondary to other maternal disease such as chronic renal disease or collagen vascular disease.

3. *Chronic hypertension with superimposed preeclampsia-eclampsia.* This category includes patients with chronic hypertension who develop

a further increase in their blood pressure accompanied by proteinuria and/or edema during the latter half of pregnancy. Approximately one fourth of patients with chronic hypertension develop superimposed preeclampsia during pregnancy.

4. *Late or transient hypertension.* In this category are patients who develop an elevation in blood pressure during the third trimester of pregnancy or within the first 24 hours after delivery but whose blood pressure returns to normal within 10 days after delivery. These patients are distinguished from those with preeclampsia by the absence of generalized edema or proteinuria.

■ What are the consequences of hypertensive disease for the pregnant patient?

Patients with chronic hypertension have a 25% chance of developing a further increase in blood pressure, together with evidence of impairment of renal function, during pregnancy. In addition, chronic hypertension is often accompanied by changes in the arteries supplying the maternal blood to the placenta, resulting in impaired placental and fetal growth and an increase in the incidence of premature delivery and low birth weight infants. There is also a two- to threefold increase in the frequency of abruptio placentae in patients with chronic hypertension.

Women who develop severe preeclampsia, eclampsia, or preeclampsia superimposed on chronic hypertension are at increased risk for the occurrence of stroke or other vascular accident or cardiac failure. Other serious complications of preeclampsia-eclampsia include impaired kidney and liver function and blood coagulation defects. The maternal blood supply to the uterus is also impaired in preeclampsia-eclampsia, and fetal growth retardation, asphyxia, and even death may occur. Preeclampsia-eclampsia may develop and progress very rapidly, and patients with this complication of pregnancy require close observation and often intensive medical care.

■ What are the critical observations in pregnancies complicated by hypertension?

The pregnant woman with elevated blood pressure should be checked immediately for the presence of hand or face edema and proteinuria. The occurrence of either of these findings suggests that preeclampsia, alone or superimposed on hypertensive disease, is present. Dependent leg edema alone is not a pathologic finding, since this may occur in a large proportion of pregnant women. The pregnant patient with generalized edema and/or proteinuria should receive prompt assessment by a specialist in obstetrics.

The hypertensive pregnant patient should also be questioned about the occurrence of severe headaches, visual disturbances, paresthesias or weaknesses, and epigastric pain. She should be examined for hyperactivity of the deep tendon reflexes (especially the knee jerks). The presence of any of these findings suggests that an eclamptic convulsion may be imminent, and immediate obstetric consultations should be obtained. In addition, the patient should be kept in quiet surroundings and stimulated as little as possible. Seizure precautions should be taken. Often preeclampsia will worsen with labor. In preeclamptic women who develop eclampsia, about one fourth will have the first convulsion during labor. One of the primary goals of treatment for preeclampsia is to prevent convulsions, for these women suffer a much greater risk of death and increased mortality of their child.

A number of regimens have been employed for the prevention and control of eclamptic seizures. Parenteral magnesium sulfate therapy has been proved to be effective and is widely used. An initial loading dose of 2 to 4 mg of 10% magnesium sulfate may be given slowly by IV route to achieve effective serum levels rapidly. This may be followed by the continuous administration of 1 to 1.5 g/hr using a constant infusion pump. A second regimen for the use of this drug begins with the IM administration of 10 g of 50% magnesium sulfate initially, followed at 4-hour intervals by repeat IM doses of 5 g. The patient receiving magnesium sulfate therapy should be monitored carefully for evidence of magnesium-induced depression of the CNS or myocardium. The most frequent sign of magnesium excess is absence of the knee jerks. Signs of greater toxicity include slowing of the respiration below 12 breaths/min or the heart rate below 60 beats/min. The finding of absent knee jerks requires only that the infusion be stopped or that the next scheduled dose of IM magnesium sulfate be delayed. CNS or cardiac depression should be reversed immediately using IV calcium gluconate. Magnesium is excreted by the kidney, and the maintenance doses of magnesium sulfate should be reduced or withheld if the urine output falls below 50 ml/hr. On the other hand, the continued presence of hyperactive deep tendon reflexes demonstrates that inadequate magnesium levels are present and indicates that an increase in the dose of magnesium sulfate is needed.

Patients with severe preeclampsia or eclampsia, alone or superimposed on chronic disease, require intensive nursing observation with careful attention to airway, intake and output, and vital signs. An obstetrician-gynecologist experienced in the management of complicated pregnancy should supervise management and be available for immediate consultation.

Although delivery "cures" preeclampsia-eclampsia, the need for intensive observation and care extends 24 to 48 hours into the postpartum period, because approximately one fourth of eclamptic seizures and other serious complications may occur during this time.

■ What is the relationship between urinary tract infection and pregnancy?

It is questionable whether pregnancy actually increases the incidence of bacterial infection of the urinary tract. The incidence of significant asymptomatic bacteriuria in pregnant women has been reported to be between 4% and 7% by many investigators, and a similar incidence has been observed in nonpregnant women. On the other hand, pregnancy does appear to increase the likelihood that a woman with a low-grade asymptomatic urinary tract infection may develop acute pyelonephritis, and this may be a severe complication for both mother and fetus.

■ What special problems accompany acute pyelonephritis during pregnancy?

The special problems of acute pyelonephritis during pregnancy relate to the effect of maternal fever on fetal well-being and to the possible occurrence of premature labor during the acute episode. The likelihood of fetal distress resulting from hyperthermia, relative hypoxia, and cardio-

vascular stress increases as the maternal temperature rises above 101° F. Thus measures to reduce maternal temperature such as physical cooling and administration of antipyretics may be part of the initial therapy of acute pyelonephritis during pregnancy. Dehydration and electrolyte imbalance should also be corrected promptly. Uterine contractions that may develop into progressive, premature labor may not be reported by the acutely ill patient and may not be noticed by medical attendants concentrating on other phases of the illness; pregnant patients with acute pyelonephritis should be observed frequently and specifically for the presence or absence of uterine contractions. Although in most patients the excessive uterine activity subsides with bed rest, hydration, and lowering of maternal fever, a few patients require specific therapy to suppress the uterine activity. Consultation with an obstetric specialist should be obtained if regular uterine contractions develop during the course of acute pyelonephritis.

■ What other medical or surgical illnesses cause problems during pregnancy?

Almost any medical or surgical disease may occur coincident with pregnancy. In the management of these intercurrent illnesses one must consider both the effect of pregnancy on the disease and the effect of the disease on pregnancy. Drugs that are known or suspected to have adverse effects on the embryo or fetus should be avoided whenever possible. Diagnostic x-ray examination, especially of the abdomen, should be performed only if necessary for the differential diagnosis or management of the patient. Maternal hypotension, blood volume deficits, and electrolyte abnormalities must be corrected promptly in order to minimize the effect of acute illness on the fetus. Administration of oxygen to the mother during episodes of maternal circulatory or respiratory embarrassment or during periods of high fever may prevent or correct fetal distress from hypoxia. In other instances these measures can sustain the fetus while preparations are being made for emergency delivery. With survival rates and long-term prognosis for premature infants improving steadily, consideration may be given to the termination of pregnancy for fetal indications at any time from 27 or 28 weeks after the LMP onward, when the abnormality producing the fetal distress cannot be corrected and the maternal condition permits.

Some of the more important medical diseases that are affected by pregnancy or that alter the management of pregnancy include diabetes, heart disease, chronic renal disease, and acute febrile illnesses.

■ **What are the major problems in diabetic pregnancy?**

Pregnancy may make latent diabetes manifest and may complicate the management of known diabetes. Nausea and vomiting in the first trimester may interfere with food intake and thus may increase the incidence of symptomatic hypoglycemia in insulin-requiring diabetic patients. Although the embryo and fetus appear to be relatively tolerant to hypoglycemia, these episodes should be recognized promptly and treated appropriately. The possibility of hypoglycemia should be kept in mind in the differential diagnosis of disturbances of consciousness and "anxiety" symptoms in early pregnancy.

Most diabetic pregnant women experience an increase in insulin requirement during the latter half of pregnancy. These patients may develop ketoacidosis when these requirements are not met or as a result of stress during an acute, intercurrent illness. Because ketoacidosis may result in death or impaired neurologic development of the fetus, the diabetic pregnant patient should be observed carefully for evidence of ketoacidosis, especially when an infection or other acute stress is present.

The incidence of intrauterine fetal death in late pregnancy is increased in diabetic patients. Measures such as fetal heart rate monitoring and estriol determinations make it possible to recognize the endangered fetus in time to prevent a fatal outcome. An obstetric consultant should thus be involved in the management of any diabetic pregnant patient.

■ **How does pregnancy complicate the management of patients with heart disease?**

The increased blood volume, heart rate, and cardiac work during pregnancy make the cardiac patient more likely to develop congestive heart failure. In general patients with class I and II cardiac disease tolerate pregnancy well, but heart failure may occur even in some of these patients during pregnancy. The pregnant cardiac patient is most likely to develop congestive failure at 28 to 32 weeks of gestation (near the end of the phase of rapid blood volume expansion), during labor and delivery, and during the first 2 days of the puerperium. Acute pulmonary edema may develop particularly rapidly during labor or immediately following delivery. Acute congestive failure may also occur at other times during pregnancy, especially if the stress of major illness or trauma is added. The management of congestive heart failure and acute pulmonary edema is the same during pregnancy as at other times.

■ **What problems does pregnancy introduce for the management of chronic renal disease?**

The patient with chronic renal disease who has minimum or absent proteinuria, no elevation of the blood urea nitrogen or creatinine levels, and no hypertension can usually tolerate pregnancy successfully. Patients with more severe renal disease are at increased risk to develop progressive deterioration in renal function during pregnancy. Normotensive patients may become hypertensive, and hypertensive patients may experience a further increase in blood pressure during pregnancy. The increasing renal impairment and hypertension may occur as a result of progression of the primary renal disease or as manifestations of a superimposed preeclampsia-eclampsia. These patients may become candidates for intensive care because of renal failure or because of a hypertensive crisis. The occurrence of either of these latter complications is usually an indication for termination of pregnancy, even if the fetus has not reached the stage of viability.

■ **What complications does pregnancy introduce into the management of acute intraabdominal disease?**

Especially during the latter half of pregnancy, the presence of the gravid uterus may alter the clinical signs of acute intra-abdominal disease (for example, the location and characteristics of pain and tenderness) and make the presence or absence of these signs less reliable in differential diagnosis. Uterine contractions may occur either as part of the primary illness or following abdominal surgery, thus adding the problems of management of impending or actual premature labor to those of the primary disease process. Fetal distress may occur when shock or high fever is part of the maternal disease process. The patient with acute abdominal disease during pregnancy thus requires extra observation directed at the early detection of increased uterine activity or fetal distress.

The bedside clinician must be aware that labor and delivery are not only possible but *likely* to occur. Vigilance for the first evidence of labor is needed for the critically ill pregnant patient who is likely to go into labor and deliver before term. This is true whether the illness is directly related to her pregnancy or not. The woman whose condition is not improving is at the greatest risk of labor. When disease or its treatment impairs the sensorium, the woman herself may be unable to communicate the sensations of labor contractions.

■ What are the warning signs of labor in the critically ill patient with an altered sensorium?

During labor uterine contractions lasting from 30 to 60 seconds usually occur at regular intervals. The following physiologic and behavioral changes may accompany uterine contractions and be observed in cyclic intervals: increased respiration rate, change in pulse rate, increase in systolic and diastolic blood pressure, restlessness, and moaning. Additional physical evidence suggesting labor and/or impending delivery are bloody vaginal discharge, rupture of the bag of waters, grunting or expulsive efforts, and bulging of the perineum.

Vaginal discharge

A clear, sticky mucous secretion is normally present in pregnancy. This may not be externally apparent until the last trimester. At times this vaginal discharge may be slightly milky colored or pale yellow. The quantity of normal vaginal discharge should not require use of a sanitary napkin. A sudden increase in the quantity of normal mucous secretion warrants further investigation. Particularly in women with first pregnancies, an increased vaginal discharge that is tinged with either brown or pinkish blood streaks may be evidence that the cervix is softening and beginning to dilate. When these signs are present, the patient should be examined for the presence of regular uterine contractions signifying labor. Bleeding from the vagina, whether old or fresh, may signify either labor or a complication and warrants immediate medical attention.

Rupture of membranes

A gush of fluid usually signifies the rupture of the fetal membranes. The fetal heart rate should be observed immediately on discovery of ruptured membranes to detect slowing or irregularity, which might signify umbilical cord prolapse and compression. When abnormal fetal heart tones are found, the mother should be placed in knee-chest or deep Trendelenburg position in an attempt to relieve cord compression. Should the maternal positioning be impossible, an attempt to displace the fetal presenting part manually should be made. In any case, oxygen should be administered to the mother and medical help obtained immediately.

When rupture of the membranes is suspected, immediate assessment should be made to determine whether labor is present, since it is possible for the membranes to rupture only a brief period of time before the delivery of the infant. The fluid has a characteristic fleshy odor and normally is a clear, watery color with specks of white vernix. However, a yellow color or a heavy "grass" green color usually indicates the presence of meconium and requires immediate obstetric consultation.

Incontinent urination should not be confused with leakage of amniotic fluid. The distinctions may be made by several tests, the simplest of which is recognition of the characteristic odor of urine, very unlike the odor of amniotic fluid. When the fluid has been collected in a container that is clean and free of soap or other foreign materials, the pH of amniotic fluid is alkaline, whereas usually the pH of urine is acid. However, it is well to remember that both protein and blood in the urine may change the pH to an alkaline reaction.

Premature rupture of membranes. The fetal membranes may rupture prior to the onset of labor. This provides a route of entrance for pathogenic organisms into the immediate environment of the fetus, which normally is sterile. The immediate recognition of leakage of amniotic fluid is important to the welfare of the fetus. There is risk of sepsis to the fetus once the sterile environment is destroyed. For this reason delivery within 24 hours of membrane rupture, by induction of labor if necessary, is often desirable if the fetus is mature (≥37 weeks). When the fetus is still premature at the time of membrane rupture, on the other hand, there is increasing evidence that delaying the delivery by 48 to 72 hours may be advantageous, resulting in a greatly reduced incidence of respiratory distress syndrome (RDS) and patent ductus arteriosus in the neonate. When expectant management is chosen, the risk of infection can be minimized by avoiding intravaginal manipulations, especially digital examination of the cervix. During expectant management, the patient should be examined regularly for evidence of amnionitis (intrauterine infection), such as gradually increasing temperature and WBC count, a rising trend in maternal or fetal heart rate, or uterine tenderness. Increasing uterine contractions may also signify amnionitis. The risk of infection increases with time. In some cases, when the history is not diagnostic of membrane rupture, it may be necessary to perform a sterile speculum examination to confirm leakage of amniotic fluid. The only equipment required is a sterile vaginal speculum, sterile ring forceps or other forceps of sufficient length to reach the cervical end of the vaginal canal, a sterile glass slide, and nitrazine or other paper suitable for testing pH. Unless pooling fluid is seen in the posterior fornix it may be necessary to collect a specimen from the vaginal pool for both pH testing and examination for ferning when the fluid dries on a glass slide; pH testing is invalid in the presence of infection or blood.

Digital vaginal examination, with palpation of the cervix, should be carried out only after the decision has been made to terminate the pregnancy.

■ **What is the significance of vena caval syndrome?**

In the last trimester of pregnancy the uterus is a large, heavy organ and lies over the inferior vena cava. This anatomic relationship may favor a diminished blood flow from the venous system into the right atrium. The diminished blood flow in turn mimics the clinical symptoms of shock caused by a serious decrease in cardiac output. The patient may exhibit a rapid thready pulse, pallor, and perspiration. A feeling of light-headedness or faintness accompanies lowered blood pressure.

When these symptoms are present without a significant blood loss or a causal relationship, the vena caval syndrome of pregnancy should be suspected. Treatment is simple and relief of all the symptoms exceedingly prompt. The patient should be turned to the left lateral position, thus allowing the shift of gravity to take the weight of the uterus off the inferior vena cava. If there are reasons why the patient cannot be turned to the side, manual displacement of the uterus to the left side of the patient may also bring about relief from these symptoms.

This syndrome is more likely to occur when the abdominal wall is well developed and in good tone, aiding in compression of the intra-abdominal organs.

SUPPORT AND COMFORT MEASURES

■ **How can the patient's anxiety be relieved?**

The presence of a calm clinician who relates to the patient in a warm, human manner does much to allay patient anxiety and fear. Although the critical care unit is completely familiar to the practitioner, the visual impact of complex equipment combined with strange noises makes this an alien and frightening environment for the patient. A simple explanation of the purpose of the equipment and orientation to the procedures should be offered to all patients. For pregnant patients additional equipment for fetal monitoring must be explained.

■ **What can be done to alleviate the mother's fears caused by her separation from the infant?**

Following delivery, the mother's physical condition prevents her from making visits to the infant. Polaroid pictures of the infant are easily made and offer the mother visual evidence of the infant's condition. Often the infant will be shown in an incubator, possibly wired to monitors. It may be well to inform the mother about such devices and their benign nature before pictures are shown. When the neonate is very ill, personal contact from the neonatal intensive care staff may be beneficial.

■ How can nurses aid bonding with the critically ill mother?

When a laboring woman is critically ill, the demands for physiologic stability could easily dominate, making it easy to overlook the importance of assisting and fostering a beginning relationship between the mother and her newborn. Should the infant be premature or ill, as often happens, the challenge is compounded. Nurses can be of great benefit to the family by deliberately including the goal of supporting a positive bonding in the daily nursing plan.

In the first few days bonding may be fostered by commenting positively and realistically about the infant and avoiding remarks that suggest the infant is unlikely to survive. It helps to mention some of the normal features of the infant, such as well formed, strong, beautiful but small. As early as possible, the baby's father or other family member should be encouraged to be with and when possible hold or touch the baby. When the mother's condition permits, arrangements can be made for her to see her infant, either by transporting her to the nursery or bringing the baby to her. While it is well to encourage and support the mother to see and touch her infant, her readiness to do so must be sought and never forced. For some women providing their own breast milk for their baby is important. They may be assured that successful nursing can begin as late as several weeks after delivery when their health has improved.

Early contact between the critically ill woman and her infant may be difficult to achieve; there is reason to believe that the foundations for the lifetime relationship between mother and child are laid in this early contact. An immediate benefit may come from the ability this gives the woman to replace her fantasy about the child with a real image, dispelling worry and fear.

■ What is the appropriate manner of dealing with the infant's death?

The death of an infant is difficult at any time. The family who bears this loss together with concern for a critically ill mother requires understanding and sympathy from the practitioners. This can be expressed by allowing them to talk about their loss and grief. The desire to talk about the infant's death is normal and a necessary part of the grieving process. Families may wish to see and hold the infant after death. Arrangements for privacy and for family members to mourn with the mother can be facilitated by the nursing personnel. The practitioner should ask the family if they wish to meet with the chaplain or have a pastor visit to provide spiritual support.

MONITORS FOR PREGNANT PATIENTS

There may be times when the intensive care unit is the most suitable location for a patient during labor. Initial provisions should include plans for the place of delivery. Under these circumstances a variety of techniques requiring special equipment may be used that are unique to pregnancy and labor. It may be advantageous to have a listing in the intensive care unit of such equipment and its location together with a description of the procedures. Suggested equipment is discussed subsequently.

The first phase of fetal monitoring is preparation. All necessary equipment and supplies must be at hand and in working condition.

The patient needs instruction and explanation of what will be done and why monitoring is valuable to her. The procedure for application may be explained as very similar to a vaginal examination. The mother might like to know that the record of the infant's heartbeat provides the best possible information about his condition. The audible heartbeat may be played at times so the mother may hear the infant. After the monitor has been functioning for a while, the alert patient may appreciate being shown a strip and given a brief explanation of the tracing.

Data collection and interpretation require skill. The practitioner must look at the strip every few minutes and recognize all deviations from normal fetal heart rate patterns.

■ **What are the techniques for monitoring during labor?**

The fetal heart may be heard by stethoscopic auscultation. Uterine contractions may be perceived objectively by palpation through the maternal abdominal wall. Direct observation by trained personnel has been the historical approach to obstetric patients. These clinical measures require constant attendance, are subject to the usual human limitations, and at best provide a minuscule sample of data. In the main there are two general approaches, using external (indirect) or internal (direct) monitoring systems. External systems do not require penetration of the maternal or fetal body. Therefore the cervix may be closed, and labor is not a prerequisite. Fetal signals are picked up through the maternal abdomen, and rupture of the amniotic sac is not required. These advantages permit the collection of data from periods as early as the eleventh week of gestation.

Direct monitoring systems employ an electrode that attaches to the fetal presenting part to pick up the fetal ECG signal and a catheter inserted via the cervix into the amniotic fluid to measure uterine contractions. These techniques are therefore applicable only after rupture of membranes in labor.

■ **What techniques of monitoring uterine activity are employed?**

Various types of tokodynamometers that record uterine activity are available. They provide continuous records of data obtained externally from equipment that encircles the woman's abdomen. Data about the frequency of uterine contractions and the relative intensity of the contractions is suggested.

Direct monitoring of uterine activity is accomplished by placing an intrauterine catheter and recording pressure changes. Intrauterine techniques measure both resting tone and the amplitude of uterine contractions. Direct techniques permit more precise data collection and allow the elimination of interfering signals. In addition, the degree of uterine activity can be deduced from the frequency, intensity, and duration of uterine contractions. Less than a minute between successive uterine contractions may indicate an excessive degree of uterine activity, and the principal practitioner should be notified immediately. If the patient is receiving oxytocin and the physician is not immediately at hand, the oxytocin should be discontinued pending the arrival of the physician. Turning the patient on her side may relieve too frequent uterine contractions occurring in the absence of uterine stimulant medication.

FETAL MONITORING

■ **How is the fetal heart rate monitored?**
Ultrasound

Ultrasound instruments, which use the Doppler principle, send a sound impulse from a transducer that also reads the reflections of the sound waves from moving surfaces such as the heart walls, valves, or even moving blood cells. Cardiac action can be heard fairly easily. The swishing sound of blood flowing through a large vessel such as the umbilical cord may be detected as well. A special transducer that can be connected to a fetal monitor may provide both an auditory and visual record of fetal cardiac action. It is necessary to have an ultrasound transmitting jelly as well as the recording instrument and the transducer.

The sounds of fetal cardiac action may be detected as early as 10 or 11 weeks of intrauterine life when ordinary auscultation is not productive. Compact portable units are available. Ultrasound methods have the advantage of external use and do not require the rupture of membranes.

Phonocardiography

Fetal phonocardiography employs a microphone held in contact with the maternal abdomen. Both a visual record and audible sounds may be obtained. Like other external techniques, it may be used prior to as well as during labor and does not require either dilatation of the cervix or ruptured membranes.

Fetal electrocardiogram (Fig. 37-1)

The fetal heart rate can often be picked up by means of skin electrodes placed on the abdomen of the mother. With a fetal heart rate monitor that is equipped to detect and process these small sig-

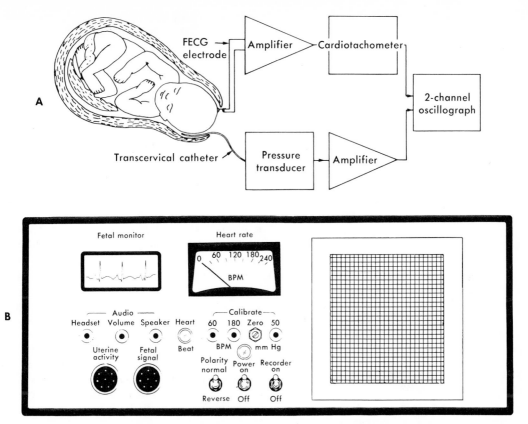

Fig. 37-1. A, Technique for fetal intensive care. Specially designed electrode is attached to presenting part of fetus to obtain FECG, which is then fed to an amplifier and signal conditioning circuit. Instantaneous cardiotachometer measures interval between successive FECG's and plots continuous graph. Output of cardiotachometer is displayed on one channel of two-channel oscillograph. Intrauterine pressure is obtained from intrauterine catheter inserted transcervically into uterus just beyond biparietal diameter of fetal head. Catheter is attached to pressure transducer, whose output is amplified and displayed beneath fetal heart rate record on other channel of oscillograph. **B,** Panel of fetal monitor, incorporating in single package components of block diagram in **A.** It can be used to obtain either indirect or direct fetal heart rate and uterine contraction monitoring techniques. (From Hon, E. H.: An introduction to fetal heart rate monitoring, New Haven, Conn., 1971, Harty Press, Inc.)

nals, the "abdominal fetal ECG" represents another external monitoring technique suitable for use before labor and with intact membranes.

The *direct* fetal ECG signal is frequently used for fetal monitoring during labor because this technique gives more reliable information than any of the external methods. An electrode is attached directly to the fetal presenting part to pick up the fetal ECG signal. The fetal QRS complex thus obtained provides a better "trigger" for the heart rate counting circuit than any of the external signal forms. The disadvantages of the direct technique are that it is "invasive" and that it can be applied only after the membranes have ruptured and at least 1 to 2 cm of cervical dilatation is present.

■ What does the fetal monitor record?

In contrast to most heart monitors used in adult intensive care, which display average heart rate and/or the form of the ECG signal, fetal heart rate monitors provide a continuous strip-chart record of the fetal heart rate and, on a second channel, the uterine contractions. With most monitors the fetal heart rate tracing is "instantaneous": that is, the rate is determined and written out for each successive pair of heartbeats. Thus in addition to *heart rate* another parameter, *heart rate variability,* can be assessed, especially when the direct fetal ECG is employed as the counting source. This continuous record of the instantaneous fetal heart rate, interpreted in relation to the uterine contraction record, provides much more information about fetal condition, and also about the probable mechanisms causing any fetal distress present, than does the average heart rate alone.

■ What are the characteristics of the normal fetal heart rate record?

The *baseline fetal heart rate* (the rate in the intervals between uterine contractions or fetal movements) is normally between 120 and 160 beats/min. Normal *baseline variability* is usu-ally indicated by the presence of fluctuations in the baseline rate, having an amplitude of 5 to 20 beats/min and occurring with a frequency of 3 to 6 cycles/min. A decrease in baseline variability may be caused by certain drugs such as atropine, tranquilizers, or magnesium sulfate, as well as barbiturates and narcotics. In the absence of drugs the baseline fetal heart rate and its variability can be considered to give information about the status of the fetus, particularly the activity of the CNS. A decrease in the baseline variability in the absence of drugs indicates depression of the CNS activity and often reflects fetal hypoxia and acidosis.

■ What fetal heart rate patterns can be expected in association with uterine contractions?

The fetal heart rate is observed during uterine contractions (Fig. 37-2). The normal fetus may show no change in heart rate or transient heart rate accelerations in response to uterine contractions. Periodic decelerations in the fetal heart rate in association with uterine contractions may in some cases be a normal feature of labor and in others indicate the occurrence of fetal stress as a result of uterine contractions. Three major types of deceleration patterns have been described by Hon[1] and others.

In the early deceleration pattern the heart rate rarely falls below 100 to 110 beats/min at the low

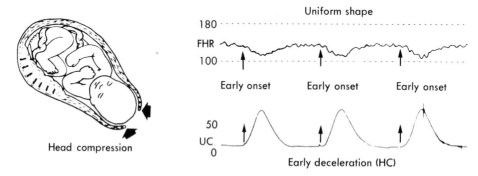

Fig. 37-2. This fetal heart rate deceleration pattern is thought to be caused by fetal head compression. It is of *uniform shape,* reflects shape of associated intrauterine pressure curve, and has its onset *early* in contracting phase of uterus. Hence it has been labeled "early deceleration." HC = head compression, UC = uterine contraction. (From Hon, E. H.: An introduction to fetal heart rate monitoring, New Haven, Conn., 1971, Harty Press, Inc.)

point of the deceleration. The heart rate has returned to the baseline level by the end of the contraction. This pattern is not associated with fetal hypoxia or depressed infants in the absence of other problems.

A second deceleration pattern is a late deceleration pattern thought to represent fetal hypoxia resulting from insufficient uteroplacental exchange (Fig. 37-3). This pattern, similar to the early deceleration pattern, tends to be uniform and U shaped. The late deceleration pattern begins relatively late, that is, 20 to 30 seconds after the onset of the uterine contraction, and the low point of the deceleration occurs near the end of the uterine contraction or even as the uterine pressure is returning to baseline levels. This pattern always indicates fetal hypoxia, and when it is associated with a flat baseline fetal heart rate, it indicates that significant fetal distress is present. When late deceleration cannot be corrected, immediate delivery is indicated.

The most common fetal heart rate pattern is variable deceleration, believed to be caused by umbilical cord compression (Fig. 37-4). This is an irregular deceleration pattern that may occur at almost any time during the contraction. The degree of deceleration frequently does not reflect the intensity of contraction. For example, several contractions of equivalent magnitude may be accompanied by variable decelerations of quite different degrees. The healthy fetus can tolerate brief episodes of cord compression lasting up to 30 or 45 seconds without distress. Longer periods of cord compression, particularly those in which the fetal heart rate falls below 60 to 70 beats/min and in which the duration of the deceleration exceeds 45 to 60 seconds, may be associated with the occurrence of progressive fetal hypoxia and acidosis. In these instances the deterioration in fetal condition will often be reflected as well in a progressive decrease in baseline variability and increase in baseline fetal heart rate.

In summary, prolonged severe variable decelerations, that is, those lasting longer than 45 to 60 seconds and with the heart rate falling to 60 to 70 beats/min or below, or late decelerations of any magnitude indicate fetal distress. When these patterns are associated with a flat baseline fetal heart rate, the situation is likely to be grave, with significant hypoxia and acidosis already present.

Periodic fetal heart rate accelerations also occur in association with uterine contractions and with fetal movement between contractions. Such fetal heart rate accelerations usually have no

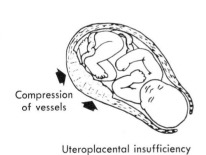

Compression
of vessels

Uteroplacental insufficiency

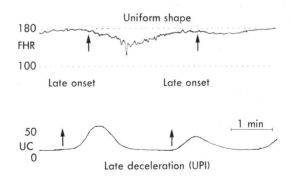

Fig. 37-3. This fetal heart rate deceleration pattern is thought to be caused by acute uteroplacental insufficiency resulting from decreased intervillous space blood flow during uterine contractions. It is also of *uniform shape* and also reflects shape of associated intrauterine pressure curve. In this case, however, in contradistinction to the early deceleration pattern of Fig. 37-2, its onset occurs *late* in contracting phase of uterus. Hence it has been labeled "late deceleration." This fetal heart rate deceleration pattern is considered indicative of uteroplacental insufficiency. UPI = uteroplacental insufficiency. (From Hon, E. H.: An introduction to fetal heart rate monitoring, New Haven, Conn., 1971, Harty Press, Inc.)

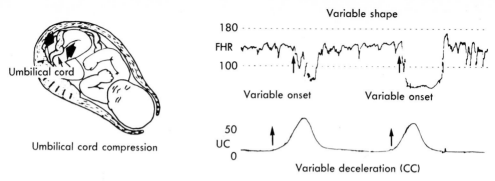

Fig. 37-4. This fetal heart rate pattern is thought to be caused by umbilical cord occlusion. It is of *variable shape,* does not reflect shape of associated intrauterine pressure curve, and its onset occurs at a variable time during contracting phase of uterus. CC = cord compression. (From Hon, E. H.: An introduction to fetal heart rate monitoring, New Haven, Conn., 1971, Harty Press, Inc.)

pathologic significance and in fact usually reflect a healthy fetus.

■ Of what use is fetal scalp blood sampling?

Another means of assessment of fetal condition during labor is fetal scalp blood sampling (Fig. 37-5). In this technique a small sample of blood is obtained from a lancet puncture in the fetal scalp and is analyzed especially for the pH, but also for carbon dioxide and oxygen tensions. Particularly in the critical care patient it may be necessary to obtain a simultaneous maternal arterial or venous blood sample in order to interpret the fetal pH, since the presence of a maternal acidosis, either metabolic or respiratory, may alter the interpretation of the fetal data. The chief role of fetal scalp blood sampling would appear to be in the interpretation of equivocal fetal heart rate patterns, although in a few centers fetal scalp blood sampling is used as the major means of assessment of fetal condition during labor. A list of the equipment necessary for fetal scalp blood sampling is found in the boxed material on p. 627 (opposite page).

Nursing care associated with fetal monitoring includes frequent observation of the tracing for the presence of periodic deceleration in the fetal heart rate or the presence of a flat baseline. Anything suspicious should be called to the physician's attention immediately. Immediate inter-

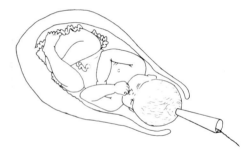

Fig. 37-5. Fetal scalp blood sampling. Endoscope is inserted transvaginally for direct visualization of fetal scalp, and light is attached to light source. (From Della Pietra, E. R.: Intrapartum maternal and fetal monitoring, Los Angeles, 1974, Postgraduate Division, School of Medicine, University of Southern California.)

vention is indicated when abnormal fetal heart rate patterns are recognized. For example, when variable decelerations are present the patient should be turned on her side in an attempt to eliminate deceleration. Repeated changes in position may be necessary to relieve cord compression. The Trendelenburg position may be necessary to eliminate deceleration patterns unaffected by turning the patient from side to side. When other decelerations are present, the patient should be turned on her side in order to remove

FETAL MONITORING

PREPARATION

It may be desirable to continue maternal care in an intensive care unit during labor. In these circumstances the obstetrician requires the following samples for fetal monitoring:

1. A functioning fetal monitoring system such as Corometrics (Fig. 37-1)
    a. A sterile unit containing a fetal scalp electrode
    b. An introducer and uterine catheter
2. A light source
3. A 30 ml container of sterile distilled water for flushing the intrauterine catheter
4. Two 5 ml syringes

IMMEDIATE ASSISTANCE IN THE EVENT OF DELIVERY

Even with diligent observation, it is still possible for labor to be undetected. Measures to ensure an immediately clear airway and provision for gas exchange, rapid drying, and prevention of chilling may mean the difference between survival of an intact infant and serious jeopardy or loss of life.

DELIVERY SUPPLIES

Preparations may be made to have a warmed incubator and a sterile pack containing two pairs of scissors, two cord clamps, a number of towels, a blanket for the infant, and a sterile bulb aspirator at hand. When possible, equipment for newborn resuscitation should be readily available.

NEWBORN RESUSCITATION

1. Laryngoscope with premature blade
2. Sterile Kole tracheal tubes, sizes 1.5, 2.0, 2.5, 3.0, and 3.5
3. DeLee aspirator
4. Infant bag for ventilation, 0.5 L with a T assembly adapter
    Where umbilical cord catheterization might be used, the following drugs may be kept at hand:
    1. 50% glucose for IV use
    2. Calcium gluconate solution
    3. H_2CO_3 ampules
    4. Epinephrine, $1:10,000$ concentration
    5. Sterile equipment for umbilical cord catheterization

FETAL SCALP SAMPLING EQUIPMENT

1. Container of ice
2. Long, heparinized capillary tubes
3. Magnet
4. Sterile supplies or disposable kit
    a. Blade holder and blade
    b. Cone-type endoscope
    c. Ring forceps
    d. Gauze pledgets
    e. Antibacterial cleansing agent
    f. Sterile towels

any element of vena caval compression with supine hypotension. In either case oxygen can be administered to the mother by face mask.

REFERENCE

1. Hon, E. H.: An introduction to fetal heart rate monitoring, New Haven, Conn., 1971, Harty Press, Inc.

BIBLIOGRAPHY

Babson, S., Pernoll, M. L., and Benda, G. I.: Diagnosis and management of the fetus and neonate at risk, ed. 4, St. Louis, 1979, The C. V. Mosby Co.

Caveness, W. F., and Walker, A. E.: Head injury, Philadelphia, 1966, J. B. Lippincott Co.

Chesley, L. C.: Hypertensive disorders in pregnancy, New York, 1978, Appleton-Century-Crofts.

Clausen, J. P., et al.: Maternity nursing today, New York, 1973, McGraw-Hill Book Co.

Della Pietra, E. R.: Intrapartum maternal and fetal monitoring, Los Angeles, 1974, Postgraduate Division, School of Medicine, University of Southern California.

Hellman, L. M., and Pritchard, J. A.: Williams obstetrics, ed. 14, New York, 1971, Appleton-Century-Crofts.

Klaus, M. H., and Kennell, J. H.: Maternal-infant bonding, St. Louis, 1976, The C. V. Mosby Co.

Martin, C. B., Jr., Ulene, A., and Guzinski, J. M.: Module, care of the pregnant patient: submodule, problems in pregnancy, Raritan, N. J., 1974, Ortho Pharmaceutical Corporation.

Matousek, I.: Fetal nursing during labor, Nurs. Clin. North Am. 1972.

Niswander, K. R., et al.: The women and their pregnancies, Philadelphia, 1976, W. B. Saunders Co.

Quilligan, E. J., and Kretchner, M., editors: Fetal and maternal medicine, New York, 1980, John Wiley & Sons, Inc.

Taber, B.-Z.: Manual of gynecologic and obstetric emergencies, Philadelphia, 1979, W. B. Saunders Co.

Woolley, A. S.: Excellence in nursing in the coronary-care unit, Heart & Lung, 1:785, 1972.

CHAPTER 38

Critical care of the neonate

Robert F. Huxtable and Mary C. Peduzi

In the past many inappropriate and sometimes misleading terms have been used to describe the neonate. They have included "premature," "postmature," "small-for-dates," "dysmature," intrauterine growth retardation," and "low birth weight."

For many years all babies weighing less than 2500 g at birth were classified as "premature." Actually a very significant proportion of those were small-for-gestational age and more mature than weight alone would suggest. These loosely applied terms, although partially accurate, fail to direct attention to the problems the baby will likely encounter. In the two examples just mentioned the infant of low birth weight is likely to have respiratory distress syndrome owing to inadequate gestation, while the small-for-gestational age infant may suffer the effects of hypoglycemia.

It is much more valuable to assign the newborn infant to one of nine categories. This provides valid comparisons with respect to mortality and morbidity statistics and helps to anticipate the problems a baby is likely to develop. Classification is based on birth weight and gestational age. *Babies above the 90th, between the 10th and 90th,* and *below the 10th weight percentile* are called *large* (LGA), *appropriate* (AGA), and *small* (SGA) for *gestational age,* respectively. Those of *less than 38, 38 to 42,* and *greater than 42 weeks'* gestation are called *preterm* (Pr T), *term* (T), and *postterm* (Po T), respectively. It is useful to classify every baby in this manner and display the classification in clear view on the bassinet or incubator.

THERMOREGULATION

■ Why is thermoregulation of such critical importance in the neonate?

Temperature regulation is based on a balance between heat loss and heat production. The newborn loses heat more rapidly and has different mechanisms for heat production than an older child. The newborn has more difficulty in maintaining body temperature, which may be a threat to survival, especially for the small infant who is ill. A body temperature change on either side of a point known as the "thermoneutral point" results in increased oxygen consumption and increased consumption of substrates for generation of heat.

■ By what mechanisms does heat loss occur?

The four mechanisms by which heat is transferred between the newborn's body and the environment are conduction, convection, radiation, and evaporation.

Heat loss by *conduction* involves the transfer of heat from a warm object to a cooler object through direct contact. This occurs when the skin is in direct contact with a surface of a different temperature such as a cold scale platform or table. Conductive heat loss can be minimized

	Pr T	T	Po T
LGA			
AGA			
SGA			

by interposing a poor heat conductor such as fabric between the infant and the cold surface.

Heat loss by *convection* involves a flow of heat from the body surface to cooler surrounding air and occurs as a result of transfer of heat into the molecules of a moving gas of lower than body temperature. This type of heat loss is dependent on the surrounding temperature and the velocity of air currents. Thus heat loss can be considerably greater in drafty rooms where a rapid flow of air enhances heat loss. The flow of cold oxygen across the face of an infant can also contribute to this type of heat loss.

Even though the air temperature is appropriate and no convection currents are present in an incubator, the infant may have heat loss by *radiation*. Radiation heat loss involves transfer of heat between two solid surfaces of different temperatures that are not in direct contact (infant to incubator walls). Therefore, if an incubator canopy is near a cold window or wall, its heat radiates to these surfaces, reducing the environmental temperature below that of the infant. The infant, in turn, radiates heat to the incubator canopy of lower than body temperature.

The fourth mechanism of heat loss is *evaporation,* which results from the conversion of a liquid to a vapor. This is a very efficient and rapid mechanism of cooling because of the large number of calories consumed to convert a unit weight of water from a liquid to a gas phase. It is probably the most important mechanism of thermal stress in the delivery room. Therefore it is imperative that the infant be dried immediately after birth to prevent heat loss by evaporation. Evaporative heat loss can also occur with bathing, thus the first bath should be delayed until the body temperature is stable.

■ How does the infant respond to a cold environment?

When exposed to a cold environment, an older child or adult is able to generate heat by increasing muscle activity or by shivering. The newborn does not possess this capability but has a unique mechanism for producing needed heat—nonshivering thermogenesis. Nonshivering thermogenesis involves a chemical reaction mediated by norepinephrine, which leads to an increase in

metabolic rate resulting in the production of heat. The major source of heat that is produced by non-shivering thermogenesis is brown fat, a unique form of adipose tissue found in most newborn mammals and described as brown because of its rich vascular supply. Brown fat is located between the scapulae, in the axillae, around the muscles and blood vessels of the neck, behind the sternum, around the kidneys and adrenal glands, and along the vertebral column. It contains fatty acids that are metabolized by norepinephrine resulting in the production of heat. In utero malnutrition results in depletion of white fat, while brown fat is preserved. Conversely, autopsies have shown that newborn infants who are well nourished at birth and are subjected to cold stress deplete brown fat, while white fat is preserved. Normally, brown fat stores gradually disappear during the first year of life, the time corresponding to the development of the shivering thermogenic mechanism.

■ What are some factors that may impair thermogenesis?

The newborn's ability to respond to cold stress may be inhibited by hypoxia associated with hyaline membrane disease, intracranial hemorrhage, hypoglycemia, cerebral malformations, and depletion of brown fat stores owing to protracted cold stress.

■ Why is thermoregulation a greater problem for preterm than term infants?

Preterm infants have a minimal supply of subcutaneous fat resulting in less fat insulation, thus limiting conservation of body heat. They also have a greater surface area in relation to body weight, which increases the amount of surface area exposed to the environment with resultant heat loss. Because of immaturity of the nervous system, preterm infants are hypotonic and unable to assume a flexed position, which preserves heat by reducing exposed surface area.

■ What are the consequences of cold stress in a newborn with or without hyaline membrane disease?

The infant responds to cold stress by increasing his metabolic rate. This requires an increase in oxygen consumption with resultant hypoxia. During hypoxia, when metabolic demands are increased, anaerobic metabolism occurs with an increase in lactic acid leading to acidosis. The acidosis, if severe, leads to peripheral vasoconstriction and pulmonary vasoconstriction. Pulmonary vasoconstriction may lead to hypoxia, intracardiac shunting through the foramen ovale, and aggravation of hyaline membrane disease if present. Hypoxia alone results from the decrease in perfusion of oxygen owing to peripheral vasoconstriction and results in increased pulmonary vascular resistance. This phenomena is more pronounced in the presence of acidemia.

Effects of hypothermia

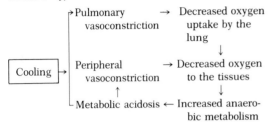

■ What is the effect of administering cold oxygen to the face of a newborn?

The thermal sensors in the skin of the face are more sensitive to cold than any other areas of skin. Exposure of the face to cold reflexly initiates production of norepinephrine resulting in an abrupt increase in metabolism and oxygen consumption. This may occur in the presence of normal environmental and core body temperatures. Oxygen must be warmed and humidified before it is delivered to the infant. At no time should dry cold oxygen be delivered directly to the infant's face.

■ What environmental temperature is recommended for neonates in various weight groups?

Suggested starting points are 34.9° C for a 1000 g baby, 33.5° C for a 2000 g baby, and 30° C for larger term infants. These are only rough guidelines and should be modified according to the infant's temperature. It is suggested that the infant's temperature be taken at least once every hour until stable and every 3 hours thereafter.

The smaller the infant, the narrower the range of environmental temperature in which heat balance can be maintained.

■ What skin temperature is recommended for the preterm and term infant?

When monitoring skin temperature with a thermistor, usually placed over the upper abdomen, the term infant's temperature should be maintained between 36.1° C and 36.5° C. Infants under 1500 g should be maintained between 36.6° C and 37° C.

■ What supplemental heat sources (other than radiant warmers and incubators) may be used under urgent circumstances?

An ordinary gooseneck lamp, heat lamps, or rubber gloves filled with warm water can be quickly and conveniently used. Care must be exercised to avoid burns of the skin. The temperature of the water for the gloves should not exceed 40° C, and they should be wrapped in diapers.

■ What precautions should be taken when rewarming a hypothermic infant?

Excessively rapid warming can cause apnea; thus a gradual process is suggested. The infant's skin temperature should be checked frequently. As needed, appropriate adjustments in the environmental temperature should be made. The difference between environmental temperature and the infant's skin temperature is 1.5° C or less.

INFECTION

■ Why are the fetus and neonate uniquely susceptible to infection?

The fetus and neonate are uniquely susceptible to infection for two principal reasons: opportunity for exposure to infection and peculiarities of immunity. It is convenient to classify infections as *transplacental* or *acquired* (during or after birth). Transplacental infections are acquired by the fetus as a result of an infection in the mother at any time during pregnancy. These infections tend to be nonbacterial and include: *cytomegalovirus, rubella, syphilis,* and *toxoplasmosis.* Transplacental cytomegalovirus can occur while the mother is asymptomatic. Rubella, on the other hand, tends to produce symptoms in the mother although these might be quite mild.

A *herpesvirus* infection might be acquired by a newborn during the process of birth as a result of contacting genital herpetic lesions in the mother.

Infections acquired during or after birth are caused mainly by *bacteria*. The risk of infection to the infant is probably increased by prolonged ruptured membranes (greater than 24 hours). When there is no evidence of infection of the mother at the time of birth and when there has not been prolonged rupture or membranes, bacterial neonatal infection does not tend to occur until after 48 hours of age.

Also, immune globulin production is unique. Of the immunoglobulins IgG, IgM, and IgA, the only one that passes freely from the mother to the fetus is IgG. During fetal life IgA and IgM remain at very low levels. The fetus can, however, produce his own IgM as a result of transplacental infection, and IgM determination in the neonate is used as a screening test for transplacental infection. Values above 20 mg/dl have diagnostic value; however, lower values are not conclusive evidence against transplacental infection. The fetus develops the ability to produce IgM in response to infection at about 20 weeks' gestation.

■ **To what bacterial organisms are newborn infants most susceptible?**

Neonatal infections are most commonly caused by gram-negative rods, *Escherichia coli* being the most common of these. Presently, there is a nationwide preponderance of group B β-hemolytic streptococcus infections, although *E. coli* remains prominent. Other gram-negative rods causing infection include *Klebsiella*, *Proteus*, and *Pseudomonas*. Remaining bacterial infections are caused principally by gram-positive cocci including staphylococci and streptococci.

■ **What is the most common mode of transmission of nursery acquired infections?**

Infecting organisms are most commonly transferred to patients on the epithelial scales from the hands of personnel attending patients. Thus the most important method of preventing spread of infections in the nursery is hand washing.

The second major source of infection is contaminated equipment.

■ **What infections most clearly justify removal of the infant from the nursery?**

Gastroenteritis owing to specific bacterial organisms (especially enteropathogenic *E. coli*) and staphylococcal disease clinically manifested by abscess formation justify removal of the infant from the nursery. Other infections can generally be handled in the nursery by "unit isolation," in which case the baby is kept in an incubator and has contact with a minimal number of personnel.

■ **What is an appropriate hand washing program for personnel in a newborn nursery?**

On entering the nursery use an antiseptic agent to scrub the hands and forearms to above the elbows for 3 minutes. Antiseptics most useful for hand washing in the nursery are iodophor or hexachlorophene-containing preparations. Following the initial 3-minute scrub there should be a 15-second scrub between handling of patients.

■ **What are the clinical signs of sepsis?**

It is important to remember that the clinical manifestations of sepsis in the newborn are subtle and often referred to as "SSS" or the soft signs of sepsis. Often the nurse feels subjectively that the baby is just "not doing well." Signs include temperature instability, poor feeding, increased gastric residuals, abdominal distention, increasing frequency of apnea and bradycardia, cyanosis, petechiae, poor muscle tone, lethargy, irritability, and jaundice. Coagulation is often impaired and platelet count depressed.

■ **What action should be taken when sepsis is suspected?**

1. When there have been prolonged ruptured membranes, but the mother and baby are both well, culture the throat and the periumbilical skin and observe.
2. When there have been prolonged ruptured membranes and the mother has signs of infection, such as fever and foul smelling amniotic fluid, culture as for a septic workup and start treatment as below.
3. When there are clinical signs of sepsis,

promptly perform a septic workup, including cultures of the throat, periumbilical skin, urine, blood, and spinal fluid. On spinal fluid also determine the cell count and differential, sugar and protein concentrations, and do a Gram stain.

Antibiotic treatment usually consists of a combination of a penicillin and aminoglycoside to cover gram-positive and gram-negative organisms. The most frequently used combination at present is penicillin or ampicillin and kanamycin or gentamicin. When the infection is thought to be hospital acquired, gentamicin is usually substituted for kanamycin. Gentamicin is effective against *Pseudomonas*, whereas kanamycin often is not.

When there is evidence of staphylococcal disease suggested by pustules or pyopneumothorax, nafcillin or methicillin is appropriately substituted for penicillin.

If after 5 days all cultures are negative and the baby is doing well antibiotics may be discontinued. If the blood cultures are positive and cerebrospinal fluid culture negative, treatment for 7 to 10 days is usually sufficient. Treatment for meningitis as proved by positive spinal fluid culture should be more prolonged in order to prevent relapse, usually in the range of 3 weeks. The value of intrathecal antibiotics for neonatal meningitis is in doubt. Newborn infants tend to metabolize and excrete antibiotic drugs more slowly than older children; therefore infections are treated with smaller and less frequent doses of drugs.

■ Is there any value in routinely culturing throats of nursery personnel?

Many of the staff members are colonized with coagulase-positive staphylococci and impose no increased risk to patients. Cultures of personnel should be performed only in connection with specific infection problems in the nursery.

■ What measures are recommended to prevent the propagation of infections in the nursery?

1. Proper hand washing techniques should be employed on entering the nursery as well as between handling infants.
2. Clean or sterilized equipment and aseptic techniques should be used for invasive procedures.
3. Visiting of unnecessary personnel in the nursery should be restricted.
4. Visiting of persons with contagious diseases should be restricted.
5. Overcrowding in the nursery should be prevented by allowing ample space for each baby.

SHOCK, ACID-BASE, AND FLUID PROBLEMS

■ What factors lead to shock in the neonate?

Any factors leading to significant disturbance in cardiopulmonary function can produce the clinical syndrome of shock. These include inadequate oxygenation (as seen in respiratory distress syndrome, pulmonary infections, central nervous system drug depression, and obstructive airway disease), hypovolemia (from hemorrhage or excessive water loss), and septicemia.

■ What are the clinical manifestations of shock?

The intense peripheral vascular constriction, a compensatory mechanism, results in extreme pallor with cyanosis around the mouth and in the nail beds. Heart rate and respiratory rate are increased. In the newborn, hypoxia produces bradycardia. Blood pressure is decreased. In contrast to the adult whose blood pressure falls early in shock the compensatory mechanisms in the newborn infant tend to sustain the blood pressure for a longer period of time. The normal mean arterial pressure of the neonate is 35 to 55 mm Hg and should be measured under conditions predisposing to shock when a central arterial catheter is in place. Indirect methods of blood pressure measurement are less reliable, but the recently available Doppler or ultrasound methods have increased the reliability of this approach.

■ What are the first steps in the treatment of shock?

Although the underlying cause must ultimately be corrected, immediate treatment is directed at relief of the compromised cardiopulmonary system and includes: (1) proper thermal regulation (Remember that oxygen consumption is increased on either side of the thermoneutral point.), (2) supplying oxygen requirements by whatever means is appropriate to the situation (See section on respiratory problems.), (3) correct acid-base balance (Very frequently the patient is acidemic and often has a combination of respiratory and metabolic acidosis.), (4) blood volume expansion in hypovolemic states, and (5) maintenance of proper fluid and electrolyte balance. It must be recognized that electrolyte concentration alone does not determine the presence of total body deficit. For example, some infants with severe water-loss diarrhea have higher than normal sodium concentrations even though there is total body sodium depletion.

■ **What is the most common form of acid-base disturbance seen in the neonate?**

The imbalance most commonly seen is that of acidemia owing to respiratory insufficiency. This is manifested by a pH <7.30, Pao_2 < 50 mm Hg, and Pco_2 > 45 mm Hg. The sum of the effects of carbon dioxide retention owing to hypoventilation and lactic acid production owing to anaerobic metabolism determines the degree of acidemia. Correction therefore must include both improvement in ventilation and oxygenation. These goals may be achieved by the proper combination of increased respiratory rate, tidal volume, ambient oxygen concentration, cardiac output, alveolar capillary diffusion rate, increased oxygen-carrying capacity of the blood, and increased blood volume in hypovolemic states.

■ **How does the fluid and electrolyte economy in a neonate differ from that in an older child or adult?**

Neonates are much more susceptible to disorders of hydration than older persons for several reasons. Early in the neonatal period renal function is immature and compensatory excretion and reabsorption mechanisms are not yet functioning efficiently. The rate of turnover of fluid per unit of body weight in a young infant is about three times that of an adult, and their body water stores can therefore be depleted much faster. An infant with diarrhea may lose more than 50 ml of fluid/kg of body weight in a single day. The percentage of total body water in the young infant is approximately 75% to 80% of the body mass as compared to 55% for the adult female. The nor-

mal newborn has a physiologic loss of 5% to 10% of body fluid during the first few days of life.

■ **What are the signs of dehydration in an infant?**

Dry skin and mucous membranes, depressed anterior fontanel, poor skin turgor, decreased urine output, increased urine specific gravity, and increased BUN are signs of dehydration in an infant.

■ **Under normal circumstances what are the fluid requirements for a term infant?**

The fluid requirements for a term infant are approximately 75 to 100 ml/kg/day in the first day of life and 100 ml/kg/day thereafter. Low birth weight infants under 1500 g require 100 to 125 ml/kg/day. An infant with respiratory problems or one exposed to increased radiant energy (under radiant warmer or phototherapy lights) may have increased insensible losses and require more than 150 ml/kg/day. The best guides are serial weight determinations and serial determinations of urine specific gravity, attempting to keep it between 1.005 and 1.015.

■ **What are the normal values and daily maintenance requirements for electrolytes in the neonatal period?**

Sodium, 135 to 145 mEq/L; potassium, 3.5 to 5.5 mEq/L; and chloride, 95 to 110 mEq/L are the normal values for electrolytes in the neonatal period. Daily requirements are sodium, 3 to 4 mEq/kg; potassium, 2 mEq/kg; and calcium, 200 mg/kg.

■ **How can the degree of fluid deficit be estimated?**

Loss of body weight of 5%, 10%, and 15% results in mild, moderate, or severe dehydration, respectively. Five percent loss results in dry skin and mucous membranes, decreased amount of urine, and slight fontanel depression. Ten percent loss results in circulatory disturbances manifested by mottled skin, tachycardia, severely reduced urine output, significantly depressed fontanel, sunken eyes, and loss of elasticity of the skin. Fifteen percent loss results in a moribund condition and demands immediate attention for survival of the patient.

HEMATOLOGIC PROBLEMS

■ **What are the more common types of hemolytic disease of the newborn (erythroblastosis fetalis)?**

The expression "erythroblastosis fetalis" has generally been replaced by the term "hemolytic disease of the newborn." The more severe type is caused by Rh sensitization of the mother. The mother who has no Rh antigen on her red cells and is therefore capable of forming Rh antibodies does so as a result of receiving transmission of very small amounts of fetal blood through the placenta. This happens during labor; therefore these cells can be destroyed by giving anti-Rh antibody to the mother shortly after birth. The more severe form of hemolytic disease occurs in the infant of a mother who has been sensitized by a previous pregnancy and received no Rh antibody. AO and BO incompatibilities are the more common types. Neither tends to be as severe as Rh incompatibility; however, BO tends to produce more severe disease than AO incompatibility. These latter types are frequently successfully treated by using phototherapy.

■ **What risks to the baby result from such a hemolytic process?**

The antibodies, produced by the mother against fetal blood, cross the placenta, enter the fetal circulation, and attach to the red cells of the fetus that carry the Rh antigen. This results in hemolysis or breakdown of the red blood cell walls and production of free hemoglobin in the circulation. There are two neonatal consequences of this: anemia and a reduced oxygen-carrying capacity in the blood. When severe enough, this can lead to heart failure (hydrops fetalis). The large amount of hemoglobin released is converted to bilirubin, and high concentrations of bilirubin can produce brain damage.

■ **How is hyperbilirubinemia clinically manifested in the neonate?**

Increased bilirubin concentration in the blood and tissue is clinically observed as jaundice or yellow color to the skin and conjunctivae of the eyes. Jaundice is not seen until bilirubin exceeds 5 to 7 mg/dl. Normal variations in color vision lead to difficulty in estimating bilirubin by inspection. It should be remembered that after a baby has been placed under the phototherapy light, estimation of bilirubin from skin color tends to be low.

■ **Is jaundice normal in the newborn?**

There is a normal rate of red cell breakdown leading to bilirubin production during fetal life. It is eliminated by way of the mother's circulation; therefore the normal newborn is not jaundiced. After delivery the mother's circulation is no longer available for elimination of bilirubin and some infants become jaundiced during early neonatal life. This "physiologic jaundice" or "icterus neonatorum" typically begins after 24 hours, peaks at 3 to 4 days, and falls to the normal value within 7 to 14 days. In contrast to this course jaundice occurring before the first 24 hours or after a week of age suggests that there is some pathologic cause that should be investigated.

■ **What types of bilirubin are found circulating in the blood?**

Bilirubin is found in the conjugated and unconjugated form. In the conjugated form bilirubin has chemically combined with glucuronic acid. This chemical reaction takes place in the liver. This conjugated form is nontoxic. The free or unconjugated form of bilirubin is lipid soluble and is toxic to the central nervous system. The unconjugated form can be bound by albumin in the circulation, reducing the concentration of unconjugated bilirubin and the probability of toxicity. The preterm baby has a less mature conjugating system in the liver and is therefore more likely to become jaundiced even when the rate of red cell destruction is not increased. Also, the preterm infant tends to have low serum protein concentration, decreasing protein binding of free bilirubin.

■ **What situations increase the likelihood of bilirubin toxicity?**

The preterm baby appears to be more subject to central nervous system bilirubin poisoning than the term infant. Exchange transfusion in the term infant is considered mandatory when the indirect or unconjugated bilirubin concentration reaches 20 mg/dl. The preterm infant who is not sick is considered a possible candidate for exchange transfusion when the unconjugated bilirubin concentration is in the range of 15 to 20 mg/dl. Certain problems in sick preterm infants increase bilirubin toxicity and lead to consideration of exchange transfusion when unconjugated bilirubin concentration is less than 15 mg/dl. When the serum albumin is low, less free bilirubin is bound and a higher concentration of the toxic form is found. The degree of binding to albumin is affected by the blood pH. When there is a high concentration of circulating hydrogen ion, albumin binding of bilirubin is reduced. Hypoglycemia results in increased circulating non-esterified fatty acids, which also displace bilirubin from albumin. Some drugs such as sulfisoxazole compete with bilirubin for albumin binding.

How is hyperbilirubinemia treated?

1. Physiologic jaundice found after the first 24 hours of age and peaking at the third to the fourth day usually does not exceed 12 mg/dl total bilirubin and requires no treatment.

2. The less severe and more slowly progressing jaundice is commonly found in preterm infants and in infants with an ABO incompatibility and can very often successfully be treated by placing the baby under phototherapy lights. The light usually used is emitted by fluorescent bulbs. Although the light appears white, the effective portion of the radiant energy acting on bilirubin is in the wavelength range of blue light. The light decomposes bilirubin by photooxidation into degradation products that are water soluble, excreted in bile and urine, and are nontoxic. During the time the baby is under the light, the eyes are covered to avoid any possible damage to the retinas. The infant should be unclothed and his position should be changed at least every 2 hours to provide exposure of all surface areas to the light. The recommended intensity of light is between 200 and 400 foot-candles. Phototherapy has been shown to reduce bilirubin concentration by an average of 1.5 to 2 mg/dl over a 12- to 24-hour period.

3. More severe and rapidly progressive forms of jaundice, as well as jaundice in sick preterm infants, are treated by exchange transfusion. This is done by placing a plastic catheter in either the umbilical artery or umbilical vein and alternately withdrawing blood and infusing donor blood. The total volume used is usually twice that of the infant's blood volume. This two-volume exchange will replace approximately 85% of the infant's blood with donor blood. Although phototherapy is not appropriate for treatment of the sick infant with the more severe forms of hyperbilirubinemia, it can reduce the need for repeated exchange transfusions.

Other than blood incompatibilities what is the single most important cause of jaundice in the newborn infant?

Bacterial or nonbacterial infections are often associated with jaundice. It is imperative that bacterial sepsis be diagnosed and treated early.

Other than Rh and ABO hemolytic disease what are the causes of anemia found in the newborn?

Blood loss from any cause results in anemia. This may occur before, during, or after the process of birth. It may result from birth trauma, placental injury, fetomaternal transfusion, or twin-to-twin transfusion. Anemia can result from late clamping of the cord when the infant is held above the level of the placenta. Hemolytic disease other than that described under Rh and ABO incompatibility may result from enzyme deficiencies of certain red blood cells, making the cells more subject to hemolysis. One of the more common of these is glucose-6-phosphate dehydrogenase.

What are normal levels of hemoglobin and hematocrit in the newborn infant?

The term infant of normal birth weight has a mean hemoglobin concentration of 17 g/100 ml of blood during the first day of life. The mean hematocrit during this time is 51%.

Are there any problems associated with excessive concentration of circulating red blood cells (hyperviscosity)?

Increased blood volume and high hematocrit levels may result from delayed clamping of the cord while the infant is held below the placental level, stripping of the cord, maternofetal transfusion, twin-to-twin transfusion, or increased red blood cell production. Central hematocrit is considered excessive and may lead to clinical problems if over 65%. The capillary hematocrit is higher than central hematocrits. Treatment decisions should be based on central hematocrit. Concentrations above this produce excessive viscosity of the blood and reduced flow. This can lead to clinical signs of respiratory distress and cardiac decompensation. Additionally, central nervous system dysfunction in the form of seizures has been observed with hypervolemia and polycythemia. Hyperbilirubinemia often follows polycythemia caused by hemolysis of the excess red blood cells.

■ **Is any treatment ever required for high hematocrit?**

It is probably wise when hematocrit is excessively high to reduce it to about 55 mg/dl by a partial exchange transfusion with albumin or plasma. This reduces blood viscosity and peak bilirubin level resulting from breakdown of the excessive number of red blood cells.

■ **What disorders of coagulation can cause problems for the newborn?**

Coagulation defects causing hemorrhage in the newborn include vitamin K deficiency, thrombocytopenia, and disseminated intravascular coagulation. Vitamin K deficiency or hemorrhagic disease of the newborn is a bleeding disorder usually occurring during the first 3 days of life. Vitamin K is necessary for the synthesis of prothrombin and other coagulation factors. Infants of mothers who had received phenobarbital or phenytoin (Dilantin) are particularly at risk for this disorder. These infants may have a generalized bleeding tendency but usually bleed from the gut. Thrombocytopenia is a platelet abnormality that can cause hemorrhage in the newborn. Platelets are necessary for an effective coagulation process. Petechiae and ecchymoses are characteristic of this disorder, which may be caused by infections, pharmacologic agents, or immunologic mechanisms. Disseminated intravascular coagulation (DIC) is a disorder found in extremely ill infants, especially those in shock and those with severe bacterial infections. There is spontaneous disseminated coagulation in the small blood vessels resulting in the consumption of platelets and blood factors normally involved in the coagulation process. Thus DIC is sometimes referred to as

"consumption coagulation." Clinical signs are variable because bleeding may occur anywhere in the body such as the skin, mucous membranes, urinary tract, or gut. Platelet count and fibrinogen levels are decreased, whereas the prothrombin time and partial thromboplastin time are prolonged. Since fibrin is formed in the coagulation process and subsequently split by enzyme action, excessive fibrin-split products in the circulating blood are also supportive of the diagnosis.

RESPIRATORY SYSTEM
■ **What is the most common reason for admission of a newborn infant to an intensive care unit?**

Approximately half of all newborn infants admitted to the intensive care unit are admitted because of respiratory difficulty.

■ **Describe the most common type of respiratory disorder leading to admission of the newborn.**

The most common respiratory disorder in the newborn is called *idiopathic respiratory distress syndrome* (RDS) or *hyaline membrane disease* and typically occurs in preterm infants. These two terms, both misnomers, are by common usage employed to describe a symptom complex that centers on pulmonary hypoperfusion, low lung compliance owing to insufficient surfactant production, and excessive extravascular pulmonary water. Insufficient surfactant results from immaturity, hypoxia, chemical or thermal injury to the surfactant-producing cells, increased surfactant utilization, or a combination of these. Surfactant is a phospholipid compound that makes it possible for alveoli to expand more easily. That is, less mechanical force is required to bring air into the alveoli of the lungs when surfactant is in the alveolar lining fluid. In the absence of the surfactant, alveoli tend to remain collapsed. The blood passing collapsed alveoli picks up little or no oxygen. Arterial blood therefore contains less than a normal amount of oxygen and the tissues become hypoxic. Metabolism of tissues continues, however, and in the absence of sufficient oxygen this metabolism produces lactic acid. Both hypoxia and acidemia act on the small blood vessels in the lung causing them to constrict. This constriction increases resistance to blood flow through the lungs causing large amounts of blood to be shunted through the ductus arteriosus and the foramen ovale, thus bypassing the lung and leading to even greater hypoxia and acidemia. The pathophysiologic process therefore tends to be self-perpetuating.

■ **From the answer to the previous question, what would be logical approaches to the prevention of respiratory distress syndrome?**

1. Prevention of preterm birth will probably ultimately become the most important method of preventing RDS. Presently, some mothers with premature labor are given alcohol to forestall active labor and steroids (betamethasone) to stimulate the elaboration of surfactant in utero.

2. Prevention of fetal hypoxia during labor and prevention of cold stress of the newborn after delivery will help in averting RDS. A surfactant production system operating at a marginal level can be so damaged by hypoxic and thermal stress as to function subnormally and lead to RDS.

3. Increasing the oxygen tension and content of circulating blood will help prevent RDS. This effort is first made by increasing oxygen concentration in the gas surrounding the baby's head. If arterial blood oxygen tension does not exceed 50 mm Hg while the infant is breathing 60% oxygen, proceed to constant positive airway pressure (CPAP) as described below.

4. When oxygen enrichment of the atmosphere alone does not result in sufficient oxygenation, measures should be taken to expand the collapsed alveoli. If the baby is breathing spontaneously, this is achieved by applying CPAP. This is usually done by intubating the infant with a 2.5 to 4 mm diameter endotracheal tube, the size depending on the baby's size, and attaching the tube to a system that does not allow the airway pressure at the end of the expiration to fall to atmospheric pressure. With this system the baby is not allowed to exhale as much gas as previously and consequently does not empty and collapse the alveoli. This establishes an increased functional residual capacity (FRC). Pressures applied are usually initially 4 to 6 cm of water and are increased or decreased depending on the baby's response. The infant who is not

breathing spontaneously is put on positive end expiratory pressure (PEEP). This expression is confusing and is generally accepted as describing respiratory assistance employing a cycling mechanical ventilatory device such as a Bird or Bourns respirator with positive end tidal pressure.

5. Acidosis is controlled by administering a buffer solution. Sodium bicarbonate is most commonly used. Less frequently tromethamine (THAM) is used. Sodium bicarbonate should be infused slowly, and usual doses should require at least 5 minutes for infusion.

■ **What are two important complications of mechanical ventilation?**

1. *Infection from contaminated equipment.* Respirator tubing and nebulizers must be changed at frequent intervals.
2. *Pneumothorax.* Equipment for emergency management of pneumothorax should be immediately at hand for any patient who is on a respirator or receiving PEEP.

■ **What happens when a term fetus in the uterus becomes hypoxic as a result of occlusion of the umbilical cord?**

The fetus becomes hypoxic, develops gasping respirations, and passes meconium into the amniotic fluid. Depending on the severity of hypoxia, meconium aspiration resulting from this process may be minimal to severe. When severe, it is referred to as the massive meconium aspiration syndrome. If the fetus has not been monitored during labor, the first clue may be meconium staining the amniotic fluid on rupture of the membranes. Amniotic fluid with meconium is sterile and produces chemical irritation in the small airways. They become partially obstructed, producing air trapping or a ball-valve effect. Meconium is an irritating foreign material that may produce a chemical pneumonitis. The volume of the chest is increased and the anteroposterior diameter may be unusually large.

■ **How should meconium aspiration be managed?**

Meconium aspiration is best managed by *prevention*. When meconium passage into amniotic fluid is suspected in the delivery room, the airway should be suctioned with a DeLee trap immediately after the head is delivered prior to the delivery of the shoulders. After the infant's body is delivered, the airway should be suctioned repeatedly through a laryngoscope and endotracheal tube until as much meconium as possible has been removed. Thereafter the best management is to provide humidified oxygen and thoracic physical therapy during the first 8 hours. The use of steroids has been suggested in the past, but there is no general agreement as to any beneficial effects.

■ **A term infant develops respiratory distress and is cyanotic immediately after birth. Amniotic fluid is normal and fetal monitoring has been normal. On inspection the abdomen appears smaller than normal and sunken (scaphoid). What is the baby's problem?**

Reduced size of the abdomen in a newborn with respiratory distress suggests *diaphragmatic hernia* in which a large proportion of the abdominal viscera has herniated through the diaphragm, occupying space that would normally be occupied by the lungs. Additionally, these infants usually have a displacement of the cardiac impulse to the opposite side of the chest and diminished breath sounds. A nasogastric tube should be inserted to decompress the stomach and minimize air distending the intestines. If resuscitation is required, a bag and mask should not be used because this would only force more air into the intestine and further compress the lung. Respiratory assistance should be given by endotracheal intubation. When this diagnosis is made, arrangements should be made for direct admission into the operating room, and the baby should be immediately placed under the supervision of the anesthesiologist and surgeon. The lungs are typically hypoplastic, and the degree of lung development is most important in the prognosis.

■ **A normal term infant regurgitates and becomes blue at the first feeding. This infant also has respiratory distress and excessive mucus. What is the most likely problem?**

Esophageal atresia and/or tracheoesophageal fistula is the most likely diagnosis. There are a variety of combinations of these lesions, but by far the most common type is esophageal atresia with a fistula between the trachea and distal esophageal pouch. Continuous suction in the upper pouch and gastrostomy to prevent aspiration of gastric contents make it possible to delay surgical repair until optimal conditions can be met.

■ **Why is it important to administer oxygen therapy to babies under very carefully monitored conditions?**

1. Injury to the retina is produced by high oxygen tension. Babies under 36 weeks' gestation and especially those under 1000 g birth weight are subject to this damage. The maximal tolerable arterial oxygen tension is not known with certainty, and small preterm infants have been known to develop retinopathy of the preterm infant (retrolental fibroplasia) even when there has been no oxygen enrichment. At present the goal of oxygen therapy is to sustain an arterial oxygen tension somewhere in the range of 50 to 70 mm Hg or a capillary oxygen tension around 35 to 45 mm Hg. The retina responds to high oxygen tension first by developing overgrowth of capillary blood vessels. This is followed by hemorrhage and scar formation causing contraction and retinal detachment.

2. Toxicity to the lung (bronchopulmonary dysplasia) is caused by high oxygen tension. Microscopically detectable damage to lung cells can be caused by breathing only moderately increased oxygen concentration for short periods of time. Oxygen lung damage is directly related to high oxygen concentrations and usually associated with breathing more than 70% oxygen for more than 2 days. The use of positive pressure ventilation (especially at high pressures) by endotracheal tube is also felt to be a predisposing factor. The duration of high oxygen concentrations and positive pressure ventilation may be implicated in the development of lung damage. Lung damage is characterized by thickening and eventual necrosis of alveolar walls and bronchiolar epithelial lining layers, atelectasis, and fibrosis. These changes impair oxygen diffusion from alveolar lumens to capillaries. This may lead to oxygen dependency, which may last from weeks to months. However after many months the lung

function and chest x-ray findings may completely return to normal.

■ **Describe some important aspects of resuscitation of the newborn infant in the delivery room.**

As soon as the infant is delivered, the nostrils and the oropharynx should be suctioned with a bulb syringe. The cord is cut and clamped and the infant is dried immediately to prevent heat loss by evaporation. The infant is placed under a radiant heat warmer and the Apgar score is assessed at 1 minute. An Apgar score of 3 or below is that of a severely depressed infant who requires immediate resuscitation. After suctioning the pharynx clear of mucus, the airway should be intubated under direct vision with a laryngoscope. Blood, mucus, and aspirated meconium should be cleared from the airway by suction, and positive pressure ventilation by bag with oxygen should be instituted. At this point oxygenation is much more important than administration of alkali. A 1-minute Apgar score of 4 to 7 is that of a moderately depressed baby who will often respond to simple stimulation to the skin or inflation of the airway by mask and bag. An Apgar score above 7 is found in nondepressed infants. Vigorous and possibly traumatic efforts to stimulate a depressed infant, such as hot and cold applications and rectal dilation, are not recommended. These maneuvers consume time that is best applied to clearing the airway and achieving proper oxygenation. The Apgar score is then evaluated at 5 minutes. The 5-minute Apgar score is more closely predictive of the long-term effects of birth anoxia.

The newborn infant does have some anatomic peculiarities that are important in resuscitation. The tongue is relatively large, the nares are narrow, the glottis is high (T4), the cricoid ring is narrow, and the mandible is short. The airway is placed in proper alignment for intubation by placing the head in the "sniffing position" with the shoulders only slightly raised and the chin protruding. This is in marked contrast to the appropriate position for the adult (hyperextension). It is important for the operator to have adequate assistance. The vocal cords can often be brought into clearer view by slight depression of the anterior neck over the laryngeal area.

If no heartbeat is heard, external cardiac massage should be initiated. This is accomplished by applying pressure with the index and middle fingers over the midsternum at a rate of 90 to 120 compressions per minute. This should be in a ratio of 3 to 1 to assisted respirations, which are given at a rate of 30 to 40 per minute. Care should be exercised to avoid injury to the sternum, liver, and spleen when applying cardiac massage.

CARDIOVASCULAR SYSTEM

■ **What types of congenital heart disease are more likely to be seen in a neonatal intensive care unit?**

Transposition of the great vessels, coarctation of the aorta, patent ductus arteriosus, and hypoplastic left heart syndrome are the congenital heart diseases most frequently seen in the neonatal intensive care unit. During the early part of the course they may be difficult to distinguish from primary lung disease.

■ **What observations might be helpful in distinguishing between heart and lung disease?**

Extreme desaturation of arterial blood owing to congenital heart disease results from large fixed right-to-left shunts. That is, the fraction of blood not flowing through the lungs is large. In this case allowing the baby to breathe high concentrations of oxygen would have a minimal effect on arterial oxygen tension. It is therefore sometimes helpful to apply the test of breathing 100% oxygen. If the oxygen tension rises appreciably, it is more likely that the baby has primary lung disease than primary congenital heart disease. There are some infants, however, with severe respiratory distress syndrome who cannot be distinguished from those with congenital heart disease by this test. In this situation the diagnostic assessment must be based on history and physical examination, x-ray findings, and echocardiograms to make the best judgment possible. When it is of extreme importance to identify heart disease for therapeutic reasons, it may be necessary to perform cardiac catheterization. Distinguishing heart and lung disease may be so difficult, even by very experienced staff, that infrequently a baby with RDS is catheterized.

■ **What are some of the common symptoms of congenital heart disease?**

Observations of feeding reveal dyspnea, choking, and coughing. Weight gain is poor. Profuse sweating, usually associated with feeding, is noted about the forehead, nasal bridge, and malar areas. Tachypnea is a cardinal sign of congenital heart disease. Tachycardia is also an important sign and is dependent on the infant's activity at the time the heart rate is determined. Cyanosis is an obvious sign of cardiac disease, and when minimal is best seen around the lips and oral mucous membrane. Arterial pulsations (brachial, radial, and femoral) can be important. Absence of femoral pulses may indicate coarctation or hypoplastic left heart syndrome. Bounding femoral pulses will indicate a patent ductus arteriosus. Murmurs may or may not be present and if present are not always an indication of heart disease.

■ **What type of supportive care should babies acutely ill with congenital heart disease be given?**

Supportive care of acutely ill babies with congenital heart disease consists of thermoregulation, optimal oxygenation, and meeting nutritional needs. Thermoregulation affects oxygen requirements and hence cardiopulmonary requirements. Oxygen should be warmed and humidified and the infant placed in a modified upright position. Oral feedings should be given to the infant with his head elevated and in frequent, small amounts. When feeding the infant, short rest periods will help ease the dyspnea and prevent aspiration. The infant should be observed closely for signs of heart failure.

■ **How is heart failure diagnosed in the newborn?**

The most useful signs in detecting heart failure in the newborn are enlarged liver, enlarged heart on chest x-ray examination, slight fullness of the anterior fontanel, moist rales in the lungs, tachypnea, and tachycardia. Peripheral edema is not an impressive sign, and fluid retention may be identified by close observation of weight. It is not necessary that a murmur be present and some of the more severe forms of congenital heart disease are not accompanied by a heart murmur.

■ **What is the treatment for congestive heart failure in the neonate?**

Treatment for congestive heart failure in the neonate consists of the following:
1. Digitalization (See charts at the end of this chapter for digoxin dosage.)
2. Temperature regulation at the thermoneutral point (Oxygen consumption is increased by either hypo- or hyperthermia.)
3. Supplementary oxygen (Care is taken to avoid overoxygenation because of the possibility of eye and lung toxicity.)
4. Control of acid-base balance
5. Sufficient fluids and electrolytes for adequate fluid balance and adequate renal function (Oral feedings should be withheld if the respiratory rate is high enough to produce the danger of aspiration.)
6. Monitoring hematocrit and correcting anemia by blood transfusion or polycythemia by partial exchange transfusion
7. Measuring blood pressures in both upper and lower extremities
8. Modified upright position to minimize the work of breathing
9. Diuretics (Furosemide is usually used if rapid diuresis is required, and a mercurial diuretic is used if a more prolonged, smoother effect is desired.)

■ **How should a neonate be monitored for digitalis toxicity?**

An ECG rhythm strip should be run prior to each dose of digoxin. Digitalis effect is assessed by its inhibition of conduction as manifested by prolongation of the P-R interval and reduction of heart rate. The next dose should generally be withheld if the rate is less than 100/min.

■ **What heart rate should be considered bradycardia in a newborn?**

A heart rate below 90/min should be considered bradycardia in a newborn.

■ **Would a heart murmur in a newborn ever be considered normal?**

Heart murmurs are very common in normal newborn infants as well as older children. The sound heard is a result of turbulent blood flow. The murmurs are often transient and rapidly changing during the neonatal period. Frequently a changing murmur is related to changing flow through the ductus arteriosus as it is closing. In the absence of associated symptoms and signs suggestive of heart disease it is best to avoid ascribing major significance to murmurs heard in early infancy and to follow the course over a longer period of time before alarming the parents.

■ **When does the ductus arteriosus usually close?**

In the healthy baby the ductus arteriosus usually closes functionally within the first 24 hours. However, anatomically it may remain open for a longer period of time, requiring, in some babies, several months for closure. The small preterm infant with respiratory distress tends to have more frequent difficulty with prolonged patent ductus arteriosus. It is not unusual for a baby of this type to require surgical ligation of the ductus arteriosus because of intractable failure and persistent need for high oxygen concentration and respiratory support.

■ **What normally causes the ductus arteriosus to close?**

Increased oxygen tension in the blood normally causes the ductus arteriosus to close. During fetal life the oxygen tension in blood flowing through the ductus is in the range of 25 to 30 mm Hg. At the time of birth the oxygen tension rises abruptly. The ductus is quite sensitive to this increase and responds by constricting. Disorders resulting in protracted hypoxemia delay closure of the ductus.

NEUROLOGIC DISORDERS

■ **Does the immaturity of the central nervous system in the preterm baby result in central nervous system abnormalities found in long-term follow-up?**

Early studies revealing that "very low birth weight babies" (1000 to 1500 g) had a high incidence (greater than 50%) of central nervous system damage suggested that the immaturity alone may have been responsible for a significant proportion of the long-term CNS deficits. With improved care provided by modern neonatal critical care units, the long-range prognosis appears to be

improving so much that this formerly held concept is probably inaccurate. Thus we are led to believe that the main causes of long-lasting central nervous system damage are hypoxia, central nervous system hemorrhage, hypoglycemia, hyperbilirubinemia, and central nervous system infections occurring before or after birth.

■ **Describe the clinical manifestations of neurologic dysfunction in the newborn.**

Observations should include abnormalities of activity, muscle tone, and alertness. Abnormal activity may be agitated (increased) or depressed (decreased). Muscle tone abnormalities include hypotonia (floppy) or hypertonia (rigidity). Alertness may vary from apathy to irritability. Abnormal behaviors may include jitteriness and seizures.

■ **What are causes of seizures in the newborn?**

Hypoxia; central nervous system hemorrhage; metabolic disorders such as hypoglycemia, hypocalcemia, hypomagnasemia, hypo/hypernatremia, pyridoxine dependency/deficiency, and aminoacidopathies; infection (meningitis/encephalitis); kernicterus from hyperbilirubinemia; narcotic withdrawal in the infant of an addicted mother; hyperviscosity (high hematocrit) syndrome; birth trauma; congenital malformations; and alkalosis (as from hyperventilation) are all causes of seizures in the newborn.

■ **How can seizures in the newborn be described?**

Seizures in a newborn may be so subtle as to be easily overlooked or may be seen only as increased muscle tone of an extremity, tremors, twitching, repetitive eye blinking, drooling, chewing movements, or apnea. More conspicuous seizure activity may be localized or may consist of generalized convulsive movements.

■ **How can seizure activity be differentiated from jitteriness?**

Jitteriness is not accompanied by abnormal gaze or extraocular movement as are seizures. Seizures are unresponsive to external stimuli, whereas jitteriness will diminish with passive flexion or external stimulation. The dominant movement of jitteriness is tremor and for seizures it is usually clonic jerking.

■ **What would be an appropriate initial workup for a neonate with seizures?**

Septic workup, including spinal fluid analysis, blood determinations of glucose, calcium, sodium, magnesium, and hematocrit, would be appropriate for a neonate with seizures. Skull x-ray films and electroencephalograms should also be done. If these are not informative, a more detailed workup may include investigations for transplacental infections, screening for inborn errors of metabolism, and administration of pyridoxine during an electroencephalogram.

■ **What is the management procedure for neonatal seizures?**

Management is aimed at elimination of the underlying cause. Immediate treatment includes maintaining a patent airway and anticonvulsant medication. Aspects of supportive care include thermoregulation, oxygenation, and meeting nutritional needs. The anticonvulsant medication of choice is phenobarbital.

INTRACRANIAL HEMORRHAGE

■ **What are the major predisposing factors for intracranial hemorrhage?**

Birth trauma, hypoxia, and preterm birth are the major predisposing factors for intracranial hemorrhage.

■ **Which infants are at greatest risk for developing intracranial hemorrhage?**

1. Infants with a history of perinatal asphyxia
2. Infants born by high- or midforceps delivery, breech extraction, or precipitous delivery
3. Preterm infants, especially those with respiratory distress syndrome and sepsis
4. Infants with maternal history of prolonged labor or cephalopelvic disproportion (especially primiparas)
5. Infants with hemorrhagic disorders

■ **What are the major clinically important types of neonatal intracranial hemorrhage?**

Subdural hemorrhage. Subdural hemorrhage results from tears of the cerebral veins and/or venous sinuses caused by birth trauma. This type of hemorrhage is more likely to occur in full-term, LGA infants in which the labor was precipitous or prolonged and the delivery was breech extraction, face or brow presentation, by forceps extraction, or rotational maneuvers. Depending on the degree of trauma, the prognosis ranges from poor to good with many survivors having neurologic deficits including hydrocephalus.

Subarachnoid hemorrhage. Subarachnoid hemorrhage is the most common type and is felt to arise from oozing capillaries and not from torn vessels. This type usually appears in preterm infants who have sustained hypoxia. In full-term infants subarachnoid hemorrhage is more likely caused by trauma and usually results in seizures with onset on day 2 of life—sometimes referred to as "the well baby with seizures." Many of the infants die, and those who survive have long-term neurologic deficits probably related to asphyxia. Hydrocephalus is the major sequela of subarachnoid hemorrhage.

Intraventricular hemorrhage. Intraventricular hemorrhage occurs more frequently in preterm infants delivered spontaneously and with a serious hypoxic event. The hypoxia, occurring either at birth or in association with respiratory distress syndrome, usually leads to venous infarctions or congestion damaging cerebral lesions and resulting in hemorrhage that may progress to rupture into the ventricles. The onset may be catastrophic deterioration or a more insidious deterioration. Most of the infants with intraventricular hemorrhage die in the immediate neonatal period. Those who survive develop hydrocephalus or have other neurologic sequelae.

Intracerebellar hemorrhage. Intracerebellar hemorrhage tends to occur more frequently in the small preterm infant. The cause is unknown but is felt to be related to hypoxic insults and extreme prematurity. Clinical details are based on autopsy findings that indicate an association with perinatal asphyxia and/or respiratory distress syndrome and a catastrophic deterioration with bradycardia, apnea, falling hematocrit, and bloody cerebrospinal fluid.

Hemorrhage into the brain substance. Hemorrhage into the brain substance is the least common type and is more often found in large term infants with precipitate or difficult delivery in which some component of hypoxia often exists. These infants are often distressed at birth, appear depressed, and a few days later show signs of agitation. Many of these infants die, but those who survive may make up a large portion of infants who are severely delayed or whose psychomotor development advances very slowly.

■ **What are some of the common clinical manifestations of intracranial hemorrhage?**

Irritability and seizure activity, lethargy, poor feeding, irregular respiration, apnea, cyanosis, pallor, decreased or absent Moro and sucking reflexes, excessive jaundice, and bulging fontanels are all clinical manifestations of intracranial hemorrhage. In preterm infants intracranial bleeding is most typically characterized by loss of muscle tone, abnormal pupils, hematocrit drop, tense fontanel, and intractable acidemia (caused by poor cardiac output).

■ **How does one manage neonatal intracranial hemorrhage?**

1. Supportive—gentle handling, thermoregulation, suction as necessary, ventilation, monitor vital signs
2. Controlling seizures
3. Monitoring hematocrit and transfuse as needed
4. CT scan (Consider subdural tap if blood localized in subdural space.)
5. Treating coagulation defect if present by giving fresh frozen plasma or blood

INFANTS OF DRUG-ABUSING MOTHERS

■ **How is the newborn affected by abusive drugs taken by the mother?**

Abusive drugs, such as heroin, barbiturates, and amphetamines, readily cross the placenta resulting in withdrawal symptoms or respiratory distress in the newborn.

■ **What are some of the common clinical manifestations of infants of drug-addicted mothers?**

Clinical signs of infants of drug-addicted mothers depend on the duration of the habit, frequency and amount of drugs taken, and the time of the last dose. Symptoms commonly seen include tremors, twitching, seizures, irritability, hyperactivity, a high-pitched shrill cry, sneezing, yawning, sucking and chewing fists, sweating, vomiting, diarrhea, temperature instability, and having a ravenous appetite with poor weight gain caused by the infants being poor feeders.

■ **What is the management of infants of drug-addicted mothers?**

Try to keep the infant quiet in a low-stimulating environment, offer a pacifier, swaddle the infant, offer frequent, small feedings, and administer sedatives. The drugs recommended for sedation are phenobarbital, chlorpromazine (Thorazine), or paregoric.

ENDOCRINE-METABOLIC DISORDERS

The endocrine and metabolic problems associated with newborns, the clinical and laboratory diagnostic signs identifying the disorder, and appropriate immediate management are summarized in Table 38-1. All of these conditions can lead to severe illness in the newborn infant.

GASTROINTESTINAL SYSTEM

■ **What is the significance of delayed passage of meconium?**

Ninety percent of babies pass meconium in the first 24 hours. Delayed passage of meconium, particularly if there is associated abdominal distention or vomiting, should lead to suspicion of obstruction somewhere in the lower intestine. Possible causes of obstruction include meconium plug syndrome, Hirschprung's disease, imperforate anus, intestinal atresia, and meconium peritonitis associated with cystic fibrosis.

■ **Is it possible to determine that blood vomited or passed rectally by the neonate is of maternal origin?**

Yes, the distinction can usually be made by an Apt test. There is a difference between susceptibility of fetal and adult hemoglobin to the effects of alkali. With the Apt test, the color will be pink for fetal hemoglobin (baby's blood) and change to yellow-brown for adult hemoglobin (maternal blood).

Table 38-1. Endocrine-metabolic problems

Endocrine-metabolic disorders	Diagnostic clues	Management
Hypoglycemia	Blood glucose level below 20 mg/dl for preterm and 30 mg/dl for term newborns; signs: irritability, jitteriness, tremors, apnea, cyanosis, lethargy, poor feeding; infants at risk: SGA, infant of diabetic mother, Rh isoimmunization, severely stressed (asphyxia, cold stress, shock)	Early feeding, intravenous glucose, adrenocortical steroids if glucose alone not effective; monitor glucose determinations; supportive nursing management
Hypocalcemia	Serum calcium level under 7 mg/dl: signs: twitching, tremors, high-pitched cry, seizures, cyanosis, apnea, hypotonia; infants at risk: LBW infant, infant of diabetic mother, stress (asphyxia), treatment of acidosis with sodium bicarbonate, exchange transfusions with citrated blood	Administration of calcium gluconate; symptomatic: 10% calcium gluconate, 0.2–0.4 ml/kg, slowly intravenously while listening to heart rate as bradycardia can occur; maintenance: 400–800 mg/kg/24 hr by IV drip; nonsymptomatic: oral calcium gluconate; calcium gluconate never to be given IM—causes sterile abscess; IV calcium administration may result in tissue necrosis; supportive management
Hypomagnesemia	Serum magnesium level under 1 mEq/L; signs: (mimics hypocalcemia) irritability, hypotonia, twitching, tremors; infants at risk: SGA, infant of diabetic mother, postexchange transfusion	Treat with 25% MgSO$_4$ 0.1 mg/kg IM; if given IV, must be given slowly with cardiac monitoring (prolonged atrioventricular conduction can occur); supportive care
Hypermagnesemia	Usually a serum magnesium level over 4 mEq/L; signs: profound CNS depression, depressed respirations, tachycardia, lethargy; found in infants of mothers treated with MgSO$_4$ for toxemia	Supportive, monitor magnesium levels, ventilatory support as needed, maintain fluid and electrolyte balance, exchange transfusion to remove excess magnesium
Late metabolic acidosis of the preterm infant	Preterm, does well first few days; after 1 or 2 weeks takes feedings poorly, fails to gain weight; low blood pH (below 7.25)	Small doses of sodium bicarbonate added to formula usually result in prompt improvement of symptoms
Galactosemia	Jaundice, sepsis, enlarged liver, cataracts, copper-reducing substance in the urine, and specific test on red cells for UDPG transferase	Control infection, reduce bilirubin by phototherapy; exchange transfusion if needed; lactose-free diet (Nutramigen, Prosobee); genetic counseling
Disorders of amino acid metabolism such as maple syrup urine disease or methylmalonic acidemia	Acidemia, difficult to control and unexplained by respiratory status; ketonemia; elevation of amino acid concentrations found on specific chromatographic tests; seizures	Buffers to modify acidemia and anticonvulsant therapy until specific dietary or vitamin therapy can be administered
Virilizing adrenal hyperplasia (adrenogenital syndrome, congenital adrenal hyperplasia)	Virilized genitalia, more conspicuous in female; vomiting followed by shock; serum potassium high (cardiac arrhythmias) and sodium low; elevated blood pregnanetriol	Intravenous sodium chloride, deoxycorticosterone for emergency treatment; adrenocortical steroids for prolonged treatment; genetic counseling
Myasthenia gravis	Infant has respiratory insufficiency soon after birth; mother has myasthenia gravis; course self-limited and usually resolves in a few weeks	Respiratory support with bag or respirator; edrophonium chloride (Tensilon) test and treatment with pyridostigmine bromide (Mestinon); taper drug as symptoms diminish

■ **A 3-week-old male infant develops projectile vomiting of nonbile-stained material, weight loss, dehydration, and scanty stools. This age, sex, and symptom complex is characteristic of what problem?**

This complex is characteristic of hypotrophic pyloric stenosis. In addition to the symptoms physical findings include impaired nutrition and hydration, gastric waves proceeding from the left to the right over the left upper and central abdomen, and a palpable mass often described as an "olive" at the position of the pylorus.

■ **A 3-week-old infant suddenly develops vomiting of bile-stained material, abdominal distention, and signs of shock. Why is it important that the correct diagnosis be made quickly?**

This clinical complex is characteristic of malrotation of the intestine and midgut volvulus. It is important to make the correct diagnosis quickly because delay can result in the loss of a large amount of bowel owing to circulatory impairment produced by the volvulus. This entity is a major contributor to the severe instances of short bowel syndrome.

■ **What are two abdominal wall defects that may interfere with functioning of the gastrointestinal system?**

Omphalocele and gastroschisis are abdominal wall defects that may interfere with functioning of the gastrointestinal system, and both require surgical repair. An omphalocele may be covered by an intact or ruptured hernia sac containing abdominal viscera occurring at the point of juncture of the umbilical cord and the abdomen. A gastroschisis is a small defect of the anterior abdominal wall lateral to the umbilicus through which the intestines eviscerate. Warm sterile sa-

TEMPERATURE EQUIVALENTS

NORMAL VALUES

Centigrade	Fahrenheit	Centigrade	Fahrenheit	Centigrade	Fahrenheit
34.0	93.2	37.2	98.9	40.4	104.7
34.2	93.6	37.4	99.3	40.6	105.1
34.4	93.9	37.6	99.6	40.8	105.4
34.6	94.3	37.8	100.0	41.0	105.8
34.8	94.6	38.0	100.4	41.2	106.1
35.0	95.0	38.2	100.7	41.4	106.5
35.2	95.4	38.4	101.1	41.6	106.8
35.4	95.7	38.6	101.4	41.8	107.2
35.6	96.1	38.8	101.8	42.0	107.6
35.8	96.4	39.0	102.2	42.2	108.0
36.0	96.8	39.2	102.5	42.4	108.3
36.2	97.1	39.4	102.9	42.6	108.7
36.4	97.5	39.6	103.2	42.8	109.0
36.6	97.8	39.8	103.6	43.0	109.4
36.8	98.2	40.0	104.0		
37.0	98.6	40.2	104.3		

To convert centigrade to Fahrenheit: $\frac{9}{5} \times$ Temperature + 32

EXAMPLE: To convert 40° centigrade to Fahrenheit
$\frac{9}{5} \times 40 = 72 + 32 = 104°$ Fahrenheit

To convert Fahrenheit to centigrade: (Temperature minus 32) $\times \frac{5}{9}$

EXAMPLE: To convert 98.6° Fahrenheit to centigrade
$98.6 - 32 = 66.6 \times \frac{5}{9} - 37°$ centigrade

NORMAL VALUES AND INFORMATION FOR NEWBORN INFANTS

Bilirubin
    10 mg/100 ml or less

BUN
    20 mg/100 ml or less

Electrolytes
    Chloride—95-110 mEq/L
    Potassium—3.5-5.5 mEq/L
    Sodium—135-145 mEq/L

Glucose
    30+ mg/dl—Hypoglycemia term infants <30 mg/dl ⎫
                Hypoglycemia preterm infants <20 mg/dl ⎬ During first 24 hr
                 ℞ IV glucose 10% solution or stronger ⎭

Hematocrit
    45-65 mg/dl—If above 65 mg/dl consider partial exchange (10% of blood volume for same volume of plasma)

Calcium
    8-10.5 mg/dl—Treat if below 7 mg/dl
                    Treat if symptomatic between 7-8 mg/dl

Phorphorus
    3.5-8 mg/dl—May be as high as 10 if calcium is low, owing to a transient hypoparathyroidism

Magnesium
    1.5-2.0 mg/dl

Blood gases (first week of life):

	Arterial	Capillary
pH	7.30-7.40	7.30-7.40
Po_2	50-70 mm Hg	35-45 mm Hg
Pco_2	35-45 mm Hg	35-45 mm Hg

Respiratory rate	35/min (range 20-60)
Heart rate	140/min (range 120-160)
Length	50 cm
Head circumference	35 cm
Weight (male)	3350 g
Weight (female)	3250 g

Retrolental fibroplasia is related to Pao_2, not FIO_2 (fraction of inspired oxygen). Any baby on any additional oxygen must be monitored with frequent blood gases (that includes babies in O_2 below 40%).

Most common antibiotic combination in neonatal sepsis is ampicillin or penicillin and kanamycin or gentamicin.

CONVERSION OF INCHES TO CENTIMETERS

Inches	Centimeters	Inches	Centimeters	Inches	Centimeters
10	25.40	15	38.10	20	50.80
10½	26.67	15½	39.37	20½	52.07
11	27.94	16	40.64	21	53.34
11½	29.21	16½	41.91	21½	54.61
12	30.48	17	43.18	22	55.88
12½	31.75	17½	44.45	22½	57.15
13	33.02	18	45.72	23	58.42
13½	34.29	18½	46.99	23½	59.69
14	35.56	19	48.26	24	60.96
14½	36.83	19½	49.53		

COMMON DRUG DOSAGES FOR THE NEONATE

Antibiotics	<1 week of age	1-4 weeks of age	Route
Ampicillin	50 mg/kg/24 hr (2 divided doses)	75 mg/kg/24 hr (3 divided doses)	IM, IV
Meningitis	100 mg/kg/24 hr (2 divided doses)	200 mg/kg/24 hr (3 divided doses)	IV
Gentamicin	5 mg/kg/24 hr (2 divided doses)	7.5 mg/kg/24 hr (2 divided doses)	IM, IV
Kanamycin	<2000 g 15 mg/kg/24 hr (2 divided doses)	<2000 g 20 mg/kg/24 hr (2 divided doses)	IM, IV
	>2000 g 20 mg/kg/24 hr (2 divided doses)	>2000 g 30 mg/kg/24 hr (3 divided doses)	IM, IV
Nafcillin	40 mg/kg/24 hr (2 divided doses)	60 mg/kg/24 hr (3 divided doses)	IM, IV
Penicillin G	50,000 U/kg/24 hr (2 divided doses)	75,000 U/kg/24 hr (3 divided doses)	IM, IV
Meningitis	100,000-150,000 U/kg/ 24 hr (2 divided doses)	150,000-250,000 U/kg/ 24 hr (3 divided doses)	IM, IV
Carbenicillin	200 mg/kg/24 hr (2 divided doses)	<2000 g 300 mg/kg/24 hr (3 divided doses)	IM, IV
		>2000 g 400 mg/kg/24 hr (4 divided doses)	IM, IV

	0-14 days age	2-4 weeks age	
Methicillin	<2000 g 50 mg/kg/24 hr (2 divided doses)	75 mg/kg/24 hr (3 divided doses)	IM, IV
	>2000 g 100 mg/kg/24 hr (4 divided doses)		IM, IV

Cardiovascular	Birth to 4 weeks of age	Route
Atropine	0.01 mg/kg/dose	IM, IV, PO, SQ
Digoxin	0.03 mg/kg total digoxin dose (give ½ total dose *stat,* remainder in 2 divided doses at 8 hr intervals)	IM, IV
	Maintenance: ⅛ of TDD q 12 hr	IM, PO

COMMON DRUG DOSAGES FOR THE NEONATE—cont'd

Cardiovascular—cont'd	Birth to 4 weeks of age	Route
Epinephrine	1 : 10,000 dilution 0.1 ml/kg/dose	IV
Furosemide (Lasix)	1-2 mg/kg/dose	PO, IV
Metabolic correction		
Calcium gluconate 10%	400-800 mg/kg/24 hr	IV
Glucagon	0.3 mg/kg/24 hr	IM
Glubionate calcium (Neo-Calglucon)	1-2 ml/kg/24 hr (3-4 divided doses)	PO
Sodium bicarbonate	Body wt (kg) × base deficit (mEq/L) × 0.35 = mEq $NaHCO_3$; give no more than 8-10 mEq/kg/24 hr	
	Stat dose: 2-3 mEq/kg/dose *slowly IV* (dilute to ½ strength prior to use)	IV
Neonatal seizures		
Phenobarbital	Stat: 4-6 mg/kg IV push, then 8-10 mg/kg/24 hr in 4 doses IM for 2 days, then 5-6 mg/kg/24 hr IM or PO; taper dosage over 7-10 days per infant tolerance	
Phenytoin (Dilantin)	5-7 mg/kg/24 hrs IV; poorly absorbed orally and may require up to 20 mg/kg/24 hr	
Diazepam (Valium)	Stat: 0.2 mg/kg, slowly, IV push	
Infant of drug-abusing mother		
Phenobarbital	8-10 mg/kg/24 hr in 4 doses IM for 2 days, then 5-6 mg/kg/24 hr IM or PO; taper dosage over 7-10 days per infant tolerance	
Chlorpromazine (Thorazine)	2-3 mg/kg/24 hr IM in 4 divided doses for approximately 4 days; then oral therapy with a gradual dosage reduction over 2-3 weeks	
Camphorated opium tincture (Paregoric)	0-2 ml q 3 hr, increase by 0.05 ml q 3 hr until a stabilizing dose is reached (It is rarely necessary to exceed 0.7 per dose.); taper dosage over 7-10 days	
Narcotic antagonists		
Naloxone (Narcan) neonatal	0.01 mg/kg/per dose IV or IM (neonatal strength 0.02 mg/ml)	

CONVERSION OF POUNDS AND OUNCES TO GRAMS

	1	**2**	**3**	**4**	**5**	**6**	**7**	**8**
0	454	907	1361	1814	2268	2722	3175	3629
1	482	936	1389	1843	2296	2750	3204	3657
2	510	964	1418	1871	2325	2778	3232	3686
3	539	992	1446	1899	2353	2807	3260	3714
4	567	1021	1474	1928	2381	2835	3289	3742
5	595	1049	1503	1956	2410	2863	3317	3771
6	624	1077	1531	1985	2438	2892	3345	3799
7	652	1106	1559	2013	2466	2920	3374	3827
8	680	1134	1588	2041	2495	2948	3402	3856
9	709	1162	1616	2070	2523	2977	3430	3884
10	737	1191	1644	2098	2552	3005	3459	3912
11	765	1219	1673	2126	2580	3033	3487	3941
12	794	1247	1701	2155	2608	3062	3515	3969
13	822	1276	1729	2183	2637	3090	3544	3997
14	851	1304	1758	2211	2665	3119	3572	4026
15	879	1332	1786	2240	2693	3147	3600	4054

Pounds across top; Ounces down side.

line sponges should be applied to the eviscerated bowel until surgical repair can be performed. Postoperative management of infants with omphalocele and gastroschisis includes thermoregulation, ventilation with oxygen if necessary, supplying nutritional needs, gastrostomy tube care, and most important the prevention of infection.

■ **A preterm infant who has had respiratory distress syndrome appears to be recovering from a respiratory problem. At 10 days of age he develops rapid onset of abdominal distention, gastric residuals, bloody stools, temperature instability, and shocklike state. What is the most probable diagnosis and what is the pathogenesis of this disease?**

The most probable diagnosis is necrotizing enterocolitis (NEC). When this clinical complex is seen, the diagnosis is supported by findings on x-ray examination of thickened bowel wall, gas in the bowel wall, free gas in the peritoneal cavity, and gas in the portal circulation. This gas is hydrogen that is generated by anaerobic bacteria in the intestines and will often disappear after feedings have been stopped. Discontinuing feedings early in the course of the disease and treating the shock are probably the most important features of successful management.

The etiology of this disease is as yet unclear. NEC has been described only in recent years. Therefore it is probably a result of one of the newer forms of management of low birth weight infants or is occurring in infants who would not formerly have survived long enough to develop the disorder. It tends to develop within 5 to 21 days of age. At the present time the most logical causes seem to include a prior period of hypoxia or infection or a combination of both of these. It has been demonstrated that aortic blood flow may be very significantly decreased by the placement of aortic catheters via the umbilical artery. This could result in reduced mesenteric artery flow, and the tips of such catheters should probably be placed no higher than the aortic bifurcation.

NEONATAL FLUID AND ELECTROLYTE NEEDS

Water requirements
    Full-term infant

First day of life	75-100 ml/kg/day
Thereafter	100 ml/kg/day
Healthy infant under 1500 g	100-125 ml/kg/day
Infant with respiratory distress syndrome under 1500 g	125-150 ml/kg/day

Electrolytes

Sodium	3-4 mEq/kg/day—maintenance
Potassium	2 mEq/kg/day—maintenance
Calcium	200 mg/kg/day—maintenance
	400-800 mg/kg/day—treatment

Caloric requirement   120-150 cal/day for growth

Colloid

Packed red blood cells	2 ml/kg/g Hb to be raised
Whole blood	6 ml/kg/g Hb to be raised
Plasma or Plasmanate	10 ml/kg

■ **What are the limitations on feeding a preterm infant with respiratory distress syndrome?**

Early feeding is considered important in preterm infants. Early feeding decreases the likelihood of hypoglycemia and the peak bilirubin level. It is wise, however, to delay feedings when the respiratory rate is excessively high. Distention of the stomach can reduce movement of the diaphragm and the possibility of regurgitation and aspiration is greater. It is usually best to delay oral feedings by nipple or gavage until the respiratory rate is below 60/min.

■ **What methods are used to provide nutrition for the sick newborn?**

1. Gavage feeding is an artificial means of providing nutrition for infants who are very ill or preterm infants less than 32 weeks' gestation who have poor suck-swallow coordination.
2. Parenterally, nutrition may be supplied by using dextrose solutions with added electrolytes or hyperalimentation solutions that contain amino acids, glucose, trace minerals, electrolytes, and vitamins.

SUMMARY

In this chapter on critical care of the neonate we have covered thermoregulation, infection, shock, acid-base, and fluid problems and have developed a body system–oriented approach to the problems, including consideration of the hematologic, respiratory, cardiovascular, neurologic, endocrine, and gastrointestinal systems.

Although problems have often been discussed individually, actual neonatal critical care often becomes very complex as a result of interwoven problems. The infant born preterm is at increased risk for infection, thermal stress, respiratory distress, cardiovascular problems (patent ductus arteriosus), eye damage (retrolental fibroplasia), lung damage (bronchopulmonary dysplasia), malnutrition, necrotizing enterocolitis, metabolic problems (hypoglycemia, hypocalcemia), and hematologic problems (hyperbilirubinemia, anemia).

Successful management of such a complex group of problems requires carefully coordinated efforts of a dedicated, well-equipped, disciplined team as well as a large financial commitment.

The role of parents is a major concern for the team caring for an infant in an intensive care unit. Parents of an infant born prematurely or with a congenital defect or serious problem experience an emotional shock that is intensified when their infant is admitted to a neonatal intensive care unit. It is the responsibility of the team to minimize the emotional stress by providing appropriate supportive measures to enhance the parent-infant relationship (see Chapter 39). On pp. 646-651 are charts covering temperature equivalents and their normal values, normal values and information for newborn infants, conversion charts, neonatal fluid and electrolyte needs, and common drug dosages for neonates.

BIBLIOGRAPHY

Aladjem, S., and Brown, A. K., editors: Clinical perinatology, St. Louis, 1974, The C. V. Mosby Co.

Avery, M. E., and Fletcher, B. D.: The lung and its disorders in the newborn infant, ed. 3, Philadelphia, 1974, W. B. Saunders Co.

Behrman, R. E.: Neonatal-perinatal medicine, ed. 2, St. Louis, 1977, The C. V. Mosby Co.

Babson, S. G., Benson, R. C., Pernoll, M. L., and Benda, G. I.: Management of high-risk pregnancy and intensive care of the neonate, ed. 3, St. Louis, 1975, The C. V. Mosby Co.

Gluck, L.: Modern perinatal medicine, Chicago, 1974, Year Book Medical Publishers, Inc.

Harper, R. G., and Yoon, J. J.: Handbook of neonatology, Chicago, 1974, Year Book Medical Publishers, Inc.

Klaus, M. H., and Fanaroff, A. A.: Care of the high-risk neonate, Philadelphia, 1973, W. B. Saunders Co.

Korones, S. B.: High-risk newborn infants, St. Louis, 1972, The C. V. Mosby Co.

Korones, S. B.: High-risk newborn infants. The basis for intensive nursing care, ed. 2, St. Louis, 1976, The C. V. Mosby Co.

Pierog, S. H., and Ferrara, A.: Medical care of the sick newborn, ed. 2, St. Louis, 1976, The C. V. Mosby Co.

Schaffer, A. J., and Avery, M. E.: Diseases of the newborn, ed. 3, Philadelphia, 1971, W. B. Saunders Co.

CHAPTER 39

Psychologic care of the critically ill newborn and family*

Rebecca Schmeeckle Brown and Melody Jacobson

This chapter presents an overview of the psychologic crisis that occurs when a newborn infant is admitted to an intensive care unit. It describes the experiences of those people directly involved: the parents, the infant, and the hospital staff who provide care. The first section explores parental reaction to the birth and subsequent events involved in the care of a critically ill infant. The kinds of stress that parents experience as well as adaptive coping mechanisms are covered. Guidelines for assessment of the parent-child relationship and support interventions are discussed. The second section describes the infant and his role in the crisis. We will examine the ways in which the critically ill and low birth weight infant differ from a healthy term baby and the impact these differences may have on the developing affectional bond between parent and child. Various infant abilities are explored and techniques for promoting responsiveness are suggested. The final section attends to the psychologic stresses experienced by the medical staff in providing comprehensive care for sick infants and their parents. Environmental and social factors are examined, indicators for maladaptive coping are outlined, and stress-reducing interventions are presented.

The first two sections are organized so as to present an overview of normal behavior necessary to the understanding of variations. Maladaptive processes are then discussed, and finally, interventions are suggested. Our goal is to provide the reader with an expanded understanding of the psychologic stresses encountered in the newborn intensive care setting and how these stresses may affect the developing infant. Additionally, we seek to improve assessment skills and promote the exploration of innovative approaches to intervention. Above all, we would like to encourage reevaluation and rethinking with regard to hospital practices in light of the expanded needs of infants and parents (Fig. 39-1).

PARENTAL REACTIONS
■ Why should special supportive care be provided to families of preterm or seriously ill newborn infants?

The birth of a child under any circumstances may be defined as a crisis.[1,2] There is a temporary disequilibrium experienced by all family members as they react to change in their lives. The dynamic balance of relationships within the family is disturbed, and each individual must adjust and become comfortable within the new family structure. This disequilibrium and readjustment process offers a unique opportunity for positive growth for all family members.

Caplan[3] states that relatively short periods of crisis in which individuals struggle to cope with stressful events seem to be of special significance for their future emotional health. Factors such as availability of resources, access to support, and

*These efforts were partially funded by National Foundation March of Dimes Grant No. C243 and Department of Health, Education and Welfare—Maternal-Child Health Services Grant No. MCT000953-05-0.

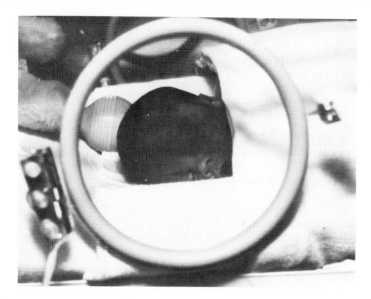

Fig. 39-1. The technology of caring for the preterm or critically ill infant may interfere with the developing affectional bond between parent and child.

previous experience with personal crisis directly affect whether the outcome is beneficial or harmful to the individual. The vulnerability that Caplan has suggested offers an opportunity for emotional growth and satisfaction versus feelings of discouragement, bitterness, and defeat. The disequilibrium of crisis has important implications for caregivers who value preventive, growth-fostering intervention. In many cases even a small amount of timely support can have a significant influence on outcome.

The delivery of a healthy term infant not only brings the challenge and promise of positive change but may also bring feelings of pride and accomplishment at having successfully completed a difficult task. The disruptive hospital stay is short and the family is able to quickly devote its energy to integrating the new member and resolving the disequilibrium. When the new infant is of low birth weight, is seriously ill, or has a congenital abnormality, the family must cope not only with the normal stress of change, but with a multitude of other severe stress factors. In addition, the state of crisis may go on for weeks or months and may become a series of crises in close

proximity to one another. In consideration of these factors, working with parents of an infant who requires intensive care is a dynamic, if somewhat dangerous, opportunity to positively affect the lives of families who find themselves in this situation.

■ **What individual processes are involved for each family member when integrating any new infant into the family group?**

For the new mother the process of developing a relationship with her infant begins in early pregnancy. As she recognizes the pregnancy, she begins to accept the changes in her own body and plans for imminent changes in her life. Frequently, this process is an ambivalent one, filled with feelings of acceptance and rejection, joyful anticipation and fearful dread. If it is the first pregnancy, she must prepare herself for an entirely new role. If it is a second or later pregnancy, all the experiences with other pregnancies may color her present feelings. She must deal with fears and hopes for the outcome of the pregnancy. She imagines what this child will be like and, finally, must prepare herself for the demands the baby will make on her time, energy, and life in general.[1,4]

Fathers, too, experience their own unique stresses throughout pregnancy and after the birth of a new baby. Phillips and Anzalone[5] report that men often react with unclear feelings about being a father when the pregnancy is confirmed. This is followed by the realization that the baby is real, usually around the time the fetus begins to move. Later, there is a period of thinking seriously about his new role and the responsibilities of fatherhood. He reacts to his wife's role change from wife and lover, to mother, wife, and lover and must prepare to share her attention with a new family member.

The addition of a new baby makes demands on the older children to adjust to the new family member and the subsequent change in family dynamics. How the siblings handle the demands of this period is largely dependent on their own developmental level. The security of their own established relationship with the parents, the preparation they have received previous to the event, and the attention and understanding they receive after the baby comes home may have a significant influence on the intensity of their stress. Acting out and regression to lower developmental levels may increase the general level of tension within the family.

■ How do the parents experience the preterm or problematic birth in contrast to the delivery of a healthy term infant?

Kaplan and Mason[6] vividly contrast the normal term birth with the preterm birth in terms of the mother's experience. Assuming the mother has accomplished the psychologic preparation for birth, she comes to term delivery both impatient to see the baby and to discharge her burden. Optimally, the atmosphere surrounding the birth is relaxed and charged with positive expectations. When events follow the expected pattern, the mother more readily feels pride in achievement and receives rewards and recognition from her husband, family, and friends, as well as the medical staff that attend her. She is encouraged to feel happy and proud, and her own emotional state of well-being enhances her first interactions with her infant.

Although she may have fears about whether the infant will be normal, the average pregnant woman may not seriously consider the possibility of a preterm birth or other delivery-related problems and may be emotionally unprepared. In addition, a shortened gestational period denies the mother adequate time to complete psychologic preparation for motherhood. Premature labor and unanticipated problems charge the delivery room with the tension of an emergency. Parents may be talked to in guarded terms and find their questions avoided or only partially answered, which further heightens their already grave concern about whether their baby will live. There may seem to be little cause for congratulations. Family and friends who visit may speak with sympathy and caution or may give unrealistic or unconvincing reassurance. Both parents may share uncertainties about the nature of the problem and what they may have done, or not done, to cause it.

If the delivery happens to be at a hospital that cannot provide the specialized care the infant may need, emergency transport is initiated. This heightens the feeling of emergency and decreases the opportunity for immediate parent-infant contact. The father is placed in the position of having to decide whether to accompany the infant to the comprehensive care center or remain with his wife and offer support. With the departure of the father and the baby, the mother may feel extremely isolated and disoriented.

The intensive care unit with its complex, buzzing equipment and tense activity level may be frightening. The child's appearance may increase parental anxiety, especially if he is emaciated, weak, and struggling for breath. At any rate, the baby frequently does not inspire pride during this early period. Lack of real contact with the infant may be frustrating and increase feelings of helplessness, confusion, disappointment, and fear. Frequently, parents are concerned over the pain the baby may be feeling and blame themselves for it.

Coming home without the baby is difficult. It may reinforce feelings of emptiness, failure, and disappointment. Frequent visiting helps, but there may be little change from day to day or the continuous stress of one crisis right after another.

When it is time to take the baby home, the mother may feel extremely anxious even though she has been anticipating the event for weeks. She may worry about her own competence in light of the expert care the baby has required.

■ What are the psychologic tasks of the parent when the baby requires intensive care?

The first major area of stress after the birth of an infant requiring intensive care concerns the infant's survival and the fledgling parent-child relationship. The parents must initially cope with uncertainty over whether the infant will live. They are faced with the dilemma of attaching to an infant who may die or detaching from an infant who may, after all, live. Kaplan and Mason[6] delineate four major tasks that mothers in this crisis must accomplish. The first of these tasks they refer to as anticipatory grief. During this stage the mother withdraws from the relationship established during pregnancy and grieves the loss of the "expected baby" while hoping simultaneously that the "real baby" will live. In a second task the mother must face her failure to produce a healthy term infant and deal with the accompanying guilt. Kaplan and Mason suggest that these tasks are optimally accomplished around the time of delivery or soon after the infant is admitted to the intensive care unit. Then as the infant begins to make progress, the mother moves to the third task. She resumes the process of relating to the infant and begins to believe that he will live and eventually join the family at home. The final task concerns the mother's understanding as to how a premature baby differs from a term or otherwise healthy infant as related to his special needs and growth patterns. In doing this she begins accepting the "real baby" and signals readiness to assume her role in mothering the child.

When the infant's hospital course increases the probability that he may be handicapped, or if the baby was born with a congenital abnormality, the last stage, acceptance of the "real baby," may be more difficult, take longer, and have different emotional characteristics than if the child was simply of low birth weight. It has been our experience that most parents of preterm or seriously ill infants worry about the child's future development. It is not unusual to find parents still concerned with this question as their child approaches school age. This may not be a continuous concern but may surface, be further resolved, and surface again throughout early childhood.

A situation that may change the process of completing the psychologic tasks just described is the number of problems the infant has during hospitalization. If he has a pendulum course, where more than once a problem is resolved only to be followed by another problem, the parents may experience a cyclic process where they grieve and hope, attach and withdraw several times during the hospitalization.

■ What additional parental stresses are present in the neonatal intensive care situation?

In addition to psychologic stresses related to the parent-child relationship, parents of an infant requiring intensive care must deal with worries over what the expensive hospitalization will mean to them financially. Even when the third party payment assists with the financial burden, dealing with the complexities of government agencies, insurance companies, and hospital billing systems can be a tremendous difficulty.

The task of maintaining a somewhat normal family life during the infant's hospitalization may be overwhelming. Other children in the family may be confused and upset by the interruption of normal routines. In coping with their own anxiety they may demand increased levels of attention, which may seem just too much for distressed parents to handle. Fathers, particularly, may face demands to return to work at a time when energy and thoughts are directed toward personal life crisis.

A final stress area that may exacerbate the trauma of this situation is the intensive care unit itself. Many parents report difficulty in coping with the equipment, lights, tubes, monitors, and the atmosphere of tension that may be present. Even the warmest, most relaxed intensive care situation is hardly the place to begin a new love relationship.

Some of the stresses and problems faced by parents of an infant who has special care needs have been delineated and specific tasks that are important in the process of adaptation have been suggested. In light of the monumental problems enumerated thus far it may seem remarkable that most parents survive this crisis and go on to develop healthy relationships with their infants. The amazing flexibility and adaptability of both parents and infants must be credited and at all times respected.

In order to provide a facilitative atmosphere for all parents and infants and therapeutic intervention for those having a particularly difficult time, it is important for nursery personnel to (1) understand the complex processes involved in a crisis of this nature, (2) develop skill in assessing healthy versus maladaptive parental reactions, and (3) gain awareness of the factors, both fixed and alterable, influencing the outcome.

■ **What are some factors that influence the manner in which parents adjust to a new parent-child relationship and cope with stress in the intensive care unit?**

Klaus and Kennell[8] describe an interactional paradigm that illustrates the effect of a multitude of influences on the outcome of the parent-child relationship. These variables can be divided into two general categories: those relatively fixed at the time of the babies' birth and those directly alterable. The infant's characteristics comprise a third category of variables that will be discussed in a later section of this chapter.

The first category consists of those factors established before the birth of the baby. These variables are considered "fixed" in the sense that they are either related to experiences that are past or to the sociocultural milieu in which the family lives. Caution is necessary when referring to "fixed" variables. Fixed is used here in the sense that the past events cannot be changed, although our understanding of them may change how we allow them to influence the present.

Each parent brings to the relationship his or her personality, which has been in process from the time of infancy. Attitudes about parenting and children and abilities to cope with change and adapt to new roles are derived from a combination of genetic endowment and past experiences. Cultural attitudes toward parenting and childrearing practices also have a significant influence on the developing parent-child relationship. If the child is ill or has a congenital mal-

formation, cultural expectations and beliefs about how and why these things occur can be either an extra support or burden for the parents within a stress situation. The quality of the marital relationship appears to be an important influence. Westbrook[2] demonstrated that women with positive marital relationships were found to have the least disturbed reactions to childbirth. Caplan[3] found that women who received support from their husbands or significant others had more positive resolutions to the crisis of premature birth.

Finally, the course and planning of the present pregnancy and experiences with previous pregnancies influence the developing parent-child relationship. Unresolved guilt and anxiety from a previous problematic birth or pregnancy may increase the negative impact of the trauma, whereas previous positive outcomes enhance confidence and coping abilities.

The second major category of variables affecting the outcome of the parent-child relationship is comprised of factors generally considered alterable by hospital and medical personnel. Included are (1) general hospital practices and rules, (2) attitudes of staff toward parents, and (3) degree of parent-child separation during the first days of life.

Hospital visitation policies including how frequently the parents may visit affects their ability to interact with their baby. Related to this is the atmosphere of the nursery when parents visit. Do they feel welcome and important, or in the way? How difficult is it for them to make personal contact with nurses and physicians? Do they feel free to ask questions and express concerns? Are parents made to feel trusted and valued for their contributions to the child's well-being?

It appears to be generally accepted that separation during the early days is not beneficial, and in instances where parents are vulnerable to parenting disorders, it can be especially damaging to the outcome of the parent-child relationship.[7,9,10] Regardless of the effect on the outcome of the relationship, parents report separation from their child as one of the most painful stresses with which they must deal. We cannot afford to let emotional detachment become a part of early hospital care. "If we separate parents and their babies physically in a way that creates emotional separation between them, we say implicitly to parents that what we can do for their babies is more valuable than what they can give."[11] We must avoid expertism that degrades the value of the parents' caring for the child.

■ **How can the parents' resolution of the crisis situation and the developing progress of the parent-child relationship be assessed?**

As with any assessment of human behavior, evaluation of the family's response to the crisis of neonatal intensive care and the developing parent-child relationship is a complex interaction of many variables. Therefore patterns of parental response must be evaluated rather than specific instances of isolated behavior that the staff may identify as unhealthy or suspect. Observation of the parents' patterns and the quality of the interaction during the visits provides valuable assessment information. It is extremely important, however, that all assessments be made within the context of the parents' own culture and background, taking into consideration the stage of crisis in which they are responding.

Fanaroff and co-workers[12] reported a higher incidence of mothering disorders among mothers who visited their hospitalized infants less than three times or who called and visited less than five times in a 2-week period. It has been our experience that very few parents visit this infrequently. This visitation pattern would indeed alert us to assess the family situation. However, there are parents who visit regularly who also may need special attention because of difficulties that they may be experiencing. From research conducted at the Harvard School of Public Health, Caplan[3] and Mason[13] have outlined patterns of response that seem to be associated with positive outcomes.

Mothers who had good outcomes were those who had moderate to high anxiety levels that were evident and openly acknowledged. They tended to worry about the baby's survival and the possibility that the baby would be abnormal and to question their own competency in caring for the infant. These mothers actively sought information about the baby's condition and opinions about his course and prognosis. Finally, they were fairly aggressive in their efforts to hear about and see the baby. In interviews with this group of mothers, strong maternal feelings were apparent. They objected to separation from their infant and seemed confident in their own motherliness. Both Caplan and Mason associated spouse and family support with positive outcomes.

Poor outcomes for the mother-infant relationship were predicted if the mother's anxiety level was low or anxiety was denied or displaced to worries other than the infant's health. Hostility toward the hospital or staff, such as that expressed by signing out against medical advice, seemed to be a significant predictor of poor outcome. Low activity levels demonstrated by passivity while on the ward, little questioning or information seeking, and infrequent visiting were additional predictors of a negative outcome. In interviews, maternal feelings were not as evident in this group of mothers. Frequently, their attitude was naive and flippant or sullen and impatient. They tended to seem unaware of the baby's needs, focusing more on their own discomforts. These mothers more frequently reported unwanted pregnancy and disappointment in the sex of the baby.

In summary, assessment of the developing parent-child relationship should include:

1. *Assessment of visiting patterns and attending to parent-infant interaction.* Does the mother focus on the infant and work to obtain responses from him? Does she actively seek and integrate information in a realistic manner?
2. *Assessment of the mother's support milieu.* What is the marital relationship like? Does she have support from her husband or some other significant person? What is the quality of this support?
3. *Assessment within the context of the parent's stage of dealing with the crisis.* An observed attitude or behavior that is perfectly normal when the baby is critically ill may be a warning signal when he is on his way to health. Again, patterns, rather than isolated behaviors, are important.

■ What are some general guidelines for providing support to parents of low birth weight or seriously ill infants?

The key to intervention during a neonatal hospitalization seems to be providing an atmosphere in which the parent can work through the emotional crisis and develop a positive relationship with the infant at his or her own rate. Initially, the atmosphere of the intensive care unit and the attitude conveyed by the staff are probably the most important support factors. Later, as the parent-child relationship develops, the infant, himself, becomes the most important tool through which to provide intervention.

Environmental interventions

From the first moments the parents have contact with intensive care unit personnel, the opportunities for intervention are present. Immediate access to the infant should be allowed to those parents who wish such contact. It is important, however, that a supportive staff member be on hand before and during the initial contact to provide information about the unit and answer questions about the baby's condition. This seems to be a particularly sensitive time in which parents need support in adjusting to the unfamiliarity of their surroundings. Parents have different levels of tolerance for the length of time they can comfortably stay during the early visits. They commonly feel guilty about leaving the infant and may remain for longer periods than are comfortable for them. By listening and observing, the support person may facilitate their leaving when tolerance limits are approached.

Parents frequently report initial anxiety about visiting the unit related to their fears of being in the way and interfering with the care of their child. Clear instructions regarding where the parent may stand or sit and what precautions are necessary decrease this discomfort. There are, of course, inopportune times for a parent visit. It is important for parents to be informed that they may be asked to leave the unit for brief periods from time to time. Similarly, parents may telephone when the nurses or physicians cannot talk with them freely because of time stresses. They appreciate the staff person who says simply

"I am sorry but I cannot talk right now, would you please call back in 30 minutes" rather than feeling rushed in their conversations.

Along similar lines, parents report frustration with receiving only the information that the baby is "fine" or "not doing too well." They often have difficulty in recognizing that the tiny infant lying in the isolette connected to tubes and equipment is a real person with individual characteristics. Personalization of the infant is enhanced by the nurse or physician who includes a description of the child's activities, "Johnny is sleeping without a care in the world," along with medical information.

The words chosen and the manner in which information about the infant's condition is conveyed may have amazingly long-term effects on the parent-child relationship. Ill-chosen words or pessimistic predictions can be particularly damaging during the early weeks before affectional bonds are firmly established. Klaus and Kennell[8] suggest that once the possibility of death or brain damage is mentioned it can never be unsaid. Alternately they suggest describing the infant's present condition, explaining that most infants survive in spite of early problems, and avoiding pessimistic predictions about future outcomes. When possible outcomes must be discussed, it is important to select words that carry as little negative connotation as possible. Judging what and how much to say at any given time is a universal problem in medicine and requires sensitivity, discernment, and compassion.

Infant interventions

Using the infant as an aid to intervention includes helping the parent to focus on the baby's attributes and abilities, overcome obstacles, and make their own contact with him. The isolette is definitely an obstacle to all the attachment behaviors that seem to be so important (Fig. 39-2). However, even while the infant is "isolated" in this way, there are some things that can be done to facilitate interaction. Eye-to-eye contact is difficult but can be accomplished if the parent is shown how to hold the baby in the isolette so that his face is parallel to the parent's face. Frequently, lifting the infant will cause him to open

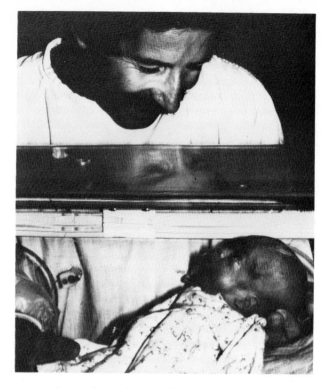

Fig. 39-2. Suggestions for handling infants inside an isolette can enhance social interaction.

his eyes and become alert. Parents can be shown how to shade the baby's eyes from intense lighting to facilitate eye opening.

Encouraging parents to bring personal items such as toys, clothing, and family photographs helps them begin to incorporate the infant into the family. Simple tasks such as rubbing lotion on the infant's dry skin, changing his position in the isolette, taking his temperature, or holding the infant while he is being gavage fed increases the parent's sense of worth to the infant and the amount of contact with him. When appropriate, feeding and bathing are important caretaking tasks for parents to perform (Fig. 39-3). Verbal reassurance is great; however, assigning parents caretaking tasks appears to have a greater impact on their belief that they have special significance to their infant.

■ What special interventions can be offered to parents of infants in intensive care?

Providing special intervention to those few parents whose behavior is perceived as being detrimental to themselves and their infant is a rather sensitive issue. Often referral for psychologic services inherently carries negative labeling. Parents of an infant in intensive care are in contact with hospital personnel because of the illness of the child. They are not there to receive psychotherapeutic services. On the other hand, hospital personnel are concerned about the future of the infant and have a professional responsibility toward the child and his family. In a very few cases the situation may be dangerous enough to take direct action in referring the family for psychologic intervention. There are, however, families whose behavior generates uneasiness among the staff,

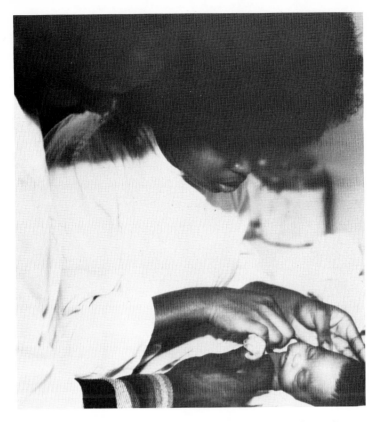

Fig. 39-3. Performing routine caretaking tasks in the nursery promotes feelings of competence in the parental role.

but because of lack of sufficient information, direct referral is contraindicated. Most intensive care units have social workers or other professionals who can be called on to make contact with these families and explore intervention possibilities. This exploration is most successful when the professional can develop a relationship with the family around a specific problem for which they themselves are seeking information or advice. Frequently, however, help can be provided these families through natural opportunities for intervention occurring in the intensive care setting before the situation deteriorates to the point where more open and active intervention is necessary. Two such opportunities are mutual support parent groups and use of the infant's own abilities as a positive point of interaction.

■ **Are parent support groups an effective means of providing support and intervention?**

Mutual support groups are becoming an increasingly popular and effective method of aiding patients and families in coping with the stresses of many types of physical illness.[14] The group setting provides opportunities for persons experiencing a particular problem to meet and interact. The mutuality of their situations is conducive to sharing feelings and solving specific problems related to the illness. Some support groups have the stated purpose of helping the patient or family member cope with problems and stress through group discussion. Other groups have an educational focus and provide information and instruction around a particular health topic, such as pre-

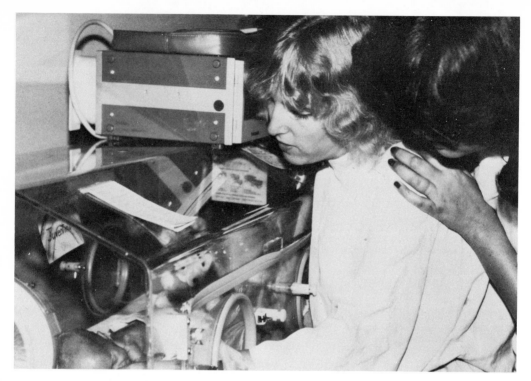

Fig. 39-4. Parents are an important source of support to each other during crisis periods.

natal birth classes. A third group approach uses graduates of a particular health crisis to provide information and support to those currently in the crisis.

The use of mutual support groups within the neonatal intensive care setting is a relatively new approach about which little has been published. Therefore the remainder of this discussion is based on personal experience and input from others who are developing similar programs.

Each of the previously described group approaches has strengths and disadvantages. Combining aspects of each has proved to be an effective group structure for the provision of support within a neonatal intensive care unit. Parents are sometimes reluctant to become involved with a group with the identified goal of helping them cope with feelings. Educational formats result in increased attendance and interest. Frequently, however, meetings that have an educational theme such as nutrition, infant abilities, or infant

development provide a comfortable forum for expressing feelings and concerns. Incorporating graduate parents into meetings provides new parents with hope. The graduate parents are concrete evidence that survival is possible. Empathetic interaction between parents results from the similarity of their experiences, and graduate parents are a source of practical information and helpful suggestions. An added benefit to incorporating graduate parents seems to be the support that they, themselves, derive from the group in working through any remaining anxieties regarding their own personal crisis experience.

■ **What are some of the problems involved in starting a new parent group?**

Any innovative approach to intervention is implemented through experimentation, evaluation, and modification. Established attitudes and methods change slowly. Change is frequently accompanied by frustration, resistance, and skepticism. Difficulties in establishing parent support groups are as varied as the settings in which they occur. Some general problems encountered are as follows:

1. Many parents are reluctant to attend meetings where they perceive they may be pressured to actively participate or reveal personal feelings. Educational formats are less threatening and provide practical information. Sharing of feelings should be invited but not expected.

2. Success of any group in providing psychologic intervention depends on group process factors that operate best in an atmosphere of familiarity. This familiarity, known as group cohesiveness, takes time to develop.[15] When the composition of the group changes from week to week as new parents join and others leave, there is little opportunity for this cohesion to develop. In its absence professionals may find themselves providing one-to-one intervention to several parents within any one session. Having a core group of graduate parents who continue to be involved provides some cohesion. This established group identity facilitates integration of new members.

3. When the parent group is implemented by professionals other than intensive care nurses or physicians, it may be difficult to obtain enthusiastic support from medical staff. The intensive care staff may feel that the need for the group is a reflection on the quality of support that they provide parents and may be anxious about the content of group sessions. Considering their concerns and involving them in the planning increases cooperation and understanding.

4. Most parents are chiefly interested in obtaining information that will help them in coping with their child's illness. If group leaders structure meetings to provide this information while retaining their own "hidden agenda" for psychologic intervention, the meetings may be negatively affected. Professionals who are unaware of their own hidden agendas may become exhausted in their efforts to provide educational experiences to the parents. Group leaders who possess the flexibility to allow the group to establish its own direction enable group needs rather than leader needs to be met.

Numerous possibilities exist for expanding the parent group into a larger network of support services. Individual parent-to-parent contact within the intensive care nurseries provides supportive opportunities for those parents who are unable or unwilling to attend group meetings. The value of parent-to-parent contact in providing supportive intervention has proved that it is more than worth the effort required to establish programs of this type.

THE INFANT'S ROLE

Until recently, parent variables were the primary focus when examining the early parent-infant relationship, as if the baby were a blank slate to be shaped solely by the parent's input and the environment. In the last 5 years there has been a blossoming of interest and exploration in the characteristics and capabilities that the newborn infant brings to the parent-infant relationship and the implications for how beginnings of this new relationship affect the future development of the child and parent.

■ **What role does the parent-infant relationship play in the future development of the child?**

In addition to the obvious need for survival, it is in this first relationship that infants learn about being in relationships for the rest of their lives. They learn skills that promote acceptance into their family and culture. They develop trust, or mistrust, in the responsiveness of their environment, which ultimately affects their own abilities to trust themselves and develop fully. The ongoing flow of the parent-infant relationship provides the infant with the raw material from which he constructs his understanding of the human experience.[16]

■ **What is the infant's impact on the parent-infant relationship?**

We have come a long way in our thinking about newborn babies. Our once held view that the neonate is a brain stem organism devoid of higher level organization has been dispelled by skilled observers using new techniques for measuring previously elusive infant behavior. New findings demonstrate that there is a much higher level of organization and competency from the very beginning. Careful observation and measurement suggest the remarkable capacity of the newborn infant to respond and interact with another human being in the early hours, weeks, and months of life. Stern[16] notes that it is within the first 6 months of life that the infant learns and develops all the basic skills for being a partner in human interaction and spends the rest of his life expanding and refining his relationship skills. Given such a monumental task to achieve so early, it is no wonder that the infant comes to the world so well equipped to begin his work.

■ **What capabilities do neonates possess that facilitate social interaction and relationship development?**

First, we must reexamine those infant behaviors and characteristics that are related to their interactive skills. A description of the capacity of a full-term healthy newborn is necessary before considering any possible deficits or disadvantages of a low birth weight or critically ill infant. It should be stated at the forefront that these capabilities and tendencies vary among individual infants and that this variability has important implications for adaptation between parent and infant.

The following description of the dimensions of infant behavior suggests that he is a fascinating and complex creature.

Spontaneity, periodicity, selectivity

Rudolph Schaffer[17] in his book *Mothering* describes the infant's spontaneity as the key feature of his sociability. Infants are not passive and inert but demonstrate order and organization, seeking out stimulation and interaction in discriminating ways. Not only are newborns selective in the type of stimuli to which they respond, but they reveal periodic and internally regulated cycles of availability.

Visual ability

Many studies demonstrate that the human newborn attends visually to his environment. Evidence indicates that an alert infant typically reacts with orientation, visual fixation, eye-widening, and reduction of motor activity to a variety of visual stimuli. Visual pursuit of an object, as well as obvious preference for contrast and complexity, is often observed in the first 3 days of life.[18] Carpenter's work[19] demonstrates visual prefer-

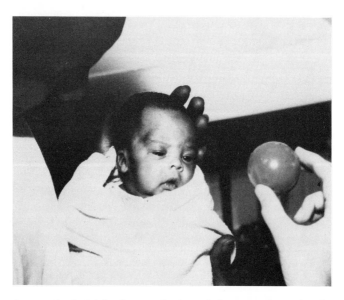

Fig. 39-5. Parents recognize their infant's strengths through demonstration and exploration of infant's abilities.

ence for mother's face by the second week of life. Early development of the visual system has important implications for social interaction. One of the earliest communications an infant has with his mother is through looking at her. The pleasurable feelings that the mother derives from having her infant look at and recognize her increase her interest in caring for and interacting with him.

Auditory functioning

At the time of birth infants are well equipped to respond to a variety of auditory stimuli. In the first days of life they demonstrate their abilities to attend to the human voice by cessation of motor activity and crying, visual searching, and head turning toward the source of stimulation. They reveal preferences for higher pitch tones characteristic of the female voice and discriminate their own mother's voice by the fourth day of life. It is no coincidence that the newborn is so well prepared to listen to this world, as hearing is one of his most powerful senses for responding to the social environment. Auditory responsiveness is a potent social releaser. It enables the infant to provide the parents with the feedback that they are recognized and sought after. The calming effect the parent's voice has on the distressed infant enhances parental feelings of competency and satisfaction.

Tactile responsiveness

Infants are tactually developed to react defensively and adaptively to a variety of stimuli. Many primitive newborn reflexes such as grasping and rooting are elicited through touch. In addition, babies are often consoled by uniform pressure and stroking applied to various areas of the body. These reflexive behaviors protect the infant from threatening events and facilitate food and oxygen intake. In addition, infants use tactual feedback to aid them in state organization. Parents receive information and communicate with their infant through tactual modes that reflect the infant's states and needs. Opportunities to enhance attentiveness and decrease levels of arousal are provided through tactual modalities including consoling and alerting techniques such as cuddling and stroking. Reflexive behaviors such as grasp-

ing and rooting are often viewed by parents as positive indicators that they are recognized and sought after by the infant.

Habituation

Infants possess the ability to decrease their response level to repeated intrusive environmental stimuli. This ability reflects the internal organization of the infant and demonstrates that he is an active selector of the stimuli to which he responds at any given time. In recognizing this adaptability, parents gain confidence and comfort in integrating the infant into their regular family routine and environment.

Cuddliness

The extent to which an infant adapts his own body posture to mold with the caregiver's body (cuddling) significantly affects the ease with which he is held and carried. Although babies vary in their responses to being held, some degree of body adjustment is usually present. Cuddling is often a pleasant experience for parents. The closeness and warmth enhances other modes of social interaction and conveys messages of affection between infant and parent.

Self-consoling maneuvers and response to consoling by others

Most newborns will initiate a variety of maneuvers to maintain or regain a lower state of arousal. Commonly this is observed by means of hand-to-mouth movements, sucking, responding to visual or auditory stimuli, or changes in body position. Caregiver consoling such as feeding, changing body position, visual, auditory, and tactile and vestibular stimulation often result in at least brief periods of decreased arousal. Infants who demonstrate self-consoling attempts, or respond to consoling by others, increase their availability to positive social interaction and cognitive stimulation. Parents often feel rewarded and competent if the infant responds by lowering his state.

State organization

Neurologists and psychologists have recently attended to states of arousal in the infant. Not only are states and how they are organized found to be important for cognitive development, but they also have been directly implicated in the social interactional process.[20] For example, infants who make smooth transitions from sleep to wakefulness, to higher levels of arousal, and back down to sleep are more predictable, often more easily soothed, and as a result are more available for positive orientation to the social and inanimate environment. Infants who have less well organized state transitions may spend more time in unavailable states. Parents of these infants may have less opportunity for social contact and may feel less effective as caretakers.

All infants vary in their organizational abilities and therefore their availability for social play and relationship building. The infant's availability and temperament may be modified or enhanced to some extent by the parent; however, the most important cue is for each individual pair to find their niche and learn from one another through sensitivity and acceptance.

■ **Along what dimensions may preterm and low birth weight infants differ from healthy full-term infants, and what impact does this have on the parent-child relationship?**

As we have stated, the infant's impact on the developing parent-child relationship is a powerful one that deserves careful consideration. It therefore becomes very important to examine the dimensions along which preterm infants differ because of their shortened gestation, illness, and extended hospitalization.

Schiffman[21] suggests that the premature infant's neurologic responses are immature because of his immature cortex. This immaturity is demonstrated along several dimensions of infant behavior that have a direct impact on early parent-infant interaction. It should be noted that the concept of immaturity, as used to describe a preterm infant, is misleading and may tempt us to dismiss behavior until its more mature version emerges. Ultimately, we are what we are, using what we have at any given time in our development. The behaviors of a 2-month-old infant are fully mature for a 2-month-old infant and the same is true of a 28-week-old infant. It is the interaction between two people and how they "work

it" together that is of primary importance and not the degree of maturity of either partner.[16] For the preterm infant, immaturity is more truly an "unpreparedness" for the complexities of the extrauterine environment.

Reflex development

Modern visitation policies bring infants and parents into close contact at a time when the infant is reflexively quite immature. The reflexive behaviors that we will now discuss have been linked to parental dissatisfaction and relationship dysfunction.[22] Many mothers of preterm infants have unsatisfactory initial experiences with their infants because their expectations for the infant's behavior are often based on full-term infant abilities. The discrepancy between the behavior they expect and what they actually experience may result in their misinterpreting the baby's behavior as a reflection on their maternal adequacy. Feeding and cuddling are important interactions that build feelings of maternal competency. Owing to reflex immaturity directly related to feeding abilities and state organization, mothers may feel they are unable to provide basic mothering to their infants and begin an avoidance pattern or inappropriate compensatory behavior.

Generally, suck-swallow coordination is not established until 32 weeks' gestation. Before this time a hyperactive gag reflex with associated choking behavior is common. For quite some time after the suck-swallow is established, it continues to be weak, less vigorous, and less efficient than that of a full-term infant. The hyperactive gag and weak sucking and swallowing often create an unsatisfying feeding experience for the new mother and rob her of a primary source of maternal satisfaction. Mothers often interpret the infant's difficulty in feeding as a reflection on their own adequacy, especially when it is apparent that nurses possess more effective feeding techniques. Often her worry and concern result in nervous tension during the feeding session and both partners miss an important opportunity for positive interaction.

This tension may demonstrate itself in an overemphasis on food intake, persisting long after it is necessitated by the infant's immediate needs for weight gain and physiologic recovery. In more extreme cases the mother may withdraw completely from the feeding interaction.

A sensitive Moro reflex, combined with hypotonicity and immature motor development results in the jerkiness and uncoordinated movements so characteristic of preterm infants. Even routine handling or spontaneous movement may cause a startle reaction. Parents often interpret this behavior as a negative reflection on themselves, feeling they frighten their infant when attempting to touch or console him. Unless this sensitivity is explained in light of the infant's immaturity, avoidance patterns and feelings of rejection may ensue.

■ **How can parents be assisted in coping with the infant's immature reflex development?**

Johnson and Grubbs[22] suggest that medical personnel can help alleviate problems related to reflexes by examining both the infant's maturity level and parental expectations for signs of discrepancy. Educating the parents regarding the behaviors they can expect and observe at the current developmental level may help them interpret their parenting skills based on their own behavior rather than the incapacity of their infant to provide the feedback they expect. In addition, demonstrating how to elicit responses within the infant's repertoire and identifying the positive feedback that the infant does provide enhance positive parental feelings. Finally, pointing out the actual abilities of the infant with the reassurance that behaviors will change with maturity provides structure that many parents need to deal with their own doubt and concern.

■ **How do preterm infants differ in sleep organization?**

Sleep is a very important issue for new parents, mostly because of their lack of it in the early weeks of the infant's life. Night wakefulness is perhaps the most intrusive aspect of an infant's behavior on an adult. Most parents can cope with the discomfort for the short time period needed for additional infant maturity; however, an abnormally long period of stress in this area is likely to decrease coping ability.

Dreyfus-Brisac[23] notes that preterm infants are known to have significantly more sleep disorganization than full-term babies. It is not until approximately 32 weeks' gestation that quiet sleep, active sleep, and wakefulness can begin to be differentiated. Even when preterm infants reach term, they do not generally display as well-organized sleep patterns as their full-term counterparts. Typically preterm infants are not awakened by hunger pangs.[24] It therefore becomes difficult to judge when to disturb them for feeding. In addition, many infants fuss or cry in the light sleep stage but often proceed back down to a lower state of arousal. Parents, particularly if they are anxious, may be too quick to respond to these brief periods of irritability and intervene, unnecessarily disturbing the baby. Another common problem is attempting to awaken a baby for a feeding during a period of quiet sleep and encountering a groggy, unresponsive infant.

■ **What are some of the other characteristics of preterm infants that may hamper social interaction between infant and parent?**

Appearance plays a crucial role in the attraction of adults to neonates. Many of the attributes of the term infant such as large head size relative to trunk size, fat cheeks, large eyes, shortened foreheads, and soft round bodies have been shown to be inherently attractive to adult humans. Preterm infants, with their frail, often emaciated appearance, probably appear very different from the expectations of the new parents.[35] Although a smaller, more vulnerable appearing infant may evoke feelings of protectiveness and nurturance from some parents, many are shocked, frightened, and perhaps even repulsed by the appearance of their preterm infant. Parents may need help in identifying aspects of their infant's appearance that are attractive. Perception of the infant as a unique person and also as a part of themselves is important to the early development of attachment. Observing various family characteristics possessed by the infant may enhance this process. Noticing nicely shaped hands and feet, dimples, hair swirls, lips, eyes, and nose helps parents look beyond the small underdeveloped infant who disappoints them.

A crucial aspect of feeling competent in caring for a young infant is the ability to assess his needs and initiate appropriate intervention. Thus far we have focused on the problem of parents evaluating their competency to provide adequate care based on the infant's underdeveloped repertoire. Just as important is the effect of this underdevelopment on the infant itself, particularly in his ability to be an active participant in a relationship. Many aspects of a preterm infant's neurologic development suggest that he may be less prepared for social interaction and relationship building.

Hypotonicity and jerky, uncoordinated movements may decrease the infant's capacity to be responsive to his parents with his body. In addition, jerky, uncontrolled body movements may interfere with attentional capacity and consolability, both of which may limit interactional participation. Inability to interpret, anticipate, and intervene with an infant's patterns may be related to parental insensitivity. However, if the problem continues beyond reasonable expectations, the difficulty may be at least partially with the infant's inability to organize himself and send readable cues to the caretaker.

■ How does acute or chronic illness affect the infant's availability?

The critically ill infant often demonstrates a decreased level of behavioral response because of the nature of the illness itself. Interference with normal biologic processes may inhibit normal levels of responsiveness to stimuli. Infants with severe illness or complications such as hyaline membrane disease, hypothermia, hypoglycemia, or infection are commonly listless, apathetic, hypotonic, and easily fatigued. Not only do sick infants appear to be less available for social interaction, but in fact they may have diminished stamina and energy with which to respond to the caregiver.

In addition to the illness, the treatment and equipment used may restrict or tire the infant. For example, the phototherapy procedure used to treat hyperbilirubinemia requires that the infant's eyes be covered to avoid damage. Although patching is a necessary precaution, it precludes spontaneous eye-to-eye contact with the parent. Other procedures require that the extremities be restrained, limiting movement and altering responses to stimuli.

■ How can demonstration of infant abilities enhance parental involvement?

Our discussion on the complex and highly sophisticated abilities and social skills of newborn infants leads us naturally to the most powerful and effective tool for cementing parents and babies together: the infant himself. There is nothing more natural for hooking the emotional involvement of parents than the responsiveness of their own infant.

We have suggested that infants vary widely in their response patterns and that especially infants who have been subjected to stress through illness and its associated treatment and hospitalization may be less available for social interaction. Preterm infants, in addition to being ill, may be disadvantaged by less mature, underdeveloped interactional abilities. However, it is an exceptional infant who does not respond in some way.

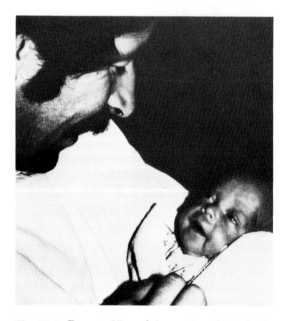

Fig. 39-6. Even at 35 weeks' gestation, this infant's social responsiveness is a powerful elicitor of parental involvement.

Even minimal responses may be enhanced by optimal interpretation.

As suggested by Brazelton,[20] the ability to present the infant in his best light and draw maximum levels of responsivity from him is developed through careful observation of infant behavior and experience in various handling techniques. A genuine interest in, and rapport with, small infants is essential.

Initially it is important to assess what parents know and believe about infant abilities. This information provides a basis for the breadth of teaching required. Many parents are expert observers of their own baby's behavior and temperament. Assessing what the parent has noticed provides information about parental sensitivity and perceptiveness, as well as attitudes toward the infant and parenthood. After exploring the parents familiarity with the infant, it is beneficial to explore with them some of the infant's abilities and characteristics.

Parents seem to understand and relate to the infant more effectively when they are able to recognize the various states of arousal. Guiding parents in identifying each state and discussing implications for responsiveness and caretaking help parents appreciate the infant's organizational abilities and apply their understanding to daily care and stimulation. Practical applications may include alerting and consoling techniques that alter states in desirable directions. General handling techniques as well as approaches based on the individual character of the infant provide parents and infants with increased opportunities for positive, satisfying interactions.

Demonstrating visual and auditory abilities is most dramatic when the infant is in a quiet alert state of attention. Sensitivity to the infant's readiness to respond, as well as optimal positioning and handling techniques that enhance attentiveness, are modeled for the parents. This may be an opportunity for expanding the parent role through including them in daily play activities.

Parents seem to be fascinated by normal reflexes such as grasping, crawling, walking, and rooting (Fig. 39-7). These behaviors are viewed as indications of "cuteness," "smartness," and "strength." How realistic these conclusions are is unimportant. What counts is the positive feelings that are promoted toward the infant.

The goal of strengthening the affectional bond through the demonstration of the infant's abilities and characteristics focuses on positive attributes and abilities of the infant and models sensitivity,

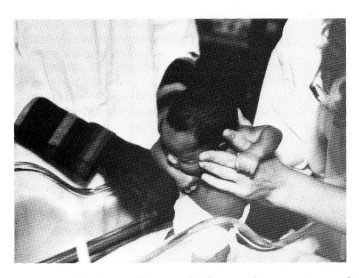

Fig. 39-7. Parents seem to be fascinated by normal reflexes such as grasping, crawling, walking, and rooting.

pacing, and patience as well as techniques for alerting and consoling. Emphasis is placed on opportunities for discovery and acceptance rather than performance. Finally, this interaction provides natural opportunities for offering positive, supportive feedback to the parents regarding their parenting skills.

■ **How does long-term developmental follow-up provide parental support and improve interaction?**

Continuing to focus on abilities and strengths as avenues to positive parent-child interactions is a valuable support before as well as after discharge from intensive care. Lingering concerns about the health and development of the child are commonly reported by parents. Periodic diagnostic screening may reassure parents of normal developmental patterns. Deviations in development may be identified early and intervention may be suggested. Homecoming of the infant and resumption of normal routines does not necessarily indicate that parents have resolved their feelings about the experience. Maladaptive patterns may emerge after discharge, or parents may be more prepared to discuss their concerns after the acute crisis is over. In any case, follow-up programs offer opportunities for professionals to continue their support of infants and parents as well as to assess developmental progress and psychologic adjustment.

PSYCHOLOGIC STRESSES OF STAFF

At a recent conference on high-risk infants, Barbara Korsch, M.D., asked this intriguing question: "Who takes care of those who care for the kids?" The development of intensive care units of all varieties shares the goal of increasing the life-saving capabilities of medical science. However, with this achievement have come new insights into the unique psychologic problems of both the critically ill patient and the professionals who care for them. A discussion of the psychologic care of parents of sick infants would be incomplete without examining the impact of working in a neonatal intensive care unit on medical and nursing staff. In the final section of this chapter we will discuss current research as well as our own experiences in this area. An intensive care unit is just what the name implies: intensive. Not only are the parents and babies affected by the psychologic atmosphere of the intensive care unit, but physicians, nurses, therapists, and other auxillary medical personnel are continuously submersed in an emotionally tense, demanding, environment.

■ **What are some of the stressful situations encountered by staff working in newborn intensive care units?**

Nursing journals abound with discussions of the stress and frustration experienced by intensive care nurses. Bilodeau[26] and Jacobson[27] offer a comprehensive overview of the frustrations commonly reported by nursing personnel. The following discussion attempts to integrate their research findings.

1. The high level of demand for patient care with its requirements for intensive observation, attention to minute details, and repetitive routines plus the need to make split-second decisions and perform highly technical procedures is as wearing as it is challenging. In light of the many demands made on staff members, the infants' and parents' immense need for support may result in feelings of inadequacy, irritation, and resentment. Worry and anxiety over the baby's condition may further deplete the nurse's energy and supportiveness at a time when the family is in greatest need. In addition, the style of the individual parent in reducing tension and coping with fear may prove very threatening to the staff. Certainly under the most pleasant working conditions it is stressful to be the focus of angry and blaming behaviors.

2. The pressure and demand for mastery of highly technical skills is often the basis for competitive, critical, and distrustful feelings among the nurses themselves, as well as between physicians and nurses. Treatment restrictions that are not based on personal skill or training level may create feelings of resentment and hostility. Restrictions as to what nurses may discuss with parents increases discomfort and may diminish the parent's trust in the nurse's professional validity.

These factors hamper team spirit and impede communication. A particularly evident example illustrating breakdown of communication is the competition between nursing shifts. Characteristically, day shift nurses have more access to physicians and direct input into treatment plans. Being "in on the action" may lead to feelings of superiority directed toward other shifts.

3. A noisy, crowded intensive care environment with its alarm-sounding equipment and barrage of people naturally increases irritability and may decrease personal effectiveness. Inadequate staffing may augment the stress by increasing responsibilities as it decreases adequate rest periods.

4. During the period of time that the nurse cares for the infant, a special relationship may develop. The nurse becomes invested in the infant and may react emotionally as the infant progresses and regresses. Jacobson[27] notes that "despite the precarious state of all infants in their care, nurses on the NICU were acutely affected by sudden changes for the worse in these babies." An even greater stress is dealing with infant death and its associated feelings of grief and detachment.

5. Intensive care nurses are placed in the difficult position of being the primary caregivers for another person's baby. They frequently find themselves competing with parents in caring for the infant. Their perceptions of the parents and how they should behave toward the child may result in negative judgments that interfere with their role in enhancing parent-infant interaction.

■ **How do nurses cope with the stress of the neonatal intensive care unit (NICU)?**

When observing nurses at work in the NICU, one would think they deal with stress quite effectively. However, when given the opportunity to share their feelings, nurses frequently relate the difficulty they have in working in the NICU. In our conversations with nurses we find they often deal with their feelings by keeping them inside or by sharing them with fellow nurses and family. In many cases nurses have difficulty in finding good listeners.

■ **What are the signs of inappropriate coping with stress?**

Strategies for coping with stress are varied and are influenced by previous experiences, individual personality styles, and the present level of personal health and emotional satisfaction.

To provide for the well-being of the patient and family, all medical and auxillary personnel must examine the appropriateness of the methods they use in coping with stress. Signs of inappropriate coping mechanisms may include:

1. Withdrawing from or avoiding the infant and/or family
2. Fostering parental overdependent behavior
3. Acting out behaviors such as calling in sick, being late, and resisting work responsibilities
4. Focusing on equipment or providing excessive technical treatment rather than attending to the infant and parents
5. Denying or repressing all feelings
6. Projecting negative feelings onto others

■ **What are effective strategies for alleviating stress within the neonatal intensive care unit?**

Bilodeau[26] suggests that frustrations and stress can be decreased through recognition of individual strengths and skills and provision of a stimulating environment. Providing opportunities for open discussion of concerns, airing of feelings, and participation in policy planning and procedural change is beneficial. Periodic rotation to less stressful assignments has proved helpful in many hospitals. In addition, promoting opportunities for the staff to have follow-up contact with their patients enhances morale and optimism in regard to their efforts. Interestingly enough, the provision of adequate facilities and services aimed at relieving parental stress has been shown to alleviate stress for medical and nursing personnel as well. Bilodeau[26] suggests that:

1. Orienting parents to the policies, equipment, and routine of the unit, both verbally and by means of a parents' handbook, helps decrease anxiety by clarifying the purpose of equipment and routines
2. Designating a comfortable area for parents

near the unit provides privacy in which they may relax, explore their feelings, and interact with other parents

3. Arranging meetings between medical staff and parents facilitates questions and expression of concerns

4. Providing parents with tangible concrete ways of helping with the care of their infant encourages the development of the parental role and decreases aimless, undirected visiting behavior

Appropriate development and use of hospital and community resources can prove very beneficial in alleviating the stress of the medical staff and family. Social workers, psychologists, chaplains, therapists, and volunteers can assist in meeting patient needs and may be useful in identifying and clarifying staff reactions to the infant's illness and the parents' behaviors and needs. With the countless alternatives to the many problems relating to stress issues, one message is perfectly clear; the need to express feelings, gain constructive feedback, debate over technique, and acknowledge personal and team achievement is absolute. With it the NICU can be a stimulating, challenging place to learn and gain satisfaction. Without it there may be irreparable psychologic damage to the patients and families as well as to those bright and highly skilled people who provide the care.

SUMMARY

Current levels of medical technology have greatly increased the number of newborn infants surviving critical illness with fewer lasting physical and mental disabilities. However, lasting deleterious psychologic effects that may accompany neonatal intensive care hospitalization have been illuminated through long-term follow-up of large groups of surviving infants. Awareness of these detrimental effects has resulted in increased attention to the quality of psychologic support given the families of these infants.

This chapter has addressed many of the issues involved in providing supportive care. The family, the infant, and the hospital staff have important roles in determining the extent to which the normal processes of attachment and the overall development of the child are disturbed. As ex-

pressed by Downey, ". . . we must eliminate the kind of care that mends the body but overlooks other impairments that linger long after scars are healed."[27]

ACKNOWLEDGMENTS

The authors wish to express appreciation to Laurence D. Becker and Mary Peduzi for their contributions to the psychologic care of the staff portion of the text and to Robert F. Huxtable, M.D. and Kenneth W. Dumars, M.D. for their support of our work with infants and families.

REFERENCES

1. Bibring, G. L., Dwyer, T. F., Huntington, D. S., and Valenstein, A. F.: A study of the psychological processes in pregnancy and of the earliest mother-child relationship, Psychoanal. Study Child **16**:9, 1961.
2. Westbrook, M. T.: The reactions to child-bearing and early maternal experience of women with differing marital relationships, Br. J. Med. Psychol. **51**:191, 1978.
3. Caplan, G.: Patterns of parental response to the crisis of premature birth, Psychiatry **23**:365, 1960.
4. Smith, N., et al.: Mothers psychological reactions to premature and full-size newborns, Arch. Gen. Psychiat. **21**:177, 1969.
5. Phillips, C., and Anzalone, J.: Fathering participation in labor and birth, St. Louis, 1978, The C. V. Mosby Co.
6. Kaplan, D. M., and Mason, E. A.: Maternal reactions to premature birth viewed as an acute emotional disorder, Am. J. Orthopsychiat. **30**:539, 1960.
7. Klaus, M., and Kennell, J.: Mothers separated from their newborn infants, Pediatr. Clin. North Am. **17**(4):1015, 1970.
8. Klaus, M., and Kennell, J.: Maternal-infant bonding, St. Louis, 1976, The C. V. Mosby Co.
9. Leifer, A., Leiderman, P., Barnett, C., and Williams, J.: Effects of mother-infant separation on maternal attachment behavior. In Rebelsky, F., and Dorman, S., editors: Child development and behavior, New York, 1974, Alfred A. Knopf.
10. Barnett, C. R., Leiderman, P. H., Grobstein, R., and Klaus, M.: Neonatal separation: the maternal side of interactional deprivation, Pediatrics **45**(2):197, 1970.
11. Brazelton, T. B.: Working with the family. In Pittnan, L., editor: The infants we care for, Washington, D.C., 1973, National Association for education of young children, chap. 2.
12. Fanaroff, A. A., Kennell, J. H., and Klaus, M. H.: Follow-up of low birth weight infants—the predictive value of maternal visiting patterns, Pediatrics **49**:288, 1972.
13. Mason, E.: A method of predicting crisis outcome for mothers of premature babies, Public Health Rep. **78**:1031, 1963.
14. Moos, Rudolf, H., editor: Coping with physical illness, New York, 1977, Plenum Medical Publishing Corp.
15. Yalom, I.: The theory and practice of group psychotherapy, New York, 1970, Basic Books, Publishers Inc.

16. Stern, D.: The first relationship, infant and mother (in the developing child series), Cambridge, 1977, Harvard University Press.
17. Schaffer, R.: Mothering (in the developing child series), Cambridge, 1977, Harvard University Press.
18. Fantz, R. S., and Nevis, S.: Pattern preferences and perceptual cognitive development in early infancy, Merrill-Palmer Q. Behav. Dev. **18:**77, 1967.
19. Carpenter, G.: Mothers' face and the newborn, New Scientist March, 1974.
20. Brazelton, T. B.: Neonatal behavioral assessment scale. Clinics in developmental medicine No. 50. Spastics International Medical Publications, Philadelphia, 1973, J. B. Lippincott Co.
21. Schiffman, W.: Neurological evaluation of the infant, Can. Nurse **57:**329, 1961.
22. Johnson, S. H., and Grubbs, J. P.: The premature infant's reflex behaviors: effect on the maternal child relationship, J. Obstet. Gynecol. Neonatal Nurs. **4**(3):15, 1975.
23. Dreyfus-Brisac, C.: Organization of sleep in prematures: implications for caregiving. In Lewis, M., and Rosenblum, L., editors: The effect of the infant on its caregiver, New York, 1974, John Wiley & Sons, Inc.
24. Parmelee, A. H., Bruck, K., and Bruck, M.: Activity and inactivity cycles during the sleep of premature infants exposed to neutral temperatures, Bilogia Neonatorum **4:**317, 1962.
25. Prugh, D.: Emotional problems of the premature infant's parents, Am. J. Nurs. **1**(8):61, 1953.
26. Bilodeau, C. B.: The nurse and her reactions to critical care nursing, Heart Lung **2:**358, 1973.
27. Jacobson, S. P.: Stressful situations for neonatal intensive care nurses, Am. J. Maternal Child Nurs. **3**(3):144, 1978.
28. Downey, G. W.: I.C.U. patients and staff are subject to emotional stress, Mod. Hosp. **117:**88, 1972.

CHAPTER 40

Critical care of infants and children after the neonatal period

Stanley M. Kegel and Melville I. Singer

■ **Why is there a need for a separate section or discussion of critical care in infants and children?**

Children are not little adults. There are major differences in the metabolic processes in adults and children. Diseases are frequently different, as are responses and toxicity with relation to medications. Drugs commonly used in adults are frequently inadequately tested for use in children, and there may be major differences in the absorption and activity of these medications between the tablet and liquid forms. Although neoplastic and degenerative diseases form a major part of adult medicine, infections, accidents, and congenital anomalies are more common in children. A knowledge of the diseases prevalent in childhood and the metabolic responses of children is essential to proper treatment.

Unexpected toxicity

A few examples will help clarify the differences between children and adults with respect to drugs. Oxygen has widely been used in the treatment of respiratory failure. High oxygen concentrations were used for many years in the treatment of premature infants with respiratory distress, resulting in the blinding of many children from retrolental fibroplasia caused by damage to the eye from oxygen. The use of chloramphenicol in small infants resulted in a shocklike state, the so-called gray babies, with many deaths until the inability of the neonate to metabolize chloram-

phenicol was demonstrated. Although adults may tolerate a wide range of fluid therapy without serious results, small errors in fluid therapy in children can result in circulatory overload, dehydration, or major electrolyte disturbances. A knowledge of the immaturity of the kidney and liver in infants and children is essential in determining the dosage and frequency of drugs detoxified or excreted by these organs.

■ **How should drug doses for children be calculated?**

Drug action, absorption, detoxification, and excretion are related to the metabolic rate of the child rather than body weight or age. Metabolic rate is most closely related to surface area.

Older rules for drug dosage such as Young's rule:

$$\frac{\text{Age (yr)} \times \text{Adult dose}}{\text{Age (yr)} + 12}$$

Fried's rule for infants:

$$\frac{\text{Age (mo)} \times \text{Adult dose}}{150}$$

or Clark's rule:

$$\frac{\text{Weight (lb)} \times \text{Adult dose}}{150}$$

are very inaccurate and usually result in infants and small children receiving ineffective doses of medication.

674

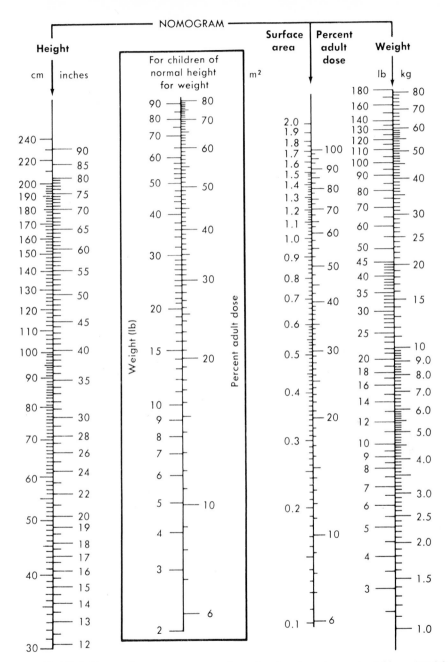

Fig. 40-1. Modified West surface area nomogram for estimating drug dosage in children. (Modified from Nelson, W. E.: Textbook of pediatrics, ed. 8, Philadelphia, 1964, W. B. Saunders Co.)

For most drugs the formula:

$$\frac{\text{Body surface area}}{1.72} \times \text{Adult dose}$$

will give a safe and effective dosage for children. In infants under 1 month of age the calculated dose should be reduced by 50%.

The nomogram derived from West's surface area nomogram can be used to calculate the portion of an adult dose a child should receive (Fig. 40-1). If the nomogram for surface areas is not used, the surface area (SA) can be calculated by the formula:

$$\text{SA (m}^2\text{)} = \frac{4 \text{ Weight (kg)} + 7}{\text{Weight (kg)} + 90}$$

For children of average height and weight the approximations in Tables 40-1 and 40-2 are helpful if it is impossible to calculate the surface area.

Table 40-1. Calculation of children's drug doses

Weight (kg)	Average adult dose (%)
0-5	$(3 \times \text{kg})$ $+3$
0-10	$(3 \times \text{kg})$
10-20	$(2 \times \text{kg})$ $+10$
20-100	kg + 30
EXAMPLE: 12 kg child	$(2 \times 12) + 10 = 24 +$
	$10 = 34\%$ adult dose
25 kg child	$25 + 30 = 55\%$ adult dose

Table 40-2. Simple guide to body surface area from weight in pounds*

Weight	BSA
6	0.2
12	0.3
18	0.4
24	0.5
30	0.6
36	0.7
42	0.75
49	0.8
56	0.9
63	1.0
70	1.1

*Up to 42 pounds, multiples of 6 plus 1; over 42 pounds multiples of 7 plus 1. Do not use over 75 pounds.

A 50 mg average adult dose is equivalent to 1 mg/kg and 30 mg/m².

■ **In the immediate treatment of acute poisoning, what are the indications and contraindications for emptying the stomach, and what means of accomplishing this should be used?**

Syrup of ipecac is the safest and most effective agent to use because it removes both the toxic agent and the emetic. The dose is 15 ml in a 1- to 5-year-old child and 30 ml in an older child, followed by a glass of water, and may be repeated in 30 minutes if vomiting has not occurred. Parenteral emetics are more dangerous and should rarely be used. Gastric lavage is less effective and is indicated primarily in the comatose child with an endotracheal tube to protect the airway or when emetics have been unsuccessful.

The induction of emesis is contraindicated if the patient is convulsing, if petroleum distillates or corrosives have been ingested, or if hematemesis has occurred. There is good evidence that the major toxicity of hydrocarbons such as cleaning fluids, gasoline and kerosene, lighter fluid, furniture polishes, and mineral sealing oils is induced by inhalation rather than ingestion. The emesis or lavage fluid should be saved for future laboratory analysis.

■ **What other measures are indicated in the acute treatment of a poisoning victim?**

Following induction of emesis or gastric lavage, activated charcoal is effective in promoting the absorption of many drugs. Activated charcoal given 30 minutes after the ingestion of aspirin, as an example, will result in a 50% reduction of maximum serum salicylate level. Charcoal is effective in the removal of most analgesics (salicylates, propoxyphene, acetaminophen); alkaloids (digitoxin, ergotamine); sedatives (barbiturates, glutethimide, ethchlorvynol); and antidepressants (chlorpromazine, imipramine, nortriptyline), as well as a variety of other commonly prescribed drugs (amphetamine, quinidine and quinine, phenytoin, primaquine, chloroquine, isoniazid).

While most effective if given within 30 minutes of ingestion, charcoal is still effective in binding poisons that have already passed through the pylorus. Charcoal is most effective against drugs that are slowly absorbed from the gastrointestinal tract.

Universal antidote, a combination of activated charcoal with magnesium oxide and tannic acid, is less effective than activated charcoal alone. Other absorbents such as evaporated milk and attapulgite are also less effective than powdered charcoal.

■ **If the poison is unknown, what signs and symptoms are helpful in making a correct diagnosis?**

1. Phenothiazines frequently are seen with a picture of "pseudotetanus" with ataxia, oculogyric crisis, and the jaws locked in an open position. This most commonly occurs with prochlorperazine.
2. Tricyclic antidepressants such as imipramine are frequently seen with cardiac arrhythmias in association with convulsions or coma.
3. Agitation, hallucinations, dilated pupils, fever, and flushed dry skin usually indicate the presence of an atropine-like agent or LSD.
4. Vomiting, hyperpnea, fever, and an odor of acetone on the breath frequently indicate salicylate intoxication.
5. Increased salivation, tearing, urination and defecation, and constricted pupils suggest organic phosphate or mushroom poisoning.
6. Constricted pupils associated with respiratory or neurologic depression should be considered indicative of narcotic poisoning until proved otherwise.
7. Confusion, agitation, blank stare, nystagmus, ataxia, hypertension, tachycardia, and increased muscle tone with myoclonic jerks is suggestive of PCP (angel dust) intoxication.
8. Hallucinations and changes in mental state associated with conjunctival injection, dry mouth, hyperphagia, and a musky odor of the breath is typical of marijuana intoxication.

■ **What are the manifestations of salicylate intoxication?**

Salicylates remain the most frequent cause of poisoning in preschool children. Over half of the cases of salicylism that require hospitalization are the result of chronic therapeutic ingestion rather than acute poisoning. Salicylate toxicity is caused by the direct effect on the gastrointestinal tract, the results of increased metabolism, the derangement of carbohydrate metabolism, the stimulation of the medullary respiratory center, and interference with blood coagulation processes.

Local gastrointestinal irritation results in vomiting, abdominal pain, and gastrointestinal bleeding. Bleeding occasionally may be severe enough to cause anemia and shock.

Salicylates stimulate the respiratory center of the CNS located in the medulla. This effect results in increased ventilation, decreased P_{CO_2} and a respiratory alkalosis. In response to the respiratory alkalosis the renal excretion of sodium, potassium, and bicarbonate is increased, reducing the body's ability to compensate for the developing metabolic acidosis.

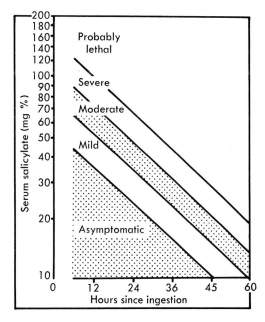

Fig. 40-2. Nomogram relating serum salicylate level to severity of intoxication after acute ingestion of single doses of aspirin. Nomogram starts at 6 hours to ensure that levels will not be interpreted before they have reached their peak. It can be used earlier if more than one level is obtained to ensure that level is declining. (From Done, A. K.: Pediatrics **26**:800, 1960.)

Salicylates also increase the metabolic rate, probably by uncoupling oxidative phosphorylation. This increases oxygen consumption, carbon dioxide formation, and heat production. Respiratory and cardiac rate and cardiac output are increased because of the increased metabolic demands. The increased heat production results in increased water loss by sweating, aggravating the water loss caused by the hyperventilation. If the aspirin was given for a febrile illness, severe hyperpyrexia may occur.

Salicylates also interfere with carbohydrate metabolism. Either hyperglycemia or hypoglycemia may occur. Hyperglycemia is in part a result of the release of epinephrine by stimulation of the hypothalamic sympathetic centers. However, salicylates also decrease aerobic metabolism and increase glucose-6-phosphatase activity, which increases the blood glucose level. Hypoglycemia may be caused by increased peripheral utilization of glucose and interference with glyconeogenesis. The brain glucose concentration may be reduced despite normal or elevated serum glucose levels by interfering with oxidative phosphorylation in the brain. Salicylates interfere with the Krebs cycle, resulting in increased fat mobilization and utilization and formation of organic acids (especially lactic, pyruvic, and acetoacetic acids), ketosis, and ketonuria.

Hyperventilation, sweating, vomiting, and diarrhea all lead to increased water and electrolyte loss. Initially urine loss is also increased as a response to the respiratory alkalosis, and further diuresis occurs as a response to the ketosis, hyperglycosuria, and metabolic acidosis. Because of the decreased extracellular water volume, effective sweating no longer occurs, increasing the hyperpyrexia and accentuating the dehydration. Intracellular shifts of potassium as well as vomiting and kaliuresis may result in severe hypokalemia that must be corrected when treating the acidosis. Shock and renal failure may occur.

Finally salicylates have prolonged effects on the coagulating mechanisms, resulting in increased capillary fragility, thrombocytopenia with impaired platelet aggregation, and decreased prothrombin and factor VII levels. Derangement of clotting may last for several weeks after a single dose of salicylates.

■ **How should salicylism be treated?**

First, further salicylate absorption must be prevented. The induction of emesis by administering syrup of ipecac should be immediately instituted if the patient is awake. If confused or comatose, gastric lavage with normal saline solution is preferable after endotracheal intubation. Lavage or emetics should be followed by the use of activated charcoal. These measures should be attempted up to 10 hours after salicylate ingestion. They are much less effective in the treatment of chronic toxicity.

If the patient is in shock, immediate expansion of the circulating blood volume is indicated. From 350 to 500 ml of a plasma expander/m² should be given in a 45- to 60-minute period. Plasmanate is most effective, but sodium bicarbonate, lactated Ringer's solution, or isotonic saline solution may be used. Dextran is contraindicated, as it may aggravate the derangement of the clotting mechanisms.

In the absence of an adequate clinical response such as improved blood pressure, pulses, and capillary filling time and increased urine production, fluids can be continued at this rate for another hour.

Once shock has been corrected and the patient regains the ability to urinate, the fluid deficit should be treated. This may require 2500 to 5000 ml/m² in the first 24 hours. A hypotonic electrolyte solution containing 5% glucose, 20 to 40 mEq of sodium, and 20 to 40 mEq of potassium/L is optimal.

Hyperpyrexia should be treated by sponging with tepid water; ice water sponging may cause cutaneous vasoconstriction, interfering with heat loss, or may cause shivering, increasing heat production, and should not be used.

Fluids should contain sufficient sodium bicarbonate to alkalinize the urine. A urine pH greater than 7.5 will increase the amount of salicylates in urine fivefold. The use of 3.5 to 5 mEq of 7.5% sodium bicarbonate/kg over a 4-hour period is usually sufficient to alkalinize the urine. Bicarbonate should be used cautiously until blood pH is obtained to ensure that the child is not in respiratory alkalosis. Acetazolamide, a carbonic anhydrase inhibitor, can be used in place of sodium bicarbonate to achieve an alkaline urine or as an adjunct to it. A single dose of 5 mg/kg is usually effective.

As the dehydration and acidosis are treated, frequent determinations of blood gas, electrolyte, and glucose levels are necessary to prevent severe hypoglycemia or hypokalemia. For hypoglycemia 10% glucose solutions are preferable. Oral potassium supplementation should be started when the patient can tolerate oral feedings.

Exchange transfusion, peritoneal dialysis, and hemodialysis are effective but should be reserved for patients with severe salicylism, coma, renal failure, or failure to respond to other means of therapy. Although hemodialysis is the most effective of these techniques, peritoneal dialysis is more generally available in the critical care unit.

Vitamin K has been widely employed to treat the coagulation disorders, although its efficacy has been questioned.

■ What are the symptoms of organic phosphate pesticide poisoning?

Organophosphorus drugs such as malathion and parathion are rapidly replacing DDT and other chlorinated hydrocarbons for pesticide control. These drugs act by inactivating acetylcholinesterase, the enzyme that hydrolyzes acetylcholine. This results in prolonged autonomic and peripheral nervous system stimulation. These drugs are not physiologically active. Toxicity depends on the relative rate of metabolic conversion to an active agent and the rate of detoxification and excretion. Drugs such as barbiturates, narcotics, phenothiazines, and theophyllines potentiate conversion and thus increase toxicity. Children appear to be especially susceptible to these drugs.

With moderate exposure to organophosphorus compounds, constriction of pupils, tearing, nasal congestion, headache, and increased salivation will occur. More severe exposure results in excessive salivation, fasciculation of skeletal muscles, abdominal cramps, diarrhea and vomiting, bronchospasm, bradypnea, respiratory paralysis, stupor, and finally shock, coma, and death. With a large dose death may occur within minutes. Most deaths occur during the first 24 hours, and patients surviving for 48 hours usually recover completely.

■ How should organic phosphate poisoning be treated?

Emesis should be induced using syrup of ipecac, and the exposed skin and eyes should be thoroughly washed. Contaminated clothing must be removed. If the patient has severe respiratory symptoms, an airway should be established with an endotracheal tube to prevent aspiration of vomitus. If the patient is stuporous or comatose, gastric lavage with saline solution should be done immediately.

Atropine blocks the action of acetylcholine. A dose of 1 to 2 mg in small children to 5 mg in adults should be given by the IV or IM route at 10- to 20-minute intervals until flushed skin, dilated pupils, and tachycardia occur. There is evidence that metaraminol (Aramine) reduces the side-effects of atropine while enhancing its effect against acetylcholine. It should be given at double the dose given of atropine.

Pralidoxime (Protopam) should be given in an IV dosage of 50 mg/kg every 12 hours. A maximum of 2 g total dosage should not be exceeded. This drug acts by breaking the covalent bond between acetylcholinesterase and the alkylphosphate, reactivating the acetylcholinesterase.

As atropine has little effect on the skeletal muscle sites, pralidoxime is more effective in relieving paralysis of the respiratory muscles. It is also effective in controlling parasympathetic symptoms but is very slow acting when compared to atropine.

If respiratory failure or bronchospasm exists, an airway and mechanical ventilation may be necessary.

Although recovery usually occurs within 48 hours, the patient will be more susceptible to these drugs for as long as 6 months. Further exposure must be prevented.

Drowning
■ What physiologic changes occur in drowning?

Ten percent of the accidental deaths in the United States are caused by drowning. Of these, 40% involve children under 5 years of age.

The physiologic changes are caused not only by the direct effects of hypoxia, but also result from the differences between the aspirated fluid and plasma. Thus the physiopathology of saltwater as compared to freshwater drowning is quite different.

The primary disturbance is acute ventilatory insufficiency with arterial hypoxia and metabolic acidosis. The presence of fluid irregularly distributed in alveoli causes a large shunting of unoxygenated blood to the pulmonary venous system. This is aggravated by pulmonary edema caused by increased capillary permeability and pulmonary hemorrhage and by decreased lung compliance.

In freshwater drowning fluid rapidly enters the circulation, resulting in hemodilution, hemolysis of red blood cells, hemoglobinemia, and hyperkalemia. The increased circulatory blood volume leads to circulatory overload, congestive heart failure, and pulmonary edema, aggravating the perfusion-diffusion defect. The pulmonary edema and decreased compliance are increased in freshwater drowning by the washing out of surfactants. Protein, sodium, and chloride are drawn into the alveolar spaces, increasing the hemodilution. The combination of asphyxia with hypoxia and hyperkalemia predisposes to ventricular fibrillation.

In saltwater drowning there is an increased concentration of electrolytes. Fluids leave the intravascular spaces, resulting in hemoconcentration and hyperelectrolytemia. The increased electrolyte concentrations act as a chemical irritant, resulting in inflammation and pulmonary edema with patchy areas of atelectasis and emphysema developing. Decreased pulmonary compliance is less severe in saltwater drowning because of the lack of damage to surfactants. The marked shift of fluids into the pulmonary spaces leads to hemoconcentration, decreased circulating blood volume, and shock. A significant drop in blood pressure is an ominous sign in saltwater drowning and is frequently preceded by a drop in central venous pressure. Serious cardiac arrhythmias are less frequent in saltwater drownings.

Hypoxia, hypercapnia, and acidosis are the major physiologic effects. The metabolic acidosis with the rise in organic acids progresses until adequate oxygen therapy is given. Bronchospasm is common. Abdominal distention is usually caused by swallowing large amounts of fluids that may be vomited later and aspirated. A tachycardia is usually present, and extrasystoles or a gallop rhythm may signify developing cardiac failure with increasing pulmonary and cardiac insufficiency. Hypoxemia and hypercapnia increase, resulting in increasing neurologic depression, seizures, and coma. Decerebrate rigidity, persistent seizures, and EEG changes frequently indicate irreversible brain injury and death follows. Persistent severe hypoxia in a patient being administered oxygen should be considered ominous.

■ **How should a drowning patient be treated?**

The primary treatment consists of maintenance of adequate ventilation and oxygenation. Oxygen should be given in adequate concentrations to achieve normal arterial oxygen levels. A patent airway must be maintained. Frequent suction may be necessary. An endotracheal tube or tracheostomy is frequently necessary to maintain the airway. Intermittent or continuous positive pressure breathing may be required to decrease pulmonary edema, to maintain an adequate oxygen diffusion, and to expand atelectatic portions of the lungs. The aspiration of gastric contents is indicated to reduce the possibility of vomiting. IV sodium bicarbonate should be used to treat the metabolic acidosis. Blood gases and electrolytes must be carefully monitored to determine the amount of ventilatory support, oxygen, and bicarbonate needed. Diuretics such as furosemide should be used to treat the marked hemodilution or cardiac failure. Digitalization is indicated in the presence of congestive failure. Isoproterenol or metaproterenol and steroids may be given by aerosol and parenterally to reduce bronchospasm. Parenteral steroids are also beneficial in preventing or reducing the cerebral edema secondary to hypoxia. Antibiotics should be given to prevent aspiration pneumonitis. In saltwater drowning a rapid infusion of plasma should be given to treat shock and restore the intracellular volume. Freshwater drowning patients may require packed cell transfusions to restore the reduced oxygen-carrying capacity caused by hemolysis and hemodilution. In the presence of severe cardiac decompensation and pulmonary edema a partial exchange transfusion using whole blood or packed cells may be necessary to prevent further overloading of the circulation. Succinylcholine

(Anectine) or curare-like drugs should be used if necessary to synchronize the patient with the respirator. Diazepam or other anticonvulsants should be given as required to control seizures. It is advisable to keep the patient normothermic in order to reduce oxygen requirements. If severe cerebral edema is suspected, hypothermia may be advisable, but shivering should be controlled by the use of parenteral chlorpromazine (Thorazine). After shock has been controlled the patient should be maintained at 1200 to 1500 ml of fluids/m^2 daily using a multiple electrolyte solution. Serum electrolytes including calcium and magnesium should be carefully monitored.

Controlled studies are now being done in several centers throughout the country to treat severely affected drowning patients who are not expected to survive with long-term cardiopulmonary bypass procedures using membrane oxygenators. Although this technique appears to be promising, it should be considered experimental at this time.

Patients who respond within 24 hours usually make complete recoveries. Patients who have been in a coma for prolonged periods occasionally completely recover but usually have extensive brain damage.

Croup and related disorders
■ What is the cause of infectious croup?

The croup syndrome is caused by inflammation or obstruction of the epiglottis, larynx, or trachea. It is manifested by inspiratory stridor, usually with hoarseness and a barking cough. It is most often caused by *Haemophilus influenzae* type B, *Corynebacterium diphtheriae,* or viruses.

■ How should viral croup be treated?

Viral croup (or laryngotracheobronchitis) usually begins with hoarseness and a barking cough that is worse at night. Mild fever and anorexia may be present. With increased swelling of the vocal cords or subglottic tissues, hoarseness becomes more severe and breathing becomes labored with inspiratory stridor. If the child becomes restless because of air hunger, becomes cyanotic, or appears to be exhausted, tracheostomy or endotracheal intubation may be necessary; however, these procedures are much less often necessary than in epiglottitis. The use of

racemic epinephrine by nebulization has been very effective in some centers in decreasing respiratory distress and reducing the necessity of tracheostomy. A mucopurulent exudate is frequently present in croup. The use of tracheostomy or endotracheal tubes is helpful not only in relieving obstruction but also in removing these secretions. Mist and oxygen are the primary initial treatment. Steroids, although never proved to be beneficial in controlled studies, are routinely used by some physicians.

■ What are other causes of croup and how should they be managed?

Spasmodic croup is most likely allergic and is characterized by minimum findings of inflammation, daytime remissions, and frequently a history of previous attacks. High humidity is usually sufficient to give relief.

Foreign bodies, angioneurotic edema of the larynx or epiglottis, and retropharyngeal abscesses may also present a crouplike syndrome.

Although many physicians use corticosteroids as anti-inflammatory agents in the croup syndrome, their efficacy has been convincingly demonstrated only in allergic states such as angioneurotic edema and spasmodic croup. Antibiotics are indicated for *Haemophilus influenzae* and *Corynebacterium diphtheriae* infections but are also used for the treatment of infections in patients with foreign bodies.

■ How should acute epiglottis be treated?

Acute epiglottis usually is seen as a severe crouplike syndrome of sudden onset. It occurs most frequently in children 3 to 7 years of age and is almost always caused by *Haemophilus influenzae* type B. *Staphylococcus aureus* and β-hemolytic *Streptococcus* type A are occasionally the offending organisms. Epiglottitis is characterized by the sudden onset of respiratory distress, barking cough, sore throat, and fever that may rapidly progress to severe respiratory obstruction. Marked drooling caused by the inability to swallow is characteristic. The cherry red swollen epiglottis can be seen on examination of the posterior pharynx. A safer means of demonstrating the swollen epiglottis is by lateral x-ray films of the neck. The difficulty in breathing is characterized by inspiratory stridor, a barking cough, and use of the accessory muscles of respiration. With increasing obstruction marked anxiety, air hunger, restlessness, increasing retractions, and cyanosis develop. Increasing cyanosis and impending exhaustion indicate death may occur unless an adequate airway is assured. In the early treatment of epiglottitis the use of high humidity and mist to decrease swelling is indicated. Oxygen should also be given. *Haemophilus influenzae* is usually responsive to ampicillin, although strains resistant to this antibiotic have appeared recently in the United States. Chloramphenicol is the alternate drug for the treatment of *Haemophilus influenzae* infections and should be considered if ampicillin-resistant strains are prevalent in the community.

In some centers routine tracheostomy is recommended for the treatment of acute epiglottitis. In other centers this procedure is delayed, providing personnel and equipment are available for an emergency tracheostomy at the bedside. Tracheostomy should not be delayed if there is increasing air hunger or restlessness, cyanosis while receiving oxygen, or a rise in arterial Pco_2 or if signs of exhaustion or mental confusion develop. It is preferable that a tracheostomy be done in the operating room following endotracheal intubation. However, in an emergency immediate tracheostomy should be carried out in the critical care unit. Recent studies have demonstrated that endotracheal intubation is as effective as tracheostomy in the treatment of epiglottitis. This must be done by an experienced intubator so that the obstruction is not acutely aggravated by trauma.

Table 40-3. Oratracheal tube specifications in pediatrics

Age	French size	Length (cm)
Newborn	11-14	3
1-6 mo	15-16	4
6-12 mo	17-18	4
12-18 mo	19-20	5
18-36 mo	21-22	5
3-4 yr	23-24	6
5-7 yr	25-26	6-7
8-9 yr	27-28	7
10-11 yr	29-30	8
12-14 yr	32-34	8

Typical tube sizes and lengths are found in Table 40-3. The advantages of intubation include a decreased risk of the procedure and a decreased duration of the artificial airway and of the hospitalization. Intubation should be continued for 48 hours.

■ **How should laryngeal diphtheria be treated?**

Laryngotracheal diphtheria, although rare today, must be considered in inadequately immunized children. The presence of a membranous tonsillopharyngitis, marked cervical adenopathy, or severe toxicity suggests the presence of diphtheria. Increasing obstruction with progressive cyanosis, coma, exhaustion, and death may occur or sudden severe hypoxia may occur from detachment and aspiration of a piece of membrane. An adequate dose of diphtheria antitoxin must be given promptly. Antibiotics are less effective but should also be used. Tracheostomy may be necessary.

Other respiratory problems
■ **How can pertussis be differentiated from croup and how is it managed?**

Pertussis (whooping cough) may be confused with croup because of the marked inspiratory stridor. Pertussis is manifested by sudden paroxysms of short rapid coughs that terminate in a prolonged inspiration with a typical high-pitched whoop. A series of coughing paroxysms and whoops may occur until a mucous plug is dislodged. Vomiting frequently follows the attack. The typical paroxysm usually does not occur until the third week of the illness. The early phase presents as an upper respiratory infection frequently with a night cough. Petechiae, subconjunctival hemorrhages, epistaxis, and subarachnoid hemorrhages are common in the paroxysmal stage and are caused by the marked increase in venous pressure. Seizures resulting from severe hypoxia may occur during paroxysms.

There is usually an elevation of the white count with the increase entirely caused by lymphocytes. At times the lymphocyte count may be as high as 100,000 and leukemia considered. The higher the white count and the younger the patient's age, the worse the prognosis.

Management includes bedrest with oxygen, humidity, and sedation. Pertussis hyperimmune globulin should be given to infants and severely ill patients. Antibiotics are less effective in decreasing morbidity and mortality but should be used to control contagiousness. To terminate a severe attack, suction of the posterior pharynx will frequently dislodge a thick mucous plug.

■ **What pulmonary problems are associated with prolonged respiratory care for hyaline membrane disease?**

Bronchopulmonary dysplasia is a pulmonary disorder seen primarily in small premature infants requiring prolonged mechanical assistance and oxygen therapy usually exceeding 10 days. Infants with bronchopulmonary dysplasia after recovering from hyaline membrane disease continue to have chronic respiratory symptoms or symptoms develop after a relatively well period. X-ray films reveal diffuse, coarse, fibrotic, and inflammatory changes with air bronchograms. Bronchopulmonary dysplasia is believed to be caused by oxygen toxicity. Similar changes are seen in animals and adults receiving oxygen concentrations greater than 60% via respirators. Superimposed pneumonia, primarily caused by gram-negative organisms, is believed to be an additional factor resulting in severe inflammation and destruction of the lung tissues. The disease slowly regresses over several years. There is no known treatment. The incidence of this illness can probably be reduced by limiting the duration of respiratory therapy, giving minimum concentrations of oxygen, closely monitoring arterial Pao_2, and intensively treating secondary infections.

■ **What other pulmonary problems are unique to premature infants?**

The Wilson-Mikity syndrome occurs in premature infants who either had no evidence of hyaline membrane disease or who had a short illness not requiring ventilatory assistance. These infants develop progressive hyperpnea, cyanosis, cough, and retractions. The illness progresses for 2 to 6 weeks and then reaches a plateau lasting several weeks. Rales appear at this time. If the infant survives the acute stage, symptoms slowly

regress and complete recovery as evidenced by clinical and x-ray examination occurs in 3 to 24 months. X-ray films reveal nonspecific interstitial thickening with patchy areas of atelectasis and multiple cystlike areas of emphysema. The cause is unknown, and there is no treatment except for supportive care using humidity and low concentrations of oxygen. Steroids and antibiotics have not been demonstrated to be helpful and are indicated only for documented complicating pneumonia.

■ **How can lobar emphysema be recognized in children?**

Congenital lobar emphysema may be noted shortly after birth but more commonly presents as respiratory distress usually associated with a respiratory infection at 1 to 2 months of age. Emphysema of a single lobe is commonly caused by a deficiency in the bronchial cartilage but may result from partial obstruction of a bronchus internally by a plug or externally by tumors or cardiovascular structures. Wheezing is usually present, and in severe cases cyanosis and retractions are prominent. Physical examination reveals evidence of overexpansion and decreased breath sounds on the affected side as well as shift of the heart and mediastinal structures to the opposite side. X-ray films confirm the radiolucent lobe, frequently with herniation of the lung to the opposite side and atelectasis of the remaining lung on that side. It can be differentiated from pneumothorax by the presence of lung markings throughout the affected lung. Early bronchoscopy is indicated. If a plug or foreign body cannot be found, surgical removal of the involved lobe may be necessary.

■ **What congenital anomalies cause obstructive respiratory disease after the newborn period?**

Tracheomalacia is a disorder consisting of tracheal rings that are too pliable and collapse easily with respiration. Although symptoms may be present from birth, they become more severe during early infancy and are frequently aggravated by respiratory infections. Clinically infants exhibit inspiratory stridor, expiratory wheezes, tachypnea, and cough. Complicating lower respiratory infections with cyanosis and distress are common. Symptoms increase during crying or feeding but are present at rest. Many infants assume an opisthotonic position that maximally opens the respiratory passageways. Bronchoscopy is indicated to rule out a laryngeal web or other surgically correctable lesion. A barium swallow esophagogram should be obtained to rule out the presence of a vascular ring. Treatment is nonspecific and consists of control of secretions by humidity and expectorants and treatment of complicating infections with antibiotics. These children usually show definite improvement by 6 months of age with complete recovery by 1 to 2 years of age.

Vascular rings present a picture of progressive stridor and wheezing usually associated with dysphagia when solid feeding is started. The presence of aberrant vessels forming a complete ring around the esophagus and trachea is demonstrable by esophagograms and confirmed by angiography. The most common aberrant vessel, an anomalous right subclavian artery, rarely produces symptoms. The most severe cases are usually associated with a double aortic arch. The rare anomalous left pulmonary artery does not produce dysphagia and is the only lesion producing an anterior constriction of the trachea. Treatment of vascular rings is surgical after clearing of secondary pulmonary infections. Symptoms frequently persist after surgery because of associated tracheomalacia.

■ What type of tracheoesophageal fistulas may not be symptomatic during the newborn period?

Tracheoesophageal fistulas without esophageal atresia (H-type tracheoesophageal fistula) usually are not diagnosed in the neonatal period. The diagnosis should be suspected in any infant with recurrent pneumonia without apparent cause or in infants who develop spells of choking, coughing, cyanosis, or respiratory distress following the ingestion of formula. Physical examination reveals evidence of pulmonary infection and usually a distended abdomen caused by air in the stomach. Infants develop repeat episodes of pneumonia, especially in the right lower lobe. Diagnosis is by esophagography via pressure injec-

tion of contrast media or by esophagoscopy or bronchoscopy. Treatment is surgical following treatment of the respiratory infection, and complete recovery can be expected.

■ What is *Pneumocystis* pneumonia and how should it be managed?

Primarily affecting premature and debilitated infants, interstitial plasma cell pneumonia is an illness caused by a protozoan, *Pneumocystis carinii*. It is also common in children with immunologic disorders such as agammaglobulinemia and thymic dysplasia and in children with leukemia or lymphomas who have received steroid or immunosuppressive therapy.

It occurs primarily between 6 and 16 weeks of age, although it is not uncommon under 1 year of age. Hospitalized children appear to be most susceptible to *Pneumocystis* pneumonia.

The onset is insidious with poor feeding, irritability, and failure to thrive preceding tachypnea, cyanosis, and respiratory distress. Fever is unusual. Auscultation of the chest may be normal or reveal scattered rales and rhonchi. X-ray films reveal a characteristic infiltration radiating bilaterally from each hilus with sparing of peripheral lung fields.

The diagnosis usually requires lung biopsy either by needle aspiration or open thoracotomy. The organism may occasionally be demonstrable in sputum or bronchial washing. Special silver stains are usually necessary to demonstrate the organism.

Treatment consists of the use of ultrasonic nebulization and oxygen therapy. Steroids, antibiotics, and gamma globulin are ineffective. Pentamidine isothionate and trimethoprim-sulfmethoxazole are the only available drugs beneficial in the treatment of *Pneumocystis* infections. The dose of pentamidine isothionate for children is 100 to 150 mg/m² daily. Trimethoprim, 20 mg/kg, and sulfmethoxazole, 100 mg/kg, are given in equally divided doses every 6 hours for 14 days. Hypoglycemia, azotemia, and liver toxicity are common in patients treated with pentamidine. Gavage feedings and IV fluid therapy are usually necessary. IV alimentation may be necessary in some children. The mortality rate associated with *Pneumocystis* pneumonia is 30% to 50%.

■ **What is the pathophysiology of bronchiolitis?**

Bronchiolitis is a severe respiratory illness affecting primarily infants, usually under 6 months of age. Most cases are caused by respiratory syncytial virus, although parainfluenza and adenovirus can produce a similar illness. Approximately 10% of infants requiring hospitalization for bronchiolitis later develop asthma. It is not known whether a predisposing tendency to asthma results in a more severe illness or whether damage to the bronchioles predisposes the patient to asthma later.

The primary lesion in bronchiolitis is bronchiolar obstruction by edema, lymphocytic infiltration, and plugs of mucus and cellular debris. As resistance to airflow in a tube is inversely proportional to the fourth power of the radius, thickening of the bronchioles in infants will cause a markedly greater increase in resistance than in the larger airways of older children and adults. Thus older children will usually have a milder respiratory illness without significant obstruction to airflow.

The bronchiolar thickening results in disturbances in air exchange. Some degree of hypoxemia is usually present even though the infant is not visibly cyanotic. Hypercapnia develops much later in the illness and is a sign of severe disease with respiratory failure.

Bronchiolitis usually starts as a mild upper respiratory infection followed in several days by a paroxysmal cough, wheeze, and difficulty in feeding. The temperature is usually normal and tachypnea and tachycardia are present. Because of obstruction to airflow, respiratory efforts increase and retractions are noted. However, retractions are less prominent than is seen in upper airway obstruction such as croup. The chest becomes overinflated, and the liver and spleen become palpable.

This combination of respiratory distress, tachycardia, and hepatomegaly is frequently misdiagnosed as congestive heart failure. Auscultation of the lungs usually reveals poor air exchange. Rales and a mild wheeze are usually present. Mild dehydration is frequently present because of the inability to feed.

Chest x-ray films reveal overexpansion with patchy areas of atelectasis that are easily misdiagnosed as pneumonia. Secondary pneumonia should be suspected when there is a fever and leukocytosis. Pneumothorax and mediastinal emphysema may occur but are rare.

■ **How should bronchiolitis be managed?**

Because hypoxemia is usually present, oxygen therapy is indicated. Concentrations above 40% are rarely necessary. Arterial Po_2 can be monitored by percutaneous arterial punctures. Although there is little evidence that high humidity decreases the bronchiolar edema, it should be used. Ultrasonic nebulizers produce much smaller droplets and are more likely to be helpful in bronchiolitis than the usual mist tent. Because of the difficulty in feeding and mild dehydration, the severely affected infant with this illness should receive IV maintenance fluids. Antibiotics should not be used unless there is evidence of secondary bacterial infection. Controlled studies have shown no beneficial effect of antibiotics as prophylaxis against bacterial complications. Steroids, although extensively used, are not beneficial except in the occasional child believed to be allergic. As these infants rarely are in congestive failure, digitalization is not usually indicated. Tracheostomy and endotracheal intubation will not relieve the obstruction. Endotracheal intubation is indicated only in the infant with severe respiratory failure requiring mechanical ventilation.

Bronchodilators such as aminophylline and isoproterenol may be helpful in some cases. A trial of 5 mg/kg of IV aminophylline is worthwhile in the infant in severe respiratory distress or if cyanosis is present during oxygen administration.

Bronchiolitis is usually self-limited. The mortality is less than 1% except in debilitated children. Complete recovery without sequelae can be expected.

Cystic fibrosis and its complications
■ **What is the earliest manifestation of cystic fibrosis?**

Meconium ileus is present in 10% to 15% of all patients with cystic fibrosis. This is a form of intestinal obstruction caused by the accumulation of abnormal puttylike meconium resulting from a lack of pancreatic enzymes. Meconium ileus may be complicated by associated intestinal atresia or stenosis, volvulus, or perforation with intestinal obstruction.

In a minority of cases the obstruction can be relieved by the use of meglumine diatrizoate (Gastrografin) enemas under careful observation by a radiologist-surgeon team. Surgery is usually required. Atretic, gangrenous, and markedly dilated areas must be resected. A Mikulicz resection with a double-barrel ileostomy or an ileostomy with a single-barrel end-to-side anastomosis is most commonly required. Pancreatic enzymes or 5% N-acetylcysteine are commonly used to irrigate the distal bowel in order to free the inspissated meconium. Total parenteral alimentation is frequently necessary in these children. Pancreatic enzymes are employed as soon as feeding can be instituted either orally or by gastrostomy. Vigorous treatment of respiratory infections and careful attention to protein, electrolyte, caloric, and blood requirements are essential during the postoperative period.

■ **What problems are associated with the sweat disturbance in patients with cystic fibrosis?**

All patients with cystic fibrosis lose excessive amounts of both sodium and chloride in their sweat. This is the basis of the pilocarpine iontophoresis sweat test for the diagnosis of cystic fibrosis. Patients with this disease have sweat chloride concentrations above 60 mEq/L and sodium concentrations above 70 mEq/L. Under conditions of increased sweating, severe hyponatremic hypochloremic dehydration may occur, and the patient may have "heat stroke," circulatory collapse, or coma. Dehydration should be suspected with fevers, during hot weather, following periods of strenuous physical activity, or while in unventilated mist tents. The hypochloremia and hyponatremia may be aggravated by the use of ultrasonic nebulization with water, as large quantities of water may be absorbed into the circulation as well as electrolytes lost into the pulmonary alveoli. When present, the electrolyte disturbance should be treated by parenteral replacement. It can usually be prevented by adding salt to the dietary intake during periods of fever or when sweating is increased. This may be in-

corporated in the preparation and seasoning of food and need not be given separately. Infants in the first year of life require 1 g of salt (¼ teaspoon) daily. In the second and third years ½ teaspoon should be given. Older children will require ¾ to 1 teaspoon supplemental salt in the diet.

■ **What is the management of the respiratory disease in the child with cystic fibrosis?**

Treatment is directed toward relieving respiratory obstruction and controlling secretions, management of the accompanying infections, and therapy for respiratory failure and other complications.

Therapy aimed at the bronchial obstruction is directed toward decreasing the viscosity of pulmonary secretions and improving the pulmonary hygiene. A water-saturated atmosphere enables the patient to mobilize secretions. Compressed air is used unless hypoxia exists. If oxygen is required, it should be given at the lowest concentration effective in relieving symptoms. Many of these patients have chronic respiratory failure with hypercapnia. In these patients the respiratory center in the medulla may be insensitive to carbon dioxide levels and driven by the hypoxia. Sudden correction of the hypoxia may result in respiratory arrest. In addition, high concentrations of oxygen may impair ciliary activity, irritate the bronchial mucosa and alveoli, and cause vasomotor changes.

The ultrasonic nebulizer is more effective than the compressed air nebulizer in increasing the deposition of water in the tracheobronchial tree. Ultrasonic nebulization can provide particles of 1 to 5 μ in size, which will reach the small bronchioles. If water is used for nebulization, large quantities of water may enter the circulation, resulting in hemodilution, hyponatremia, and hypochloremia. Circulatory overload and congestive failure may occur. Dilute saline (0.25 to 0.5 normal) solutions should be used to prevent this complication. A 10% propylene glycol solution can be used in air compressor nebulization to stabilize particle size. Acetylcysteine has been used by nebulization to thin secretions but must be used very cautiously because it is irritating and will frequently result in a marked increase in pulmonary secretions. The cautious use of this drug, especially for the treatment for localized disease under direct vision during bronchoscopy, can be very effective in selected patients with increasing respiratory failure despite intensive conservative management.

Chest physical therapy and postural bronchial drainage are important adjuncts in the treatment of pulmonary disease. These procedures should be done before meals or at least 1 to 2 hours after eating. They are especially effective at bedtime to help clear the airways and reduce nocturnal coughing. Two to four treatments per day are optimal. Procedures that help loosen secretions and facilitate bronchial drainage include clapping, deep breathing, assisted coughing, thoracic squeezing, and vibration. With localized lung disease the drainage of the affected bronchi should precede that of uninvolved areas. With generalized disease the lower lobes are drained first, followed by the middle lobe, the lingula, and the upper lobes. The order should be reversed in infants and postoperative patients.

Intermittent positive pressure breathing may be effective in relieving obstruction and in administering antibiotics and other medications. However, this procedure is not without risk and must be used with caution, as it may spread pulmonary infection or cause air trapping or pneumothorax. Short periods of therapy are advisable and pulmonary function studies should be monitored. Saline solution, bronchodilator drugs, antibiotics, and enzymes can be given by this means. The use of β-2-adrenergic agents such as isoetharine (Bronkosol) are preferable to isoproterenol or epinephrine because of their reduced cardiac effects. The simultaneous aerosol and systemic administration of antibiotics may be especially effective in *Pseudomonas* and staphylococcal infections. Local irritation, toxicity, and allergic reactions can result from the aerosol administration of antibiotics.

Penicillin (100,000 to 200,000 units), methicillin (250 to 500 mg), neomycin (100 to 200 mg), kanamycin (50 to 100 mg), polymyxin (4 mg), colistin (10 to 20 mg), gentamicin (10 to 20 mg), and carbenicillin (250 to 500 mg) can be administered daily by aerosol therapy. Mucolytic agents such as acetylcysteine may be of value in selected patients but more frequently result in an increased production of secretions and prolonged morbidity and duration of the hospitalization. In patients with progressive respiratory disease and pulmonary failure the use of endotracheal tubes, tracheostomy, or bronchoscopy may be necessary to remove secretions and provide ventilatory support.

■ **How should pulmonary infection be treated in cystic fibrosis?**

Patients with cystic fibrosis must be assumed to have mixed infections caused by resistant organisms. *Staphylococcus aureus* and gram-negative rods, especially *Pseudomonas aeruginosa* and *Klebsiella pneumoniae*, remain the most common pulmonary pathogens. The current trend is to use antibiotics intermittently for the treatment of exacerbations rather than to use continuous antibiotic therapy. Adequate cultures and sensitivity studies are imperative prior to instituting antimicrobial therapy. Until these studies are reported, a combination of antibiotics should be chosen, based on the sensitivity patterns of pathogens in the local community. Usually initial treatment will consist of a penicillinase-resistant penicillin such as oxacillin with a drug effective against gram-negative organisms such as colistin or carbenicillin. Maximum therapeutic dosages are necessary and in the acutely ill patient should be given parenterally.

Typical dosages that can be given are found in Table 40-4 on p. 688.

■ **What is cor pulmonale and how can it be recognized in cystic fibrosis?**

Continuous or intermittent obstruction of the airways causes pulmonary vasoconstriction as a result of hypoxia and acidosis. The occurrence of airway obstruction from early infancy may retard maturation of the pulmonary arterioles, with retention of thick, reactive arteriolar musculature. The acute development of more severe obstruction may then result in severe vasoconstriction. If the right ventricle cannot eject the required cardiac output against the increased afterload, right ventricular dilatation and acute right heart failure ensue. With chronic respiratory failure, intimal changes occur, resulting in obstructive pul-

Table 40-4. Dosages of antibiotics used for cystic fibrosis patients

Drug	Route	Dose/day	Maximum dose/day
Penicillin	Oral, IV, IM	50,000 U/kg	20,000,000 U
Methicillin	IV, IM	100-200 mg/kg	4-6 g
Ampicillin	Oral, IM	100-200 mg/kg	3-4 g
Amoxicillin	Oral	40-50 mg/kg	1-2 g
Oxacillin	Oral, IV	100-200 mg/kg	4-6 g
Carbenicillin	Oral, IV	300-400 mg/kg	20-25 g
Cephalothin	IM, IV	50-100 mg/kg	4-12 g
Chloramphenicol	Oral, IV	50-100 mg/kg	2-4 g
Erythromycin	Oral	50-100 mg/kg	2-4 g
Kanamycin	IM	15 mg/kg	1-1.5 g
Lincomycin	IM, IV	20-30 mg/kg	1.5-2 g
Streptomycin	IM	20-40 mg/kg	1-2 g
Colistin	IM	4-7 mg/kg	200-300 mg
Gentamicin	IM	4-7 mg/kg	200-300 mg
Tetracycline	Oral, IV	50-100 mg/kg	2-4 g

Table 40-5. Normal respiratory values in children

	Newborn	Infants	Children
Respiratory frequency	40-60	20-30	20-30 to 6 yr, 15-20 over 6 yr
pH	7.30-7.40	7.30-7.40	7.35-7.45
$Paco_2$	30-35	30-35	35-45
Pao_2	60-90	80-100	80-100
Tidal volume (cc/kg)	5-6	7-8	7-8
Dead space (cc/kg)	2	2	2

monary hypertension, right ventricular hypertrophy, and eventually chronic right heart failure. Small thrombi or emboli may aggravate these changes. The airway obstruction may be in the upper or lower respiratory tract. Children with cystic fibrosis may have upper respiratory obstruction as a result of nasal polyps or enlarged adenoids and tonsils severe enough to cause hypoxia and pulmonary vasoconstriction.

Heart failure may be difficult to distinguish in cystic fibrosis patients with chronic respiratory disease. The emphysema may displace the liver inferiorly, suggesting hepatomegaly. Visible neck vein distention may be present. Rales, dyspnea, and tachycardia are seen with acute respiraotry disease. Poor nutrition or absorption may result in significant hypoproteinemia with resulting ascites and peripheral edema. An acute fluid overload from oral or parenteral intake or absorption of fluids from aerosol therapy may result in circu-

latory overload and heart failure in the absence of cor pulmonale.

The ECG is frequently of value in the diagnosis of cor pulmonale. In the emphysematous patient without cor pulmonale deep S waves in the right precordial lead are typical. This is frequently misdiagnosed as left ventricular hypertrophy. With acute right heart failure, a significant shift of the frontal QRS complex of at least 60 degrees is typical. With chronic right heart failure, the typical right ventricular hypertrophy and peaked P waves suggesting right atrial enlargement are found. Chest x-ray films usually reveal cardiac enlargement with dilatation of the large central pulmonary arteries tapering to small pulmonary arteries peripherally. In active infection pulmonary vascular disease may not be readily distinguishable. Echocardiography will reveal right ventricular dilatation, paradoxic motion of the ventricular septum, and increased thickness of the right ventricle wall. The pulmonary valve echocardiogram frequently demonstrates a flat E-F slope, absence of the a wave, and early systolic closure resulting in the flying-W pattern. Satisfactory echos are frequently difficult to obtain in the presence of emphysema. Hypoxia and acidosis are present. In cor pulmonale the pH and Pao_2 are reduced, and the $Paco_2$ is elevated. The pH is frequently reduced greater than the elevation of $Paco_2$ because of associated metabolic acidosis. Normal respiratory values for children may be found in Table 40-5. With chronic cor pulmonale, polycythemia and clubbing are typical.

■ What is the treatment for cor pulmonale?

Since the basis of cor pulmonale is obstructive disease of the airways with hypoxemia and acidosis, the primary treatment is the improvement of ventilation. If there is upper airway obstruction, removal of enlarged nasal polyps, adenoids, and tonsils may result in significant improvement in cardiac function. Steroids have been used to shrink nasal polyps or prevent their recurrence. Vigorous management of the lower respiratory disease and impaired ventilation is necessary. Oxygen therapy should be initiated to improve the hypoxemia. It must be remembered that in children with chronic respiratory failure and chronic hypercapnia, the central respiratory center may be insensitive to the Pco_2 elevation, and the hypoxemia may provide the only stimulus to maintain respiration. The administration of oxygen to these children may decrease respirations, resulting in increased carbon dioxide narcosis and respiratory arrest. Assisted ventilation will be necessary in these children and should not be delayed, being performed if necessary with endotracheal intubation or tracheostomy.

As acidosis also increases pulmonary vasoconstriction, this should be corrected with the use of sodium bicarbonate or tromethamine (THAM). While many authors recommend THAM in these patients because plasma bicarbonate is already high, it offers no advantage over bicarbonate and is more apt to result in respiratory arrest.

Some studies have suggested that tolazoline (Priscoline) may be of value in lowering the pulmonary vascular resistance. It is more apt to be of value in acute hyperactive cor pulmonale than in the more chronic obstructive form. Further studies of this and other pulmonary vasodilators are necessary.

Digitalis glycosides, by their positive inotropic effect on the heart, improve the efficiency of the heart in patients with cor pulmonale. Digoxin (Lanoxin) is most commonly used in children because of its rapid action and short duration of toxicity. Since a therapeutic response to digitalis may be difficult to distinguish because of the pulmonary disease, serum digoxin determinations may be necessary to determine the adequacy of digitalization and the presence of toxicity.

Salt restriction and diuretics are also useful in improving cardiac function but must be used cautiously because of increased salt losses in the sweat in these patients. Because of the increased vascular and extracellular fluid volume in heart failure and the tendency to hyponatremia and hypochloremia in cystic fibrosis, water restriction is important in these children. It must be remembered that a low serum sodium level is not indicative of low total body sodium. Furosemide has replaced mercurial diuretics as the drug of choice in heart failure in children. Salt restriction should be moderate. Potassium replacement is necessary when diuretics are used unless spironolactone (Aldactone) is used as a second diuretic. Replacement of chloride by oral ammonium chloride may be necessary with the frequent use of diuretics but should be used cautiously because it will increase the acidosis. Hypokalemia and hypochloremia may be avoided by using diuretics every other day rather than daily.

Anemia aggravates the congestive heart failure by decreasing the oxygen-carrying capacity, thus increasing the necessary cardiac output to meet the metabolic requirements. The cyanotic patient in chronic respiratory failure should be polycythemic. A "normal" hematocrit or hemoglobin in these patients indicates a significant anemia and should be treated. Small transfusions of packed red blood cells should be considered. If large transfusions are necessary, a partial exchange transfusion with packed cells may prevent severe cardiac decompensation. Albumin transfusions may be necessary if significant hypoproteinemia is present.

The correction of the pulmonary insufficiency remains the most important goal in the treatment of right heart failure caused by cor pulmonale, the other measures being only supportive.

■ What is the pathogenesis of disseminated intravascular coagulation?

Disseminated intravascular coagulation (DIC) is a disease process caused by the consumption of plasma clotting factors and platelets, resulting in thrombi in small vessels followed by a hemorrhagic diathesis.

DIC commonly occurs in infections by bacteria that form endotoxins. It occurs most frequently in meningococcal infections and sepsis caused by gram-negative rods but may be seen in other infections, including streptococcal and staphylococcal disease, varicella, rickettsial infections, and generalized vaccinia. DIC may also be seen in patients with cyanotic congenital heart disease, especially during surgery using the pump oxygenator; severe burns or trauma; malignancies; snake bites; drug intoxications; anaphylactic reactions; and giant cavernous hemangiomas.

The process in infections caused by endotoxin-producing bacteria is believed to be direct damage to the vascular endothelium and activation of Hageman factor. In burns or trauma tissue thromboplastin is formed. In patients with giant hemangiomas platelets aggregate and release platelet thromboplastin. Each of these defects initiates a series of reactions resulting in the conversion of prothrombin to thrombin, which activates fibrinogen into fibrin, the formation of intravascular thrombi, and the depletion of platelets and plasma clotting factors. Factors depleted during the process include antihemophilic factor, proaccelerin, prothrombin, and fibrinogen. As fibrin is deposited, fibrinolysins are activated and split fibrin into products that act as anticoagulants until they are removed by the reticuloendothelial system.

These processes result in thrombi and emboli that produce tissue ischemia and necrosis, depletion of clotting factors, and the effects of fibrin products, which lead to widespread hemolysis, hemolytic anemia caused by red blood cell fragmentation by fibrin strands in peripheral vessels and, if severe, shock and death.

The diagnosis is made by the demonstration of abnormalities of coagulation, including low platelet count, prothrombin time, and partial thrombo-

plastin time, and by the presence of fibrinolysins and fibrin split products. The euglobulin lysis time and cryofibrinogen tests are valuable in determining the presence of these latter two groups. Specific determination of multiple factors may be necessary for differentiation of DIC from other hemorrhagic diatheses.

■ What is the treatment of DIC?

Heparin is the drug of choice in DIC. It is given by IV route in doses of 1 to 1.5 mg (100 to 150 units)/kg every 4 to 6 hours. This is continued until coagulation factors return to normal. In severe cases the replacement of depleted factors by transfusion of platelet concentrates and fresh-frozen plasma should also be used. Antifibrinolytic agents such as ϵ-aminocaproic acid (Amicar) should not be used in the treatment of DIC.

Survival depends on the correction of causative factors and shock and on the extent of damage to major organs. Specific antibiotics for the bacterial infection are necessary. Shock must be vigorously treated with fluids and colloids. Large dosages of steroids are indicated in endotoxic shock. The correction of anemia, dehydration, acidosis, and other metabolic disturbances may be required, as may the use of peritoneal dialysis or hemodialysis if renal failure develops.

The mortality remains high despite heparinization and adequate correction of the coagulopathy.

VOMITING
■ What is the most common cause of severe vomiting in infants and how should it be managed?

Congenital hypertrophic pyloric stenosis is the most common cause of upper gastrointestinal obstruction in children. It is eight times more frequent in males than females, is frequently familial, and most often occurs in the firstborn child. It is characterized by vomiting, usually beginning in the second or third week of life and becoming progressively more frequent and projectile in nature. Weight loss and dehydration ensue, and death may occur if treatment is delayed. The obstruction is caused by thickened pyloric musculature. The vomiting is of gastric fluids containing hydrochloric acid and potassium, resulting in a metabolic alkalosis. The thickened muscle is usually palpable as an "olive" in the right upper quadrant, and visible gastric peristaltic waves are usually seen. Laboratory studies reveal an elevation of pH and plasma carbon dioxide content and decreased serum chloride and potassium. Hemoconcentration is frequently present.

The initial treatment is directed toward correction of the dehydration and alkalosis. The IV administration of saline solutions with supplemental potassium chloride (20 to 40 mEq/L) should be used rather than prepared multiple electrolyte solutions such as Isolyte P or M, as these solutions are constituted for the treatment of acidosis. Gastric replacement solution or other acidifying solutions such as ammonium chloride are rarely necessary. When the dehydration and electrolyte derangement are corrected, surgery is indicated. The Fredet-Ramstedt procedure consists of splitting the thickened pyloric muscles. Recovery is rapid, and oral feedings are usually initiated as soon as the infant awakens from the anesthesia. Glucose water is usually given for the first few feedings, followed by increasing amounts of formula.

■ What are the other common causes of severe vomiting in infancy and early childhood?

Adrenogenital syndrome, intussusception, gastroenteritis, Reye's syndrome, and increased intracranial pressure owing to meningitis, brain tumor, lead intoxication, subdural hematoma, or pseudotumor cerebri, should be considered in any infant with severe or prolonged vomiting.

■ What is the adrenogenital syndrome?

Adrenogenital syndrome is more easily diagnosed in female infants because of the ambiguous genitalia. In the male the genitalia may appear large or abnormally pigmented but are usually considered normal. The salt-losing form of adrenogenital syndrome occurs in about one fourth of all cases. When salt loss is present, the infant is usually between 1 and 3 weeks of age with severe vomiting, weight loss, diarrhea, anorexia, and evidence of dehydration. In the 11-hydroxylase variety of adrenogenital syndrome significant hypertension is present. These children frequently are in shock. Laboratory studies readily distinguish these children from the child with pyloric stenosis as hyponatremia, hypo-

chloremia, hypercalcemia, acidosis, and frequently hyperkalemia are present. A definitive diagnosis is made by urinary steriod studies. All forms have an elevation of 17-ketosteroids. In the common 21-hydroxylase form there is a marked elevation of pregnanetriol. The rare 3-hydroxysteroid form has an elevation of Δ 5-pregnanetriol. The hypertensive form has a marked increase in tetrahydro-S and only moderate elevation of pregnanetriol.

■ How is it treated?

Initial treatment is the restoration of body fluids. If the patient is in shock, a colloid solution such as plasma or normal albumin should be given at the rate of 350 ml/m² over the first hour. This should be followed by 0.9% NaCl and 5% dextrose in water at a rate of 2500-3000 ml/m²/day. Hydrocortisone sodium succinate (Solu-Cortef), 1.5 gm/m²/day, can be added to the IV. Desoxycorticosterone acetate in oil, 1 to 4 mg IM, can be given daily instead of intravenous hydrocortisone.

After initial hydration, intravenous fluids can usually be discontinued. 2 to 8 g of sodium chloride should be added to the daily formula. At this time, the infant is usually started on desoxycorticosterone acetate, 1 mg IM daily, and cortisone acetate, 80 to 100 mg/m² daily.

■ What is intussusception and how is it treated?

Intussusception is an invagination or telescoping of a portion of the intestine into an adjacent part. Most start at the ileocecal region and occur between 1 and 12 months of age. Intussusception is more common in males. It occurs frequently in patients with Schönlein-Henoch purpura and with Meckel's diverticulum and is a common complication in older children with cystic fibrosis. As the intestine invaginates into a distal portion, it pulls along the mesentery. With time this compromises the circulation, resulting in strangulation and gangrene.

Intussusception typically is seen with a sudden onset of cramplike pain associated with straining, vomiting, and restlessness. The patient is usually asymptomatic between paroxysms. Blood and mucus usually appear in the stools within 12 hours, and the stools frequently have the typical currant jelly appearance. Later a high fever and a shocklike state may develop. The abdomen is soft at first but becomes distended and tender. An elongated sausage-shaped tumor is usually palpable, most frequently in the right upper quadrant, and the right lower quadrant feels empty (Dance's sign). At times a portion of the intussusceptum may prolapse through the anus.

The immediate treatment is the treatment of shock and electrolyte fluid balance. The intussusception should then be reduced as soon as feasible. In early cases without evidence of peritonitis, reduction can be attempted by barium enema using hydrostatic pressure. This should be done by an experienced radiologist or surgeon. If the intussusception cannot be easily reduced or if signs of peritonitis, fever, or shock are present, immediate surgical reduction is necessary. The recurrence rate is 1% to 3% with either form of therapy.

REYE'S SYNDROME
■ What is Reye's syndrome?

Reye's syndrome (pronounced "rye," as in the grain) is a virus-associated encephalopathy first described by Dr. R. D. J. Reye. The clinical diagnosis is made when the following criteria are fulfilled:

1. Prodromal viral illness
2. Protracted vomiting within a week after the onset of the viral illness
3. Delirium and stupor beginning soon after the onset of vomiting
4. Absence of focal neurologic signs
5. Abnormalities of liver function as demonstrated by elevated enzyme (particularly SGOT) levels, increased blood ammonia, and abnormal prothrombin time
6. No (or slight) jaundice
7. Normal cerebrospinal fluid protein and cell count
8. Fatty infiltration of the liver (usually found at autopsy)

■ What is the clinical picture of Reye's syndrome?

Lovejoy and associates in 1974 proposed a system of clinical staging that would allow inter-

pretation of the therapeutic effectiveness of different modes of therapy. They described stage 1 as being associated with vomiting, lethargy, liver dysfunction, and a mildly abnormal EEG. Stage 2 is associated with delirium, combativeness, hyperventilation, hyperactive reflexes, liver dysfunction, and a somewhat more severely abnormal EEG. The third stage is associated with obtundation or coma, evidence of decortication, liver dysfunction, and also a moderately severe abnormal EEG. Stage 4 represents a deepening coma, decerebration, a cephalocaudal progression of brain stem dysfunction, and often improvement in liver dysfunction associated with a severely abnormal EEG. Finally stage 5 is associated with seizures, loss of reflexes, respiratory arrest, correction of liver dysfunction, and an isoelectric EEG. Lovejoy and associates believed that stages 1 through 3 were compatible with full recovery, but a poor outcome was predicted when there was rapid passage through the first three stages, the presence of seizures in stage 2, a presenting blood ammonia concentration of greater than 300 μg/100 ml, increased spinal fluid pressure in stage 3, a markedly increased prothrombin time in stage 3, or a severely abnormal EEG.

■ Which viral infections lead to Reye's syndrome?

In 1974 about 350 cases of Reye's syndrome were reported to the Center for Disease Control in Atlanta. Of these, 55 followed type B influenza, 25 were apparently secondary to chickenpox, another 20 succeeded nonupper respiratory infection, and the remainder followed various upper respiratory illnesses. Those cases associated with influenza B and upper respiratory infections, shared another characteristic. The median age of incidence was 11 years for both, with peak rates clustered in children aged 12 to 15 years. In contrast, in the 25 patients whose encephalopathy followed chickenpox the median age was 6 years.

The mechanism by which viral infections are linked to Reye's syndrome is unknown. The viral infection may be related to direct damage to the liver, CNS or secondary toxic damage, or a postviral immunologic reaction.

■ What is the treatment of Reye's syndrome?

There are many unanswered questions with regard to Reye's syndrome relative to etiology, optimum therapeutic management, and subsequent capability to prevent this disorder. Until further information is available, the correct therapeutic approach is not known. It does appear from recent information that therapy to reduce cerebral edema may be an important facet in treatment. Measurement of intracranial pressure, either using the Richmond bolt technique or by placement of an interventricular catheter, appears necessary to monitor cerebral edema. Measures utilized for controlling cerebral edema include administration of mannitol, dexamethasone, diuretics, restriction of fluid intake, hypothermia, and administration of barbiturates in relatively large doses. Other therapeutic measures that may be utilized include the oral administration of nonabsorbable antibiotics and maintenance of normoglycemia.

HEMOLYTIC UREMIC SYNDROME
■ What is the hemolytic uremic syndrome and what causes it?

The hemolytic uremic syndrome is the most common cause of acute renal failure in infants. The sexes are affected equally. There is usually a seasonal incidence, with the peak occurring in late summer or early fall. Involvement of more than one member of the family has been reported on several occasions. Definite evidence for infection as a cause of this condition has largely been negative, although several viruses have been isolated in individual cases.

■ What are the clinical features of the syndrome?

The disease attacks infants who previously were well; more rarely it occurs in older children. There is a predromal stage that lasts from a few hours to several days. The most common symptoms in this stage are gastrointestinal disorders, diarrhea is quite characteristic, and there may be abdominal pain, vomiting, and occasionally hematemesis. Fever occurs in about half the cases; temperature is usually moderate (38° to 39° C). There may be enlargement of the lymph nodes or rash. The syndrome may also develop without any prodromal symptoms. The principal signs of the disease in the acute phase are the simultaneous appearance of hemolytic anemia, hematuria or anuria, and thrombocytopenia.

■ Is the hemolytic anemia severe?

Hemolytic anemia is rapid in onset and very severe and may worsen in subsequent exacerbations. The red blood cell count may fall to 2 million/mm^3 in 24 hours. The hemolytic nature of this anemia is demonstrated by a high level of reticulocytes in circulating blood and an increase in erythroblastosis in the bone marrow with the passage of normoblasts in the peripheral blood. Generally the serum bilirubin level is only slightly elevated. The red blood cells are very deformed, and there are numerous schistocytes. Although the deformities are not specific, they are a constant feature of this syndrome.

■ Are there disturbances of coagulation?

Coagulation disorders are almost a constant feature, often appearing at the onset of the disease, and are manifested by purpura, cutaneous ecchymosis, and gastrointestinal bleeding. Cerebral hemorrhage is rare but has been seen. The bleeding time is frequently prolonged, and in nearly every case there is considerable thrombocytopenia with a platelet count below 100,000. The half-life of the platelets is diminished. The thrombocytopenia rarely persists for more than 8 days. There is a variability in the coagulation factors from patient to patient and from day to day. However, these factors suggest that localized intravascular coagulation does play a part in the pathophysiology of the syndrome.

■ What are the renal manifestations?

The renal manifestations appear at the same time as the anemia and are manifested either by signs of acute glomerulonephritis with or without a decrease in urine output or by total anuria. When the urine output is maintained, there is nearly always hematuria (often macroscopic) and proteinuria that may be sufficient to produce the nephrotic syndrome with edema. The blood urea nitrogen is nearly always elevated on the first examination. Anuria at the onset is very common in infants. The few milliliters of urine that are passed contain a very large number of red blood cells, and there is a special risk of hyperkalemia in these infants because of hemolysis.

■ How are the cardiovascular system and CNS affected?

Blood pressure is elevated in more than half of the cases. The hypertension may appear in the initial stages. It is generally moderate with systolic blood pressures of 140 mm Hg but rarely may be more severe and can lead to cardiac failure. Neurologic signs are particularly common in infants. Convulsions may occur at the onset of the disease. The cerebrospinal fluid is generally normal.

■ What is the prognosis of this condition?

The majority of children under the age of 2 years recover without ill effects. In children more than 2 years of age the prognosis is not as good. Two thirds of these cases proceed to progressive renal failure with malignant hypertension. There has never been demonstrated a relapse of the hemolytic uremic syndrome after recovery or a deterioration in renal function in patients clinically cured after the acute episode. However, hypertension and later neurologic complications have been reported.

■ How is the syndrome treated?

In the absence of precise etiology the specific treatment is based on the hypothesis that there is a process of intravascular coagulation in the hemolytic syndrome. The logical treatment is to use heparin to prevent the formation of new fibrin deposits or to accelerate the process of fibrinolysis by plasminogen activators. Heparin therapy has been used for some years. It is impossible to be certain that the treatment is effective in view of the unpredictable course of the untreated disease and the absence of any controlled trials. Despite this, heparin is widely used. The daily dose of heparin in infants is 8 to 10 mg/kg/24 hours injected continuously into a vein by means of an infusion pump. The therapy is controlled by measuring the clotting time twice a day using micromethods. Treatment is generally continued for 10 to 15 days. If there is a risk of hemorrhage from a therapeutic maneuver such as peritoneal dialysis, the action of heparin should be neutralized by protamine immediately before the particular procedure and the heparin therapy resumed immediately afterward. Therapy by fibrinolysis activators such as streptokinase and urokinase has been used, but there is no real proof of effectiveness.

Anemia is cautiously corrected by transfusion. Hypotensive drugs are used to control blood pressure. Steroid therapy is ineffective.

■ How is renal failure treated?

Early and intensive treatment of the acute renal failure has considerably improved the prognosis of the hemolytic uremic syndrome of infants. This includes the control of hyperkalemia by oral or rectal administration of exchange resins and/or varied and successive IV infusions, limitation of fluid administration, and peritoneal dialysis.

■ How is peritoneal dialysis performed?

There are many techniques of peritoneal dialysis that have been utilized. The following is a brief outline of one method of management that can be utilized in the critical care unit.

Patients may be premedicated, depending on their state of awareness. Skin, subcutaneous tissues, and peritoneum are anesthetized with 1% procaine or lidocaine at a site lateral to the rectus muscle. If the liver is enlarged, the right upper quadrant is avoided; otherwise upper and lower quadrants on either side are suitable. A No. 18 lumbar puncture needle is inserted into the peritoneal cavity and connected to the dialysis administration set. Approximately one third of the calculated volume of dialysis fluid, warmed to body temperature, is administered and the lumbar puncture needle is removed. A 0.5 cm incision is then made in the skin, and an adult-size disposable catheter with a self-contained trocar is advanced until the peritoneal cavity is entered. This is indicated by a sudden decrease in resistance. The trocar is then removed, and the catheter is advanced toward the pelvis. The correct position of the catheter is confirmed by the influx of the previously infused fluid. No sutures are required, and the catheter is kept in place with adhesive tape.

■ Why inject fluid before placing the catheter?

The intraperitoneal administration of dialysis fluid prior to insertion of the catheter facilitates the flow by allowing the catheter to lie free within the peritoneal cavity.

■ What kind of and how much dialysis fluid is used?

The dialysis fluid utilized will vary with the requirements, and it may be necessary to add heparin in a dose of 5 mg/L. The fluid is administered over 10 to 15 minutes. Prophylactic antibiotics are not required. The fluid is allowed to equilibrate over 30 minutes and then is drained in 10 to 15 minutes. In children 6 to 14 years of age 1 L fluid exchanges are performed. In younger children and infants 50 to 100 ml/kg exchange is recommended. The length of dialysis and the total amount of fluid exchanged depends on the requirements of the patient.

■ What causes hyperkalemia?

Increased serum potassium occurs as a result of inadequate renal excretion (acute renal failure) or the accidental administration of potassium.

■ How is hyperkalemia controlled?

In the presence of renal failure a slow rise in serum potassium can usually be controlled with ion-exchange resins. In an emergency a level of 8 to 9 mEq/L may be corrected as indicated subsequently. A serum potassium level of 7 mEq/L not responding to conservative management is an indication for dialysis. The emergency treatment of elevated serum potassium includes the following measures:

1. Slow IV infusion of sodium bicarbonate (3 ml/kg) up to a total of 50 ml
2. Administration of 25% to 50% glucose to provide a dose of 0.5 g of glucose/kg/hr by slow IV drip with 1 unit of regular insulin added to each 2 g of glucose

For the slow increase in serum potassium caused by renal failure sodium polystyrene sulfonate (Kayexalate) resin may be given orally in a dose of 1 g/kg up to 20 g mixed with 50 to 75 ml of water or a dose of 2 g/kg up to 40 g mixed with 100 ml of water as a retention enema. Repeat doses of Kayexalate resin should be based

on determinations of the serum potassium level.

The T wave of the ECG provides a means of observing changes in cellular potassium without serum determinations. As the potassium concentration increases, the T wave increases in height and becomes sharply spiked.

■ What are hypoxic spells?

One of the complications of cyanotic congenital heart disease is the so-called hypoxic spells, also known as blue spells, anoxic spells, paroxysmal dyspnea, syncopal attacks, and paroxysmal hyperpnea. These spells are characterized by an increasing rate and depth of respiration with increasing cyanosis often associated with crying, progressing to limpness and syncope, and occasionally ending in convulsions, cerebrovascular accidents, and/or death. Cerebrovascular accidents are most likely to occur in infants with relative iron deficiency anemias or in infants with hematocrits over 70%. These episodes occur in the tetralogy of Fallot, pulmonary atresia, tricuspid atresia, and similar cyanotic congenital defects, but are rarely if ever found in transposition of the great arteries.

■ What causes hypoxic spells?

The precise etiology of these episodes is not clear. Several theories have been proposed to explain them, and indeed the true etiology may be a combination of all these theories. Hyperpnea or an increase in the depth and rate of respiration appears to be crucial to the beginning of the spell. In normal individuals hyperpnea will increase arterial oxygen saturation. However, in patients with right-to-left shunts hyperpnea causes a decrease in arterial oxygen saturation. Similarly, in the normal individual hyperpnea leads to increased cardiac output of both right and left ventricles, whereas in patients with a fixed resistance to the flow of blood into the lungs, there is an increase in systemic blood flow without a similar increase in pulmonary flow. This leads to a decrease in arterial Po_2 and pH and an increase in Pco_2. These changes tend to stimulate respiration and a vicious cycle is begun.

Another theory of the etiology of these spells suggests that they are caused by obstructive spasm of the right ventricular infundibulum, which may occur as a result of the release of catecholamines. This increase in infundibular obstruction thus decreases pulmonary blood flow and leads to similar changes that result in an increase in respiratory activity. Other explanations of the spells are related to a sudden decrease in systemic vascular resistance or in the development of metabolic acidosis secondary to hypoxia.

HYPOXIC SPELLS
■ When do these spells occur?

The onset of the symptoms may be as early as the first month of life but may occur as late as 12 years of age or older. The peak incidence is between 2 and 3 months of age. In the more severely cyanotic infants the attacks may occur at any time of the day, but in patients with only occasional episodes the attacks commonly occur in the morning after a full night of sleep. Crying, defecation, and feeding are frequent precipitating events. Curiously the attacks are not restricted to patients with severe cyanosis. They have been observed in patients with normal arterial saturations at rest, and some patients with severe desaturation do not develop spells. However, the arterial oxygen saturation during a spell is always low.

■ How is the spell treated?

The treatment of a hypoxic spell requires placement of the child in the knee-chest position, administration of oxygen, and IM administration of morphine sulfate in a dose of 0.1 to 0.2 mg/kg of body weight. Propranolol, 0.1 to 0.2 mg/kg IV, is also effective in aborting a hypoxic spell. Occasionally the IV administration of sodium bicarbonate in a dose of 1 to 3 mg/kg will combat metabolic acidosis.

Some patients with relative anemia will require the transfusion of packed red blood cells or the administration of iron to increase the oxygen-carrying capacity of the blood. In patients with severe polycythemia a partial exchange transfusion with plasma to reduce the hematocrit to 70% may be necessary. Propranolol in a dose of 1 mg/kg given every 6 hours night and day may prevent hypoxic episodes. Usually one hypoxic episode is an absolute indication for some type of surgery to improve pulmonary blood flow.

CONGESTIVE HEART FAILURE
■ What is heart failure?

Heart failure is defined as the state in which the heart fails to maintain an adequate circulation for the needs of the body despite a satisfactory venous filling pressure. The heart compensates for the increased demands of the body by changing the strength of cardiac contraction and varying the heart rate. The strength of cardiac contraction for short-term needs is increased by adrenaline, sympathetic tone, and increased diastolic filling of the ventricles. For long-term needs increased cardiac contraction is maintained by cardiac hypertrophy. Drugs such as digitalis also increase the strength of cardiac contraction. (The effect on the strength of cardiac contraction by a drug is known as an inotropic effect.) An increase in heart rate increases cardiac output until a critical rate is reached (about 180 beats/min). Above the critical rate cardiac output falls because the decrease in diastolic time prevents adequate filling of the ventricles. At this point coronary flow becomes inadequate, and the mechanical efficiency of the heart falls. Cardiac failure occurs when the previously mentioned mechanisms fail and the ventricles become overdistended in diastole. Cardiac failure may occur with high cardiac output such as in thyrotoxicosis, anemia, and arteriovenous fistula, but it is more commonly seen with low cardiac output. The increased diastolic pressure of the failing ventricle raises left atrial and pulmonary venous pressure, increasing lung volume. The increased right atrial and peripheral venous pressure rises, distending the liver and peripheral veins. Cerebral and coronary circulation are maintained at almost normal levels initially, but renal blood flow is reduced, leading to oliguria, salt and water retention, and edema. Cardiac failure may occur as a result of increased pressure work of the heart, such as with valvular stenosis; increased volume work of the heart, such as with left-to-right shunts; or damaged ventricular muscle, such as in myocarditis or cardiomyopathy. In the postoperative period cardiac failure may occur from an overloaded vascular system, as with overtransfusion of blood or other fluids, sudden onset of arrhythmias, or anoxemia.

■ What are the signs and symptoms of heart failure?

The manifestations of heart failure are related to impaired myocardial performance and systemic and pulmonary venous congestion.

■ What are the signs of an impaired myocardium?

Cardiac enlargement on chest x-ray films is a most consistent sign of decreased cardiac function and is produced by ventricular dilatation. Tachycardia above 160 beats/min in infants and above 120 beats/min in older children is commonly seen with heart failure. Rates above 220 beats/min should raise the question of paroxysmal supraventricular tachycardia, which may be the cause of congestive heart failure rather than its result. A gallop rhythm is frequently heard in infants and children with congestive heart failure. Cold extremities with weakly palpable peripheral pulses and lowered blood pressure are commonly seen. Bounding arterial pulses in the presence of congestive heart failure are suggestive of a high output state such as patent ductus arteriosus or systemic arteriovenous fistula.

■ How is systemic venous congestion manifested?

The signs of systemic venous congestion include enlargement of the liver, which is usually tender with a rounded edge, and neck vein distention, which can be readily seen in the older child. In the infant this is difficult to assess because of the short neck. Peripheral edema is a rare finding in cardiac failure in infants and young children. Facial edema is more common in a child. Ascites and anasarca are rare except in older children with restrictive pericardial disease or severely compromised myocardial function.

■ How is pulmonary venous congestion manifested?

Tachypnea is a common sign of pulmonary congestion, and respiratory rates greater than 60 respirations/min are not uncommon in infants. Wheezing is a frequent sign of left ventricular failure in infants and may be confused with bronchiolitis. Rales are usually not heard in infants and young children with congestive heart failure.

Sweating, growth failure, and chest deformity are frequently seen in patients with long-standing chronic congestive heart failure.

■ How is heart failure treated?

The treatment of congestive heart failure is directed toward improving myocardial performance and reversing the deranged function of other organ systems. Frequent clinical reappraisal is necessary during treatment to reach the optimum degree of improvement in myocardial performance.

Digitalis is the drug of choice for the management of congestive heart failure. Digoxin is the most widely used digitalis glycoside for infants and children and is available in oral and parenteral preparations. One must be aware of the varying response of patients to this drug and be prepared to adjust the dose depending on the reaction of the individual. This is particularly true in patients with inflammatory disease of the myocardium where there is an increased sensitivity to digitalis glycosides. Orders for the use of digitalis must be explicitly written to include the type of glycoside, the route of administration, the dose in milligrams or micrograms, and the number of milliliters containing this dose. It is important to realize that the oral preparation of digoxin (Lanoxin) contains 0.05 mg/ml, whereas the parenteral form contains 0.25 mg/ml, and the pediatric parenteral form contains 0.1 mg/ml. Recent reports have indicated a variation in the effectiveness of differing digoxin preparations, and it is recommended that only the Burroughs Wellcome brand of digoxin, Lanoxin, be used in infants and children.

■ How is digoxin administered?

The total digitalizing dose for a given patient is calculated on the basis of body weight and age; the following list may serve as a guide:

Birth to 2 mo	0.05 mg/kg
2 mo to 2 yr	0.075 mg/kg
2 yr to 5 yr	0.06 mg/kg
Over 5 yr	0.05 mg/kg

An alternate dosage schedule is 0.6 mg/m^2 for term infants under 1 month of age and premature infants under 2 months of age and 0.9 mg/m^2 for older infants, children, and adults. One half of the digitalizing dose is given immediately and the remainder in two equal doses at 4- to 6-hour intervals. In extremely urgent situations or if perfusion is severely impaired, the initial dose may be given by the IV route, but more commonly digitalization is accomplished by the IM route. This route should not be used in patients with significant peripheral edema or patients in circulatory collapse because of delayed and irregular absorption of the drug. The patient must be watched for evidence of digitalis toxicity, and evaluation of the heart rate and rhythm are particularly necessary prior to the administration of the last one fourth of the digitalizing dose. Adequacy of the total digitalization should be evaluated 4 to 6 hours following the administration of the calculated total digitalizing dose, and if digitalization is complete without evidence of toxicity, orders should then be written for maintenance digitalis, which may be given orally or parenterally. The daily maintenance digoxin dose is one fourth of the total digitalizing dose and is given in two equal doses at 12-hour intervals. Orders should always be written indicating that a dose should be withheld and the patient reevaluated if the heart rate falls below 100 to 120 beats/min for infants and 60 to 80 beats/min in older children or if irregularity is noted. Digitalis toxicity should be treated by immediate cessation of administration, followed by frequent ECG monitoring. With mild intoxication the signs of toxicity will usually disappear in 2 to 3 days. With evidence of severe toxicity or in the presence of hypokalemia the administration of potassium by slow IV infusion at a dose not to exceed 0.5 mEq/kg/24 hr in a patient who has voided is most effective. Phenytoin is an effective drug in the treatment of digitalis-induced tachy- or bradyarrhythmias. Lidocaine, procainamide, and propranolol are effective in treating tachyarrhythmias owing to digitalis. Severe bradyarrhythmias usually are effectively treated with atropine but may require electrical pacing.

■ **Why and how are diuretics used?**

Since abnormal salt and water retention are major manifestations of congestive heart failure, and since the overloaded circulation further hinders myocardial performance, diuretic therapy occupies an important place in the management of congestive heart failure. Furosemide (Lasix) is the most effective diuretic agent available and can be administered by either IV or IM route in a dose of 1 to 2 mg/kg.

Common oral diuretics used in infants and children include chlorothiazide (Diuril), which is given in a dose of 25 mg/kg/day to a maximum of 250 mg/day in two divided doses, and spironolactone (Aldactone), which is given in a dose of 0.7 mg/kg/day in two divided doses.

Other therapeutic measures useful in the treatment of acute congestive failure include elevation of the head and shoulders to an angle of 45 degrees, bedrest, reduction in feedings, decreased intake of sodium, administration of oxygen in up to 50% concentrations with increased humidity up to 80%, and administration of antibiotics if infection is suspected. In acute pulmonary edema, sedation with morphine sulfate (0.1 mg/kg) and tourniquets on three extremities rotated every 10 to 15 minutes may be helpful. If pulmonary edema has been precipitated by rapid infusion of fluids or blood, removal of blood by venipuncture may be of value.

ARRHYTHMIAS

Abnormal cardiac rhythm in the pediatric patient is of importance when it affects the cardiac output, and in a postoperative patient it can lead to ineffective cardiac pumping. Anoxia, drugs, uremia, or surgical trauma to the conducting system must be considered as possible causes of arrhythmias. The diagnosis of arrhythmia must be made by interpretation of the ECG and may be classified into ectopic beats, tachycardias, and heart block.

■ **What is the significance of ectopic beats?**

Single ectopic beats may originate in the atrium, junctional or nodal area, or ventricle. They may occur singly or in a repetitive fashion associated with normal beats such as in a bigeminy or trigeminy. Those ectopic beats arising in the atrial or nodal areas usually do not require treatment. Ventricular premature beats, if they are frequent or if they occur from more than one focus, may be a prelude to more severe ventricular arrhythmias. Digitalis toxicity often leads to ventricular arrhythmias. Treatment is most often effective with lidocaine, procainamide, quinidine, and propranolol.

Frequent unifocal ventricular ectopic beats including bigeminy may occur in children with no heart disease. Treatment is usually not necessary.

■ **What are tachycardias and how are they treated?**

Tachycardias include sinus tachycardia, paroxysmal supraventricular tachycardia, and ventricular tachycardia. Sinus tachycardia is usually present at rates between 150 and 200 beats/min. The rate will usually vary slightly in the ECG, and each ventricular complex is preceded by P waves. Treatment should be directed to the cause of sinus tachycardia, such as fever or congestive heart failure.

Paroxysmal supraventricular tachycardia is very common in infants but can occur at any age. Heart rates are usually in excess of 160 beats/min and frequently above 220 beats/min. There may be a history in an older patient of recurrences of tachycardia. The ECG demonstrates the tachycardia occurring at an extremely regular rate without variation. P waves are frequently not visible, but in the rare instance when they are present, there is usually a prolonged P-R interval. The physiologic effect of the tachycardia is to shorten diastole, leading to inadequate cardiac filling and the development of congestive heart failure. The treatment of choice in children is the administration of digitalis, which will cause a reversal of the tachycardia. Cardioversion is effective in restoring normal heart rate and rhythm and is the treatment of first choice in some institutions.

Ventricular tachycardia, which is recognized by the widened abnormal ventricular beats, is of major significance because of the inadequate ventricular filling produced, the resultant diminished cardiac output, and the tendency for ventricular tachycardia to proceed to ventricular fibrillation. Immediate treatment is indicated and the IV administration of lidocaine first as a bolus and then as a drip is usually the first modality utilized. Procainamide and propranolol can be used by IV route. Cardioversion may be necessary to restore normal rhythm. Should the tachycardia proceed to ventricular fibrillation, cardiopulmonary resuscitation and electrical defibrillation are needed.

Atrial fibrillation or flutter, which is occasionally seen in the pediatric age group, is usually associated with a rapid ventricular rate. Initial treatment usually consists of the administration of digitalis to slow the ventricular response and the subsequent administration of quinidine to correct the fibrillation "flutter" to sinus rhythm.

■ **What is heart block?**

Heart block occurs in three degrees. First-degree heart block, which is manifested by prolongation of the P-R interval on the ECG, indicates a delay in the transmission of electrical impulse from the sinus pacemaker through the internodal area. It may be present in rheumatic fever as well as toxic states and is sometimes found in congenital cardiac abnormalities, including endocardial cushion defects or corrected transposition. It occurs after digitalis administration but does not indicate toxicity.

Second-degree heart block is manifested by the failure of an occasional sinus beat to be followed by a ventricular response. This may occur on a regular basis or may be demonstrated by an increasing P-R interval with final failure of the ventricular response (Wenckebach phenomenon).

Third-degree heart block describes a condition where there is no relationship between the atrial and ventricular beats. It may be congenital in origin, secondary to surgical interruption of the bundle of His, or induced by drugs such as digitalis or quinidine. The ventricular rate usually ranges from 30 to 45 beats/min and can produce symptoms related to insufficient cardiac output. Emergency treatment of complete heart block may require the administration of isoproterenol (Isuprel), temporary cardiac pacing, or a permanent pacemaker.

■ **How does the treatment of cardiac arrest differ in infants and children?**

Cardiac arrest is in a sense a severe form of cardiac arrhythmia in which there is failure of the heartbeat. It requires immediate cardiopulmonary resuscitation, including establishment of an airway, ventilation of the patient, and closed chest cardiac massage. It is important to remember in the establishment of an airway in a child that overextension of the head can compress the trachea and close it. Ventilation is most effectively provided by mouth-to-mouth resuscitation, but in a critical care unit intubation and bag ventilation can be effectively performed. Closed chest resuscitation in a newborn or small infant requires the use of two-finger pressure over the midsternum, gradually increasing to one-hand pressure on the lower portion of the sternum in an older child. The sternum should be massaged at a rate of 80 to 100 times/min, with one respiration for about every five chest movements. Sodium bicarbonate should be administered as soon as possible, since acidosis develops rapidly. An ECG should be obtained to determine whether ventricular fibrillation is present, and electrical defibrillation should be done. Other drugs useful in stimulating the arrested heart include isoproterenol, epinephrine, and calcium chloride.

It should be pointed out that resuscitation of a child with cyanotic congenital heart disease is very difficult and seldom successful because of the inability to oxygenate the patient's blood caused by the right-to-left shunt and/or obstruction of the flow of blood to the lungs as a result of the cardiac defect.

■ **What is the etiology of severe hypertension in children?**

Essential hypertension is very rare in children, and a specific etiology must be investigated in every child. The most common cause is renal parenchymal disease such as streptococcal or lupus glomerulonephritis. Surgically correctable lesions such as coarctation of the aorta, unilateral renal disease, renal artery stenosis, or tumors such as pheochromocytoma, neuroblastoma, or Wilms' tumors must be excluded. Significant increase in hypertension is frequently seen postoperatively after the repair of coarctation of the aorta and must be adequately treated because of the danger of mesenteric thrombosis. Increased intracranial pressure caused by space-occupying lesions such as tumor, lead intoxication, or pseudotumor cerebri should be considered. Cushing's disease, primary aldosterone, familial dysautonomia, ingestion of excessive amounts of licorice, and chronic administration of glucocorticoids, oral contraceptives, or androgens should also be considered. Whenever possible, the investigation into the cause of hypertension should be completed before therapy is initiated. In the acute hypertensive crisis this may not be possible, but as much of the investigation as is feasible should be done.

■ **What is the treatment of severe hypertension in children?**

Malignant hypertension, hypertensive encephalopathy, and acute left ventricular failure occur as life-threatening emergencies in the hypertensive patient, and rapid reduction in blood pressure is necessary. The vasodilator drugs are the most effective rapidly acting antihypertensive drugs. Diazoxide must be given by rapid IV push and is not effective if injected slowly. It is usually effective for 4 to 6 hours. Diazoxide has a sodium retention property and requires the concurrent use of a diuretic. Sodium nitroprusside must be given by continuous pump infusion. An initial rate of 0.1 mg/kg/min is slowly increased until the desired effect is obtained or to a maximum of 10 mg/kg/min. The usual effective dose is 1 to 3 mg/kg/min. Sodium nitroprusside is converted to thiocyanate in the body, and cyanide poisoning has occurred with its use. Serum thiocyanate levels should be monitored and the drug discontinued if the serum level is greater than 12 mg%. Cyanide poisoning may be prevented by the concurrent use of hydroxycobalamin (Vitamin B_{12a}). Hydralazine, although less effective than diazoxide or nitroprusside, has been safely and effectively used in children for many years and is the preferred drug in many centers.

Magnesium sulfate, 50% IM, was frequently used in the past to rapidly reduce blood pressure. However, it is rarely used today because of marked irritation and pain locally, respiratory depression, and occasional severe hypotension.

Diuretics are frequently used as the primary drug in the treatment of mild hypertension. They are a valuable adjunct to more effective drugs in hypertensive crises. Chlorothiazide and furosemide are the most commonly used diuretics. Chlorothiazide is usually preferred because of its more prolonged action. Chlorothiazide and furosemide result in a potassium diuresis. Spirono-lactone, a very mild diuretic with potassium-retaining properties, may be used as second diuretic, or potassium supplements should be given. Fluid restriction may be valuable. Marked sodium restriction is usually not necessary when potent diuretics are being used.

■ What is pseudotumor cerebri?

Pseudotumor cerebri is a condition causing increased intracranial pressure in children, often mimicking the findings in a brain tumor. It should be considered in any child with symptoms of increased intracranial pressure, such as nausea and vomiting, severe headaches, and transient visual disturbance. On physical examination, papilledema is usually present. Blood pressure may be elevated and pulse and respiratory rates reduced. In infants a bulging fontanel and increasing head size are usually present. In older children nuchal rigidity or separation of the sutures is present. Cerebrospinal fluid pressure is markedly elevated without cellular or chemical abnormalities. CAT scanning or pneumoventriculography reveals normal or small ventricles. It is often the result of an aseptic occlusion of one of the lateral sinuses or the longitudinal sinuses. Pseudotumor cerebri may follow a viral infection or a minor head injury, but it has been frequently associated with the use of drugs in children. Tetracycline, nalidixic acid, hypervitaminosis A, and the chronic use of corticosteroids have been most frequently implicated. It can also follow the rapid withdrawal of corticosteroids after several months of use. Hypoparathyroidism and Addison's disease are rare causes of this syndrome. Reye's syndrome and lead poisoning should be considered in children with increased intracranial pressure.

■ What is the treatment of increased intracranial pressure in children?

The most effective treatment of increased intracranial pressure is the removal of the primary cause when this is possible. This can be the removal of an intracranial mass, evacuation of a subdural or epidural hematoma, or decrease of ventricular enlargement by a shunt procedure.

If there is a rapid or progressive neurologic deterioration or signs of impending herniation, rapid reduction in intracranial pressure is necessary. The initial step in treatment is immediate hyperventilation by mask or endotracheal tube to rapidly reduce Pco_2. Elevation of Pco_2 produces potent cerebral vasodilation. Hyperventilation results in cerebral vasoconstriction, decreasing intracerebral volume and pressure. In the infant with an open fontanel or the child with a burr hole, prompt evacuation of a few milliliters of ventricular fluid is a very effective means of reducing pressure. Lumbar puncture for removal of fluid is contraindicated in these patients because of the danger of herniation through the foramen magnum.

Osmolar diuretics and steroids are used extensively to reduce intracranial pressure. Mannitol is the most widely used agent; 1.5 to 2 g/kg of 20% mannitol is given IV over 30 to 60 minutes every 6 hours. Mannitol remains in the extracellular space and is rapidly excreted by the kidneys. It is preferable to urea as there is less rebound effect between doses. The rebound phenomenon can be reduced by water restriction. When used with fluid restriction, serum hyperosmolarity and hyperkalemia may develop, especially if renal function is impaired. Without fluid restriction, the increased blood volume can result in fluid overload and frank congestive heart failure. Osmotic diuretics therefore must be used with caution. Fluid restriction is usually the safer course. Maintenance fluids should be limited to 1000 ml/m²/day.

Glycerol is an osmotic diuretic that can be given orally; 1.5 to 2 g/kg can be given two to four times daily. It is mixed with fruit juices to decrease nausea and vomiting. There are more fluctuations in pressure between doses than with mannitol and urea, which limits its use. It is, however, a useful adjunct in patients receiving irradiation for cerebral tumors or for outpatient maintenance of the patient with pseudotumor cerebri. Obesity is a common complication of prolonged usage since a 50 kg child receives 650 calories per day from the glycerol. It can also lead to nonketogenic hyperglycemia and glycosuria. Acetazolamide is a useful adjunct to the osmolar diuretics but may result in a metabolic acidosis. Serum electrolytes and blood gases should be monitored when acetazolamide is used.

Corticosteroids are the most widely used drugs for the treatment of increased intracranial pressure. Dexamethasone, 0.25 to 0.5 mg/kg/day to a maximum of 16 mg daily, is the preferred steroid. Improvement is usually delayed 8 to 24 hours after initiation of therapy. Therefore osmotic diuretics are usually started in conjunction with dexamethasone for the acutely ill child.

Hypothermia is a useful adjunct in the treatment of cerebral hypertension, especially for head trauma and acute cerebral edema following hypoxia from drowning or cardiac arrest. Shivering should be prevented in the hypothermic patient. Chlorpromazine is effective in preventing shivering in hypothermic patients. General supportive measures are imperative. The airway must be maintained and ventilatory assistance may be necessary. Frequent suctioning of the airway and emptying of the gastric contents by nasogastric tube are important. Vital signs must be monitored closely. Anticonvulsants may be necessary to control seizures. Recent studies have indicated that large doses of barbiturates may be effective in reducing increased intracranial pressure.

An indwelling urethral catheter may be necessary to prevent urinary retention and to accurately measure intake and output. Acid-base and electrolyte status should be monitored. A central venous catheter is often useful in the management of fluid balance.

■ **What are the sources of lead poisoning in children?**

The ingestion of lead-containing paint remains the major source of lead poisoning in children. The sale of paint containing more than 0.5% lead has been banned for home use in the United States since 1973. However, the incidence of lead-containing paints in homes remains high, especially in low socioeconomic areas. Inhaled airborne lead is an additional hazard especially in urban areas as a result of automobile emission from ethyl-containing gasoline. Lead poisoning can follow the burning of lead battery casings and is not uncommon in residents living near lead smelters. Lead poisoning is common in Scotland where lead tanks and pipes result in a high lead content in home drinking water. Lead poisoning has also been reported from the ingestion of the paint on pencils or colored illustrations such as those used in comic books and newspapers. The safety of canned foods, especially fruit juices, has been a concern as a source of lead. This has been less of a problem since the Food and Drug Administration began monitoring the lead content of canned foods and the manufacturers' safety efforts.

■ **What are the symptoms and findings of lead poisoning in children?**

Lead poisoning should be considered in any child with evidence of increased intracranial pressure and any child with a history of pica.

Acute lead poisoning is rare. Nausea, vomiting, and abdominal pain are usually followed by paresthesia, muscle pain, weakness, and pallor. Anemia, hemoglobinuria, and renal damage is common. Death is usually from shock.

Chronic lead poisoning may be asymptomatic or be seen as a severe encephalopathy. Symptoms may follow a mild infection caused by release of lead from bones during infections. Mild symptoms include weakness, pallor, irritability, anorexia, weight loss, pica, vomiting, coliclike abdominal pain, and insomnia. More severe symptoms include peripheral motor paralysis, joint pain, muscular incoordination, hypertension, seizures, stupor, and coma. Encephalopathy is common in children. Abdominal colic is much more common in adults.

Physical examination usually reveals pallor. A lead line may be seen on the gums. The optic disc may reveal edema, and in infants separation of the sutures and a bulging fontanel may be present.

X-ray films of the long bones may reveal a lead line. Lumbar puncture reveals increased intracranial pressure. Protein may be elevated but few cells are present. Albuminuria, hematuria, glycosuria, and aminoaciduria may be present and indicate renal tubular damage.

The diagnosis of lead poisoning is made by an elevated presence of lead in whole blood and increased urine excretion. Urine coproporphyrins are elevated as is the free erythrocyte protoporphyrins. There is usually a moderate microcytic hypochromia, anemia, and basophilia stippling of the red cells. In equivocal cases measurement of increased lead excretion following a single dose of ethylenediaminotetraacetate (EDTA) is diagnostic.

■ What is the treatment of lead poisoning?

Treatment of lead encephalopathy consists of prevention of continued absorption, increase in excretion of lead as well as an increasing deposition in bone, and treatment of the encephalopathy. All sources of lead must be removed from the environment. If acute ingestion is suspected, large amounts of milk are given to form insoluble lead salts in the intestines.

Treatment of lead encephalopathy by correc-

tion of the increased intracranial pressure is immediately initiated using hyperventilation, corticosteroids, and osmotic diuretics. Frequent removal of small quantities of cerebrospinal fluid by lumbar puncture must be used cautiously because of the danger of herniation.

The primary treatment in lead poisoning is the use of chelating agents. Calcium disodium EDTA, British anti-lewisite (BAL), and penicillamine are available for this use. Salts of EDTA form a nonionized chelate with lead, which is excreted in the urine; 75 mg/kg/day is given intravenously, intramuscularly, or subcutaneous-

Table 40-6. Drug dosages and therapeutic measures not given in the text

Agents	Dosage
Diuretics	
Chlorothiazide (Diuril)	10-40 mg/kg/day PO in 2 divided doses
Furosemide (Lasix)	1-2 mg/kg/dose, PO or IV, 1-3 times daily
Spironolactone (Aldactone)	2-3 mg/kg/day PO
Mannitol	1 g/kg by slow IV drip
Urea	800 mg/kg/day IV
Acetazolamide (Diamox)	5 mg/kg/day PO
Antihypertensive agents	
Sodium nitroprusside (Nipride)	1-10 μg/kg/min IV
Diazoxide (Hyperstat)	5 mg/kg rapid IV push
Hydralazine (Apresoline)	0.75-5 mg/kg/day in 4-6 doses PO; 0.15 mg/kg/dose IM or IV
Reserpine (Serpasil)	0.02-0.15 mg/kg/day PO; 70 μg/kg/dose, 1-6 times daily IM
Methyldopa (Aldomet)	10-65 mg/kg/day in 3-4 doses PO; 2-10 mg/kg/dose IV
Magnesium sulfate, 50%	0.2 ml/kg IM
Cardiotonic drugs	
Epinephrine	0.5 μg/kg/min IV drip
In cardiac arrest	1-4 ml of 1:10,000 dilution by slow IV push
Isoproterenol (Isuprel)	1 mg in 250 ml 5% glucose in water to make 4 μg/ml given as IV drip and titrated to heart rate; start with 0.05 μg/kg/min
Calcium chloride	1-4 ml 10% by slow IV push
Dopamine (Intropin)	2-5 μg/kg/min starting dose to maximum 50 μg/kg/min; 200 mg in 250 ml fluid to make 0.8 mg/ml
Antiarrhythmic agents	
Lidocaine (Xylocaine)	1 mg/kg IV every 3-5 min by bolus as loading dose, then 50 ml 2% in 200 ml 5% glucose in water to make 4 mg/ml; start with 0.04 mg/kg/min as continuous drip
Procainamide	2-2.5 mg/kg by slow IV push as loading dose, then 0.04-0.08 mg/kg/min; 30 mg/lb/day PO
Quinidine	12-30 mg/kg/day
Propranolol (Inderal)	0.1 mg/kg by slow IV push, 0.5-2 mg/kg/day in 3-4 divided doses PO
Sodium bicarbonate	1-5 mEq/kg IM, repeated at 5-10 min intervals
Atropine	0.01 mg/kg/dose
Phenytoin (Dilantin)	3-5 mg/kg by slow IV push 4 times daily
Cardioversion or electrical defibrillation	2-5 watt-seconds/kg (if >50 kg, 400 watt-seconds)

ly in four to six divided doses, after a test dose of 200 mg in 200 ml 5% dextrose in water IV over an hour. EDTA should not be used if lead is still present in the intestinal tract as it facilitates absorption of lead from the intestines. EDTA is usually given for 5 to 7 days. If the serum lead level is greater than 80 mg%, BAL, 24 mg/kg/day, is given IM in divided doses. Although BAL increases urinary excretion of lead, it does not affect the body tissue levels and is never used alone in the treatment of lead intoxication. BAL is discontinued after 3 days and a second course given 1 to 2 weeks later if necessary. Penicillamine, 30 to 40 mg/kg, given orally between meals is used for long-term chelation in children who have elevated serum lead levels after parenteral administration. Permission of the FDA is required for this use.

A high intake of calcium, phosphorus, and vitamin D diminishes the solubility of lead and increases its deposition in the bone. Acidosis increases ionization of lead and decreases bone deposition. Correction of acidosis is important in the treatment of lead poisoning. Sodium citrate, 1 to 2 g, orally three times a day not only is effective in control of acidosis but forms a soluble complex with lead that is excreted in the urine, resulting in a lowered blood lead level. Infections must be adequately treated because of the mobilization of lead from bone during infectious illnesses.

Table 40-6 indicates drug dosages and therapeutic measures not given in the text.

SHOCK
■ What is shock?

Shock is a term used to describe a syndrome in which the patient exhibits a number of characteristic signs. These include ashen skin; oral mucous membranes that are pale and dry; cold, clammy extremities; decrease in temperature; a fast, thready pulse; low blood pressure; CNS depression or restlessness; thirst; and decreased or absent urinary flow. These signs are either caused by the decreased blood flow that is a major part of shock or are the result of compensatory sympathetic activity. Shock is not a single entity but may be caused by a variety of factors and mechanisms. The common denominator is a reduction in blood flow and resulting abnormalities

of tissue metabolism. Shock may be produced by a loss of blood volume (hypovolemia), such as in acute blood loss with hemorrhagic or traumatic shock; a loss of plasma, such as in burn shock or dehydration; secondary to a disturbance in cardiac filling, such as pericardial tamponade, or cardiac emptying, such as in myocardial disease or inflammation; abnormalities of the blood vessels, such as in neurogenic shock, which is a mild form of shock that may be caused by certain humeral influences on blood vessels; and bacteria, which is known as endotoxic shock or septic shock. Shock can be produced by respiratory failure secondary to hyaline membrane disease. It can also be caused by the positive pressure of ventilation used to treat this condition, if used to excess, which can interfere with the filling of the heart. It can occur secondary to a ruptured omphalocele or to hemorrhage caused by DIC.

When the insult causing shock is not severe, various compensatory mechanisms can serve to maintain the cardiovascular system. If the shock is severe and of prolonged duration, the circulation deteriorates and the shock condition is said to be decompensated. Continuation of the shock condition leads to irreversible shock and death.

■ What is the pathophysiology of shock?

The pathophysiology of shock is best illustrated by blood loss. Following reduction of blood volume, compensation occurs by a decrease in venous capacity and an increase in cardiac emptying. There is vasoconstriction of the blood vessels in the limbs, splanchnic organs, and kidneys, so that there is preferential blood circulation to the heart and brain. Initially the sympathetic nervous system helps to maintain the arterial blood pressure. The vasoconstriction of the splanchnic and renal vessels leads to metabolic acidosis, and the acidosis results in the decreased ability of the cardiovascular system to respond to catecholamines, the mediating agent of the sympathetic nervous system. As acidosis increases, capillary sphincter tone decreases, and this leads to an increase of blood flow into the capillary beds, which results in an engorgement of capillaries and transudation of fluid into the extracellular space. In general when the blood volume is reduced to 60% to 70% of normal, signs of shock are clearly evident. If these volume deficiencies remain uncorrected, the reductions of volume, pressure, and flow, instead of being minimized by compensatory mechanisms, may become progressively more severe.

■ **What parameters should be monitored in shock?**

In the management of the patient with shock it is important to monitor central venous pressure, blood pressure, cardiac output if possible, blood gas concentrations, urinary output, body weight, hematocrit and white blood cell count, sodium, potassium, chloride, blood urea nitrogen, and creatinine concentrations, and in the newborn, glucose levels.

■ **How is shock treated?**

Treatment of the condition involves first treating the primary causes, if known. Respiratory assistance with tracheostomy or an endotracheal tube may be necessary. In shock associated with increased central venous pressure myocardial failure must be considered, and treatment utilizing digitalis and diuretics would be indicated. Abnormal heart rhythm or rates must be controlled. Acidosis must be corrected. In the patient with shock and low venous pressure the replacement of blood or electrolytes is mandatory. In patients with a mild decrease in urinary output the use of mannitol is sometimes helpful. Isoproterenol (Isuprel) or dopamine given by IV drip is sometimes helpful in improving myocardial function and peripheral perfusion. Antibiotics are indicated if there is evidence of infection. Steroids may be of benefit in endotoxic and anaphylactic shock.

FLUID AND ELECTROLYTE THERAPY

■ **Why is fluid balance so important in infants and children?**

Even in health the amounts of water, electrolytes, and calories are relatively greater in children than in adults. Water constitutes a greater proportion of the body of a child and the daily turnover of fluid is greater. Infections that bring about increased losses of water are more common in childhood, and the body's responses to them are more violent. Fever, vomiting, and diarrhea

are more frequent and relatively more severe. Therefore in children and infants the maintenance or restoration of normal fluid and electrolyte balance often overshadows specific therapy in importance. This applies to the greatest extent in diarrheal disease, but the fluid management of other conditions associated with fever or vomiting, severe burns, and many surgical conditions is a necessary part of any plan of therapy.

■ **What are the clinical features of dehydration?**

The clinical assessment of dehydration is of great importance. It should be remembered that the usual electrolyte studies give information as to the concentration of electrolytes, and only by inference based on clinical observation and history can one judge abnormalities in the total amounts of electrolytes and fluid. In the infant signs of dehydration are sunken fontanel, sunken eyes, and skin that has lost its elasticity. The last is most easily demonstrated on the skin of the abdomen, which, when picked up, remains in sharp folds. In cases in which water loss has been predominant and the retention of electrolytes has occurred, a doughy thick consistency of the skin may be noted. In older children the severity of dehydration may be difficult to evaluate clinically. In severe cases in which there is poor peripheral circulation the skin is often gray and the extremities are cold and blue. In the child where the loss of water is greater than the loss of electrolytes, there will be elevated levels of sodium and chloride in the serum. As dehydration progresses, renal function diminishes and the dehydration produces high fever, further augmenting the water loss. In severe case signs of CNS dysfunction are frequent, with convulsions that do not respond to calcium or measures taken to reduce the fever. This type of dehydration is known as hypernatremic dehydration.

■ **What types of fluid are available for parenteral therapy?**

Solutions available for parenteral fluid and electrolyte therapy include glucose and water, which is usually given in concentrations of 5% or 10%; sodium chloride, most commonly used as physiologic saline solution (0.85% sodium chloride); Ringer-type solutions, which are essentially sodium chloride with trace minerals added; and poly-ionic solutions such as Darrow's, Butler's and lactated Ringer's or Hartman's solution. Potassium chloride is available to be added to infusions, and alkalinizing solutions such as sodium bicarbonate and sodium lactate are available for the correction of acidosis.

■ **How are parenteral fluids administered?**

Fluids are most efficiently administered by the IV route. This can be by means of a scalp vein needle or a butterfly needle, which is a short segment of straight needle of varying sizes from 18 to 25 gauge connected to a piece of plastic tubing through which the IV solution can be administered. The advantage of these scalp vein needles is that they can be immobilized readily and maintained in a vein. The most frequent sites for administration are in the scalp veins or veins in the hand, wrist, ankle, or foot. IV fluids can also be administered by direct cannulation of larger veins with a metal or plastic needle; they can be given via a cutdown, most commonly in the ankle; recently in children over 15 pounds, we have been introducing a large plastic catheter into the femoral vein by percutaneous Seldinger technique and advancing this into the inferior vena cava for both the administration of fluid and electrolytes and the measurement of central venous pressure.

■ **How are the electrolyte and water requirements estimated?**

Calculation of the fluid used to treat dehydration and electrolyte imbalance consists of two parts: maintenance, which is the intake required by a well infant or child of the same age and size, and replacement, which is the amount required to replace abnormal fluid or electrolyte losses that have occurred and may still be going on.

■ **How are the maintenance requirements calculated?**

Maintenance requirements in an infant or child are most accurately calculated on the basis of the rate of metabolic turnover and are based on the metabolism of 100 calories. Water and electrolyte needs can be determined from caloric turnover. The basic formula for water maintenance by

caloric needs is 100 ml/kg for the first 10 kg, 50 ml/kg for the next 10 kg, and 25 ml/kg for each kilogram more than 20 kg. Corrections must then be utilized for changes in body temperature and activity. Less exact but clinically effective calculations can be obtained from formulas using surface area or body weight. For all infants from age 1 week to adult life the normal requirements per square meter are as follows: water, 1500 to 2000 ml; sodium, 35 to 50 mEq; and potassium, 30 to 40 mEq. These requirements can also be estimated on the basis of body weight. For infants under 1 year of age 150 ml/kg of body weight is the maintenance water requirement. From ages 1 to 2 years the requirement is 125 ml/kg, and from 2 to 4 years of age 100 ml/kg is needed. After the age of 4 years the amount gradually decreases to 70 ml/kg at 10 years of age. The requirements for sodium of an infant 1 to 6 months of age are 15 mEq/day, for 6 months to 2 years of age they are 22 to 30 mEq/day, and for older children 30 to 60 mEq/day is required. Requirements for potassium of infants weighing up to 10 kg are 3 mEq/kg/day; for children weighing 10 to 20 kg the requirements are 1 to 2 mEq/kg/day; and for children weighing 20 to 70 kg 1 mEq/kg/day is required.

■ **How is replacement therapy calculated?**

Replacement therapy is estimated on the basis of the patient's body weight. The amount of fluid lost is estimated from the following considerations: loss of 5% of the body weight in fluid is the smallest amount clinically detectable, and loss of 20% is about the maximum compatible with life. Children moribund from dehydration are therefore estimated to have lost 10% of their body weight. Moderately dehydrated children are estimated to have lost 10% of their body weight. In mild dehydration the weight loss is assumed to be 5% of body weight. Fluid used for replacement therapy is essentially saline solution modified to include potassium if there is potassium deficiency and bicarbonate or lactate if there is acidosis. In a patient in a moribund state and in circulatory collapse the initial fluid should be isotonic saline solution, plasma, albumin solution, or blood. The primary object in this case is to restore circulating blood volume. In this instance 20 to 30 ml/kg or 350 ml/m² is injected over the first hour. At the end of this time the rate of administration is changed to permit normal replacement. Essentially calculations are made for the total needs of the infant based on maintenance plus replacement therapy. This is given over a 24-hour period, depending on the infant's condition. The initial therapy may be given more rapidly if there is circulatory embarrassment. In a patient with hypernatremia it is essential to correct electrolyte and fluid imbalance slowly so as not to produce cerebral edema or changes in brain volume.

■ What is hypernatremia and how is it treated?

Hypernatremia or hyperelectrolytemia is caused by fluid loss in excess of electrolytes and/or excessive intake of electrolytes. It results in a higher mortality and morbidity than other forms of dehydration. It occurs frequently in infants with diarrhea, especially if treated with boiled skim milk or family-prepared electrolyte solutions.

In hypernatremia most of the fluid loss is intracellular. Therefore the patient appears much less dehydrated than he actually is. The skin, especially on the abdomen, may feel doughy or scleremic. The infants are usually lethargic with a high-pitched cry and twitching. Convulsions are common.

In hypernatremia the high extracellular osmotic pressure draws fluid from the intracellular fluid into the circulation. This results in stretching and rupture of intracerebral vessels passing from the brain to the dura and may result in subdural hematomas or hygromas and permanent CNS damage.

The treatment of hypernatremic dehydration must be slow. Too rapid correction of hypernatremia may result in water intoxication, rapid increase in intracranial pressure owing to fluid leaving the circulation and entering the intracellular compartment, seizures, and often brain damage.

If the patient is in shock, plasma or albumin, 350 ml/m², should be given in the first 30 to 60 minutes. For the next 24 hours a solution of 5% dextrose in approximately one-fourth normal saline should be given. When urination is established, potassium chloride, 15 to 40 mEq/L, should be added. A multiple electrolyte solution such as Isolyte P can be used. A severely dehydrated child should receive 3000 ml/m², a moderately dehydrated child 2500 ml/m², and a mildly dehydrated child 2000 ml/m² on the first day. After the first day, 2000 ml/m² for excessive fluid loss by diarrhea or vomiting can be given. This regimen should correct the dehydration and electrolyte imbalance in 48 to 72 hours.

If seizures or other signs of water intoxication occur during treatment, 3% sodium chloride solution, 6 ml/kg, can be slowly infused. If overhydration has also occurred from too rapid infusion of fluids, furosemide, 1 mg/kg IV, should be given with the hypertonic saline solution.

■ What is the cause of water intoxication in children and how is it treated?

Water intoxication most often occurs from inappropriately large volumes of hypotonic solutions given intravenously. It can also occur if large volumes of nonelectrolyte-containing fluids are given orally to a child with diarrhea or vomiting. It is occasionally seen in the inappropriate antidiuretic hormone syndrome (ADH) and following the frequent use of potent diuretics combined with salt restriction. It can also occur after too rapid treatment of hypernatremia. In this case the serum sodium level may be normal or high.

Normal daily maintenance for a newborn infant is approximately 300 ml. A 250 ml bottle of fluid allowed to run over a shift will result in severe fluid overload. Infants should have a plastic reservoir in the tubing holding 50 to 100 ml, which limits the fluid the infant can receive. The tubing should be calibrated to 60 drops/ml rather than 15 drops/ml, which is usually used in adults. The reservoir should not contain more fluid than the child is to receive in an 8-hour shift.

Inappropriate ADH in children occurs most frequently after neurosurgery, especially surgery for midbrain tumors. It may occur in patients with head injuries, meningitis, encephalitis, Guillain Barré syndrome, pituitary tumors, and occasionally pneumonia. It can be a side-effect of many drugs including diuretics, diazoxide, antineoplastic drugs, or analgesics. It may be seen after cardiopulmonary bypass or other major surgery. Inappropriate ADH should be suspected in a hyponatremic patient if urine osmolality is higher than serum osmolality. Urine volume may be low in spite of administration of diuretics.

Symptoms of water intoxication are confusion, delerium, stupor or coma, and convulsions. Although total body fluids are increased, frank edema may not be present.

The primary treatment is water restriction. Daily fluid intake should not exceed insensible loss (350 to 500 ml/m²) plus urine volume. Dextrose, 5% in 0.45 to 0.9 NaCl, should be used. If hypokalemic or normokalemic, potassium chloride, 20 to 40 mEq/L, should be included.

If convulsions or other significant neurologic symptoms are present, hypertonic saline solutions can be used; 6 to 12 ml/kg of 3% sodium chloride will increase the serum sodium level 5 to 10 mEq%. This should be given slowly over a 30- to 60-minute period. Furosemide, 1 mg/kg IV, should be given with the hypertonic solution to induce a rapid diuresis. After the infusion, total oral and intravenous fluids should be limited to 125 ml/m² over the next 6 hours.

Replacement rules in pediatrics

2.5 ml/kg whole blood will raise the hemoglobin 1 g%.

1.5 ml/kg packed cells will raise the hemoglobin 1 g%.

0.75 ml/kg 7.5% sodium bicarbonate will decrease the base deficit 1 mEq/L.

4 ml/kg ⅙M lactate will decrease the base deficit 1 mEq/L.

1 ml/kg 0.3M tris buffer will decrease the base deficit 1 mEq/L.

A 10 mEq/L correction of the base deficit will raise the serum pH 0.15 units.

In respiratory acidosis an increase in Pco_2 of 10 torr will decrease the pH 0.08 units.

1 ml/kg 7.5 sodium bicarbonate will raise the pH 0.02 units.

1.2 ml/kg 3% sodium chloride will raise serum sodium 1 mEq/L.

0.7 ml/kg 5% sodium chloride will raise serum sodium 1 mEq/L.

2 g/kg rectal Kayexalate will decrease serum potassium 1 mEq/L.

0.6 mEq/kg potassium will raise serum potassium 1 mEq/L.

PATENT DUCTUS ARTERIOSUS

■ Why is patent ductus arteriosus common in premature infants?

In the fetus the ductus arteriosus provides a channel allowing 50% to 60% of the cardiac output to be ejected into the descending aorta without first passing through the lung vessels. At birth there is a sudden rise in systemic vascular resistance caused by the closure of the placental circulation and a drop in pulmonary vascular resistance caused by expansion of the lungs with dilatation of the pulmonary vessels. Thus almost immediately after birth the systemic and pulmonary resistances are approximately equal, and there is little or no flow through the ductus arteriosus in either direction. The ductus arteriosus in the term infant is exquisitely sensitive to the rise in oxygen concentration, resulting in constriction of the ductus followed by structural closure in the first few days of life.

It has been long recognized that the ductus arteriosus frequently remains patent in premature infants and may not close spontaneously for many months. Animal studies have demonstrated that the response of the ductus musculature to oxygen concentration depends on the gestational age of the fetus. It has been estimated that two thirds of all infants with birth weights less than 1750 g have delayed closure of the ductus arteriosus and that the ductus is patent in virtually all infants with birth weights under 1000 g. Suggested causes have included the high threshold of ductus tissue to oxygen, lower pulmonary capillary Po_2 as a result of inadequate ventilation because of weak respiratory musculature or pathologic processes such as hyaline membrane disease, and immature development of the ductus musculature. The latter cause is unlikely, as the ductus can be demonstrated to constrict quite readily with the infusion of acetylcholine and other drugs. The higher incidence of patent ductus arteriosus (PDA) in both term and premature infants born at high altitudes certainly results from the lower Po_2 at high altitudes.

■ How is PDA seen in the premature infant?

The pattern of presentation is closely related to the size of the infant. In infants weighing over 1750 g PDA is seen in a pattern similar to term infants. Usually no murmur or other abnormal findings are noted until 4 to 6 weeks of age. At that time a soft systolic ejection-type murmur is usually heard along the left sternal border. Over the next several weeks to months the murmur becomes louder, the pulses become bounding, and the maximum location of the murmur moves higher to the area of the second intercostal space at the left midclavicular line. In early infancy the findings frequently suggest an interventricular septal defect. The typical machinery murmur extending into diastole may not be present until 6 months to 1 year of age. Some of these infants with large ductus and low pulmonary vascular resistance develop evidence of congestive heart failure, gain weight slowly, or develop recurrent lower respiratory tract infections. Most remain asymptomatic except for the physical findings indicating PDA.

In infants weighing between 1500 and 1750 g the findings usually occur earlier. These infants typically have little if any respiratory distress and appear to be doing well until 1 to 2 weeks of age when a systolic murmur is heard at the upper left sternal border. Over the next several days the murmur becomes louder and more prolonged frequently extending into diastole, and the pulses are noted to be brisk to bounding. The precordium may be hyperactive, and a third sound is frequently noted at the apex. Many of the infants will develop mild respiratory distress at this time. In most infants after 2 to 3 weeks the murmur becomes shorter and softer, pulses diminish, and by 6 weeks of age there is no further evidence of PDA. However, some infants develop evidence of congestive heart failure, and occasionally apneic spells occur. The earlier findings in premature infants appear to be caused by a more rapid fall in pulmonary vascular resistance than occurs in term infants.

Infants with birth weights between 1000 and 1500 g usually have moderate to severe respiratory distress from birth. The infant usually begins to improve after several days and may no longer require oxygen or respiratory assistance. Typically 5 to 8 days after birth a systolic murmur will be heard over the pulmonic area in these infants and may be heard only intermittently for the first few days. The murmur becomes louder and longer, frequently extending into diastole, and pulses become bounding. There is usually an increase in respiratory effort with sternal retractions, indicating the development of congestive heart failure. Increased oxygen is required to prevent hypoxia, and the infant usually requires continuous positive air pressure (CPAP) to maintain adequate pulmonary functions. Increasing end-expiratory pressures become necessary, and frequently the infant will have apneic spells requiring stimulation or the frequent use of respiratory assistance. The heart may be larger than on previous x-ray examinations, but pulmonary vascularity is difficult to differentiate from pulmonary disease.

Infants weighing less than 1000 g almost always have respiratory distress from birth and may require a respirator to assist in breathing. Findings of PDA usually develop at 3 to 5 days of age. If the infant is breathing spontaneously, the development of apneic spells, increasing retractions, a hyperactive precordium, and an increase in the required end-expiratory pressure usually indicate the presence of a significant PDA. If the infant is on a respirator, increasing pressures will usually be required for the maintenance of adequate ventilation to prevent a rising Pco_2. Occasionally a murmur is present. However, murmurs usually cannot be heard if the infant is on a respirator or receiving CPAP therapy. Pulses usually become stronger, and if an arterial catheter is in place, a wide pulse pressure is noted.

■ **How can congestive heart failure caused by PDA be distinguished from progressive pulmonary disease in the premature infant?**

The diagnosis of congestive heart failure is usually not difficult in the term or premature infant without respiratory distress. However, there is little in the physical examination that can readily distinguish whether the symptoms are caused by the cardiac or pulmonary disease. The bounding pulses and murmurs present only confirm that the ductus is patent. Rales are frequently present in either condition, and the liver is usually not markedly enlarged even in the presence of congestive heart failure. X-ray films usually reveal evidence of hyaline membrane disease with a vascularity that is not distinguishable. The heart may be mildly to moderately enlarged.

If an arterial catheter is in place in the upper to midthoracic descending aorta, a single film aortogram can be obtained by rapidly hand-injecting 2 ml of half-strength sodium diatrizoate (Renografin-76) and obtaining a posteroanterior chest film at the end of the injection. If the infant is in congestive heart failure with a large left-to-right shunt, marked filling of the pulmonary arteries will usually be seen. Centers experienced in obtaining echocardiograms on infants have been impressed with the use of measures of left atrial size by this technique to determine the significance of PDA. Normally in infants weighing less than 1300 g the left atrial dimension is 4 to 5 mm, those weighing between 1300 and 2000 g, 5 to 9 mm, and those weighing over 2000 g, 9 to 12 mm. If the left atrial diameter is over 9 mm in premature infants weighing less than 1300 g, over 14 mm in infants weighing from 1300 to 2000 g, or over 17 mm in infants weighing over 2000 g, significant left-to-right shunt with congestive heart failure can be assumed. The ratio of the left atrium to aortic size can also be used. In normal term or premature infants the left atrial:aortic ratio is 0.71 ± 0.13. In infants in congestive failure the left atrial:aortic ratio will be 1.19 ± 0.18 or greater.

Several precautions are necessary in using echocardiograms in infants. It is important that a transducer of the proper size be used. The transducer should measure 5 MHz or greater with a diameter of no more than 3/8 inch. Infants who are undergoing retractions or who have chest deformities will usually have a pancaked left atrium. The usually obtained echocardiogram transecting the pulmonary outflow tract, aortic valve, and left atrium will reveal a normal-sized left atrium and normal left atrial:aortic ratios even in the presence of severe congestive heart failure. To obtain accurate measurements in these infants, the transducer must be placed in the suprasternal notch and directed down and slightly to the left. In this position the beam will transect the right pulmonary artery, arch of the aorta, left atrium, and mitral valve and will give accurate measurements of aortic and left atrial size. Evidence of the accuracy of this method of determining heart failure in these infants can be demonstrated by the rapid fall in left atrial size and left atrial:aortic ratio measurements in those infants who respond to digitilization, the rapid fall to normal of these measurements after surgery in

infants with clinical improvement, and the lack of improvement with surgery in those infants undergoing surgery who had normal left atrial measurements.

■ **How should the older infant with PDA be managed?**

The asymptomatic infant at 2 weeks to 6 months of age with findings typical of PDA needs no treatment. Surgery can be done electively at 1 year of age if the ductus does not close spontaneously.

The infant with evidence of congestive heart failure should be digitalized. Term infants over 1 month of age usually require 60 to 75 μg/kg of digoxin (Lanoxin) as a digitalizing dose. Premature infants are more sensitive to digitalis glucosides than larger infants. A dose of 40 μg of digoxin/kg of body weight is usually adequate for digitalization in these infants. Maintenance requirements are usually 10 to 15 μg/kg given in two divided doses. In acute heart failure salt restriction and diuretics are also helpful. SMA S:26 and Similac PM 60:40 (not regular Similac) have the lowest sodium content of the readily available formulas. Lonolac, a formula very low in sodium, should not be used because of failure to gain weight. Infants on solid feedings should have foods strained in a blender rather than canned baby food, which has a very high sodium content. Many commercial baby food manufacturers are now reducing the sodium content of their products. In the hospitalized infant with congestive heart failure furosemide (Lasix), 1 mg/kg, should be given parenterally. Less ill infants can be given chlorothiazide oral suspension (Diuril), 15 mg/pound/day, or furosemide (Lasix) oral suspension, 1 mg/kg/day. The infant with severe congestive heart failure may be improved significantly by a course of catecholamines administered by a constant infusion pump. Epinephrine, 0.2 to 0.4 mg/kg/min, dopamine, 2 to 5 μg/kg/min, or isoproterenol, 0.1 to 0.25 mg/kg/min, can be given for several hours to prepare the child for cardiac catheterization or surgery as soon as failure and infections are controlled. Cardiac catheterization is indicated only in those infants in whom the diagnosis is in doubt or a second lesion is suspected.

■ How should the premature infant with early evidence of PDA be managed?

The larger premature infant who develops evidence of PDA at 7 to 14 days of age without symptoms requires no treatment. If the infant is anemic, small transfusions should be given until the hematocrit is 40% to 45%. Raising the hematocrit is frequently associated with closure of the ductus within 1 or 2 days. If congestive failure develops, this should be treated and the infant should be taken to surgery as soon as the condition stabilizes. The infant with apneic spells should also have surgical closure of the PDA if a significant left-to-right shunt can be demonstrated by echocardiography, cardiac catheterization, or aortography.

The management is more difficult in the younger infant with respiratory distress, as it is difficult to distinguish the part played by the ductus from that of the respiratory disease. Transfusions, digitalization, diuretics, and oxygen are indicated, and respiratory assistance may be necessary. Indications for surgery differ in centers throughout the country. There is no doubt that many of these infants with large left-to-right shunts caused by PDA will survive without surgery. However, these infants will frequently require long periods of respiratory support and high oxygen concentrations and are likely to develop bronchopulmonary dysplasia. It is in this group of infants that the use of echocardiography using the suprasternal notch approach is of most value.

Those infants in which the left atrial size fails to decrease following digitalization or those having a significant increase in left atrial size following a good response to conservative management should have surgical closure of the ductus performed as soon as possible. Surgery usually is not indicated in those infants without left atrial enlargement, as their symptoms are probably caused by the pulmonary disease.

Cardiac catheterization prior to surgery is indicated only if there is a question of a more complex cardiac lesion or if adequate echocardiographic studies are not available. Cardiac catheterization carries a significant risk in an ill premature infant requiring respiratory assistance, and if necessary, a rapid study sufficient to make a diagnosis is preferable to a complete physiologic study.

Prevention of hypothermia and acidosis during catheterization is important. Minimum amounts of contrast media should be used, as these drugs are very hypertonic and will draw large amounts of fluid into the circulation, resulting in severe overloading of the circulation and an increase in congestive heart failure and pulmonary edema. There is usually a rapid improvement in premature infants with large left-to-right shunts caused by PDA following surgery, and respiratory assistance and oxygen therapy can usually be gradually discontinued over a short period of time.

There has been considerable enthusiasm recently over medical closure of the ductus by the use of prostaglandin synthetase inhibitors. Aspirin has been used to close the patent ductus arteriosus, but indomethacin has become the drug of choice. The usual dosage is 0.1 to 0.3 mg/kg given orally or rectally and repeated in 12 to 24 hours if necessary. While the results have been impressive in many centers, this method should be considered experimental at this time.

HYPERVISCOSITY
■ What is the hyperviscosity syndrome?

Neonates may be severely polycythemic because of excessive placental-fetal transfusion at birth or maternal-fetal or twin-to-twin transfusions. Severe polycythemia is also seen in dysmaturity and small-for-date infants believed to be the result of chronic hypoxia in utero. It has been well recognized that these polycythemic infants have a high incidence of hypoglycemia and hypocalcemia with seizures, lethargy, vomiting, and feeding problems. It is less well recognized that these infants frequently have a course suggesting transposition of the great vessels or other forms of severe cyanotic heart disease, and the syndrome is frequently not recognized until after a normal cardiac catheterization and angiocardiographic study. The infant is plethoric and cyanotic with the cyanosis in the legs frequently appearing greater than that in the arms and face. Respiratory distress may be present. A loud single second sound is heard at the upper left sternal border. A systolic murmur may be present at the lower left sternal border. The liver may be enlarged. The syndrome is seen only in infants with hematocrits above 70%, and the average hematocrit in symptomatic infants is 77%. Polycythemic blood has high viscosity. This results in a decrease in the rate of blood flow and by physical factors alone increases pulmonary vascular resistance to a greater extent than systemic resistance. This results in pulmonary hypertension and a reversal of flow through the ductus arteriosus. The resulting hypoxemia further increases pulmonary vascular resistance by vasoconstriction and prevents closure of the ductus. The high pulmonary pressure is transmitted to the right ventricle, which must act against an increased afterload to eject its contents. Right ventricular end-diastolic pressure increases and with it there is an increase in right atrial pressure that becomes higher than left atrial pressure. This causes the foramen ovale to open and a right-to-left shunt occurs at this level as well. Thus there is a persistence of the fetal circulation in these children. Blood gas determinations reveal a very low Po_2 and oxygen saturation. It must be remembered that sampling from a catheter in the low thoracic or abdominal aorta includes blood that has been shunted right to left through the ductus.

Treatment is by erythropheresis, that is, phlebotomy with replacement of the same quantity of plasma. Enough blood should be removed to reduce the hematocrit to 65%. Symptoms caused by the pulmonary hypertension and persistent fetal circulation will usually be rapidly improved. Lethargy and other evidences of CNS depression are also frequently improved unless resulting from hypocalcemia or hypoglycemia. Serum glucose and calcium levels should be monitored and glucose or calcium given if low. Recognition of this syndrome can prevent unnecessary cardiac catheterization in these ill infants as well as rapidly curing their illness.

BIBLIOGRAPHY

Avery, M. E.: The lung and its disorders in the newborn infant, ed. 2, Philadelphia, 1968, W. B. Saunders Co.

Coleman, A. B., and Alpert, J. J.: Poisoning in children, Pediatr. Clin. North Am. 17:471, 1970.

Cooke, R. E.: Biologic basis of pediatric practice, New York, 1968, McGraw-Hill Book Co.

Guide to diagnosis and management of cystic fibrosis, Atlanta, 1971, Cystic Fibrosis Foundation.

Kendig, E. L., Jr.: Pulmonary disorders. In Kendig, E. L., Jr., editor: Disorders of the respiratory tract in children, vol. 1, ed. 2, Philadelphia, 1972, W. B. Saunders Co.

Lovejoy, F. H., Jr., et al.: Clinical staging in Reye's syndrome, Am. J. Dis. Child. 128:36, 1974.

Reece, R. M.: Manual of emergency pediatrics, ed. 2, Philadelphia, 1978, W. B. Saunders Co.

Rowe, R. D., and Mehrizi, A.: The neonate with congenital heart disease, Philadelphia, 1968, W. B. Saunders Co.

Royer, P., Habib, R., Mathiew, H., and Broyer, M.: Pediatric nephrology, Philadelphia, 1974, W. B. Saunders Co.

Rudolph, A. M.: Congenital diseases of the heart, Chicago, 1974, Year Book Medical Publishers, Inc.

Shirkey, H. C.: Pediatric dosage handbook, ed. 2, Washington, D.C., 1973, American Pharmaceutical Corporation.

Shirkey, H. C., editor: Pediatric therapy, ed. 6, St. Louis, 1980, The C. V. Mosby Co.

CHAPTER 41

Pathophysiology and treatment of circulatory shock

Clayton H. Shatney and Richard C. Lillehei

The definition of shock has always been a source of controversy among investigators. This problem has stemmed in part from the lack of knowledge of the precise pathophysiology of shock. The various types of shock and its many presentations have also added fuel to the debate. Finally, there has been a tendency for each investigator to define shock in terms of the particular aspect under investigation in that laboratory or hospital. Despite these problems, one description of circulatory shock has come to be generally accepted: shock occurs when perfusion of the bodily tissues is inadequate to sustain normal physiologic function.

■ What are the causes of shock?

There are three basic types of circulatory shock: (1) cardiogenic, (2) hemorrhagic (traumatic or oligemic), and (3) septic. Anaphylactic shock is a systemic hypersensitivity reaction, a response to allergen exposure. Although such a reaction can produce some of the classic manifestations of circulatory shock (pallor, hypotension, obtundation), anaphylactic "shock" is usually not considered a form of true shock. It is usually readily managed by the combination of *transient* circulatory and respiratory support and antihistamines. In addition, problems associated with the true shock states, such as coagulation disorders and pulmonary dysfunction, do not generally follow an episode of anaphylactic shock.

Cardiogenic shock occurs when the heart is unable to pump a sufficient volume of blood to the tissues. The most common antecedent event is a massive myocardial infarction, following which there is an inadequate amount of functioning myocardium to meet the circulatory needs of the body. Cardiogenic shock can also occur after open-heart surgery or secondary to severe congestive heart failure caused by coronary artery, valvular, or myocardial disease. Although heart disease is the leading cause of death in the United States, cardiogenic shock is the second most common form of circulatory collapse. Because of its genesis, this form of shock is prevalent in the middle and older age groups.

Hemorrhagic or hypovolemic shock is the most common type of circulatory collapse in our society. Profound hemorrhage is the usual etiology of this form of shock, but it can also occur in patients who become severely dehydrated. Hemorrhagic shock is seen in patients of all ages, but because the most frequent antecedent event is trauma, oligemic shock tends to be most prevalent in the younger, more active age groups.

Septic shock is the third most frequently encountered form of shock, but its incidence is on the rise. It occurs in all age groups and is most prevalent in postoperative patients. Since it is caused by an overwhelming systemic infection, the aged and debilitated are most commonly affected with this condition. Although often used synonymously, a distinction should be made between endotoxin shock and septic shock (Table 41-1). Endotoxin shock is a form of circulatory collapse produced in experimental animals by the

Table 41-1. Comparison of endotoxin and gram-negative shock

Parameter	Cause of shock	
	Endotoxins	Gram-negative bacteria
Mean arterial pressure	Low	Normal-low
Central venous pressure	Low	Low
Total peripheral resistance	High	Low
Cardiac index	Low	High
Arterial O_2 tension	Normal	Low
Pulmonary arteriovenous admixture	Normal	High
Lactic acidemia	High	High

systemic injection of endotoxin, a lipopolysaccharide derived from the cell wall of gram-negative bacteria. Septic shock occurs in man and can be produced by gram-negative or gram-positive bacteria, fungi, yeast, and possibly viruses. Most instances in man are caused by gram-negative bacteria.

■ **What parameters are used to evaluate and treat patients in shock?**

In the past shock was equated with hypotension. However, with the advent of the intensive care unit and the resultant close monitoring of critically ill patients, most investigators realized that there was more to circulatory collapse than simply a decreased blood pressure. As we have become increasingly more sophisticated in the management of these patients, a host of hemodynamic and metabolic disturbances besides hypotension are now known to occur.

The hemodynamic parameters most frequently employed to describe and treat shock are the mean blood pressure, the cardiac output, and the total peripheral vascular resistance. These variables are interrelated by the formula:

$$P = F \times R$$

where P is the mean arterial blood pressure, F represents the systemic blood flow (that is, cardiac output), and R is the total peripheral vascular resistance. Both the mean blood pressure and the cardiac output are directly measurable. The total peripheral resistance (TPR, in dynes-sec/

cm^5), however, is a derived function, that is obtained using the expression:

$$TPR = \frac{\overline{BP} - RAP}{CO} \times 80$$

where $\overline{BP}$ is the mean arterial blood pressure, RAP is the right atrial pressure, CO represents the cardiac output, and 80 is the standard conversion factor in the formula.

Using these hemodynamic variables and other measurable parameters, one can obtain many derived indices that are useful in evaluating and treating the patient in shock. One such function is the systemic oxygen consumption (SOC, in ml/min), which is determined by the following expression:

$$SOC = CO \times (Ao_2 - Vo_2)$$

where Ao_2 and Vo_2 are the arterial and venous oxygen contents, respectively. The SOC indicates the amount of oxygen utilized by the body each minute and thus gives an indication of the aerobic metabolic state.

Another helpful variable, contained in the previous formula, is the arteriovenous oxygen difference, $Ao_2 - Vo_2$. This value is indicative of not only the state of oxygen uptake by the tissues but also the amount of tissue perfusion. Further manipulation of these parameters results in a formula describing the oxygen extraction ratio $\frac{(Ao_2 - Vo_2)}{Ao_2}$, the oxygen availability ($Ao_2 \times CO$), and a number of other variables that help to describe the hemodynamic-metabolic status of the patient in shock. Despite the ready availability of sophisticated equipment and analyses, one must never forget that there is no substitute for frequent, careful clinical assessment of the patient.

■ **What is the pathophysiology of shock?**

Although in the late stages there are many similarities among the various types of shock, the fundamental pathophysiology early in shock differs with each form of circulatory collapse.

Cardiogenic shock

The advent of coronary care units has reduced the incidence of death caused by arrhythmias in the early postinfarction period.[1] However, there has been no change in the incidence of power failure and shock in these patients.[2] In fact, cardiogenic shock is more frequently encountered today because the prevention of deaths from rhythm disturbances has increased the population at risk. At least 15% of patients hospitalized for acute myocardial infarction develop cardiogenic shock.[3]

Cardiogenic shock occurs when there is an insufficient amount of residual functioning myocardium to adequately perfuse the body. Page et al.[4] demonstrated that at least 40% of the left ventricular mass must be lost for shock to occur. This amount of destruction may occur either with a massive acute myocardial infarction or following a succession of smaller infarcts. There does not appear to be a crucial area of the left ventricle that is necessary for proper myocardial function,[5,6] although some studies have demonstrated a high frequency of apical infarction in

patients who develop shock.[4,7] It is most likely that the *total area* of left ventricular damage is the determining factor in the development of shock.

Because of the association between the size of the infarct and the occurrence of cardiogenic shock,[8] there has been a recent renewal of interest in the concept of infarct extension. A number of studies have demonstrated an ischemic zone surrounding a fresh infarct.[4,9] This perimeter of marginally viable or ischemic tissue has the potential to undergo necrosis, thereby extending the area of the original infarct. Reid et al.[10] demonstrated that some infarct extension occurs in 85% of patients following acute myocardial infarction. Through such extension a patient may develop cardiogenic shock several days after the acute insult. In fact, such a delay in the onset of cardiogenic shock is a frequent occurrence in patients with this form of circulatory collapse.

The initiating pathophysiologic event in cardio-

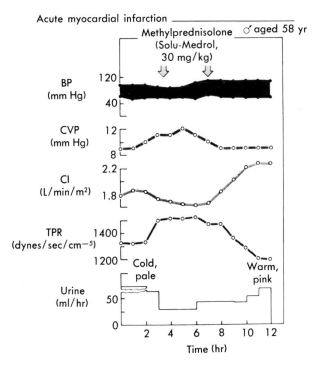

Fig. 41-1. Hemodynamic presentation of cardiogenic shock and the response to methylprednisolone (Solu-Medrol).

genic shock is the acute inability of the heart to adequately perfuse the body. Cardiac output is markedly reduced because of a decrease in myocardial contractility[11] (Fig. 41-1). Coronary blood flow is reduced, and there is a compensatory increase in myocardial oxygen extraction. Myocardial oxygen consumption can vary, but it is usually reduced. Because of the diminished supply of oxygen and nutrients, anaerobic metabolism occurs in the myocardium, as evidenced by excess lactate and lysosomal enzymes in the coronary sinus blood and by an increase in NADH in the ischemic tissue.[11-13] Under the stimuli of hypoxia and acidosis the coronary arteries dilate in an attempt to divert blood to the ischemic myocardium.[14] Delivery of blood to the ischemic tissue, however, may be limited by obstructive disease in the vessels supplying this region.

Within seconds after the onset of ischemia there is a loss of contractile function in the involved myocardium. Intracellular acidosis is thought to be responsible for this change,[15] which probably represents an attempt by the endangered tissue to preserve itself by reducing its metabolic needs. Another compensatory cellular response by the myocardium is the use of glycolysis, rather than the usual oxidation of fatty acids, to generate ATP and maintain cellular viability. These myocardial responses occur immediately after the onset of ischemia. If the hypoperfusion is brief, there is little or no permanent tissue damage. However, with prolonged ischemia myocardial cells in the affected zone are forced to operate with only a limited supply of ATP. With a reduction in blood flow to and lymph and blood flow from the ischemic area,[16] nutrients cannot enter and metabolic waste products cannot leave the cells. Insufficient lymph drainage also causes edema in the ischemic tissue and further compromises the blood supply. Ultimately ion transport is impaired, intracellular metabolic processes are further reduced, and the process of autolysis

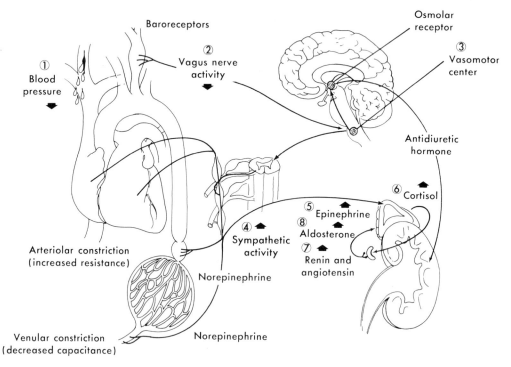

Fig. 41-2. Sympathoadrenal response to circulatory collapse. Circled numbers indicate sequence of events after initiation of sympathoadrenal response.

begins. The point at which myocardial cells become irreversibly damaged is unknown but is thought to be related to the inability of mitochondria to resume ATP synthesis following reperfusion.[17] The influx of calcium into the cell may be related to this mitochondrial inhibition.[18] When the level of ATP generated is insufficient to maintain membrane integrity, lysosomal disruption and cellular autolysis occur.

In addition to these myocardial responses to injury, a number of systemic compensatory changes occur when myocardial contractility is sufficiently reduced to cause a significant drop in the cardiac output (Fig. 41-1). With the fall in cardiac output the blood pressure initially declines. This reduction in systemic perfusion pressure is detected by pressure-sensitive baroreceptors in the aortic arch and carotid sinus (Fig. 41-2). Through a combination of neurologic and humoral (epinephrine and norepinephrine) reactions mediated by the sympathetic nervous system, the body attempts to raise the systemic blood pressure in order to provide a sufficient head of pressure for adequate perfusion. The net result of these neurologic and chemical inputs is an increase in the total peripheral vascular resistance, that is, systemic vasoconstriction in arterioles and venules (Fig. 41-3). The increased total peripheral resistance, which is a systemic compensatory response, further increases the ischemia of the heart by increasing the "afterload," or force required by the heart to expel blood from the left ventricle (Fig. 41-4).

Despite the measurable increase in the total systemic vascular resistance, the caliber of *all* blood vessels is not reduced. Since the distribution of α-receptors, which primarily receive the vasoconstrictor commands of the sympathetic nervous system, is not universal, some vascular beds are not constricted (Fig. 41-5). The heart and brain, for example, contain few α-receptors, and the vessels supplying these vital organs are

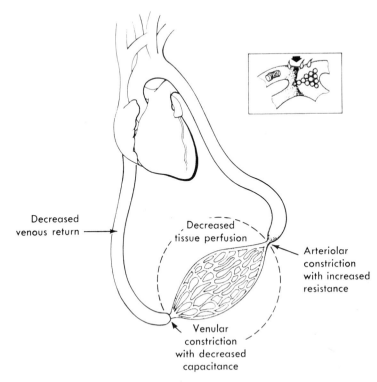

Decreased venous return

Decreased tissue perfusion

Arteriolar constriction with increased resistance

Venular constriction with decreased capacitance

Fig. 41-3. Representation of the pathophysiology of ischemic anoxia in the capillary bed.

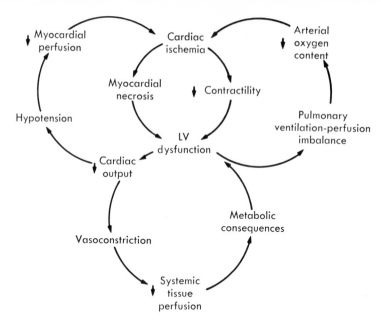

Fig. 41-4. Hemodynamic-metabolic interrelationships creating "vicious cycle" of cardiogenic shock.

largely spared from the early generalized vasoconstriction. Consequently, these organs preferentially receive more blood than other parts of the body during cardiogenic shock.

Shortly after the onset of the initial pathophysiologic changes the secondary effects of cardiogenic shock become evident. As a result of the heightened activity of the sympathetic nervous system and elevated levels of circulating catecholamines, the heart rate increases. The combination of tachycardia and a reduction in cardiac output results in a decreased stroke volume. At this point all indices of left ventricular work are reduced. Depending on the state of hydration of the patient and the magnitude of the pump failure, the central venous pressure and/or the pulmonary artery pressure may rise, and the patient may become dyspneic. Moreover, pulmonary arteriolar and venular constriction further impedes the flow of blood through the lungs and the heart.[19] The reduction in blood flow in the splanchnic circulation produces a drop in the urine output and promotes the release of a pancreatic myocardial depressant substance, which can further impair cardiac contractility.[20,21] Vaso-

constriction in the cutaneous circulation, together with the generalized sympathetic discharge, produces a pale, cool, clammy quality in the skin. The poor perfusion of large areas of the body ultimately results in a decreased oxygen extraction and consumption, accompanied by metabolic acidosis. In the majority of patients the respiratory system initially compensates for this acidosis, but with unrelenting circulatory collapse uncompensated metabolic acidosis eventually occurs.

The hallmarks of cardiogenic shock are therefore hypotension, low cardiac output, elevated peripheral and pulmonary vascular resistance, tachycardia, oliguria, and acidosis. The patient is cold, clammy, and often obtunded. Pulmonary edema is a common finding. The mortality rate in most series is in excess of 80%.[3,11,22]

Hemorrhagic shock

Following the loss of more than 20% of the circulating blood volume, the signs of hypovolemic shock appear. Because of the reduction in intravascular fluid volume, venous return to the heart is decreased.[23] The cardiac output consequently

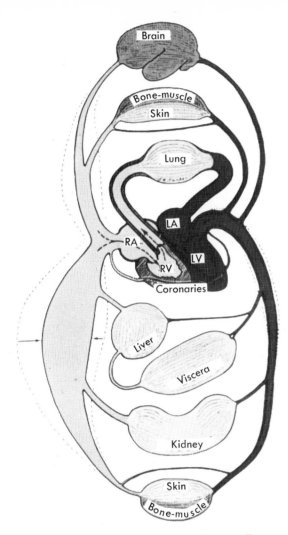

Fig. 41-5. Tissue sensitivity in circulatory collapse. Light-shaded are structures primary target organs affected early in shock.

falls, and, mediated by the baroreceptor system,[24] a sequence of physiologic compensatory events like that in cardiogenic shock occurs.

To maintain a systemic blood pressure sufficient for adequate perfusion, the total peripheral vascular resistance rises.[25,26] Through the combination of a reduction in cardiac output and a decrease in the caliber of the systemic blood vessels, blood flow to the splanchnic, pulmonary,

cutaneous, and muscle beds is sharply reduced.[27-29] Because of local autoregulatory mechanisms, however, not all organs are equally affected.[30] Blood flow in the kidney and liver is not significantly depressed until late in the course of hemorrhagic shock.[29,31-33] After an initial vasoconstrictor response, the blood flow to the muscle mass rises as a result of autoregulatory "escape" from the sympathetic neurohumoral influence.[30] This competition between sympathoadrenal vasoconstriction and autoregulatory dilatation in various organs of the body is the normal physiologic compensatory mechanism that attempts to divert blood flow preferentially to the most vital organs. The net result is that in early hemorrhagic shock there is a redistribution of the cardiac output favoring the heart, brain, kidneys, liver, and adrenal glands.[29,34,35]

The onset of oligemic shock also promotes the redistribution of body fluids in an attempt to increase the circulating intravascular volume. With the exception of muscle,[36] interstitial fluid is transferred from organs to the intravascular compartment at a rate approaching 1 L/hr.[37] Through the combination of a redistribution of renal blood flow within the kidneys and an increase in the circulating level of antidiuretic hormone (ADH), the renal excretion of water is markedly reduced.[38] Although the bowel is capable of normal secretion during early hypovolemic shock,[39] the dramatic reduction in superior mesenteric artery blood flow prevents this potential "third-space" fluid loss within the gastrointestinal tract. The entire organism therefore becomes oriented toward not only retaining fluid but also transferring that fluid to the intravascular compartment.

These volume-regulating compensatory responses are capable of transiently sustaining life and even promoting survival if the duration of shock is brief. With continued blood loss or delayed or inadequate volume replacement, however, the pronounced systemic vasoconstriction and hypovolemia produce ischemia and stagnant hypoxia in the viscerocutaneous circulation. The results of this decreased systemic perfusion are anaerobic cellular metabolism, lactic acidosis, and cell death, all of which further compromise the organism (Fig. 41-6).

It has long been observed that myocardial

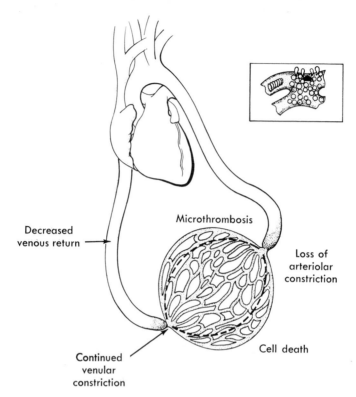

Fig. 41-6. Stagnant anoxia resulting from severe initial stress or prolonged shock states.

function deteriorates in prolonged oligemic shock. The initial fall in cardiac output following hemorrhage is strictly caused by the reduction in venous return to the heart as a result of the loss of circulating blood volume. With persistent blood loss or inadequate treatment there is a further reduction in cardiac output as a result of the inability of the cardiovascular compensatory mechanisms (increased heart rate, increased peripheral resistance) to keep up with the loss of intravascular volume. Although there are individual variations, coronary blood flow essentially parallels the systemic flow pattern in hemorrhagic shock. Ultimately blood flow during systole far exceeds that in diastole, and coronary filling and flow become persistently reduced.[40] With the onset of myocardial ischemia, cardiac function begins to deteriorate, and myocardial oxygen availability and consumption fall.[41]

In addition to the detrimental effects of these coronary perfusion abnormalities on cardiac function, there is evidence that a myocardial depressant factor (MDF) may be present in the circulation of animals and man during hemorrhagic (and septic) shock.[42,43] This peptide has been isolated from the venous effluent of the ischemic pancreas and has been shown to depress contractility in isolated cat papillary muscle. The existence or importance of MDF in shock is still controversial, however, since other investigators have either been unable to detect it or have attributed the myocardial depressant activity in shock serum to electrolyte disturbances or to endotoxin released into the systemic circulation from ischemic bowel.[44-46] The existence or importance of circulating endogenous endotoxin in hemorrhagic shock is yet another highly controversial subject, however.[47] Regardless of the precise mechanisms involved, hemorrhagic shock is associated with an absolute reduction in cardiac performance, especially late in the course of circulatory collapse.

During the past decade the cellular effects of hypovolemic shock have been extensively studied. Because the ultimate pathophysiology is similar, many of these findings also apply to cardiogenic shock.

An early effect of hypotension and hypoxia is the shift of cellular metabolism from aerobic to less efficient anaerobic metabolic pathways.[48] The end product of cellular metabolism thus changes from carbon dioxide and water to lactic acid, which reduces intracellular pH. Hobler and Carey[49] have shown that in normotensive dogs excess lactate begins to accumulate when the arterial oxygen tension falls below 36 mm Hg. An abrupt decrease also occurs in the systemic oxygen consumption, reflecting the cellular utilization of anaerobic metabolic pathways. With hypotension superimposed on hypoxia and acidosis, less oxygen is delivered to the cells, enhancing the rate of appearance of anaerobic metabolism.

Although anaerobic metabolism is capable of temporarily sustaining the majority of the cells of the body, it is much less efficient than aerobic metabolism. Thus tissue adenosine triphosphate (ATP) levels progressively decline with continued hemorrhagic shock.[50,51] Because the cyclic nucleotides (cAMP, cGMP) are derived from ATP, their cellular concentrations also decline.[52-54] Since these cyclic nucleotides are thought to be the intracellular "messengers" that directly regulate the quality and quantity of cellular metabolic processes, the reduction in their generation has profound effects on cell function in general.

The combination of acidosis, hypoperfusion, and hypoxia results in significant functional and morphologic changes in the intracellular organelles[55] (Fig. 41-7). Baue and Sayeed[56] found a reduction in the functional capacity of mitochondria in hemorrhagic shock. Not only was the oxidation of substrates reduced, but the efficiency of the electron transport system was also impaired, owing to inhibition of mitochondrial enzymes (adenosinetriphosphatase, ATPase) involved in oxidative phosphorylation.[57] Rhodes et al.[58] showed that α-ketoglutarate oxidation is more sensitive to ischemic injury than succinate oxidation.

Baue and associates[59] also demonstrated that mitochondrial concentrations of sodium and calcium increased, whereas the levels of potassium and magnesium decreased. Since the changes in mitochondrial function are reversed by correction of these electrolyte abnormalities, it appears that electrolyte disturbances are intimately involved in the observed functional impairment of mitochondria during hypovolemic shock.[60] Free intracellular lysosomal enzymes may also be involved in the disruption of mitochondrial structure and function in shock.[61] The ultimate consequences of depressed mitochondrial activity are reductions in the tissue levels of the high-energy compound ATP as well as the intracellular messengers derived from ATP. Chaudry et al.[62] have recently shown that the extent of the decrease in adenine nucleotides during shock may be directly related to the metabolic activity of each organ. Hence the reduction in ATP and creatine phosphate during hemorrhagic shock is greater in the diaphragm, liver, and kidney than in resting soleus muscle.

Another organelle profoundly affected during hemorrhagic shock is the lysosome. This structure becomes very fragile in the face of hypotension, hypoxia, or acidosis. With prolonged oligemic shock an increasing number of lysosomes rupture and discharge their contents into the cell. The concentration of these substances in the serum progressively rises with the duration of circulatory collapse.[63-65] Although the primary site of lysosomal enzyme release during hemorrhagic shock is the gastrointestinal tract, substantial amounts have also been detected in the venous effluent from other splanchnic tissues.[63,64] Once released from the cell of origin, lysosomal enzymes possibly exert detrimental effects on the morphology and function of other cells and intracellular organelles.[66] As with MDF, the role of circulating lysosomal enzymes in shock is still a controversial subject. Glenn et al.[67] reproduced the hemodynamic profile of circulatory shock in normal dogs by infusing homogenized liver tissue, which contains high amounts of lysosomal enzymes. Mason and Wangensteen,[68] however, noted no effect in the normal dog from the ad-

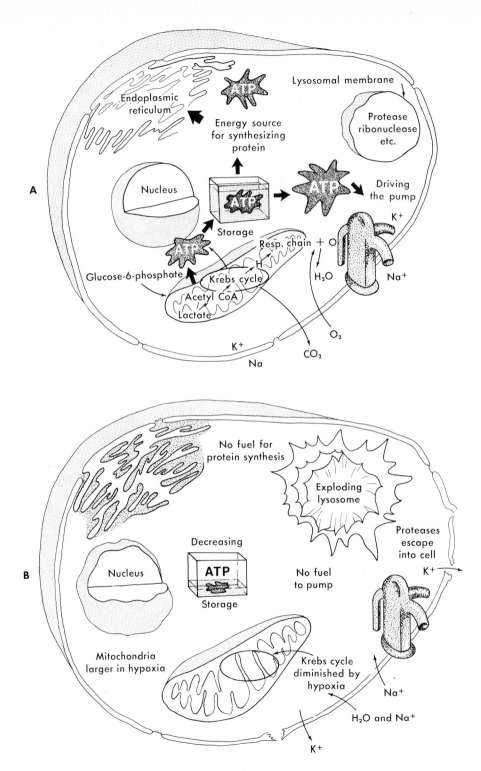

Fig. 41-7. A, Normal cell. **B,** Cell in shock.

ministration of purified cathepsin D, and they criticized earlier studies that did not employ pure lysosomal enzyme preparations.

The observed changes in the structure and function of cells and intracellular organelles in hemorrhagic shock have been linked by membrane physiologists to profound alterations in the integrity of cell membranes. Studies by a number of investigators[69-73] on skeletal muscle, vascular smooth muscle, liver, and lung have shown increases in intracellular water and sodium and a decrease in potassium during hypovolemic shock. A concomitant decrease in extracellular fluid and calcium and an increase in interstitial potassium and magnesium are observed.[74] Preceding these changes is a marked reduction of the resting cell membrane potential in liver and muscle, followed by a decrease in the amplitude of the muscle action potential and a prolongation of both depolarization and repolarization times.[71,75] Although the exact cause of these electrical changes during hemorrhagic shock is unknown, the findings have been interpreted as reflecting either changes in the transport properties of cells or a reduction in the efficiency of the active sodium pump. Similar data have been obtained in the kidney, connective tissue, and red blood cells.[76,77] Interestingly, ischemia alone does not affect muscle transmembrane potential difference.[78] Thus there are other factors specific to the shock state that are responsible.

The pathologic cellular alterations in hypovolemic shock are abundantly reflected in the changes seen in many important clinical parameters used to evaluate and treat patients. The ultimate appearance of metabolic acidosis caused by the production of excess lactic acid by cells undergoing anaerobic metabolism has already been discussed. Depending on the state of the kidneys and the lungs, however, many patients seen in early hemorrhagic shock may have a normal blood pH or may even be slightly alkalotic as a result of adequate compensatory mechanisms (principally hyperventilation).[79] With prolonged circulatory collapse and the associated visceral vasoconstriction, the compensatory ability of the kidneys is markedly reduced. In addition, the capacity for compensation of systemic acidosis by the lungs is severely restricted because of a num-

ber of changes that can occur in this organ during hemorrhagic shock. Thus with sustained shock acidosis is an almost universal finding.

In sum, the primary characteristics of hemorrhagic shock are hypotension and reductions in the cardiac output, stroke work, pulmonary artery pressures, circulating blood volume, and oxygen consumption. Early compensatory (secondary) changes are tachycardia, systemic and pulmonary vasoconstriction, increased myocardial contractility, an elevated oxygen extraction, and a shift to cellular anaerobic metabolism. With prolonged shock oxygen extraction and myocardial contractility are reduced, and systemic acidosis occurs. Initially the circulating blood volume is redistributed to preferentially perfuse the brain, heart, kidneys, and liver. In late shock the absolute and relative flow to all organs is decreased, and cellular energy generation is minimal.

Septic shock

In the face of an overwhelming infection a patient may suddenly experience a fever spike, mental confusion, tachypnea, oliguria, and tachycardia. The skin may be cool and clammy, or it may be warm and pink. Hypotension may or may not be present. The cardiac output is either normal or high, and the total peripheral vascular resistance is reduced. This constellation of signs and symptoms of septic shock in its early stage (Table 41-1) differs markedly from that following hemorrhage or myocardial infarction. In later stages these differences tend to disappear.

Unlike cardiogenic or traumatic shock, septic shock appears to pass through at least three fairly distinct stages.[80-82] The usual initial presentation consists of a hyperdynamic cardiovascular and metabolic picture. The blood pressure is generally normal, and the cardiac output is high. Since hypotension is not a common feature in early septic shock, there is frequently a delay in the diagnosis of this condition. If one is attuned to the initial symptoms, especially mental confusion, and the clinical setting of bacteremic shock, the diagnosis and treatment can be established quite early in the course of the disease.

The patient can remain in the early, hyperdynamic stage of septic shock for some time (up to several days) before signs of deterioration appear.

As shock progresses, the cardiovascular status changes to a normodynamic pattern. The heart rate remains elevated, but the cardiac output is now in the normal range. The blood pressure is somewhat reduced, and the peripheral vascular resistance remains below normal. The patient continues to hyperventilate, and respiratory assistance is frequently necessary because of a progressively declining arterial Po_2. The urine output remains low, and frank renal shutdown is common. This middle stage of bacteremic shock is usually of brief duration (several hours), and patients not responding to treatment soon experience profound cardiovascular decompensation.

Late, or preterminal, septic shock is almost invariably manifested by a hypodynamic cardiovascular picture, since cardiac insufficiency is the rule. It is in this stage of bacteremic shock that the "classic" signs and symptoms of circulatory collapse exist: hypotension, low cardiac output, and high total peripheral resistance. The heart rate continues to be elevated, and urine output is scanty at best. The stroke index, left ventricular stroke work, and other parameters of cardiac performance rapidly deteriorate. The central venous and pulmonary artery wedge pressures rise. Mechanical respiratory assistance may be unable to correct either the profound hypoxia or the metabolic acidosis. Patients who remain in this decompensated state for more than a few hours fail to survive.

The reason(s) for these physiopathologic differences between septic shock and the other forms of circulatory collapse is unknown and will remain so until an acceptable, reproducible experimental model of human septic shock is developed. Steps have been taken in this direction,[83] and hopefully the mysteries of septic shock will soon be unraveled. Meanwhile, we can only speculate on the mechanisms underlying the pathophysiology of this condition.

One obvious difference between septic shock and shock from other causes is the presence of infection. The responsible pathogens not only can elaborate vasoactive toxins, but they also create a focus of inflammation. Hopkins and Damewood[84] showed that a nonseptic inflammatory lesion produces a high-flow, low-resistance state with a decreased arteriovenous oxygen difference. Endo-toxin, on the other hand, creates a low-flow, high-resistance picture. Thus it would appear that the inflammatory reaction accompanying the septic state is at least partly responsible for the hemodynamic presentation in septic shock. It is quite possible that the interrelationship between inflammatory influences and those caused by endotoxin dictates the type of hemodynamic presentation of patients in septic shock, as well as the magnitude and duration of each type of hemodynamic profile. For example, in early clinical septic shock inflammatory factors may predominate, while in late shock endotoxin-related abnormalities may assume control of hemodynamic and metabolic events.[85] The accumulative metabolic effects of endotoxin, as well as the progressive reduction of endotoxin clearance (and detoxification) by the host, would be a likely explanation for this potential sequence of events.[86]

Another mechanism behind the pathophysiology of septic shock may be that various vasoactive substances are liberated at different times or in different amounts than in hemorrhagic or cardiogenic shock. In addition, the activity of these substances may be modified by the presence of endotoxin or inflammation. For example, large amounts of the potent vasodilators, histamine and kinins, are released into the circulation in early endotoxin shock[87-89] but are found in insignificant amounts late in shock. Since the pattern of the release of these substances follows the hemodynamic profile in septic shock, it is tempting to speculate that these events are related.

In addition to the hemodynamic differences between septic shock and cardiogenic and hypovolemic shock, there are significant metabolic differences resulting from cellular and systemic actions of bacteria and their toxins. A striking finding in patients in early septic shock is profound systemic vasodilatation, usually associated with a very high cardiac output. Although cellular metabolic factors may play a role in the genesis of the elevated cardiac index, thus making vasodilatation more secondary than primary, most evidence indicates that the converse is true.[90,91] In other words, it appears that the high cardiac index is primarily the result of the decreased systemic resistance caused by vasodilatation and/or shunting in several regions of the body. Finley et al.[92] have shown a direct relationship between cardiac output and muscle capillary blood flow in patients with sepsis. Since they could not demonstrate anatomic shunting in this vascular bed, they postulated that the increased muscle blood flow in sepsis was a response to the heightened metabolic needs of the body. In starvation and in sepsis skeletal muscle is the main source of the protein used for gluconeogenesis. Hence skeletal muscle blood flow—and cardiac output—may be increased in septic patients in order to provide a conduit for the systemic delivery of substrates needed to maintain viability.

Another consistent finding during the early and middle stages of bacteremic shock is a decrease in the pulmonary and systemic arteriovenous oxygen difference, indicative of shunting in these circulatory systems[81,93,94] (Fig. 41-8). As a result of

these shunts, much of the blood passing through the lungs is not oxygenated. In addition, vast areas of the body are either not perfused with blood or receive poorly oxygenated blood. These underperfused tissues soon become hypoxic, and anaerobic metabolism with lactic acid production ensues. Oxygen extraction and consumption decline, and metabolic acidosis occurs[95] (Fig. 41-9). As a result of specific depressant action(s) of endotoxin and hypoxia on carbohydrate metabolism, cellular glucose utilization is markedly reduced.[96-99] Lysosomal enzymes become elevated in the systemic circulation and may add further insult to the tissue injury caused by bacterial toxins and ischemia.[100]

Initially the lungs can compensate for the metabolic acidosis by reducing the arterial carbon dioxide tension. Thus patients in early septic shock are usually mildly alkalotic and hypocap-

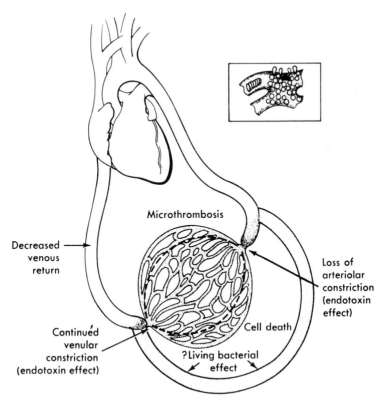

Decreased venous return

Microthrombosis

Loss of arteriolar constriction (endotoxin effect)

Continued venular constriction (endotoxin effect)

Cell death

?Living bacterial effect

Fig. 41-8. Cellular anoxia in septic shock is associated with venular constriction and severe arteriovenous shunting thought to be caused by an inflammatory effect of living bacteria.

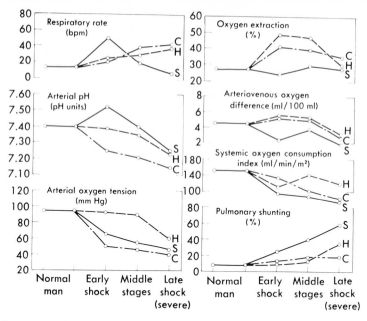

Fig. 41-9. Progressive changes in systemic oxygenation in untreated shock. *C,* Cardiogenic shock; *H,* hemorrhagic shock; *S,* septic shock.

nic. With time, however, bacterial toxins exert pronounced detrimental effects on pulmonary structure and function. Pulmonary edema and cytoplasmic swelling of alveolar type I and II cells are histologically evident early in bacteremic shock.[101,109] These changes are caused in part by hypotension but mostly by a direct action of endotoxin and other circulating vasoactive substances on pulmonary capillaries, resulting in an increase in membrane permeability.[103] The consequences of these pulmonary cellular changes are a decreased oxygen-diffusing capacity of the lung, a reduced pulmonary compliance, and an increase in the work of breathing. Systemic hypoxia occurs and is frequently resistant to increasing concentrations of oxygen in the inspired air. Initially only the ability of the lungs to oxygenate blood is impaired, but ultimately the arterial Pco_2 also increases. The net result of these pulmonary events is a reduction in the delivery of oxygen to the tissues and a decrease in the buffering capability of the lungs. Thereafter anaerobic metabolism totally supports the organism, and metabolic acidosis worsens.[104] As a result of the severe re-

duction in the functional capacity of the respiratory system, uncompensated metabolic acidosis eventually occurs, leaving the patient in a preterminal state.[80]

The decreased ability of patients to extract sufficient oxygen from both the inspired air and the blood are early, persistent abnormalities in septic shock. In addition, there are adverse changes in the oxygen-carrying capacity of the blood. Red blood cell 2,3-diphosphoglycerate (DPG) concentration is reduced, and the oxyhemoglobin dissociation curve is shifted to the left.[105,106] Thus hemoglobin has less tendency to release oxygen, and consequently the transfer of oxygen to those tissues being perfused is reduced. Intravascular coagulation associated with fibrin deposition and platelet aggregation and the ultimate deterioration of cardiac function, perhaps aided by MDF, further decrease the delivery of oxygen to the tissues.[107,108]

In summary, current evidence strongly suggests that the basic pathophysiology of septic shock is markedly different from that in circulatory failure following hemorrhage or myocardial infarction. Whereas in the latter two forms of circulatory collapse hemodynamic alterations precede metabolic changes, in bacteremic shock cellular derangements apparently precede and may form the etiology of cardiovascular abnormalities.[92] As a result of the combined effects of cellular and hemodynamic aberrations, however, the late state of septic shock is remarkably similar to that found in hemorrhagic and cardiogenic shock, consisting of hypotension, vasoconstriction, low cardiac output, hypoxia, and acidosis.

■ What are the metabolic changes in shock?

References have already been made to some of the profound metabolic alterations that occur during circulatory collapse. This section will integrate this information, define the various interrelationships involved, and demonstrate those aspects that may be unique to a given type of shock.

In shock the organism must contend with a reduction in or a maldistribution of systemic perfusion. To compensate for the decrease in blood flow and the reduction in oxygen and nutrient delivery, a number of hemodynamic and metabolic reactions are set in motion. One compensatory mechanism is the shift of cellular metabolism to anaerobic pathways. Another related compensatory action is the outpouring of several hormones and the suppression of the secretion of other potentially metabolically active substances.

The release of epinephrine from the adrenal medulla and norepinephrine from the sympathetic nerve terminals has been discussed in an earlier section. This catecholamine response has been demonstrated in all forms of circulatory collapse and is an early event following the onset of shock. Carey et al.[109] showed that the increase in epinephrine secretion was dependent on the rate of hemorrhage. A much greater response was elicited with rapid blood loss than with slow hemorrhage of an equal amount. Clowes and associates[97] found that patients with low output septic shock had significantly higher levels of circulating catecholamines than those with the high output version. Hence there is some variability in the magnitude of the catecholamine response to circulatory failure.

Serum cortisol concentration significantly rises in all types of shock. In contrast to the catechol-amine response in hemorrhagic shock, the rate of blood loss does not affect the onset of enhanced cortisol secretion. Herman et al.[110] demonstrated that as long as adrenal blood flow does not fall below a critical level (1 ml/min in the dog), the cortisol secretory rate remains elevated for a considerable period of time. After 12 hours of shock, despite maintenance of previously adequate adrenal perfusion, there is a progressive decrease in corticosteroid secretion.

Growth hormone levels are also strikingly elevated following shock and trauma in man.[111] Similarly, the serum glucagon concentration is increased following hemorrhage in man[112] and during endotoxin shock in the dog[113] and sepsis in man.[114] Meguid et al.[115] showed that the rise in serum glucagon and cortisol levels is more pronounced when trauma has been severe. The concentration of circulating gastrin is also significantly increased during hemorrhagic shock.[116] Serum insulin concentration, however, remains normal or is decreased during hemorrhagic shock and after trauma in man[117] as well as in many experimental animals.[109,117-119] Meguid and colleagues[120] found that the magnitude and/or duration of the insulin response was a function of the severity of the trauma and the duration of the illness. Both Moss et al.[118] and Hiebert and associates[119] demonstrated that there is a reduction in insulin secretion by the pancreas in shock and after trauma. This decrease in insulin production is primarily caused by the combined effects of hypoperfusion and catecholamines on the pancreas.[118,121] Thus decreased production, not increased utilization, accounts for the low levels of circulating insulin in hemorrhagic and endotoxin shock.[122] Dykes et al.[123] reported an abnormal insulin response to tolbutamide stimulation in patients with cardiogenic shock. According to studies by Clowes and associates,[97] the insulin response of patients in septic shock varies with their cardiovascular status. Patients with high flow septic shock have elevated serum insulin levels, while those with low output shock have low levels. It thus appears that, both metabolically and hemodynamically, patients with low output (usually late) septic shock are pathophysiologically similar to patients in hemorrhagic or cardiogenic shock.

The hormonal changes in circulatory collapse have profound metabolic effects and vice versa. Patients in shock present a picture of carbohydrate intolerance, which is manifested by hyperglycemia, a reduction in glucose utilization, and the lack of an appropriate insulin response to the elevated levels of circulating blood glucose. The hyperglycemia of shock is due to many factors. Jordan et al.[124] noted that traumatized patients who sustained an episode of shock became hyperglycemic, while those who did not develop circulatory collapse remained normoglycemc. Thus *shock,* not trauma per se, is related to the increased circulating blood glucose. Carey and associates[117] demonstrated that hyperglycemia develops within minutes after the onset of hypovolemic shock and that the magnitude of the hyperglycemic response is related to the severity of shock. They also noted that the relative hypoinsulinism of hemorrhagic shock does not resolve following resuscitation of the patient.

Printen et al.[125] showed that changes in serum glucose (and free fatty acid) concentration during shock are mediated by a pathway more complex than just a response to hypotension. Many investigators have demonstrated that the high concentration of circulating catecholamines is instrumental in creating the hyperglycemia of shock. Carey and colleagues[109] found a close correlation between changes in blood glucose and epinephrine secretion in pigs with hemorrhagic shock. Furthermore they were able to produce hyperglycemia with epinephrine infusions in normal pigs. Hanson et al.[126] demonstrated a hyperglycemic response to norepinephrine infusion in man before or following hemorrhage. Catecholamines promote hyperglycemia during shock through several mechanisms: by inducing glycogenolysis in the liver, by decreasing pancreatic release of insulin, and by adversely affecting glucose metabolism in peripheral tissues.[127,128] Studies by Hiebert et al.[121] however, have revealed that additional factors also contribute to the reduction in peripheral glucose utilization during shock. Hinshaw and associates[129] showed that endotoxin may directly exert adverse effects on glucose uptake by circulating white blood cells. Wright and Henderson[128] found that the liver contributes to the hyperglycemia of circulatory collapse not only by enhanced glucose mobilization but also by decreasing utilization owing to diminished glucose phosphorylation.

The reason(s) for the reduction in cellular glucose utilization in shock is not known. Under normal conditions the transport of glucose across the cell membrane involves a carrier that takes glucose down the concentration gradient that exists across the cell membrane. Insulin markedly enhances the rate of glucose transport into the cells by increasing the amount, the availability, or the mobility of the carrier. The concentration gradient across the cell membrane is maintained by the continuous delivery of glucose to the cell and by the constant utilization of glucose, via phosphorylation, within the cell. In shock this entire pattern of glucose metabolism is disrupted.

As previously stated, intracellular glucose utilization is reduced in circulatory failure. Thus unused glucose may accumulate within the cell and lower the transmembrane concentration gradient. Furthermore despite the elevated levels of glucose in the blood, the reduction in tissue perfusion during shock decreases the delivery of glucose to the cell. This perfusion defect also lowers the transmembrane glucose concentration gradient. The decrease in the amount of circulating insulin also impedes the transport of glucose into the cell. In addition to these factors, recent studies in animals in shock have shown a tissue insulin resistance, which is not due to steroid or catecholamine effects or to an alteration of the inherent glucose carrier mechanism.[130] Ryan et al.[131] have found that tissue insulin resistance persists for as long as 1 week after recovery from hemorrhagic shock. Thus multiple factors alter the body's capability to use glucose during circulatory collapse, despite its ready availability in the blood.

The reduction in glucose availability and utilization during circulatory failure means that other substrates must be used to sustain the body's metabolic needs. Most studies in experimental cardiogenic, endotoxin, and hemorrhagic shock have shown decreases in the levels of circulating free fatty acids once the shock state is established.[113,125,132,133] Clowes et al.[97] have also demonstrated this phenomenon in clinical septic shock. Not only is serum free fatty acid concentration diminished during shock, but free fatty acid turnover and lipolysis are decreased as well. These findings suggest that the normal antilipolytic action of insulin is retained during shock, that is, the previously described tissue insulin resistance does not apply to fat.[97] The antipolytic activity of insulin is aided by the reduction in adipose tissue perfusion during circulatory collapse and by the high level of circulating lactic acid.[133]

Since utilization of both fat and carbohydrate is impaired in shock, a net deficit in cellular fuel exists. This substrate deficiency is made up, partially, by oxidation of branched chain amino acids derived from protein. The increased use of protein as a substrate in shock is suggested by many observations. It is well known that the muscle mass progressively decreases following trauma and during sepsis or starvation.[97] This observation suggests that muscle protein is being broken down and, presumably, utilized for fuel. The finding that muscle is the primary source of the elevated blood lactate in shock also supports this contention.[134] Further substantiation is provided by the increased levels of certain amino acids, especially alanine and glycine, found in shock.[135-138] Finally, Daniel et al.[133] demonstrated an increased urea production in both endotoxin and cardiogenic shock and showed that protein oxidation was doubled.

Using the above information, it is now possible to assemble many of the pieces of the metabolic puzzle in circulatory failure. As suggested clinically and hemodynamically, there is a difference between the metabolic patterns of patients in early (high flow) septic shock and those with late septic shock or with cardiogenic or hemorrhagic shock. Patients with high output septic shock have elevated levels of blood glucose, insulin, and lactate; low amounts of circulating free fatty acids; and high urinary nitrogen excretion.[97,139] Muscle perfusion is increased in direct proportion to the increase in cardiac output.[92] Muscle free fatty acid uptake and glucose utilization are reduced, and muscle proteolysis with oxidation of branched chain ketogenic amino acids is substantially increased.[97,136] Other amino acids from muscle protein, such as alanine and glycine, are transported to the liver, where they serve as sub-

strates for gluconeogenesis.[140] Owing to the elevated serum alanine concentration, as well as other factors, the pancreatic alpha cells secrete increased amounts of glucagon, which also stimulates hepatic gluconeogenesis. Thus, although hepatic glycogen stores are depleted, the liver continues to produce glucose and maintains a slightly elevated oxygen consumption during high flow septic shock.[141] As long as the patient remains in high output septic shock, these metabolic adjustments are sustained.

Patients in low output septic shock and in circulatory collapse caused by hemorrhage or myocardial infarction present a different metabolic picture, however. Although the blood glucose level may initially be elevated, with time hypoglycemia develops. The serum insulin concentration remains low. Free fatty acid levels are variable[97,115] but are usually low. The concentrations of circulating catecholamines are much higher than in high output septic shock. Hence not only is peripheral glucose utilization low, but hepatic gluconeogenesis is also low because of the decreased ability of the liver to form glucose from precursors.[135,142] Thus blood lactate levels and urinary nitrogen loss are greater than in high output septic shock,[97] while systemic and hepatic oxygen consumption are much lower. Eventually the ability of the liver to produce glucose is impaired, and hypoglycemia develops. The reductions in circulating glucose and free fatty acids substantially reduce myocardial metabolism. In hemorrhagic and septic shock cardiac insufficiency appears; in cardiogenic shock myocardial performance further deteriorates. Consequently the peripheral perfusion and metabolic defects are accentuated, paving the way for the onset of refractory shock. In sum, the metabolic, as well as the clinical and hemodynamic, presentations of cardiogenic, hemorrhagic, and late septic shock are quite similar.

■ How do specific organs respond to shock?

Owing to autoregulatory factors, the response patterns of the various organs differ during shock. Some organs, such as the skin, undergo remarkable changes early in the course of circulatory collapse. Other structures, such as the heart, are not significantly affected until late in shock. Major sequential changes in organ structure and function during circulatory collapse will be described in the following section.

The lung

Patients dying from shock or massive trauma exhibit pathologic changes in the lungs more frequently than in any other organ.[143] Involvement of the lung in the shock process produces a characteristic clinical picture, variously termed "shock lung" or "wet lung." Posttraumatic pulmonary insufficiency syndrome or respiratory distress syndrome (RDS) are more proper designations.

The diagnostic features of this syndrome are marked respiratory distress and hypoxia (arterial oxygen tension less than 50 mm Hg) with associated pulmonary infiltrates and/or consolidation (Fig. 41-10). RDS can occur with any type of severe injury or sepsis, with or without attendant or antecedent shock. However, respiratory insufficiency following trauma is more common in patients who exhibit shock and hypoxia when initially seen.[144] The syndrome is insidious in onset and thus is not usually diagnosed prior to the ap-

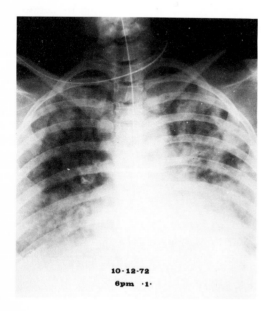

10-12-72
6pm ·1·

Fig. 41-10. Radiologic findings in posttraumatic pulmonary insufficiency syndrome.

pearance of severe symptoms. The reported mortality in this condition has been as high as 50% to 90%.[145]

Besides hypoxia and tachypnea, several other systemic and pulmonary aberrations have been noted in these patients. Until the late stages, the arterial carbon dioxide tension is generally normal or only slightly decreased because of the increased respiratory rate. Likewise, the pH is normal or slightly alkalotic in the early phase. The cardiac index and systemic oxygen consumption vary widely early in the course of the syndrome but generally decrease with time. Virtually all patients exhibit reduced pulmonary compliance, increased physiologic dead space, increased pulmonary arteriovenous shunting, and abnormal ventilation-perfusion ratios.[146-148] In the few patients in whom pulmonary diffusing capacity was measured, it was reduced.[147]

The pathologic findings in the lungs vary with the duration of the syndrome. The initial changes consist of scattered petechial hemorrhages and areas of consolidation and atelectasis in the lower lung fields. Under light microscopy there is capillary engorgement, atelectasis, interstitial edema, and thromboemboli in the small pulmonary blood vessels.[146,147] With time, hemorrhagic consolidation of the lung occurs. There is severe pulmonary venous congestion and interstitial edema with peribronchial, perivascular, and intra-alveolar hemorrhage. Ultimately the lungs grossly resemble liver. Microscopically there are hyaline membranes in the alveoli and diffuse hemorrhage, congestion, and bronchopneumonia.[146]

The etiology of posttraumatic pulmonary insufficient is unknown, but a number of factors have been implicated. The contributing factors in the development of posttraumatic pulmonary insufficiency are as follows:

Abnormal hemodynamics of shock (increased pulmonary vascular resistance)

Circulating endogenous vasoactive substances (catecholamines, histamine, serotonin, bradykinin, lysosomal enzymes, prostaglandins)

Pulmonary infection

Nonpulmonary sepsis

Pulmonary microemboli and sequestration of leukocytes and platelets

Fat emboli

Endotoxin or bacterial interactions
Fluid overload
Oxygen toxicity
Cerebral ischemia
Decreased surfactant synthesis

Certainly shock itself with the attendant acidosis, reduced pulmonary blood flow, and increased pulmonary vascular resistance (caused by arteriolar and venular vasoconstriction) plays a role.[149-152] However, low blood flow is not the sole cause, since the lung is capable of withstanding short periods of ischemia without apparent damage.[153] Thromboemboli in the pulmonary vascular tree caused by intravascular coagulation and the administration of blood products have been implicated in the shock lung syndrome.[146,154] In addition, fibrin degradation products, resulting from tissue trauma or intravascular coagulation, have been shown to be toxic to the respiratory system.[155-156] High levels of circulating catecholamines, histamine, and serotonin have also been entertained as factors.[157-159] Other investigators have stressed the injurious effects of fat emboli,[160,161] since respiratory insufficiency following trauma is more common in patients sustaining long bone fractures.[144] The origin of the fat emboli may be from the marrow of fractured long bones or from the extensive fatty acid mobilization that occurs in severe stress.[162] Oxygen toxicity has also been cited as a contributing influence in the genesis of RDS, since a large number of these patients have required mechanical respiratory support with high inspired oxygen concentrations from the time of injury.[163,164]

Lastly the work of Moss[165] has suggested a relationship between cerebral ischemia and the development of posttraumatic pulmonary insufficiency. Dogs undergoing carotid artery perfusion with hypoxemic blood develop the classic signs, symptoms, and pathologic changes of RDS. Spinal cord section (that is, interruption of nervous pathways from the brain to the lungs) prevents the pulmonary abnormalities.

Over the past decade much of the investigative work—and debate—on posttraumatic pulmonary insufficiency has been concentrated on the influence of the type and/or volume of IV fluids used in resuscitating traumatized patients. Although RDS was recognized as long ago as World War I,

it became much more frequently seen and hence popularized during the conflict in Vietnam. Advances in patient transport and resuscitation allowed victims who had previously died to live long enough to sustain the pulmonary complications of shock. Most of the patients in these early series of posttraumatic pulmonary insufficiency had received massive amounts of IV fluids and blood products during resuscitation, and it was suggested that perhaps RDS was iatrogenic.[166] Despite the report of Simmons and associates[167] that severely traumatized soldiers receiving massive amounts of IV fluids did not exhibit overexpansion of their blood volume, there was an outpouring of research into the effects of various resuscitative fluids on lung structure and function.

Magilligan et al.[168] and Fulton and Fischer[169] showed in dogs that resuscitation from hemorrhagic shock with normal saline solution resulted in an increase in pulmonary extracellular water and pulmonary dysfunction, suggesting that the sodium load was an etiologic factor. With the use of hypertonic saline solution Fulton and Fischer[169] found that the functional and morphologic pulmonary changes were reduced, indicating that a large fluid volume increased the sodium-induced collection of fluid in the lungs. Although initial studies in baboons by Seigel and Moss[170] revealed no functional pulmonary impairment following saline resuscitation from hypovolemic shock, subsequent work in their laboratory demonstrated the accumulation of sodium and fluid in the pulmonary interstitium of these animals.[170-173] Thus large volumes of sodium-containing fluids can be a factor in the etiology of posttraumatic pulmonary insufficiency.

Just as excessive amounts of crystalloids can be associated with respiratory insufficiency, massive blood replacement is also a factor in its genesis.[174] Pulmonary trapping of platelet and leukocyte aggregates has been demonstrated in shock and trauma,[156,175,176] and a relationship exists between these collections and the development of pulmonary shunting and systemic hypoxemia.[175] However, such entrapment is unrelated to changes in physiologic dead space, pulmonary vascular resistance, or lung compliance.[176] Dacron-wool filtration of infused blood decreases the pulmonary pathology by eliminating most of the platelet and leukocyte microaggregates,[177] but large amounts of even filtered blood may be injurious to the lungs.[178] It appears that the pulmonary manifestations of the sympathoadrenal response to shock, arteriolar and venular vasoconstriction, reduce the lungs' ability to tolerate large volumes of *any* IV replacement fluid.

The latest culprit in the etiology of RDS is sepsis. While it has long been recognized that pneumonitis predisposes a patient to respiratory failure, it has only recently been appreciated that sepsis outside the lung is also a significant factor. In 1975 Fulton and Jones[179] reviewed the case histories of 399 patients with major injuries. Forty-four patients developed respiratory insufficiency. RDS occurred in half of the patients with sepsis, and more than 90% of the patients who developed posttraumatic pulmonary insufficiency had sepsis. In 55% of the patients the primary focus of infection was extrapulmonary. The contribution of sepsis to the development of RDS in patients with trauma or hemorrhagic shock was further demonstrated experimentally by Esrig and Fulton[180] and clinically by Clowes et al.[181] As suggested by the report of Walker and Eiseman,[182] there are some differences between posttraumatic pulmonary insufficiency following hemorrhagic shock and the RDS associated with sepsis. The former appears within 24 to 48 hours after the insult, and with aggressive treatment most patients recover. RDS caused by sepsis tends to occur 5 or more days following injury and is quite lethal.

As with posttraumatic pulmonary insufficiency, the specific cause of respiratory failure in the face of sepsis is unknown. Pulmonary and systemic hypoperfusion, as well as most of the insults previously listed are probably contributing factors. Pulmonary sequestration of platelets and leukocytes occurs in septic shock to an even greater degree than in hemorrhagic shock, and in experimental studies either these collections or endotoxin can be shown to directly injure the pulmonary endothelium.[183,184] Such injury leads to increased capillary permeability and to the interstitial edema found in animals with endotoxin shock[185] and patients with sepsis.[186] Although the

studies of Siegel and Farrell[187] and Hechtman et al.[188] minimize the influence of pulmonary edema on the development of fulminant pulmonary insufficiency, one should, nevertheless, bear in mind the fact that every pulmonary insult in shock is additive.

In addition to controversy over the etiology of posttraumatic pulmonary insufficiency, there is also debate concerning the pulmonary pathology necessary to produce the syndrome. Both Bryant et al.[189] and Wilson et al.[190] reported functional respiratory impairment out of proportion to the morphologic changes observed in the lungs of dogs following hemorrhagic shock. These findings led some investigators to conclude that the functional pulmonary changes were not significant in determining irreversibility in shock and that respiratory insufficiency was the result of vigorous resuscitation in the face of reversible pulmonary injury. Other investigators, however, have demonstrated marked functional and structural respiratory impairment resulting from hemorrhagic shock alone.[157,190,191] Studies by Northrup and Humphrey[192] and by Fischer et al.[159] have demonstrated that hemorrhagic shock alone produces significant increases in the permeability of the pulmonary vasculature and in lung water. Henry et al.[193] found that pulmonary pathology progressively increased during the recovery period. Pulmonary congestion was the earliest change, and this picture progressed with time to peribronchial and perivascular edema and hemorrhage. Patchy atelectasis and consolidation occurred during the third and fourth hours after shock. These studies indicate that hemorrhagic shock itself can be responsible for creating significant damage to the lungs and that other injurious factors are probably superimposed on the initial pathology caused by the shock or trauma.[194]

From the data currently available a sequence of events can be outlined in the development of shock lung. With the onset of circulatory collapse both the systemic and pulmonary artery pressure and blood flow decline, and pulmonary vascular resistance increases. Because of these hemodynamic changes the distribution of pulmonary blood flow is altered so that the dependent portions of the lungs are preferentially perfused.

With continued hypotension, pulmonary blood flow first shifts to the previously underperfused, less dependent areas and then is ultimately distributed throughout the lungs in a pattern similar to that in the preshock period.[195,196] In response to the hypoperfusion and under the influence of acidosis, hypoxia, histamine, serotonin, or endotoxin the permeability of pulmonary capillaries increases, and fluid collects in the interstitium. There is also a loss of albumin that further increases edema through a decrease in the colloid osmotic pressure of the blood. Interstitial edema causes the lungs to become relatively stiff, and pulmonary compliance decreases while dead space increases. The combination of local acidosis, edema, ischemia, and hypoxia promotes bronchoconstriction, which increases airway resistance, produces atelectasis, and creates ventilation-perfusion abnormalities and pulmonary shunting.

With continued shock, overly vigorous resuscitation, or the onset of sepsis these early changes progress. The integrity of the pulmonary capillary endothelial membrane becomes disrupted, and interstitial edema increases. Pericapillary and peribronchial extravasation of red blood cells occurs. Scattered areas of atelectasis appear and increase the ventilation-perfusion defect. Destructive changes occur in types I and II alveolar cells, and surfactant synthesis is impaired.[197-199] The consequent reduction in intra-alveolar surface tension accentuates the atelectasis and thus reduces the surface area available for gas exchange. The diffusing capacity for oxygen is reduced, and systemic hypoxia occurs. The decreased ability of the lungs to exchange gases also creates progressive hypercapnia, and uncompensated metabolic acidosis ultimately occurs. Superimposed on this pathophysiologic scheme are the effects of microemboli from contused soft tissue, intravascular coagulation, infused blood and pulmonary platelet and leukocyte entrapment; fat emboli from coalescing fatty acids in the blood and/or extremity fractures; high oxygen concentrations in the inspired air; and fluid overload. These additional factors are capable of converting initial, potentially reversible pulmonary changes to a life-threatening situation.

The kidney

As indicated previously, the kidney is one of the primary target organs in shock. Renal dysfunction occurs with almost the same frequency as respiratory insufficiency. With the onset of circulatory collapse, a host of hemodynamic and metabolic changes occur in the kidney. Owing to its autoregulatory capacity, however, the kidney's response to shock may be variable, especially in the early stages of circulatory decompensation.[31,200]

Stone and Stahl,[32] using normal volunteers, studied the renal response to the rapid removal of 15% to 20% of blood volume (approximately 2 units of blood). Both cardiac output and systemic blood pressure fell, and total peripheral vascular resistance rose. There were decreases in renal blood flow, renal vein pressure, urine output, and urine sodium and potassium concentrations, but there was no change in renal vascular resistance. Urine osmolality and plasma renin levels doubled. Thus with mild to moderate hemorrhage, local autoregulatory factors prevent a renal vasoconstrictive reaction. Nevertheless, there is still a drop in urine output, which is primarily caused by reductions in renal blood flow and perfusion pressure. In severe hemorrhagic shock, endotoxin shock, cardiogenic shock, and low output septic shock, renal vascular resistance rises, and renal blood flow and urine output fall dramatically. That these changes are primarily due to the sympathoadrenal response to circulatory collapse is shown by their prevention or reduction by α-adrenergic blockade.[201,202]

Not only does renal blood flow decrease in hemorrhagic, cardiogenic, and endotoxin shock, but the *distribution* of blood flow within the kidney changes considerably. Even in the early phases of circulatory collapse, blood is diverted from the renal cortex, while medullary flow is kept fairly constant.[203-205] As shock progresses, the cortex becomes increasingly ischemic, but the medulla is perfused as long as possible. The purpose of this autoregulatory redistribution of renal perfusion is most likely to preserve the function of the juxtamedullary nephrons. These nephrons are essential to the function of the countercurrent system, which is responsible for concentrating the urine. If the duration of shock is brief, the kidney has a good chance of recovering function. With prolonged shock, however, continued cortical ischemia, with concomitant reduction in sodium resorption, produces a failure in the countercurrent mechanism, owing to the loss of solute input into the system. The urine is then dilute, and creatinine and osmolar clearances are markedly reduced.[206] Acute renal failure soon occurs and is frequently associated with acute tubular necrosis. The exact mechanism by which acute tubular necrosis occurs in shock is unknown.

As with many other physiologic variables, the renal response in patients with septic shock may deviate from the pattern just described. Again, the response of a patient with sepsis is related to the hemodynamic presentation. Patients with low output shock generally have a renal response similar to that of patients with hemorrhagic or cardiogenic shock.[206] Patients with high output septic shock, however, may exhibit a syndrome of polyuria without azotemia. In this syndrome the glomerular filtration rate and renal plasma flow are slightly depressed, but renal blood flow is increased and varies directly with the cardiac output.[207] These data suggest that early sepsis is associated with renal vasodilatation. Since the high urine flow occurs in the face of hypotension and an inadequate circulating blood volume, it has been termed "inappropriate" diuresis. Because this diuresis occurs at the expense of an effective circulating blood volume, it appears that in early septic shock the normal renal homeostatic mechanisms are not operative. The cause of this high output renal reaction (not failure) to septic shock is unknown, but it may be related to such factors as the redistribution of renal blood flow, osmotic diuresis, or selective renal tubular dysfunction.[204,208] Toxic metabolites of bacteria or circulating or fixed tissues may also be involved.[208] The clinical significance of this syndrome lies in the need to replace the volume lost via the kidneys. If this inappropriate volume loss is not replenished, systemic hypovolemia will occur, and acute renal failure will result.[207]

Another renal response to shock, high output renal failure, is being seen with increasing frequency.[209] In this form of renal failure the urine output is inappropriately elevated, but, unlike the nonazotemic polyuric response to sepsis, there is azotemia. High output renal insufficiency can occur following all types of circulatory collapse. As in oliguric renal insufficiency, patients with high output renal failure have a low glomerular filtration rate, high serum creatinine, and low renal osmolar clearance. The cause of high output renal insufficiency is unknown but is probably related to the increasing success in the early resuscitation of patients with circulatory collapse. Thus the duration of insult(s) to the kidneys is shortened, and oliguria is prevented. As with nonazotemic polyuria in septic patients, the renal volume loss must be restored in patients with high output renal failure, or oliguric renal insufficiency will develop. This potential progression of events must be avoided, since patients with high output renal failure are not only easier to manage but also have a much greater chance of survival than their oliguric counterparts.[207]

The stomach

Clinicians involved in the care of critically ill patients are very aware of the fact that the stomach is a target organ in shock. Patients with major trauma, sepsis, or hemorrhage have a high incidence of upper gastrointestinal bleeding secondary to "stress" gastritis. Both experimental[210] and clinical[211,212] studies have demonstrated the appearance of lesions in the gastric mucosa during the early stage of illness. The typical location of such erosive lesions is the fundus and/or corpus. The antrum is usually spared from this process. The earliest changes that occur during shock are mucosal edema associated with signs of extravasation and capillary stasis.[210] Under electron microscopy aggregates of thrombocytes can be seen in mucosal capillaries, and mitochondrial dilatation is present in the cells at the neck region of the mucosal glands. With progression of shock these early changes become more prominent, and mucosal hemorrhage appears. The involved mucosa then undergoes exfoliation and necrosis. Again, cells in the gastric mucosal glands seem to be preferentially involved in this pathologic process.[210] Ultimately, bleeding mucosal ulcerations occur.

With the onset of hemorrhagic or endotoxin shock, both total gastric blood flow and mucosal blood flow are substantially reduced.[213,214] This flow response is primarily mediated through the sympathoadrenal system, since it is abolished by gastric sympathectomy.[215] The reduction in mucosal blood flow is not a generalized phenomenon, however, the decrease in flow to the fundus and corpus is much greater than that to the antrum.[213,216,217] It thus appears that mucosal ischemia is related to the development of erosive "stress" lesions, since both occur in the same regions of the stomach. Furthermore, even after successful resuscitation, with restoration of normal systemic and total gastric blood flow, the mucosa of the fundus and corpus remains underperfused.[216] Associated with this gastric ischemia are reductions in myoelectric activity[218] and acid secretion.[213]

Although mucosal ischemia plays an important role in the genesis of erosive gastritis in shock, the precise etiology of these lesions has not been defined. It is well known that intraluminal acid is important in the production of stress ulcers during shock.[219] Skillman, Silen, and associates[220,221] have suggested that acid does not directly injure the mucosal surface, but that "back-diffusion" of hydrogen ions from the lumen through the mucosa somehow causes the damage. This concept of a breakdown in the gastric mucosal barrier by acid or associated hydrogen ion back-diffusion has little substantiation, however.[214,219,222,223] Other factors that may be involved in the formation of erosive gastritis are refluxed bile[224] and endotoxin.[214,217] Endotoxin poses a dual threat: it causes mucosal ischemia via its systemic hemodynamic effects, and it directly reduces mucosal blood flow, despite the maintenance of normal systemic pressure and flow.[225]

None of these factors, by itself, satisfactorily explains the mechanism of erosive stress gastritis. Even ischemia is not the universal common denominator in the formation of these lesions, since in septic shock acute erosive gastritis can occur in the face of an increase in total gastric and mucosal blood flow.[226] The single common pathophysiologic denominator with all of the insults previously mentioned is a mucosal energy deficit, which is progressive and of sufficient magnitude to cause cellular necrosis. Menguy and Masters[227] showed that within 15 minutes after the onset of hemorrhagic shock gastric mucosal ATP concentration dropped 75%. Furthermore, compared to liver and muscle the stomach was peculiarly vulnerable to the metabolic effects of shock. The creation of a mucosal energy deficit by fasting produced stress lesions. Lastly, intraluminal bile salts had an adverse effect on mucosal cellular metabolism. It this appears that cellular energy derangements are ultimately responsible for the genesis of acute stress-related erosive gastritis. Although acid, bile, endotoxin, and decreased mucus production enhance mucosal injury during shock, ischemia is the most important pathogenetic factor in the development of gastric stress lesions.[228]

The liver

In recent years the hepatic response to shock has received increasing attention from clinicians. It has long been recognized that the liver is a target organ in shock, but in the past few patients survived long enough to manifest the hepatic complications of circulatory collapse. Today this is no longer true. We have reached the state of acute and chronic resuscitative expertise, where patients are living long enough to develop—and die from—the hepatic consequences of shock.

The liver is a unique organ in that it has a dual blood supply. It is perfused by blood from the hepatic artery and the portal vein. The total hepatic blood flow in the average individual is approximately 1500 ml/min or 1 ml/g of liver tissue. This flow represents 20% to 25% of the cardiac output. Normally the portal vein supplies 75% of the total blood flow, while the hepatic artery delivers about 25%. Under certain conditions either of these vessels can compensate to some extent for a reduction in pressure or flow in the other.[229] Because of the higher oxygen saturation of arterial blood, more than one third of the oxygen supply to the liver is delivered by the hepatic artery. The majority of the substrates for liver metabolism arrive via the portal vein, which drains most of the extrahepatic intra-abdominal viscera. Thus, when evaluating the hepatic changes in shock, one must consider the effects on both the systemic and portal circulation.

In the presence of circulatory collapse the pressure and flow in both the hepatic artery and portal vein fall, and a vasoconstrictor response is initiated. Hypoxemia, acidosis, and hypercarbia soon become evident in the portal vein blood.[230]

Hepatic mitochondria swell, and the endoplasmic reticulum begins to dilate.[231] Hepatic oxygen consumption decreases, and dramatic changes occur in liver metabolism. Circulatory collapse also leads to a hepatic outflow block, believed to be due to constriction of venous sphincters in response to hepatic hypoxia.[232] Hepatic sinusoids, especially those in the region of the central veins, begin to enlarge, and red blood cell aggregates appear.[33] The resultant stasis in the sinusoids creates a further impedance to portal blood flow and enhances hepatic hypoxia.[230] In patients who sustain a prolonged episode of circulatory collapse generalized intracellular edema appears, and the hepatic plates are compressed. The central veins, portal tracts, and lymphatics become dilated. The sinusoids are congested with erythrocytes. Ultimately, the cells around the central veins become necrotic and disappear. This centrilobular necrosis is the classic pathologic feature of the liver in shock.[33]

All patients will have some microscopic evidence of hepatocellular injury following an episode of shock.[231] However, as with other aspects of circulatory failure, the extent of the damage depends on the severity and/or the duration of shock. In addition, preexisting hepatic disease predisposes the liver to a greater insult during circulatory collapse.[233] Champion et al.[231] noted that serum enzyme levels indicative of hepatocellular injury tend to reflect the magnitude of the insult. Patients with mild shock or with minimal microscopic evidence of hepatic damage did not exhibit a rise in LDH or SGOT. Patients who were successfully resuscitated from severe hemorrhagic shock generally exhibited increases in the serum LDH and SGOT concentrations within a few hours. In the absence of further hepatic insult the levels of these enzymes returned to normal over the ensuing 3 to 4 days. A rise in serum biliburin concentration, owing to liver injury and massive transfusion, occurred 8 to 10 days after the insult. Indices of intrahepatic cholestasis (serum alkaline phosphatase and gamma glytamyl transpeptidase) also increased at this time. In patients experiencing no further complications the hepatic chemical and morphologic abnormalities gradually returned to normal. Frequently, however, there were further increases in these variables, owing to the onset of sepsis, hypotension, or the need for surgical intervention.[231] Sepsis, in particular, tended to precipitate a deterioration in hepatic function. This adverse influence of gram-negative bacteria on the liver has also been demonstrated experimentally.[234]

As with many aberrations in shock, the cause of hepatic insufficiency is unknown. Most investigators have cited ischemia, hypoxia, and acidosis as the probable culprits. However, the assessment of the relative influence of each factor has been hampered by uncertainty over what constitutes the best indicator of acute hepatic dysfunction. Using liver lactate concentration and mitochondrial respiration as end points, Farkouh and associates[235] determined that the maximal safe period of normothermic ischemia in the canine liver was 40 minutes. Rangel and colleagues[236] found that the dog could tolerate hepatic ischemia for 30 minutes before significant increases in lysosomal enzymes appeared in the circulation. Clermont et al.[237] noted that the canine liver could withstand hemorrhagic shock for 2 hours before there was a significant elevation in acid phosphatase in the effluent blood and lymph. Carlson and Lefer[238] evaluated the relative influences of acidosis, hypoxia, and ischemia on hepatic function in an isolated perfused cat liver preparation. Utilizing perfusate lysosomal enzyme concentrations and reticuloendothelial clearance as indicators, they found that hypoxia was the most significant insult. However, White et al.[239] using mitochondrial morphologic changes as end points found that hypoxia alone was not responsible for the mitochondrial abnormalities seen in shock.

In sum, the precise mechanism of liver injury in circulatory collapse is not yet known. What is fact, however, is that the liver is a target organ in shock. As methods of acute resuscitation and multisystem support continue to improve, the hepatic consequences of circulatory failure will be encountered with increasing frequency.

The intestine

Since the classic work of Lillehei[240,241] 20 years ago, the intestine has been recognized as a primary target organ in shock, especially in experimental animals. With the onset of circulatory collapse following hemorrhage or endotoxin administration, there is a significant decline in intestinal blood flow and a concomitant increase in the degree of vasoconstriction.[242] These flow and resistance changes are most likely due to both a loss of circulating blood volume and an increase in the secretion of catecholamines. Hemorrhagic shock, for example, causes a 70- to 100-fold increase in the serum epinephrine concentration and a 10- to 20-fold increase in the norepinephrine level.[242] Compared with other organs, the mesenteric circulation in the dog suffers the largest reduction in blood flow, regardless of the etiology of shock.[242] Thus in circulatory collapse blood is diverted from the bowel to preferentially perfuse organs more vital to immediate survival.

The earliest histologic lesion seen in the intestine during shock is the development of subepithelial spaces near the tips of the villi.[243] This defect, Gruenhagen's space, is formed by the rupture of the basal portion of the cells lining the tips of the villi. With time the epithelial damage extends toward the mucosal crypts, and eventually there is separation and sloughing of the mucosa.[244] Transmural necrosis with hemorrhage may also be observed. Accompanying these histologic events, there is a significant decline in mucosal ATP content and oxygen utilization and a rise in serum acid phosphatase, RNAse, and β-glucuronidase—indicative of lysosomal damage.[243,245] Ultimately, the absorptive capacity of the bowel is interrupted, and in the end-stage of circulatory failure there is secretion and sequestration of fluid in the bowel lumen. Chiu et al.[243] noted that the pace with which these histologic, biochemical, and functional abnormalities developed was dependent on the magnitude of the reduction in blood flow. However, Haglund and associates,[246] using an isolated perfused bowel preparation, found that hypoxia, not flow per se, was the pathogenetic factor.

The significance of these intestinal abnormalities in circulatory failure goes beyond the concept of organ failure. The work of Lillehei and colleagues[240-242] demonstrated that in the dog the intestine plays a major role in determining the reversibility of shock. These investigators found that if superior mesenteric artery pressure and flow were maintained at normal levels during shock, the animal would survive. This discovery

led to the hypothesis that the ischemic bowel elaborated toxic substances, which adversely affected the structure and function of other organs. Indeed, recent work by Rangel et al.[232] and Haglund et al.[247] verifies that injurious substances are released into the circulation by ischemic bowel. The normal liver is capable of detoxifying this material and preventing the appearance of abnormal cardiovascular indices.[232] In shock, however, liver function is impaired, and hence these agents can exert their full potential on the systemic circulation. Although at one time it was thought that endogenous endotoxin was the responsible agent,[248] this theory is no longer generally accepted. In addition to the effects of toxic substances on cardiovascular dynamics, it is now appreciated that the volume deficit caused by the loss of fluid into the intestinal lumen plays a substantial role in the lethality of shock.[249]

In summary, the bowel is adversely affected by the sympathoadrenal response to circulatory collapse. As a result of this damage, intestinal "failure" occurs. In contrast to pulmonary, renal, or hepatic failure, however, the major significance of the bowel pathology in shock lies not in the loss of gastrointestinal absorptive capacity (intestinal failure) but in the elaboration into the circulation of substances harmful to the organism and in the sequestration in the bowel lumen of large volumes of fluid.

The heart

Because of its obvious central position in the cardiovascular system, the heart has often been entertained as the determinant factor in the development of irreversibility in circulatory collapse owing to hemorrhage or sepsis. During the past decade, however, numerous studies have shown not only that myocardial dysfunction is a relatively late event in the course of hemorrhagic and septic shock but also that heart failure is not the mysterious point of no return in the shock process. The sequential changes in the heart during the progression of hemorrhagic and septic shock will be discussed here. Myocardial responses in cardiogenic shock have been discussed in an earlier section.

With the onset of hemorrhagic shock, coronary artery blood flow falls considerably, and coronary vascular resistance initially rises.[140,141] Cardiac output falls dramatically, primarily because of the profound reduction in venous return. These hemodynamic events are accompanied by progressive ST-T wave changes consistent with myocardial ischemia.[41] Concomitant with the fall in coronary blood flow, myocardial oxygen extraction increases, while oxygen consumption declines. Glucose and free fatty acid extraction fall markedly, and the heart begins to produce pyruvate.[41,250] These events precede any measurable functional deficit. With continued shock, however, there is a progressive reduction in myocardial contractility.[251] Left ventricular end diastolic pressure rises, and left ventricular dP/dt_{max} falls.[252] Coronary blood flow continues to decrease and, along with the drop in hematocrit, results in a drop in myocardial oxygen availability. Ultimately, coronary blood flow during systole exceeds that during diastole, and effective myocardial perfusion is further diminished.[40] There is a progressive loss of myocardial compliance, which further impedes left ventricular performance.[253] Eventually, frank heart failure occurs and can contribute to the demise of the organism.

As with noncardiac organ failure, numerous studies have been conducted in an attempt to elucidate the reason(s) for the development of heart failure in hemorrhagic shock. For a time it was thought that MDF was the culprit,[43] but its role has now been reduced to that of a potentially minor contributor in late shock. Although acidosis[251,254] and the loss of circulating red blood cells[255] certainly have adverse effects on cardiac performance, most investigators agree that myocardial ischemia is the critical factor.[252] Lee and Downing[251] found a highly significant correlation between oxygen availability and left ventricular dP/dt_{max}, an indicator of ventricular contractility. Wilson et al.[44] noted that as long as coronary blood flow and blood gas and electrolyte concentrations were normal, no depression of myocardial function occurred during hemorrhagic shock. Raymer and colleagues[256] have also shown that inadequate coronary perfusion is primarily responsible for the reduction in cardiac function. Not only is total coronary perfusion decreased in hemorrhagic shock, but there is also an inequitable distribution of coronary blood flow,

such that the subendocardium is preferentially underperfused.[257,258] Thus this tissue becomes more ischemic than the rest of the myocardium. Furthermore, with the reestablishment of adequate coronary blood flow (that is, during resuscitation) the subendocardium does not tend to reperfuse as well as other areas of the left ventricle—a manifestation of the "no-reflow phenomenon."[259] Despite these seemingly catastrophic changes in cardiac structure and function, however, the heart has the capacity to return to normal function even in late hemorrhagic shock.[260] Thus deterioration of cardiac performance is not the factor that prevents recovery from irreversible hemorrhagic shock.

Since the study of Solis and Downing,[261] who showed that endotoxin administration reduced left ventricular contractility in the cat, there has been considerable interest in and debate on the role of the heart in endotoxin and septic shock. Studies by Siegel[82,91] and Cann[262] have clearly demonstrated that cardiac failure occurs in the intermediate and late stages of clinical septic shock. When Hinshaw et al.[263] and then Geocaris and associates[264] found that endotoxin did not adversely affect myocardial function in early (up to 4 hours) shock in the dog and the baboon, the potential role of MDF in endotoxin shock was enhanced.[108] However, in 1972 Hinshaw et al.[265] showed in an isolated heart preparation that heart failure did occur in late endotoxin shock (6 to 9 hours). Whereas in early endotoxin shock the depressed cardiac performance could be explained by the decreased venous return, the heart failure seen in late shock appeared to be intrinsic. Subsequent investigation by Greenfield[266] revealed similar findings in primates. Cross-circulation studies failed to demonstrate a direct myotoxic effect by either endotoxin or MDF.[267] Thus the reductions in left ventricular dP/dt, power, compliance, and work in endotoxin shock are related to the state of circulatory inadequacy itself and not to the etiologic agent.

Recent work has substantially clarified the mechanism by which cardiac failure occurs in septic shock. As in hemorrhagic shock, insufficient coronary perfusion during sepsis appears to be the primary determinant of myocardial performance.[268] If adequate coronary blood flow is maintained during endotoxin shock, the heart continues to function normally even in late shock. With decreased coronary perfusion, there is a marked reduction in myocardial oxygen consumption and a deterioration in the indices of myocardial function. As in hemorrhagic shock, the subendocardium is preferentially underperfused during sepsis,[258] and myocardial cellular edema occurs.[269] This swelling further impairs the delivery of oxygen and substrate to the cells, which potentially increases the consequences of ischemia. Thus the heart is intimately involved in the pathophysiology of endotoxin and septic shock. Once again, however, transplantation studies have shown that the derangements in cardiac structure and function are not irreversible even in late shock.[270] Hence the heart is not the determinant of irreversibility in endotoxin —and probably septic—shock.

The brain

Compared to our understanding of the functional impairment in other organs, little is known about the response of the brain in shock. That cerebral function is impaired in circulatory collapse is demonstrated by the observable changes in mental status in patients experiencing circulatory decompensation. Virtually every clinician has seen such patients progress (or regress) from mental alertness to confusion, obtundation, and finally coma. Yet little is known about the mechanism behind these developments. With the availability of more accurate techniques to measure the events occurring in the brain, we are slowly learning more about the responses of this important organ during shock.

Early studies suggested that the brain was a privileged organ in circulatory failure—that cerebral blood flow was maintained at the expense of perfusion of other organs.[165] The reason for this misconception was that few studies were of sufficient duration or quality to demonstrate significant changes in flow. Using radioactive microspheres, Slater and associates[271] showed that there is a slight decrease in cerebral blood flow in early hemorrhagic shock. Since there is a profound reduction in cardiac output at this time, the fraction of cardiac output flowing to the brain is increased. Thus in early hemorrhagic shock the

brain does receive blood flow at the expense of other organs. Later in the course of hemorrhagic shock both the absolute and relative cerebral blood flow are reduced. In contrast, in endotoxin shock there is an early and persistent decrease in cerebral blood flow.[272] Although Slater[271] found that the reduction in blood flow to the brain was universal and of equal distribution, Kovach[273,274] noted that shock resulted in a redistribution of flow. The midbrain and cerebellum were relatively underperfused, while flow in the cerebral cortex was moderately decreased. Flow to the medulla oblongata was essentially normal. In other words, this redistribution of blood flow within the brain ensures that those portions of the brain most vital to survival remain relatively well perfused. Kovach also noted areas scattered throughout the brain that were devoid of flow.[275] Pertinent histologic changes were ischemia of the cerebral cortex, disruption of the normal capillary pattern, and intravenous sludge formation.

The reason for these cerebral changes during shock has not been clearly defined. Although it is traditionally accepted that the brain is not highly sensitive to α-adrenergic stimulation, Kovach[273] showed that pretreatment with phenoxybenzamine significantly increased cerebral blood flow during hemorrhagic shock. Thus in some way the sympathetic nervous system and/or circulating catecholamines have a strong influence on the blood flow changes seen during circulatory collapse. Other factors affecting brain perfusion during shock are the fall in Pco_2, which would tend to reduce cerebral blood flow.[271] Since there appears to be a redistribution of blood flow within the brain during shock, it is probable that unknown local autoregulatory factors also affect brain perfusion.

The reduction in blood flow to the brain during circulatory collapse means that eventually the brain becomes ischemic and hypoxic. The brain, like other tissue, turns to anaerobic metabolism when oxygen availability reaches a critically low level, and lactate concentration begins to rise.[276] Glucose consumption falls,[272] and the availability of energy (ATP) necessary to maintain cellular integrity and central nervous system function declines. Energy production is further impaired by the onset of hypoglycemia, which decreases glucose availability. With prolonged shock cerebral cell damage and death are demonstrable.[277] By this time, however, it is likely that factors other than brain dysfunction have produced a state of irreversibility.

The blood

The constituents of blood, the liquid organ, undergo many changes during circulatory collapse. Some of these alterations and the way they potentially relate to lung function in shock have already been discussed. This section will examine the effects of shock on the components of blood, as well as the means by which alterations in the constituents of blood can interfere with each other and with other organs.

An obvious change in hemorrhagic shock is the reduction in the number of circulating red blood cells. As mentioned previously, the loss of erythrocytes reduces the oxygen-carrying capacity of the blood. Proctor et al.[278] showed that the removal of half the red cell mass and replacement with crystalloid solution resulted in a 16% drop in available oxygen. In contrast to septic shock[106] hemorrhagic shock causes no change in red cell 2,3-DPG concentration, which also can affect the ability of the blood to transport oxygen. In septic shock not only is red cell 2,3-DPG concentration reduced and the oxyhemoglobin curve shifted to the left, but in 30% to 50% of patients the circulating red cell volume is significantly reduced.[107] This decrease in hematocrit is primarily due to occult blood loss, especially in the gastrointestinal tract.

Surprisingly, little data are readily available on the status of the white blood cells in circulatory collapse. In studies on hemorrhagic shock we have noted an increase in the leukocyte count during acute shock, followed by a profound decrease during resuscitation.[279] In both phases there was a predominant granulocyte response, with severe depression of the lymphocyte count. Similar findings on the lymphocyte response were reported by Bauer et al.[280] in traumatized patients. While intravascular dilution by resuscitative fluids may explain the reduction in leukocytes, evidence suggests that other, selective factors may be involved. Dinbar and associates[281] noted a profound, persistent fall in the white

blood cell count in monkeys given endotoxin, and Hammon et al.[282] made similar observations in baboons following *E. coli* infusion. Milligan and colleagues[107] found a variable pattern in the leukocyte response in patients in septic shock. In some patients the white cell count remained normal or was depressed, while in others there was a rise in the leukocyte count. No comment was made regarding the possible relationship between the white blood cell response and survival. In our experience patients who cannot mount a leukocyte response to sepsis tend to fare poorly, presumably because they are more susceptible to lethal infection. Altura and Hershey[283] noted in endotoxin-treated animals that survivors had a progressive decrease in the lymphocyte-granulocyte ratio, while the ratio remained unchanged among those that died. Again, the suggestion is present that organisms capable of mounting a granulocyte response to sepsis fare better than those who cannot. The reasons for a reduction in the white blood cell population during septic shock are numerous. A great many leukocytes are undoubtedly destroyed in combatting the offending microorganisms. Endotoxin causes toxic damage to neutrophils and also increases neutrophil adherence characteristics, which may contribute to their effective removal from the circulation.[284,285] Another factor in the genesis of neutropenia is the sequestration of white cells in the lung during shock.[175] Finally, it is possible that shock somehow impairs white blood cell release from the marrow.

The majority of the research on the hematologic response to circulatory collapse has been concentrated on the coagulation changes of shock. Both patients and experimental animals exhibit coagulation abnormalities in cardiogenic, hemorrhagic, and septic shock and following trauma[107,286-290] (Table 41-2). The superimposition of sepsis on a traumatized patient increases the likelihood of coagulopathy.[289] In general, there are elevations in the prothrombin, activated partial thromboplastin, and whole blood clotting times. The platelet count falls markedly, as does the serum fibrinogen level. In septic shock there is also a decline in serum complement concentration.[287,291,292] When coagulation factors are assayed serially, decreased levels of factors V, VII,

Table 41-2. Laboratory findings in disseminated intravascular coagulopathy

Assay	Normal values	Status in DIC
Whole blood clotting time	7-18 min	Prolonged-incoagulable
Partial thromboplastin time	30-45 sec	Prolonged-incoagulable
Quick one-stage prothrombin time	12-15 sec	Elevated
Thrombin time	12-15 sec	Prolonged-incoagulable
Fibrin split products	Negative	Strongly positive
Bleeding time	2-7 min	Usually prolonged
Platelet count	150,000-400,000/mm³	Low
Fibrinogen	200-400 mg%	Low
Factor V	70%-140%	Very low
Factor VIII	50%-200%	Low
Factor XII	60%-170%	Often low in sepsis
Vitamin K–dependent factors		
Factor X	70%-140%	Low
Factors VII and IX	60%-170%	Reduced
Plasminogen	2-4 U/ml	Low

IX, X, and XI and plasminogen are found. Increased amounts of fibrin degradation products are noted, indicative of ongoing intravascular coagulation. Such coagulation abnormalities potentially place the patient at a greater risk of spontaneous bleeding and microembolism. The latter can contribute to both the hepatic and pulmonary dysfunction seen in patients after traumatic shock.[293,294]

String et al.[288] reported a strong correlation between the magnitude of the coagulation changes and the severity of trauma and suggested that intravascular coagulation plays a detrimental role in circulatory collapse. Attar and associates,[290] however, reported that although significant alterations in the coagulation and fibrinolytic systems are demonstrable in patients in shock, DIC does not play a major role in determining irreversibility. They based their conclusions on the lack of evidence of fibrin deposition in the organs of 52 patients examined carefully at autopsy. Similar observations have also been made in septic baboons by Hammon et al.[282] Although these findings are at odds with the experimental data of Holcroft and associates,[295] the conclusion of Attar[290] is in keeping with the knowledge that fulminant DIC is a near-terminal event in shock.

The reason(s) for the development of intravascular coagulation in circulatory failure is not entirely known. Garcia-Barreno et al.[287] studied this question in dogs subjected to endotoxin and hemorrhagic shock. They noted that in endotoxin shock there was no relationship between the hemodynamic-metabolic changes and the appearance of coagulopathy. Rather, it appeared that endotoxin directly initiated the coagulopathy by producing thrombocytopenia and by activating the coagulation system—a conclusion previously reached in baboons by Horwitz and associates.[286] In hemorrhagic shock (and cardiogenic shock) intravascular coagulation appears to be a secondary phenomenon, possibly a result of changes in vascular endothelium or microcirculatory abnormalities, which set the coagulation mechanism in motion. This observation fits well with the fact that DIC can occur in patients sustaining major trauma without shock. The role of platelets in initiating or perpetuating intravascular coagulation is not well defined. It is thought that platelet aggregates might participate in the DIC syndrome by releasing activating substances or by plugging capillaries in the microcirculation.[295-297] However, studies in thrombocytopenic animals have shown that the presence of platelets is not determinative of the pathogenetic events in shock.[298,299]

In summary, significant hematologic alterations occur during all forms of circulatory collapse. While DIC has attracted most of the attention in recent years, it appears that, in general, these coagulation changes are of minor clinical significance. Fulminant DIC is a very late finding in patients experiencing circulatory collapse and thus does not determine irreversibility in the shock process. In addition to anemia, probably the most significant hematologic change that can occur from a clinical standpoint is lymphopenia, since this state appears to render the host more susceptible to lethal infection.

The reticuloendothelial system and the immune mechanism

While not an organ per se, the reticuloendothelial system (RES) and the immune apparatus function like an organ system. Since these two mechanisms share several interrelated functions, they will be discussed together.

The RES has two cellular components. The major portion consists of sessile macrophages in the liver, spleen, and bone marrow. These macrophages are in direct contact with the blood. This strategic location gives them an ideal opportunity to monitor the constituents of the blood and to clear foreign and endogenous particulate matter (damaged erythrocytes and platelets, fibrin split products, immune complexes, cell debris, bacteria) and toxic substances from the blood. The majority of the work done by the sessile component of the RES is performed by the hepatic Kupffer cells, which comprise 80% to 90% of the total phagocytic activity.[300] The reason for the yeoman job by the Kupffer cells is that they have a high phagocytic capacity and they are located in an organ that receives a large blood flow (25% to 30% of cardiac output).

In addition to this sessile arm of the RES, there is a mobile component consisting of wandering macrophages in the blood, pulmonary alveoli, peritoneal cavity, and other tissue spaces. The locations of these cells also place them in ideal sites for the clearance of particulate and toxic substances from the body. There is a third component of the RES, opsonin. Opsonin is a serum factor identified as an α_2 SB glycoprotein. While the precise mechanism of action of opsonin is unknown, it somehow prepares either the RES or particulate matter itself for phagocytosis.

There is a considerable body of evidence linking the RES to the pathophysiology of shock. It is well known that reticuloendothelial function is depressed in hemorrhagic, endotoxin, septic, and traumatic shock.[300-302] The degree of RES impairment is directly related to the severity of the insult. Animals that survive various degrees of hemorrhagic shock, for example, demonstrate early depression of reticuloendothelial function, followed in a few days by transient hyperfunction.[303] Nonsurviving animals exhibit persistent RES depression.[304] Similar RES changes have been observed in surviving and nonsurviving trauma patients.[300]

Blockade of the RES with large doses of particulate matter increases the susceptibility of the host to insults by endotoxin, hemorrhage, or trauma.[305-307] On the other hand, stimulation of the RES (for example, zymosan) results in increased phagocytic capability and produces a greater resistance to sepsis, intestinal ischemia, and endotoxin or hemorrhagic shock.[302,307-309] This "tolerance" to shock is associated with a marked hypertrophy and hyperfunction of the RES.[310] To a large extent, animals made tolerant to one form of shock exhibit cross-tolerance to other insults.[311] The establishment of tolerance in this fashion is also associated with an increase in the functional capability of the RES. These findings have led some investigators[302,303,307] to suggest that the RES may represent the critical common pathway in the pathogenesis of shock.

Further evidence for a pivotal role of the RES in circulatory collapse comes from the relationship between RES function and survival. Rangel et al.[312] observed that the systemic injection of endotoxin produces a more severe hypotension than does injection into the portal vein. This finding suggests that in the latter situation endotoxin is removed from the circulation and detoxified by the hepatic RES. Olcay and colleagues[313] studied the response of the RES to hepatic ischemia in baboons. They found that those animals that developed phagocytic depression ultimately died, whereas those with minor changes in reticuloendothelial function survived. Scovill and associates[314] reported that restoration of normal plasma opsonin levels in patients with sepsis reversed RES depression and produced dramatic clinical improvement. Thus it appears that reticuloendothelial function is intimately related to the pathophysiology and the ultimate consequences of circulatory collapse.

The mechanism(s) behind the RES changes seen during circulatory failure are still poorly understood. Although Fine's group[248,315] has championed a role for endogenous endotoxin in the pathophysiology of all forms of shock, studies by Zweifach et al.[316] and by Olcay and associates[317] have ruled out an influence on the RES by endotoxin in nonseptic shock. Similarly, lysosomal enzymes have been eliminated as adverse influences on the RES, since reticuloendothelial depression occurs prior to shock-induced cellular injury.[318] Since hepatic and splenic blood flow are decreased in circulatory collapse, hypoperfusion of a crucial arm of the RES seems to be a factor in the depression of reticuloendothelial function.[319] In addition, there is evidence that vasoactive substances, such as histamine, serotonin, and bradykinin, liberated during circulatory collapse adversely affect reticuloendothelial function.[320] To date, the most important variable relating to RES function is plasma opsonin, a glycoprotein that seems to enable the RES to discriminate between self- and nonself-material. Loegering and Carr[321] found a close temporal relationship between the level of circulating opsonin and depression of the phagocytic index during hemorrhagic shock, suggesting that serum opsonin mediates reticuloendothelial function. Saba[322] noted a similar relationship in rats following surgical trauma. He was able to prevent the postoperative depression in reticuloendothelial function with opsonin treatment. Similar results were noted in traumatized patients by Scovill et al.[314] Thus of all the factors that can affect reticuloendothelial function during circulatory failure the serum opsonin concentration is presently the most influential. The following are adverse influences on the RES during circulatory collapse:

Opsonin depletion
Hepatic ischemia
Hypotension
Hypoxia
Acidosis
Vasoactive substances (RES depressants)
Colloid therapy

Antibiotics and other drugs
Anesthesia
Surgery
Blood products
Infection
Bacteremia, endotoxin
DIC

While changes in reticuloendothelial function during shock have been extensively investigated, the influence of circulatory collapse on the immune mechanism has received little attention. It is now appreciated that there is a heightened risk of serious infection in patients sustaining shock and/or trauma.[323] This association implies that circulatory failure produces a breakdown in the host defense mechanisms. From the foregoing discussion we know that macrophage phagocytic activity is depressed in shock. Likewise, the potential role of granulocytopenia and lymphopenia in the reduction of host defenses has been mentioned. In addition to the potential decline in the *number* of the circulating white blood cells that participate in cell-mediated immunity, there is evidence that trauma can reduce their *function*.[324] MacLean et al.[325,326] found a close correlation between infection, septicemia, and death and a reduction in cell-mediated immunity in seriously ill and traumatized patients. The presence of cutaneous anergy, a crude measure of cell-mediated immunity, was predictive of the development of infectious complications in these patients. Furthermore, restoration of delayed hypersensitivity responses was correlated with clinical improvement.[327] Although little else is presently known about the effects of shock on immune mechanisms, it appears that abnormalities can occur in this important system and that such dysfunction can have lethal consequences.

A number of important conclusions can be reached from this section on organ dysfunction in shock. First, circulatory collapse is a total-body phenomenon. As such, virtually every organ is adversely affected at some time during the course of the disease. Second, different organs have varying degrees of sensitivity to shock. Hence, the magnitude of the histologic and biochemical changes and the timing of organ failure is different for each organ. Third, there are many interrelationships among the organ systems, such that one cannot focus on the impairment of a given structure as though it existed in a vacuum. Lastly, it is apparent that the development of irreversibility in circulatory collapse cannot be attributed to the failure of any one organ or component of a given system. On the contrary, deterioration in the status of a patient in circulatory failure is associated with increasing dysfunction in many organ systems. Only with this understanding of the shock process can the clinician begin to treat the condition properly.

■ What is the treatment of shock?

The proper management of the patient with circulatory collapse depends on an accurate initial assessment and frequent reassessment of the ongoing pathophysiologic processes. Although the specific treatment program varies with both the type of shock and the individual patient, the method of patient evaluation and many of the treatment modalities are common to all forms of shock.

The initial step in evaluating the patient in shock is to obtain a good history and perform a thorough physical examination. As with any other disease, the history and physical examination will indicate the etiology of circulatory collapse in the majority of patients. Particular attention should be given to the respiratory status of the patient, and if necessary an airway and assisted ventilation should be employed.

Because of the possibility of sepsis as the cause of shock, all IV and urinary catheters and tubing should be removed, cultured, and replaced. A closed-drainage urinary catheter system is mandatory in order to reduce the incidence of subsequent urinary tract infection. Samples of blood, sputum, urine, and drainage are obtained for Gram stain and culture. An arterial catheter is inserted, usually into a brachial or radial artery, for accurate measurement of blood pressure and for use in determining cardiac ouput with dye dilution curves. A balloon-tipped catheter (Swan-Ganz) is customarily introduced into a major vein and advanced into the pulmonary artery to measure pulmonary pressures and to determine cardiac output by thermodilution. Blood samples

are drawn for the determination of arterial gases, hemoglobin, leukocyte count, electrolyte levels, proteins, glucose, creatinine, and clotting studies. An ECG and chest x-ray film are obtained, and the initial set of hemodynamic measurements is made.

Using this systematic approach to the evaluation of patients in shock, it is possible to establish the type of shock and to determine the hemodynamic and metabolic status of the patient within the first 30 to 60 minutes after the onset of circulatory collapse. The importance of obtaining such studies, which enable the practitioner to tailor treatment to the patient's needs, cannot be overemphasized. In extremely urgent circumstances it may be necessary to forego some of these initial assessments and begin treatment more promptly. As soon as the patient's condition has stabilized, however, a complete hemodynamic and metabolic evaluation should be undertaken.

Since the basic pathophysiology of shock varies with the cause of the circulatory collapse, there are some differences in the manner in which each type of shock is treated. As already indicated, attention should first be directed to the respiratory status of the patient, since potential pulmonary abnormalities are an integral part of any form of circulatory collapse. As soon as proper steps have been taken to correct the respiratory and acid-base disturbances, other measures are initiated in line with the etiology of the shock process.

Hemorrhagic shock

In hypovolemic shock the basic defect is the lack of an adequate circulating blood volume. The essence of treatment is the replacement of the patient's fluid losses, which in most instances eventually involves the use of whole blood (Table 41-3). Since some delay is experienced in obtaining properly matched blood for transfusion, the patient must be initially supported by nonerythrocyte-containing solutions. In the past there was considerable debate over not only the merits of colloid versus crystalloid solutions but also over the relative values of the various kinds of colloid and crystalloid solutions used. Much of this

Table 41-3. Treatment of traumatic shock

Condition to be corrected (restored)	Treatment
Hypovolemia	Control of hemorrhage; blood, plasma fractions, dextran, crystalloids
Stagnant anoxia, membrane integrity	Synthetic glucocorticosteroids (methylprednisolone, dexamethasone)
Oncotic pressure	Albumin
Oliguria	Furosemide
Hypoxemia	Respirator (volume type, positive end-expiratory pressure), oxygen
Persistent hypoperfusion	Dopamine, phenoxybenzamine, glucagon, and glucose

controversy has been resolved in recent years, and current evidence indicates that the patient in hemorrhagic shock can be hemodynamically supported during the initial phase of resuscitation with Ringer's solution, normal saline solution, low molecular weight dextran, plasma, or a 5% albumin solution.[328,329] Reich and Eiseman[330] have demonstrated normal tissue oxygenation following resuscitation with Ringer's solution. Contrary to previous belief, the use of lactated Ringer's solution does not increase serum lactate concentration and contribute to metabolic acidosis.[328,331] Both Litwin[332] and Matsuda and Shoemaker[333] have shown increased oxygen transport and consumption following the use of dextran 40 in hemorrhagic shock. We prefer a balance of crystalloid and colloid solutions to avoid any disadvantages of each type of fluid.[334] Warming the fluid to at least room temperature prior to administration is of some benefit, especially if the fluids are given rapidly.[335]

Although the immediate steps in the resuscitation of the patient in hypovolemic shock are directed toward correcting the respiratory and circulatory deficits, another initial concern should be to discover and control the source of the fluid loss, in most instances bleeding. Pressure is applied to obvious external bleeding points. Surgery is usually required to control internal sites of hemorrhage. In patients with pelvic fractures and shock a G suit may significantly decrease blood loss and improve survival.[336] Whatever the source, it is imperative that any major bleeding be controlled early in order to reduce the duration of circulatory collapse and the likelihood of subsequent complications.

When the source of bleeding is obscure in trauma patients, a peritoneal lavage using 1 L of 5% glucose instilled through a dialysis catheter may be of help. If the returning fluid is grossly bloody or if it contains more than 100,000 red blood cells/mm³, then a laparotomy should be done to find the source of bleeding. Similarly, if the white blood cell count of the fluid is greater than 500 cells/mm³, a perforated viscus must be suspected.

Although blood and IV fluids are the cornerstones of treatment, in many instances of hemorrhagic shock or multisystem trauma merely restoring the blood volume may not be enough to successfully resuscitate the patient. Under these circumstances certain other maneuvers may be helpful. Exogenous glucose, for reasons that are not clear, improves hemodynamics and survival in experimental oligemic shock.[337,338] Glucagon increases the cardiac output and stroke volume and lowers the total peripheral resistance and the splanchnic resistance in experimental hypovolemic shock.[339] In addition, glucagon appears to stimulate the hepatic conversion of lactic, amino, and fatty acids to glucose and it possibly increases ATP production.[340] Recent experiments suggest that the administration of 50% glucose with glucagon enhances the inotropic effect of the drug.[341] We have not found glucagon to be a beneficial agent clinically, however. The administration of high-energy compounds (ATP $MgCl_2$) is beneficial in experimental hemorrhagic shock,[342-344] but the treatment has not been clinically evaluated. Phenoxybenzamine and dopamine, by reducing peripheral resistance and improving renal blood flow, may be helpful in hypovolemic shock.[202,345]

In our experience the most successful agents in the treatment of refractory (to volume replacement) hemorrhagic shock have been the corticosteroids. Numerous studies[346-351] have documented that the use of massive doses of glucocorticosteroids may correct many of the hemody-namic and cellular disturbances of shock.

EFFECTS OF CORTICOSTEROIDS IN PHARMACOLOGIC DOSES IN SHOCK

INCREASES IN
Visceral organ blood flow
Cardiac index
Coronary blood flow
Systemic oxygen consumption
Lactic acid metabolism
Glucose metabolism

DECREASES IN
Sympathetic nerve transmission
Arteriolar and venular resistance
Platelet aggregability
Leukocyte destruction and sequestration
Extravascular lung water
Myocardial infarct size
Complement fixation by endotoxin
Kinin production

RESTORATION OF
Vascular membrane integrity in lung, intestine, and
forelimb

STABILIZATION OF
Lysosomal membranes in lung, intestine, pancreas,
heart, liver, kidney, and forelimb

PREVENTION OF
Fat embolism to lung in multisystem trauma

We use 30 mg/kg of methylprednisolone sodi-um succinate (Solu-Medrol) or 6 mg/kg of dexa-methasone (Decadron) given IV over a 10-min-ute period. This same dose may be repeated once or twice in the first 12 to 24 hours and then is stopped abruptly. This regimen allows for all of the beneficial effects of these protean substances without producing any of the side-effects that may come from chronic use.

We frequently use furosemide (Lasix) in shock patients to improve urine output. Doses of 20 to 40 mg are given initially for oliguria or anuria, and if there is no response, 100 to 500 mg may be given. A patient who is producing urine—even dilute urine—is easier to manage than one who is anuric.

In the treatment of hemorrhagic shock there are many agents that should probably be avoided. It used to be thought that patients in hemor-rhagic shock were always acidotic and that the administration of IV bicarbonate should be bene-ficial. However, recent studies have shown that

there is less need for such buffering agents, and they are now reserved for patients with a pH be-low 7.40.[352,353]

Norepinephrine was formerly used in the treat-ment of all forms of shock, but we now know that this potent vasoconstrictor causes damage to the visceral organs, especially the lungs and kid-neys.[202] Norepinephrine increases the mean sys-temic blood pressure at the expense of increas-ing vascular resistance. It also increases the work of the heart. Vasopressors more often improve the practitioner's sense of well-being than that of the patient, since the survival of patients in whom they are used is not improved. Dopamine, another catecholamine that increases blood pres-sure and lowers peripheral resistance, also does not improve survival in experimental hypovole-mic shock.[354] Isoproterenol seems to have a lim-ited potential in these patients, since its use is contraindicated in patients with heart rates in ex-cess of 120 beats/min.

The essentials of the treatment regimen for hemorrhagic shock are, therefore, regulation of the respiratory and acid-base status, stopping the blood loss, appropriate volume replacement, and, in some patients, the use of corticosteroids and di-uretics. With early, vigorous treatment of hemor-rhagic shock the mortality of this condition can be under 10%.[352,353]

Cardiogenic shock

The basic defect in cardiogenic shock is an in-effective blood pump. The heart has become too weak to circulate a sufficient blood volume for the body's needs. The treatment of this form of shock, therefore, centers around attempts to improve the pumping ability of the heart (Table 41-4). There are two means by which this aim is currently accomplished: the administration of certain agents to increase the contractility of the myocar-dium and the use of measures designed to re-duce the pressure against which the heart must pump blood (afterload).

The first step in resuscitation should always be directed at the regulation of the respiratory (and acid-base) status of the patient. The circulatory status is the next concern, since hypovolemia may occur in patients with cardiogenic shock.[355] Moreover, an optimum response to all other ther-

Table 41-4. Treatment of cardiogenic shock

Condition to be corrected (restored)	Treatment
Hypovolemia	Plasma fractions, dextran, crystalloids, blood (occasionally)
Stagnant anoxia, membrane integrity, infarct size	Synthetic glucocorticosteroids (methylprednisolone, dexamethasone)
Substrate deficiency	Glucose-insulin-potassium
Oncotic pressure	Albumin
Oliguria	Furosemide
Pulmonary edema	Digitalis
Myocardial contractility	Glucagon(?), digitalis, α-blockers, dobutamine(?)
Hypoxemia	Respirator (volume type, positive end-expiratory pressure), oxygen

apeutic maneuvers will not occur in the face of a circulatory deficit. The central venous and pulmonary artery pressures and urine output serve as guides to proper fluid replacement. In general, the pulmonary artery wedge pressure should not be allowed to exceed 18 mm Hg, since overaggressive fluid therapy can promote pulmonary edema.[356] The central venous pressure alone is not a reliable guide to fluid replacement in cardiogenic shock,[357] but when pulmonary artery wedge pressures are unavailable, the cautious use of the central venous pressure and urine output in gauging fluid administration is superior to the use of clinical judgment alone.

The treatment of cardiogenic shock primarily centers around the use of pharmacologic agents to assist the failing heart. Although at one time there was considerable controversy over the use of vasopressors versus vasodilators, it is now generally accepted that vasodilator therapy is the treatment of choice. There is ample evidence in the literature that vasopressors such as epinephrine, levarterenol, and metaraminol do not improve the survival of patients in cardiogenic shock.[358,359] These agents do increase the blood pressure, but at the expense of an increased peripheral resistance, with a consequent reduction in tissue perfusion and an increased oxygen demand on the already hypoxic myocardium. Posi-

tive inotropic agents, such as glucagon and isoproterenol, are also ineffective in the treatment of cardiogenic shock[360-362] (Fig. 41-11). Dopamine, a substance that increases blood pressure and cardiac output and reduces peripheral resistance,[363,364] was expected to enhance patient survival. Such has not been the case, however.[365] Furthermore, both dopamine and isoproterenol may increase the extent of ischemic injury in acute myocardial infarction.[366,367] Digitalis should be used if congestive heart failure is present, but should not be administered prophylactically. It should be emphasized that care must be taken with the use of pharmacologic agents in patients with acute myocardial infarction to ensure that these maneuvers do not increase the size of the infarct.[368]

At the present time the most effective pharmacologic agents in the management of cardiogenic shock are the corticosteroids (Figs. 41-11 to 41-14). A dose of 30 mg/kg of methylprednisolone or its equivalent is recommended, and this amount is administered once as an IV bolus. In patients who either do not respond to a single injection or deteriorate after temporary improvement, we administer a second bolus. Under no circumstances should routine multiple doses of corticosteroids, constant infusions of these agents, or tapering dosage schedules be employed in patients with cardiogenic shock, or adverse effects on myocardial structure may result.[369] Methylprednisolone has a stabilizing influence on cell membranes and causes peripheral vasodilatation. By decreasing afterload and/or by a direct myocardial effect, corticosteroids may decrease infarct size.[370] Although corticosteroids usually produce significant improvements in hemodynamics (Fig. 14-13), in some cases it may be necessary to transiently employ a positive inotropic agent, such as dobutamine, to further augment cardiac output. The use of massive doses of corticosteroids has increased the survival rate in both experimental and clinical cardiogenic shock from 20% to 60%.[3,371-373]

Patients who do not respond to pharmacologic agents are candidates for mechanical circulatory support. The mechanical assist devices basically fall into two categories: the series units, which reduce left ventricular pressure work, and

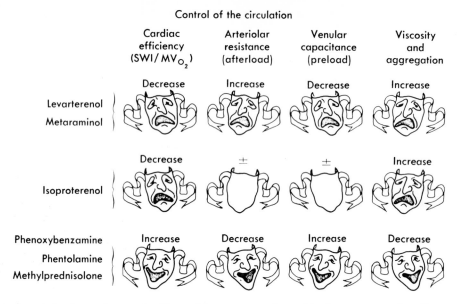

Fig. 41-11. Cardiac and systemic effects of drugs commonly used in the treatment of cardiogenic shock. SWI (stroke work index) = MSP (mean systolic pressure) − LVEDP (left ventricular end-diastolic pressure) × CI (cardiac index) ÷ Heart rate. MV_{O_2}, Mean oxygen utilization.

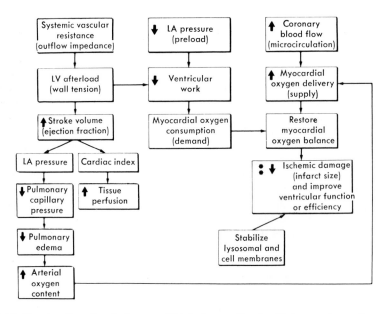

Fig. 41-12. Therapeutic rationale for use of high-dose corticosteroid therapy in cardiogenic shock.

Low output syndrome   Myocardial infarction

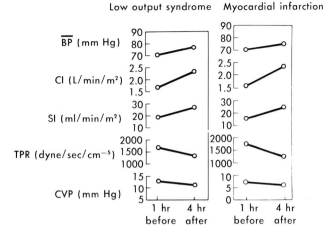

Fig. 41-13. Hemodynamic changes in cardiogenic shock following methylprednisolone administration (30 mg/kg).

Low output syndrome Myocardial infarction

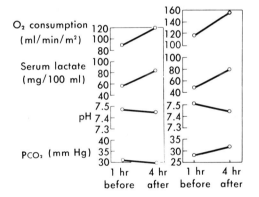

Fig. 41-14. Metabolic effects of methylprednisolone (30 mg/kg) in cardiogenic shock.

Table 41-5. Effect of intra-aortic balloon pumping on survival in cardiogenic shock

	No. of patients	Unable to insert balloon	Survival	%
Acute myocardial infarction	8	1	0	0
Low output syndrome	14	3	1	7
TOTAL	22	4	1	5

Table 41-6. Influence of external counterpulsation on survival in cardiogenic shock

	No. of patients	Survival	%
Acute myocardial infarction	3	1	33
Low output syndrome	7	2	29
TOTAL	10	3	30

the parallel devices, which decrease volume work. The intra-aortic balloon pump and the external counterpulsation machine are examples of the former. Both maneuvers augment the systemic pressure and organ perfusion during diastole.[374] In addition, by increasing the runoff during diastole, the heart has less of a pressure head against which it must pump during systole. Although both hemodynamic and metabolic improvement have been observed following the use

of these series devices, patient survival has not been enhanced unless there is a surgically correctable lesion causing shock.[375-377] (Tables 41-5 and 41-6). Thus, at present, the series units are primarily used to support patients resistant to pharmacologic agents until emergency aortocoronary bypass surgery can be performed.[378] The parallel devices, which pump blood during systole and thereby reduce the volume handled by the left ventricle, are still beset with problems and not available for widespread clinical use.

Of primary importance in the use of mechanical circulatory assistance is the need to use these devices early in the course of circulatory collapse rather than many hours or days later when many of the complications of shock have occurred. Usually the clinician can determine in a few hours whether volume-drug-respirator support will resuscitate the patient. If not, the assistance devices should be used immediately.

Although cardiogenic shock is still the most lethal form of circulatory collapse, advances are slowly being made in our understanding of this condition. Hopefully this knowledge will eventually be translated into improved patient survival. From a practical standpoint, the most promising treatment of cardiogenic shock is its prevention by the use of appropriate agents to limit the size of myocardial necrosis during infarction. In the future cardiac transplantation or replacement may be realistic considerations in these patients. At present, our therapeutic results are hampered by the limited number of successful interventions available and by many physiologic factors beyond our control (Table 41-7).

Septic shock

Unlike cardiogenic and hemorrhagic shock, the basic pathophysiologic defect in septic shock is unknown. These patients all have overwhelm-

Table 41-7. Prognostic indicators in patients with cardiogenic shock

Poor prognosis	Favorable prognosis
Prior myocardial infarction	Mean arterial pressure > 74 mm Hg
Hypertension	Stroke index > 25 ml/beat/m²
Prior heart failure	Cardiac index > 1.8 L/min/m²
Age over 65	Diastolic pressure > 55 mm Hg
Pulmonary edema	Pulmonary wedge pressure < 20 mm Hg
Late onset of shock after myocardial infarction	Cardiac work > 3 kg-m/min
Late admission to hospital after myocardial infarction	Left ventricular filling pressure < 15 mm Hg
Resistance to pharmacologic treatment	Urine output > 60 ml/hr
Lack of surgically correctable lesion	Lactate < 3.5 moles
Unable to wean from balloon pump	Pco_2 > 41 mm Hg
Persistent sinus tachycardia	pH > 7.300
Atrioventricular block	Hematocrit > 48

Table 41-8. Treatment of septic shock

Condition to be corrected (restored)	Treatment
Hypovolemia	Plasma fractions, dextran, crystalloids, blood
Stagnant anoxia, membrane integrity, endotoxin activation	Synthetic glucocorticosteroids (methylprednisolone, dexamethasone)
Substrate deficiency	Glucose-insulin-potassium
Oncotic pressure	Albumin
Oliguria	Furosemide
Congestive heart failure	Digitalis, glucose-insulin-potassium, nitroprusside, nitroglycerin
Sepsis	Antibiotics, elimination of source
Arteriovenous admixture	Respirator (volume type, positive end-expiratory pressure)
Hypoxemia	Oxygen
Gastric erosions	Cimetidine, antacids

Table 41-9. Sources of infection in 43 patients with septic shock at the University of Minnesota Hospitals

Site of infection	No. of patients
Lung	27
Urinary tract	23
Wound	10
Peritoneum	9
Intra-abdominal abscess	6
IV catheter	6
Biliary tract	3
Uterus	3
Chest cavity	2
Abdominal wall abscess	2
Pancreatic pseudocyst	1
Liver abscess	1
Colon	1
Esophagus	1

ing systemic infections, but the mechanism by which the microorganisms produce shock is not clear. The uncertainties regarding the etiology and treatment of septic shock and the frequent failure to diagnose the condition in its early stages have contributed to the high mortality in the past. In recent years significant advances have been made in the treatment of this condition.

Once control of the patient's respiratory status has been accomplished, the circulatory needs should be evaluated (Table 41-8). Most of these patients are either absolutely or relatively volume deficient, and a large number will show considerable clinical improvement following the administration of IV fluids. Since anemia and defective tissue oxygenation are common in septic shock, the administration of blood or blood products is often necessary.[91,107] Hypoalbuminemia is also a frequent finding, and if present, appropriate amounts of albumin should be given.[379] Concomitant with fluid therapy, large amounts of parenteral antibiotics should be given. Appropriate agents are used when positive cultures or smears

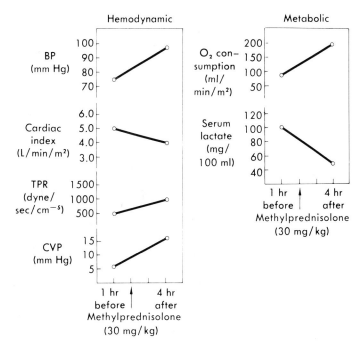

Fig. 41-15. Hemodynamic-metabolic effects of methylprednisolone (30 mg/kg) in septic shock.

are available. In the absence of a known pathogen we customarily employ the combination of cephalothin, gentamicin, and clindamycin in an attempt to provide coverage against the anaerobes and aerobes that are most commonly cultured from patients in septic shock. A localized infection should be drained if possible (Table 41-9) to prevent continued seeding of the patient's

Table 41-10. The influence of corticosteroids on the treatment of gram-negative septic shock in man

R̷	No. patients	No. survived
Standard without glucocorticosteroids (*Spink—U. Minnesota*)	300	90 (30%)
Standard with one or more doses methylprednisolone (Solu-Medrol), 30 mg/kg IV (*Lillehei—U. Minnesota*)	52	36 (70%)
Standard without glucocorticosteroids (*Schumer—U. Illinois*)	160	92 (53%)
Standard with one or more doses methylprednisolone (Solu-Medrol), 30 mg/kg IV, or dexamethasone (Decadron), 3 mg/kg IV (*Schumer—U. Illinois*)	168	144 (86%)
Standard without glucocorticosteroids (double blind study [*Schumer—U. Illinois*])	86	53 (62%)
Standard with one or more doses methylprednisolone (Solu-Medrol), 30 mg/kg IV, or dexamethasone (Decadron), 3 mg/kg IV	86	77 (90%)

circulation with bacteria and their products.

As emphasized in the section on pathophysiology, the hemodynamic presentation of septic shock can be quite variable and is to a large extent dependent on the time at which the patient is seen after the onset of shock. Thus the use of cardiotonic and vasoactive agents can produce diverse effects in these individuals. Although various hemodynamic changes can be effected by the use of such agents,[365,380,381] there is no evidence in large series of patients that survival is improved.[382,383]

Naturally, certain individuals with specific complications such as arrhythmia or congestive heart failure are benefited by the judicious use of some of these drugs.

At present the best results in the treatment of septic shock have been obtained with the use of massive IV doses of corticosteroids in combination with the general supportive measures already described. Pharmacologic doses of the synthetic glucocorticosteroids improve both the hemodynamic and metabolic status of the septic patient (Fig. 41-15) and, more importantly, greatly enhance survival.[382] Corticosteroids are the only agents in the treatment of shock that have been subjected to a controlled, double-blind study to establish the most important aspect of clinical efficacy, survival[384] (Table 41-10). There is now little doubt as to their value in septic shock. With the advent of corticosteroid therapy, survival in bacteremic shock has risen from 20% to 35% to over 80%.[385-387] Survival can exceed 90% if glucocorticosteroids are administered early in the course of septic shock[384] (Table 41-11).

Although the overall survival in patients with septic shock is improved, it should be noted that there are certain patients (Table 14-12) who presently tend to have an unfavorable prognosis. Such patients require extra special attention if they are to be saved.

Table 41-11. Results of corticosteroid therapy in septic shock

	Patients treated early	Patients treated late	Totals
Survived shock	25 (92.5%)	10 (62.5%)	35 (81.4%)
Died	2 (7.5%)	6 (37.5%)	8 (18.6%)
Discharged or 30-day survivors	15 (55.6%)	3 (18.8%)	18 (41.9%)

SUMMARY

Shock occurs when tissue perfusion is inadequate to sustain normal physiologic function. The three types of circulatory collapse, in order of prevalence, are hemorrhagic, cardiogenic, and septic shock. The primary physiologic hallmarks of hypovolemic and cardiogenic shock are hypotension, vasoconstriction, and low cardiac output. The patient is cool, clammy, tachycardic, oliguric, and frequently acidotic. Patients in septic shock initially have mental confusion, tachypnea, oliguria, and alkalosis. The blood pressure is usually low-normal, the total peripheral resistance is low, and the cardiac output is elevated. The pathophysiology of late bacteremic shock is similar to that of oligemic and cardiogenic shock. Anaerobic cellular metabolism is common in all types of circulatory collapse. Pulmonary insufficiency can occur with any form of shock, and its incidence is increased in patients who develop sepsis.

The treatment of circulatory collapse should be tailored to the type of shock and the needs of the patient. Adequate respiratory support and proper volume replacement are essential. Corticosteroids have an important place in the treatment of all types of circulatory collapse, since significant improvement in survival has been associated with their use. Various cardiotonic and vasoactive drugs may be useful, depending on the needs of the patient. With early, vigorous treatment the survival rates of hemorrhagic and septic shock can approach 90% and the salvage rate in cardiogenic shock can be 60%.

Table 41-12. Influence of the source of sepsis and other factors on prognosis in septic shock

Favorable	Unfavorable
Genitourinary tract	Lung
Pelvic abscess	Extensive burn
Gastrointestinal or biliary fistula	Subdiaphragmatic abscess
Wound infection	Immunosuppressed patient
Heart	Elderly patient
Gynecologic system	Debilitated patient
Infected CVP catheter	Delay in diagnosis
Infected extremity	Generalized peritonitis
Subcutaneous or ano-rectal abscess	Prior history of organ failure (especially heart)

REFERENCES

1. Sloman, G., Stannard, M., and Goble, H. J.: Coronary care unit: a review of 300 patients monitored since 1963, Am. Heart J. **75**:140, 1968.
2. Sobel, B. E.: The cardiac care unit in 1973, Hosp. Pract. Feb., 1973, p. 115.
3. Scheidt, S., Ascheim, R., and Killip, T., III: Shock after acute myocardial infarction, Am. J. Cardiol. **26**:556, 1970.
4. Page, D. L., et al.: Myocardial changes associated with cardiogenic shock, N. Engl. J. Med. **285**:133, 1971.
5. McQuay, N. W., Edwards, J. E., and Burchell, H. B.: Types of death in acute myocardial infarction, Arch. Intern. Med. **97**:1, 1955.
6. Malach, M., and Rosenberg, B. A.: Acute myocardial infarction in a city hospital. III. Experience with shock, Am. J. Cardiol. **5**:487, 1960.
7. Soloff, L. A.: Coronary artery disease and the concept of cardiac failure, Am. J. Cardiol. **22**:43, 1968.
8. Sobel, B. E., et al.: Estimation of infarct size in man and its relation to prognosis, Circulation **46**:640, 1972.
9. Maroko, P. R., et al.: Precordial ST-segment mapping: an atraumatic method for assessing alterations in the extent of myocardial ischemic injury. The effects of pharmacologic and hemodynamic interventions, Am. J. Cardiol. **29**:223, 1972.
10. Reid, P. R., et al.: Myocardial-infarct extension detected by precordial ST-segment mapping, N. Engl. J. Med. **290**:123, 1974.
11. Mueller, H., Ayres, S. M., and Gregory, J. J.: Hemodynamics, coronary blood flow, and myocardial metabolism in coronary shock; response to l-norepinephrine and isoproterenol, J. Clin. Invest. **49**:1885, 1970.
12. Ricciutti, M. A.: Myocardial lysosome stability in the early stages of acute ischemic injury, Am. J. Cardiol. **30**:492, 1972.
13. Mills, S. A., Jobsis, F. F., and Seaber, A. V.: A fluorometric study of oxidative metabolism in the in vivo canine heart during acute ischemia and hypoxia, Ann. Surg. **186**:193, 1977.
14. Kirklin, J. W., and Archie, J. P.: The cardiovascular subsystem in surgical patients, Surg. Gynecol. Obstet. **139**:17, 1974.
15. Williamson, J. R., Schaffer, S. W., Ford, C., and Safer, B.: Contribution of tissue acidosis to ischemic injury in the perfused rat heart, Circulation **53**(Suppl. I):3, 1976.
16. Feola, M., Merklin, R., Cho, S., and Brockman, S. K.: The terminal pathway of the lymphatic system of the human heart, Ann. Thorac. Surg. **24**:531, 1977.
17. Trump, B. F., Mergner, W. J., Kahng, M. W., and Saladino, A. J.: Studies on the subcellular pathophysiology of ischemia, Circulation **53**(Suppl. I):17, 1976.
18. Jennings, R. B., Ganote, C. E., and Reimer, K. A.: Ischemic tissue injury, Am. J. Pathol. **81**:179, 1975.
19. Romero, L. H., Motsay, G. J., Schultz, L. S., and Lillehei, R. C.: Precapillary and postcapillary resistances in the

pulmonary microcirculation in cardiogenic shocked dogs, Surg. Forum **22:**36, 1971.

20. Okuda, M., and Yamada, T.: Activity of a myocardial depressant factor and associated lysosomal abnormalities in experimental cardiogenic shock, Circ. Shock **1:**17, 1974.

21. Spath, J. A., Jr., Reed, E. A., and Lefer, A. M.: Influence of increased circulating levels of splanchnic lysosomal enzymes on the response to myocardial ischemia, Ann. Surg. **181:**813, 1975.

22. Ross, J. Jr.: Hemodynamic changes in acute myocardial infarction, Hosp. Pract. Mar., 1972, p. 125.

23. Kerr, A. B., and Kirklin, J. W.: Changes in canine venous volume and pressure during hemorrhage, Surgery **68:**520, 1970.

24. Guss, R., Badder, E. M., Seaton, J. F., and Harrison, T. S.: Cardiac output following adrenomedullary deprivation, Surg. Gynecol. Obstet. **145:**545, 1977.

25. Brobmann, G. F., et al.: Early regional vascular responses to hemorrhage and reinfusion in dogs, Surg. Gynecol. Obstet. **131:**409, 1970.

26. Chien, S., and Usami, S.: Effects of hemorrhage on anesthetized dogs: role of the sympathetic system, Am. J. Physiol. **216:**1322, 1969.

27. Barton, R. W., Reynolds, D. G., and Swan, K. G.: Mesenteric circulatory responses to hemorrhagic shock in the baboon, Ann. Surg. **175:**204, 1972.

28. Roding, B., and Schenk, W. G.: Mesenteric blood flow after hemorrhage in anesthetized and unanesthetized dogs, Surgery **68:**857, 1970.

29. Slater, G. I., et al.: Sequential changes in distribution of cardiac output in hemorrhagic shock, Surgery **73:**174, 1973.

30. Ludbrook, J.: The interaction between vasoconstriction and autoregulation after hemorrhage, Surg. Clin. North Am. **49:**637, 1969.

31. Selkurt, E. E.: Current status of renal circulation and related nephron function in hemorrhage and experimental shock. I. Vascular mechanisms, Circ. Shock **1:**3, 1974.

32. Stone, A. M., and Stahl, W. M.: Renal effects of hemorrhage in normal man, Ann. Surg. **172:**825, 1970.

33. Vanecko, R. M., Szanto, P. B., and Shoemaker, W. C.: Microcirculatory changes in primate liver during shock, Surg. Gynecol. Obstet. **129:**995, 1969.

34. Rutherford, R. B., Balis, J. V., Trow, R. S., and Graves, G. M.: Comparison of hemodynamic and regional blood flow changes at equivalent stages of endotoxin and hemorrhagic shock, J. Trauma **16:**886, 1976.

35. Zinner, M. J., Gurll, N. J., and Reynolds, D. G.: The effect of hemorrhagic shock and resuscitation on regional blood flow in Cynomulgus monkeys, Circ. Shock **4:**291, 1977.

36. Fronek, A., and Witzel, T.: Hemodynamics of the terminal vascular bed in canine hemorrhagic shock, Surgery **75:**408, 1974.

37. Carey, L. C., Lowery, B. D., and Cloutier, C. T.: Hemorrhagic shock, Curr. Probl. Surg., p. 3, Jan., 1971.

38. Chien, S., and Usami, S.: Rate and mechanism of release of antidiuretic hormone after hemorrhage, Circ. Shock **1:**71, 1974.

39. Bacalzo, L. V., et al.: Effect of prolonged hypovolemic shock on jejunal fluid and sodium transport, Surg. Gynecol. Obstet. **134:**399, 1974.

40. Granata, L., et al.: Left coronary hemodynamics during hemorrhagic hypotension and shock, Am. J. Physiol. **216:**1583, 1969.

41. Heimbach, D. M., et al.: Myocardial blood flow and metabolism during and after hemorrhagic shock in the dog, Surg. Gynecol. Obstet. **137:**243, 1973.

42. Lovett, W. L., et al.: Presence of a myocardial depressant factor in patients in circulatory shock, Surgery **70:**223, 1971.

43. Lefer, A. M., and Spath, J. A.: Pancreatic hypoperfusion and the production of a myocardial depressant factor in hemorrhagic shock, Ann. Surg. **179:**868, 1974.

44. Wilson, J. M., Gay, W. A., and Ebert, P. A.: The effects of oligemic hypotension on myocardial function, Surgery **73:**657, 1973.

45. Wangensteen, S. L., Crampton, R. S., and Ferguson, W. W.: Myocardial depressant factor in cardiogenic shock, J.A.M.A. **228:**1638, 1974.

46. Tamakuma, S., et al.: Demonstration of a lethal endotoxemia of intestinal origin in refractory non-septic shock, Ann. Surg. **173:**219, 1971.

47. Herman, C. M., et al.: The relationship of circulating endogenous endotoxin to hemorrhagic shock in the baboon, Ann. Surg. **179:**910, 1974.

48. Schumer, W.: Localization of the energy pathway block in shock, Surgery **64:**55, 1968.

49. Hobler, K. E., and Carey, L. C.: Effect of acute progressive hypoxemia on cardiac output and plasma excess lactate, Ann. Surg. **177:**199, 1973.

50. Chaudry, I. H., Sayeed, M. M., and Baue, A. E.: Depletion and restoration of tissue ATP in hemorrhagic shock, Arch. Surg. **108:**208, 1974.

51. Blackwood, J. M., et al.: Tissue metabolites in endotoxin and hemorrhagic shock, Arch. Surg. **107:**181, 1973.

52. Rutenburg, A. M., et al.: Adenosine 3',5'-monophosphate metabolism in the liver in experimental hemorrhagic shock, Surgery **74:**660, 1973.

53. McArdle, A. H., Chiu, C. J., and Hinchey, E. J.: Cyclic AMP response to epinephrine and shock, Arch. Surg. **110:**316, 1975.

54. Chaudry, I. H., and Baue, A. E.: Depletion and replenishment of cellular cyclic adenosine monophosphate in hemorrhagic shock, Surg. Gynecol. Obstet. **145:**877, 1977.

55. Holden, W. D., et al.: Ultrastructural changes in hemorrhagic shock, Ann. Surg. **162:**517, 1965.

56. Baue, A. E., and Sayeed, M. M.: Alterations in the functional capacity of mitochondria in hemorrhagic shock, Surgery **68:**40, 1970.

57. Mela, L. M.: Oxygen's role in health and shock. The organ in shock. Kalamazoo, 1977, Scope Publications, p. 8-15.

58. Rhodes, R. S., DePalma, R. G., and Druet, R. L.: Reversibility of ischemically induced mitochondrial dysfunction with reperfusion, Surg. Gynecol. Obstet. **145:**719, 1977.

59. Baue, A. E., Wurth, M. A., and Sayeed, M. M.: The dynamics of altered ATP-dependent and ATP-yielding cell processes in shock, Surgery **72:**94, 1972.

60. Mela, L. M., Miller, L. D., and Nicholas, G. G.: Influence of cellular acidosis and altered cation concentrations on shock-induced mitochondrial damage, Surgery **72:**102, 1972.

61. Mela, L., et al.: Role of intracellular variations of lysosomal enzyme activity and oxygen tension in mitochondrial impairment in endotoxin and hemorrhagic shock in the rat, Ann. Surg. **178:**727, 1973.

62. Chaudry, I. H., Sayeed, M. M., and Baue, A. E.: Alterations in high-energy phosphates in hemorrhagic shock as related to tissue and organ function, Surgery **79:**666, 1976.

63. Clermont, H. G., Williams, J. S., and Adams, J. T.: Liver acid phosphatase as a measure of hepatocyte resistance to hemorrhagic shock, Surgery **71:**868, 1972.

64. Clermont, H. G., and Williams, J. S.: Lymph lysosomal enzyme acid phosphatase in hemorrhagic shock, Ann. Surg. **176:**90, 1972.

65. Berman, I. R., et al.: Thoracic duct lymph in shock: gas exchange, acid base balance and lysosomal enzymes in hemorrhagic and endotoxin shock, Ann. Surg. **169:**202, 1969.

66. Bell, M. L., et al.: Role of lysosomal instability in the development of refractory shock, Surgery **70:**341, 1971.

67. Glenn, T. M., et al.: Circulatory responses to splanchnic lysosomal hydrolases in the dog, Ann. Surg. **176:**120, 1972.

68. Mason, M. S., and Wangensteen, S. L.: The effects of purified cathepsin D infusions in intact animals, Am. J. Surg. **134:**278, 1977.

69. Cunningham, J. N., Shires, G. T., and Wagner, Y.: Cellular transport defects in hemorrhagic shock, Surgery **70:** 215, 1971.

70. Shires, G. T., et al.: Alterations in cellular membrane function during hemorrhagic shock in primates, Ann. Surg. **176:**288, 1972.

71. Trunkey, D. D., et al.: The effect of hemorrhagic shock on intracellular muscle action potentials in the primate, Surgery **74:**241, 1973.

72. Sayeed, M. M., Chaudry, I. H., and Baue, A. E.: Na$^+$-K$^+$ transport and adenosine nucleotides in the lung in hemorrhagic shock, Surgery **77:**395, 1975.

73. Day, B., and Friedman, S. M.: Intracellular sodium and potassium changes in vascular smooth muscle during hemorrhagic shock, Surg. Gynecol. Obstet. **147:**25, 1978.

74. Trunkey, D., Holcroft, J., and Carpenter, M. A.: Calcium flux during hemorrhagic shock in baboons, J. Trauma **16:**633, 1976.

75. Baue, A. E., Wurth, M. A., Chaudry, I. H., and Sayeed, M. M.: Impairment of cell membrane transport during shock and after treatment, Ann. Surg. **178:**412, 1973.

76. Essiet, G. S., and Stahl, W. M.: Water and electrolyte content of tissues in hemorrhagic shock and surgical trauma, Surg. Gynecol. Obstet. **137:**11, 1973.

77. Johnson, G., and Baggett, C.: Red-cell fluid and electrolytes during hemorrhagic shock in the monkey, Ann. Surg. **178:**655, 1973.

78. Arango, A., Illner, H., and Shires, G. T.: Role of ischemia in the induction of changes in cell membrane during hemorrhagic shock, J. Surg. Res. **20:**473, 1976.

79. Lowery, B. D., Cloutier, C. T., and Carey, L. C.: Blood gas determinations in the severely wounded in hemorrhagic shock, Arch. Surg. **99:**330, 1969.

80. MacLean, L. D., et al.: Patterns in septic shock in man—a detailed study of 56 patients, Ann. Surg. **166:**543, 1967.

81. Shoemaker, W. C., et al.: Use of sequential physiologic measurements for evaluation and therapy of uncomplicated septic shock, Surg. Gynecol. Obstet. **131:**245, 1970.

82. Siegel, J. H., Goldwyn, R. M., and Friedman, H. P.: Pattern and process in the evolution of human septic shock, Surgery **70:**232, 1971.

83. Perbellini, A., Shatney, C. H., MacCarter, D. J., and Lillehei, R. C.: A new model for the study of septic shock, Surg. Gynecol. Obstet. **147:**68, 1978.

84. Hopkins, R. W., and Damewood, C. A.: Septic shock: hemodynamics of endotoxin and inflammation, Am. J. Surg. **127:**476, 1974.

85. Seyfer, A. E., Zajtchuk, R., Hazlett, D. R., and Mologne, L. A.: Systemic vascular performance in endotoxin shock, Surg. Gynecol. Obstet. **145:**401, 1977.

86. Gans, H., and Wendell, G.: Evaluation of the possible role of serum factors in the clearance of endotoxin from blood, J. Surg. Res. **21:**415, 1976.

87. Altura, B. M., and Halevy, S.: Circulatory shock, histamine, and antihistamines: therapeutic aspects. In Silva, M. R., editor: Handbook of experimental pharmacology, Berlin, 1977, Springer-Verlag, pp. 575-602.

88. Lowry, P., Blanco, T., and Santiago-Delpin, E. A.: Histamine and sympathetic blockade in septic shock, Am. Surg. **43:**12, 1977.

89. Nies, A. S., Forsyth, R. P., Williams, H. E., and Melmon, K. L.: Contribution of kinins to endotoxin shock in unanesthetized Rhesus monkeys, Circ. Res. **22:**155, 1968.

90. Wilson, R. F., et al.: Hemodynamic measurements in septic shock, Arch. Surg. **91:**121, 1965.

91. Siegel, J. H., Greenspan, M., and DelGuercio, L. R. M.: Abnormal vascular tone, defective oxygen transport, and myocardial failure in human septic shock, Ann. Surg. **165:**504, 1967.

92. Finley, R. J., et al.: Capillary muscle blood flow in human sepsis, Surgery **78:**87, 1975.

93. Archie, J. P., Jr.: Anatomic arterial-venous shunting in endotoxic and septic shock in dogs, Ann. Surg. **186:**171, 1977.

94. Cohn, J. D., et al.: Arteriovenous shunting in high output shock syndromes, Surg. Gynecol. Obstet. **127:**282, 1968.

95. Duff, J. H., et al.: Defective oxygen consumption in septic shock, Surg. Gynecol. Obstet. **128:**1051, 1969.

96. Gimpel, L., Hodgins, D. S., and Jacobson, E. D.: Effect of endotoxin on hepatic adenylate cyclase activity, Circ. Shock **1:**31, 1974.

97. Clowes, G. H. A., Jr., O'Donnell, T. F., Jr., Ryan, N. T., and Blackburn, G. L.: Energy metabolism in sepsis: treatment based on different patterns in shock and high output stage, Ann. Surg. **179:**684, 1974.

98. Harken, A. H., Lillo, R. S., and Hufnagel, H. V.: Direct influence of endotoxin on cellular respiration, Surg. Gynecol. Obstet. **140:**858, 1975.

99. Lefer, A. M., and Galvin, M. J.: Comparison of the cytotoxic actions of hypoxia and endotoxin in the perfused cat liver, Circ. Shock **5:**145, 1978.

100. Clermont, H. G., Williams, J. S., and Adams, J. T.: Steroid effect on the release of the lysosomal enzyme acid phosphatase in shock, Ann. Surg. **179:**917, 1974.

101. Wilson, J. W.: Treatment or prevention of pulmonary cellular damage with pharmacologic doses of corticosteroid, Surg. Gynecol. Obstet. **134:**675, 1972.
102. Wilson, J. W.: Pulmonary factors produced by septic shock: cause or consequence of shock lung? J. Reprod. Med. **8:**307, 1972.
103. Motsay, G. J., et al.: Effects of massive doses of corticosteroids in experimental and clinical gram-negative septic shock. In Forscher, B. K., Lillehei, R. C., and Stubbs, S. S., editors: Shock in low- and high-flow states, Amsterdam, 1972, Excerpta Medica Foundation.
104. Schumer, W., and Sperling, R.: Shock and its effect on the cell, J.A.M.A. **205:**215, 1968.
105. Miller, L. D., et al.: The affinity of hemoglobin for oxygen: its control and in vivo significance, Surgery **68:**187, 1970.
106. McConn, R., and DelGuercio, L. R. M.: Respiratory function of blood in the acutely ill patient and the effect of steroids, Ann. Surg. **174:**436, 1971.
107. Milligan, G. F., et al.: Pulmonary and hematologic disturbances during septic shock, Surg. Gynecol. Obstet. **138:**43, 1974.
108. Wangensteen, S. L., et al.: Relationship between splanchnic blood flow and a myocardial depressant factor in endotoxin shock, Surgery **69:**410, 1971.
109. Carey, L. C., Curtin, R., and Sapira, J. D.: Influence of hemorrhage on adrenal secretion, blood glucose and serum insulin in the awake pig, Ann. Surg. **183:**185, 1976.
110. Herman, A. H., Mack, E., and Egdahl, R. H.: The relationship of adrenal perfusion to corticosteroid secretion in prolonged hemorrhagic shock, Surg. Gynecol. Obstet. **132:**795, 1971.
111. Carey, L. C., Cloutier, C. T., and Lowery, B. D.: Growth hormone and adrenal cortical response to shock and trauma in the human, Ann. Surg. **174:**451, 1971.
112. Skillman, J. J., Hedley-White, J., and Pallotta, J. A.: Hormonal, fuel and respiratory relationships after acute blood loss in man, Surg. Forum **21:**23, 1970.
113. Garcia-Barreno, P., and Balibrea, J. L.: Metabolic response in shock, Surg. Gynecol. Obstet. **146:**182, 1978.
114. Rocha, D. M., Santeusanio, F., Faloona, G. R., and Unger, R. H.: Abnormal pancreatic alpha-cell function in bacterial infections, N. Engl. J. Med. **233:**700, 1973.
115. Meguid, M. M., et al.: Hormone-substrate interrelationships following trauma, Arch. Surg. **109:**776, 1974.
116. Terry, R. B., and Turner, M. D.: Effect of acute hemorrhage on gastrin secretion rate and blood levels of gastrin and insulin in normal dogs and in dogs after vagotomy, Surg. Gynecol. Obstet. **142:**353, 1976.
117. Carey, L. C., Lowery, B., and Cloutier, C. T.: Blood sugar and insulin response of humans in shock, Ann. Surg. **172:**342, 1970.
118. Moss, G. S., Cerchio, G., and Siegel, D. C.: Decline in pancreatic insulin release during hemorrhagic shock in the baboon, Ann. Surg. **175:**210, 1972.
119. Hiebert, J. M., McCormick, M. J., and Egdahl, R. H.: Direct measurement of insulin secretory rate: studies in shocked primates and postoperative patients, Ann. Surg. **176:**396, 1972.
120. Meguid, M. M., Aun, F., and Soeldner, J. S.: Temporal characteristics of insulin: glucose ratio after varying degrees of stress and trauma in man, J. Surg. Res. **25:**389, 1978.
121. Hiebert, J. M., Sixt, N., Soeldner, J. S., and Egdahl, R. H.: Altered insulin and glucose metabolism produced by epinephrine during hemorrhagic shock in the adrenalectomized primate, Surgery **74:**223, 1973.
122. Manny, J., Rabinovici, N., and Schiller, M.: Insulin response to continuous glucose load in endotoxin shock in the dog, Surg. Gynecol. Obstet. **145:**198, 1977.
123. Dykes, J. R. W., Saxton, C., and Taylor, S. H.: Insulin secretion in cardiogenic shock, Br. Med. J. **2:**498, 1969.
124. Jordan, G. L., Jr, Fischer, E. P., and Lefrak, E. A.: Glucose metabolism in traumatic shock in the human, Ann. Surg. **175:**685, 1972.
125. Printen, K. J., Keefe, W. E., Foster, E., and Brown, W.: Fluxes in serum glucose and free fatty acid in early endotoxemia and hemorrhage, Surg. Gynecol. Obstet. **138:**686, 1974.
126. Hanson, E. L., Brennan, M. F., O'Connell, R. C., and Moore, F. D.: Response of glucose, insulin, free fatty acid, and human growth hormone to norepinephrine and hemorrhage in normal man, Ann. Surg. **177:**453, 1973.
127. Rhodes, R.: The effect of mitochondrial dysfunction on glucose metabolism during shock, Circ. Shock **5:**203, 1978.
128. Wright, P. D., and Henderson, K.: Cellular glucose utilization during hemorrhagic shock in the pig, Surgery **78:**322, 1975.
129. Hinshaw, L. B., et al.: Glucose utilization and role of blood in endotoxin shock, Am. J. Physiol. **233**(2):E71, 1977.
130. Chaudry, I. H., Sayeed, M. M., and Baue, A. E.: Insulin resistance in experimental shock, Arch. Surg. **109:**412, 1974.
131. Ryan, N. T., George, B. C., Egdahl, D. H., and Egdahl, R. H.: Chronic tissue insulin resistance following hemorrhagic shock, Ann. Surg. **180:**402, 1974.
132. Coran, A. G., Cryer, P. E., Horwitz, D. L., and Herman, C. M.: Changes in serum free fatty acids during experimental live escherichia coli septicemia, Surg. Gynecol. Obstet. **135:**417, 1972.
133. Daniel, A. M., Pierce, C. H., Shizgal, H. M., and MacLean, L. D.: Protein and fat utilization in shock, Surgery **84:**588, 1978.
134. Daniel, A. M., Shizgal, H. M., and MacLean, L. D.: The anatomic and metabolic source of lactate in shock, Surg. Gynecol. Obstet. **147:**697, 1978.
135. Groves, A. C., et al.: Impaired gluconeogenesis in dogs with E. coli bacteremia, Surgery **76:**533, 1974.
136. O'Donnell, T. F., Jr., et al.: Proteolysis associated with a deficit of peripheral energy fuel substrates in septic man, Surgery **80:**192, 1976.
137. Kuttner, R. E., and Spitzer, J. J.: Gluconeogenesis from alanine in endotoxin-treated dogs, J. Surg. Res. **25:**166, 1978.
138. Woolf, L. I., Groves, A. C., and Duff, J. H.: Amino acid metabolism in dogs with E. coli bacteremic shock, Surgery **85:**212, 1979.
139. Clowes, G. H. A., Jr., et al.: Blood insulin responses to blood glucose levels in high output sepsis and septic shock, Am. J. Surg. **135:**577, 1978.
140. Imamura, M., Clowes, G. H. A., Jr., et al.: Liver metabo-

lism and glucogenesis in trauma and sepsis, Surgery **77**:868, 1975.

141. Imamura, M., Clowes, G. H. A., Jr.: Hepatic blood flow and oxygen consumption in starvation, sepsis and septic shock, Surg. Gynecol. Obstet. **141**:27, 1975.

142. Holtzman, S., and Balderman, S. C.: Comparison of lactate and pyruvate during endotoxic shock, Surg. Gynecol. Obstet. **145**:677, 1977.

143. Martin, A. M., et al.: Pathologic anatomy of the lungs following shock and trauma, J. Trauma **8**:687, 1968.

144. Simmons, R. L., et al.: Respiratory insufficiency in combat casualties: IV hypoxemia during convalescence, Ann. Surg. **170**:53, 1969.

145. Geiger, J. P., and Gielchinsky, I.: Acute pulmonary insufficiency, Arch. Surg. **102**:400, 1971.

146. Blaisdell, F. W., Lim, R. C., and Stallone, R. J.: The mechanism of pulmonary damage following traumatic shock, Surg. Gynecol. Obstet. **130**:15, 1970.

147. McLaughlin, J. S.: Physiologic consideration of hypoxemia in shock and trauma, Ann. Surg. **173**:667, 1971.

148. Germon, P. A., et al.: Shunting following trauma, J. Trauma **8**:724, 1968.

149. Kim, S. I., and Shoemaker, W. C.: Role of acidosis in the development of increased pulmonary vascular resistance and shock lung in experimental hemorrhagic shock, Surgery **73**:723, 1973.

150. Shapiro, B. J., Simmons, D. H., and Linde, L. M.: Pulmonary hemodynamics during acute acid-base changes in the intact dog, Am. J. Physiol. **210**:1026, 1966.

151. Gerst, P. H., et al.: The effects of hemorrhage on pulmonary circulation and respiratory gas exchange, J. Clin. Invest. **38**:524, 1959.

152. Sealy, W. C., et al.: Functional and structural changes in the lung in hemorrhagic shock, Surg. Gynecol. Obstet. **122**:754, 1966.

153. Buckberg, G. D., and Dowell, A. R.: The effects of hemorrhagic shock and pulmonary ischemia on lung compliance and structure in baboons, Surg. Gynecol. Obstet. **131**:1065, 1970.

154. Barrett, J., et al.: Pulmonary microembolism associated with massive transfusion: II. The basic pathophysiology of its pulmonary effects, Ann. Surg. **182**:56, 1975.

155. Luterman, A., Manwaring, D., and Curreri, P. W.: The role of fibrinogen degradation products in the pathogenesis of the respiratory distress syndrome, Surgery **82**:703, 1977.

156. Peer, R. M., and Schwartz, S. I.: Development and treatment of post-traumatic pulmonary platelet trapping, Ann. Surg. **181**:447, 1975.

157. Wyche, M. Q., et al.: Lung function, pulmonary extravascular water volume and hemodynamics in early hemorrhagic shock in anesthetized dogs, Ann. Surg. **174**:296, 1971.

158. Berk, J. L., et al.: Pulmonary insufficiency caused by epinephrine, Ann. Surg. **178**:423, 1973.

159. Fischer, P., Millen, J. E., and Glauser, F. L.: The pulmonary alveolar capillary membrane during hemorrhagic hypotension in dogs, Surg. Gynecol. Obstet. **146**:383, 1978.

160. Derks, C. M., and Peters, R. M.: The effect of shock and fat embolus on pulmonary mechanics and gas exchange, Surg. Gynecol. Obstet. **138**:413, 1974.

161. Derks, C. M., and Peters, R. M.: The role of shock and fat embolus in leakage from pulmonary capillary, Surg. Gynecol. Obstet. **137**:945, 1973.

162. Herndon, J. H., and Riseborough, E. J.: Alterations in serum lipid concentrations following skeletal trauma, Surg. Gynecol. Obstet. **146**:244, 1978.

163. Greenfield, L. J., McCurdy, W. C., and Coalson, J. J.: Pulmonary oxygen toxicity in experimental hemorrhagic shock, Surgery **68**:662, 1970.

164. Lee, C. J., Lyons, J. H., and Moore, F. D.: Cardiovascular and metabolic responses to spontaneous and positive-pressure breathing of 100 percent oxygen at one atmosphere pressure, J. Thorac. Cardiovasc. Surg. **53**:770, 1967.

165. Moss, G.: Shock lung: a disorder of the central nervous system? Hosp. Pract. Aug., 1974, pp. 77-86.

166. Collins, J. A.: The causes of progressive pulmonary insufficiency in surgical patients, J. Surg. Res. **9**:685, 1969.

167. Simmons, R. L., Heisterkamp, C. A., III, Moseley, R. V., and Doty, D. B.: Postresuscitative blood volumes in combat casualties, Surg. Gynecol. Obstet. **128**:1193, 1969.

168. Magilligan, D. J., et al.: Pulmonary intravascular and extravascular volumes in hemorrhagic shock and fluid replacement, Surgery **72**:780, 1972.

169. Fulton, R. L., and Fischer, R. P.: Pulmonary changes due to hemorrhagic shock resuscitation with isotonic and hypertonic saline, Surgery **75**:881, 1974.

170. Siegel, D. C., Cochin, A., and Moss, G. S.: The ventilatory response to hemorrhagic shock and resuscitation, Surgery **72**:451, 1972.

171. Moss, G. S., et al.: Effects of saline and colloid solutions on pulmonary function in hemorrhagic shock. Surg. Gynecol. Obstet. **133**:53, 1971.

172. Moss, G. S., et al.: Morphologic changes in the primate lung after hemorrhagic shock, Surg. Gynecol. Obstet. **134**:3, 1972.

173. Moss, G. S., et al.: Effect of hemorrhagic shock on pulmonary interstitial sodium distribution in the primate lung, Ann. Surg. **177**:211, 1973.

174. Swank, R. L., Connell, R. S., and Webb, M. C.: Dacron wool filtration and hypotensive shock: an electron microscopical study, Ann. Surg. **179**:427, 1974.

175. Hechtman, H. B., Lonergan, E. A., and Shepro, D.: Platelet and leukocyte lung interactions in patients with respiratory failure, Surgery **83**:155, 1978.

176. Hechtman, H. B., et al.: Pulmonary entrapment of platelets during acute respiratory failure, Surgery **83**:277, 1978.

177. Hallett, J. W., Sneiderman, C. A., and Wilson, J. W.: Pulmonary effects of arterial infusion of filtered blood in experimental hemorrhagic shock, Surg. Gynecol. Obstet. **138**:517, 1974.

178. Schloerb, P. R., et al.: Pulmonary edema after replacement of blood loss by electrolyte solutions, Surg. Gynecol. Obstet. **135**:893, 1972.

179. Fulton, R. L., and Jones, C. E.: The cause of post-traumatic pulmonary insufficiency in man, Surg. Gynecol. Obstet. **140**:179, 1975.

180. Esrig, B. C., and Fulton, R. L.: Sepsis, resuscitated hemorrhagic shock and "shock lung," Ann. Surg. **182**:218, 1975.

181. Clowes, G. H. A., Jr., et al.: Septic lung and shock lung in man, Ann. Surg. **181**:681, 1975.

182. Walker, L., and Eiseman, B.: The changing pattern of post-traumatic respiratory distress syndrome, Ann. Surg. **181**:694, 1975.

183. Balis, J. U., Gerber, L. I., Rappaport, E. S., and Neville, W. E.: Mechanisms of blood-vascular reactions of the primate lung to acute endotoxemia, Exper. Molec. Pathol. **21**:123, 1974.

184. Myrvold, H. E., and Svalander, C.: Pulmonary microembolism in early experimental septic shock, J. Surg. Res. **23**:65, 1977.

185. Snell, J. D., Jr., and Ramsey, L. H.: Pulmonary edema as a result of endotoxemia, Am. J. Physiol. **21**(1):170, 1969.

186. Finley, R. J., Holliday, R. L., Lefcoe, M., and Duff, J. H.: Pulmonary edema in patients with sepsis, Surg. Gynecol. Obstet. **140**:851, 1975.

187. Siegel, J. H., and Farrell, E. J.: A computer simulation model to study the clinical observability of ventilation and perfusion abnormalities in human shock states, Surgery **73**:898, 1973.

188. Hechtman, H. B., et al.: The independence of pulmonary shunting and pulmonary edema, Surgery **74**:300, 1973.

189. Bryant, L. R., Trinkle, J. K., and Dubilier, L.: Acute respiratory pathophysiology after hemorrhagic shock, Surgery **68**:512, 1970.

190. Wilson, J. W., et al.: The lung in hemorrhagic shock, Am. J. Pathol. **58**:337, 1970.

191. Wilson, J. W.: Treatment or prevention of pulmonary cellular damage with pharmacologic doses of corticosteroid, Surg. Gynecol. Obstet. **134**:675, 1972.

192. Northrup, W. F., III, and Humphrey, E. W.: The effect of hemorrhagic shock on pulmonary vascular permeability to plasma proteins, Surgery **83**:264, 1978.

193. Henry, J. N., et al.: A study of the acute and chronic respiratory pathophysiology of hemorrhagic shock, J. Thorac. Cardiovasc. Surg. **54**:666, 1967.

194. Garvey, J. W., Hagstrom, J. W. C., and Veith, F. J.: Pathologic pulmonary changes in hemorrhagic shock, Ann. Surg. **181**:870, 1975.

195. Tieffenbrun, J., and Shoemaker, W. C.: Sequential changes in pulmonary blood flow distribution in hemorrhagic shock, **174**:727, 1971.

196. Tieffenbrun, J., Kim, S. I., and Shoemaker, W. C.: The relation of the distribution of pulmonary blood flow to lung function during hemorrhagic shock, Surg. Gynecol. Obstet. **138**:557, 1974.

197. Henry, J. N.: The effect of shock on pulmonary alveolar surfactant, J. Trauma **8**:756, 1968.

198. Gilder, H., and McSherry, C. K.: Mechanisms of oxygen inhibition of pulmonary surfactant synthesis, Surgery **76**:72, 1974.

199. Moss, G. S., Newson, B., and Das Gupta, T. K.: The normal electron histochemistry and the effect of hemorrhagic shock on the pulmonary surfactant system, Surg. Gynecol. Obstet. **140**:53, 1975.

200. Stein, J. H., and Fadem, S. Z.: The renal circulation, J.A.M.A. **239**:1308, 1978.

201. Feigen, L. P., Coleman, B., and Glaviano, V. V.: Effects of alpha-adrenergic blockade on renal function in hemorrhagic shock, Am. J. Physiol. **232**:F409, 1977.

202. Bell, G., and Lister, G. D.: The effect of noradrenaline and phenoxybenzamine on the renal response to hemorrhage, Surg. Gynecol. Obstet. **130**:813, 1970.

203. Passmore, J. C., Neiberger, R. E., and Eden, S. W.: Measurement of intrarenal anatomic distribution of krypton-85 in endotoxic shock in dogs, Am. J. Physiol. **232**:H54, 1977.

204. Cronenwett, J. L., and Lindenauer, S. M.: Distribution of intrarenal blood flow during bacterial sepsis, J. Surg. Res. **24**:132, 1978.

205. Neiberger, R. E., and Passmore, J. C.: Intrarenal blood flow distribution during endotoxemia in dogs, Circ. Shock **5**:339, 1978.

206. Strauch, M., et al.: Effects of septic shock on renal function in humans, Ann. Surg. **165**:536, 1967.

207. Lucas, C. E., Rector, F. E., Werner, M., and Rosenberg, I. K.: Altered renal homeostasis with acute sepsis, Arch. Surg. **106**:444, 1973.

208. Ravikant, T., and Lucas, C. E.: Renal blood flow distribution in septic hyperdynamic pigs, J. Surg. Res. **22**:294, 1977.

209. Rosenberg, I. K., et al.: Renal insufficiency after trauma and sepsis, Arch. Surg. **103**:175, 1971.

210. Collan, Y., Kivilaasko, E., Kalima, T. V., and Lempinen, M. L.: Ultrastructural changes in the gastric mucosa following hemorrhagic shock in pigs, Circ. Shock **4**:13, 1977.

211. Altemeier, W. A., Fullen, W. D., and McDonough, J. J.: Sepsis and gastrointestinal bleeding, Ann. Surg. **175**:759, 1972.

212. LeGall, J. R., et al.: Acute gastroduodenal lesions related to severe stress, Surg. Gynecol. Obstet. **142**:377, 1976.

213. Shirazi, S. S., Mueller, T. M., and Hardy, B. M.: Canine gastric acid secretion and blood flow measurement in hemorrhagic shock, Gastroenterology **73**:75, 1977.

214. Zinner, M. J., Gurll, N. J., and Reynolds, D. G.: The effects of endotoxemia and fluid expansion on gastric hemodynamics and mucosal permeability in the baboon, J. Surg. Res. **22**:605, 1977.

215. Hottenrott, C., Seufert, R. M., Kühne, F. W., Büsing, M.: Experimental gastric sympathectomy. An effective prophylaxis of gastric stress lesions, Ann. Surg. **186**:762, 1977.

216. Gurll, N. J., Zinner, M. J., Reynolds, D. G., and Shirazi, S. S.: Effects of hemorrhagic shock and resuscitation on regional gastric blood flow in monkeys, Circ. Shock **5**:195, 1978.

217. Richardson, R. S., Norton, L. W., Sales, J. E. L., and Eiseman, B.: Gastric blood flow in endotoxin-induced stress ulcer, Arch. Surg. **106**:191, 1973.

218. Kowalewski, K., and Zajac, S.: Effect of hemorrhage on myoelectric activity of stomach and duodenum in dogs, Surg. Gynecol. Obstet. **141**:237, 1975.

219. Zinner, M. J., Turtinen, L., and Gurll, N. J.: The role of acid and ischemia in production of stress ulcers during canine hemorrhagic shock, Surgery **77**:807, 1975.

220. Skillman, J. J., Gould, S. A., Chung, R. S. K., and Silen, W.: The gastric mucosal barrier: clinical and experimental

studies in critically ill and normal man, and in the rabbit, Ann. Surg. **172:**564, 1970.

221. Kivilaasko, E., Fromm, D., and Silen, W.: Relationship between ulceration and intramural pH of gastric mucosa during hemorrhagic shock, Surgery 84:70, 1978.

222. Ritchie, W. P., Jr.: Ischemia and the gastric mucosal barrier: a note of caution, Surgery 76:363, 1974.

223. Moody, F. G., and Aldrete, J. S.: Hydrogen permeability of canine gastric secretory epithelium during formation of acute superficial erosions, Surgery 70:154, 1971.

224. Fischer, R. P., Peter, E. T., and Ritchie, W. P., Jr.: The role of bile in antral mucosal disruption during hemorrhagic shock, Ann. Surg. **180:**892, 1974.

225. Cheung, L. Y., Reese, R. S., and Moody, F. G.: Direct effect of endotoxin on the gastric mucosal microcirculation and electrical gradient, Surgery 79:564, 1976.

226. Lucas, C. E., Ravikant, T., and Walt, A. J.: Gastritis and gastric blood flow in hyperdynamic septic pigs, Am. J. Surg. **131:**73, 1976.

227. Menguy, R., and Masters, Y. F.: Gastric mucosal energy metabolism and "stress" ulceration, Ann. Surg. **180:**538, 1974.

228. Hottenrott, C., Seufert, R. M., and Becker, H.: The role of ischemia in the pathogenesis of stress induced gastric lesions in piglets, Surg. Gynecol. Obstet. **146:**217, 1978.

229. Ternberg, J. L., and Butcher, H. R.: Blood-flow relation between hepatic artery and portal vein, Science **150:**1030, 1965.

230. Hankins, J. R., et al.: Use of the umbilical vein to study the splanchnic and portal beds in shock and trauma: II. Metabolic studies, Ann. Surg. **180:**110, 1974.

231. Champion, H. R., et al.: A clinicopathologic study of hepatic dysfunction following shock, Surg. Gynecol. Obstet. **142:**657, 1976.

232. Rangel, D. M., et al.: Cross transfusion of effluent blood from ischemic liver and intestines, Surg. Gynecol. Obstet. **130:**1015, 1970.

233. Yamamoto, M., et al.: Obstructive jaundice and hemorrhagic shock, Circ. Shock **5:**235, 1978.

234. Utili, R., Abernathy, C. O., and Zimmerman, H. J.: Effects of Salmonella enteritidis endotoxin on the excretory function of the isolated perfused rat liver, Proc. Soc. Exper. Biol. Med. **155:**184, 1977.

235. Farkouh, E. F., Daniel, A. M., Beaudoin, J. G., and MacLean, L. D.: Predictive value of liver biochemistry in acute hepatic ischemia, Surg. Gynecol. Obstet. **132:**832, 1971.

236. Rangel, D. M., et al.: Enzymatic evaluation of hepatic preservation using cell-stabilizing drugs, Surg. Gynecol. Obstet. **129:**963, 1969.

237. Clermont, H. G., Williams, J. S., and Adams, J. T.: Liver acid phosphatase as a measure of hepatocyte resistance to hemorrhagic shock, Surgery 71:868, 1972.

238. Carlson, R. P., and Lefer, A. M.: Hepatic cell integrity in hypodynamic states, Am. J. Physiol. **231:**1408, 1976.

239. White, R. R., IV, et al.: Hepatic ultrastructure in endotoxemia, hemorrhage, and hypoxia: emphasis on mitochondrial changes, Surgery 73:525, 1973.

240. Lillehei, R. C.: The intestinal factor in irreversible shock, Surgery 42:1043, 1957.

241. Lillehei, R. C., and MacLean, L. D.: Intestinal factor in irreversible endotoxin shock, Ann. Surg. **148:**513, 1958.

242. Longerbeam, J. K., Lillehei, R. C., Scott,. W. R., and Rosenberg, J. C.: Visceral factors in shock, J.A.M.A. **181:**878, 1962.

243. Chiu, C. J., et al.: Intestinal mucosal lesion in low-flow states. I. A morphological, hemodynamic, and metabolic reappraisal, Arch. Surg. **101:**478, 1970.

244. Santiago-Delpin, E. A., Vivoni, V., Suarez, A., and Roman-Franco, A. A.: Protection of organs during experimental ischemia, Surg. Gynecol. Obstet. **147:**740, 1978.

245. Bounous, G., and McArdle, A. H.: Release of intestinal enzymes in acute mesenteric ischemia, J. Surg. Res. **9:**339, 1969.

246. Haglund, U., et al.: The intestinal mucosal lesions in shock. I. Studies on the pathogenesis, Eur. Surg. Res. **8:**435, 1976.

247. Haglund, U., et al.: The intestinal mucosal lesions in shock. II. The relationship between the mucosal lesions and the cardiovascular derangement following regional shock, Eur. Surg. Res. **8:**448, 1976.

248. Cuevas, P., and Fine, J.: Demonstration of a lethal endotoxemia in experimental occlusion of the superior mesenteric artery, Surg. Gynecol. Obstet. **133:**81, 1971.

249. Chiu, C. J., Scott, H. J., and Gurd, F. N.: Volume deficit versus toxic absorption: a study of canine shock after mesenteric arterial occlusion, Ann. Surg. **175:**479, 1972.

250. Goodyer, A. V. N., Hammond, G. L., Gross, C. C., and Kabimba, J.: Myocardial production of pyruvate in hemorrhagic shock, J. Surg. Res. **11:**501, 1971.

251. Lee, J. C., and Downing, S. E.: Myocardial oxygen availability and cardiac failure in hemorrhagic shock, Am. Heart J. **92:**201, 1976.

252. MacDonald, J. A. E., Milligan, G. F., Mellon, A., and Ledingham, I. M.: Ventricular function in experimental hemorrhagic shock, Surg. Gynecol. Obstet. **140:**572, 1975.

253. Alyono, D., Ring, W. S., and Anderson, R. W.: The effects of hemorrhagic shock on the diastolic properties of the left ventricle in the conscious dog, Surgery 83:691, 1978.

254. Cingolani, H. E., et al.: Depression of human myocardial contractility with "respiratory" and "metabolic" acidosis, Surgery 77:427, 1975.

255. Geha, A. S.: Coronary and cardiovascular dynamics and oxygen availability during acute normovolemic anemia, Surgery 80:47, 1976.

256. Rayner, A. V. S., Lambert, G. E., Fulton, R. L.: Cardiac function during hemorrhagic shock and crystalloid resuscitation, J. Surg. Res. **24:**235, 1978.

257. Archie, J. P., Jr., and Mertz, W. R.: Myocardial oxygen delivery after experimental hemorrhagic shock, Ann. Surg. **187:**205, 1978.

258. Adiseshiah, M., and Baird, R. J.: Correlation of the changes in diastolic myocardial tissue pressure and regional coronary blood flow in hemorrhagic and endotoxic shock, J. Surg. Res. **24:**20, 1978.

259. Jones, C. E., Smith, E. E., DuPont, E., and Williams, R. D.: Demonstration of nonperfused myocardium in late hemorrhagic shock, Circ. Shock **5:**97, 1978.

260. Culpepper, R. D., Kondo, Y., Hardy, J. D., and Turner, M. D.: Successful orthotopic allotransplantation of hearts

from dogs in irreversible shock, Surgery **77:**126, 1975.

261. Solis, R. T., and Downing, S. E.: Effects of *E. coli* endotoxemia on ventricular performance, Am. J. Physiol. **211:**307, 1966.

262. Cann, M., Stevenson, T., Fiallos, E., and Thal, A. P.: Depressed cardiac performance in sepsis, Surg. Gynecol. Obstet. **134:**759, 1972.

263. Hinshaw, L. B., Archer, L. T., Greenfield, L. J., and Guenter, C. A.: Effects of endotoxin on myocardial hemodynamics, performance and metabolism, Am. J. Physiol. **221:**504, 1971.

264. Geocaris, T. V., Quebbeman, E., Dewoskin, R., and Moss, G. S.: Effects of gram-negative endotoxemia on myocardial contractility in the awake primate, Ann. Surg. **178:**715, 1973.

265. Hinshaw, L. B., et al.: Precipitation of cardiac failure in endotoxin shock, Surg. Gynecol. Obstet. **135:**39, 1972.

266. Greenfield, L. J., et al.: Cardiopulmonary effects of volume loading of primates in endotoxin shock, Surgery **76:**560, 1974.

267. Greenfield, L. J., McCurdy, J. R., Hinshaw, L. B., and Elkins, R. C.: Preservation of myocardial function during cross-circulation in terminal endotoxin shock, Surgery **72:**111, 1972.

268. Elkins, R. C., McCurdy, J. R., Brown, P. P., and Greenfield, L. J.: Effects of coronary perfusion pressure on myocardial performance during endotoxin shock, Surg. Gynecol. Obstet. **137:**991, 1973.

269. Hinshaw, L. B.: Role of the heart in the pathogenesis of endotoxin shock, J. Surg. Res. **17:**134, 1974.

270. Kondo, Y., Culpepper, R. D., Hardy, J. D., and Turner, M. D.: Heart transplantation in endotoxin shock, Surg. Gynecol. Obstet. **140:**252, 1975.

271. Slater, G., et al.: Sequential changes in cerebral blood flow and distribution of flow within the brain during hemorrhagic shock, Ann. Surg. **181:**1, 1975.

272. Raymond, R. M., and Emerson, T. E., Jr.: Cerebral metabolism during endotoxin shock in the dog, Circ. Shock **5:**407, 1978.

273. Kovach, A. G. B., et al.: Control of organ blood flow following hemorrhage, Adv. Exper. Med. Biol. **33:**1, 1973.

274. Kovach, A. G. B., and Sandor, P.: Cerebral blood flow and brain function during hypertension and shock, Ann. Rev. Physiol. **39:**571, 1976.

275. Kovach, A. G. B.: Importance of nervous and metabolic changes in the development of irreversibility in experimental shock, Fed. Proc. **20:**122, 1961.

276. Yashon, D., et al.: Brain, CSF, and blood lactate levels during hemorrhagic shock, Surg. Forum **22:**23, 1971.

277. Tamura, H., et al.: The nervous system in experimental hemorrhagic shock, J. Trauma **12:**869, 1972.

278. Proctor, H. J., Lentz, T. R., Johnson, G., Jr.: Alterations in baboon erythrocyte 2,3-diphosphoglycerate concentration associated with hemorrhagic shock and resuscitation, Ann. Surg. **174:**923, 1971.

279. Shatney, C. H., and Formeister, J. F.: Unpublished data.

280. Bauer, A. R., Jr., et al.: The depression of T lymphocytes after trauma, Am. J. Surg. **136:**674, 1978.

281. Dinbar, A., et al.: Hematologic effects of endotoxin on the macaque monkey, Surgery **70:**596, 1975.

282. Hammon, J. W., et al.: The role of fibrin formation in the pathogenesis of bacteremic shock in the primate, Surg. Gynecol. Obstet. **146:**535, 1978.

283. Altura, B. M., and Hershey, S. G.: Endotoxemia in the rat: role of blood coagulation and leukocytes in the progression of the syndrome, Circ. Shock **1:**113, 1974.

284. Cline, M. J., et al.: Mechanism of endotoxin interaction with human leukocytes, Br. J. Haematol. **15:**539, 1968.

285. MacGregor, R. R.: Relationship between granulocyte adherence and granulocyte kinetics, Clin. Res. **23:**308A, 1975.

286. Horwitz, D. L., Moquin, R. B., and Herman, C. M.: Coagulation changes of septic shock in the sub-human primate and their relationship to hemodynamic changes, Ann. Surg. **175:**417, 1972.

287. Garcia-Barreno, P., Balibrea, J. L., and Aparicio, P.: Blood coagulation changes in shock, Surg. Gynecol. Obstet. **147:**6, 1978.

288. String, T., Robinson, A. J., and Blaisdell, F. W.: Massive trauma, Arch. Surg. **102:**406, 1971.

289. Hirsch, E. F., et al.: Coagulation changes after combat trauma and sepsis, Surg. Gynecol. Obstet. **133:**393, 1971.

290. Attar, S., et al.: Intravascular coagulation: reality or myth? Surgery **68:**27, 1970.

291. McCabe, W. R.: Serum complement levels in bacteremia due to gram-negative organisms, N. Engl. J. Med. **288:**21, 1973.

292. Heideman, M., Kaijser, B., and Gelin, L. E.: Complement activation early in endotoxin shock, J. Surg. Res. **26:**74, 1979.

293. Blaisdell, F. W., Lim, R. C., Jr., and Stallone, R. J.: Mechanism of pulmonary damage following traumatic shock, Surg. Gynecol. Obstet. **130:**1, 1970.

294. Nunes, G., Blaisdell, F. W., and Margaretten, W.: Mechanism of hepatic dysfunction following shock and trauma, Arch. Surg. **100:**546, 1970.

295. Holcroft, J. W., Blaisdell, F. W., Trunkey, D. D., and Lim, R. C.: Intravascular coagulation and pulmonary edema in the septic baboon, J. Surg. Res. **22:**209, 1977.

296. Myrvold, H. E., and Lewis, D. H.: Platelets, fibrinogen, and pulmonary haemodynamics in early experimental septic shock, Circ. Shock **4:**201, 1977.

297. Rowe, M. I., et al.: The mechanisms of thrombocytopenia in experimental gram-negative septicemia, Surgery **84:**87, 1978.

298. From, A. H. L., Fong, J. S. C., Chiu, T., and Good, R. A.: Role of platelets in the pathogenesis of canine endotoxin shock, Infect. Immun. **13:**1591, 1976.

299. Lefer, A. M., Bridenbaugh, G. A., and Flynn, J. T.: Effect of induced thrombocytopenia on experimental circulatory shock, J. Surg. Res. **21:**429, 1976.

300. Saba, T. M.: Reticuloendothelial defense: its relevance to cardiopulmonary function in septic surgical trauma, and burn patients, Contemp. Surg. **14:**64, 1979.

301. Hershey, S. G., and Altura, B. M.: Function of the RES in experimental shock and combined injury, Anesthesiology **30:**138, 1969.

302. Fine, J., Rutenberg, S., and Schweinberg, F. B.: The role of RES in hemorrhagic shock, J. Exp. Med. **110:**547, 1959.

303. Altura, B. M., and Hershey, S. G.: Sequential changes in RES function after acute hemorrhage, Proc. Soc. Exp. Biol. Med. **139:**935, 1972.

304. Zweifach, B. W., and Benacerraf, B.: Effects of hemorrhagic shock on the phagocytic function of Kupffer cells, Circ. Res. **6:**83, 1958.

305. McKenna, J. M., and Zweifach, B. W.: Reticuloendothelial system in relation to shock, Am. J. Physiol. **187:**263, 1959.

306. Zweifach, B. W., and Thomas, L.: Influence of RES on response to hemorrhage and trauma, RES Bull. **3:**31, 1957.

307. Zweifach, B. W., Benacerraf, B., and Thomas, L.: The relationship between the vascular manifestations of shock produced by endotoxin, trauma and hemorrhage. II. The possible role of RES in resistance to each type of shock, J. Exp. Med. **106:**403, 1957.

308. Filkins, J. P., Lubitz, J. M., and Smith, J. J.: The effect of zymosan and glucan on the RES and on resistance to traumatic shock, Angiology **15:**465, 1964.

309. Joyce, L. D., et al.: Evaluation of the mechanism of zymosan-induced resistance to experimental peritonitis, Surgery **83:**717, 1978.

310. Zweifach, B. W.: Contribution of RES to the development of tolerance to experimental shock. IV. Relationship of RES to stress, organic metabolism and growth processes, Ann. N.Y. Acad. Sci. **88:**203, 1960.

311. Lillehei, R. C., and MacLean, L. D.: Increased resistance to hemorrhagic shock in epinephrine-tolerant dogs, Fed. Proc. **18:**415, 1959.

312. Rangel, D. M., et al.: The hepatic response to endotoxin shock; hemodynamic and enzymatic observations, J. Surg. Res. **10:**181, 1970.

313. Olcay, I., et al.: Reticuloendothelial function: determinant for survival following hepatic ischemia in the baboon, Surgery **76:**643, 1974.

314. Scovill, W. A., et al.: Opsonic surface binding glycoprotein therapy during sepsis, Ann. Surg. **188:**521, 1978.

315. Schweinberg, F. B., and Fine, J.: Evidence for a lethal endotoxemia as the fundamental feature of irreversibility in three types of traumatic shock, J. Exp. Med. **112:**793, 1960.

316. Zweifach, B. W., Gordon, H. A., Wagner, M., and Reyniers, J. A.: Irreversible hemorrhagic shock in germ free rats, J. Exp. Med. **107:**437, 1958.

317. Olcay, I., et al.: Reticuloendothelial dysfunction and endotoxemia following portal vein occlusion, Surgery **75:**64, 1974.

318. Loegering, D. J., and Carr, F. K.: Plasma cathepsin activity and reticuloendothelial phagocytic function during hemorrhagic shock, Circ. Shock **5:**61, 1978.

319. Glass, K., Palmerio, C., and Fine, J.: Further evidence of the role of the RES in the maintenance of vascular integrity, Surgery **66:**709, 1969.

320. Blattberg, B., and Levy, M. N.: Vasoactive substances and reticuloendothelial function, Am. J. Physiol. **210:**569, 1966.

321. Loegering, D. J., and Carr, F. K.: Humoral factor activity and carbon clearance rate during the early stages of hemorrhagic shock, J. Reticuloendothel. Soc. **21:**263, 1977.

322. Saba, T. M.: Prevention of liver reticuloendothelial systemic host defense failure after surgery by intravenous opsonic glycoprotein therapy, Ann. Surg. **188:**142, 1978.

323. Schimpff, S. C., Miller, R. M., Polakavetz, S., and Hornick, R. B.: Infection in the severely traumatized patient, Ann. Surg. **179:**352, 1974.

324. Howard, R. J., and Simmons, R. L.: Acquired immunologic deficiencies after trauma and surgical procedures, Surg. Gynecol. Obstet. **139:**771, 1974.

325. MacLean, L. D., et al.: Host resistance in sepsis and trauma, Ann. Surg. **182:**207, 1975.

326. Pietsch, J. B., Meakins, J. L., and MacLean, L. D.: The delayed hypersensitivity response: application in clinical surgery, Surgery **82:**349, 1977.

327. Meakins, J. L., et al.: Delayed hypersensitivity: indicator of acquired failure of host defenses in sepsis and trauma, Ann. Surg. **186:**241, 1977.

328. Lowery, B. D., Cloutier, C. T., and Carey, L. C.: Electrolyte solutions in resuscitation in human hemorrhagic shock, Surg. Gynecol. Obstet. **133:**273, 1971.

329. Moss, G. S., et al.: A comparison of asanguineous fluids and whole blood in the treatment of hemorrhagic shock, Surg. Gynecol. Obstet. **129:**1247, 1969.

330. Reich, M. P., and Eiseman, B.: Tissue oxygenation following resuscitation with crystalloid solution following experimental acute blood loss, Surgery **69:**928, 1971.

331. Coran, A. G., et al.: The effect of crystalloid resuscitation in hemorrhagic shock on acid-base balance: a comparison between normal saline and Ringer's lactate solutions, Surgery **69:**874, 1971.

332. Litwin, M. S.: Comparison of effects of dextran 70 and dextran 40 in postoperative animals, Surgery **71:**295, 1972.

333. Matsuda, H., and Shoemaker, W. C.: Cardiorespiratory responses to dextran 40, Arch. Surg. **110:**296, 1975.

334. Giordano, J. M., Campbell, D. A., and Joseph, W. L.: The effect of intravenously administered albumin on dogs with pulmonary interstitial edema, Surg. Gynecol. Obstet. **137:**593, 1973.

335. Copping, J. W., Mather, G. S., and Winkler, J. M.: Physiologic responses to the administration of cold, room temperature, and warm balanced salt solutions in hemorrhagic shock in dogs, Surgery **71:**206, 1972.

336. Batalden, D. J., et al.: Value of the G suit in patients with severe pelvic fracture, Arch. Surg. **109:**326, 1974.

337. McNamara, J. J., et al.: Effect of hypertonic glucose in hypovolemic shock in man, Ann. Surg. **176:**247, 1972.

338. Gump, F. E., et al.: Exogenous glucose as an energy substrate in experimental hemorrhagic shock, Surg. Gynecol. Obstet. **136:**611, 1973.

339. Bower, M. G., et al.: Hemodynamic effects of glucagon, Arch. Surg. **101:**411, 1970.

340. Schumer, W., et al.: Metabolic and microcirculatory effects of glucagon in hypovolemic shock, Arch. Surg. **107:**176, 1973.

341. Drucker, M. R., et al.: The interactions of glucagon and glucose on cardiorespiratory variables in the critically ill patient, Surgery **75:**487, 1974.

342. Massion, W. H.: Value of high energy compounds in the treatment of shock, Am. J. Surg. **110:**342, 1965.

343. Chaudry, I. H., Sayeed, M. M., and Baue, A. E.: Effect of

adenosine triphosphate–magnesium chloride administration in shock, Surgery **75:**220, 1974.

344. Chaudry, I. H., Sayeed, M. M., and Baue, A. E.: Evidence for enhanced uptake of ATP by liver and kidney in hemorrhagic shock, Am. J. Physiol. **233**(3):R83, 1977.

345. Latts, J. R., and Goldberg, L. I.: Dopamine in the management of shock, Drug. Ther. **4:**25, 1979.

346. Altura, B. M., and Altura, B. T.: Vascular actions of glucocorticoids and their relationship to protection in circulatory shock, Fed. Proc. **33:**394, 1974.

347. Kusajima, K., Wax, S. D., and Webb, W. R., Effects of methylprednisolone on pulmonary microcirculation, Surg. Gynecol. Obstet. **139:**1, 1974.

348. Schumer, W., and Nyhus, L. M.: Corticosteroid effect on biochemical parameters of human oligemic shock, Arch. Surg. **100:**405, 1970.

349. Vargish, T., et al.: Dose-response relationships in steroid therapy for hemorrhagic shock, Am. Surg. **43:**30, 1977.

350. Sladen, A.: Methylprednisolone. Pharmacologic doses in shock lung syndrome, J. Thorac. Cardiovasc. Surg. **71:**800, 1976.

351. Lozman, J., Dutton, R. E., English, M., and Powers, S. R., Jr.: Cardiopulmonary adjustments following single high dosage administration of methylprednisolone in traumatized man, Ann. Surg. **181:**317, 1975.

352. Cloutier, C. T., Lowery, B. D., and Carey, L. C.: Acid-base disturbances in hemorrhagic shock, Arch. Surg. **98:**551, 1969.

353. Collins, J. A., et al.: Acid-base status of seriously wounded combat casualties. II. Resuscitation with stored blood, Ann. Surg. **173:**6, 1971.

354. Dagher, F. J., Seaton, J. F., and Harrison, T. S.: Lack of effect of dopamine in experimental hypovolemic shock, Surg. Gynecol. Obstet. **130:**717, 1970.

355. Loeb, H. S.: Hypovolemia in shock due to acute myocardial infarction, Circulation **11:**653, 1969.

356. Johnson, S. A., and Gunnar, R. M.: Treatment of shock in myocardial infarction, J.A.M.A. **237:**2106, 1977.

357. Toussaint, G. P. M., Burgess, J. H., and Hampson, L. G.: Central venous pressure and pulmonary wedge pressure in critical surgical illness; a comparison, Arch. Surg. **109:**265, 1974.

358. Binder, M. J.: Effect of vasopressor drugs on circulatory dynamics in shock following myocardial infarction, Am. J. Cardiol. **16:**834, 1965.

359. Dietzman, R. H., et al.: Relation of cardiac work to survival in cardiogenic shock in dogs, J.A.M.A. **199:**825, 1967.

360. Gunnar, R. M., et al.: Ineffectiveness of isoproterenol in shock due to acute myocardial infarction, J.A.M.A. **202:**64, 1967.

361. Deraney, M. F.: Glucagon? One answer to cardiogenic shock, Am. J. Med. Sci. **261:**149, 1971.

362. Smith, H. J., et al.: Hemodynamic studies in cardiogenic shock: treatment with isoproterenol and metaraminol, Circulation **35:**1084, 1967.

363. Beregovich, J., et al.: Dose-related hemodynamic and renal effects of dopamine in congestive heart failure, Am. Heart J. **87:**550, 1974.

364. Goldberg, L. I., Hsieh, Y. Y., and Resnekov, L.: Newer catecholamines for treatment of heart failure and shock: an update on dopamine and a first look at dobutamine, Prog. Cardiovasc. Dis. **19:**327, 1977.

365. Loeb, H. S., et al.: Acute hemodynamic effects of dopamine in patients with shock, Circulation **44:**163, 1971.

366. Shatney, C. H., MacCarter, D. J., and Lillehei, R. C.: Effects of infusion of dopamine and nitroprusside on size of experimental myocardial infarct, Chest **73:**850, 1978.

367. Ramanathan, K. B., et al.: Contrasting effects of dopamine and isoproterenol in experimental myocardial infarction, Am. J. Cardiol. **39:**413, 1977.

368. Hillis, L. D., and Braunwald, E.: Myocardial ischemia, N. Engl. J. Med. **296:**1034, 1977.

369. Kloner, R. A., et al.: Mummification of the infarcted myocardium by high dose corticosteroid, Circulation **57:**56, 1978.

370. Shatney, C. H., and Lillehei, R. C.: Effects of allopurinol and methylprednisolone and propranolol on experimental myocardial infarction site, Am. J. Cardiol. **37:**572, 1976.

371. Dietzman, R. C., Beckman, C. B., and Lillehei, R. C.: Pharmacologic and mechanical support for managing cardiogenic shock, Geriatrics **28:**69, 1973.

372. Dietzman, R. H., et al.: Corticosteroids as effective vasodilators in the treatment of low output syndrome, Chest **57:**440, 1970.

373. Motsay, G. J., et al.: Effects of corticosteroids on the circulation in shock: experimental and clinical results, Fed. Proc. **29:**1861, 1970.

374. Bhayana, J. N., Scott, S. M., Sethi, G. K., and Takaro, T.: Effects of intraaortic balloon pumping on organ perfusion in cardiogenic shock, J. Surg. Res. **26:**108, 1979.

375. Bardet, J., et al.: Clinical and hemodynamic results of intraaortic balloon counterpulsation and surgery for cardiogenic shock, Am. Heart J. **93:**280, 1977.

376. Beckman, C., et al.: Hemodynamic evaluation of external counterpulsation in surgical patients, Surgery **74:**846, 1973.

377. Scheidt, S., et al.: Intra-aortic balloon counterpulsation in cardiogenic shock, N. Engl. J. Med. **288:**979, 1973.

378. Mundth, E. D., et al.: Circulatory assistance and emergency direct coronary-artery surgery for shock complicating acute myocardial infarction, N. Engl. J. Med. **283:**1382, 1970.

379. Vito, L., et al.: Sepsis presenting as acute respiratory insufficiency, Surg. Gynecol. Obstet. **138:**896, 1974.

380. Cerra, F. B., Hassett, J., and Siegel, J. H.: Vasodilator therapy in clinical sepsis with low output syndrome, J. Surg. Res. **25:**180, 1979.

381. Manny, J., et al.: Effect of glucose-insulin-potassium on survival in experimental endotoxin shock, Surg. Gynecol. Obstet. **147:**405, 1978.

382. Nishijima, H., Weil, M. H., Shubin, H., and Cavanilles, J.: Hemodynamic and metabolic studies on shock associated with gram negative bacteremia, Medicine **53:**287, 1973.

383. Wilson, R. F., Sarver, E. J., and Rizzo, J.: Hemodynamic changes, treatment, and prognosis in clinical shock, Arch. Surg. **102:**21, 1971.

384. Schumer, W.: Steroids in the treatment of clinical septic shock, Ann. Surg. **184:**333, 1976.
385. Neely, W. A., et al.: Septic shock: clinical, physiological, and pathological survey of 244 patients, Ann. Surg. **173:**657, 1971.
386. Weil, M. H., Shubin, H., and Biddle, M.: Shock caused by gram-negative microorganisms. Analysis of 169 cases, Ann. Intern. Med. **60:**384, 1964.
387. Winslow, E. J., et al.: Hemodynamic studies and results of therapy in 50 patients with bacteremic shock, Am. J. Med. **54:**421, 1973.

CHAPTER 42

Hepatic encephalopathy

Bertram F. Felsher

Among the five major manifestations of severe liver disease—jaundice, ascites, hepatomegaly, variceal hemorrhage, and encephalopathy—only the latter two are urgently life-threatening. Hepatic coma, an extreme form of encephalopathy, is the most common terminal event in patients with fulminant hepatitis or severe chronic liver disease. It is a frequent contributory or direct cause of death following variceal hemorrhage. It predisposes to physical injury, aspiration, decubitus ulcer, infection, fluid and electrolyte abnormalities, and malnutrition. An ominous condition, hepatic encephalopathy is, nevertheless, potentially reversible. Thus knowledge of the clinical manifestations and treatment of hepatic encephalopathy is of paramount importance in the effective management of critically ill patients with liver disease.

■ What is the definition of hepatic encephalopathy?

Hepatic encephalopathy is the neuropsychiatric syndrome caused by liver disease. It has various manifestations of altered sensorium but is essentially characterized by cerebral dysfunction, abnormal behavior, impaired intellect, and disturbed neuromuscular function. Several terms have been applied to this condition, including hepatic coma, hepatic precoma, portal-systemic encephalopathy, nitrogenous encephalopathy, and hyperammonemia. The term "hepatic failure" should not be used synonymously with hepatic encephalopathy, as the former refers to the existence of any overt clinical sign of hepatic dysfunction such as jaundice, which is not necessarily associated with encephalopathy.

■ What are the clinical manifestations of hepatic encephalopathy?

Hepatic encephalopathy comprises a broad clinical spectrum that ranges from almost undetectable mental impairment to unarousable coma (Table 27-1). The early manifestations usually consist of mild changes in memory, mood, and mental alertness. At this stage the patient may appear lethargic, apathetic, depressed, irritable, or euphoric. More advanced stages are marked by further deepening of the mental obtundation and the development of asterixis. Asterixis refers to the inability to sustain a prolonged muscular contraction and is usually demonstrated by having the patient hyperextend the hands with fingers spread and arms outstretched. This produces a typical flapping motion ("liver flap") with a frequency of 1/1 to 3 sec. Asterixis also can be elicited in the eyelids, tongue, and feet. A maniacal phase may intervene, especially in patients with fulminant hepatitis, that not infrequently leads to the inappropriate admission of the patient to a psychiatric unit.

Other common neurologic findings include slurred speech, dysphasia, ataxia, apraxia, rigidity, and hyperreflexia with ankle clonus. Less common late manifestations are involuntary movements of the face and limbs, hemiparesis, and positive plantar reflexes. Hepatic fetor, a musty "garliclike" breath odor, is a reliable sign of severe hepatic failure and therefore is frequently associated with encephalopathy.

In the last stage of encephalopathy the patient is deeply comatose and unresponsive to painful stimuli. Breathing is often stertorous. Preterminally there may be decerebrate rigidity and convulsions.

The course of encephalopathy varies according to whether the liver disease is acute or chronic. In acute cases the course is usually rapid and the ultimate outcome is reached within 10 days. In contrast, in patients with chronic liver disease the course is ordinarily gradual, fluctuating, and lasts several days to a few weeks. Chronic encephalopathy is found only in patients with chronic liver disease who either have undergone a portacaval shunt operation or have unusually large natural portal-systemic anastomoses. Patients with chronic encephalopathy may develop progressive ataxia and choreoathetosis (non-Wilsonian hepatocerebral degeneration) or spastic paraparesis.

■ Are there any pathognomonic signs of hepatic encephalopathy?

The signs of mental impairment associated with hepatic encephalopathy are nonspecific. Other causes for cerebral dysfunction must be considered in the evaluation of patients with liver disease and apparent encephalopathy. Among these are subdural hematoma, brain tumor, brain abscess, hypoglycemia, acute alcoholic withdrawal, chronic alcoholic brain syndrome, and drug intoxication. Because localizing neurologic signs are unusual manifestations of hepatic encephalopathy, their appearance should suggest a space-occupying intracranial lesion. Hypoglycemia may be a complication of alcoholism, acute or chronic liver failure, and primary liver cell carcinoma. The tremor usually occurring in the alcoholic withdrawal syndrome is an important diagnostic feature. It is sometimes more difficult to decide whether the dementia and psychologic signs are produced by chronic alcoholism per se or result from hepatic failure. When these signs persist for several weeks despite appropriate therapy for encephalopathy in an alcoholic patient who had not previously undergone a portacaval shunt, chronic alcoholic brain syndrome is a more likely diagnosis even in the presence of obvious liver disease. If asterixis is present, the diagnosis

of hepatic encephalopathy is strongly favored. The other less common causes of asterixis, namely, uremia, diabetic ketoacidosis, carbon dioxide narcosis, heart failure, sedative overdose, and myxedema coma, are easily distinguished from hepatic failure.

■ What are the most useful tests for the diagnosis of hepatic encephalopathy?

There are no specific tests for hepatic encephalopathy. In patients with chronic liver disease the usual tests of liver function are not reliable indications of encephalopathy. However, in patients with acute hepatic necrosis, a prothrombin activity of less than 10% is almost invariably associated with some degree of encephalopathy.

The employment of auxiliary tests may be helpful when encephalopathy is subclinical or is not clearly attributable to liver failure. The Reitan trailmaking test, EEG pattern, and levels of blood ammonia and cerebrospinal fluid glutamine provide psychometric, electrophysiologic, and biochemical data that may complement the clinical findings.

The usual clinical assessment of mental state permits detection of only gross encephalopathy. Subclinical encephalopathy may be detected by the Reitan trailmaking test, which is objective, simple, inexpensive, and quick. This test has supplanted the less reliable patient's signature and five-pointed star tests.

In a majority of patients with hepatic encephalopathy there is an abnormal EEG pattern characterized by bursts of high amplitude slow waves (1½ to 3 sec) occurring synchronously and beginning in both frontal areas. In later stages these slow (delta) waves spread and may eventually become generalized. The appearance of blunted triphasic activity interspersed with periods of flattening portends a fatal outcome in patients with acute hepatic failure. Usually as the patient's level of consciousness improves, the EEG changes revert to normal, but occasionally despite clinical remission, they persist for many days to several weeks. These EEG abnormalities can occur in other conditions associated with severe metabolic derangements and therefore are not specific for liver disease.

The blood ammonia determination, despite decreasing acceptance of its diagnostic applicability, remains as the most commonly employed biochemical test for hepatic encephalopathy. The lack of correlation of the blood ammonia level with the degree of hepatic encephalopathy is the primary reason for rejection of this test. Moreover, elevated levels may occur in patients with chronic liver disease in the absence of encephalopathy, and normal levels may be found in patients with advanced encephalopathy. It has been argued that a major cause for this absolute lack of correlation is the lag period required for the establishment of an equilibrium between peripheral tissue and blood ammonia. This disequilibrium is accentuated by a rise in blood pH that favors the conversion of the ammonium ion to free ammonia, which more readily passes through cell membranes. Thus the brain ammonia level, which is the actual determinant of CNS toxicity, will temporarily exceed the blood level. In addition, the neurologic expression of increased cerebral ammonia concentration may not occur immediately, accounting for a normal mental state in the face of elevated blood ammonia.

As a group, patients with liver disease show a poor correlation between the degree of encephalopathy and the level of blood ammonia. In the individual patient, however, if allowance is made for a lag period of as much as 72 hours, the ammonia levels reflect the state of consciousness. Therefore a persistently normal blood ammonia level is good evidence against encephalopathy, and a change from an elevated to a normal value in conjunction with clinical improvement supports a diagnosis of encephalopathy. Depending on the analytic method used, the maximum normal adult value ranges from 40 to 150 μg/100 ml whether in the arterial or venous blood. However, even moderate physical activity of the forearm muscles may produce a substantial increase in the antecubital venous blood concentration. Furthermore, the ingestion of protein increases the blood ammonia level. It is therefore recommended that to avoid spurious results the determination of blood ammonia should be made on arterial blood with the patient in a rested, fasted state. Elevated blood ammonia levels may occur in individuals, usually children, with a primary metabolic, as opposed to gross morphologic, dis-

turbance of the liver as in the congenital urea cycle enzyme defect syndrome and in Reye's syndrome.

A more reliable test of hepatic encephalopathy is measurement of the cerebrospinal fluid glutamine level. This test appears to be better correlated with the degree of encephalopathy. It is unusual to find normal levels in patients with liver disease and any degree of encephalopathy. A value of 35 mg/100 ml is diagnostic of encephalopathy in patients with underlying liver disease but no respiratory failure, another cause for elevated glutamine levels. The cerebrospinal fluid α-ketoglutaramate concentration, initially considered to be a more specific biochemical indicator of encephalopathy, is also increased in patients with respiratory failure.

■ Are there any pathologic changes correlated with hepatic encephalopathy?

The morphologic changes found in the brains of patients with hepatic encephalopathy are nonspecific and appear to vary according to the duration of cerebral dysfunction. In patients with fatal acute massive hepatic necrosis and a telescoped course of coma, cerebral edema is a major complication, causing death in 13% to 22%. In patients with chronic liver disease and a longer duration of encephalopathy, hypertrophy and hyperplasia of the protoplasmic astrocytes of the cerebral cortex are commonly found. More severe neuropathic changes, including axonal degeneration and demyelination in the brain and spinal cord, have been described in patients with very prolonged, severe irreversible hepatic encephalopathy. It is difficult to explain the clinical manifestations of reversible encephalopathy or of encephalopathy in patients with acute liver failure on the basis of these observed pathologic changes. The clinical expression of this syndrome prior to the development of fixed neurologic deficits is more likely to be caused by biochemical rather than structural abnormalities.

■ What is the physiologic basis for hepatic encephalopathy?

Hepatic encephalopathy results from the metabolic disturbance produced by a combination of hepatic dysfunction and shunting of portal blood away from functional liver cells and into the systemic circulation. Portal-systemic shunting may result from anatomic anastomoses or functional shunts within the liver caused by the imbalance of hepatocellular function and sinusoidal perfusion. In patients with chronic liver disease, large extrahepatic portal-systemic anastomoses contribute toward the development of encephalopathy. However, portal-systemic anastomoses rarely cause encephalopathy in the absence of underlying liver disease. Hepatocellular dysfunction and portal-systemic shunting act in concert to alter the metabolic exchange between liver and blood. This situation could lead to either a toxic accumulation of substances normally metabolized by the liver or a deficiency of factors produced by the liver that are necessary for normal cerebral function. Actually the latter hypothesis is virtually untested. On the other hand, there is abundant evidence supporting the concept of cerebrotoxicity.

A vast array of substances have been implicated in the pathogenesis of hepatic encephalopathy. This is not surprising considering the magnitude of the biochemical activity of the liver and the likelihood of multiple metabolic alterations occurring in the diseased liver. Thus elevated levels of various "candidate cerebrotoxins" have been found in the blood, cerebrospinal fluid, and urine of patients with encephalopathy. In most instances, however, supportive evidence of their pathogenic role was not obtained. Determination of the encephalopathogenic potential of these substances has been hampered by the lack of a suitable animal model. None of the putative chemical substances proposed thus far appears to be the sole cerebrotoxin causing encephalopathy. It is possible of course that the etiology of this condition is multifactorial. Moreover, it is unclear whether different biochemical mechanisms are involved in the different forms of encephalopathy. At the present time ammonia, short-chain fatty acids, mercaptans, biogenic amines, and aromatic amino acids are the leading candidates for circulating chemical mediators of encephalopathy.

Ammonia appears to play a prominent role in the pathogenesis of hepatic encephalopathy. Supporting this concept are the following lines of evidence: (1) Elevated blood and cerebrospinal fluid ammonia concentrations are found in most patients with hepatic encephalopathy. (2) Therapeutic measures designed to reduce hyperammonemia are clinically effective. (3) Administration of ammonia or its precursors to patients with liver disease or animals elicits the syndrome. (4) In children, hyperammonemic states caused by enzyme defects in the urea cycle are associated with a syndrome similar to hepatic encephalopathy.

In man the major source of ammonia is the intestines, where about 4 g is produced daily, and all but 50 mg is absorbed. This accounts for the five times greater concentration of ammonia in the portal vein as compared to the systemic circulation. The ammonia produced in the intestines is derived mainly from urea secreted into the intestines and hydrolyzed by gastrointestinal ureases but also from nonurea nitrogenous sources. An increased intake of protein leads to augmented ammonia production primarily by enhancing urea synthesis. Although most of this urease activity is of bacterial origin, a small fraction is contained within the intestinal mucosa. Of all the ammonia produced in the intestines, three fourths is derived from the colon and one fourth from the small intestine. A pH effect governing the transport of ammonia has been demonstrated for the colon but not the small intestine. That is, lowering the pH of the colonic contents reduces the absorption of ammonia (NH_3) because of the conversion to the less diffusible ammonium ion (NH_4^+).

Under normal conditions the ammonia absorbed from the gastrointestinal tract is taken up by the liver and then reconverted back to urea. In patients with liver disease ammonia may accumulate in the systemic circulation because of portal-systemic shunting as well as impaired hepatic synthesis of urea.

Short-chain fatty acids, such as butyric, valeric, and octanoic acids appear to play a contributing but not a primary role in the cerebrotoxicity of hepatic encephalopathy. Mercaptans, like short-chain fatty acids, cause reversible coma in animals and act synergistically with ammonia. Mercaptans are the likely cause for fetor hepaticus. Further information is needed to clarify the pathogenetic significance of these compounds.

A recent extension of the cerebrotoxic theory of hepatic encephalopathy is the displacement of normal neurotransmitters in the brain by amines acting as false neurotransmitters. This hypothesis is supported by the finding of elevated levels of octopamine in the blood and urine of patients with hepatic encephalopathy and in the brain of animals with experimentally induced hepatic coma. This amine is apparently synthesized in the brain from amino acids or from tyramine, which is produced in the intestine by the action of bacterial enzymes. Although octopamine levels correlate with the degree of hepatic encephalopathy in patients with acute or chronic hepatic failure, it is probably not cerebrotoxic. Whether any false neurotransmitters actually cause encephalopathy remains to be proved.

The aromatic amino acids, phenylalanine, tyrosine, and tryptophan have been implicated as being directly or indirectly cerebrotoxic. In patients with encephalopathy and chronic liver disease, the plasma levels of phenylalanine, tyrosine, methionine, aspartate, and glutamate are increased, while the branched chain amino acids are reduced. In patients with acute liver failure all the plasma amino acids except the branched chain amino acids are increased. The branched chain amino acids compete with the aromatic acids for transport through the blood-brain barrier. A reduced ratio of branched to aromatic amino acids in plasma favors entry of the latter into the brain. Tyrosine can be converted to octopamine via tyramine. Tryptophan is a precursor of serotonin, which is increased in the brain of animals with experimental hepatic coma. When given separately to animals, none of these amino acids induce coma. The concept that these amino acids are cerebrotoxic is still speculative. The changes in plasma amino acid patterns in patients with hepatic encephalopathy may be epiphenomena rather than causal factors.

Neither the mechanism nor site of action of the putative cerebrotoxins is known. Theoretically, encephalopathy may be caused by impaired neurotransmission, disturbed cellular metabolism, or damaged cell membrane. The defects in oxidative metabolism of the brain associated with hepatic encephalopathy are probably not pathogenetically significant. Mercaptans and short-chain fatty acids may cause impairment of neuronal membrane activity by inhibiting brain Na^+, K^+-ATPase.

■ **What is the contribution to the development of hepatic encephalopathy by nonhepatic factors?**

Besides the previously discussed primary determinants of hepatic encephalopathy, certain nonhepatic factors are known to promote the development of encephalopathy in patients with chronic liver disease. Common precipitating factors of hepatic encephalopathy are as follows:

Azotemia
Gastrointestinal hemorrhage
Diuretics
Drugs causing CNS depression
Excessive nitrogenous intake
Hypokalemic alkalosis
Infection
Constipation
Rapid paracentesis

These factors by themselves are insufficient to cause the syndrome, but when superimposed on a background of underlying liver disease, they may precipitate or aggravate encephalopathy. In general these factors act by one or two physiologic mechanisms: (1) enhancing the cerebrotoxin (especially ammonia) level of the brain or (2) lowering the encephalopathic threshold of the cerebrotoxins. The cerebrotoxic level in the brain is raised by overproduction in nonhepatic sites as well as by local factors promoting entry into neuronal cells. The intake of nitrogenous substances, especially in the intestines, is a critical factor affecting ammonia and perhaps biogenic amine production. Thus increased dietary protein, ingestion of ammonium salts, and hemorrhage into the intestines are important secondary causes of encephalopathy. An additional cause for increased ammonia production is enhanced urea formation and secretion into the intestines because of protein degradation (starvation, infection, neoplasm) and azotemia. A decreased plasma insulin:glucagon ratio leading to enhanced gluconeogenesis promotes the formation of ammonia in patients with cirrhosis. Constipation may cause increased intestinal absorption of ammonia. Potassium depletion and acidosis augment ammonia production from the kidneys. Any factor that causes hypovolemia and prerenal azotemia (diuretics, rapid paracentesis, blood loss) has the potential for precipitating encephalopathy. Hypokalemic alkalosis promotes the entry of ammonia into neuronal cells of the brain. Any factor that further compromises brain function (drug, hypoglycemia, anoxia, carbon dioxide narcosis) may lower the encephalopathic threshold to ammonia or other cerebrotoxins. Tranquilizers, sedatives, anesthetics, and analgesics may precipitate or aggravate encephalopathy by causing CNS depression or anoxia. The deleterious effect of diuretics is attributable to multiple effects: transient hypovolemia with consequent azotemia and decreased hepatic or cerebral blood flow, potassium depletion and alkalosis, increased renal ammonia production, and reduction in plasma branched chain : aromatic amino acid ratio.

■ What is the conventional treatment of hepatic encephalopathy?

The rationale for the conventional therapeutic regimen for hepatic encephalopathy, which has been in effect for more than a decade, is reduction in the production and absorption of ammonia from the intestines and removal of precipitating factors. The first goal is accomplished by restricting dietary protein, cleansing the gastrointestinal tract with oral purgatives and/or high enemas, and reducing the fecal flora of urea-splitting bacteria with poorly absorbed antibiotics given orally or by retention enema. In general, dietary protein is restricted to 0 to 20 g/day for acute encephalopathy, but in cases of chronic encephalopathy it is titrated according to the patient's clinical response. In cleansing the gastrointestinal tract an effective oral purgative is magnesium sulfate. It is preferable to use acidic cleansing enemas to minimize ammonia absorption. The most commonly used agent to reduce the fecal flora is neomycin in a total daily dose, including oral and rectal administration, of 2 to 3 g/day. It is best not to exceed this dose, as neomycin is absorbed slightly and excreted in the urine. It can cause oto- and nephrotoxicity as well as intestinal malabsorption, diarrhea, and staphylococcal enterocolitis. There is no evidence that the

larger doses sometimes recommended are more effective. Alternatives to neomycin are other broad-spectrum antibiotics and nonabsorbable sulfonamides such as succinylsulfathiazole (Sulfasuxidine). These other antibacterial agents may be useful in cases of neomycin hypersensitivity or renal failure.

The common precipitating factors to be considered in every patient with hepatic encephalopathy are indiscretionary protein intake; hemorrhage in the gastrointestinal tract; diuretic therapy; renal failure; drugs that act on the CNS or are ammonia precursors, such as methionine; metabolic imbalances, especially hypokalemic alkalosis; infection (pneumonia, spontaneous peritonitis, or gram-negative septicemia); and constipation. Many of these factors can be eliminated. Variceal hemorrhage and functional renal failure (hepatorenal syndrome) are the least reversible of the precipitating factors and therefore commonly produce fatal hepatic coma.

In addition to these specific therapeutic measures, general supportive therapy for the other complications of hepatic failure such as coagulation defects, malnutrition, electrolyte disturbances, hypoglycemia, and hypoxemia, as well as provision of adequate caloric intake, should be instituted. Agitation should obviously not be treated with drugs. In cases of chronic active hepatitis the liver disease itself may be ameliorated by corticosteroid therapy.

■ What are the newer or less conventional forms of treatment of hepatic encephalopathy?

A more direct approach to reducing intestinal ammonia production has been the use of the urease inhibitor acetohydroxamic acid. Although preliminary studies showed reduction in the blood ammonia levels after oral administration of the drug to patients with encephalopathy, associated clinical improvement was not observed. Similarly, a transient induction of antibodies to urease was achieved by the injection of jack bean urease to patients with encephalopathy, but again clinical improvement did not consistently parallel the reduction in blood ammonia, and some toxic reactions were observed. The feeding of *Lactobacillus* in the attempt to replace the colonic flora with nonurease-producing bacteria is not by itself clinically effective but may be of some use as adjunctive therapy.

Lactulose appears to be at least as effective as neomycin in the treatment of acute as well as chronic encephalopathy. This agent is a synthetic disaccharide that is neither absorbed nor metabolized in the small intestine but is converted by colonic bacterial enzymes to acetic and lactic acid, which causes acidification of the bowel contents. It can be given orally or by enema. Its mechanism of action is thought to be related primarily to the effect of fecal acidification in reducing ammonia and amine absorption as well as by its direct cathartic activity. A recently proposed alternative mechanism is that it acts as a bacterial substrate, which leads to diminished generation and increased uptake of ammonia by bacteria. This drug may be a useful substitute for neomycin in the treatment of patients with encephalopathy that is chronic or associated with renal failure.

Another approach to the treatment of encephalopathy is reduction or neutralization of circulating cerebrotoxins. Dialysis, exchange transfusions, total body washout, and extracorporeal animal liver perfusion have not improved the survival rate in patients with encephalopathy caused by chronic liver disease or fulminant viral hepatitis. Exchange transfusions may be beneficial in the treatment of hepatic coma resulting from Reye's syndrome, but vigorous reduction of cerebral edema with dexamethasone and surgical reduction of intracranial pressure are the most effective means of reducing mortality. Dramatic permanent reversal of hepatic coma has been reported in patients with fulminant toxin-induced hepatitis treated with the establishment of cross-circulation to human volunteers. Ethical considerations limit the applicability of this rather heroic measure. An artificial liver would certainly be a more acceptable form of therapy. A major step in that direction was seemingly achieved by early studies showing that hemoperfusion through columns of activated charcoal effectively reverses hepatic coma in patients with acute or chronic liver disease. However, later experience indicates that the available artificial liver support systems do not improve mortality from fulminant liver failure.

In an attempt to counteract the possible effect of false neurotransmitters, levodopa, a precursor of dopamine, has been used in the treatment of hepatic encephalopathy. So far the reports of the effectiveness of this treatment have been inconclusive. Gastric irritation and bleeding and other side-effects may limit its usefulness. The efficacy of bromocriptine, a specific dopamine receptor agonist, has not been proved.

In a preliminary study administration of keto-analogues of essential amino acids to patients with hepatic encephalopathy was associated with clinical improvement as well as reduction of plasma glutamine and ammonia.

The infusion of an amino acid mixture with a high concentration of branched chain amino acids was associated with normalization of the plasma amino acid pattern and clinical improvement in a group of patients with cirrhosis and encephalopathy. Controlled studies are needed to determine whether this form of treatment is actually beneficial.

In patients with compensated cirrhosis therapeutic elevation of the insulin : glucagon ratio by glucose feedings leads to increased protein tolerance and slight reduction of blood ammonia concentration. On the other hand, hyperinsulinism, theoretically, might adversely affect hepatic encephalopathy because it selectively causes reduction of the branched chain amino acids, thereby promoting entry of the aromatic amino acids, potential cerebrotoxins, into the brain.

An extreme method to reduce the colonic formation of cerebrotoxins is colonic resection or bypass. The mortality rate for this procedure in patients with chronic liver disease is 25%. Therefore this treatment should be reserved only for patients with spontaneous, refractory, and chronic or recurrent encephalopathy present for at least 6 months and with otherwise good liver function. Good results have been reported for patients with postshunt encephalopathy.

Finally, the most direct and perhaps most dramatic form of treatment of hepatic encephalopathy is liver transplantation, which presently is still being developed and therefore reserved only for select patients with severe chronic liver disease. Hopefully further progress in the field of transplantation technology and immunotherapy will allow expansion of the indications for this treatment in the near future.

BIBLIOGRAPHY

Conn, H. O.: Current diagnosis and treatment of hepatic coma, Hosp. Prac. **8:**65, 1973.

Conn, H. O.: Trailmaking and number connection tests in the assessment of mental state in portal systemic encephalopathy, Am. J. Dig. Dis. **22:**541, 1977.

Fischer, J. E., et al.: The effect of normalization of plasma amino acids on hepatic encephalopathy in man, Surgery **80:**77, 1976.

Gazzard, B. G., et al.: Charcoal haemoperfusion in the treatment of fulminant hepatic failure, Lancet **1:**1301, 1974.

Kennedy, J., Parbhoo, S. P., MacGillivray, B., and Sherlock, S.: Effect of extracorporeal liver perfusion on the electroencephalogram of patients in coma due to acute liver failure, Q. J. Med. **42:**549, 1973.

Maddrey, W. C., et al.: Effects of keto analogues of essential amino acids in portal-systemic encephalopathy, Gastroenterology **71:**190, 1976.

Rikkers, L., et al.: Subclinical hepatic encephalopathy: detection, prevalence, and relationship to nitrogen metabolism, Gastroenterology **75:**462, 1978.

Schenker, S., Breen, K. J., and Hoyumpa, A. M.: Hepatic encephalopathy: current status, Gastroenterology **66:**121, 1974.

Summerskill, W. H. J., and Wolpert, E.: Ammonia metabolism in the gut, Am. J. Clin. Nutr. **23:**633, 1970.

Walker, C., Petertson, W., and Unger, R.: Blood ammonia levels in advanced cirrhosis during therapeutic elevation of insulin: glucagon ratio, N. Engl. J. Med. **291:**168, 1974.

Zieve, L.: Amino acids in liver failure, Gastroenterology **76:** 219, 1979.

Zieve, L., and Nicoloff, D. M.: Pathogenesis of hepatic coma, Ann. Rev. Med. **26:**143, 1975.

CHAPTER 43

Gastrointestinal bleeding

Stephen R. Severance

Hemorrhage from the gastrointestinal tract is a common and serious problem[1-9] accounting for at least 1% of all hospital admissions and ranking second only to cardiovascular disease as a reason for emergency hospitalization. The overall mortality from this condition ranges from 5% to 30%, but if only cases of *massive* bleeding (estimated loss of at least 20% of blood volume) are considered, the mortality ranges from 25% to 50%. Increased mortality is clearly related to delay in appropriate diagnosis and treatment. Therefore nowhere in the field of critical care is a well-organized, systematic, multidisciplinary approach more important. This chapter outlines such an approach.

■ What are the common causes of gastrointestinal bleeding?

The advent of fiberoptic endoscopy has greatly increased the accuracy of the diagnosis of gastrointestinal bleeding. Between 85% and 90% of gastrointestinal bleeding originates from a lesion proximal to the ligament of Treitz (*upper* gastrointestinal bleeding); another 5% to 10% from lesions distal to this point (*lower* gastrointestinal bleeding); and finally, in 5% to 10%, despite extensive diagnostic procedures, the exact site of bleeding cannot be established. Bleeding into the gastrointestinal tract may, in fact, originate from anywhere in the gastrointestinal tract, as well as from communicating (pancreas or biliary tree) or contiguous (aorta or spleen) organs. Potential sources of gastrointestinal bleeding are given in the following list:

Sources of gastrointestinal hemorrhage*

Upper gastrointestinal bleeding
  Inflammatory
    Duodenal ulcer
    Gastritis
    Gastric ulcer
    Esophagitis
    Stress ulcer
    Pancreatitis
  Mechanical
    Hiatus hernia
    Mallory-Weiss syndrome
    Hematobilia
  Vascular
    Esophageal or gastric varices
    Aortointestinal fistula
    Hemangioma
    Rendu-Osler-Weber syndrome
    Mesenteric vascular occlusion
    Blue nevus bleb
  Systemic
    Blood dyscrasias
    Collagen diseases
    Uremia
  Neoplasms
    Carcinoma
    Polyps—single, multiple, Peutz-Jeghers syndrome
    Leiomyoma
    Carcinoid
    Leukemia
    Sarcoma
Lower gastrointestinal bleeding
  Inflammatory

---

*Modified from Sleisinger, M., and Fordtran, J.: Gastrointestinal disease: pathophysiology, diagnosis, and management, Philadelphia, 1973, W. B. Saunders Co.

Ulcerative colitis
Diverticulitis
Enterocolitis—regional (Crohn's disease)
    tuberculous, radiation, bacterial, toxic
Mechanical
    Diverticulosis
Neoplasms
    Carcinoma
    Polyps—adenomatous and villous, familial
        polyposis, Peutz-Jeghers syndrome
    Leiomyoma
    Sarcoma
    Lipoma
    Metastatic (melanoma)
Anomalies
    Meckel's diverticulum
Vascular
    Hemorrhoids
    Aortoduodenal fistula
    Aortic aneurysm
    Hemangioma
    Mesenteric thrombosis
    Hereditary hemorrhagic telangiectasia
    Blue nevus bleb
Systemic
    Blood dyscrasias
    Collagen diseases
    Uremia

Among these, four account for approximately 90% of upper gastrointestinal bleeding episodes: peptic ulceration (gastric or duodenal), diffuse erosion (esophagitis, gastritis, or duodenitis), esophageal varices, and gastroesophageal tears (*Mallory-Weiss syndrome*). Peptic ulcer disease is by far the most common cause of gastrointestinal bleeding in this country.

One of these causes of upper gastrointestinal bleeding, the gastroesophageal tear, or Mallory-Weiss syndrome, deserves special mention. This lesion, usually the result of abrupt elevation of intra-abdominal pressure by forceful vomiting or other means, has been considered to be a very rare, nearly always catastrophic event invariably requiring surgery. However, recent studies[10,11] employing fiberoptic endoscopy have proved this syndrome to be far more common than previously thought, accounting for 5% to 15% of cases of upper gastrointestinal hemorrhage. Furthermore, only one fifth of these patients require surgery, and a substantial number do not even require transfusion.[11]

■ **What are the causes of lower gastrointestinal bleeding?**

The necessity for time-consuming preparation limits the fiberoptic endoscopic localization of the site of lower gastrointestinal bleeding in the acute situation. Carcinoma of the colon, usually on the left side, remains the most common cause of rectal bleeding. This condition together with (in order of frequency) diverticulosis, ulcerative colitis, and polyps accounts for 90% to 95% of the cases. Interestingly, if analysis is restricted to those patients with bleeding severe enough to require transfusion, diverticulosis becomes most common, accounting for approximately 70% of the cases.[12]

■ **What are the clinical features seen in patients with gastrointestinal bleeding?**

Rectal bleeding and hematemesis or melena are the most common complaints of patients with lower and upper gastrointestinal bleeding, respectively. Hematemesis occurs in about one half to two thirds of patients with upper gastrointestinal bleeding. Blood exposed for a significant period of time to either acid or bacterial action turns black, explaining the frequent clinical observations of "coffee-ground" emesis or shiny black "tarry" stools (melena). Melena is almost always a sign of upper gastrointestinal bleeding, occurring in two thirds of such patients. Under normal conditions a minimum of approximately 100 ml of blood introduced into the stomach will produce melanotic stools. However, in conditions of diminished bacterial action (for example, neomycin therapy) or increased intestinal motility (blood within the gastrointestinal tract has a strong cathartic effect), upper gastrointestinal bleeding may result in the passage of actual red or more commonly "maroon-colored" blood via the rectum. Conversely, in conditions of stasis or diminished intestinal motility such as an obstructing carcinoma, lower gastrointestinal bleeding may produce black stools or so-called *pseudomelena*. Oral preparations containing either iron or bismuth may produce black stools in the absence of gastrointestinal bleeding. Such stools usually lack the shiny or tarry appearance produced by actual blood and yield a negative or weakly positive chemical reaction for blood. Truly melenic stool should invariably produce a strong (that is, 4+) chemical reaction for blood.

In addition to these overt symptoms of bleeding, approximately half of the patients with gastrointestinal bleeding will describe less specific symptoms such as weakness, faintness, fatigue, or abdominal pain. A few patients with acute and many with chronic bleeding have one of these symptoms alone.

■ **What specific information should always be obtained from the patient with gastrointestinal bleeding?**

Ideally a complete traditional medical history and systems review should be obtained from every patient with gastrointestinal bleeding. Unfortunately the presence of severe bleeding or even shock may make this impractical early in the patient's hospital course. However, even under these circumstances there are a few pertinent questions that provide invaluable information and should never be omitted.

Any prior history of gastrointestinal disease or surgery should be noted. In Palmer's large series[13] nearly half the patients were already known to have a gastrointestinal lesion capable of producing bleeding. Such a history, while obviously very valuable, should not lead to diagnostic over-complacency, since 40% of these patients were in fact bleeding from lesions other than those previously diagnosed.

Pain may suggest peptic ulcer, pancreatitis, or biliary disease (hematobilia); prior vascular surgery may lead to a diagnosis of aortoenteric fistula; and protracted wretching or vomiting of clear material *followed by* bloody emesis may indicate a gastric or gastroesophageal tear (Mallory-Weiss syndrome). Symptoms of liver disease should be sought, and careful questioning may be required to elicit a description of symptoms suggestive of bleeding diathesis. Although the symptoms of the more severe dyscrasias (for example, hemophilia) are commonly volunteered spontaneously, an almost forgotten difficult dental extraction may be the only clue to a mild one (for example, von Willebrand's disease).

Finally, and perhaps most important, a meticulous drug history is indispensable in any case of gastrointestinal bleeding. Salicylates and alcohol are by far the most common offenders, causing bleeding in their own right (that is, hemorrhagic erosive gastritis) as well as potentiating bleeding from independent lesions, especially peptic ulcer. More equivocal evidence has linked drugs such as indomethacin, phenylbutazone, corticosteroids, reserpine, nicotine, and the antimetabolites to either peptic ulcer formation, gastrointestinal bleeding, or both. The association of anticoagulants such as warfarin with gastrointestinal bleeding should be obvious. Less appreciated is the fact that the great majority of patients who bleed while on anticoagulant therapy do so from a distinct, usually independent anatomic lesion, for example, an ulcer or diverticulum.

When taking a drug history, it is important to recall that many nonprescription over-the-counter preparations, including innumerable aspirin-containing compounds, may not be classified as "medicines" by the patient and therefore may not be mentioned unless asked about specifically. Nowhere in the medical history is careful circumspection more important than in the detection of alcohol abuse. Witness the patient who is patently "tipsy" at 9:00 in the morning who drinks only "socially!" Questions regarding alcohol intake should always be casual and nonaccusatory in nature, possibly appended in an offhand manner to inquiries about nonprescription medications. When doubt exists, tactful questioning of family members is appropriate and may be helpful.

■ **What elements of the physical examination are particularly useful in the evaluation of patients with gastrointestinal bleeding?**

As in the case of the medical history, a complete examination is ideal, but not always immediately practical. The abdominal examination is obviously important, and the presence or absence of tenderness, peritoneal signs, succussion splash, or bruits as well as the relative activity of bowel sounds should be carefully noted. Hepatic or splenic enlargement, as well as other signs suggestive of liver disease or chronic alcoholism, such as palmar erythema, Dupuytren's contracture, spider telangiectasis, parotid enlargement, gynecomastia, and peripheral neuropathy, should be carefully sought.

The oronasopharyngeal area should never be

overlooked in the physical examination. Silent bleeding in this area may be manifested by hematemesis alone (so-called *paradoxical hematemesis*) with unfortunate (and embarrassing) consequences if not detected.

Some of the most useful clues, and seemingly the most easily overlooked, occur in the skin. A partial list of mucocutaneous disorders associated with gastrointestinal bleeding is reproduced here:

Mucocutaneous disorders associated with gastrointestinal bleeding[*]
Hereditary hemorrhagic telangiectasia
Universal angiomatosis
Blue rubber bleb nevus syndrome
Multiple phlebectasia
Pseudoxanthoma elasticum
Ehlers-Danlos syndrome
Homocystinuria
Polyarteritis nodosa
Atrophying papulosis of Degos
Neurofibromatosis
Kaposi's sarcoma
Peutz-Jeghers syndrome
Carcinoid syndrome

■ What is hereditary hemorrhagic telangiectasia?

The most common mucocutaneous disorder associated with gastrointestinal bleeding is hereditary hemorrhagic telangiectasia, or the Osler-Weber-Rendu syndrome.[14] The *telangiectasia* seen in this syndrome are dilated superficial capillary-venous vessels that may appear anywhere on the skin or in the mucous membrane of the gastrointestinal tract from the nasopharyngeal orifice to the anus. The telangiectasia may be restricted to the gastrointestinal tract with sparing of the skin, and unless suspected, they are easily missed on endoscopic examination. These lesions never appear on x-ray films. Although they appear to be hereditary, the lesions are not usually manifested until middle age. Bleeding tends to be chronic and seldom well-localized enough to be amenable to surgery. Oral iron therapy alone may be inadequate, and parenteral iron therapy may be necessary to maintain even a low normal he-

[*]Modified from UCLA Interdepartmental Conference: Ann. Intern. Med. **71**:993, 1969.

moglobin level. *Acute massive bleeding* is uncommon in a patient with this disorder and should lead to a search for an associated localized arteriovenous malformation or an unrelated source of bleeding such as peptic ulcer.

■ How is the severity of bleeding most accurately assessed?

The rate of blood loss is as important as the total quantity lost in determining the clinical manifestations. Loss of more than half the circulating blood volume over a period of several weeks or months may produce only mild pallor and weakness, whereas the acute loss of 2 or 3 units of blood may result in syncope with many of the clinical signs of hypovolemia. The hypotension, tachycardia, mental confusion, clammy skin, and constricted veins of *shock* are reliable but rather insensitive signs, usually indicating relatively acute loss of at least 2000 ml of blood. Perhaps the most sensitive bedside indication of acute blood loss is *postural changes* in pulse or blood pressure, so-called *vasomotor instability*.[15] Under normal conditions a change from the supine to the sitting or standing position initiates complex cardiovascular compensatory responses mediated by both neurogenic and humoral mechanisms that maintain blood pressure and pulse with minor changes. When hypovolemia caused by a deficit in blood or other fluids is present, these compensatory responses may be required to maintain normal blood pressure and pulse *even in the supine position*. In such a case, a change in position will result in abnormal changes in these values. The tilt test, utilizing a specially designed table to provide various angles of elevation, has been recommended as a sophisticated, although somewhat impractical, method of quantitating these changes. Nearly as much information may be obtained simply by determining blood pressure and pulse first in the supine and then in the sitting position. A drop in systolic pressure of 10 mm Hg or more or an increase of 20 beats/min or more in pulse indicates a minimum blood loss of 1000 ml in the average patient and even less in the older patient with diminished vascular tone. In the patient who already has hypotension in the supine position, this simple test adds little information and indeed may be dangerous.

■ **How do hemoglobin or hematocrit values correlate with the results of blood loss?**

The hemoglobin or hematocrit values immediately after acute blood loss, no matter how massive, will be virtually unchanged, since the blood remaining will be identical in composition to that lost. However, in an effort to restore intravascular volume, complex homeostatic mechanisms are initiated, resulting in renal conservation of fluid and electrolytes and in gradual shifts of fluid from extra- to intravascular compartments. These compensatory changes and the fall in hemoglobin and hematocrit that accompanies them are gradual, requiring more than 24 hours to be complete. *Hemoglobin and hematocrit are therefore unreliable indices of acute blood loss.* However, the IV infusions of fluid restore intravascular volumes as effectively and much more rapidly than the body's homeostatic mechanisms, and once fluids sufficient to eradicate any postural change in blood pressure or pulse have been infused, hemoglobin or hematocrit values reflect quantitative blood loss more accurately, each 4% drop in hematocrit reflecting a loss of approximately 1 unit of blood.

■ **What initial diagnostic studies should be obtained?**

A hemoglobin or hematocrit determination should be performed immediately. Stool and gastric aspirate, if not grossly bloody, should be tested for blood using guaiac or benzidine reagents. Complete blood count, urinalysis, and serum amylase, electrolyte, and liver function tests should be ordered. Assessment of the coagulation system is desirable in all patients and essential in any patient with liver disease or a history suggestive of a bleeding diathesis. Prothrombin and partial thromboplastin times, fibrinogen level, and platelet count or qualitative assessment of platelets on peripheral smear constitute an adequate coagulation "screen," with more sophisticated testing to elucidate any initial abnormalities. In addition, routine x-ray films of the chest and abdomen should be obtained. Because myocardial infarction, often "silent," occurs in 1% to 2% of patients with gastrointestinal hemorrhage, an ECG is indicated for older patients and those with coronary risk factors or massive bleeding. It

is recommended that a gastrointestinal bleeding flow sheet similar to that shown in Fig. 43-1 be utilized at the bedside.

■ **What should be included in the initial treatment of patients with gastrointestinal bleeding?**

Since diagnostic procedures such as endoscopy or radiography are more hazardous when the patient's condition is unstable, the goal of initial treatment should be the *resuscitation* and stabilization of the patient's condition. IV therapy should be initiated using a large-bore (14- or 16-gauge) IV cannula (for example, Medicut or Intracath). A catheter for monitoring central venous pressure (CVP) should be placed in any patient with hypotension or shock and continued blood loss, and should be strongly considered in older patients or those with a history of cardiovascular disease in whom more than modest fluid and blood replacement is anticipated. In addition, oxygen therapy is indicated for any patient with hypotension or significant anemia. Most of these patients will be extremely apprehensive, and in all except those with definite shock, an appropriate sedative, such as phenobarbital, may be given parenterally. A vitamin K preparation such as phytonadione, 10 to 20 mg, may be given by IM or IV route to any patient with a prolonged prothrombin time. Since this medication is relatively harmless unless given in excessive dosages and requires several hours to begin generating prothrombin, it is not necessary to await laboratory results in patients with known cirrhosis, malnutrition from any cause, or a history of heavy salicylate use, which may also depress the prothrombin time.

Finally, a nasogastric tube should be placed in any patient with suspected upper gastrointestinal bleeding or with rectal passage of blood that is not clearly lower gastrointestinal in origin. Since a significant number of bleeding duodenal ulcers will present solely with rectal bleeding, this simple and harmless procedure may avoid considerable frustration and embarrassment.

Even in the presence of continuous bleeding from the duodenum, a closed pylorus may prevent the reflux of blood into the stomach, except at inconstant intervals. A significant number of

The stomach and duodenum
Gastrointestinal bleeding: flow sheet

Date: 4/17/73
Clinical:

Times:	1 AM	1³⁰	2³⁰				
Mental status	Confused		clear				
Pulse	140	120	100				
Blood pressure Supine	90/60	100/70	110/76				
Upright	—	70/50	100/70				
CVP	1	2	6				
Gastric lavage	bloody	brown	clear				
Stool	bloody		500 cc black				
Laboratory: Hg/Hct	7/20		8.5/25				
WBC	20,000	—	—				
BUN/creatinine	45/1.8						
Prothrombin (sec)	14						
Arterial pH and gases							
Blood electrolytes	NA 140 K 3.7						
Diagnostic: Note endoscopy barium studies, angiography, string test, intubation, etc.	Esophagoscopy NEG.		X-Ray D.U.				
Therapy: Blood products	—	1500 Blood	whole →				
Fluids (IV and PO)	1000 Ringers						
Electrolytes	"						
Pharmacologic dose	20 u. PiTressin						
Tamponade with pressure							
Comments:							

Name   Bleeder, G.I.

Hosp. No.   .000 000

Fig. 43-1. Flow sheet of stomach and duodenum. (Modified from Sleisinger, M., and Fordtran, J.: Gastrointestinal disease: pathophysiology, diagnosis and management, Philadelphia, 1973, W. B. Saunders Co.)

lesions of the stomach that have stopped bleeding will rebleed early in the hospital course. Finally, distention as well as acidity aggravates the bleeding of erosive gastritis. For these reasons, except in the case of probable lower gastrointestinal bleeding, the nasogastric tube should not be removed following an initially negative aspiration, but rather taped in place and attached to intermittent or continuous suction for a period of several to 24 hours.

If the initial gastric aspirate is bloody or "coffee ground" in appearance, gastric lavage (*gavage*) using an iced solution should be begun. The purpose of this procedure is twofold. First, it reduces gastric blood flow by 50%[16] and will stop bleeding, at least temporarily, in approximately two thirds of patients with upper gastrointestinal hemorrhage.[13] Second, it allows removal of retained secretions, blood, and large clots, all of which interfere with the performance or interpretation of diagnostic procedures such as endoscopy or gastrointestinal x-ray films. Unfortunately this procedure may lose effectiveness if performed improperly. The most common mistake is the use of the relatively small nasogastric tube rather than a large tube (at least No. 36 French). A large tube is easier to position, less likely to become clogged, and allows removal of blood clots too large to pass through the small tube. Large double-lumen[17] or triple-lumen[18] tubes have been especially designed for this purpose, but in their absence an Ewald tube attached to a simple Y connector may be used. Using rubber tubing, one branch of the Y leads to an *irrigation bag* or similar receptacle for instillation of fluid, while the other branch leads to a pail or basin where the fluid may drain from the stomach by gravity. When one branch is in use, the other should be clamped with a hemostat. The tube is passed through the mouth or nose into the stomach and the patient placed in the prone or left lateral position at an angle of elevation that places the feet higher than the head. Proper positioning of the tube is then ensured by adjusting it until at least 40 ml of lavage solution can be aspirated after 50 ml is instilled.

Since varying degrees of absorption may occur during this procedure, there has been some dis-agreement over the recommended composition of the solutions used.[19] Very rarely, electrolyte abnormalities such as hyponatremia have been attributed to the use of iced *water* solutions, while the absorption of sodium chloride from *saline* solutions may lead to volume excess in susceptible patients who are not significantly volume depleted from bleeding. Isotonic sodium sulfate solutions have been used to minimize (although not eliminate) sodium absorption. In reality the choice of solution is probably irrelevant unless massive volumes are used in a patient with medical problems predisposing to fluid and electrolyte disturbances (for example, hyponatremia in the cirrhotic patient or volume overload in the patient with heart disease or renal failure). One or two liters of the solution chosen is placed over ice in a large basin, and approximately 300 ml at a time of the resultant mixture is instilled into the stomach. After each instillation the stomach is allowed to drain by simple gravity, but in order to dislodge blood clots, the tube should be irrigated frequently using a 50 ml irrigating syringe. Care should be taken to avoid unduly forceful suction, which may produce gastric artifacts difficult to distinguish from erosive gastritis if gastroscopy is performed later. Cessation of bleeding is indicated by a persistently clear or faint pink return from the stomach, and lavage should not be considered unsuccessful unless continued for a minimum of 1 hour without such clearing. Since iced lavage may cause shivering and discomfort, at times actually lowering the body temperature, the patient should be covered as warmly as possible during the procedure.

■ What type of fluid should be used for IV replacement in the presence of gastrointestinal bleeding?

Obviously the types and quantities of fluid used must be tailored to meet the specific needs of the individual patient. For example, the needs of the patient with minimum or slow bleeding and chronic congestive heart failure differ immensely from those of the patient with more rapid blood loss and preexisting dehydration from intractable vomiting.

In general IV therapy has two major objectives. The first is restoration of intravascular volume (reflected in blood pressure and pulse), which may be accomplished by infusion of either blood products or nonsanguineous fluids such as saline or albumin solutions. The second is restoration of oxygen-carrying capacity (reflected in the hemoglobin or hematocrit values), which can be accomplished solely through the use of blood products. Both practical and theoretical considerations govern the choice of preparations used to achieve these objectives. Practically speaking, the sophisticated methods involved in the modern "type and cross match" may require as much as an hour or more, making nonsanguineous solutions the mainstay of early resuscitation. In the small hospital with limited blood bank reserves or in the patient with a rare blood type, this delay may be even greater. In the rare circumstance of massive bleeding with shock and critically reduced oxygen-carrying capacity from the outset, *type-specific* blood can usually be provided in 10 minutes or less. If blood of the patient's specific type is not immediately available, O-negative blood may serve as the "universal donor" in this circumstance. A less important practical consideration is cost. A liter of saline solution costs a little over $1, a similar quantity of 5% albumin in saline solution over $50, and a unit of blood $25 to $50.[21]

In a more theoretical vein, studies in both man and animals have shown that acute blood loss is followed by a reduction not only in intravascular volume but in extravascular volume as well, and that replacement of blood alone will not restore extravascular volume. Studies in experimentally bled animals have shown that animals treated with their lost blood plus nonsanguineous solutions such as saline or plasma solutions have twice the survival of those treated with the lost blood alone.[22] Similar, although less well-controlled, observations have been made in man.

The type of nonsanguineous solution to be used remains a subject of controversy.[21,23,24] *Crystalloid* solutions such as saline or Ringer's lactate solution have economy and relatively greater availability to recommend them. On the other hand, the recent theoretical implication of a fall in plasma oncotic pressure in the development of *posttraumatic respiratory insufficiency,* or *shock lung,* following the treatment of shock states has created a bias toward the use of *colloid* solutions such as albumin or plasma. Whether using crystalloid, colloid, or both, sodium bicarbonate should be added when systemic acidosis is present. In addition, solutions containing some glucose may be preferable in alcoholic patients, who occasionally develop hypoglycemia. (Dextrose-containing solutions may agglutinate the red blood cells in banked blood and therefore should never be infused simultaneously through the same IV line with blood.)

Blood may be administered in its whole form or as packed blood cells (with the plasma removed). Packed blood cells have the advantages of conserving other components such as plasma or clotting factors for use elsewhere and reducing the volume load for patients with marginal cardiac, renal, or liver function. In addition, packed blood cells contain considerably less ammonia than whole blood, possibly of importance in patients with severe liver disease. Whether whole blood or packed cells are used, transfusion therapy should be adequate not only to restore oxygen-carrying capacity sufficiently to maintain normal functions, but also to allow some reserve in case of recurrent blood loss. Under ordinary circumstances the return of the hematocrit to approximately 30% (or hemoglobin to about 10%) will achieve these objectives. Both packed cells and whole blood donated more than 24 hours before use are deficient in several clotting factors. Therefore every fifth or sixth unit transfused should be fresh (less than 24 hours old) whole blood. Banked blood is prevented from clotting by the addition of *citrate* to bind calcium, which is an essential factor in normal coagulation. For this reason, even though most hematologists believe that frank tetany will occur before ionized calcium is depressed sufficiently to effect clot formation, intermittent IV calcium infusion is a common practice during massive transfusion therapy.

Finally, the majority of commonly encountered clotting abnormalities will respond readily to adequate quantities, where indicated, of fresh-frozen plasma, platelet packs, or both. Clotting factor concentrates (for example, Konyne) carry an inordinate risk of hepatitis, may precipitate intravascular coagulation (especially in patients with liver disease),[25,26] and therefore should rarely, if ever, be used.

■ What diagnostic approach should be followed to localize exactly the site of upper gastrointestinal bleeding?

A step-by-step systematic approach to the diagnosis of gastrointestinal bleeding has been devised[27] and should be extremely helpful as long as the importance of individualizing each case is remembered. The major diagnostic alternatives are barium contrast radiography, fiberoptic endoscopy, and selective or superselective abdominal arteriography.

With occasional dissent,[28] it is now generally agreed that barium contrast radiography, once the mainstay of diagnosis, has little if any diagnostic usefulness *in the presence of active upper gastrointestinal bleeding*. First, when compared with fiberoptic endoscopy, it is inaccurate, failing to detect many lesions even in well-prepared non-bleeding patients. For example, as many as 50% of esophageal varices,[29] 11% to 14% of benign gastric ulcers, 4% to 12% of gastric cancers, 6% to 17% of duodenal ulcers, and 50% of marginal ulcers are missed by the upper gastrointestinal series.[30] In unprepared patients with intraluminal blood and clots the degree of inaccuracy will be even greater. Although a special air contrast technique has recently been described for the detection of gastric erosions, gastric varices, and gastric or esophageal tears, these lesions will be detected by conventional barium studies in *less than 5%* of the cases. In addition, the detection of a lesion with bleeding potential on barium studies *does not establish that lesion as the site of present bleeding*. Among 1313 patients with upper gastrointestinal bleeding described by Palmer,[12] 2024 actual or potential bleeding lesions were found by endoscopy. More than 50% of the patients with cirrhosis, definite esophageal varices, and upper gastrointestinal bleeding were bleeding from a lesion other than the esophageal varices.[31,32] Finally, contrast material in the intestinal tract precludes the effective use of fiberoptic endoscopy for several hours and of arteriography for 24 to 48 hours after a barium contrast study.

With rare exceptions,[33,34] gastroenterologists seem to agree that fiberoptic endoscopy is the diagnostic procedure of choice in the patient with active upper gastrointestinal bleeding and no contraindications to the procedure.[13,35-37] Endoscopy is more fruitful if performed within the first 24 to 48 hours of hospitalization,[37] and if it is properly performed should yield a positive diagnosis in over 80% of the cases. The complication rate of the procedure is probably less than 1 in 300, with an overall mortality of less than 1 in 4000.[30]

There are relatively few contraindications to endoscopy. Since cooperation on the part of the patient is a prerequisite, it should not be performed in the combative or delirious patient. The comatose patient not only lacks cooperativeness but carries a higher risk of aspiration as well and should never undergo endoscopy unless endotracheal intubation has been performed. The patient's condition should always be stabilized prior to endoscopy, as morbidity and mortality are drastically increased in the presence of shock or vasomotor instability. Similarly, patients with acute cardiac or pulmonary conditions such as acute myocardial infarction or respiratory failure should not undergo endoscopy. Alternative diagnostic procedures should be strongly considered in cases of pancreatitis or possible perforated viscus, since either condition may be aggravated by endoscopy. Finally, since most institutions lack the facilities for actual sterilization of the endoscope itself, the procedure should be avoided if at all possible in cases of active tuberculosis or hepatitis B antigenemia.

The procedure may be carried out at the bedside or, more conveniently, in a specially equipped room. It should always be preceded by a thorough gastric lavage. Atropine or propantheline is administered parenterally prior to the procedure to reduce secretions and motility and minimize the risk of vagal reactions. Sedation should be adequate but minimal. Parenteral diazepam, phenobarbital, or meperidine (Demerol) alone or in various combinations has been used. The pharynx is usually anesthetized with a gargle of lidocaine viscous (2%) or anesthetic lozenges.

Examination following these preparations should disclose the precise lesion responsible for the bleeding in the majority of patients. In cases of torrential bleeding the lesion itself may be obscured by blood, and only the area involved can be stated with certainty. Conversely, bleeding may be slow enough to escape detection by conventional endoscopy. In the latter instances, examination using an ultraviolet light source immediately following the IV injection of fluorescin has been recommended.[38]

The most important complications of endoscopy are cardiorespiratory in nature, ranging from minor arrhythmias to apnea or cardiac arrest during the procedure. Rarely the instrument may perforate a viscus, most commonly the upper esophagus. An easily overlooked complication is pulmonary aspiration of gastric or oral secretions. One study[39] showed that variable quantities of radiopaque fluid introduced into the mouth during the examination were visible in the pulmonary tree on subsequent chest x-ray films in 25% of the patients. Fortunately none of these patients developed symptoms, but symptomatic aspiration has been reported.[40] The appearance of unexplained fever or respiratory symptoms following endoscopy should always suggest the possibility of this complication.

Selective or superselective arteriography should be considered in any case where endoscopy is contraindicated or fails to identify the site of bleeding.[41] The current disagreement concerning its diagnostic efficacy probably arises from its use in cases where the rate of bleeding is insufficient for visualization. In the experimental animal, blood loss of at least 0.5 ml/min, the equivalent of less than 1 L/24 hr in man, was necessary for arteriographic visualization. Many clinical investigators, however, believe that blood loss of less than 2 ml/min or approximately 3 L/24 hr will seldom be demonstrated arteriographically.[42] Obviously, quantitating blood loss precisely in the average clinical situation is impossible. In one study[42] arteriography successfully localized the bleeding point in 85% of the patients receiving 5 units or more of blood in the 24 hours prior to study and in 80% of those manifesting shock at any time prior to examination.

The major complications of arteriography are vascular difficulties, including thrombosis, hemorrhage, and perforation. These can be minimized by careful assessment of the patient's clotting status prior to the procedure and by examination of the peripheral pulse both before and at frequent intervals after the maneuver.

■ What about the diagnosis of lower gastrointestinal bleeding?

The lower gastrointestinal tract is obviously more difficult to prepare for study than the upper. For this reason barium contrast radiology is even more difficult to interpret, and the exact role, if any, of fiberoptic endoscopy (colonoscopy) remains undefined. With few exceptions, the initial procedure should be proctosigmoidoscopy. If the history suggests the possibility of inflammatory mucosal disease such as ulcerative colitis or amebiasis, this procedure should be performed with minimum or no preparation to avoid the production of mucosal artifacts by enemas. Anoscopy, using a slotted instrument, should always precede sigmoidoscopy. Occasionally large internal hemorrhoids are seen and suspected as the site of bleeding but are not bleeding at the time of examination. In such a case, suspicion may often be confirmed simply by repeating the examination after asking the patient to "bear down" forcefully. Sigmoidoscopy should be performed whether anoscopy is positive or not. If no source of bleeding is observed, the presence or absence of blood coming from beyond the furthest penetration of the instrument should be noted. If sigmoidoscopy is nondiagnostic in the face of continued bleeding at a rate judged sufficient to allow visualization, arteriography should be considered.[43] As in the case with upper gastrointestinal bleeding, arteriography is of questionable value if barium contrast studies have been performed in the previous 24 to 48 hours. However, since bleeding from diverticula is commonly noted to cease following a barium enema,[44] barium contrast studies probably have a greater place in lower rather than upper gastrointestinal bleeding.

■ Other than iced lavage, what nonsurgical methods can be used to control bleeding?

The lack of any single consistently effective treatment is attested to by the multiplicity of those recommended.[45] With few exceptions, studies of these treatments have been uncontrolled. Usually the effectiveness of a given treatment in the initial control of bleeding is promising. Quite often, however, the incidence of recurrent bleeding or the number of patients eventually requiring surgery or another form of treatment is not clearly reported. Because many of the reported methods are new, the incidence of complication remains undefined. Especially for those procedures requiring special skill, the reported incidences of complications may vary widely from institution to institution.

Nowhere are these problems more apparent than in the treatment of bleeding esophageal varices. An effective method for at least temporary control of variceal bleeding is the infusion of pitressin, 20 units in 100 ml of dextrose and water, over a period of 20 minutes. The mechanism of this treatment is a reduction in portal blood flow. In one study[46] bleeding was arrested in over half of the patients so treated as compared to none in a control group treated with placebo injections. In the same study the overall mortalities of the treated and control group were 93% and 80%, respectively. Esophageal tamponade in some form or another has been used since 1930, and yet controversy over its effectiveness and safety still rages. For example, the reported incidence of major complications resulting directly from the use of the Sengstaken-Blakemore tube ranges from 8.6%[47] to 35%.[48] Deaths *directly attributable* to the use of the tube occurred in from 5.7%[47] to 22%[48] of the patients in whom it was used. Yet esophageal tamponade will arrest bleeding initially in 50% to 80% of the cases.

The major complications of esophageal tamponade are rupture or erosion of the esophagus, occlusion of the airway by the balloon, or aspiration of secretions resulting from inadequate drainage of the occluded esophagus. Each of these complications can be minimized by meticulous attention to the details of the procedure and a healthy respect on the part of all involved personnel for its malignant potential. Either a Sengstaken-Blakemore or a Linton tube may be used.

The Linton tube has a single large (400 cc) gastric balloon that is inflated in the stomach and drawn back snugly against the cardioesophageal sphincter by traction on the tube proximally. Lumens for aspiration distal to the balloon in the stomach and proximally in the esophagus allow for continuous monitoring of bleeding and aspiration of pooled secretions in the esophagus.

The Sengstaken-Blakemore tube has two balloons. The distal or gastric balloon holds only 200 cc and is designed less for tamponade than for simply anchoring the tube in its proper position. If bleeding continues once it is anchored snugly in place at the cardioesophageal junction, control is usually achieved by inflation of the proximal or esophageal balloon (Fig. 43-2). The volume in the esophageal balloon is less important than the pressure, which is measured by connecting its inflow tube to a sphygmomanometer and maintained at the minimum required to control bleeding, *no more than 40 mm Hg.* As with the Linton tube, a lumen distal to the gastric balloon allows monitoring of stomach contents. Difficulty in aspirating this lumen in either tube may be caused by its entrapment under the gastric balloon and may be corrected by deflating the balloon and readjusting the tube prior to reinflation. The Sengstaken tube has no lumen for esophageal aspiration and a regular Levine-type tube *must be passed for this purpose.* This second tube may be tied to the Sengstaken tube just above the esophageal balloon using suture material, or it may be passed separately through the opposite nostril.

The effectiveness and overall complication rate of these two tubes is probably very similar. The Linton tube has the advantage of being somewhat simpler to use and exerts its primary effect at the area most commonly involved in variceal bleeding—the cardioesophageal junction. The extra lumen for esophageal aspiration is an added convenience. (Sengstaken tubes with esophageal lumens are available, but considerations of size limit this extra lumen to an impractically small diameter.) The major disadvantage of the Linton tube is its greater dependency on traction and, with it, a greater risk of erosion or pressure necrosis. The Sengstaken tube, on the other hand, carries a greater risk of respiratory complications such as airway occlusion or aspiration.

Whichever tube is used, it should be inserted

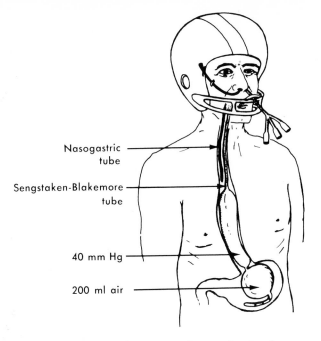

Nasogastric
tube

Sengstaken-Blakemore
tube

40 mm Hg

200 ml air

Fig. 43-2. Sengstaken-Blakemore tube in place. Both balloons inflated with nasogastric tube placed through external nares into position just above esophageal balloon.

by someone skilled in its use, preferably a gastroenterologist or surgeon. Each balloon should be tested by installing air prior to insertion. Smaller leaks can be detected by holding the balloon under water. To avoid the additional hazard of aspiration, topical anesthesia of the pharynx should be avoided when possible. The tube should be passed through the nose (preferably) or mouth *to its full length;* 50 to 100 cc of air instilled; and the balloon pulled up until the resistance of the cardioesophageal junction is encountered. The distance from mouth to cardioesophageal junction is amazingly constant from one individual to another, and if the tube is properly positioned, its 40 cm mark should be just visible at the patient's nose or mouth. At this point, unless bleeding is truly exigent, a plain x-ray film should be taken to assure proper positioning. The tube should then be advanced a few centimeters, the full quantity of air (200 cc for the Sengstaken, 400 cc for the Linton) instilled, and the balloon once again drawn snugly against the cardioesopha-

geal junction, gentle traction then being applied.

The use of orthopedic gravity traction, although popular, is to be deplored. Should continued bleeding occur despite adequate traction on the gastric balloon, the esophageal balloon of the Sengstaken tube should be inflated. Channels to the balloon should be double clamped with rubber-shod clamps to avoid inadvertent use during subsequent irrigation. The patient should be in an intensive care area with constant observation for signs of respiratory embarrassment. A pair of scissors should be kept in a clearly visible spot near the bedside so that the tube may be cut should this occur. In addition to continuous suction on the esophageal tube, pharyngeal and tracheal suction should be performed as frequently as possible.

Some experts leave the balloon tubes inflated for only a few hours after hemostasis is achieved; others leave them for 24 hours. The tubes should never be inflated continuously for more than 24 hours.

■ **What is the role of vasoconstrictor infusion in the treatment of gastrointestinal hemorrhage?**

The most commonly infused vasoconstrictor is the posterior pituitary hormone vasopressin (Pitressin), which reduces both mesenteric and portal blood flow when given either intravenously or intra-arterially.[49,50] Side-effects include abdominal cramps, diarrhea, hyponatremia, peripheral vasoconstriction, hypertension, decreased cardiac output, angina, and arrhythmias.[51] In hopes of minimizing some of these side-effects as well as enhancing the therapeutic effects, infusion directly into the arteries supplying the bleeding point has been recommended in the past. In the case of esophageal varices (which are veins, not arteries) the superior mesenteric artery, which contributes most to portal blood flow, was selected. However, both experimental[52,53] and more recently clinical evidence[54] suggest that, in the case of esophageal varices at least, continuous intravenous infusion is no less effective and causes no greater side-effects than intra-arterial administration. In fact, owing to the hazards of arterial catheterization, the complication rate was actually somewhat higher for intra-arterial infusion.[54] For these reasons, superior mesenteric artery infusion has been abandoned in favor of continuous intravenous infusion in the treatment of bleeding varices. Pending further investigation, intra-arterial administration continues to be favored for other sources of bleeding.

■ **Exactly how is vasopressin administered?**

Whichever route is chosen, a solution of 200 units of vasopressin in 500 ml of D5W is most commonly used. Using an Ivac unit, or better still a Harvard pump, this solution is infused at a maximum rate of 1 ml (or 0.4 units) per minute. In the case of intra-arterial infusion the major reported local complication has been infarction, often fatal, of infused areas of gut.[55] This complication can be minimized by repeating arteriography 20 to 30 minutes after the maximum rate of infusion is established to assess for angiographic evidence of ischemia. The only reported local complication of intravenous infusion is soft tissue necrosis (treated essentially like a third-degree burn) following subcutaneous infiltration

at the intravenous site.[56] A central venous line, when already present, is therefore preferred for intravenous infusion. If peripheral veins are fragile (as is often the case in older patients) or access tenuous and the central venous line is not already present, one should probably be established for this purpose. Even if the peripheral intravenous site appears secure and the vein nonfragile, it should never be obscured by dressings and good nursing care should include hourly checks for *any* signs of infiltration.

Since vasopressin exerts a strong antidiuretic hormone–like effect, varying degrees of hyponatremia may occur. The administration of hypotonic solutions should be avoided and serum sodium measured frequently. The effect of reduced hepatic blood flow in cirrhotic patients treated with vasopressin has not yet been determined.

■ **What is the best treatment for hemorrhagic gastritis?**

Hemorrhagic erosive gastritis poses a particular problem, since there is no completely satisfactory surgical approach should medical therapy fail. Fortunately bleeding will be arrested by iced lavage in nearly 90% of these patients. Several other methods have been reported to be successful in refractory gastric bleeding from gastritis or other causes. Bleeding was controlled in 23 of 25 patients treated with quantities of antacid sufficient to maintain gastric pH at 7.0 or above.[57,58] Given alone or in combination with antacid therapy the new H_2-receptor antagonists such as cimetidine may also be useful in the treatment[59] or prophylaxis[60] of gastrointestinal bleeding. Intragastric administration of 8 or 16 mg of levarterenol in 100 or 200 ml of saline solution temporarily controlled bleeding in 7 of 13[61] and 11 of 12[62] patients, respectively. Levarterenol, 8 to 16 mg in 500 ml or more of saline solution, has also been administered intraperitoneally[62] with varying success in both upper and lower gastrointestinal bleeding. This technique has even been extended to *continuous* intraperitoneal infusion of levarterenol.[63] More anecdotally, a "thrombin cocktail" (also known as "magic mud") consisting of several thousand units of topical thrombin and a cup of Gelfoam mixed with antacid or saline solution may be instilled into the stomach. Gastric hypothermia, or cooling of the stomach by a cold alcohol solution run through a special intragastric balloon, has fallen into disrepute but still has its proponents.[64] Even a treatment as exotic as daily injections of human growth hormone has been alleged to control bleeding.[65] Finally, intra-arterial vasopressin infusion has been used almost as successfully in gastritis as it has in more localized lesions.[66]

■ When should surgical intervention be considered?

Obviously the answer to this question will depend on the general condition of the patient as well as the etiology of bleeding and its potential for surgical correction. Reported mortality for emergency surgery in peptic ulcer disease ranges from 10% to 25% as opposed to 50% to 75% for variceal bleeding.[67] Prediction of mortality through "indices"[67,68] based on the presence or absence of various laboratory or clinical findings is of questionable value to the individual patient. In general a previous history of bleeding ulcer, recurrent bleeding during the current hospitalization, blood loss requiring 6 or more units of blood following the initiation of medical therapy, or continuous bleeding for 48 hours or more requiring 4 or more units of blood are all indications for surgical intervention in the duodenal ulcer patient. Criteria may be less strict for the patient with gastric ulcer, since many still consider surgery the treatment of choice for this condition whether bleeding is present or not. When considering surgery, it should be remembered that older patients or those with other conditions adding to surgical risk are also often those least likely to withstand the insult of unabated bleeding.

■ What new developments can be anticipated in the treatment of gastrointestinal bleeding?

With the increasing refinement of instruments a more definitive approach to specific lesions will become more and more feasible. Bleeding polyps have already been removed endoscopically from the upper gastrointestinal tract,[69] and endoscopic electrocoagulation has been used in the successful treatment of a variety of lesions.[70] Hemostasis has been achieved in the canine stomach using an endoscopically conducted laser beam, and human studies with this modality are projected in the near future.[71] In the field of arteriography, bleeding has been successfully controlled by embolization of the artery, supplying the bleeding site with the patient's own clotted blood.[72-74]

REFERENCES

1. Sleisinger, M., and Fordtran, J.: Gastrointestinal disease: pathophysiology, diagnosis and management, Philadelphia, 1973, W. B. Saunders Co.
2. U.C.L.A. Interdepartmental Conference: Diagnosis and management of gastrointestinal bleeding, Ann. Intern. Med. **71:**993, 1969.
3. Dagradi, A. E.: Management of gastrointestinal bleeding, Am. J. Gastroenterol. **46:**309, 1966.
4. Sedgwick, C. E., and Vernon, D. K.: Gastrointestinal bleeding: diagnosis and management, Surg. Clin. North Am. **48:** 523, 1968.
5. Malt, R.: Control of massive upper gastrointestinal hemorrhage, N. Engl. J. Med. **286:**1043, 1972.
6. Palmer, E.: Upper gastrointestinal hemorrhage, J.A.M.A. **231:**853, 1975.
7. Crook, I.: Upper gastrointestinal bleeding, Ann. Surg. **175:**771, 1972.
8. Myren, J., and Semb, L. S.: New trends in diagnosis and treatment of upper gastrointestinal bleeding, Scand. J. Gastroenterol. **5:**415, 1974.
9. Sedgwick, C. E., and Reale, V. F.: Upper gastrointestinal bleeding: diagnosis and treatment, Surg. Clin. North Am. **56:**695, 1976.
10. Dagradi, A., et al.: The Mallory-Weiss lesion: an endoscopic study of thirty cases, Gastrointest. Endosc. **13:**18, 1967.
11. Watts, H. D., and Adnurand, W. H.: Mallory-Weiss syndrome: a reappraisal, J.A.M.A. **230:**1674, 1974.
12. Moen, R., et al.: Rectal hemorrhage: moderate and severe, Ann. Surg. **155:**794, 1962.
13. Palmer, E.: The vigorous diagnostic approach to upper-gastrointestinal tract hemorrhage: a 23-year prospective study of 1400 patients, J.A.M.A. **207:**1477, 1969.
14. Holpern, M., Turner, A. F., and Citron, B. F.: Hereditary hemorrhagic telangiectasia, Radiology **90:**1143, 1968.
15. Bookman, L. B., and Simoneau, J. K.: The early assessment of hypovolemia: postural vital signs, J. Emergency Nurs. **3:**43, 1977.
16. Waterman, N. G., and Walker, J. L.: Effect of a topical adrenergic agent on gastric blood flow, Am. J. Surg. **127:** 241, 1974.
17. Stempien, S. T., and Dagradi, A. E.: A double lumen tube for gastroesophageal lavage, Gastrointest. Endosc. **13:**26, 1966.
18. Tielman, P. R., and Yanek, S. X.: New tube for the diagnosis and treatment of upper gastrointestinal hemorrhage, Am. J. Surg. **127:**771, 1974.
19. Bryant, L. R., et al.: Comparison of ice water with iced saline solution for gastric lavage in gastroduodenal hemorrhage, Am. J. Surg. **124:**570, 1972.

20. Blumbert, N., and Bove, J. R.: Un-cross-matched blood for emergency transfusion: one year's experience in a civilian setting, J.A.M.A. **240:**2057, 1978.
21. Moss, G.: An argument in favor of electrolyte solution for early resuscitation, Surg. Clin. North Am. **52:**3, 1972.
22. Gillon, J., et al.: A bioassay of treatment of hemorrhagic shock, Arch. Surg. **93:**537, 1966.
23. Weaver, D. W., et al.: Pulmonary effects of albumin resuscitation for severe hypovolemic shock, Arch. Surg. **113:**387, 1978.
24. Getzen, L. C., et al.: The effect of fluid infusions upon serum protein concentrations during hemorrhagic shock, Surg. Gynecol. Obstet. **146:**745, 1978.
25. Ratnoff, O.: Prothrombin complex preparation: a cautionary note, Ann. Intern. Med. **81:**852, 1974.
26. Lewis, M. D., et al.: Coagulation factor concentrates in the treatment of the hemorrhagic diathesis of fulminant hepatic failure, Gut **15:**993, 1974.
27. Hedberg, S. E.: Endoscopy in gastrointestinal bleeding: a systematic approach to diagnosis, Surg. Clin. North Am. **54:**549, 1974.
28. Allam, R. N., Dykes, B. W., and Toy, D. K.: Diagnostic accuracy of early radiology in acute gastrointestinal haemorrhage, Br. Med. J. **4:**281, 1972.
29. Dagradi, A. E., Skorneck, A. B., and Stempien, S. J.: The problem of diagnosis of esophageal varices: a radiologic and endoscopic study, Gastrointest. Endosc. **8:**2, 1961.
30. Cotton, P. B.: Fibreoptic endoscopy and the barium meal—results and implications, Br. Med. J. **2:**161, 1973.
31. Dagradi, A. E., Tan, D. J., and Stempien, S. J.: Sources of upper gastrointestinal bleeding in patients with liver cirrhosis and large esophagogastric varices, Am. J. Gastroenterol. **54:**458, 1970.
32. Waldran, R., et al.: Emergency endoscopy after gastrointestinal haemorrhage in 50 patients with portal hypertension, Br. Med. J. **4:**94, 1974.
33. Sandlow, L. J., et al.: A prospective randomized study of the management of upper gastrointestinal hemorrhage, Am. J. Gastroenterol. **61:**282, 1974.
34. Morrissey, J. F., and Winans, C. S.: The emergency endoscopy controversy, Dig. Dis. **22:**534, 1977.
35. Koton, R. M., and Smith, F. W.: Panendoscopy in the early diagnosis of acute upper gastrointestinal bleeding, Gastrenterology **65:**728, 1973.
36. Sugawa, C., et al.: Early endoscopy, Arch. Surg. **107:**133, 1973.
37. Forrest, J. A., Finlayson, N. D., and Shearman, D. J.: Endoscopy in gastrointestinal bleeding, Lancet **2:**394, 1974.
38. Smith, B. H., and Berk, J. E.: Ultraviolet endoscopy in the diagnosis of upper gastrointestinal bleeding, Am. J. Gastroenterol. **60:**549, 1973.
39. Prout, F. J., and Metreweli, C.: Pulmonary aspiration after fibre-endoscopy of the upper gastrointestinal tract, Br. Med. J. **4:**269, 1972.
40. Taylor, P. A., et al.: Pulmonary complications after oesophagogastroscopy using diazepam, Br. Med. J. **1:**666, 1972.
41. Athonasoulis, C. A., et al.: Angiography: its contribution to the emergency management of gastrointestinal hemorrhage, Radiol. Clin. North Am. **XIV:**265, 1976.
42. Stanley, R. J., and Wise, L.: Arteriography in diagnosis of acute gastrointestinal tract bleeding, Arch. Surg. **107:**138, 1973.
43. Casarella, W. J., et al.: Lower gastrointestinal tract hemorrhage: new concepts based on arteriography, Am. J. Roentgenol. Radium Ther. Nucl. Med. **121:**351, 1974.
44. Adams, J. T.: The barium enema as treatment for massive diverticular bleeding, Dis. Colon Rectum **17:**430, 1974.
45. Boyce, H. W.: Nonsurgical treatment for gastrointestinal hemorrhage, J.A.M.A. **231:**1065, 1975.
46. Merigar, T. C., Jr., Plotkin, G. R., and Davidson, C. S.: Effect of intravenously administered posterior pituitary extract on hemorrhage from bleeding esophageal varices, N. Engl. J. Med. **266:**134, 1962.
47. Bauer, J. L., Kreel, I., and Kark, A.: The use of the Sengstaken-Blakemore tube for immediate control of bleeding esophageal varices, Ann. Surg. **179:**273, 1974.
48. Conn, H. O., and Simpson, J. A.: Excessive mortality associated with balloon tamponade of bleeding varices, J.A.M.A. **202:**587, 1967.
49. Conn, H. O., et al.: Intraarterial vasopressin in the treatment of upper gastrointestinal hemorrhage: a prospective controlled clinical trial, Gastroenterology **68:**211, 1975.
50. Athanasoulis, C. A., et al.: Mesenteric arterial infusions of vasopressin for hemorrhage from colonic diverticulosis, Ann. Surg. **129:**212, 1975.
51. Serinek, K. R., and Thomford, N. R.: Isoproterenol in offsetting adverse effects of vasopressin in cirrhotic patients, Ann. Surg. **129:**130, 1975.
52. Barr, J. W., LaRin, R. C., and Rosch, J.: Similarity of arterial and intravenous vasopressin on portal and systemic hemodynamics, Gastroenterol. **69:**13, 1975.
53. Freedman, A. R., et al.: Primate mesenteric blood flow: effect of vasopressin and its route of delivery, Gastroenterol. **74:**875, 1978.
54. Johnson, W. C., et al.: Control of bleeding varices by vasopressin: a prospective randomized study, Ann. Surg. **186:**369, 1977.
55. Berardi, R. S.: Vascular complications of superior mesenteric artery infusion with pitressin in treatment of bleeding esophageal varices, Am. J. Surg. **127:**757, 1974.
56. Greenwald, R. A., et al.: Local gangrene: a complication of peripheral Pitressin therapy for bleeding esophageal varices, Gastroenterol. **74:**744, 1978.
57. Curtis, L. E., et al.: Evaluation of the effectiveness of controlled pH in management of massive upper gastrointestinal bleeding, Am. J. Surg. **125:**474, 1973.
58. Hastings, P. R., et al.: Antacid titration in the prevention of acute gastrointestinal bleeding, N. Engl. J. Med. **298:**1041, 1978.
59. Dykes, P. W., et al.: Treatment of upper gastrointestinal haemorrhage with cimetidine, Second International Symposium on H$_2$-receptor antagonists, Exerpta Med. 337-344, 1977.
60. Bailey, R. J., MacDougall, B. R. D., and Williams, R.: A controlled trial of H$_2$-receptor antagonists in prophyloxis of bleeding from gastrointestinal erosions in fulminant hepatic failure, Lancet **1:**617, 1977.
61. Kiselow, M. C., and Wagner, M.: Intragastric instillation of levarterenol, Arch. Surg. **107:**387, 1973.
62. Douglass, H. O.: Levarterenol irrigation: control of massive

gastrointestinal bleeding in poor-risk patients, J.A.M.A. **230:**1653, 1974.

63. Oliveira, G. G., et al.: Long-term intraperitoneal infusion of norepinephrine in the control of massive bleeding from stress ulcers, Crit. Care Med. **2:**262, 1974.

64. Sandlow, L. J., and Spellberg, M. A.: Gastric hypothermia for control of upper gastrointestinal bleeding, Am. J. Gastroenterol. **59:**307, 1973.

65. Winamer, S. T., et al.: Beneficial effect of human growth hormone on stress ulcers, Arch. Intern. Med. **135:**569, 1975.

66. Athanasoulis, C. A., et al.: Intrarterial posterior pituitary extract for acute gastric mucosal hemorrhage, N. Engl. J. Med. **290:**597, 1974.

67. Kim, U., et al.: Factors influencing mortality of surgical treatment for massive gastroduodenal hemorrhage, Am. J. Gastroenterol. **60:**24, 1974.

68. Wirthlein, L. S., et al.: Prediction of surgical mortality in patients with cirrhosis and nonvariceal gastroduodenal bleeding, Surg. Gynecol. Obstet. **139:**65, 1974.

69. Dagradi, A. E., Ruiz, R. A., and Alaama, A.: Endoscopic duodenal polypectomy, Am. J. Gastroenterol. **61:**379, 1974.

70. Papp, T.: Endoscopic electrocoagulation in upper gastrointestinal hemorrhage, J.A.M.A. **230:**1172, 1974.

71. Dwyer, R. M., et al.: Laser induced hemostasis in the canine stomach, J.A.M.A. **231:**486, 1975.

72. Rosch, J., Dotter, C. T., and Brown, M. J.: Selective arterial embolization: new method for control of acute gastrointestinal bleeding, Radiology **102:**303, 1972.

73. Seto, R., et al.: Management of diffuse hemorrhage from gastric mucosa pathophysiology and microcirculatory responses in diffuse gastric hemorrhage controlled by arterial embolization, Int. Surg. **59:**103, 1974.

74. Grace, D. M., Pitt, D. F., and Gold, R. E.: Vascular embolization and occlusion by angiographic techniques as an aid or alternative to operation: collective review, Surg. Gynecol. Obstet. **143:**469, 1976.

CHAPTER 44

Pancreatitis

Stephen R. Severance

■ Where is the pancreas located and what is its function?

The pancreas is an oblong organ 15 cm in length and weighing about 85 g. It is located in an area called the "retroperitoneal space," anterior to the spine but posterior to the stomach, colon, and small bowel, crossing the spine horizontally somewhere between the first and third lumbar vertebra. This relatively obscure location in close contiguity to such vital structures as the portal vein, inferior vena cava, splenic artery, and aorta makes difficult both diagnosis and treatment of pancreatic disorders. Pancreatic carcinoma, for instance, is almost invariably incurable by the time of discovery (Fig. 44-1).

The major biologic functions of the pancreas are classified as either *endocrine* or *exocrine*. The endocrine function, residing in specialized areas called the Islets of Langerhans, involves the production of the hormones insulin and glucagon, which are essential to the regulation of a number of vital metabolic processes, including maintenance of normal levels of the sugar glucose in the blood. Relative or absolute deficiency in this function results in the condition known as diabetes mellitus.

The exocrine function of the pancreas, occurring throughout the organ in glandular structures called acini, involves the production of a number of enzymes, including trypsin, chymotrypsin, lipase, amylase, phospholipase, elastase, and others,[1] all of which are involved in the digestion of various proteins, fats, and carbohydrates in the diet. Under ordinary circumstances these en-zymes are released from the acini into the ducts of the pancreas in inactive forms known as *zymogens* and remain in this inactive state until they have traveled through the main pancreatic duct into the small intestine. There, through the action of another enzyme known as enterokinase, they are converted to their potent active forms. Deficiency in the exocrine function of the pancreas is one of several causes of the condition known as steatorrhea, characterized by voluminous diarrhea and weight loss.

■ What is pancreatitis and what are its causes?

As the name implies, pancreatitis is a condition characterized by diffuse inflammation of the pancreas gland.[2-6] This condition has a number of causes, with their relative importance dependent largely on the incidence of alcoholism in the hospital studied. Overall, perhaps 40% of cases are the result of alcohol abuse, usually for a period of 3 or more years prior to the first attack. Another 40% or so will be associated with gallstones, very often being passed from the gallbladder into the intestines at the time of the attack.[7,8] The remaining 20% of cases have a variety of causes that are listed below.

Causes of pancreatitis

Alcohol
Biliary disease
Drugs
  Thiazides
  Furosemide (?)
  Sulfa drugs

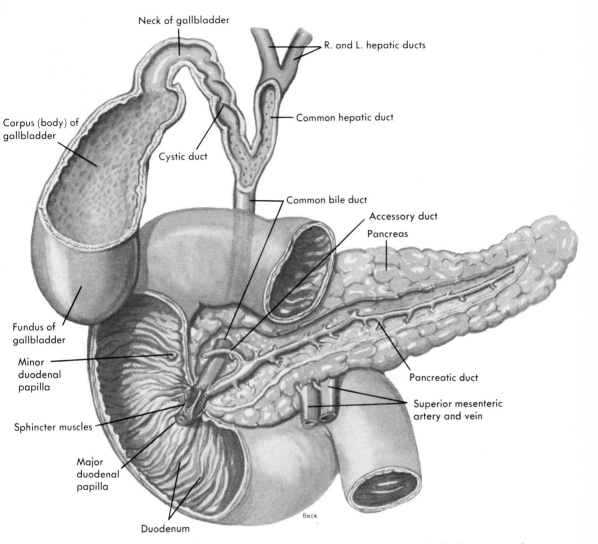

Neck of gallbladder

R. and L. hepatic ducts

Common hepatic duct

Corpus (body) of
gallbladder

Cystic duct

Common bile duct

Accessory duct

Pancreas

Fundus of
gallbladder

Minor
duodenal
papilla

Pancreatic duct

Sphincter muscles

Superior mesenteric
artery and vein

Major
duodenal
papilla

Duodenum

Beck

Fig. 44-1. The pancreas. (From Anthony, C. P., and Thibodeau, G. A.: Textbook of anatomy and physiology, ed. 10, St. Louis, 1979, The C. V. Mosby Co.)

Tetracycline
Corticosteroids
Oral contraceptives
Immunosuppressives
Antimetabolites
INH
Sulfasalazine
Methanol
Phenformin
Toxins

Scorpion bite
Anticholinesterases
Metabolic
  Hypercalcemia
  Hyperlipidemia
  Acidosis
  Hypothermia
  Pregnancy
  Hemochromatosis
Infectious

Mumps
Rubella
Coxsackievirus
Hepatitis
Mononucleosis
PPLO
Typhoid
Scarlet fever
Leptospirosis
Clonorchis
Ascaris
Mechanical
Trauma
Surgery
Duodenal disease
Electric shock
Vascular
Vasculitis
Atherosclerosis
Hereditary

■ **How do these diverse and seemingly unrelated precipitants cause pancreatitis?**

Common to all causes of pancreatitis is the activation of the potent digestive enzymes within the pancreas itself,[9] where they are normally in their inactive zymogen form. Theories abound, but the exact mechanism of this activation is not known for any of the common precipitants. The result of this premature activation has been referred to as "autodigestion." In about 90% to 95% of cases the predominant effect of this process is the production of hyperemia and edema, and the resultant clinical picture is referred to as *edematous pancreatitis*. Since repeated bouts of edematous pancreatitis may lead to either endocrine or exocrine insufficiency, scattered cell death must occur, but frank necrosis is not grossly apparent. In the remaining 5% to 10% of cases frank necrosis with hemorrhage predominates pathologically, and the resultant clinical picture is referred to as *hemorrhagic* or *necrotizing pancreatitis*. Since the mortality rate for edematous pancreatitis is 5% to 10%, as opposed to more than 50% for hemorrhagic pancreatitis, the early distinction between these two clinical forms is of more than academic significance.

■ **How then does one distinguish between hemorrhagic and edematous pancreatitis?**

The blood present in the retroperitoneal space of hemorrhagic cases may in a small percentage produce a blue "bruiselike" discoloration of the flanks. This has been referred to as "Turner's sign." A similar discoloration around the umbilicus, which may occur also in ruptured ectopic pregnancies, has been referred to as "Cullen's sign." While fluid rich in enzymes (that is, "pancreatic ascites") may occur within the peritoneal cavity in both hemorrhagic and edematous forms, aspiration will yield *blood-tinged* fluid only in the hemorrhagic form. Finally, *methemalbumin*, an end product of pancreatic enzymatic digestion of hemoglobin, appears in the blood of patients with hemorrhagic pancreatitis but is absent in those with edematous pancreatitis. This test[10] is helpful but not specific, since it also occurs with intravascular hemolysis from any cause as well as in other instances of intraperitoneal bleeding such as bowel infarction or ruptured ectopic pregnancy.

■ **What are the symptoms and signs of acute pancreatitis?**

The most consistent symptom of pancreatitis, present in nearly 100% of the patients, is abdominal pain. In about 50% of the patients the pain will be centered in the periumbilical or epigastric area, being described as "boring" in quality, radiating straight through to the back, and alleviated by leaning forward or even doubling or curling up. This description is not specific for pancreatitis but does suggest retroperitoneal pathology, occurring also, for instance, with retroperitoneal lymphoma. The remaining patients will have less specific pain patterns, some (about 5%) even complaining of pleuritic pain.

Other commonly observed symptoms include nausea and vomiting (92%), anorexia (83%), hematemesis (12%), fever and chills (12%), and abdominal swelling (4%).[2]

On physical examination tachycardia is quite common, reflecting hypovolemia, pain, or both. Surprisingly, systemic hypertension, possibly related to vasoactive substance released into the blood, is common, occurring in 40% to 90% of the cases. Hypotension is less common and suggests a less favorable prognosis. As in cases of gastrointestinal hemorrhage, patients should be tested for postural changes in vital signs. Ten to twenty percent of patients will have a temperature of more than 101°, which does not necessarily signal infection. Abdominal tenderness is present in almost all patients and may be accompanied by rigidity and guarding. Bowel sounds will be absent in 50% of the patients. Indeed, abdominal examination in more severe cases may yield findings indistinguishable from acute surgical emergencies such as bowel infarction or perforated ulcer. These conditions together with acute cholecystitis, leaking abdominal aneurysm, ruptured ectopic pregnancy, and perforated diverticulum must always be considered in the differential diagnosis. Signs of ascites may occur in 10% to 20% of the cases.

■ How does one establish the diagnosis of pancreatitis?

Under ordinary circumstances small quantities of each of the enzymes elaborated by the pancreas are detectable in the serum. In the research laboratory, assays have demonstrated increased serum levels of almost all of these enzymes, often in the active form, during bouts of acute pancreatitis. However, only the assays for serum amylase and lipase have provided reproducibility and practicality sufficient to gain widespread clinical use. According to one study of patients with acute pancreatitis,[11] *admission* serum amylase was elevated in 70%, admission lipase in 63%, admission levels of one or both in 83%, with *serial* assays indicating elevation of at least one of these enzymes at least once in almost all cases. This same study failed to confirm earlier suggestions that lipase rose later than amylase, instead revealing a more or less simultaneous rise. Interestingly the degree of elevation of these enzymes does not correlate well with the severity of the disease. Indeed, one study[12] suggested a more or less *inverse* correlation. While these two serum assays used simultaneously and serially thus have a high degree of *sensitivity*, their *specificity* is less easy to establish. The pancreas is anatomically inaccessible enough that only laparotomy or autopsy can confirm the validity of any test, and neither of these occurs often in milder cases (where a specific test is most desirable). Of the two enzymes, amylase has been most widely studied.[12-13] This enzyme is found not only in the pancreas but also in the salivary glands, small bowel, fallopian tubes, and probably in the lung. Elevated serum levels may occur in disorders of all of these organs. Salivary amylase is the most common cause of confusion, and as many as 50% of elevations in alcoholics may originate from the salivary glands.[14] Special assays can distinguish salivary from pancreatic amylase,[15] but these are not generally available to the clinician. Amylase entering the serum from any of these organs is excreted in the urine, so that renal disease may also produce elevations. A summary of the disorders associated with an elevation of serum amylase may be found in the outline below. In addition to these specific causes, an occasional chronic and consistent elevation of serum amylase will defy explanation.[16-18]

Causes of hyperamylasemia and/or hyperamylasuria*

A. Pancreatic disease
1. Pancreatitis
   a. Acute
      (1) Common causes (alcoholism, gallbladder disease, and so on)
      (2) Uncommon (vasculitis, uremia, and so on)
      (3) Drug-induced
      (4) Viral
         (a) Hepatitis
         (b) Other
      (5) Postendoscopy
      (6) Postoperative
      (7) Renal transplantation
   b. Chronic
   c. Complications
      (1) Pseudocyst
      (2) Ascites
      (3) Abscess
2. Pancreatic carcinoma
3. Pancreatic trauma
B. Disorders of nonpancreatic origin (mechanism known)
1. Renal insufficiency
2. Salivary-type hyperamylasemia
3. "Tumor" hyperamylasemia
4. Salivary gland lesions
   a. Mumps
   b. Calculus
   c. Irradiation sialadenitis
   d. Maxillofacial surgery
   e. Drugs
5. Macroamylasemia
C. Disorders of complex origin (mechanism unknown or uncertain)

*From Salt, W. B., II, and Schenker, S.: Medicine **55**(4):269, 1976. Copyright © 1976, The Williams & Wilkins Co.

1. Biliary tract disease
2. Intra-abdominal diseases other than pancreatitis
   a. Perforated peptic ulcer
   b. Intestinal obstruction
   c. Ruptured ectopic pregnancy
   d. Mesenteric infarction
   e. Afferent loop syndrome
   f. Aortic aneurysm with dissection
   g. Peritonitis
   h. Acute appendicitis
3. Cerebral trauma
4. Burns and traumatic shock
5. Postoperative hyperamylasemia
6. Diabetic ketoacidosis
7. Renal transplantation
8. Pneumonia
9. Acquired bisalbuminemia
10. Prostatic disease
11. Pregnancy
12. Drugs

Possibly because of a defect in tubular reabsorption of the enzyme, amylase is excreted more rapidly into the urine during an attack of acute pancreatitis.[19] This as yet unexplained phenomenon has led to the measurement of urinary amylase as a test for acute pancreatitis.[20] Urinary excretion can be expressed (in order of increasing sensitivity and specificity) as simple concentration (units per milliliter), as a function of time (units per 2 hours), or as a ratio of amylase clearance to creatinine clearance. Elevated urinary amylase was once felt to be highly specific for acute pancreatitis,[20] but this specificity has recently been challenged,[21,22] and elevations have also been described in severe burns, diabetic ketoacidosis, severe renal failure, and following open-heart surgery. Nevertheless its measurement remains useful in certain situations. It rises earlier and falls later than serum levels in acute pancreatitis, so it should be ordered when pancreatitis is strongly suspected and serum levels return within normal range. Hyperlipemia, which causes pancreatitis in a small number of cases and which occurs as a secondary phenomenon in 10% to 20% of cases,[23-26] may cause falsely normal depression of the serum amylase[27] but less frequently (if at all) affects urine levels. (This interference may also be circumvented by diluting the serum.[28]) In recurrent or chronic cases of pancreatitis, not infrequently *only* the urine amylase will be abnormal, and in rare cases even this may remain normal, with only nonspecific indicators such as the white blood count or erythrocyte sedimentation rate to suggest the presence of pancreatic inflammation.

■ **What other tests should be included in the initial evaluation of the patient with suspected pancreatitis?**

Laboratory tests should include serum methemalbumin, calcium, electrolytes, BUN, creatinine, glucose, CBC, urinalysis, and liver profile with prothrombin time. In cases of obscure etiology lipids should also be measured. If elevated, repeat levels during a later asymptomatic interval will be necessary to determine whether this elevation was secondary or actually causative. Abdominal x-ray films, although seldom specific, will be abnormal in the majority of cases[29,30] and will help to exclude such worrisome possibilities as perforated peptic ulcer or bowel infarction. Chest x-ray films should be included. In severe cases and in all older patients electrocardiography should be done. Arterial blood gases should be done in severe cases also.

■ **How is acute pancreatitis treated?**

All but mild cases of acute pancreatitis should be managed in an intensive care area. Aprotinin (Trasylol),[31] a trypsin inhibitor, and glucagon, a physiologic inhibitor of pancreatic secretion,[32] have been used in Europe with equivocal[33] success. Except for these no therapy specific for the inflammatory process itself has been suggested, and conventional treatment is directed instead at the *results* of this inflammation. The overwhelming majority of early deaths result from irreversible shock, so that early and adequate fluid replacement is essential.[34] The potent pancreatic enzymes produce the equivalent of a retroperitoneal "burn" with sequestration or "third-spacing" of large volumes of nearly isotonic, alkaline fluid rich in protein. Thus in severely ill hypotensive patients an average of 6 L of crystalloid (Ringer's lactate or saline) and colloid (Plasmanate, and so on) solution was infused during the first 24 hours.[34] In older patients or in severe cases of any age, a central venous catheter or Swan-Ganz catheter is essential to successful management of fluids. Female patients have compared the pain of pancreatitis unfavorably to the pain of childbirth, so that analgesia is also essential to early therapy. Unfortunately, all effective analgesics including morphine, meperidine, and pentazocine cause marked elevations in biliary pressures,[35] a theoretical disadvantage usually outweighed by the severity of the pain. However, since a single narcotic injection in a normal human volunteer may produce as much as a tenfold elevation in serum levels of pancreatic enzymes,[36] diagnostic confusion may be avoided by withholding analgesia at least long enough to obtain initial laboratory tests. The main physiologic stimuli to pancreatic secretion are dietary fats and protein plus gastric acid. With the theoretical rationale of putting the pancreas "at rest" the patient with pancreatitis is made NPO, and gastric acid is removed by nasogastric suction. Like a great many medical concepts that have historically "made great sense," the latter treatment, at least, has failed the acid test of scientific scrutiny. Controlled clinical studies[37] have now demonstrated that the only statistically significant effect of nasogastric suction in pancreatitis is to increase the duration of ileus. Since these studies included a large proportion of mild to moderate cases, omission of nasogastric suction is probably justifiable in less severe cases (unless inordinate nausea and vomiting are present). Pending more specific studies, we still use it in more severe cases. If nasogastric suction is not employed, frequent antacid administration makes sense. Use of an H_2-receptor antagonist such as cimetidine would also seem logical, but this drug worsens experimental pancreatitis in animals,[38,39] and preliminary human clinical studies suggest that it prolongs the elevation of serum amylase.[40] We therefore reserve its use for those patients (20%) with gastrointestinal bleeding or concomitant peptic ulcer. Anticholinergic drugs are favored by some, but these, too, have recently failed the test of scientific scrutiny.[41]

Finally, while most early deaths result from hypovolemic shock, late mortality is invariably the result of extrapancreatic effects, with prominent causes of death including septicemia, gastrointestinal hemorrhage, and pulmonary or renal failure.[42] Diagnostic and therapeutic "tunnel vision" should therefore be avoided, with meticulous attention being directed to these other organ systems from the very outset. Careful monitoring of urine output and, when appropriate, central venous or pulmonary pressures, vigorous pulmonary toilet, prophylactic antacids, and compulsive vigilance for signs of infection are all essential to successful management. Malnutrition probably contributes significantly to mortality, and parenteral or "enteral" hyperalimentation should be considered early in complicated cases.[43]

■ What about pancreatic pseudocysts and abscesses?

At the risk of oversimplifying, a pancreatic pseudocyst might be described as a large "blister" arising from the pancreas during an attack of pancreatitis.[44] It is a free collection of pancreatic juice and enzymes that dissects along "the path of least resistance," most often into an area behind the stomach known as "the lesser sac" and less commonly extending to areas as improbable as the groin or the mediastinum.[45,46] The term "pseudo" is both appropriate and of therapeutic significance, since this collection initially has no well-defined wall or boundary of its own, being limited only by the resistance of surrounding structures. Over a period variously estimated as several days to 6 weeks, the inflammatory response elicited by its potent enzymes produces a well-defined fibrous capsule, and the cyst is said to be "mature."

Depending on how they are defined and how carefully they are sought, the reported incidence of pseudocyst formation in acute pancreatitis has ranged from 8% to 50%.[47,48] Its presence should be suspected in any patient with unusually prolonged symptoms, protracted serum or urine enzyme elevation, or both. A palpable abdominal mass will be present in about 50% of pseudocysts, and 75% will produce suggestive compression of the stomach or small bowel on upper gastrointestinal contrast studies. They are most accurately and economically diagnosed by abdominal ultrasound with the incidence of false negative and false positive examinations each being in the range of 5% to 10%.[47] Those few missed by ultrasound, usually located in the tail of the pancreas, are detectable by abdominal computed tomography, which should be ordered only if sonography is negative and suspicion is high. Sophisticated studies such as endoscopic retrograde pancreatography have been recommended[49] but are rarely necessary and may be hazardous.

There are four common complications of pseudocyst formation: (1) rupture, which may be catastrophic or more chronic ("pancreatic ascites"), (2) hemorrhage, (3) infection, and (4) mechanical effects—bile duct obstruction with jaundice, gastric outlet or bowel obstruction, splenic infarct, portal vein compression with variceal hemorrhage, and so forth. Such complications are reported to occur eventually in only one third or less of cysts, but the reported mortality of these complications (25% to 50%) is sufficient to favor treatment of all persistent pseudocysts. While the necessity for such treatment is widely accepted, both the timing and nature of this treatment are the subject of much discussion.[50-53] To begin with, the natural course of these cysts has not been clearly defined. For instance, the reported incidence of spontaneous resolution of these cysts ranges from 8% to 85%.[48,54] The exact true incidence will probably be soon defined by more prospective sonographic studies, but what is important is that in some as yet undefined proportion of patients spontaneous resolution is uncontestably possible. Most agree that when spontaneous resolution does occur it will be apparent within the first 2 to 3 weeks. This, in itself, would seem to make some delay in surgical therapy desirable. Even more important, early surgical intervention is felt by most to be accompanied by a prohibitive risk. In one study[55] the mortality for surgery performed before 6 weeks was 60% compared to a perioperative mortality of only 9% when surgery was delayed until after 6 weeks. (As in many uncontrolled surgical series, one must ask *why* the patients in the first group required early surgery in order to properly interpret this data.) This inordinate risk for early surgery is probably related to the "maturation" process of the cyst.

As to the nature of surgery performed, some form of "internal" drainage is probably prefer-able—most often drainage into the stomach ("cystgastrostomy") or jejunum ("cystjejunostomy"). The exception is the infected cyst that should be drained externally and generously.

The incidence of pancreatic abscess[56-60] in acute pancreatitis is 2% to 4%. Infection may be primary, arising in necrotic pancreatic tissue; secondary, arising in a pseudocyst; or on occasion may be introduced by surgery. As one would expect, enteric bacteria predominate, with multiple organisms found in 50% of the cases. This is a serious condition with reported mortality rates as high as 50%. Unfortunately four prospective controlled studies[61-64] have failed to show benefit from prophylactic antibiotics (although these studies all utilized ampicillin, which may not be the most logical choice of antibiotic given the flora most commonly involved). Diagnosis is problematic. Since pancreatitis is an inflammatory condition, both fever and leukocytosis are to be expected and do not always herald infection. In most (but not all) uncomplicated cases these parameters normalize within a few days. The "classical" abscess patient may actually improve initially, with recurrence of fever and leukocytosis in the second or third week signalling infection. Thus either persistence of fever and leukocytosis beyond the first few days or their recurrence at a later time should prompt frequent blood cultures, chest x-ray examination, and daily abdominal x-ray examinations. Twenty-five percent of abscesses will cause diagnostic extraluminal "soapsuds" (a dyshomogeneous collection of gas, liquid, and solid) on abdominal flat plate. Sometimes diagnosis may be made by abdominal ultrasound, but in our experience the admittedly much more expensive computed tomographic (CT) scan is more reliable in this instance. In severe cases of pancreatitis even this examination may reveal simply an amorphous retroperitoneal mass, failing to distinguish between abscess and sterile "phlegmon" owing to enzymatic digestion. Gallium citrate scanning has been used successfully,[65] but false positive examinations may occur with severe pancreatic inflammation, so that results must be interpreted in the context of other clinical tests. Each clinician has a different "threshold" of anxiety for the introduction of "empirical" antibiotic therapy, but this may be moot, since this is basically a surgical disease. In fact, 30% of those surviving initial surgery will require a second surgery for residual infection.

■ What are the other complications of acute pancreatitis?

The other complications of acute pancreatitis are numerous,[66] affecting virtually every major organ system in the body. They may be classified both as *early* or *late* and as *local* or *distant*. Limitations of space preclude individual discussion of each of these complications, which are outlined with appropriate references below.

Complications of pancreatitis

I. Early or acute
  A. Local
    1. Jaundice—rarely cholangitis[67-70]
    2. Pseudocyst
    3. Abscess
    4. Splenic vein thrombosis[71]
    5. Portal vein thrombosis
    6. Bowel obstruction[72]
    7. Gastric outlet obstruction[73]
    8. Gastrointestinal bleeding[74]
  B. Nonlocal
    1. Cardiovascular
      a. Systemic hypertension[75]
      b. Electrocardiographic abnormalities[76,77]
    2. Neurologic
      a. Organic mental syndrome ("pancreatic encephalopathy")[78]
    3. Renal
      a. Acute renal failure[79]
    4. Hematologic
      a. Disseminated intravascular coagulation[80]
      b. Hypercoagulability[81]
    5. Metabolic
      a. Hypocalcemia[82-90]
      b. Hypomagnesemia
      c. Hyperlipemia[23-26]
    6. Dermatologic
      a. Subcutaneous nodules[91-94]
    7. Musculoskeletal
      a. Arthritis[95,96]
      b. Aseptic necrosis[97]
      c. Bone lesions[98]
    8. Pulmonary[99,100]
      a. Pulmonary hypertension[100]
      b. Atelectasis
      c. Pleural effusion[101] (more often left-sided)
      d. Pneumonia
      e. Pulmonary embolus
      f. Adult respiratory distress syndrome ("shock lung")[102-104]
II. Late or chronic[105]
  A. Chronic pancreatitis
  B. Pancreatic calcification
  C. Diabetes mellitus (endocrine insufficiency)
  D. Steatorrhea (exocrine insufficiency)[106]
  E. Hypercoagulability[81]
  F. Aseptic necrosis
  G. Bone lesions

One or two do deserve mention, since they represent pitfalls in therapy. Surprisingly, in a condition characterized by volume depletion, both systolic and diastolic hypertension are reported to occur during the course of acute pancreatitis in 80% of the cases. It is probably related to enzyme-induced release of vasoactive kinins. Moderate elevations are probably not deleterious. Treatment at worst may be harmful and even at best may confuse volume replacement by distorting a useful parameter.

Hypocalcemia is a common event, occurring to some degree in two thirds of the patients. Mild depression in many may be factitious, being associated with hypoalbuminemia and normal levels of *ionized* (biologically active) calcium. Depression in others may be both profound and resistant to therapy, a finding associated with poorer outcome and increased mortality. Several mechanisms have been suggested to explain the fall: (1) The digestion of retroperitoneal fat by the pancreatic enzyme lipase precipitates large quantities of calcium in the form of soaps. (2) Levels of parathyroid hormone may be low or, if "normal," inappropriate for the degree of hypocalcemia. (3) Glucagon released from the pancreas may stimulate release of thyrocalcitonin from the thyroid gland. (4) Lowered serum magnesium, common in pancreatitis, is known to depress release of calcium from the bone. Each or all of these may be operative in any given case, but in clinical practice only the last can be easily treated. Serum magnesium may be measured or, in absence of renal failure, 2 ml of 50% magnesium sulfate may be given IV or IM every 6 to 8 hours for the first few days. It should be remembered that calcium is a cofactor in the activation of trypsin.

Therefore, if it is to be administered at all in the absence of clinical signs of hypocalcemia, it should be given with caution.

Unless the cause of acute pancreatitis is removed, most patients will have recurrent bouts of acute pancreatitis and eventually develop calcifications in the pancreas, exocrine insufficiency (steatorrhea), or endocrine insufficiency (diabetes). The alcoholic patient with a history of 10 or more years of alcohol abuse will manifest an average of two of these, while a history of 20 years or more of alcohol abuse in the patient with pancreatitis is usually associated with all three.[105]

■ Outside of the treatment of pseudocyst or abscess, what is the role of surgery in acute pancreatitis?

There have been some animal studies,[107] occasional anecdotal case reports,[108] and a few uncontrolled clinical series,[109-111] but this important question has not been subjected to controlled human studies. Any benefit in edematous pancreatitis would seem unlikely, but in the case of hemorrhagic or necrotizing pancreatitis, where medical therapy has proved so unsatisfactory, its use makes theoretical sense. Certainly this is the only intra-abdominal condition in which the presence of necrotic or devitalized tissue is commonly tolerated without almost automatic surgical extirpation. Controlled studies are urgently needed. Unfortunately in the absence of such studies the present tendency is to employ surgery as a "last resort," while animal studies[107] suggest beneficial results only *early* in the disease. Peritoneal lavage is a promising and somewhat less drastic modality that also deserves further study.[112]

■ What about follow-up care in these patients?

The causative agent should be eliminated when at all possible. In the case of gallstones this implies surgery, which should be done as early as feasible, since the incidence of recurrent attacks is high.[113] Some formal program of alcoholic rehabilitation, often overlooked, should be encouraged when indicated. The gallbladder should be studied at least once in every patient.[114] Since gallstones and alcoholism each afflict 10% of the population, a history of alcohol abuse does not obviate this need. Gallbladder visualization by oral cholecystography may be impaired by pancreatitis itself,[114,115] but recent prospective studies[116,117] reveal a normal incidence of visualization if the study is deferred until oral feeding is resumed.

Patients should arbitrarily be kept on a low-fat diet for 6 to 8 weeks after discharge and much longer in selected cases.

REFERENCES

1. Hadorn, B.: Pancreatic proteinases. Their activation and the disturbances of this mechanism in man, Med. Clin. North Am. **58**(6):1319, 1974.
2. Olsen, H.: Pancreatitis. A prospective clinical evaluation of 100 cases and review of the literature, Dig. Dis. **19**(12):1077, 1974.
3. Geokas, M. C.: Acute pancreatitis, Calif. Med. **117**:25, 1972.
4. Geokas, M. C.: Acute pancreatitis, Ann. Intern. Med. **76**: 105, 1972.
5. Carey, L. C.: Acute and chronic pancreatitis, Surg. Clin. North Am. **55**:(2):325, 1975.
6. Acosta, J. M., and Ledesma, C. L.: Gallstone migration as a cause of acute pancreatitis, N. Engl. J. Med. **290**: 484, 1974.
7. Acosta, J. M., Rossi, R., and Ledesma, C. L.: The usefulness of stool screening for diagnosing cholelithiasis in acute pancreatitis. A description of the technique, Dig. Dis. **22**(2):168, 1977.
8. Tuzhilin, S.: The clinical features of pancreatic inflammation, Am. J. Gastroenterol. **61**(2):97, 1974.
9. Geokas, M. C., and Rinderknecht, H.: Free proteolytic enzymes in pancreatic juice of patients with acute pancreatitis, Dig. Dis. **19**(7):591, 1974.
10. Geokas, M. C., et al.: Methemalbumin and acute pancreatitis, Ann. Intern. Med. **81**:483, 1974.
11. Lifton, L. J., et al.: Pancreatitis and lipase. A reevaluation with a five-minute turbidimetric lipase determination, J.A.M.A. **229**:47, 1974.
12. Adams, J. T., Libertino, J. A., and Schwartz, S. I.: Significance of an elevated serum amylase, Surgery **63**:877, 1968.
13. Salt, W. B., II, and Schenker, S.: Amylase—its clinical significance: a review of the literature, Medicine **55**(4): 269, 1976.
14. Berk, E. J., Fridhandler, L., and Webb, S. F.: Does hyperamylasemia in the drunken alcoholic signify pancreatitis? Am. J. Gastroenterol. **71**(6):557, 1979.
15. Berk, E. J.: New dimensions in the laboratory diagnosis of pancreatic disease, Am. J. Gastroenterol. **69**(4):417, 1978.
16. Berk, E. J., et al.: Macroamylasemia: serum and urine amylase characteristics, Am. J. Gastroenterol. **53**:223, 1970.
17. Warshaw, M. D., and Lee, K. H.: Macroamylasemia and other chronic nonspecific hyperamylasemias: chemical oddities or clinical entities? Am. J. Surgery **135**:488, 1978.

18. Jam, I., et al.: Elevated serum amylase activity in the absence of clinical pancreatic or salivary gland disease, Am. J. Gastroenterol. **70**:480, 1978.

19. Johnson, S. G., Ellis, C. J., and Levitt, M. D.: Mechanism of increased renal clearance of amylase/creatinine in acute pancreatitis, N. Engl. J. Med. **295**(22):1212, 1976.

20. Warshaw, A. L., and Fuller, A. F., Jr.: Specificity of increased renal clearance of amylase in diagnosis of acute pancreatitis, N. Engl. J. Med. **292**(7):325, 1975.

21. Bindrich, D., Dürr, H. K. D., and Bode, J. C.: Amylase/creatinine clearance ratio of little diagnostic value in macroamylasemia and acute pancreatitis, Scand. J. Gastroenterol. **12**:701, 1977.

22. Levitt, M. D., and Johnson, S. G.: Clinical trends and topics. Is the ^{C}am/^{C}cr ratio of value for the diagnosis of pancreatitis? Gastroenterology **75**:118, 1978.

23. Cameron, J. L.: Lipid abnormalities and acute pancreatitis, Hosp. Prac. **12**(4):95, 1977.

24. Farmer, R. G., et al.: Hyperlipoproteinemia and pancreatitis, Am. J. Med. **54**:161, 1973.

25. Greenberger, N. J.: Pancreatitis and hyperlipemia, N. Engl. J. Med. **289**:586, 1973.

26. Cameron, J. L., et al.: Acute pancreatitis with hyperlipemia. Evidence for a persistent defect in lipid metabolism, Am. J. Med. **56**:482, 1974.

27. Fallat, R. W., Vester, J. W., and Glueck, C. J.: Suppression of amylase activity by hypertriglyceridemia, J.A.M.A. **225**:1331, 1973.

28. Lesser, P. B., and Warshaw, A. L.: Diagnosis of pancreatitis masked by hyperlipemia, Ann. Intern. Med. **82**:795, 1975.

29. Stein, G. N., et al.: An evaluation of the roentgen changes in acute pancreatitis: correlation with clinical findings, Gastroenterol. **36**:352, 1959.

30. Moreno, G., and Rivera, H. H.: Evaluation of the gastrocolic space in 100 cases of acute pancreatitis, Radiology **118**:535, 1976.

31. Trapnell, J., et al.: A controlled trial of Trasylol in the treatment of acute pancreatitis, Br. J. Surg. **61**:177, 1974.

32. Knight, M. J., Condon, J. R., and Smith, R.: Preliminary communications. Possible use of glucagon in the treatment of pancreatitis, Br. Med. J. **2**:440, 1971.

33. Editorial: Death from acute pancreatitis, Lancet **2**:632, 1977.

34. Facey, L. F., Weil, M. H., and Rosoff, L.: Mechanism and treatment of shock associated with acute pancreatitis, Am. J. Surg. **111**:374, 1966.

35. Greenstein, A. J., Kaynan, A., Singer, A., and Dreiling, D. A.: A comparative study of pentazocine and meperidine on the biliary passage pressure, Am. J. Gastroenterol. **58**:417, 1972.

36. Bogoch, A., Roth, J. L. A., and Bockus, H. L.: The effects of morphine on serum amylase and lipase, Gastroenterol. **26**(5):697, 1954.

37. Levant, J. A., et al.: Naogastric suction in the treatment of alcoholic pancreatitis, J.A.M.A. **229**(1):51, 1974.

38. Hadas, N., et al.: Cimetidine in pancreatitis, N. Engl. J. Med. **299**(9):487, 1978.

39. Hadas, N., Wapnick, S., Grosberg, S. J., and Sugaar, S.: Cimetidine induced mortality in experimental pancreatitis, Gastroenterology **76**(5):1148, 1979.

40. Meshkinpour, H. M. D., et al.: Cimetidine in the treatment of acute alcoholic pancreatitis: a randomized, double blind study, Gastroenterology **76**(5):1201, 1979.

41. Cameron, J. L., Mehigan, D., and Zuidema, G. D.: Evaluation of atropine in acute pancreatitis, Surg. Gynecol. Obstet. **148**:208, 1979.

42. Storck, G., Pettersson, G., and Edlund, Y.: A study of autopsies upon 116 patients with acute pancreatitis, Surg. Gynecol. Obstet. **143**:241, 1976.

43. Blackburn, G. L., et al.: New approaches to the management of severe acute pancreatitis, Am. J. Surg. **131**:114, 1976.

44. Winship, D., and Trenbeath, M.: Clinical gastroenterology conference. Pancreatitis: pancreatic pseudocysts and their complications, Gastroenterology **73**:593, 1977.

45. Christensen, N. M., Demling, R., and Mathewson, C., Jr.: Unusual manifestations of pancreatic pseudocysts and their surgical management, Am. J. Surgery **130**:199, 1975.

46. Edell, S. L., and Good, L. I.: Mediastinal pancreatic pseudocyst, Am. J. Gastroenterol. **71**:78, 1979.

47. Gonzalez, A. C., Bradley, E. L., and Clements, J. L., Jr.: Pseudocyst formation in acute pancreatitis: ultrasonographic evaluation of 99 cases, Am. J. Roentgenol. **127**:315, 1976.

48. Sankaran, S., and Walt, J.: The natural and unnatural history of pancreatic pseudocysts, Br. J. Surg. **62**:37, 1975.

49. Andersen, B. N., et al.: The diagnosis of pancreatic cyst by endoscopic retrograde pancreatography and ultrasonic scanning, Ann. Surg. **185**(3):286, 1977.

50. Bradley, E. L., III, and Clements, L. J.: Spontaneous resolution of pancreatic pseudocysts. Implications of timing of operative intervention, Am. J. Surg. **129**:23, 1975.

51. Pollak, E. W., Michas, C. A., and Wolfman, E. F., Jr.: Pancreatic pseudocyst management in fifty-four patients, Am. J. Surg. **135**:199, 1978.

52. Ravelo, H. R., and Aldrete, J. S.: Analysis of forty-five patients with pseudocysts of the pancreas treated surgically, Surg. Gynecol. Obstet. **148**:735, 1979.

53. Elechi, E. N., Callender, C. O., Leffall, L. D., Jr., and Kurtz, L. H.: The treatment of pancreatic pseudocysts by external drainage, Surg. Gynecol. Obstet. **148**:707, 1979.

54. Czajan, A. T., Fisher, M., and Marion, G. A.: Spontaneous resolution of pancreatic masses (pseudocysts?) aggravating after acute alcoholic pancreatitis, Arch. Intern. Med. **135**:558, 1975.

55. Carilli, J., and Faris, T. D.: Pancreatic pseudocysts: delayed versus immediate treatment, Surgery **61**:541, 1967.

56. Camer, S. J., Tan Eric, G. C., Warren, K. W., and Braasch, J. W.: Pancreatic abscess. A critical analysis of 113 cases, Am. J. Surg. **129**:426, 1975.

57. Holden, J. L., Berne, T. V., and Rosoff, L.: Pancreatic abscess following acute pancreatitis, Arch. Surg. **111**:858, 1976.

58. Ranson, J., and Spencer, F. C.: Prevention, diagnosis, and treatment of pancreatic abscess, Surgery **82**(1):99, 1977.

59. Owens, B. J., III, and Hamit, H. F.: Pancreatic abscess and pseudocyst, Arch. Surg. **112**:42, 1977.

60. Paloyan, D., Simonowitz, D., and Bates, R. J.: Guidelines in the management of patients with pancreatic abscess, Am. J. Gastroenterol. **69**:97, 1978.

61. Trapnell, J.: The natural history and prognosis of acute pancreatitis, Ann. R. Coll. Surg. Engl. **38**:265, 1966.

62. Howes, R., Zuidema, G., and Cameron, J. L.: Evaluation of prophylactic antibiotics in acute pancreatitis, J. Surg. Res. **18**:197, 1975.

63. Craig, R. M., Raidal, E., and Myles, L.: The use of ampicillin in acute pancreatitis, Ann. Intern. Med. **83**:831, 1975.

64. Fuich, W. T., Sawyers, J. L., and Schenker, S.: A prospective study to determine the efficacy of antibiotics in acute pancreatitis, Ann. Surg. **183**:667, 1976.

65. Kennedy, T. D., Morten, N. L., Robinson, R. G., and Preston, D. F.: Identification of and infected pseudocysts of pancreas with 67-Ga-Cetratin. Case report, J. Nucl. Med. **16**:1132, 1975.

66. Lukash, W. M.: Complications of acute pancreatitis. Unusual sequelae in 100 cases, Arch. Surg. **94**:848, 1967.

67. Snape, W. J., Jr., et al.: Liver physiology and disease marked alkaline phosphatase elevation with partial common bile duct obstruction due to calcific pancreatitis, Gastroenterology **70**:70, 1976.

68. Warshaw, A. L., et al.: Persistent obstructive jaundice, cholangitis, and biliary cirrhosis due to common bile duct stenosis in chronic pancreatitis, Gastroenterology **70**:562, 1967.

69. Schulte, W., et al.: Chronic pancreatitis: a cause of biliary structure, Surgery **82**(3):303, 1977.

70. Gremillion, D. E., Jr., et al.: Biliary obstruction a complication of chronic pancreatitis diagnosed by endoscopic retrograde cholangiopancreatography (ECRP), Dig. Dis. Sci. **24**(2):145, 1979.

71. Hastings, O. M., et al.: Intrasplenic pancreatic pseudocyst complicating severe acute pancreatitis, Am. J. Gastroenterol. **69**:182, 1978.

72. Grodsinsky, C., and Ponka, J. L.: The spectrum of colonic involvement in pancreatitis, Dis. Colon Rectum **21**(1):66, 1978.

73. Rheingold, O. J., Walker, J. A., and Barkin, J. S.: Gastric outlet obstruction due to a pancreatic pseudocyst, Am. J. Gastroenterol. **69**:92, 1978.

74. Bank, S., Marks, I. N., Kiywm, J. H., and Farman, J.: Peptic ulceration and gastrointestinal bleeding in pancreatitis, Gut **8**:253, 1967.

75. Sankaran, S., Lucas, C. E., and Walt, A. J.: Transient hypertension with acute pancreatitis, Surg. Gynecol. Obstet. **138**:235, 1974.

76. Pollock, A. V., and Bertrand, C. A.: Electrocardiographic changes in acute pancreatitis, Surgery **40**(5):951, 1956.

77. Fulton, M. C., and Marriott, H. J. L.: Acute pancreatitis simulating myocardial infarction in the electrocardiogram, Ann. Intern. Med. **59**(4):730, 1963.

78. Johnson, D. A., and Tong, T.: Pancreatic encephalopathy, South. Med. J. **70**(2):165, 1977.

79. Goldstein, D. A., Llach, F., and Massry, S. G.: Acute renal failure in patients with acute pancreatitis, Arch. Intern. Med. **136**:1363, 1976.

80. Greipp, P. R., Brown, J. A., and Gralnick, H. R.: Defibrillation in acute pancreatitis, Ann. Intern. Med. **76**:73, 1972.

81. Tuzhilin, S. A., and Dreiling, D. A.: Cardiovascular lesions in pancreatitis, Am. J. Gastroenterol. **63**:381, 1975.

82. D'Souza, A., and Floch, M. H.: Calcium metabolism in pancreatic disease, Am. J. Clin. Nutr. **26**:352, 1973.

83. Peoples, J. B., Webster, M. W., Jr., and Carey, L. C.: Mechanisms of hypocalcemia in acute hemorrhagic pancreatitis, Surg. Gynecol. Obstet. **141**:724, 1976.

84. Condon, J. R., Ives, D. Knight, M. J., and Day, J.: The aetiology of hypocalcaemia in acute pancreatitis, Br. J. Surg. **62**:115, 1975.

85. Norberg, H. P., DeRoos, J., and Kaplan, E. L.: Increased parathyroid hormone secretion and hypocalcemia in experimental pancreatitis: necessity for an intact thyroid gland, Surgery **77**(6):773, 1975.

86. Weir, G. C., et al.: The hypocalcemia of acute pancreatitis, Ann. Intern. Med. **83**:185, 1975.

87. Canale, D. D., and Donabedian, R. K.: Hypercalcitoninemia in acute pancreatitis, Clin. Endocrinol. Metab. **40**:738, 1975.

88. Peoples, J., Eberlein, T., and Webster, M. W.: Prevention of hypocalcemia by administration of homologous plasma during experimental hemorrhagic pancreatitis in the pig, Am. J. Surg. **133**:42, 1977.

89. Sowa, M., Appert, H. E., and Howard, J. M.: The hypocalcemia activity of pancreatic tissue homogenate in the dog, Surg. Gynecol. Obstet. **144**:365, 1977.

90. Robertson, G. M., Jr., et al.: Inadequate parathyroid response in acute pancreatitis, N. Engl. J. Med. **294**(10):512, 1976.

91. Bennett, R. G., and Petrozzi, J. W.: Nodular subcutaneous fat necrosis. A manifestation of silent pancreatitis, Arch. Dermatol. **111**:896, 1975.

92. Forstrom, L., and Winkelmann, R. K.: Acute, generalized panniculitis with amylase and lipase in skin, Arch. Dermatol. **111**:497, 1975.

93. Hughes, P., Apisarnthanarax, P., and Mullins, J. F.: Subcutaneous fat necrosis associated with pancreatic disease, Arch. Dermatol. **111**:506, 1975.

94. Bennett, R. G., and Petrozzi, J. W.: Nodular subcutaneous fat necrosis: a manifestation of silent pancreatitis, Arch. Dermatol. **111**:896, 1975.

95. Tannenbaum, H., Anderson, L. G., and Schur, P. H.: Association of polyarthritis, subcutaneous nodules, and pancreatic disease, J. Rheumatol. **2**:1, 1975.

96. Gibson, T. J., et al.: Arthropathy, skin and bone lesions in pancreatic disease, J. Rheumatol. **2**:1, 1975.

97. Achord, J. L., and Gerle, R. D.: Bone lesions in pancreatitis, Am. J. Dig. Dis. **11**(6):453, 1966.

98. Bank, S., et al.: Case reports: further observations on calcified medullary bone lesions in chronic pancreatitis, Gastroenterology **51**(2):224, 1966.

99. McWilliams, H., and Gross, R.: Pancreatitis and the lungs, Am. Surg. **40**:448, 1974.

100. Halmagyi, D., et al.: Pulmonary hypertension in acute hemorrhagic pancreatitis, Surgery **76**(4):637, 1974.

101. Light, R., and Ball, W. C., Jr.: Glucose and amylase in pleural effusions, J.A.M.A. **225**(3):257, 1973.

102. Hayes, M. F., Jr., et al.: Adult respiratory distress syndrome in association with acute pancreatitis. Evaluation of

positive end expiratory pressure ventilation and pharmacologic doses of steroids, Am. J. Surg. **127**:314, 1974.

103. Rovner, A. J., and Westcott, J. L.: Pulmonary edema and respiratory insufficiency in acute pancreatitis, Radiology **118**:513, 1976.
104. Troyer, A. D., et al.: Impairment of pulmonary function in acute pancreatitis, Chest **73**:3, 1978.
105. DiMagno, E. P., Malagelada, J. R., and Go, V. L. W.: Relationship between alcoholism and pancreatic insufficiency, Ann. N. Y. Acad. Sci. **252**:200, 1975.
106. Arvantitakis, C., and Cooke, A. R.: Diagnostic tests of exocrine pancreatic function and disease, Gastroenterology **74**:932, 1978.
107. Henry, L. G., and Condon, R. E.: Ablative surgery for necrotizing pancreatitis, Am. J. Surg. **131**:125, 1976.
108. Dritsas, K. G.: Near total pancreatectomy in the treatment of acute hemorrhagic pancreatitis, Am. Surg. **42**:44, 1976.
109. Lawson, D. W., et al.: Surgical treatment of acute necrotizing pancreatitis, Surgery **172**:605, 1970.
110. Jonsell, G., and Boutelier, P.: Observations during treatment of acute necrotizing pancreatitis with surgical ablation, Surg. Gynecol. Obstet. **148**:385, 1979.
111. Grana, W., and Wise, L.: Role of emergency laparotomy in acute pancreatitis, Am. J. Surg. **42**(2):128, 1976.
112. Ranson, J. H. and Spencer, F. C.: The role of peritoneal lavage in severe acute pancreatitis, Ann. Surg. **187**:565, 1978.

113. Paloyan, D., Samonowitz, D., and Skinner, D. B.: The timing of biliary tract operations in patients with pancreatitis associated with gallstones, Surg. Gynecol. Obstet. **141**:737, 1975.
114. Burrell, M. I., et al.: Diagnostic imaging procedures in acute pancreatitis. Comparison of ultrasound, intravenous cholangiography, and oral cholecystography, J.A.M.A. **242**(4):342, 1979.
115. Palogan, D., and Samonowitz, D.: Diagnostic considerations in acute alcoholic and gallstones pancreatitis, Am. J. Surg. **132**:329, 1976.
116. Roller, R. J., et al.: Oral cholecystography after alcoholic pancreatitis, Gastroenterology **73**:218, 1977.
117. Roller, R. J., et al.: Oral cholecystography in acute pancreatitis, Gastroenterology **74**:964, 1978.

BIBLIOGRAPHY

Cameron, J. L.: Clinical trends and topics of chronic pancreatic ascites and pancreatic pleural effusions, Gastroenterol. **74**:134, 1978.
Cochran, J. W.: Pancreatic pseudocyst presenting as massive hemothorax, Am. J. Gastroenterol. **69**(1):84, 1978.
Kaye, M. D.: Pleurapulmonary complications of pancreatitis, Thorax **23**:297, 1968.
Mann, S. K., and Mann, N. S.: Pancreatic ascites, Am. J. Gastroenterol. **71**:186, 1979.

CHAPTER 45

Instrument safety

Paul E. Stanley

All of recorded history indicates that man has been interested in the health of his neighbor and has always been ready to suggest favorite remedies for whatever the illness might be. One of the earliest of the recorded rules and regulations concerning the health of the individual as well as the health of the public is to be found in the early books of the Bible, the so-called Mosaic Law, which was written about 1500 BC.

Some instrumentation was developed over the years, but it remained for men of the 20th century to bring forth modern medical devices. Referring to the results of developments, Dr. John D. Porterfield III, director of the Joint Commission on Accreditation of Hospitals, recently remarked that "the patient has somehow learned to expect the difficult to be routine, the impossible to be frequent, and the miraculous to be something only slightly less than frequent."[1] These changes are the result of the application of engineering and technology to health care and medical problems.

■ Have engineering and technology made contributions to health care services?

As early as 1747 Benjamin Franklin observed that electricity passing through a muscle caused it to "convulse."[2] A few years later Fontana of Bologna discovered that electricity was involved in the functioning of the heart. It was in 1887 that Waller displayed the electrical activity of the heart,[3] but it was not until 1912 that Einthoven was able to produce a useful ECG.[4] Electronic medical devices were introduced late in World War II, and the computer is now in operation in many hospitals. In 1969 about $25 million was spent on cardiac monitoring devices. In 1975 the figure was in the neighborhood of $75 million, with the total medical instrumentation sales approaching $1.6 billion[5] (Fig. 45-1).

Tiny transistorized radios, miniaturized computers, instant-on color television sets, and microwave ovens are constant reminders of the contributions of electrical technology to the quality of our everyday lives. Similarly, the care of the ill has been aided by technologic advances that are the result of the application of engineering and technology to the problems of the diagnosis and treatment of diseases. Probably the effect has been more prominent in the care of critically ill patients than anywhere else. Cardiac monitors, cardiac pacemakers, respirators, and even automatic blood gas analysis instruments are but a few of the many devices now used in the critical care areas of the modern hospital.

While technologic advances provide assurance that critically ill patients will receive every possible assistance in their efforts to return to health, they also contribute problems.

■ Has engineering affected nursing?

To a very great extent the responsibility for the safe use of medical instrumentation and equipment falls on the attending critical care technician. Often a specialist in the operation of the ECG may be dispatched from the hospital's central services to connect a machine to a patient and take an ECG recording. The staff in the critical

800

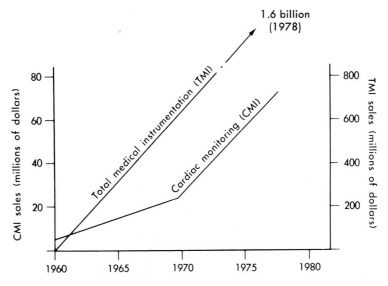

Fig. 45-1. Electronic medical device sales. *CMI*, cardiac monitoring instrumentation; *TMI*, total medical instrumentation.

care unit will have training along similar lines.

But it is especially important for critical care practitioners to be aware of the technical changes that have occurred and are occurring. They should be informed not only of the medical implications of such developments, but of the safety factors involved. In addition, the development of new electromedical devices is so rapid that a continuing program of learning is needed. This chapter has been prepared as a partial step in this education.

■ **How does instrumentation introduce problems?**

In the home, problems arising from failure of one of the multitude of appliances are usually no more than nuisances. However, in a hospital critical care unit, device failure can bring discomfort, injury, or even death to the patient. These hazards are many but can be brought together in two general classes: instrument effectiveness and instrument system safety. It is therefore apparent that everyone in anyway associated with critical care should be well informed of the hazards as well as the benefits of the vast array of instruments and devices in current use.

■ **What does the term "instrument effectiveness" mean?**

Instrument effectiveness can be said to be simply that the data obtained from the meter readings are accurate and truly indicate what the practitioner who ordered the use of the instrument wanted. A precise reading of the oxygen content of the blood (Po_2) is of no value if the desired information is the pH. Nor is a precise value of an average of the systolic and diastolic pressures of importance when the peak values of both are desired for the diagnosis of the condition. Whether or not a device does what it is intended to do may be described as its effectiveness.

■ **What are some examples of ineffectiveness?**

In the *Report of the Inter-Society Commission for Heart Disease Resources* (1971) it is pointed out that all models of one brand of defibrillator failed to deliver the energy indicated.[6] In a recent test program four defibrillators of identical make and model delivered from 55% to 93% of the indicated or stored energy, while another delivered 444 watt-seconds when set at the 400 watt-second level.[17]

If a patient should receive 400 watt-seconds (joules) of defibrillation energy, he may fail to respond to 55% of 400 (or 220) watt-seconds received from a faulty defibrillator. The result may be death—death caused by an ineffective device.

A similar condition has been known to exist in pacemakers in that the figures on the dial have been found to not correspond to the current delivered by the device. In numerous instances "noise" or artifacts on the screen of a cardiac monitor obscure the ECG, thus making the monitor ineffective.

Such failure of instruments to perform effectively may be caused by poor design, poor maintenance, or improper use of the device. Because of the importance of continued effective and safe operation, both the engineers and the technicians acquainted with the design, manufacture, and care of the devices are needed in hospitals to ensure that the medical devices used anywhere, and especially in critical care areas, perform their functions effectively and safely.

■ What is meant by the term "instrument safety"?

Although effective instrument or apparatus operation is of the utmost importance and a part of safety, no other hazards must ensue from the use of the equipment. The patient must not suffer electric shock, burns, undue pain, or other trauma caused by any part of the electromedical system in operation. This safety must extend to the operator and other personnel as well as to the patient.

The hazards from the unsafe operation or use of devices are many. Since most of the devices are electrically operated, electric shock is usually the hazard considered most likely to occur. It is important, but electric devices may start fires or ignite explosive gas mixtures, or they may not function properly when there is "too little" electricity, that is, when the voltage is lowered, as during a "brown out." Many situations may occur that require engineering analysis for solution, and for that reason these will not be treated here. Since the analysis of the electric shock hazard is quite straightforward, it will be examined rather fully.

■ What is an electric current?

It is not the purpose of this chapter to discuss the whole of the science and engineering of electricity. One text dealing with the basics of electricity is given in the references.[8] However, a few of the principles can be expressed very briefly.

There are two requisites for the flow of an electric current: (1) a voltage source and (2) a closed circuit that includes the voltage source.

The character of the voltage source is determined in part by the potential difference between its two poles. For the dry cell flashlight battery this is 1.5 volts; the voltage of an x-ray unit will be in the thousands or even hundreds of thousands of volts.

Also of importance in the voltage source character is its frequency. A *direct* current source is one that "pushes" continually in one direction. The unit of current is the ampere. It may be said to be at 0 frequency as compared with an *alternating* current source, having a frequency greater than 0, most commonly, 60 cycles per second, or 60 hertz (Hz). The usual household supply and that of the hospital room is a 120 V, 60 Hz alternating current.

The character of the circuit is a bit more complicated and must be described in terms of three kinds of elements: resistance, inductance, and capacitance. These combine into an overall characteristic called impedance. For simplicity we shall use resistance only and will represent it by R. The unit of resistance is the ohm. Current is represented by I (Fig. 45-2) and voltage by V. The relationship between these quantities is known as Ohm's law and is as follows:

$$I = \frac{V}{R}$$

The circuit may be closed by any conductor, including the human body; in the latter case electric shock hazards occur.

Resistances (or impedances) may occur at many places in the circuit, and all must be taken into account in evaluating the possible hazards. One resistance component exists within the voltage source itself. For example, a 1.5 V No. 6 dry cell will generate a current of more than 30 amperes through an ammeter, which is essentially a

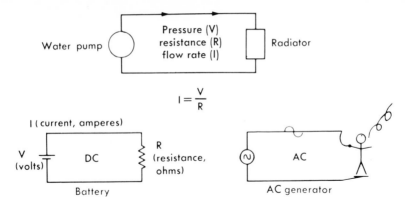

$$I = \frac{V}{R}$$

Fig. 45-2. Schematics of electric circuits.

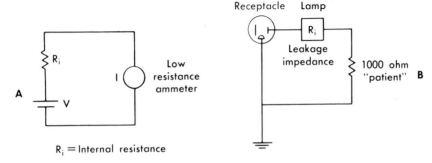

R_i = Internal resistance

Fig. 45-3. A, Internal resistance and internal impedance. **B,** Leakage impedance.

short circuit; that is, it has zero resistance. This means that the resistance of the cell is:

$$R_1 = \frac{1.5}{30} = 0.05 \text{ ohm}$$

On the other hand, an AA size 1.5 V dry cell will generate less than 3 amperes. This means its resistance is:

$$R_1 = \frac{1.5}{3} = 0.5 \text{ ohm}$$

Fig. 45-3 illustrates a voltage source caused by "leakage" of an alternating current lamp. It has a voltage of 120 V, yet it will generate less than 1 microampere of current through a 1000 ohm "patient." By Ohm's law this means that the internal leakage resistance is 120 megohms (120 million ohms). This is so high that it will cause a volt-meter to read incorrectly, showing only 80 V or even less.

Body resistance

It is to be noted that a "patient" was indicated as having a resistance of 1000 ohms. A precise value is very difficult to specify. With the use of needle electrodes and low voltage direct current, measurements seem to indicate that the minimum body resistance may range from 100 to 1000 ohms, depending on the distance between the electrodes. A conservative value of 1000 ohms should be used in most calculations, especially when one of the electrodes may be a cardiac catheter.[9]

Skin resistance is a function of the thickness of the callous skin on the surface, the amount of other dead tissue, the oiliness of the surface, and the amount of moisture in the skin. For dry, cal-loused hands the skin resistance may be as high as 500,000 ohms or more. After scrubbing with soap and thorough soaking in water, the same hand skin may drop to a resistance of 500 to 1000 ohms or less. Similar low resistances may occur when the skin is cleansed with alcohol and cov-ered with an electrode paste or lotion before at-taching an ECG electrode, for example. Thus it is apparent that the body resistance, including skin, may be quite low, and that a value of 1000 ohms is a safe and conservative assumption for skin-to-skin-to-electrode resistance (Fig. 45-4).

The effect of frequency on the current flow in the human body and its physiologic reaction is simulated by paralleling the 1000 ohms with an-other resistor and a capacitor (Fig. 45-5).

■ What is electric shock?

Benjamin Franklin's analysis of the "convul-sion" of the muscle caused by the flow of elec-tricity through it has been alluded to. This is elec-tric shock. In itself this electrical contraction of the muscles, if brief and not too violent, does little if any harm. Some pain may be felt and the ex-perience is frightening, but little else. However,

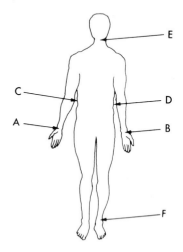

Fig. 45-6. Macrocurrent shock. Current flows between points on surface of body, for example, *A* to *F*.

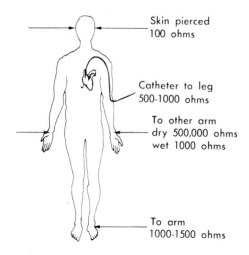

Fig. 45-4. Typical body resistance.

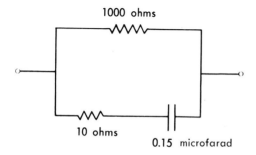

Fig. 45-5. The "patient" simulator.

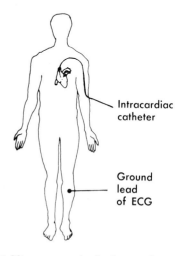

Fig. 45-7. Microcurrent shock. Current flows directly to heart through catheter to ECG ground lead.

the conditions under which the shock occurs may result in other phenomena that are serious.

Two general categories of electric shock are recognized: (1) the macrocurrent or gross shock situation, wherein a current passes through the body of the subject and (2) the microcurrent shock, wherein a current passes directly through the heart wall from a conductor in the heart (Figs. 45-6 and 45-7).

■ What are macrocurrent shock hazards?

The macrocurrent shock may be considered as a stimulus causing an involuntary reaction (Fig. 45-8). Almost everyone jumps at the slightest shock. The threshold of sensitivity varies greatly with individuals, but for some persons currents as small as ½ milliampere (ma) will be unpleasant and may cause a reaction. Such convulsive reactions have led to fatal falls, and it does not take much imagination to conceive of situations in the hospital wherein a reaction to shock could have serious consequences. Therefore it is included here as one of the several lethal effects of the electric current.

Dalziel conducted numerous experiments to determine perception and "let-go" currents.[10] Continued investigations have shown that for man the average current for which the subject can just let go is about 16 ma. For children and those debilitated by disease, the let-go level may be 4 ma or less. If the current is only slightly larger than this value, the muscle "freezes" and the subject is unable to move the part of the body through which the current flows. The sensation is very painful, and if for no other reason than

fright, there appears to be an almost complete paralysis of the body. Obviously if the current flow is through the chest muscles, respiration stops and the subject will undergo asphyxiation in a few minutes. If the circuit is broken in time, rsepiration will spontaneously begin again.

However, there is one form of respiratory arrest that may persist after the current ceases to flow. Called permanent respiratory arrest, it results when the current flows through the medulla of the brain where the respiratory control is centered. This means that the current must flow through the head and neck to some point on the body. Very little data exist concerning the magnitude of current that will cause this phenomenon, but it is probable that a current of a few milliamperes will be hazardous. Larger currents may cause permanent and often fatal damage to the nervous system.

Artificial respiration is the most obvious treatment for the person who has suffered permanent respiratory arrest. Here more than in any other circumstance prolonged respiratory assistance may result in recovery, even after several hours of seemingly useless effort.

Burns of electrical origin constitute a considerable hazard. Low frequency currents may produce deep burns that can lead to the loss of a limb or even to death. These are most likely to occur when the person comes in contact with a high voltage source, because quite large currents are required. However, electrical burn injuries do occur in the hospital because of the high frequency currents used in cautery and surgical procedures.

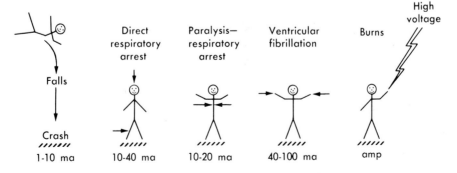

Fig. 45-8. Possible effects of gross or macrocurrent shock.

By far the largest portion of electrical deaths occur as a result of ventricular fibrillation.

■ How much voltage is dangerous?

A question often asked is, How much voltage is required to cause death or serious injury? The answer comes from the application of Ohm's law to the data just given on current and resistance. If the circuit through which the current passes runs from a cardiac catheter in the heart to a well-applied ground electrode on the right leg, the resistance can be seen to be of the order of 1000 ohms. If a current in excess of 50 microamperes is considered to be hazardous, 50 mv from a low impedance source would be a lethal voltage. On the other hand, for the calloused 500,000 ohm hands a voltage of 100 V would cause a very small current to flow and probably no harm would result. Of course when the voltage is several hundred volts, other effects such as burns occur; these are not to be considered here.

Since the hand-to-hand resistance may be as low as 1000 ohms and if 10 ma or so may cause sudden involuntary muscular reactions that could lead to a fall or other undesirable results, a potential difference of approximately 10 V could be considered hazardous.

■ How does electric shock cause ventricular fibrillation?

The heart consists of a large number of muscle cells that possess the properties of excitability, contractibility, and conductivity. Briefly, these arise from the electrolytic makeup of the cells, which results in a potential difference of some 90 mv between the inside and outside of the cell across the membrane that makes up the cell wall. An electrical stimulus (or even a mechanical or chemical stimulus) will cause a flow of ions across the cell wall, giving rise to the conductivity aspect, and will cause a contraction. The flow of ions is a current whose effect is observed on the body surface as one phase of the ECG. The current flow changes the potential difference across the cell wall and puts the cell in a "depolarized" state for a fraction of a second, after which it slowly repolarizes again.

In the right atrium of the heart there is a small mass of special tissue called the sinoatrial node that serves as a pacemaker for the heart. It has

the property of self-excitation, so that about 70 times/min it sends out an electrical pulse that causes the muscles of the atria to contract in a wavelike manner. The result of this contraction forces the blood from the atria into the ventricles. When this wave reaches the group of cells known as the atrioventricular node, the accompanying electric currents trigger the node, causing it to send out a signal through highly conducive lines called the bundle of His and the Purkinje fibers to all parts of the ventricle muscles, causing them to contract and drive the blood out into the arteries.

The P wave of the ECG is the sum of the contraction and associated current flow of the atrial muscles of the heart. The QRS complex comes from the contraction of the ventricles, whereas the T wave is the repolarization of these muscles.

For a short time after a cell has been excited and contracts it is incapable of responding to further excitation. This is true of the ventricular muscles just after the QRS complex has been generated. However, soon after, in the S-T interval, some cells will be repolarizing, so that if an external stimulus is applied just about the time of the T wave, another contraction of the ventricles will occur. Such an action is called premature ventricular contraction (PVC). If the stimulus is a small 60 Hz current applied at this sensitive time, a series of PVC's may result. Often the frequency of occurrence of the PVC will increase, and the heart action degenerates into ventricular fibrillation. This is a state of random quivering of the heart muscle with no pumping action; hence unless the condition is corrected soon, death results.

If a flow of electric current occurs through the body, a small portion of it will pass through the heart and may cause the heart to fibrillate. This is the condition referred to as "macrocurrent shock" or macroshock because the magnitude of current required to produce harmful results is of the order of a thousand times larger than the hazardous current level when there is a direct electrical connection to the heart muscle.

Because the mechanism of death from electric shock was not understood, especially when ventricular fibrillation appeared to have been induced, King at Columbia University undertook to conduct a systematized study of the problem.[11] During a 6-year period over a thousand animals, ranging in size from rabbits to calves and sheep, were subjected to carefully controlled electric shocks. Anesthetized animals were used, and starting with a small current, repeated shocks of increasing strength were applied until ventricular fibrillation resulted. The investigation resulted in a wealth of data, but only limited conclusions were drawn. Among them was the observation that once fibrillation was induced in a heart, it seldom, if ever, spontaneously reverted to normal action. Furthermore, the heart was found to be most sensitive if it was shocked between the termination of the T wave and the beginning of the QRS complex. Few conclusions were drawn as to the magnitude of current that would induce fibrillation. However, this work as extended by others in association with King remained the landmark in this area for some 20 years. Kouwenhoven and his associates at Johns Hopkins University, using more sophisticated measuring devices, carried on an investigation somewhat similar to King's, but with the objective of determining the minimum fibrillating current as an additional parameter.[12]

Dalziel at the University of California at Berkeley, as already noted, conducted a study of the magnitude of the just perceptible and the maximum let-go currents and developed a statistical technique for analyzing the results. He applied this technique to the King data and deduced from it a threshold fibrillating current for man that incorporated the concept that it was dependent on the weight of the man. Later, using Kouwenhoven data, Dalziel proposed the following equation:

$$I = \frac{K}{\sqrt{T}}$$

where I is the current in milliamperes, T is the time in seconds, and K is a constant (approximately 100 ma/sec$^{1/2}$). This leads to the conclusion that 100 ma flowing for 1 second from arm to arm in an adult will probably induce ventricular fibrillation.[13]

In some cases it appears that cardiac arrest occurs when large currents flow through the chest. This situation probably would require the current to flow for some minutes so that death occurs as a result of the cessation of circulation. There is some probability that, if the current flow is for just a second or so, the heart rhythm might start spontaneously after the current flow stops, somewhat in the manner observed after defibrillation.

Until relatively recent times, these macroshock situations were the only electric shock hazards against which care had to be taken.

■ **What is microshock?**

When an electrical conductor connects directly to the heart wall, all of the current flowing in it will pass through the heart. The current required to cause fibrillation will be quite small, measured in millionths of amperes, or microamperes. This condition is called microshock, in contrast to macroshock, wherein the current is measured in thousandths of amperes, or milliamperes.

In 1962 Weinberg and associates published a report of studies of electric shock hazards in cardiac catheterization, concluding that currents as low as 35 microamperes could produce ventricular fibrillation in the dog when the current passed through the heart wall.[14] Other studies indicate that a current as low as 12 microamperes at 60 Hz has been known to produce fibrillation in the canine ventricle. One case is reported in which 180 microamperes produced fibrillation in a human being. More recently the evidence is that usually larger heart currents are required to produce fibrillation in human beings. However, in the interest of safety a value of 10 to 20 microamperes is considered to be the maximum safe current through the heart wall (Fig. 45-9).

■ **How serious is the electric shock hazard?**

There have been many articles about the hazards of electricity in hospitals and the number of fatalities that result. Most of them have no basis in fact. Although there are no hard data available, the number of fatalities caused by electric shock in hospitals is probably less than 10 annually. But even one is too many, because most, if not all, such accidents can be eliminated. The methods are relatively simple and will be discussed later.

■ **Where do the hazards originate?**

First, most electrical energy in the United States is provided by means of a two- (or three-) wire system in which one (or two) of the wires may be at or near ground potential and the other

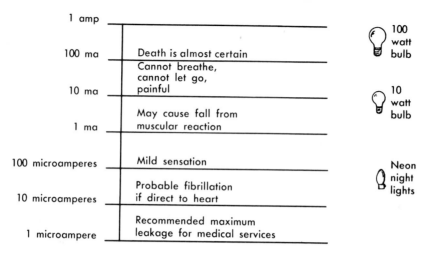

Fig. 45-9. Electric current shock hazard. NOTE: This is an approximation. Many other factors affect the result.

(the live conductor) at the line voltage—nominally 120 V. A current will flow through a circuit (or a human being) connected from the "live" wire to the ground, which may be either of the other circuit wires, or a water pipe, or a wet floor. Several possibilities exist for the development of a hazardous situation whenever electrical equipment is used on this electrical supply system.[15]

Second, an important consideration is that the electrical system includes not only the instrumentation and devices but also the wiring of the building. If it is not installed properly many hazardous conditions may result.

Third, the equipment used may be the source of the hazards. For example, a very common fault in electrical equipment is the failure of the ground connection in the power cord. The design of many types of plugs is such that the ground wire breaks in the plug after a few months of use. When this happens, that piece of equipment is ungrounded and a hazard could exist.

A fourth hazard is generated if, because of wear and improper maintenance or because of a flaw in design or manufacture, the live wire is exposed or touches the ungrounded frame of a lamp, instrument, or bed. A person touching the electrically live wire or frame and ground will provide a conducting path through which a danger-

ous or lethal current may flow. Obviously the current could be large enough to be hazardous in the macroshock category. If the current passes through a catheter directly into the heart, death would almost certainly result.

Fifth, whenever two electrical conductors are in close proximity, a capacitive coupling exists between them. This means simply that it is possible for a small quantity of electric charge to pass through the insulation from one conductor to the other. If the voltage between the conductor is alternating, an alternating current will flow. Thus if one of the conductors is the hot wire of the electrical supply to a piece of equipment, a current will flow through the capacitive coupling to the frame and to ground through any available path. This path could be the human body. The current is called the leakage current and should be measured as it flows through a 1000 ohm resistance. Resistive and inductive coupling may also contribute to the leakage current.

A sixth source of hazardous electric shock is the failure of the personnel using the equipment to understand that misuse can result in danger. Most equipment offered on the market today is safe if well maintained and properly used. However, the simplest of devices can kill if faulty operation is not recognized or if the unit is misused.

A seventh hazard may be termed "intentional" for want of a better word. It is most likely to occur with children who put hairpins or paper clips into receptacle slots, but many persons "play" with electric devices and may do the wrong thing.

■ What are some examples of sources of electric shock hazards?

In one of the earliest reports of the induction of ventricular fibrillation by the flow of current through a catheter in the heart, Mody and Richings[16] found that the ground wire opened in the distribution box as the result of a loose screw. This could have been prevented by a good testing and maintenance program in the hospital.

In a second case sufficient voltage and low enough leakage impedance existed between the x-ray tube mounting over the table used in cardiac catheterization and the cable so that 25 microamperes would flow through 1000 ohms connected between them. The problem was that the ground wire had never been connected to the ground bus. Although some problems with 60 Hz noise had been observed during angiography, this condition had been allowed to go uninvestigated for the 3 years after the installation had been "completed" in the new hospital. Had a serious incident occurred, it could have been credited to poor workmanship, inspection, and testing, but more importantly, to poor reporting of the problem on the part of the physicians and nurses.

In still another case an ECG was to be used in a regular hospital room. As a matter of course, the wall outlet was checked for polarity and ground continuity. The grounding wire was found to be broken, although it had been "good" some time in the past. Inspection showed the wire had been nicked in removing the insulation, and building vibration had caused the failure. Here a testing procedure may have prevented a serious incident.

In a coronary care unit in which five of the eight patients had indwelling intracardiac catheters, all of the monitors had leakage currents in excess of 25 microamperes.[17] Pulsing in the leakage currents of up to 48 microamperes was observed on one monitor, evidently caused by a faulty grounding system and coupling between the monitor and other electric devices. This is an example of faulty design and faulty testing and maintenance.

These are probably enough examples to give an indication of the varied nature of the problems that can arise from improper wiring of the hospital building accentuated by poor reporting and testing procedures.

Some hazards are equipment problems. They may arise from improper maintenance and use, but many will result from poor quality control or poor design on the part of the manufacturer of the instrument. Here are examples, some of them mere statements of observed facts.[7]

A leakage current of 120 microamperes was measured in the injector used in angiography. A recorder used in the cardiac catheterization laboratory had a leakage current of 45 microamperes. A leakage current of 5 milliamperes was measured in ultrasonic generators used in the physiotherapy section. These are examples of poor design of the equipment. However, the shortcomings of the design can be offset by making certain that the grounding wires of the instruments are in good condition. This is a matter for the maintenance technicians to check regularly.

An example of the need for the engineer and technician to be involved in checking and replacing the plugs on the power cords of the instruments follows. One hospital engineer reported that a survey of 300 molded-on plugs cut off of hospital equipment such as electric beds, portable suction pumps, hypothermia machines, etc. revealed the following conditions on detailed examination: (1) Fifty-five percent of the plugs had no ground prong. The ground prongs had been removed because they were broken in "normal" hospital use or were bent and could not be inserted in receptacles. (2) Forty-five percent of the plugs had all three prongs apparently intact. Visual inspection showed *apparently* safe plugs.[17] When the plugs with apparently intact prongs were tested with a continuity meter, it was found that only 15% of the plugs were actually safe. Often when such a situation occurs in the critical care area, artifacts will be seen on the monitor. It becomes the duty of the practitioner to report it, but the best remedy is a good testing and maintenance program.

A final example of both faulty equipment and

improper building wiring is that of a cardiac patient who was shocked sufficiently to be thoroughly frightened when he touched the pendant nurse call button. He was on a cardiac monitor. Investigation showed that the call button was not insulated but was grounded and the monitor was faulty in that it had a partial short of the live wire to the chassis and was not grounded. These are both design and maintenance faults.

But the users of the equipment are often at fault. Because the attached cord was too short, a two-wire extension was used for 2 months on an injector in angiography.[17] The leakage current on the injector was high, resulting in the ungrounded machine-induced fibrillation of a number of patients before the cause was detected and repaired. No physician, nurse, or technician should ever allow the use of a two-wire cord on an instrument that has a three-wire power cord. In another case an inexpensive two-wire extension cord was found on an ECG machine "because the regular three-wire cord would not work."

Two examples will suffice to show that several items may be involved. A 53-year-old patient was thrown into ventricular fibrillation when the control mechanism of the electrically operated bed was immersed in urine.[18] Analysis of this case revealed the following situation: The patient, having a mild left hemiparesis, had elevated the backrest of the electrically operated bed to the vertical position, leaving the control mechanism resting on the lap. While attempting to return the urinal to the bedside table with the paretic left arm, the patient lost control of the heavy bottle and spilled most of its content over the bed, thereby immersing the control mechanism in the urine. The control mechanism, in turn, carried current from a conventional 120 grounded power line to the motor operating the bed mechanism. The patient was connected to ground by one of the ECG monitor electrodes taped to the anterior chest wall, its connecting cable terminating at the chassis of the monitor grounded through the third wire of the power cord. Thus current from the control mechanism passed through the urine, the patient's buttocks, the chest electrode to the chassis of the monitor, and from there to ground via ground wire. Only the quick action of a resident who observed the appearance of a 60 Hz sig-

nal on the remote monitor at the nurses' station prevented the accident from becoming fatal.

In another case a 52-year-old male patient was on an external cardiac pacemaker connected to the power line. A transvenous bipolar catheter electrode was placed through the right jugular vein into the right ventricle of the heart. Later the patient was found dead. An examination revealed that the instrument grounding system (third prong) was eliminated by use of a 10-foot two-wire extension cord. Leakage current of the instrument (including the 8-foot three-wire power cord of the instrument and the 10-foot two-wire extension cord) measured 54 microamperes.[19]

This accident could have been avoided if (1) a three-wire, instead of a two-wire, extension cord had been used on the pacemaker, (2) the patient had no access to any conductor to ground, (3) the pacer lead had had a current-limiting device of 5 microamperes, or (4) a battery-powered pacemaker had been used. However, the primary cause was an improper procedure—the use of the two-wire extension cord.

An incident of the "intentional" type occurred in a pediatric ward when a child found a hairpin and inserted it into the "live" slot of a receptacle. He then tried to pull it out with his teeth. His nose touched the grounded metallic plate surrounding the receptacle, resulting in a circuit from the hairpin through the lips to the nose and the plate. He suffered severe burns of the mouth and lips.[18]

To sum up and repeat for emphasis, the electric shock incidents just reviewed were caused by one or a combination of the following: (1) poor design of the wiring system or equipment; (2) poor maintenance of the wiring system or the equipment; (3) improper use of a device; and (4) carelessness on the part of the designer, manufacturer, or user or lack of knowledge as to how to use the instruments.

These examples do not exhaust the list of ways in which electric shock accidents can occur. Instead they merely point out that the conditions that lead to shock are almost as varied as the number of possible combinations of people, devices, and wiring systems. They indicate that the only way to avoid accident is to be "eternally vigilant." However, certain basic principles can be applied that will help reduce the hazards of electric shock.

In the preceding paragraphs, examples of electric shock incidents have been described. However, it should be pointed out that the agencies responsible for writing electric safety standards have recognized the hazards and have continuously moved toward safer system specifications. The medical equipment manufacturers have taken these recommendations seriously so that many of the incidents described would probably not occur today. Nevertheless, it is important that the effort to produce a safe electrical environment, including the design of the electrical power supply system and the patient-related instruments, be continued. Further, it is important that the devices be well maintained, and that they be used properly by an informed medical and nursing staff.

A final paragraph about static electricity is in order. A static electric charge is generated when two insulated materials are separated. An example is that of a sheet being removed from a bed or another is that of walking across a carpet. While the voltages built up may be several thousand volts, the total energy is usually quite small. Thus it is quite probable that the spark discharge noticed when a patient is touched will not be harmful. It will be disturbing, however. It is a good practice therefore to touch the bed or other metallic object before touching the patient. The use of antistatic materials in laundering linens will help to keep the annoying static spark from occurring. Similar materials may be used on carpets in some cases. Higher relative humidities sometimes aid in reducing the generation of static electricity. However, this is often not helpful when synthetic cloth is used.

■ How is electric shock prevented?

From an earlier discussion it would seem that protecting a patient from the probability of electric shock is quite simple in principle. The reduction of hazardous currents can be achieved by:

1. Preventing a voltage difference from occurring in such a way that the patient or other person cannot close the circuit and thus allow a current to flow (Fig. 45-10, *A*)

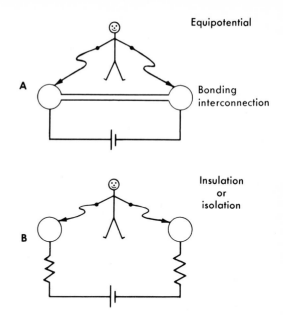

Fig. 45-10. Preventing electrical shock by, **A,** equipotential bonding or grounding or, **B,** inserting high resistance in circuit.

2. Putting a high resistance in all circuits that could include the patient, thus reducing the current to less than hazardous levels (Fig. 45-10, *B*).

However, the implementation of these procedures is quite difficult, especially when the human factor is included.

It has been pointed out that the values contributed by electric instruments far outweigh the hazards they introduce. Nevertheless, accidents do occur and they can result in discomfort, injury, or death to the patient, nurse, or physician, but almost all are preventable. To assist in the task of providing for conditions that will result in reasonable safety, many groups are working on codes and standards that help establish recommended safe practice.

For all patients all devices designed and manufactured in accordance with standards adopted by the electrical manufacturing associations and maintained by regular inspection and repair will be safe, if properly used. This will include having acceptable wiring in the area where such devices are to be used. The minimum wiring system is a three-wire grounded system with a ground conductor separate from the conduit.

The acceptable wiring system combines the minimum with the grounding of exposed conductive surfaces such as water pipes and construction metal.

The grounding system may have additional features added, such as the insulation of all exposed metal or the use of isolated power systems. Further detail on the design and installation of such systems is appropriate to an engineering manual and will not be treated here. However, great care must be exercised in the use of equipment in the presence of the patient. Perhaps foremost is the assurance that the equipment is properly designed, that it is the right equipment for the purpose, and that it has been well maintained.

An important part of the purchase of any device is preparation of a set of specifications for it. These specifications should be prepared by a committee consisting of members of the medical and nursing staffs who will be involved in the use of the apparatus and members of the engineering and technical staffs who can determine the electrical safety features of the device. Such a committee should determine the availability of repair and calibration services and many other features in addition to the medical functions that the device may fulfill.

If possible, the engineering members of the committee should have the opportunity to make prepurchase inspections and tests on the device, and the medical and user staff members should be permitted to check its operational features.

Once the device is ordered and received at the hospital, a series of inspections and tests should be established for it. These will include (1) preacceptance testing, (2) preventive maintenance procedures, (3) preuse testing under certain critical circumstances, (4) postrepair testing, and (5) postmisuse testing.[20]

To expand further on the preceding discussion, the first testing and inspection of a device may come when a unit has been brought to the hospital for demonstration and possible purchase. It should be there only on the approval of the appropriate engineer, who will have examined the specifications prior to the approval for demonstration. When it comes to the hospital, perhaps brought by a salesman, it should go directly to the engineer and engineering staff for acceptance testing. After this and only after this should it go to a floor to be used or demonstrated.

Much of the acceptance test procedure may be circumvented in some cases by the use of the work done in Philadelphia by The Emergency Care Research Institute.* However, this does not eliminate examination of a particular piece of equipment in a particular hospital.

One of the things to be looked for in this first test is how many little-used knobs are on the front panel—knobs that can disturb the functioning of the equipment if not correctly adjusted. For example, one moment of panic occurred in the open-heart surgery room when the patient's blood pressure as shown on the scope was very low. The actual situation was that the technician had turned the wrong knob, intending to raise the pattern on the screen. Instead the knob he turned unbalanced the pressure transducer bridge. Other prepurchase tests should include calibration frequency response where important. For example, a small square wave applied to an ECG machine can give a good indication of excessive filtering or damping in the recording part of the machine or its quality of performance.

Once the prepurchase acceptance tests are completed, the decision on what instrument or device to buy is made and the order placed, the engineering staff now waits for the arrival of the equipment. Once again, inspection and testing are in order. Equipment can be damaged in shipment, maybe not visibly, but as far as safety or performance is concerned. A dropped box may break a fuse holder in such a manner that the hot wire touches the ungrounded case, yet no damage may show externally.

Once the equipment is accepted and in use in the hospital, continued and regular preventive maintenance tests specifically designed for each device should be performed. Records of these tests and any corrective repairs made should be kept by the hospital.

Sometimes it becomes important to make tests that combine the characteristics of the power system and the instrumentation and to separate

---

*The Emergency Care Research Institute, 5200 Butler Pike, Plymouth Meeting, Pa. 19462.

them if they combine in an adverse fashion. For example, I recently had occasion to test the leakage of a piece of equipment that the hospital planned to use on an isolated power system. The hospital tests showed the leakage exceeded the specifications by 50% and the engineer refused to accept the device. However, a test on the same unit made in the hall outside the electronics laboratory on a conventional grounded power supply showed a lower leakage current within specifications. The problem was in the very high leakage of the isolated system and the method of measurement.

Test protocols should include provision for testing immediately prior to any difficult and dangerous procedure such as cardiac catheterization and extensive surgery. These may be simple go–no go tests that can be performed by the nurse or medical technician, or they may be more instrumented measurements made by the medical equipment technician or engineer.

The remarks just made may seem to be more detailed and technical than necessary in a book such as this. However, since critical care practitioners are most involved with the use of all manner of electromedical devices, it is important that they be informed on what is required to have a safe, effective instrumentation system. This includes the acceptance of responsibility, specific tasks, participation in planning and implementation, and awareness and reporting.

Acceptance of responsibility for environment

The most important thing critical care practitioners can do to ensure the safety of their patients as far as the instrumentation is concerned is to recognize that they must accept responsibility for the entire environment of the patient. This means that the patient must receive the best possible care with the minimum of discomfort commensurate with the situation. Obviously an electric shock, even a slight one, cannot be tolerated, nor can burns, excessive pressures, or whatever unnecessary effects occur to disturb the patient.

Specific tasks

At the risk of repetition, to be involved in a continuing education program is the next most important thing critical care practitioners can do in

the instrument safety field; this means to be informed. They should not only have studied these notes, but should have read some of the references listed in the bibliography. They should have read very carefully the operation manuals on the devices they are likely to be called on to use. They should give special attention to any precautionary notes in the operation manuals.

Planning and implementation

Being involved in the planning and implementation of the instrumentation program is also important. Although architects and engineers are the usual sources for designs of hospitals, the medical and nursing staff are the users. In an area where the design and the installation of the instrumentation are such an important part of the functioning of the system, critical care practitioners should have input into the design. Furthermore, they should have an opportunity to plan the ways in which the system is to be used. This means they should ask for and accept membership on planning committees, safety committees, and so on.

Awareness and reporting

To recognize and report any incidents, observations, or accidents involving the instrumentation may be lifesaving. The observation of artifacts, stray "noise," extra-wide baseline, or any other effect on an oscilloscope or recording device may be an indication of possible hazardous conditions in electrical devices or they may merely mean that the electrodes are not making contact with the patient. In any case, their cause should be investigated, and if the problem is not immediately recognized and remedied, help should be obtained. The nursing supervisor and/or the engineer or technician should be called. The problem may be simple and the solution equally simple, but it could result in a fatality.

If a tingling sensation is felt, or someone thinks that it is, the occurrence should be reported to the technical staff and they should investigate it immediately.

Sometimes an instrument is dropped accidentally or a fluid is spilled over it. Unless the device is a life-support instrument, it should be unplugged and the incident reported. Anyone may experience an accident, and there should be no penalty. But the failure to report it could be reason for severe penalty.

SUMMARY

This chapter is in itself a brief summary of a subject that has blossomed into volumes of continuing growth. Briefly, the nature of electricity and its associated hazards have been reviewed. The prevention of accidents involving these hazards is the responsibility of many persons—engineers, manufacturers, hospital administrators, technicians, and nurses. For all these persons, and especially for the critical care practitioner, the whole safety problem can be summed up in two very brief statements:

1. Be informed.
2. Be involved.

REFERENCES

1. Porterfield, J. D., III: To the defense of the system, hospitals, J. Am. Hosp. Assoc. **48:**49, 1974.
2. Smyth, A. H., editor: The life and writings of Benjamin Franklin, vol. 2, New York, 1905, Macmillan Inc.
3. Waller, A.: On the electromotive changes connected with beats of the mammalian heart, and the human heart in particular, Trans. R. Soc. Lond. **180:**169, 1889.
4. Einthoven, W.: The different forms of the human electrocardiogram and their signification, Lancet **1:**853, 1912.
5. A.A.M.I. News, **13,** no. 3, March-April, 1978.
6. Intersociety Commission for Heart Disease: Electronic equipment in critical care areas, Circulation **43:**A-97, 1971.
7. Stanley, P. E.: Personal notes.
8. Karselis, T.: Descriptive medical electronics and instrumentation, Thorofare, N.J., 1973, Charles B. Slack.
9. Safe use of electricity in patient care areas of health care facilities, Tentative Standard 76BT, Boston, Mass., 1973, National Fire Protection Association.
10. Dalziel, C. F.: Threshold 60 cycle fibrillating currents, Trans. Am. Inst. Electrical Engineers **79:**667, 1960.
11. King, B. G.: Effect of electric shock on heart action with special reference to varying susceptibility in different parts of the cardiac cycle, Doctoral thesis, Columbia University, New York, 1934, Aberdeen Press.
12. Kouwenhoven, W. B., Knickerbocker, G. G., Chestnut, R. W., Milnor, W. R., and Soss, D. J.: A-C shocks of varying parameters affecting the heart, A.I.E.E. Trans. E.E. **78:**163, 1959.
13. Dalziel, D. F., and Lee, W. R.: Re-evaluation of lethal electric currents, I.E.E.E. Trans. IGA **4:**467, 1968.
14. Weinberg, D. L., Artley, J. L., Whalen, R. E., and McIntosh, H. D.: Electric shock hazards in cardiac catheterization, Circ. Res. **11:**1004, 1962.
15. Bruner, J. M. R.: Hazards of electrical apparatus, Anesthesiology **28:**396, 1967.
16. Mody, S. M., and Richings, M.: Ventricular fibrillation resulting from electrocution during cardiac catheterization, Lancet **2:**698, 1962.
17. Lubin, D.: Molded-on attachment plug caps can create hazardous electrical situations in the hospital, report to the American Society of Hospital Engineers, Committee on Electrical Safety in Hospitals, 1968, American Society of Hospital Engineers.
18. Aronow, S., Bruner, J. M. R., Siegal, E. F., and Sloss, L. J.: Ventricular fibrillation associated with an electrically operated bed, N. Engl. J. Med. **281:**31, 1969.
19. Von der Mosel, H. A.: Accident case history, Med. Electronics Data **1:**74, 1970.
20. Stanley, P. E.: Safety in the electromedical equipment system, National Safety News **110:**No. 5, 71; No. 6, 90; **111:** No. 1, 87, 1975.

BIBLIOGRAPHY

California Hospital Association: Hospital electrical safety manual, Sacramento, 1972.
Link, J. J., and Feinberg, B.: Electrical safety in hospitals, Erie, Pa., 1976, American Sterilizer Co.
Roth, H. H., Teltscher, E. S., and Kane, I. M.: Electrical safety in health care facilities, New York, 1975, Academic Press, Inc.
Spooner, R. B., editor: Hospital instrumentation care and servicing for critical care units, Pittsburgh, 1977, Instrument Society of America.

CHAPTER 46

Assessment and rehabilitation of the patient recovering from stroke*

Laura Wall and James F. Toole

Stroke is a major illness of our time. Ranking third as the cause of death in the United States today, stroke claims more than 275,000 lives each year. But the impact of stroke is not measured by mortality alone. Roughly one half of all stroke victims survive, and at any given time there are 2½ million stroke victims living in our country.[1] The morbidity within this group is significant. Of every 100 stroke survivors, only 10 reach full recovery, 40 suffer a mild disability, another 40 are so disabled that they require special care, and 10 need institutional care.[2] If mortality and morbidity caused by stroke are surprising, the costs are astounding. The annual cost of medical care alone is estimated at $1.2 billion, and costs attributed to man hours lost exceed $3 billion yearly.[1] The sad thing is that these figures, although impressive, cannot begin to compare with the amount of sorrow, personal loss, and disruption of family life caused by stroke.

Ideally, prevention of stroke is more desirable than treatment after the fact. Much is being done in the area of public education regarding stroke risk factors by volunteers working with the American Heart Association. Emphasis on preventive aspects, such as promotion of good general health plus detection and treatment of stroke-prone individuals, is a focal point for family practice centers, hypertension clinics, and other outpatient facilities.

Still, stroke patients are admitted daily to hos-

pitals all over our country. These patients deserve optimal supportive care and thorough assessment of their rehabilitative potential. This chapter describes the multidisciplinary approach to stroke patient care and points out that rehabilitative measures begin during the acute phase of illness. Emphasis is placed on the responsibilities of the nurse in a team approach to assessment and care of the patient recovering from stroke.

■ What is a stroke?

Stroke is a word used to describe the sudden onset of neurologic signs and symptoms caused by damage to brain tissue following interruption of its blood supply by obstruction or hemorrhage. The most common cause of stroke, accounting for about 75%, is occlusion of the arteries supplying the brain by atherosclerosis with superimposed thrombosis. Cerebral infarction caused by atherothrombosis classically occurs during periods of decreased activity, such as sleeping, when blood pressure tends to be low. It also occurs when emboli from these atherothrombotic lesions occlude distal arteries. Abrupt occlusion of cerebral arteries by embolism occurs during periods of normal or increased activity. A common source of large cerebral emboli is the heart. Myocardial infarction, valvular disease following rheumatic fever, bacterial endocarditis, and atrial fibrillation all encourage formation of blood clots, which are potential cerebral emboli.

Cerebral hemorrhage caused by hypertension and subarachnoid hemorrhage following rupture

*Supported by USPHS Contract RFP, NIH-NINCDS 78-02.

of an aneurysm are also causes of stroke. Brain damage from the forceful jet of blood during hemorrhage, infarction of the area distal to vessel rupture, increased intracranial pressure from cerebral edema, and the mass effect of an intracranial hematoma contribute to the catastrophic result of hemorrhagic stroke. This type of stroke occurs 25% of the time.

■ What are stroke syndromes?

Groups of signs and symptoms that predictably follow damage in specific arterial distributions of the brain are called stroke syndromes. Understanding stroke syndromes depends on a basic knowledge of the arterial supply to the brain (Fig. 46-1).

Carotid system

The carotid system is one of two arterial systems that supply the brain with oxygenated blood. The right common carotid artery arises from the innominate artery, and the left common carotid

artery is the second large artery to branch from the aortic arch. These vessels travel up the anterior neck and divide into internal and external branches. The external carotid arteries supply the face and scalp, while the internal carotid arteries enter the cranium anteriorly to serve the brain. At the base of the brain, the internal carotid arteries branch to form the anterior and middle cerebral arteries. Connections between the anterior cerebral arteries of the two carotid arteries form part of the circle of Willis.

Internal carotid artery syndrome. Gradual occlusion of the internal carotid artery may not produce symptoms if collateral circulation through the circle of Willis is sufficient. The first symptoms may be transient in nature. By definition, transient ischemic attacks (TIA's) are episodes of focal neurologic deficit lasting a few minutes or hours but no longer than 24 hours that disappear, leaving the patient neurologically normal. TIA's are usually caused by small emboli from atherosclerotic plaques at the bifurcation of the carotid

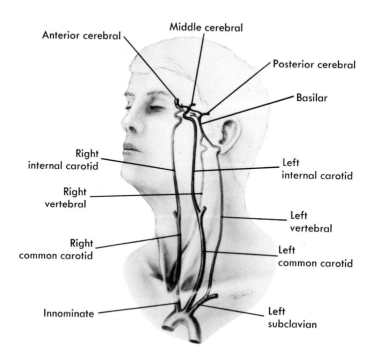

Fig. 46-1. The carotid and vertebrobasilar artery systems supply the brain with oxygenated blood.

artery in the neck. They result in loss of vision in the ipsilateral eye, weakness on the contralateral side, aphasia if the dominant hemisphere is affected, and varying degrees of altered consciousness.

Middle cerebral artery syndrome. The middle cerebral artery syndrome is the most common of the stroke syndromes because the middle cerebral artery transports more blood and is occluded more often than the other cerebral arteries. Occlusion at its origin produces a contralateral hemiplegia with sensory loss. Paralysis of the face and arm is marked and improves more slowly than that of the leg. If the dominant hemisphere is affected, the patient will exhibit expressive and receptive aphasia. Homonymous hemianopia sometimes occurs. The main difference between this and the internal carotid syndrome is episodic loss of vision in one eye in the latter.

Anterior cerebral artery syndrome. Infarction in the distribution of the anterior cerebral artery produces a contralateral hemiplegia with the leg weaker than the arm. If the dominant hemisphere is affected, the patient sometimes exhibits expressive aphasia. Less commonly seen are deterioration of intellectual function and bowel and bladder incontinence. This artery is affected in less than 10% of ischemic strokes.

Vertebrobasilar system

The right and left vertebral arteries branch from their respective subclavian arteries at the base of the neck. They travel up the neck within the transverse processes of the cervical vertebrae and enter the cranium posteriorly through the foramen magnum. Intracranially the vertebral arteries merge to form the single basilar artery that supplies the brain stem. The basilar artery terminates by dividing into the two posterior cerebral arteries and by joining the circle of Willis.

Vertebrobasilar syndrome. Stenosis of the vertebral and basilar arteries caused by atherosclerosis and compression of the vertebral arteries by osteoarthritic cervical vertebrae are causes of vertebrobasilar insufficiency. Head turning, hyperextension of the neck, and transient postural hypotension exaggerate the symptoms. The signs and symptoms caused by vertebrobasilar insufficiency are myriad. The most common ones include vertigo, tinnitus and hearing change because the vertebrobasilar system supplies the inner ear (an important point to remember is that the carotid system supplies the eye and the vertebrobasilar system supplies the ear), diplopia, homonymous hemianopia, cerebellar signs, nausea and vomiting, and dysarthria. Infarction in the distribution of the basilar artery causes fixed and constricted pupils, quadriplegia, and coma. The prognosis for a patient in this state is grave.

Wallenburg syndrome. Occlusion of the posterior inferior cerebellar artery (PICA) causes severe vertigo, nausea, and vomiting, dysphagia, and ataxia. Horner's syndrome (constricted pupil and ptosis) of the ipsilateral eye is sometimes seen, as is loss of pain and temperature sense in the face on the side of the lesion and in the trunk and extremities on the contralateral side.

Posterior cerebral artery syndrome. Occlusion of the posterior cerebral artery deprives the visual cortex in the occipital lobe of the cerebrum and results in homonymous hemianopia.

■ How does the nurse plan care for the stroke patient?

The degree and type of disability after stroke depends on the area and extent of brain damage and so varies widely from one patient to another. *Recovery* is dependent on the above plus the age and general health of the patient, his personality and emotional state, the support of those dear to him, and, of course, the care he receives.

With this many variables, it is easy to see that planning care for the stroke patient must be individualized and patient oriented. Nurses are familiar with the phrase, "patient-oriented nursing care." In fact, the phrase is used so often it sometimes seems a cliché. After all, isn't care given to a specific patient oriented just to him? Not necessarily. Care is disease or disability oriented unless time is taken to recognize that the patient is a person with a family and place in society who because of illness has special needs.

To identify these needs there are several questions to consider, and the family or the patient himself can supply the answers. First, what was his personality like before the stroke? Was he independent and productive or was the patient weak and dependent on his family or society?

Was he optimistic or depressed, friendly or reclusive? Is there history of emotional instability? All of these questions are important because strokes can mask or magnify personality traits and increase emotional lability.

The nurse needs information about the patient's family. How much support can the family offer the patient? Is the spouse healthy? Are there children? Do the children live near the patient or are they distantly scattered? Will other family members or friends be involved with care after hospitalization?

Understanding the patient's role in society before the stroke is essential because a change in daily responsibility can be the most difficult adjustment for the patient and his family unit. Appropriate questions are: What was the patient's occupation? What skills are required in his job? Is he able to read and write? What are his primary interests? Was the patient the primary provider for his family? Does the patient have obligations to or affiliations with church, social, or professional groups?

Evaluating the patient's general health by noting his past medical history and health habits completes the picture of what he was like prior to the stroke. Is there a history of other health problems such as heart disease, hypertension, or diabetes? Does the patient smoke or have signs of chronic lung disease? Has he had major surgical procedures in the past? Is he obese? Has he been on a special diet? What medications was the patient taking at the time of his stroke?

When the nurse knows the patient's personal and medical history, it is time to assess the effects of the stroke itself.

■ How does the nurse assess the patient's neurologic status?

Frequent and accurate patient assessment is a natural role for the critical care nurse. Evaluation of nervous system function is basic to care of the stroke patient and can be accomplished easily if approached in a systematic way.

Cerebral functions

The patient's level of consciousness is the most important single indicator of his neurologic state. Any change in the level of consciousness is important. There are numerous scales by which the

patient can be evaluated, but generally it is agreed that the normal patient is alert and oriented, and as his neurologic status deteriorates he becomes drowsy, disoriented, stuporous, semicomatose and responsive to pain only, and finally, comatose and nonresponsive.

Noting the patient's general behavior and emotional state should be second nature to the empathetic nurse. These observations are especially meaningful for the stroke patient because bizarre behavior, short attention span, and mood swings can be signs of organic disease as well as reactions to stress.

His intellectual function can be partially determined by observing his cooperation and interaction with others. Does he follow directions easily? Does he recognize people that should be familiar to him? Is his response to social cues normal, that is, does he smile or nod when greeted? Even the patient with a speech disorder will be able to do these things. More specific assessment of intellectual function depends on normal speech function. The patient's memory for recent and remote events is important. Does he remember what he ate for breakfast? Can he tell you the year he was born or details of his first job? To assess the patient's general knowledge, ask him to name the president or tell you about prominent current events. Having him calculate mathematical problems or interpret proverbs like, "A rolling stone gathers no moss," are other ways of testing intellectual function. Of course, all these assessments are made with the patient's educational and social background in mind. Formal psychologic testing is beneficial when the patient reacts abnormally to these simple tests.

Speech disorders that are common after stroke include dysarthria and aphasia. Dysarthria is a slurred dysrhythmic speech caused by weakness and incoordination of the muscles of articulation. It is easily detected by simply listening to the patient as he speaks. Aphasia is a speech disorder characterized by the inability of the patient to use the spoken or written word for communication. The patient with expressive (motor, Broca's) aphasia, the most common type, is unable to verbalize what he wants to say. This disorder is easily detected by observing absence of speech or use of the wrong words when the patient does try to express himself. The patient with receptive (sensory, Wernicke's) aphasia is unable to understand what is said to him. This disorder is identified by observing that the patient does not follow directions or does so only after directions are repeated with the use of gestures.

Cranial nerve function

Cranial nerve dysfunction after stroke causes visual disturbances, paralysis of facial muscles, and difficulty swallowing. The nurse begins to assess cranial nerve function by taking a close look at the face. Having the patient exaggerate facial movement by telling him, "Show me your gums," will make weakness more obvious. Does his face move and wrinkle symmetrically or does one cheek look flat and expressionless? Does his mouth droop at the corner? Is he able to open and close his eyes normally? Ask the patient to raise his eyebrows and look for symmetric movement and wrinkling of the forehead. Weakness of the lower face denotes a central facial palsy, while weakness of the entire face on one side is due to peripheral facial nerve palsy.

Most nurses are accustomed to examining the eyes by noting pupillary size, equality, and reaction to light. Visual acuity can be measured by having the patient read small print. The patient with a visual field defect such as homonymous hemianopia (loss of the corresponding half of the visual field in each eye) may tend to disregard the affected side or he may turn his head so as to scan his environment. Both of these observations can be made by the nurse at the bedside. To test the visual fields by confrontation, stand directly in front of the patient and ask him to look at your nose. Tell the patient to cover one of his eyes while you cover the corresponding eye to serve as a control. Move your finger from the periphery of each quadrant of his vision toward the center. Ask the patient to tell you when he first sees your finger. He should be able to see it at about the same time you do. Eye movement is evaluated by noting if the eyes move in a conjugate manner on side-to-side, upward, and downward gaze. This is also a good time to observe for nystagmus.

Dysphagia (difficulty in swallowing) is not a very common result of stroke, but when it does occur, it creates a major problem for the patient. If the patient drools or chokes on his saliva, he should be checked carefully before being fed. Ask him to say, "ah," and look for a symmetric rise of the soft palate. Attempt to elicit a gag reflex by touching the oropharynx with a tongue depressor. If the patient is able to speak, listen carefully for hoarseness. Finally, give him a sip of plain water to see if he can swallow. If he coughs suddenly or regurgitates the water through his nose, he must not be allowed anything by mouth.

Motor function

Muscular weakness or paralysis is a common result of stroke. To assess the degree of dysfunction, muscles on one side are compared to corresponding muscles on the other side. To evaluate strength in the upper extremities, test the patient's grip and flexion and extension of the elbow and shoulder to opposition. If possible, have the patient stand to evaluate the lower extremities. First, ask him to walk and observe his gait. In normal gait, the stride is even and rhythmic and the arms swing slightly. Hemiplegic gait, caused by stroke, is characterized by circumduction and dragging the weak leg and absence of arm swinging. Next, ask the patient to walk on his heels and toes and do a deep knee bend.

Muscle tone is measured by noting resistance while taking a joint through passive range of motion. Words that describe abnormal muscle tone are flaccid, rigid, and spastic.

■ What rehabilitative measures are required during acute care?

The acute phase of the stroke patient's illness is measured not in hours or days but by the length of time that he has unstable vital signs, decreased level of consciousness, or the need for respiratory support. Rehabilitative measures during this phase are aimed only at maintenance of bodily functions and prevention of complications until he is ready for a formal rehabilitative program.

Turning and careful positioning are needed every 2 hours. A schedule for turning the patient alternately from his unaffected side, supine, and three-quarters prone maximizes circulation, alveolar ventilation, and drainage of secretions and minimizes pressure on the skin of any body part.

The skin should be examined for reddened areas each time the patient is turned. Massaging his back and pressure areas with lotion promotes circulation and is soothing to the patient. The routine use of foam pads on bony prominences and heel and elbow protectors is a good preventive measure.

Flaccid extremities must be kept in proper alignment by the use of pillows, sandbags, and foam pads. Supporting the shoulder at 30- to 45-degree abduction with the elbow only slightly flexed helps prevent shoulder and elbow contractures. Elevating the arm and hand slightly on a pillow helps prevent dependent edema and wrist contracture. A 4-inch roll can be used to keep the hand in a normal grip position with the thumb and forefinger opposed. Positioning of the affected leg is aimed at prevention of external rotation of the hip and hip and knee contractures. When the patient is supine, the legs should lie flat without pillows under the knees. Padded sandbags or trochanter rolls at the hips and knees prevent external hip rotation. In the side-lying or three-quarter prone position, pillows or foam pads are used to support the affected leg in a slightly flexed position. Positioning the foot against a footboard prevents a plantar flexion deformity caused by heel cord tightening. If the patient is comatose or bedridden for a prolonged period, the foot and ankle can be supported by a splint that will hold the foot in a functional position.

Passive range of motion exercises of each joint in the affected extremity should be done at least twice and preferably three times daily. The idea is not to force movement or move the joint beyond the point of pain but simply to keep the joint mobile within its normal range of motion. The unaffected side can be used as a guide to determine what is normal for the individual patient. These simple passive exercises, performed consistently, can prevent the deformity and pain of contractures. The nurse is responsible for these exercises even though a physical therapist is actively involved in patient care.

Special bowel and bladder care is needed for those stroke patients who are comatose or otherwise unable to control elimination. A plan for care is based on knowledge of the patient's elimination habits prior to the stroke and assessment of function afterwards.

Bowel care

Constipation is a common problem because patients in the age group most affected by stroke often have a history of poor bowel habits and some are laxative dependent. Also, bedrest and alteration of diet and fluid intake tends to decrease bowel function. Expecting the patient to have a bowel movement every day is probably unrealistic. However, if the patient does not have a bowel movement in 3 days or if he passes liquid stools, the nurse should check his rectum for fecal impaction. Rectal suppositories or small tap water enemas can be used to stimulate bowel function every second or third day. Cleansing enemas and digital removal of stool from the rectum should be reserved for relief of impaction only. As the patient's condition improves, he will be able to take an active role in a bowel program based on proper hydration, a diet with adequate bulk, timing, and regular activity. In the beginning the patient should be given the opportunity and privacy to defecate at the same time of day according to his prior habits. After breakfast and before the bath is an especially good time to plan for bowel elimination. After supper and before retiring is another good time depending on what is usual for the patient. If possible, the patient should be helped from the bed to the bathroom or bedside commode because the upright position enhances bowel action. If a bedpan must be used, help the patient sit upright and lean forward to encourage use of the abdominal muscles. The time allowed for defecation should not exceed 30 minutes because of the danger of exhausting the patient and also because it is unlikely that he will have a movement if he has not done so in 30 minutes time. Eventually, the patient will establish his own bowel routine without the regular need for laxatives, suppositories, or enemas.

Diarrhea with fecal incontinence is usually a short-term problem caused by improper diet, use of antibiotics, fecal impaction, or excessive laxative use. Treatment consists of determining and eliminating the cause.

Bladder care

Because urinary incontinence is an invitation for skin breakdown, special nursing measures are necessary. It is essential that the skin be kept clean and dry. External collecting devices, such as the condom catheter, are useful for the male patient, and incontinence pads help absorb the urine of the incontinent female patient. Use of an indwelling Foley catheter should be reserved for those patients who have urinary retention owing to a flaccid bladder or prostatic obstruction or whenever the patient's medical condition requires strict measurement of intake and output. When the patient's overall condition improves, the catheter is removed so that he can take an active part in a bladder program based on proper hydration, timing, and motivation. The patient should be given the opportunity to void on awakening in the morning and every 2 to 3 hours throughout the day. Fluid intake should be increased during waking hours, especially during the morning, and tapered off during the early evening. Allowing the patient to empty his bladder just before bedtime will often prevent nighttime wetting.

■ What are the most common problems requiring rehabilitation after stroke?
Decreased motor function

The most obvious sign of stroke is loss of motor function on one side of the body. Picture, in your mind's eye, the stroke patient. You may have seen him while shopping, at church, or at a sporting event. He is the person who holds one arm and hand to his body in a flexed position and walks with a circumductive gait. He may be wearing a short leg brace on one leg and holding a cane in the opposite hand. This person is functioning in spite of his disabilities because he has been taught to focus on his abilities! He is a product of rehabilitation. This illustration is not meant to simplify or stereotype stroke, although it is based on the clinical picture of the most common type of stroke, which is infarction in the distribution of the middle cerebral artery. The point is that between the time the patient is bedridden because of vascular insult to his brain until he is upright and mobile again, many weeks or months pass during which he progresses through a step-by-step program of rehabilitation.

A formal program planned by the physician, nurse, and physical therapist working together begins as soon as the patient is conscious and free of medical problems such as hypotension or cardiac dysfunction. The beginning is not marked by a single event but is a normal progression of care with the patient taking an active role. For instance, the range of motion exercises that were once performed passively by the nurse gradually become a patient activity as he learns to assist. The patient also learns how to become mobile in the bed by helping to turn himself and come to a sitting position.

Before he can be taught more independent activities, the patient must achieve sitting balance on the side of his bed. This is not as simple as it might seem because most hemiplegics tend to lean toward the involved side, and some patients, especially those with right brain damage, actually have difficulty determining a vertical line. Balance training begins by helping the patient sit on the side of the bed adjacent to his uninvolved side. He is instructed to place his strong leg under the weak one and swing them over the edge of the bed while pulling up on a side rail with his unaffected arm. His first attempts may be assisted by a firm hand to his back. When the patient achieves an erect sitting position, he is instructed to place his unaffected hand flat on the bed and lean toward his strong side. Although this encourages overcorrection, it also gives the patient control over his posture and promotes self-confidence. With practice, the patient will be able to sit comfortably for increasing periods of time.

The next step is to achieve standing balance in preparation for transfer activities. Some patients will accomplish this easily on the first attempt, but when balance problems are anticipated, the nurse can fasten a balance belt around the patient's waist before he tries to stand. To begin, the patient sits on the side of his bed with both feet on the floor. He comes to a standing position by pushing himself up with his strong arm while bearing weight on his strong leg. The nurse assists by standing directly in front of the patient and helps to steady him by means of his balance belt. She is reminded that this is a patient activity and her role is to promote balance, not to support the patient's weight.

The hemiplegic who can sit and stand with minimal help will have little difficulty mastering transfer activities. The bed-to-chair or bed-to-wheelchair transfer is the most basic and usually the first one learned. The chair is brought to the side of the bed adjacent to the patient's unaffected side. The patient stands, reaches for the outer arm of the chair with his strong arm, pivots on his strong leg, and eases himself to a seated position. Transfer from the chair back to bed is accomplished by moving the chair around so that the patient's unaffected side is nearest the bed and the technique is repeated. Chair-to-toilet and other transfers are accomplished in much the same way with the strong side always leading. Being able to leave his bed with relative ease is emotionally satisfying to the patient. Increased independence reassures him and improves his self-image. Increased activity stimulates his mind, his appetite, and bodily functions such as circulation and peristalsis. So the patient should be encouraged, within his tolerance, to get out of bed several times a day.

For the patient to increase his activity level safely, he may need additional support of the joints on the affected side. Ideally a physical therapist should evaluate the patient's particular needs and help plan his care. When he is in an upright position, the downward pull of an unsupported flaccid arm can cause subluxation of the shoulder joint. In the beginning, when he sits for brief periods only, the flaccid arm should be supported with a pillow under the elbow and forearm. Later, when he spends more time out of bed, a properly fitted sling can support the arm in a functional position. The sling should be removed when he returns to bed so that the arm and shoulder can be exercised and supported in an abducted position. Even before he is able to ambulate, the patient may bear weight on the affected leg or attempt a step during transfer activities. This is the time to assess his need for a short leg brace so that injury owing to poor ankle support is prevented.

Gait training begins when the patient achieves standing balance and is medically able to tolerate more strenuous activity. The personnel and facilities required depend on the patient's individual needs and expectations. The patient who has little return of motor function but is highly motivated will profit from gait training by a physical therapist using the most up-to-date facilities and techniques. Even the severely disabled patient, who expects to spend part of each day in a wheelchair, can raise his level of mobility by learning to take the few steps necessary to overcome structural barriers outside his home. He too deserves referral to a physical therapist. On the other hand,

the patient who has rapid return of motor function needs only limited instructions from a physical therapist and relies on the nurse to help him practice ambulation before discharge from the hospital.

Regardless of who is primarily responsible for gait training, there are some basic measures with which the nurse should be familiar. To begin, the patient should be fitted with sturdy, low-heeled shoes. Bedroom slippers or socks do not provide the support needed for walking and can cause the patient to slide and fall. Most patients who need gait training also require some type of walking aid. A cane is used primarily for balance but can support some weight. The simple straight cane is used for the patient who needs minimal assistance, while the three- or four-pod cane offers maximum stability. The length of the cane is determined by measuring the patient from the greater trochanter of his hip to the floor. The cane is held in the unaffected hand and advanced with the step of the affected foot. The patient is instructed to lean slightly toward his strong side and use his cane for balance. If his weight is allowed to shift to the affected side, the patient finds it extremely difficult to reestablish balance and can fall. Until he learns to lean consistently or is able to overcome balance errors, a nurse or family member should stand at his affected side while he walks. The idea is not to grasp his plegic arm or otherwise support the patient but to be there in case he loses his balance. A walker is useful for the patient who needs more support than is provided by a cane.

Speech disorders

The word "aphasia," which by definition means absence of speech, is often used interchangeably with the word dysphasia, which describes varying degrees of speech dysfunction. The aphasic patient has difficulty understanding and using the spoken or written word as symbols for meaning. Symbolic use of numbers is also disturbed and interferes with counting, mathematical calculation, and telling time.

Aphasia is caused by damage to the speech centers in the dominant hemisphere of the cerebrum, which is most commonly, but not exclusively, the left. When the speech center in the frontal lobe, Broca's area, is affected, the patient exhibits expressive or motor aphasia. He understands but is unable to say what he wants to say or express himself through writing. Damage to the speech center in the temporal lobe, Wernicke's area, results in receptive or sensory aphasia. The patient is unable to understand what he hears or reads. Most aphasic patients exhibit a combination of these two disorders, although one is usually more evident than the other.

Because communication is a basic human need, inability to understand or express ideas, desires, and social comments is exceedingly frustrating. This explains why many aphasic patients become anxious, angry, and depressed and why the nurse must promote communication even before return of speech function. Words are only one vehicle for sending messages; others include gestures, facial expressions, and touching. Basic guidelines for the nurse to follow when working with an aphasic patient include the following:

1. When talking to the patient, face him and see that you have his attention before speaking.
2. Use short simple sentences. Long sentences and detailed information confuses even the patient with moderate receptive abilities.
3. Use questions that can be answered with a simple "yes" or "no." A great deal of information can be exchanged when the patient is able to respond in this manner.
4. Speak in an adult manner with normal volume and pitch. Aphasia does not interfere with hearing so there is no reason to shout. Speaking in a high, overly protective voice sounds like "baby talk" and is demeaning to the patient, especially when he cannot understand what is said.
5. Include the patient in social conversation. Even the patient who exhibits severe receptive abilities deserves a pleasant greeting and an appropriate thank-you.
6. Avoid talking about the patient in his presence unless you want him to hear you. He may understand more than you think or he may misunderstand what is said.
7. Use gestures and visual aids such as pic-

tures or drawings to help convey your message.
8. Accept whatever words the patient is able to say without ridicule, even if they do sound bizarre. If the patient says "sit in chat" and points to a chair, accept his words and help him transfer to a chair. Remember, communication is more important than words.
9. Do not be alarmed if the patient swears. This is a result of emotional frustration and automatic speech and is very common.
10. If, after repeated attempts, the patient is not able to get his message across, share some of the responsibility and say, "I can't understand, let's try again later," instead of, "You aren't talking right, say it again."
11. Remember, your facial expression and other body language conveys as much as words to the aphasic patient.

Dysarthria refers to slow, slurred, dysrhythmic speech caused by weakness and incoordination of the muscles of articulation. The degree to which this speech disorder interferes with communication and the amount of frustration or embarrassment suffered by the patient is variable. Evaluation and treatment by a speech therapist helps the patient to focus on the articulation abilities that remain. He also learns how to compensate for paretic muscles by speaking at a rate that allows him to practice articulation. In addition to the actual treatment, the patient profits from contact with a speech therapist because this specialist best understands the anxieties generated by speech and communication problems.

Visual and spatial perceptual problems

Visual and spatial perceptual problems are not as obvious to the observer as motor or speech deficits but can interfere significantly with rehabilitation of the stroke patient.

Perception of one's environment is dependent on normal transmission of sensory input from the end-organ through the peripheral nerves, spinothalamic tracts, and thalamus to the sensory cortex in the parietal lobe of the cerebrum. The sensory cortex integrates and interprets this input. When the cerebrum is damaged by stroke, sensory input is disrupted at the integrative level.

The patient fails to perceive his environment normally and may not even be aware of his problem.[3]

The most common visual problem caused by stroke is homonymous hemianopia or loss of one half of the visual field in each eye. This visual field defect can be simulated by wearing a pair of goggles with the corresponding half of each lens covered with tape. The patient with this problem does not see beyond midline on the affected side. If the patient realizes that he has a visual deficit, he can be taught to compensate by turning his head so as to scan the area of visual loss. In fact, some patients automatically do this. On the other hand, some patients ignore the affected side and fail to scan in that direction even after repeated instruction to do so. They ignore activity and conversation of people outside their diminished field of vision. These patients may even disregard their affected arm or leg as if the extremities were not their own. This disorder is called one-sided neglect and cannot be explained simply by the presence of homonymous hemianopia or loss of tactile sense. The problem is one of perception and is due to injury of the sensory cortex. One-sided neglect can occur on either side of the body but is seen more often with left-sided paralysis.[4]

The left hemiplegic also has spatial perceptual problems that interfere with his ability to judge distance and size. The patient may walk into a doorframe because he failed to perceive how close he was to it or try to wheel his chair through a space too narrow for passage. Because of difficulty determining vertical and horizontal lines, the patient may not be able to tell if he is leaning or standing upright and therefore has difficulty with balance. His altered recognition of shapes and the relationship of parts to wholes can cause the patient to confuse tops with bottoms and insides with outsides of clothing. This makes dressing himself a major task. Also, the left hemiplegic often has a behavior pattern marked by a short attention span, impulsiveness, and overestimation of his abilities. On a positive note, this patient usually has good understanding and command of speech functions. Therefore verbal or written instructions can help him cope with his disabilities when he is learning a new skill such as one-handed dressing technique. He should be encouraged to slow down and perform activities in a step-by-step fashion. It may be helpful for the patient to "talk himself" through tasks because his own words give feedback and reassurance. To help him cope with altered visual perception, his surroundings should be uncluttered and well lighted. Full-length mirrors and bold vertical lines painted beside doorways and at the ends of halls provide useful visual cues.

As a rule, the patient with right hemiplegia has more difficulty with speech function than with tasks requiring visual spatial judgment. Still, his behavior often suggests altered perceptive abilities. His actions are slow and cautious, and the patient's performance may seem to be below par to his apparent abilities. He approaches familiar activities, such as dressing or grooming himself, in a disorganized fashion and may fail to complete even simple tasks. The patient who behaves in this manner needs constant reassurance and feedback. Verbal or written instructions should be kept to a minimum. One or two word cues such as "good," "fine," or "try again" used with appropriate facial expressions give him the feedback he needs.

■ When should the family become involved in the stroke patient's care?

The family should become involved in the stroke patient's care from the beginning. Discharge planning that includes involvement of the family in patient care must begin early. No matter how sophisticated the care and no matter the number of specialists involved in his care, the patient's famiy is his most important long-term support system. The amount of family support available to the patient is more dependent on the stability and proximity of its members than its size. The extent to which support is developed is largely dependent on an ongoing plan of patient-family education. Family members are naturally interested and want to help but they are also affected by his illness and can be overwhelmed if not given necessary information and guidance.

As soon as the diagnosis is made, there are certain things the patient and his family need to know. They need to know what a stroke is, what caused it, and how it affected the patient. The physician should give initial information regarding diagnosis, but the nurse is responsible for helping the patient and his family understand this information. From this point, patient-family education is a continuing process that proceeds according to a plan based on individual needs. Formulation of a teaching plan is primarily a nursing responsibility. This does not mean the nurse is the only person involved in teaching. Patient-family education is part of total care and is a multidisciplinary team effort. The physician continues to give information throughout the patient's care. As he progresses, other specialists such as the dietician and physical, speech, and occupational therapists contribute to his care and are resources for patient-family education. Written materials, such as those prepared by the American Heart Association for the family of a stroke patient, also help facilitate learning.[5,6,7] Still the nurse is more readily available for day-to-day questions than any other team member and for this reason is best able to plan, coordinate, and evaluate the effectiveness of patient-family education.

Involvement in the patient's physical care is emotionally satisfying to his family members. It is also the best way to help them learn how to care for the patient in preparation for his discharge from the hospital. The nurse should encourage involvement in bedside care such as turning and positioning the patient. Family members should also be shown how to perform range of motion exercises and allowed to demonstrate their learning. When the patient is transported to the physical therapy department for gait training, someone from the family should accompany him and learn the technique. Likewise, patient sessions with the speech therapist and dietician should be attended by a family member.

When the patient progresses to the point of learning activities of daily living (ADL), the family must learn how to give him the time and opportunity to take care of himself. The goal of ADL practice is to promote independence of the patient in bathing, grooming, dressing, and other activities essential for daily self-care. The occupational therapist is expert in this area and helps the patient learn how to use special techniques or self-help devices to compensate for his disabilities. The occupational therapist also helps family members learn how to support the patient in his efforts toward independence. Sometimes, the most difficult thing for the family to learn is how not to help too much.

Finally, family members may need help in keeping care of the patient in healthy perspective to their own needs. Caring family members are only too willing to put the needs of the patient first and foremost. In the beginning this attitude probably serves a good purpose and satisfies their need to be helpful or feel useful, but on a long-term basis, the practice of always putting the patient first is exhausting and can lead to serious emotional conflicts within the family unit. Dr. I. S. Cooper, in his book, *Living with Chronic Neurological Disease,* points out that family members must learn how to reduce stress and preserve some joy in their own lives.[8] This subject is best raised while the patient is still in the hospital so the family can think ahead and develop a reasonable plan for care at home. It may be helpful for the nurse to assist a key family member to formulate a written plan. One simple way to begin is to develop a list of specific patient needs. A second list identifies equipment the family needs to acquire for home care and a third lists people who are available to help. A written plan is especially helpful because it does not require the family, which is already under stress, to commit to memory the details of home care.

SUMMARY

Although efforts at prevention are increasing, stroke continues to be a leading cause of death and disability in our country. The medical community must be informed and have a positive attitude about stroke in order to give the patient and his family the support they deserve.

The team approach, with the physician, nurse, and other specialists working together, provides optimum assessment and treatment of the patient as well as evaluation of the care he receives. The nurse has a unique opportunity in that as the patient progresses from the acute to the intermediate and rehabilitative phases of his care, she is ever-present. While the physician initiates the overall plan of care and the physical, speech, and occupational therapists give periodic input, it is the nurse who is available to the patient for day-to-day care.

The patient's family deserves special consideration because it is his most important source of long-term support. This support is developed through an ongoing plan of patient-family education that begins during the early phases of his illness. Early involvement of the family in the stroke patient's care is emotionally satisfying and prepares the family for care of the patient after discharge from the hospital.

REFERENCES

1. Toole, J. F., and Patel, A.: Cerebrovascular disease, ed. 2, New York, 1974, McGraw-Hill Book Co.

2. Sahs, A. L., et al.: Guidelines for stroke care, Department of HEW, Publication No. (HRA) 76-14017, 1976.
3. Burt, M.: Perceptual deficits in hemiplegia, Am. J. Nurs. **70**(5):1026, May 1970.
4. Fowler, R., and Fordyce, W. E.: Stroke: why do they behave that way? American Heart Association, 1974.
5. Strokes—a guide for the family, American Heart Association, Publication No. 50-025A, 1969.
6. Aphasia and the family, American Heart Association, Publication No. 50-002A, 1969.
7. Strike back at stroke, American Heart Association, Publication No. 50-024A.
8. Cooper, I. S.: Living with chronic neurological disease, New York, 1976, W. W. Norton & Co., Inc.

CHAPTER 47

Rehabilitation of the patient with coronary atherosclerotic heart disease*

Arlene La Baw Niccoli

Heart disease is America's number one killer! Death from cardiovascular disease is, in fact, among the leading causes of death in the United States. The actual number of persons afflicted with coronary atherosclerotic heart disease is immense; it is not only a disease of the elderly but one that afflicts those in their most productive years of life as well. Consequently, the impact, individually and economically, is outstanding and the prevention and management of this disease are now receiving wide attention by both professionals and lay persons.

Acute care or critical care is only part of the total care of people with cardiac disease. Nurses would be negligent if they did not consider the comprehensiveness and long-term aspects of this disease. That is what this chapter will be directed to—the long-term care, the rehabilitation of people with coronary atherosclerotic heart disease. The practical discussion will be directed toward several primary objectives: (1) to stimulate a comprehensive care approach to the cardiac patient; (2) to assist in developing an understanding of the philosophy, principles, and fundamentals of cardiac rehabilitation; (3) to assist the nurse in becoming knowledgeable regarding the coronary

atherosclerotic heart disease process and potential sources of disability, which the nurse can detect and manage or assist in management; (4) to present the basis for rational progression of activity both in and out of the hospital; (5) to help the nurse become knowledgeable regarding her role in cardiac rehabilitation; and (6) to stimulate and support the performance of the nurse as a competent, interested patient advocate.

There have been major advances in the critical care of patients with coronary atherosclerotic heart disease in the past decade and a half that have helped decrease mortality from this disease. Consequently, the number of patients who are candidates for cardiac rehabilitation has grown. The art and science of cardiac rehabilitation have improved greatly over the past years as well, and, gratifyingly, we have seen the advancement and spread of the rehabilitation approach to these patients over recent years. Fifteen years ago the patient with a myocardial infarction was hospitalized approximately 1 month receiving almost total care so that by the time he went home he was practically an invalid as a result of inactivity. In 1970 the average hospital stay was approximately 3 weeks; now at the beginning of the 80's the average hospitalization of an acute myocardial infarction patient has decreased to an average of 10 days to 2 weeks.

Considering the concept of care, Groden recog-

*Supported by a Research and Training Center Grant (16-P-56815) from the National Institute of Handicapped Research, Department of Education, Washington, D.C.

nized that standard medical management is often inadequate to cope with the threatening situations presented to a patient who has had a coronary occlusion, thus permitting the development of disability through mounting fear or anxiety.[1] Standard care in the past has often involved primarily crisis intervention, medical and surgical decision making, medication adjustment, and has had a case- or disease-oriented focus. In short, one could describe standard care as being incomplete. In contrast, rehabilitation is comprehensive care, total person care.

■ What is comprehensive care?

Comprehensive care or rehabilitation is simply an approach to the care of a patient with a disease or disability. It is obviously not specific to people with cardiac disease. It is a care approach that should be offered to all people with chronic diseases and disabilities. The discussion of comprehensive care in this chapter, however, is specific to the patient with coronary atherosclerotic heart disease.

Cardiac rehabilitation is longitudinal care; it is open-ended. It starts when the disease is first diagnosed and continues until that person dies or is no longer accessible to your care. Comprehensive care should be personalized—individualized to the patient, his family, community setting, and all those who interact with the patient. In other words, the care should be directed to the patient in consideration of all that affects him in his life—total person-oriented care.

Recognizing the total patient aspect, attention must also be given to the management of potential sources of disability—the three primary ones being physiologic, psychosocial, and vocational sources. Major components of comprehensive care include restoration, optimization, and maintenance. As an early pioneer of cardiac rehabilitation, Naughton presented this concise definition of cardiac rehabilitation: "The process of restoring and maintaining a patient at his optimal physiologic, psychologic, vocational and social status."[2] Important also to the effectiveness of comprehensive care is that it be participatory. The patient and his family must be included as active participants in the care process and be considered as key members of the cardiac rehabilitation

team. Individualization of care and active participation by the patient are the key factors to rehabilitation success.

The preventive aspect of comprehensive care is also significant. Until recently prevention had been almost totally ignored—certainly not in the best interest of the patient. Prevention is mainly accomplished through management and modification of coronary risk factors and disease or illness complications, all of which involve a variety of entities such as education and motivation of the patient. Primary prevention is the prevention of the coronary atherosclerotic disease process or the prevention of myocardial infarction or other clinical events in those who have no documented disease. Secondary prevention, however, is the prevention of future clinical events and progression of the disease in those who already have documented disease. Thus secondary prevention is the one emphasized in cardiac rehabilitation, whereas primary prevention should be practiced in childhood and early adult life and thereafter.

Considering the principles of comprehensive care, certain rehabilitation program aspects can be elicited to guide professionals in the practice of cardiac rehabilitation. In 1958 White listed five rehabilitation program components that serve to illustrate a practical philosophy of cardiac rehabilitation:

1. Evaluate the patient's medical, psychological, social and vocational status.
2. Individualize management including diet, drugs, physical activity, emotional stress, environmental stress, etc.
3. Discuss with the patient the nature of his disease, the treatment and prognosis, as well as the assessment of his capacities, and how he can best arrange his life to fit his needs.
4. Make every effort to eliminate the patient's fear of heart disease.
5. Encourage him to live the best life possible within the limits (if any) imposed by his disease.[3]

Clearly, more than 20 years ago White concisely outlined the basics of rehabilitative care for us. It is the nurse's responsibility to fulfill these program components through such roles as patient advocate, nurse clinician, educator, counselor, and administrator. An awareness of the comprehensive care approach to cardiac patients is important in our nursing roles, but an understanding of some of the fundamentals specific to cardiac rehabilitation further improves nursing performance and enhances interest and advocacy.

■ What are the fundamentals of cardiac rehabilitation?

Cardiology is a comprehensive specialty in itself, but there are a few specific fundamentals of cardiac rehabilitation that can be identified:

Anatomy and physiology of the cardiac system
The coronary atherosclerotic heart disease process
Causes of disability
Healing of infarction
Energy cost of activities
Types of exercise
Activity counseling
Potential for modifying natural history

Some of these will be discussed in this chapter, but the anatomy, physiology, and pathology of the cardiac system should be reviewed in detail elsewhere. To be an effective educator, the nurse must personally be well-educated regarding the cardiovascular system so that she feels comfortable and confident in assisting the patient and family in their understanding of coronary atherosclerotic heart disease.

Coronary atherosclerotic heart disease process

When one thinks of coronary atherosclerotic heart disease, most often it is in the context of clinical events such as myocardial infarction, angina, or coronary artery bypass surgery. Commonly, the disease itself is not considered. This pathologic condition causes narrowing of the coronary arteries of the heart with critical clinical events being manifested as a consequence of this process. Nurses must recognize also that the coronary atherosclerotic heart disease process begins early in life. It is not a disease that suddenly occurs late in life or at the time of the critical event. It has been developing over many years. Neither does one particular cause seem evident. The process results from multivariate causes commonly known as the risk factors that are thought to contribute to the disease. It is a progressive disease, not an acute disease that can be

cured. Even with appropriate preventive and management measures the disease continues over a lifetime, and the possibility of progression is always present. Another aspect that frequently is not considered is that the disease process is invisible and any limitations or disability suffered by the patient may not be obvious to others as would a disability restricting a patient to a wheelchair.

Coronary atherosclerotic heart disease can therefore be described as a disabling, life-threatening, chronic disease. Realizing the scope of this illness helps one to better understand the disease and perhaps be able to more quickly and easily accept what has happened and begin to adjust. With this insight both the nurse and the patient should be better prepared to actively approach rehabilitation from a constructive, positive viewpoint.

Causes of disability

Disability from any disease results from three primary sources: physiologic causes, psychosocial aspects, and vocational problems. Physiologic sources specific to coronary atherosclerotic heart disease are chest pain, left ventricular failure, and cardiac arrhythmias. These causes, discussed in detail in other sections of this text, are of real concern in the management of this disease. Psychosocial and vocational sources can be just as significant and are considered in this chapter as they relate to cardiac rehabilitation.

In addition to the impact of the chronic aspect of coronary atherosclerotic disease the acute aspect of the illness must be understood. The initial awareness of the disease may be a sudden traumatic clinical event. An acute myocardial infarction is certainly a crisis event when one realizes that it threatens not only life itself but the general health of a person, his self-esteem, pleasures, income, job, and role in his family. In fact, there is hardly an aspect of his life or life-style that is not affected. The most common initial responses are those of anxiety, depression, denial and fear of death, disability, and recurrence. There can be family problems related to the role reversal resulting at least temporarily from the illness and the overall effect of emotional stress on the patient and his family. The diversity and complexity of the acute psychosocial responses dramatically illustrate the need for immediate and individualized attention.

Initial patient responses may even have an effect on rehabilitation potential. Those who are more aggressive are usually more prone to denial and less willing to change. The rehabilitation of this type of individual is usually rather frail. Often it seems that education is not making any difference in them, but the key in taking care of this type of patient is persistence. They do learn and accept some of what is taught that may make a difference in their care, and if education and follow-up care are regularly provided, even though denial remains, it seems that some progress can be made. Patients who have a regressive response, usually demonstrated by those who are rather dependent individuals, frequently are unable to make a good adjustment to their illness. It is often thought that rehabilitation is difficult or next to impossible in this type of person. Early rehabilitation, however, might make a difference through the approach of encouraging independence early in the course of the illness. A constructive response to an illness is of course the most advantageous. This type of individual can learn to adapt to the illness; he is willing to work with the program and try to change as much as possible. This demonstrates a good rehabilitative effort. A comprehensive rehabilitation approach should help develop a more constructive response in a large number of individuals.

Healing of infarction

The actual stages of the healing of infarction provide some direction in the timing of the approach to the return of physical activity for the patient. Historically, it had been thought that one must rest during the healing process because of the belief that exertion would cause arrhythmias, reinfarction, ventricular aneurysm formation, or myocardial rupture. A review of the stages of the healing of infarction, as described by Mallory, White, and Salcedo-Salgar,[4] supports the fact that low-level physical activity might be safe at an earlier time in the healing process. As they described it, the first stage of leukocytic infiltration takes place during the first week after myocardial damage. This is the period of time that the myocardi-

um is weakest and is the time in which activity should be limited. During the second week after damage there is removal of necrotic tissue. Active scar formation actually begins in the third week after damage and continues on for full scar maturation up to 12 weeks after damage, depending on the size of the infarcted area. This would lend credence to the fact that low-level activity could be permitted after the first week of damage with a progressive increase in activity over the next 3 months.

A recent review by Brammell[5] of early ambulation and progressive activity points out that generally there is no evidence that early mobilization is harmful for most patients, but that it must certainly be individualized and that vocational and psychosocial viability are enhanced by early rehabilitation. With the realization and acceptance over the years that progressive in-hospital activity can be both safe and valuable, rehabilitation activity goals have been defined and programs designed to meet them.

Simply, in-hospital activity goals should be to prevent deconditioning and to begin to establish the idea of reconditioning for the patient; the activity goal for out-patient rehabilitation should be to promote conditioning.

Energy cost of activities

Before discussing actual cardiac progressive activity programs, it is important that the nurse has an understanding of the energy cost of activities so she can help the patient understand activity restrictions and prescriptions. The basic measurement of energy or the one most commonly used today is the metabolic equivalent (met), which is equal to the amount of oxygen consumed per kilogram of body weight per minute. One met is the amount of oxygen consumed at rest, seated, and is approximately 3.5 cc O_2/kg of body weight/min. Energy cost is expressed in multiples of this measurement. In the past the calorie has been a common measurement of energy cost and is still used by some today. The large calorie (kilocalorie) of energy represents the heat (energy) required to raise the temperature of 1 kg of water from 0° to 1° C. A person lying quietly consumes approximately 1 calorie (cal) of energy or 200 cc O_2/min. Since calories are based on total

Table 47-1. Caloric expenditure or metabolic equivalents of energy required for miscellaneous activities for 70 kg man*

Activity	Cal/min	Mets	Activity	Cal/min	Mets
Hospital			Vocational		
Bedrest	1.0	1	Watch repairing	1.6	1.5
Sitting	1.2	1	Radio assembly	2.7	2.5
Dangling feet, 5 min	1.5	1	Sewing/machine	2.9	2.5
Standing/relaxed	1.4	1	Bricklaying	4.0	3.5
Eating	1.4	1	Plastering	4.1	3.5
Conversing	1.4	1	Wheeling barrow, 115 lb/2.5 mph	5.0	4.0
Dressing/undressing	2.3	2	Carpentry	6.8	5.5
Washing hands/face	2.5	2	Mowing lawn/hand	7.7	6.5
Using bedside commode	3.6	3	Felling tree	8.0	6.5
Walking, 2.5 mph	3.6	3	Shoveling	8.5	7.0
Showering	4.2	3.5	Ascending stairs, 17 lb load/27 feet/min	9.0	7.5
Using bedpan	4.7	4	Recreational		
Walking downstairs	5.2	4.5	Painting/sitting	2.0	1.5
Walking, 3.5 mph	5.6	5.5	Playing piano	2.5	2
Propulsion/wheelchair	2.4	2	Driving car	2.8	2
Ambulation/braces, crutches	8.0	6.5	Canoeing, 2.5 mph	3.0	2.5
Housework			Horseback riding/slowly	3.0	2.5
Sewing/hand	1.4	1	Playing volleyball	3.0	2.5
Sweeping floor	1.7	1.5	Bowling	4.4	3.5
Sewing/machine	1.8	1.5	Cycling, 5.5 mph	4.5	3.5
Polishing furniture	2.4	2	Running	5.0	4
Peeling potatoes	2.9	2.5	Swimming, 20 yd/min	5.0	4
Scrubbing/standing	2.9	2.5	Jogging, 5 mph	5.6	7-9
Washing small clothes	3.0	2.5	Walking briskly, 3.5 mph	5.6	5-7
Kneading dough	3.3	2.5	Dancing	5.5	4.5
Scrubbing floors	3.6	3	Gardening	5.6	4.5
Cleaning windows	3.7	3	Playing tennis	7.1	6
Making beds	3.9	3	Riding horse/trotting	8.0	6.5
Ironing/standing	4.2	3.5	Spading	8.6	7
Mopping	4.2	3.5	Skiing	9.9	8
Hanging wash	4.5	3.5	Playing squash	10.2	8.5
			Cycling, 13 mph	11.0	9

*Modified from Zohman, L. R., and Tobis, J. S.: Cardiac rehabilitation, New York, 1970, Grune & Stratton, Inc., pp. 46-47.

oxygen consumption for total body weight with most tables based on the values for a 70 kg man, mets seems to be a better measurement to use in that it is based on body weight per kilogram. Therefore persons of different sizes can be given an activity prescription in mets that really provides the same relative amount of energy for the activity. Table 47-1 lists various activities with the required expenditures. There are numerous references that can be helpful in determining appropriate activities for specific energy levels.[5-8] Energy levels can also be associated with the functional class of cardiac patients, as indicated in Table 47-2. Activity can thus be prescribed by matching the patient's functional capacity with activities requiring similar energy expenditure, but it is important also to consider other factors that might affect the person's level of perfor-

Table 47-2. The relationship between functional classification, mets, and oxygen consumption*

Functional class	Mets	VO$_2$ (cc/kg/min)
I. No limitations; no symptoms with ordinary activity	7 & >	24.5 & >
II. Slight limitation, comfortable at rest, symptoms with ordinary activity	5-6	17.5-21.0
III. Marked limitation, comfortable at rest, symptoms with less than ordinary activity	3-4	10.5-14.0
IV. Discomfort with any activity, may have symptoms at rest	1-2	3.5-7.0

*Modified from New York Heart Association Functional Classification.

mance, such as his personality, emotional stresses, and the environment.[5]

Energy cost of activities is certainly an important fundamental to the progressive activity programs of cardiac rehabilitation. It will be utilized in the outpatient reconditioning phase as well, and other fundamentals such as types of activities and activity counseling will be further discussed with that phase.

CARDIAC REHABILITATION: INPATIENT PROGRAM

Since cardiac rehabilitation is a program of comprehensive care that should be individualized to the cardiac patient and the community, there is no one recommended cardiac rehabilitation program. There are, in fact, a number of inhospital programs that have been developed over the years and that are in practice throughout the nation. Information presented in this chapter is from the program at the University of Colorado Health Sciences Center, Denver, Colorado.

The design and goals of this program are derived from the philosophy and principles of comprehensive care described earlier in this chapter. There are three main components of the inpatient program of the University of Colorado Health Sciences Center: (1) progressive mobilization, (2) patient education, and (3) psychosocial and vocational evaluation and intervention. The goals of

this comprehensive care program are basically twofold: The first is to improve the *quality* of life through educating the patient and his family about the disease process and how to best care for himself, by attempting to maintain psychosocial integrity, and by helping return the patient to activities and work as early as possible. The second main goal is to extend life or to improve the *quantity* of life. This is primarily achieved through risk factor identification and modification and through the optimization of medical and/or surgical treatment of the patient, both of which should also contribute to improvement of the quality of life.

■ Who are candidates for cardiac rehabilitation?

Any person with coronary atherosclerotic heart disease should be a candidate for comprehensive care with the inhospital and outpatient phases individualized according to his needs. This would include those who suffer an acute event such as myocardial infarction or angina or coronary artery bypass surgery for example. Outpatient candidates include those who have had a critical cardiac medical or surgical event and really any person who is at high risk of acquiring or suspected to have coronary atherosclerotic heart disease.

Cardiac rehabilitation team

The cardiac rehabilitation team is a group of professionals working together to provide comprehensive care to a person with cardiac disease. The members of the team are determined primarily by those individuals available in the community setting to provide this care. The patient is a key member of the team. Whatever is done should be directed to his benefit. The physician is the best one to direct the program both for the medical/legal aspects involved and for relationships with the medical community. He is responsible for directing the medical/surgical management of the patient and can be very helpful in the total aspects of the program. The nurse is a clinician, educator, and administrator and is usually the coordinator of the program and the patient's care. A physical therapist and occupational therapist are especially helpful in assisting with inhospital progressive activities, patient education, and outpatient reconditioning. Other valuable team members are the clinical psychologist or psychiatrist, medical social worker, vocational rehabilitation counselor, dietitian, exercise physiologist, and any other professional who may be identified to contribute to the care of a particular patient at any time. It is important that these members meet together on a regular basis to discuss the patients being followed and to continue their own education so that the philosophy and care approaches are consistent and optimal for the patient.

Progressive activity programs

Progressive activity programs must be individualized according to the prevailing critical care practices and philosophies in each community. The activity programs of the University of Colorado Health Sciences Center are purposely designed to be simple, progressive mobilization type activity programs, utilizing activities of daily living and walking. The activities for the acute myocardial infarction patient, the patient with unstable angina, and the postcoronary artery bypass surgery patient are all similar except the time of initiation of activities varies owing to the different lengths of hospitalization. The average stay of the bypass patient is approximately 7 to 10 days, and the average hospital stay for the angina patient is 5 days, depending on his condition and needs for medical management. The program for the acute myocardial infarction patient is usually longer, approximately 10 to 14 days, to allow time for early healing of the myocardial necrosis. The programs are designed to safely mobilize the patient after an acute clinical event, while monitoring his responses to the increased activities and educating the patient about these responses and his management.

Post myocardial infarction progressive mobilization

The activities of the acute myocardial infarction progressive activity program (see boxed material, p. 834) are divided into three main phases: the first is the acute phase during the stay in the coronary care unit; the semiacute phase begins with transfer out of the coronary care unit; and the third phase is the convalescent or predis-

charge phase, which allows for increased activity as tolerated by the patient. They are all comprised of low-level activities, progressing to a maximum of approximately 5 mets and provide an appropriate amount of activity to prevent deconditioning of the patient. The educational approach is directed toward developing the idea of reconditioning and providing activity guidelines for the patient to follow the first 2 weeks out of the hospital.

As one can see from the daily care activities, the patient is allowed or actually encouraged to be independent and help take care of himself as soon as his condition permits. This early independence is very important in preventing depression and developing an awareness that the individual will soon be able to return to as normal an active life as possible.

Actually, independent activities often require less energy expenditure than the old total care approach. It is much easier, for example, for the patient to sit up in the chair at the bedside, rather than to be rolled about in the bed while one makes an occupied bed for him. Use of the bedside commode is another activity that is much less stressful than the terribly unnatural act of using a bedpan in the bed. Feeding oneself is another way of decreasing the stress compared to being "spoon-fed" by the nurse. The key is to remember that we are trying to assist the patient to temporarily limit energy expenditure and the work load on his heart. Considering the patient's personality and his condition, his care should be approached in whatever way possible to limit physical and emotional stress. It is also our responsibility to help the patient and his family understand the need for decreased work load on the heart during the early phase in order to reduce their anxiety and ensure their cooperation and participation in the program.

The activity form is kept on a clipboard at the foot of the patient's bed so that it is easily accessible, and everyone is encouraged to write comments regarding the patient's activities and responses to activity in order to optimize the individual plan of care. The patient and his family are also involved in the activity plan and are encouraged to record activity responses and pulse rates when they monitor his activity. Physical thera-

University of Colorado Health Sciences Center

ACUTE MYOCARDIAL INFARCTION
CARDIAC REHABILITATION PROGRESSIVE ACTIVITY PROGRAM

Type/location of event _____ Date of event _____

	Date	Hr	Activity/comments	Instructions

Acute phase (1-4 days)—coronary care unit (1-2 mets)
Complete bedrest until pain remits
  1. Orientation to rehabilitation program
  2. Bedside commode
  3. Feed self
  4. Active foot exercises
  5. Sit at bedside for meals and partial AM care (wash hands, face, brush teeth)
  6. May sit in chair for bedmaking and stand to be weighed
  7. Sit in chair up to 3 times daily*				

Semiacute phase (4-10 days)—transfer to ward (2-3 mets)
First day out of CCU
  1. Walk to bathroom
  2. Up in chair 3-4 times daily*
  3. Sponge bath seated
  4. Walk in room
  5. Bedside exercises
Second day out of CCU
  1. Up in chair as tolerated
  2. Sponge bath seated or standing*
  3. Walk in room ad lib
  4. Walk in hall
  5. Bedside exercises
Third day out of CCU
  1. Sponge bath or shower*
  2. Walk in hall
  3. Bedside exercises
Fourth day out of CCU
  1. Sponge bath or shower*
  2. Walk in hall
  3. Bedside exercises
Fifth day out of CCU
  1. Tub bath or shower
  2. Continue all prior activities*				

Discharge phase (10-14 days)—ward (3-5 mets)
Sixth day through discharge
  1. Continue activities   3. Activity counseling
  2. Stairs before discharge

Progressive activity will be individualized according to patient's needs and condition and should be increased as tolerated using signs and symptoms and heart rate guidelines: maximum heart rate increase of 16 to 20 beats/min over resting heart rate for any activity. Specific exercise instructions (intensity, frequency, duration) will be given each patient.

Absolute/relative contraindications: shock, CHF, uncontrolled ventricular arrhythmias, angina.

*As tolerated or instructed.

pists and occupational therapists are responsible for monitoring the patients and introducing all of these activities as well as educating the patient regarding these activities, his care, the coronary atherosclerotic disease process, and return to activities. Whoever is monitoring the patient should have knowledge of untoward symptoms and be experienced in the recognition of any signs and symptoms of intolerance to activity, including resting heart rate increase and signs of congestive heart failure, angina, orthostatic intolerance, and arrhythmias. They should also be able to take blood pressures and apical heart rates and be certified in cardiopulmonary resuscitation. It is very important that the patient and his family also be trained to observe for any untoward symptoms.

As indicated on the progressive activity sheet, the progressive activity will be individualized according to the patient's needs and condition and will be increased as tolerated using signs and symptoms and the heart rate guideline of a maximum heart rate increase of 16 to 20 beats/min over resting heart rate for any activity. This heart rate guideline is also followed by the patient during the 2 weeks of recovery at home until an actual clearance heart rate can be determined by an exercise evaluation. A progressive mobilization program safely assists the patient in his return to activities after an acute event and concomitantly provides a means for educating him regarding his disease and his rehabilitation.

Education program

Another major component of the inhospital rehabilitation program is education. To actively participate in the rehabilitation process one must be well informed regarding the disease and rehabilitation itself; as previously indicated this applies to everyone on the "team" including the patient. Education of the patient and family is certainly one of the primary responsibilities of the nurse—and one of the most challenging and rewarding. The "how to" of patient education is not discussed in this chapter but the principles, fundamentals, and practices of teaching and learning are vitally important, and it is the nurse's responsibility to learn how to be an effective educator. I encourage further reading of the many excellent articles written for nurses on patient education in the bibliography.

The focus of this chapter is the information useful to one involved in cardiac rehabilitation. For clarification, when patient education is discussed, it is understood that this includes education of the family—or anyone included in, affecting, or affected by this person's life.

The question of what to tell the patient was asked so often that an outline of information important to the understanding of coronary atherosclerotic heart disease and rehabilitation was developed (see boxed material on pp. 836 and 837). It was designed in simple outline form so as not to require a lot of "charting" time yet to provide an overview of content that could be easily individualized and utilized for a patient. The form, along with the progressive activity form, is kept on a clipboard at the foot of the patient's bed where it can be used easily and shared with the patient and family. The suggested topics of information are listed in outline form but this does not mean that the sections must be discussed in that sequence. Education must always be individualized to the patient and his readiness. The overview can also serve as a stimulus for the patient to ask questions.

In addition to one-on-one and group education, a variety of materials, both written and audiovisual, can be used to help educate the patient. There are useful pamphlets from the American Heart Association as well as a number of books published especially for the lay person. The important point is that the patient should have continued, consistent information, that there is ample time for reinforcement, and that it is presented in a way in which it is understood and can be used by him. This education process begins in the coronary care unit at a level appropriate to the patient and his condition. Many believe that the education should not be started while the patient is in the coronary care unit, but since there are many anxieties at this time education is important to the beginning rehabilitation process if only to help relieve the immediate anxieties. This information may have to be reinforced at a later time. Often, the family may be the ones who need the most contact at first. It is evident also that as the patient begins to feel better in the coronary care unit he usually asks questions about his return to activities. These should be answered as realistically as possible with the explanation that

CORONARY ATHEROSCLEROTIC HEART DISEASE
TEACHING OUTLINE

	Dates of		Comments
	Initial discussion	Rein-forcement	
I. General medical information			
A. The coronary atherosclerotic heart disease process			
B. The acute clinical event			
1. Myocardial infarction			
2. Angina pectoris			
3. Coronary artery bypass surgery			
C. Related anatomy and physiology to help understanding of how the heart functions in health and disease			
D. The healing process			
E. Patient's and family's concept and reaction			
II. Rehabilitation overview			
A. Definition			
B. Goals			
1. Comfortable, independent convalescent by hospital discharge			
2. Quality of life			
3. Quantity of life			
C. Rehabilitation team			
D. Duration of hospitalization			
E. Activity progression inhospital			
F. Activity modification			
G. Posthospital rehabilitation			
H. Outlook for continued employment			
III. Psychosocial aspects			
A. Reactions to acute event			
1. Intervention to assist with coping			
B. Financial considerations			
C. Family adjustments			
D. Individual problems and needs			
IV. Risk factor identification and modification			
A. Age, sex, heredity			
B. Smoking			
C. Hypertension			
D. Obesity			
E. Blood fats			
F. Diet			
G. Physical inactivity			
H. Personality/behavior			
I. Diabetes			
J. List patient's risk factors			
K. Specific recommendations			
V. Diet			
A. Cholesterol/saturated fats			
B. Triglycerides (carbohydrates and sugars)			
C. Calories			
D. Sodium			
E. Caffeine			
F. Alcohol			

CORONARY ATHEROSCLEROTIC HEART DISEASE
TEACHING OUTLINE—cont'd

	Dates of		Comments
	Initial discussion	Rein-forcement	
VI. Medications			
A. List patient's medications			
1. For each give: name, dose, schedule, action and purpose, side-effects			
B. Nitroglycerin			
1. Discuss how and when to use			
2. Action and side-effects			
VII. Activity guidelines			
A. Plan for return to activities			
B. Pulse taking and heart rate response			
C. Pacing activities			
D. Work simplification			
E. What to avoid			
F. Exercise			
1. Theory and benefits			
2. Types of exercise			
3. Warm-up exercise			
4. Individual prescription			
G. Specific activities			
1. Driving			
2. Altitude			
3. Sex			
4. Hobbies			
5. Chores			
6. Other			
VIII. Special information			
A. Warning symptoms			
B. Emergency care			
C. Follow-up appointment			
D. Community resources			
IX. Vocational aspects			
A. Return to work			
B. Employer/employee relationships			
C. Work modifications			
D. Special considerations			
X. Long-term management			
A. Prevention of another clinical event; improvement of preevent status			
B. Causes of disability			
1. Angina			
2. Pump failure			
3. Arrhythmias			
4. Psychosocial			
C. Diagnostic procedures			
D. Medical management			
E. Surgical management			

this information will be discussed later as well. It is not good to put off the answer to a question by saying it will be discussed later after he is out of the coronary care unit. This just creates or adds to the anxiety he may have at this time. Whenever a patient asks a question, he is indicating a concern or fear and a need for some information or explanation at that time.

General medical information

The first section of the teaching outline is very comprehensive in that it includes the anatomy and physiology of the heart and the disease process. The patient and his family need to understand what has happened to him, what happened to his heart and how it heals, and the coronary atherosclerotic heart disease process. An understanding of these facts and an awareness of their reactions to this illness will help provide a foundation for further learning about themselves and this disease.

Rehabilitation overview

The rehabilitation overview is often the section that is first discussed because first contact with the patient in the coronary care unit involves discussion of the rehabilitation team, progressive activity and education, and an explanation of what rehabilitation means. It is very important, both for their reassurance and cooperation, that the patient and his family have an idea of what to expect during the next few weeks.

Psychosocial aspects

The psychosocial aspects of cardiac disease are immense and can even be of greater importance in rehabilitation than physical limitations. Because of the diversity and impact of psychosocial responses to cardiac illness—both acute and chronic—the third main component of the in-hospital program is identified as psychosocial and vocational assessment and intervention. The nurse, through her frequent interactions with the patient, assumes a key and initial responsibility in this aspect of care and must be effective and comfortable in this position.

A very useful reference for nurses is an excellent article reviewing behavioral responses following an acute myocardial infarction written by Cynthia Scalzi.[9] She identified three main phases of adaptation: The first phase is shock and disbelief, which includes behavioral responses such as anxiety, denial, and aggressive sexual behavior. The second phase is the developing of awareness during which depression and anger are frequently manifested. Resolution is the third phase during which the patient may experience all of the previous behavioral responses. It is very important that nurses understand these behavioral responses so they can assist the patient and his family in understanding why they are responding as they are and so they can better intervene to assist the family in coping with these responses to illness. Nurses must help patients understand that many of these responses are normal and a natural consequence of an acute event. It is also the nurse's responsibility to identify the need for others such as a social worker, clinical psychologist, or psychiatrist to assist in the process of assessment and intervention.

Practically speaking, the problems facing the patient recovering from an event such as a myocardial infarction include the patient's ability to accept and deal with his illness, family crises and changes, financial considerations, and problems surrounding the patient's work and the entire scope of quality of life. The patient and his family must be approached in a very individual way so that their identified problems and needs can be dealt with in a pragmatic and timely manner. A successful rehabilitative effort demands that nurses be understanding of what might occur in response to an illness, know how to deal with these responses, and be appropriate in their request for others to assist them and the patient and family in dealing with the psychosocial aspects of acute and chronic cardiac disease.

Risk factor identification and modification

Risk factor modification should be part of the treatment and prevention program of every patient with coronary atherosclerotic heart disease. Risk factor identification and modification can be easily initiated during the inpatient phase of rehabilitation. In fact, one should capitalize on the acute event phase because it provides a situation in which the patient's environment is controlled to some extent, and as a result of such an acute threat to life, the person usually has a sense of need to do something to prevent such an occurrence again. Therefore the patient should receive education as early as possible regarding the factors that are felt to contribute to his disease, and he should be assisted in identifying the particular factors that he needs to modify. Special attention should be given to the three major coronary risk factors—cigarette smoking, hypercholesterolemia, and hypertension. Not only is this a time during which no smoking and a judicious diet can be enforced, but the patient has the time to learn how he can participate in his care. Hopefully, nurses can utilize the early convalescent phase to motivate the patient to participate in a risk factor modification program in his behalf. Obviously, there are some risk factors that cannot be corrected or modified, but it is important that nurses identify those that the patient might have that can be changed and assist the patient in working on modifying these. It is important to help him keep in mind that it will not happen overnight and without a lot of effort; a continual effort over an extended period of time is required.

Of particular interest is the recognition of the importance of the person's personality or behavior or the way he responds to stresses. This personality was described by Friedman and Rosenman[10] as the type A personality and also identified as coronary prone behavior.[11] The type A person is frequently characterized as one who is very competitive, hard-driving, time conscious, often tense and anxious, and eager to gain recognition and status. Friedman recently wrote the following, "Most Type A behavior—especially the sense of time urgency and free-floating hostility—cannot be modified unless the subjects either avoid or learn how to respond in a different way to many of the struggle-inducing factors in their socioeconomic environments."[12] In line with this statement the current trend to modifying this personality type is through behavior modification or stress management. Personality or behavior can certainly be one of the most difficult risk factors to modify because it has been learned and practiced over many years time. But it is felt that new behavior can be learned and "old" behavior "unlearned" as a means of assisting this type person to modify a possible coronary risk factor.

In addition to helping the patient understand himself and his behavior, nurses can offer continued encouragement, support, and reinforcement.

Diet

Diet is also discussed with the emphasis being on a judicious diet that usually is a moderately low cholesterol, low triglyceride, and low calorie one. If a person is in need of specific dietary management, then a diet prescription is written and the patient and spouse are counselled by a dietitian. The American Heart Association's dietary pamphlets are very helpful handouts for the patient. Weight loss for the obese patient is generally very difficult and may require enrollment in a group weight-loss program. It certainly is a factor necessitating continued reinforcement and assistance from the health care team. A sodium-restricted diet may be prescribed for those patients suffering from left ventricular failure; otherwise, general recommendations such as seasoning food only lightly in cooking, adding no salt at the table, and avoiding highly salted foods are adequate for most patients. Moderate use of caffeine and alcohol is usually okay for most patients. Patients need to understand that caffeine is a stimulant and can cause increased heart rate, blood pressure, and arrhythmias. For the patient who is used to drinking coffee all day while he works, decaffeinated coffee should be substituted if he cannot decrease his intake. Alcohol in excess can decrease cardiac contractility, but occasional and moderate use of alcohol is acceptable. Patients taking tranquilizers, sedatives, or other such drugs should be cautioned regarding intake of alcohol.

Medications

Another important item listed on the outline is that of medications. It is the nurse's responsibility to make sure that the patient knows every medication that he is taking and what its purpose is and what the side-effects might be. While he is in the hospital, he should learn to identify them as he takes them. In line with the philosophy that the patient be an active participant in rehabilitation, he must therefore understand his medical management so that he can be a good observer of how he is responding to the medication prescribed and can identify problems early should they occur. Most every patient should have nitroglycerin on hand and know how to use it, when to use it, and what its action and side-effects are. He must also know about its proper storage and replacement. There are many ways and aids to help patients learn about their medications, but, again, the key is individualization. Medication cards are helpful. A daily time sheet with the medications set out for the day is a useful aid for those who have difficulty remembering whether they have taken their medications. Certainly if the patient himself is not responsible, the one helping take care of him and administering the medications should be taught about them.

Activity guidelines

Preparing the patient for return to activities of work, recreation, and reconditioning while he is in the hospital can alleviate a lot of anxieties and unknowns for the patient when he returns home. The old recommendation of "Take it easy" is simply inadequate and inconsiderate. The patient needs specific guidelines (a simple handout is very useful) plus an understanding of the physiologic responses to exercise, other activities, and stresses so he can use his own judgment in situations that arise so that he will not feel anxious about every move he makes. By the time of discharge from the hospital, the patient should know how to take his pulse, know his heart rate guidelines, and know the warning signs and symptoms. The patient needs to understand that the next few weeks at home are a continuation of his convalescence, that the healing process of his heart is continuing, and that it is a period of regaining strength and activity tolerance. In addition to the specifics of exercise, it is worthwhile to help the patient understand work simplification measures and pacing of activities. The key point is that this period of reduced activity is temporary and that he will gradually return to his usual activities plus prescribed reconditioning activities.

Special information

The best preparation for discharge is to make sure that all the patient's questions have been answered, that he has been given specific instructions, that education has been reinforced adequately, and that the patient demonstrates understanding of important guidelines and seems confident in his ability to manage his continued recovery at home. The patient and his family should have a person to contact with any questions or problems that might arise. They should also have information on how to obtain emergency care, and the family should be given suggestions as to what to do in case of an emergency. The patient should be given an appointment for his first outpatient visit and know what the next steps in his rehabilitation program will be. Those in need of other assistance should certainly be helped in contacting community resources available to them.

Vocational aspects

Return to work is commonly one of the early and major concerns of the patient. Even though the outcome, or full recovery, may not be known for a while, one can usually expect a patient to return to his previous employment or other work about 70% to 90% of the time after a myocardial infarction. Perhaps the only need might be to assist in communicating with the employer so that he can appreciate what has happened to his employee and know the anticipated time of return to work. The vocational rehabilitation counselor can be of great assistance with this aspect of rehabilitation. Sometimes there may need to be some modifications in the patient's job, maybe only temporarily, but this should be approached early with the employer so that he can understand and be supportive and helpful to the patient. Only occasionally will someone be unable to return to his previous employment. If this is the case, the vocational counselor can assist the patient in acquiring other employment, new training, or even education for new employment. Whichever the case, this is another facet of rehabilitation in which each patient needs to be individually managed and all special considerations approached for the benefit of the patient. Again, the quality of the patient's life and therefore the quality of his work should be considered. It is important that he enjoy as much as possible what he is doing and that it not be a stress that might be detrimental to his rehabilitation or continued lifestyle. Recognizing this, long-range follow-up counseling and management in the vocational aspects can be of significant value.

Long-term management

The last topic listed on the outline is included because education of the patient and his family is open-ended and continual. Nurses need to think of the long-term management and long-range goals, part of which is the prevention of another clinical event and the continued improvement of the preevent status, primarily through the risk-factor modifications. Other things listed, such as the causes of disability, diagnostic procedures, medical management, and surgical management, should be discussed as they come up in the patient's case or can be discussed just so he knows some of the terms and conditions that he might hear or read about. Again, it is part of the comprehensive approach to helping him understand coronary atherosclerotic heart disease.

• • •

This teaching outline, or any other type of teaching guideline, can be a useful educational tool. The point to be made is that there needs to be some organized, consistent approach to the education of the patient and his family during the inhospital cardiac rehabilitation program as well as during the outpatient program. The education must be individualized and must be continually reinforced. Even though education is a major component of the inpatient program, one should not expect patients to fully retain what has been taught or be able to recall all of what is regarded as important. Generally, the information becomes personalized as it is incorporated in practice during the first weeks out of the hospital. Education, both informal and formal, continued during the outpatient program and every time the patient is seen in follow-up visits is a significant, essential component of comprehensive care. Hopefully, at the time of discharge the patient will be an independent, motivated individual prepared to participate in his continued rehabilitation.

CARDIAC REHABILITATION: OUTPATIENT PROGRAM

Rehabilitation of the patient with coronary atherosclerotic heart disease after discharge from the hospital is a continuation of the comprehensive rehabilitation care program. The goals of the open-ended outpatient cardiac rehabilitation program are therefore the same as the overall program: to improve both the quality and quantity of the patient's life. Every time a patient is seen as an outpatient is a time to continue education and assessment of psychosocial adjustment. Evaluation of exercise tolerance and progressive exercise reconditioning are initiated during this phase. Vocational assessment and plans for return to work are pursued as well. Risk factor modification and optimization of medical/surgical management as needed are continued with immediate and long-term goals identified.

The first few months following an acute cardiac event are very important to the patient. It is the optimum time for teaching the patient how to participate in his own care and prevention program, to motivate him to modify his risk factors, to assist him in developing a positive attitude toward himself and his rehabilitation, and to assist him in attaining the best possible quality of life. Actually, this is a period of time for intensifying the approach to all the components of comprehensive rehabilitation. As with the inpatient program, there is no one specific way of doing this. The critical factor is the philosophy of comprehensive rehabilitation, whether it be approached by an individual practitioner or through an organized formal rehabilitation team and program. It is the nurse's responsibility to assist and to motivate the patient in every way possible to assume responsibility in his long-term management. In summary, every effort should be made to restore and maintain each individual with heart disease at his optimal physiologic, psychologic, social, and vocational status.

■ Who is a candidate?

Every person with coronary atherosclerotic heart disease should receive individualized outpatient rehabilitation care. In the past the advisability of the reconditioning component has been questioned. However, everyone can safely be evaluated to determine an individualized exercise prescription for activities of work, play, and reconditioning—no matter how limited his functional capacity. This determination can then be utilized to counsel the patient regarding activities and to develop a safe plan for reconditioning—

whether it be slow walking, just enabling a patient to resume activities of daily living if that be all he is capable of, or a regular aerobic exercise reconditioning program.

■ When should a patient be seen?

The timing of outpatient follow-up care will vary according to individual patient needs and conditions as well as the community practices and resources. Ideally, the patient should have had adequate preparation for the first weeks of convalescence at home during his hospital stay, and he should have someone available to contact for questions or problems; he should be seen as an outpatient approximately 2 weeks after discharge (or about 1 month after his acute event). An exercise evaluation to approximately 75% of age-corrected maximum heart rate or symptoms should be performed at this time. Succeeding visits, including exercise evaluations, should be 1 month later when the target heart rate should be limited to 85% of maximum or symptoms and then after another month, which would be 3 months after the acute event. At this time the myocardium should be fully healed to permit a symptom limited or maximally tolerated exercise evaluation. After each evaluation, an updated exercise prescription should be given the patient. Follow-up evaluation is recommended at 6 months after the acute event and every 6 months thereafter. This timetable for outpatient visits has proved to be safe, practical, and effective for the University of Colorado Health Sciences Center program; however, it is recognized that follow-up care will have to be adjusted according to available resources and patient needs. Basically, a patient should receive regular follow-up care of a comprehensive nature that is individualized to his person, his needs, and his condition. The patient should have an appointment made for his next regular visit at the end of each visit and educated to call if there is ever any change in his condition or any problem or concern identified.

Fundamentals of outpatient rehabilitation

No matter what kind of outpatient rehabilitative care or program is provided, the primary fundamentals of the overall cardiac rehabilitation program, just as with the philosophy and goals, apply. The additional fundamentals that are important to this phase of the program relate to the principles of exercise evaluation and exercise itself. Specific fundamentals or principles to be considered for outpatient rehabilitation include exercise evaluation, the exercise prescription, and exercise conditioning and guidelines.

The current consensus is that regular exercise enhances the quality of life and that it can be a safe, effective component of cardiac rehabilitation. A variety of potential direct or indirect benefits of exercise, ranging from the preventive aspects to those contributing to the improvement of quality of life, have been identified. Specifically, some of these are (1) improved exercise and work tolerance or increased functional capacity; (2) improved energy, productivity, and endurance or stamina; (3) improved ability to tolerate or cope with stress and tension; (4) its "tranquilizer" effect; (5) its prevention or treatment of depression; (6) decreased food intake or an aid to proper selection of foods eaten; (7) enhanced self-image; (8) an incentive to prudent living habits; and (9) its "ripple" effect. Regardless of objective results, from my experience appropriate exercise subjectively seems to make patients "feel better." Basically, the reconditioning or conditioning aspect of the rehabilitation process is one of the most "active" ways to help the patient modify risk factors and attain a desired quality of life whether the physical conditioning alone contributes to reducing the risk of inactivity and a sedentary lifestyle per se or whether it is through the "ripple" effect of assisting the patient to work on other risk factors such as weight loss and reduction of body fat and blood fats as well as the reduction of tension and stress. It has not yet been proved that exercise can modify the natural history of coronary atherosclerotic heart disease (improve the quantity of life); however, supportive evidence for its preventive value, whether it be due to a direct effect or from its secondary effects, seems to be increasing.

Recognizing the value of exercise and increased activity for patients with coronary atherosclerotic heart disease, it is imperative that health care professionals, and patients as well, understand the principles and techniques of exercise conditioning in order that it be a safe and effective component of the rehabilitation program.

Evaluation of exercise tolerance

An evaluation of exercise tolerance is required to determine the level of physical activity or exercise that is appropriate for a cardiac patient in regard to his clinical and functional status. As stated by the Committee on Exercise of the American Heart Association, "Exercise tolerance testing is the observation and recording of an individual's cardiovascular responses during a measured exercise challenge in order to determine his capacity to adapt to physical stress."[13] A number of objectives or indications for exercise testing are as follows: (1) to diagnose ischemic heart disease, (2) to evaluate functional capacity, (3) to evaluate chest pain or other anginal symptoms, (4) to evaluate arrhythmias, (5) to evaluate blood pressure or other clinical signs, (6) to educate the patient regarding symptoms or clinical signs, (7) to assess medical or surgical treatment, (8) to motivate an individual to exercise or adhere to a program of exercise, and (9) to determine appropriate parameters for an individualized exercise prescription.

Exercise testing obviously has many uses in the rehabilitation setting, but it must be administered by specially trained, knowledgeable, experienced professionals and monitored or closely supervised by a qualified physician. The exercise test can be individualized to the patient and objective by using one of a variety of protocols and methods. The most commonly used device is the motor-driven treadmill; other tests are designed to use steps, or bicycle or arm-cranking ergometers. The following are recommended principles and standards for exercise testing modified from the Committee on Exercise of the American Heart Association[14,15] and as practiced in the Cardiac Rehabilitation Laboratory at the University of Colorado Health Sciences Center:

1. Immediately prior to the test, a physical and cardiovascular examination and history should be done and a 12-lead resting electrocardiogram should be taken and interpreted.

2. Informed consent of the patient should be obtained prior to testing.
3. Emergency equipment, including a defibrillator, and appropriate drugs for emergency care must be in the room.
4. Personnel should be certified in cardiopulmonary resuscitation.
5. Although other parameters might also be monitored, the minimal requirements include heart rate, ECG, blood pressure, and symptoms and clinical signs, monitored at rest, every minute during exercise, and during recovery.
6. Multilevel work load tests as opposed to single level tests should be used and the amount of the work should be quantifiable.
7. A test should allow for a period of warm-up and begin at a work level below the estimated level of impairment.
8. The number of minutes at each stage of work load should be adequate to ensure that the individual's responses are stabilized.
9. Work loads should be progressively increased.
10. Commonly used criteria for terminating a test include:
    a. Attainment of maximum tolerated performance
    b. Attainment of an end point based on emergence of adverse signs or symptoms (symptom-limited performance)
    c. Attainment of a predetermined end point or target, such as a percentage of heart rate or arbitrary work load or diagnostic parameter

Exercise evaluation is a very useful yet complex tool that must be administered only by physicians and other professionals properly trained and experienced in this specialty. Only a general introduction to acquaint the reader with evaluating exercise has been presented. (See the bibliography for the specifics of testing protocols, reasons for stopping, contraindications to exercise, and interpretation of findings.)

Familiarity with the procedure will aid the nurse in properly preparing the patient for the evaluation and allaying his anxiety. From experience, use of the term "exercise evaluation" has seemed to be better accepted and understood by the patient as opposed to exercise test or stress test because the word "test" inappropriately implies a pass or fail performance. The safety, value, and technical aspects of the procedure as well as the reason for doing it and what the patient might expect and what to report should all be discussed.

After the evaluation, the results should be thoroughly explained to the patient; this can be an excellent learning and motivational experience for him. The findings also enable the physician to better manage and plan his patient's care.

The exercise prescription

Based on the results of the exercise evaluation, an individualized prescription can be written for activities for work, leisure, and exercise. It is important that health care professionals, as well as the patient, understand that the same principles that apply to prescription of medication should be followed. Exercise is a therapeutic agent designed to provide beneficial effects and, as such, has specific indications and contraindications and possible adverse reactions.[16] Four specific factors that must be considered in the exercise prescription are intensity, duration, frequency, and type of exercise or activity.

Intensity

Heart rate is the easiest and best measurement to use in developing the exercise prescription. Some of the reasons why heart rate is a desirable variable for controlling the intensity of exercise were discussed by Wilmore.[17] The heart rate represents a physiologic parameter that can be easily monitored by the individual and provides insight into the amount of metabolic and myocardial stress. The heart rate is independent of environmental factors. In other words, if an added stress, such as a temperature extreme or altitude, is encountered, the heart rate increase will reflect this, requiring the work load to be decreased in order to maintain the prescribed heart rate. In addition, since the heart rate response for a standardized amount of exercise decreases with training, the measured heart rate will reflect this change and permit a natural progression in actual work as exercise training continues.

The individualized heart rate prescription for measuring intensity is determined from the clearance heart rate established from the exercise evaluation and is called the target heart rate or training heart rate. The clearance heart rate is the maximum safe heart rate for any activity or exercise. It is the level at which the parameters of blood pressure, electrocardiographic repolar-

ization and rhythms, and symptoms are normal or within acceptable limits. Then, to allow for a margin of safety, 85% of the clearance heart rate is established as the peak target heart rate for exercise or any activity. The recommended intensity for exercise is a target heart rate within the range of 70% to 85% of the individual's clearance heart rate.

Duration

The exercise session should consist of three phases: a warm-up period of 5 to 10 minutes; a workout or aerobic exercise phase within the target heart rate range for 20 to 40 minutes; and a cool-down period of about 5 minutes. The duration of the exercise session should also be individualized by taking into account a person's physical capacity, including muscular and joint fitness and limitations, as well as cardiovascular fitness and limitations or symptoms.

Frequency

The frequency of exercise conditioning sessions should be three to five times a week.

Type of exercise

Exercises that increase metabolic functions and improve cardiorespiratory endurance are recommended for a physical conditioning program. Aerobic and isotonic exercises are of this type. Aerobic or dynamic exercise results in increased oxygen consumption through increased heart rate and systolic blood pressure and is the form of exercise most commonly utilized in conditioning programs. Aerobic activities include walking, jogging, running, bicycling, bench stepping, swimming, rhythmic calisthenics, rope jumping, and some types of sports, games, and dancing. Isotonic exercise involves the same muscle tone through a full range of joint motion, and when the weight or resistance is kept at a low level, the physiologic effects are similar to those of aerobic exercise. Low weight and frequent repetitions are necessary when using dumbbells and pulley-weights. Sit-ups and pull-ups are other common examples of isotonic exercises. A third type of exercise is isometric or static exercise, which involves exertion against a high or fixed resistance and results in little or no motion. Lifting heavy weights, Charles Atlas–type of exercises, and working with arms over the head involve isometric work. Isometric activities do not improve cardiovascular function, and because of the marked increase in both systolic and diastolic blood pressure and only slight or moderate increase in heart rate, isometric activities should be avoided by people with heart disease.

Conditioning programs

Whenever possible, it is recommended that patients with coronary atherosclerotic heart disease begin their exercise reconditioning program under medical supervision. Experience with the reconditioning program at the University of Colorado Health Sciences Center has shown that group exercise under close supervision and leadership and with telemetry monitoring during the early convalescent period of 1 to 3 months after a clinical event is safe and provides extremely valuable information for both the physician and the individual patient. The individualized exercise prescription, updated at monthly intervals, is carefully monitored and controlled while patients learn the principles of exercise. The camaraderie of the group and the informal educational setting, which includes a weekly group education class as well as individual education, are very beneficial

---

University of Colorado Health Sciences Center

CARDIAC REHABILITATION UNIT EXERCISE GUIDELINES

INTENSITY

Walk (jog) _____ mile(s) in _____ minutes. Your average heart rate should be from _____ to _____. These numbers are 70% and 85% of your maximum safe heart or clearance heart rate of _____ determined by your treadmill evaluation.

FREQUENCY

Exercise at least three to five times per week.

DURATION

Maintain your exercise 20 to 30 minutes at least.

TYPES OF EXERCISE RECOMMENDED

Walking, jogging, bicycling, and swimming are recommended. (Do not start until your doctor okays the exercise.) These are aerobic exercises—they help in your conditioning.
Avoid isometrics or static exercise (exertion without movement).

NOTE

To measure your heart rate count your pulse for 10 seconds and multiply by 6.
Do not exceed your clearance heart rate of _____.
Always "warm-up" 3 to 5 minutes. See warm-up exercises.
Allow for "cooling down" period—while you take your pulse move your legs in a walking motion while standing in place. Then, walk slowly 3 to 5 minutes before stopping.
Do not exercise soon after eating—wait approximately 2 hours.
Avoid exercising out-of-doors when the weather is severe—too cold or too hot. An indoor shopping mall is a good place to walk when the weather is bad.
No maximal efforts of any kind should be attempted.
Acceptable exercise sensations include moderate breathlessness, moderate fatigue, moderate sweating, and a *pleasant* sense of muscular fatigue.
Warning symptoms: Stop if you note chest pain, excessive shortness of breath, fatigue (more than expected for a particular activity), dizziness, light-headedness, irregular heartbeat, or nausea.

to these patients. As a result of the 8-week program, the patients have seemed better motivated and better educated to continue their exercise program in an unsupervised setting or to participate in other group programs.

Even though the number of supervised conditioning programs is increasing, many patients will not have the advantage of such a program. Reconditioning exercise should still be recommended to these patients, but they must be thoroughly educated on the principles of exercise and given individualized written guidelines (see boxed material on p. 845).

In general, the same principles and guidelines for exercise conditioning apply to both the supervised and unsupervised exercise settings. In addition to being appropriately individualized, exercise should be fun, have variety, and be acceptable and practical for the patient. A number of authors have published very useful information regarding the physiology, principles, and programs of exercise conditioning (see the bibliography). Nurses are in a key position to encourage and educate patients in this aspect of cardiac rehabilitation and with proper training can effectively coordinate, direct, assist, or participate in exercise conditioning programs for patients.

In summary, an individualized approach to the prescription of exercise is a safe, practical, and valuable component of cardiac rehabilitation. Two key factors in ensuring the success of individualized exercise, according to Wilmore,[18] are the provision of adequate education and the generation of the motivation needed to carry out the initial program with an appreciation that exercise is a lifetime pursuit.

SUMMARY

An overview of the rehabilitation of the patient with coronary atherosclerotic heart disease was presented in this chapter with the intent to stimulate an interest in and advocacy for the comprehensive care approach to the cardiac patient. A philosophy of comprehensive rehabilitation and some fundamentals of inpatient and outpatient cardiac rehabilitation programs were discussed to assist the nurse in becoming more knowledgeable of her role in cardiac rehabilitation. From my experience the practice of cardiac rehabilitation is as challenging, exciting, and rewarding as any

acute or critical care program. It fully utilizes all of one's talents and skills in nursing and interpersonal relationships and requires an understanding and appreciation of the entire natural history of coronary atherosclerotic heart disease. Through the art and science of comprehensive rehabilitation it is possible to improve the quality and hopefully the quantity of the lives of individuals with coronary atherosclerotic heart disease. Individualization of care is a prevailing factor and is a key to the success of a cardiac rehabilitation program. To accomplish this satisfactorily the nurse must learn about the patient as an individual person. It behooves one to follow Osler's advice to "Learn not only what kind of sickness this man has, but what kind of man has this sickness."[3]

REFERENCES

1. Groden, B. M.: Return to work after myocardial infarction, Scot. Med. J. **12:**297, 1967.
2. Naughton, J. P., and Hellerstein, H. K., editors: Exercise testing and exercise training in coronary heart disease, New York, 1973, Academic Press, Inc., p. 337.
3. White, P. D.: Rehabilitation of the cardiovascular patient, New York, 1958, McGraw-Hill Book Co., pp. 115-116.
4. Mallory, G. K., White, P. D., and Salcedo-Salgar, J.: Speed of healing of myocardial infarction: a study of the pathologic anatomy in seventy-two cases, Am. Heart J. **18:**647, 1939.
5. Brammell, H. L.: Early rehabilitation of the post infarction patient. In Long, C., editor: Prevention and rehabilitation in ischemic heart disease, Baltimore, The Williams & Wilkins Co. In press.
6. Colorado Heart Association: Exercise equivalents. Cardiac reconditioning and work evaluation unit, Denver, Colorado, 1970.
7. Exercise testing and training of individuals with heart disease or at high risk for its development: a handbook for physicians, The Committee on Exercise, American Heart Association, 1975, pp. 42-43.
8. American College of Sports Medicine: Guidelines for graded exercise testing and exercise prescription, Philadelphia, 1975, Lea & Febiger.
9. Scalzi, C. C.: Nursing management of behavioral responses following an acute myocardial infarction, Heart Lung **2**(1): 62, 1973.
10. Friedman, M., and Rosenman, R.: Type A behavior and your heart, New York, 1974, Alfred A. Knopf.
11. Glass, D. C.: Behavior patterns, stress and coronary disease, New Jersey, 1977, Lawrence Erlbaum Associates, pp. 23-24.
12. Friedman, M.: Modifying "type A" behavior in heart attack patients, Primary Cardiology, p. 11, Jan., 1978.
13. Exercise testing and training of individuals with heart disease or at high risk for its development: a handbook for

physicians, The Committee on Exercise, American Heart Association, 1975, p. 11.

14. Exercise testing and training of individuals with heart disease or at high risk for its development: a handbook for physicians, The Committee on Exercise, American Heart Association, 1975.

15. Exercise testing and training of apparently healthy individuals: a handbook for physicians, The Committee on Exercise, American Heart Association, 1972.

16. Exercise testing and training of individuals with heart disease or at high risk for its development: a handbook for physicians, The Committee on Exercise, American Heart Association, 1975, p. 24.

17. Wilmore, J. H.: Individualized exercise prescription. In Amsterdam, E. A., Wilmore, J. H., and DeMaria, A. N., editors: Exercise in cardiovascular health and disease, New York, 1977, Yorke Medical Books, p. 270.

18. Wilmore, J. H.: Individualized exercise prescription. In Amsterdam, E. A., Wilmore, J. H., and DeMaria, A. N., editors: Exercise in cardiovascular health and disease, New York, 1977, Yorke Medical Books, p. 273.

BIBLIOGRAPHY

Abdellah, F. G.: The physician-nurse team approach to coronary care, Nurs. Clin. North Am. 7:423, 1972.

Amsterdam, E., Wilmore, J., and DeMaria, A., editors: Exercise in cardiovascular health and disease, New York, 1977, Yorke Medical Books.

Baden, C. A.: Teaching the coronary patient and his family, Nurs. Clin. North Am. 7:563, 1972.

Boggs, B., Malone, D., and McCulloch, C.: A coronary teaching program in a community hospital, Nurs. Clin. North Am. 13(3):457, 1978.

Burch, G. E., and DePasquale, N. P.: Potentials and limitations of patients after myocardial infarction, Am. Heart J. 72: 830, 1966.

Cay, E. L., Vetter, N. J., and Phillips, A. E.: Practical aspects of cardiac rehabilitation: psychosocial factors, G. Ital. Cardiol. 3:646, 1973.

Dock, W., et al.: Physician's roundtable: five experts spell out post-MI communication, Patient Care, July 1, 1975.

Exercise testing and training of apparently healthy individuals: a handbook for physicians, The Committee on Exercise, American Heart Association, New York, 1972.

Exercise testing and training of individuals with heart disease or at high risk for its development: a handbook for physicians, The Committee on Exercise, American Heart Association, New York, 1975.

Farquhar, J. W.: The American way of life need not be hazardous to your health, New York, 1978, W. W. Norton & Co., Inc.

Fox, S. M., III, Naughton, J. P., and Haskell, W. L.: Physical activity and the prevention of coronary heart disease, Ann. Clin. Res. 3:404, 1971.

Frank, K. A., Heller, S. S., and Kornfeld, D. S.: A survey of adjustment to cardiac surgery, Arch. Intern. Med. 130:735, 1972.

Friedman, M., and Rosenman, R. H.: Type A behavior and your heart, New York, 1974, Alfred A. Knopf.

Garrity, T. F., and Klein, R. F.: Emotional response and clinical severity as early determinants of six-month mortality after myocardial infarction, Heart Lung 4:730, 1975.

Gentry, W. D., and Haney, T.: Emotional and behavioral reaction to acute myocardial infarction, Heart Lung 4:738, 1975.

Gorlin, R.: Coronary artery disease, Philadelphia, 1976, W. B. Saunders Co.

Heinzelmann, F., and Bagley, R. W.: Response to physical activity programs and their effects on health behavior, Public Health Rep. 85:905, 1970.

Holland, J. M.: Cardiovascular nursing: prevention, intervention, and rehabilitation, Boston, 1977, Little, Brown & Co.

Holub, N., Edlund, P., and Keenan, P.: Family conferences as an adjunct to total coronary care, Heart Lung 4:767, 1975.

Hurst, J. W., Logue, R. B., Schlant, R. C., and Wenger, N. K.: The heart, ed. 4, New York, 1978, McGraw-Hill Book Co.

Kos, B. A.: The nurse's role in rehabilitation of the myocardial infarction patient, Nurs. Clin. North Am. 4:593, 1969.

Naughton, J. P., and Hellerstein, H. K., editors: Exercise testing and exercise training in coronary heart disease, New York, 1973, Academic Press, Inc.

Netter, F. H.: The CIBA collection of medical illustrations. The heart, Vol. 5, CIBA Pharmaceutical Company, 1969.

Phibbs, B.: The human heart: a guide to heart disease, ed. 4, St. Louis, 1979, The C. V. Mosby Co.

Rahe, R. H., Scalzi, C., and Shine, K.: A teaching evaluation questionnaire for postmyocardial infarction patients, Heart Lung 4:759, 1975.

Redman, B. K.: The process of patient teaching in nursing, ed. 3, St. Louis, 1976, The C. V. Mosby Co.

Sonnenblick, E. H., and Lesch, M., editors: Exercise and heart disease, New York, 1977, Grune & Stratton, Inc.

Stocksmeier, U., editor: Psychological approach to the rehabilitation of coronary patients, International Society of Cardiology Scientific Council on Rehabilitation of Cardiac Patients, Berlin, 1976, Springer-Verlag.

Tobis, J., and Zohman, L. R.: Rehabilitating the coronary patient, Postgrad. Med. 47:139, 1970.

Wenger, N. K., editor: Exercise and the heart, Philadelphia, 1978, F. A. Davis Co.

Wenger, N. K., and Hellerstein, H. K., editors: Rehabilitation of the coronary patient, New York, 1978, John Wiley & Sons, Inc.

Wilson, P. K.: Adult fitness and cardiac rehabilitation, Baltimore, 1975, University Park Press.

Wishnie, H., Hackett, T. P., and Cassem, N. H.: Psychological hazards of convalescence following myocardial infarction, J.A.M.A. 215:1292, 1971.

Zander, K. S., et al., editors: Practical manual for patient-teaching, St. Louis, 1978, The C. V. Mosby Co.

Zohman, L. R., and Tobis, J. S.: Cardiac rehabilitation, New York, 1970, Grune & Stratton, Inc.

CHAPTER 48

Dark skins: recognizing and interpreting color changes

Lora B. Roach

Mr. Cy N. Otic was just admitted to the critical care unit following major trauma to the chest and abdomen. He is suspected of having "internal injuries," therefore the nurses will be observing him closely for evidence of internal hemorrhage (ruptured spleen and/or liver), cardiac tamponade, and pulmonary bruising. The nurses begin their initial assessment with dismay. His skin is coal-black; how will they ever recognize the pallor, cyanosis, or abdominal ecchymoses that are such important clues for the suspected disorders?

Assessment problems comparable to the one just described are commonly encountered by nurses, physicians, and paramedics in critical care areas and at the scenes of accidents because a substantial number of trauma victims and critically ill persons have darkly pigmented skin. These assessment problems are not as troublesome as they seem, however, because a person who has the ability to discriminate color variations in light skin can learn to recognize color changes in heavily pigmented skin.

■ Why is the skin called a "mirror for disease"?

The skin is a large and highly visible organ, encompassing approximately 1.5 to 2 m² of tissue (adult). The outer layer (epidermis) is thin and normally translucent, allowing the colors of the underlying layer (dermis) to be seen. The reddish and bluish color tones are reflections of the blood in the superficial capillaries and venous plexuses of the dermis. Disease conditions that change the character and quality of the blood and blood vessels are accordingly mirrored by the skin as color changes (pallor, cyanosis, flushing, purpura). Conditions that disturb the genetically determined balance of melanin, melanoid, and carotene deposits will be mirrored by the skin as increased, decreased, or irregular pigmentation. Abnormal pigments such as bilirubin, methemoglobin, silver, and quinacrine are also visible under the epidermis.

■ How does dark skin differ from light skin?

Except for genetic anomalies such as the albino, people of all races have approximately the same number of melanocytes (the cells that produce melanin). However, these cells, which are located along the junction of the dermis and epidermis, produce melanin in varying amounts in response to genetic, hormonal, or environmental stimuli. Genetic control determines whether the skin will have large amounts of dark pigment (Negro race), a lesser amount of brown pigment (Indian, Latin races, and others), or the yellowish pigment of Oriental races. Hormonal and environmental stimuli (especially exposure to sunlight) can cause increased production and irregular distribution of melanin.

At birth, pigmentation is very light, but it gradually darkens until it reaches maximum intensity at 6 to 8 weeks of age. Persons with heavily pigmented skin generally have a normal distribution of melanin similar to that of lighter pigmented skin. Most persons have evenly distributed pigmentation, but some display nonpathogenic irregularities (for example, freckles, chloasma, vitiligo). Skin areas exposed to the elements and those with a heavier layer of subcutaneous tissue are usually darker than the thinner and protected areas. Heavy pigmentation conceals the normal reddish skin tone, but its presence provides a healthy glow that becomes particularly noticeable in its absence.

Even in persons with very heavily pigmented skin, there are areas with little or no melanin deposits. The palms and soles of the feet (except in the creases) are relatively free of melanin, but if they are calloused, heavy deposits of carotene and carotenoid may obscure the underlying red and blue tones. Nail beds are usually free of melanin, but some blacks have irregular deposits that may impede color evaluation or may be mistaken for petechiae. Similarly, some blacks have patchy deposits of melanin in the mucous membranes (conjuctiva, sclera, oral mucosa), although these areas are usually free of pigmentation. Full-blooded Negroes often have a normal bluish coloration of the gums, distributed evenly or in irregular patches. Some dark-skinned people, particularly of Mediterranean origin, have distinctly blue lips, giving the appearance of cyanosis.

■ Are specialized skills needed for assessing color changes in dark skin?

Good *color sensitivity* is essential in identifying color changes in any kind of situation. Color blindness will severely impair the ability to recognize early, subtle pallor of preshock and the first bluish tints of developing cyanosis. Some persons have no physiologic disturbance in color identification, but they lack *color awareness*. These individuals need to make frequent deliberate observations of skin and mucosal color to develop a greater sensitivity to color changes.

A good *memory* for the patient's normal color is also necessary in recognizing subtle changes. Again, deliberate practice will prove helpful because people are more likely to remember the degree of darkness (for example, black, brown, tan) than the *total* color, which includes the underlying reddish tone. *Change in this normal reddish tone is the most frequent visible warning of impending danger to a patient.*

Palpation is a useful complement to inspection because many color changes are accompanied by other signs. For example, the pallor of vasoconstriction is usually accompanied by cooling and increased moisture of the skin and perhaps a less perceptible pulse. The redness of inflammation is accompanied by heat and swelling. Sensitive fingertips may be used to determine changes in contour, texture, elasticity, and moisture of the skin. The top (dorsal) surface of the fingers should be used for checking skin temperature differences because it is more sensitive to heat and cold than the palmar surface.

■ What equipment is needed for assessing skin color?

Sunlight provides the best light source for accurate color interpretation, but its use is impractical in most intensive care units. Some units have lighting systems that simulate daylight, but the majority have fluorescent lights that may vary in color, some causing a rather bluish tint to the skin and others a yellowish or greenish tint. It is important to know the limitations of the basic light source and to have supplemental sources available. Stand lights with bulbs of at least 60 watts are useful in nullifying the false color of fluorescent light. Flashlights with fresh batteries and a diffusing lens, rather than a spot lens, are very useful for examining less accessible areas such as inside the mouth.

Other useful supplies include a glass slide, magnifying glass, or piece of firm clear plastic that can be pressed against the skin for inspection (diascopy) of noncompressible color and for assessing capillary filling time. A small lighted magnifying lens (or an otoscope) can be helpful for distinguishing small hemorrhagic lesions (petechiae) from natural pigmentation of the conjunctiva, oral mucosa, and nail beds.

■ What variables complicate the interpretation of skin color?

In addition to the degree of color sensitivity and the quality of the light source, a large number of factors may influence the accuracy of skin color interpretation. Psychologic factors such as fear and anger may cause peripheral vasoconstriction that produces a false pallor; embarrassment may result in a flushing that masks pallor or produces a false erythema. Excessive warmth (for example, a light source that produces heat) also produces a concealing vasodilatation. A chilly environment (for example, an air conditioned room or cold examining table) and cigarette smoking cause marked peripheral vasoconstriction with pallor and cooling of the terminal extremities, which, in turn, reduces the accuracy of nail bed color and the capillary filling test. Marked vasoconstriction will also prevent cyanosis even though serious hypoxemia is present.

The force of gravity has a distinct effect on skin color. In the presence of adequate circulation, prolonged elevation of an extremity will produce a slight normal pallor and coolness that must be considered when checking for circulatory integrity. The extremity positioned lower than heart level will normally have slightly distended veins, increased redness, and obvious warmth when compared to the extremity resting at heart level.

Prolonged inactivity of an extremity (for example, an arm immobilized by an intravenous infusion) will result in slowed circulation and lowered cellular metabolism of the part. The skin will be cool and pale, and nail beds will be pale with a slightly prolonged capillary filling time.

Edema reduces the intensity of skin color because the excess fluid lies between the skin surface and the pigmented and vascular layers. The resultant pallor may be misleading and will obscure early evidence of cyanosis, jaundice, and erythema. Always check for the presence of edema when observing for color change.

Extraneous products such as cosmetics, dust, and stains may obscure color changes, and unskilled removal of these products may add to the problem causing erythema, excoriation, or rash. Prevent these complications by minimizing the use of friction and irritant chemicals. For example, use cream or lotion to remove lipstick with a minimum of friction.

To accurately interpret color change, you need to prevent or control as many of the distracting variables as possible. The first step is to be astutely aware of their actual or potential presence. Most of the undesirable environmental situations can be corrected easily once they are rec-

ognized. The psychologic problems require a special sensitivity for recognition. Once you recognize them, spend a little time and effort to provide the needed information, reassurance, distraction, or privacy for surprisingly successful results.

■ **What is the significance of pallor?**

Pallor in the dark-skinned patient is a manifestation of diminished vascular perfusion of the skin and mucous membranes. The diminished perfusion may be a relatively insignificant problem such as peripheral vasoconstriction owing to a cold environment, cigarette smoking, or fear. More often, pallor of a degree perceptible in darkly pigmented skin signifies serious problems such as anemia, shock, or local arterial insufficiency (arterial spasm, obstruction, or disease). Pallor may be diffuse or localized, as determined by systemic or local disruption of perfusion.

■ **How do you assess pallor in dark-skinned patients?**

Even when a patient's skin is heavily pigmented, pallor can be detected by anticipatory observation for the characteristic changes:

BLACK SKIN: Color becomes ashen-gray, losing the healthy glow of the underlying reddish tone.
BROWN SKIN: Color becomes a dull, yellowish brown.

Both types of color changes have a distinctly unhealthy appearance.

Generalized pallor

When you suspect diffuse pallor in a newly admitted patient or when you cannot remember a patient's former color accurately, one or more of the following procedures may prove helpful.

1. Compare the color of the patient's conjunctiva with a healthy person's. Expose the entire lower conjunctiva for inspection, otherwise the lighter color near the inner canthus may be misinterpreted as pallor.
2. Check the color of the nail beds. Be sure the patient is supine with hands (or feet) near heart level and that environmental factors are not causing peripheral vasoconstriction.
3. Determine the capillary filling time of the nail bed by one of the following procedures:

   procedure Briefly press the free edge of the second or third fingernail (or the large toenail) to blanch the nail bed. Following release, the color normally returns within 1 second. A prolonged filling time indicates impaired circulation or vasomotor function. (If you cannot place the extremity at heart level, allow for the normal slightly prolonged filling time.) When the color of the nail bed is difficult to see, enhance the color by placing gentle pressure against the finger pad.

procedure If there are deposits of pigmentation in the nail beds or nail polish covering the nails, do the capillary (or venous plexus) filling test on the finger pad, mucous membrane, or a lightly pigmented skin area. Press the skin or mucous membrane firmly for a few seconds to cause blanching. Better visibility is possible if a glass slide, a piece of firm clear plastic, or a magnifying glass is used to create pressure. Color should return uniformly from below and the periphery of the blanched area within 1 to 2 seconds. Delay, especially with an irregular pattern, is consistent with arterial insufficiency.

4. Observe for adjunctive signs. Pallor of impending shock is accompanied by cool clammy skin, apprehension, increasing pulse rate, and restlessness. Pallor of anemia may be accompanied by a variety of signs. Persons with severe anemia may manifest easy fatigability, anorexia, dizziness, chilliness, rapid pulse, dyspnea on exertion, and impaired mental function. "Spoon" (concave) nails commonly indicate chronic iron deficiency anemia.

Localized pallor

To identify pallor, compare the color and capillary filling time of the pallid area or extremity with another area of the patient's body. In addition, observe for adjunctive signs such as the numbness and/or pain, coldness, and possibly reduced arterial pulsation that accompany localized vascular insufficiency.

Pallor localized to an extremity is usually caused by arteriocapillary insufficiency; therefore postural changes may provide additional information by enhancing the pallor and/or producing other color changes. If postural changes are *not contraindicated,* try the following procedure after having the patient at rest in a comfortably warm environment for at least one-half hour.

1. With the patient in the horizontal position, inspect the color of the extremity, comparing it with the other one and acquiring an accurate mental picture of the differing skin tones.

2. Support both extremities in an elevated position (15 to 45 degrees, as determined by the patient's condition) for 5 to 15 minutes. Pallor will become visible or increase noticeably if there is vascular insufficiency of the extremity. If the color remains the same and pallor is still suspected, have the patient flex his feet (or open and close his fists) repeatedly for a minute or so, then lower the extremities to heart level and inspect for increased pallor of the sole of the foot (or palm), which indicates the presence of reduced arterial circulation.

3. Support both extremities in a dependent position (30 to 90 degrees) for 5 minutes. A pink flush, best seen in the nail beds or the plantar/palmar skin surfaces, will occur normally within 10 seconds. An irregular, patchy color return that is delayed 45 seconds or longer indicates arterial insufficiency. If the color becomes reddish blue (cyanotic) with continuation of the dependent position, it indicates capillary stagnation caused by poor vascular tone (or serious varicosities).

■ What is the significance of cyanosis?

The dusky bluish color of cyanotic skin and mucous membranes is caused by an excess of reduced (deoxygenated) hemoglobin in the superficial capillaries. A minimum of 5 g % of reduced hemoglobin (or 6 to 7 vol % of unsaturated arterial blood) is necessary for clinical cyanosis. This degree of cyanosis is usually discernible in the mucous membranes and nail beds but not in darkly pigmented skin; a much larger quantity of deoxyhemoglobin is necessary for visibility in dark skin.

Central cyanosis is caused by inadequate arterial oxygenation such as may occur when too little oxygen is available (for example, suffocation or airway obstruction), when gas exchange is impaired (for example, bronchopneumonia, chronic emphysema, or pneumothorax), or when a major arteriovenous shunt dilutes the oxygenated blood with venous blood (for example, congenital cardiac anomalies or pulmonary fistulas).

Peripheral cyanosis results from increased reduction of oxyhemoglobin (to 11 to 13 vol % of unsaturated blood) in the capillaries during circulatory stagnation. The stagnation may be caused by venous obstruction (for example, thrombosis, compression of large vein by tumor, or trauma), arterial obstruction (for example, arteriosclerosis or atherosclerosis), or circulatory failure (for example, congestive heart failure, coronary disease with arterial hypertension, or mitral stenosis). Some types of peripheral cyanosis are localized. For example, in Raynaud's disease, vasospasm will cause cyanosis of the fingers; in chest trauma with mediastinal hemorrhage, compression of the superior vena cava will cause a striking facial cyanosis.

The presence of methemoglobin (1.5 g %) or sulfhemoglobin (0.5 g %) in the blood will cause color changes similar to cyanosis. Small amounts of methemoglobin (oxidized hemoglobin) in the blood are normal, but excessive exposure to certain chemicals or drugs may increase the amount beyond the body's capacity to reduce it to hemoglobin. Newborns are particularly susceptible because of their immature metabolic enzyme systems. Substances known to cause methemoglobinemia include nitrites, nitrates, sulfones, phenacetin (for example, APC, Empirin Compound, Stanback), acetanilid (for example, Bromo-Seltzer), lidocaine, benzocaine, resorcinol, and aniline dye (for example, shoe dye, marking ink, and wax crayons).

Sulfhemoglobin is not normally present in the blood but may be produced when an oxidizing drug (especially phenacetin or acetanilid) is taken in excessive amounts. Once sulfhemoglobin is formed, it cannot be converted to hemoglobin; consequently the affected erythrocytes remain nonfunctional until their natural destruction.

Although the cyanotic coloration of sulfhemoglobinemia and methemoglobinemia may be intense, symptoms of hypoxemia are rare; more commonly the patient manifests drug-related symptoms such as bromide intoxication.

■ When the skin is heavily pigmented, how can you recognize cyanosis?

Cyanosis changes the underlying skin tones in much the same way as pallor. Black skin remains dark and takes on a dull, lifeless appearance; brown skin assumes a dusty, grayish look. As with pallor, the skin appears distinctly unhealthy. Unless the cyanosis is acute and severe, the skin changes may be too subtle to be recognized. For this reason, if cyanosis is suspected or anticipated, make frequent inspections of the nail beds, oral mucosa, and conjunctiva. The same techniques for identifying pallor may be used in checking for cyanosis, but good color discrimination and memory for color are especially essential for successful recognition.

Central cyanosis is usually visible in the mucous membranes as well as the skin and nail beds, so in the presence of dark pigmentation, inspect the nails, lips, oral mucosa (especially under the tongue), and the conjunctiva. This kind of cyanosis intensifies with exercise. When an infant's cyanosis intensifies with crying, it indicates a cardiovascular rather than a pulmonary or neurogenic basis for the cyanosis.

Peripheral cyanosis occurs predominantly in the distal extremities, so inspect the nail beds, palms, or soles of the feet. Also, check the skin temperature; it will feel distinctly cool in contrast to normal in central cyanosis. Unless peripheral cyanosis is caused by local arterial insufficiency, gentle warming or massage of the cyanotic tissue will restore a pinkish color; there will be no change if the cyanosis is central in origin. Do not attempt such testing if arterial insufficiency is suspected, because gangrene may be precipitated. A safer procedure would be, first, to check the severity of the cyanosis by applying firm pressure with a glass slide. Failure of the color to blanch is a criterion for irreversible cyanosis (that is, necrosis or gangrene will result). If the color blanches and returns, *cautiously* use the position changes described for evaluating pallor. A more intense cyanosis, especially during brief elevation of the extremity, strongly suggests local arterial insufficiency.

Differentiating methemoglobinemia and sulfhemoglobinemia from cyanosis is accomplished by laboratory studies. Although the bluish tint has more gray or brown undertones than true cyanosis, the difference is extremely difficult to recognize in persons with dark skin. Obtain a careful history of ingestion or contact with causative agents whenever a patient has generalized cyanosis with no symptoms of hypoxemia.

■ What are the implications of erythema and hemorrhagic lesions?

Erythema is an intense redness of the skin caused by an excess of blood (hyperemia) within the superficial vessels. Hyperemia of the skin may be classified as active or passive.

In *active hyperemia* there is an increased blood supply *to* the area, causing engorgement primarily of the arterioles and capillaries. The color is the bright pinkish red of oxyhemoglobin. The etiology of active hyperemia (of the skin) may be paralysis of the vasoconstrictor (sympathetic) nerves, stimulation of the CNS vasodilator mechanism (for example, in fever and blushing), or a reflex nerve response (to local heat, irritation, or tissue damage). The presence of carboxyhemoglobin (30 vol % or more) in carbon monoxide poisoning will cause a bright cherry-red erythema particularly of the face and upper torso.

The increased skin temperature that accompanies some types of erythema is caused by an increased rate of blood flow through the superficial vessels. Inflammation and fever are the most common causes of heat and redness; the most important causes of redness without heat are hypersensitivity reactions and poisoning (for example, certain drugs and carbon monoxide).

In *passive hyperemia* there is a decreased flow of blood *from* the area, causing engorgement primarily of the capillaries and venules. This stasis of flow results in the dull bluish red color of deoxyhemoglobin. The etiology of passive hyperemia (of the skin) may be obstruction (for example, direct pressure, increased hydrostatic pressure, or venous thrombosis) or atony of capillaries and venules (for example, advanced shock or severe tissue hypoxia). Severe local passive hyperemia is often a transient prelude to necrosis, as commonly seen in the developing decubitus ulcer.

Hemorrhagic lesions may be the result of trauma, coagulation disorders, capillary damage (for example, bacterial toxins or hypoxia), and an imbalance between capillary fragility and intracapillary pressure. *Petechiae* are tiny, punctate (pinpoint) red/purple/brown discolorations of the skin, and their presence indicates capillary bleeding. In systemic disorders (for example, meningococcemia or subacute bacterial endocarditis) petechiae may be distributed in the skin, mucous membranes, and nail beds, whereas in local disorders (for example, damage to fragile capillaries) the petechiae will be limited to a localized area. Blacks commonly have petechiae with rashes, particularly with varicella.

Ecchymoses are larger, diffuse patches of capillary bleeding commonly called bruises. The color begins as reddish purple and changes to a brownish, greenish, and then yellowish color. A localized ecchymosis may also be evidence of a superficial hematoma (which can be palpated and possibly seen as a swelling) or of deep bleeding such as from splenic rupture or hemorrhagic pancreatitis. When the ecchymotic and petechial lesions are numerous and extensive, such as in generalized disorders (for example, thrombocytopenia, scurvy, Waterhouse-Friderichsen syndrome), the condition is referred to as *purpura*.

■ Can erythema and hemorrhagic lesions be seen and differentiated when the skin is darkly pigmented?

Mild erythema and minor hemorrhagic lesions are completely concealed by black and very dark brown pigmentation; a bright erythema and dark bruising will cause a localized darkening of the already dark skin. Moderate to light pigmentation will allow the colors of erythema and bruising to show through. Unless the skin is exceedingly dark, petechiae may be seen by close inspection and diascopy, and they are easily detected in the mucous membranes and nail beds.

Constant awareness of skin temperature will assist in recognizing erythema. Develop the habit of regularly touching the skin (with the dorsal surface of your fingers) over areas with a high potential for inflammation, such as a vein being used for intravenous infusion, the bony prominence of a patient on bedrest, and tissue surrounding a surgical incision. Remember that when a patient is turned, the skin that has been resting against the mattress may feel excessively warm, so allow several minutes of exposure to comfortably warm air before checking the skin temperature.

In addition to checking for warmth, feel for the "slick," tight skin and firm underlying tissue of inflammatory edema. The patient may also have discomfort or pain during palpation. A hardened and exquisitely tender vein suggests phlebitis even when erythema is imperceptible. The cherry-red erythema of carbon monoxide poisoning can be seen in the oral mucosa and fingernails when pigmentation obscures the skin color. Skin temperature is not increased in carbon monoxide poisoning or in most rashes (unless accompanied by fever).

The following examination techniques are especially helpful in locating and differentiating lesions of darkly pigmented skin.

1. Lightly palpate the skin with a brushing motion of the fingertips to locate papules, hematomas, or edema. Petechiae and ecchymoses are not palpable unless there is an associated inflammatory edema as in trauma or vasculitis.
2. Use side lighting in a dimly lighted room to create observable shadows of small inconspicuous papules.
3. Examine the skin closely with a bright light and magnifying lens to discover the presence of petechiae, discrete macules, or papules. Examine the nail beds, conjunctiva, and oral mucosa for petechiae.
4. Use diascopy to inspect and evaluate the skin color. Gently press a glass slide or magnifying lens against the skin (or stretch the skin between your fingers) to cause a slight blanching. The pressure should be about one half the strength needed for a capillary filling test of the skin.

When pigmentation does not completely obscure erythema, this technique will help differentiate certain lesions. Macules that result from dilated, congested blood vessels (for example, rubella or early rubeola lesions) will blanch on pressure, whereas lesions containing extravasated blood (for example, petechiae, advanced rubeola lesions, varicella, or some insect bites) will remain visible during pressure. Some allergic rashes require considerably more pressure for blanching the underlying punctate macules than the surrounding erythema.

When pigmentation completely obscures the underlying color, but a darkened area suggests erythema or ecchymosis, diascopy will reduce the color of erythema but not of ecchymosis.

■ What causes jaundice?

Jaundice is a yellow or yellowish green discoloration of the skin and mucous membranes caused by an increased serum bilirubin (2 mg % or higher). Hyperbilirubinemia is commonly attributed to liver and biliary tract disorders, but it may also result from acute cardiopulmonary problems such as a pulmonary infarction with resultant cor pulmonale. When increased hemolysis is accompanied by a marked decrease in cardiac output, the compromised liver is unable to eliminate the bilirubin as rapidly as it is produced, and acute-onset jaundice develops. A concomitant cyanosis from circulatory stagnation may produce an alarming olive-green color.

Pseudojaundice may be caused by carotenemia, many industrial chemicals, and certain drugs (quinacrine, picric acid). Carotene is a yellow pigment obtained principally from yellow vegetables and is a fat-soluble precursor of vitamin A. In carotenemia the excess carotene is deposited in fatty tissue and the cornified layer of the epidermis (especially calloused hands and feet). The mucous membranes and sclerae are not discolored, but the fatty deposits in the scleral and palpebral conjunctivae will be quite yellow, often giving the appearance of jaundice.

Industrial products stain exposed skin areas. The mucous membranes and sclerae will not be yellow unless the frequently hepatotoxic chemicals have damaged the liver and produced a combination of staining and jaundice.

Quinacrine produces a diffuse yellow or greenish yellow color that is accentuated in the exposed areas and folds of the skin. Unless the color is intense, the mucous membranes and sclerae are not usually discolored. Excessive use of picric acid (which is rarely used now because of its toxicity) colors the skin, mucous membranes, and sclerae a distinct yellow.

■ How do you detect jaundice in dark-skinned patients?

Moderate to dark pigmentation conceals jaundice very effectively; nevertheless, the diffuse systemic nature of jaundice makes it readily detectable in other locations. With a very good light (preferably nonglare daylight), inspect the sclerae, conjunctivae, hard palate, and palms. When inspecting the sclera, look at the *naturally* exposed portion. The yellowish fatty deposits are heavier under the eyelids and tend to be misinterpreted as jaundice. The palpebral conjunctivae may also be examined for jaundice, but more skill is needed for recognizing it there than in the posterior hard palate. Despite the mechanical difficulties of inspecting the hard palate, it is one of the best areas for detecting early jaundice. The palms and possibly soles of the feet reveal jaundice, but the color is often distorted in adults by other factors such as increased deposits of carotene and intense thickening and staining of the epidermis.

Scratch marks and complaints of itching may be suggestive of jaundice, but many unrelated problems also cause itching, and three fourths of the people with jaundice do not have itching.

Pseudojaundice is distinguished from true jaundice by laboratory determination of serum bilirubin values, but discriminating observations by the nurses may determine the need for prompt diagnostic differentiation. For example, patients with yellowing of the palms and soles of the feet or with other patterns of yellow discoloration that do not include the sclera and hard palate probably have pseudojaundice. The patient's urine may also provide clues: orange to red urine accompanies picric acid abuse; red to brown urine (hemoglobinuria) is associated with hemolytic jaundice; normal yellow urine and darkly colored stools are seen in hemolytic jaundice complicated by severe hepatic insufficiency.

■ Are you certain to see color changes that are visible?

In general, our habits and cultural mores impede effective observation. We tend to disregard or underestimate the value of things to which we have become accustomed, and we are so accustomed to seeing the skin that we can look directly at it without perceiving the color or other characteristics. Moreover, most of us were taught as children that it is impolite to "stare" at people, and as a result, we often merely glance at a person or look in his general direction rather than study his facial expression and color. I found in a small informal survey that nurses who had just admitted a patient to a children's unit frequently could not describe the color of the patient's skin; some could not recall whether the patient was Negro or Caucasian. This lack of color awareness in otherwise observant nurses is not at all uncommon.

To ensure that you *will* see visible color changes, develop your own plan of "sensitivity training." Practice color assessment on each patient you encounter. Perhaps you would prefer to obtain your mental picture of the patient's basic color while interviewing him or while doing a procedure such as checking the TPR for the admission record. Rather than staring off into space while counting the pulse or waiting for the thermometer to register, study the patient's color, using a consistent, organized approach. For example, check the general color of the skin (black, brown, and so forth), degree and quality of undertone, irregularities of color in the face (circumoral, butterfly area, and so forth), and color of the lips, sclera, and nail beds. Then a quick inspection of the palpebral conjunctivae and oral mucosa will complete the minimum basic assessment for color; other areas of skin should be inspected when possible and particularly when a pathologic state is present or suspected. Once you have completed the basic color assessment, do a "review" *each* time you encounter the patient by deliberately looking at his face, eyes, lips, and nails (include other specific areas and/or other examination procedures as appropriate). Furthermore, while doing procedures that may cause color change (for example, tracheal suctioning may cause cyanosis), watch the patient's color closely throughout the procedure. You should discover a very satisfying heightened awareness of color following conscientious application of such a "sensitivity training" program.

BIBLIOGRAPHY

Bauer, J.: Differential diagnosis of internal disease, ed. 3, New York, 1967, Grune & Stratton, Inc.

Braunwald, E., et al.: Cyanosis, hypoxia, and polycythemia. In Thorn, G. W., et al., editors: Harrison's principles of internal medicine, ed. 8, New York, 1977, McGraw-Hill Book Co.

Cartwright, G. E.: Methemoglobinemia and sulfhemoglobinemia. In Thorn, G. W., et al., editors: Harrison's principles of internal medicine, ed. 8, New York, 1977, McGraw-Hill Book Co.

Hopps, H. C.: Principles of pathology, ed. 2, New York, 1964, Appleton-Century-Crofts.

Jeghers, H., and Mescon, H.: Pigmentation of the skin. In MacBryde, C. M., editor: Signs and symptoms, ed. 4, Philadelphia, 1964, J. B. Lippincott Co.

Roach, L. B.: Color changes in dark skin, Nursing '77 **7:**48, 1977.

CHAPTER 49

Introduction to human sexuality for critical care professionals

Karen Lee Fontaine and Raymond A. Fontaine

In recent years the helping professions have reaffirmed the holistic approach to people in health and illness; however, at the same time, patients and clients have nearly always been considered to be asexual. This is evidenced by critical care professionals who rarely discuss with their patients the effects that illness, surgery, or hospitalization will have on their sexuality. Patients on every unit of the hospital have sexual problems that no one helps them solve. The majority suffer in silence. Health professionals need to be specifically educated to recognize the problems and intervene in a therapeutic manner.

Furthermore, nurses and physicians are frequently the first professionals to whom patients turn with their sexual questions and problems, and these patients are entitled to informed answers. Many of them do not require in-depth sexual counseling, but they do need someone with whom they can openly and honestly discuss their concerns—someone who is able to give understanding support and accurate information.

■ What is meant by sexuality?

Sexuality is both easy and difficult to define. It is the life force and biologic urge that we share with most of animate creation. (It turns out, after all, that the pistils and stamens of flowers are really their genitalia.) In biology we distinguish between sexual and asexual reproduction; however we also know that sexuality is much more than reproduction.

The most important sex organ is the brain and, given a moment's thought, most people recognize that. Many have learned and/or relearned that sexuality and sensuality are so closely related that at times they are indistinguishable. Electronic and printed media, in both helpful and harmful ways, keep sexuality before us to such a degree that it is impossible to escape, even if one wanted to.

Sexuality is also an integral part of one's self-concept and as such is intrinsically involved in one's body image and self-esteem. It can be best understood as a life force or as an important aspect of all of one's feelings and behavior. In our culture sexuality is rarely appreciated and promoted in positive ways; instead, it has been a source of conflict and guilt. Resolution of this conflict and guilt must be accomplished in order to move on to the view that sex and sexuality enhance our feelings about ourselves as persons and help us relate more comfortably and positively to other people.

There is much talk and head-shaking these days about the sexual revolution that is taking place. If there is a sexual revolution, it is that some are now at ease with the subject of sex, have opportunities to ask questions without embarrassment, and may request help for sexual distresses without fear of being thought improper. However, even with this change in atmosphere, many people are no more comfortable with or knowledgeable about sexuality than were members of previous generations.

■ When does "sex" begin and end for a person?

Every individual is a sexual person from the day of birth until the day of death. This is evident by a person's sexual activity throughout life. Children, even in infancy, clearly respond to sexual stimuli. Infants of both sexes seem to experience pleasure from the stimulation of the genitalia and other areas of the body that are commonly recognized as erogenous zones. Male infants respond with erection and female infants respond with lubrication of the vagina.[1] The Kinsey studies showed that orgasmic experiences may occur in infants and children throughout the preadolescent period and that the percentage of children able to reach climax increases with age.[2]

The child entering adolescence cannot be said to be sexually mature; however he* is reproductively and genitally mature and capable of reproduction. In our culture this becomes a stressful period. Difficulty in obtaining helpful information from parents, teachers, or other adults about the physical and emotional changes and experiences that they face constitutes a serious problem for the adolescent.

In early adolescence masturbation becomes a central concern for both males and females. Their anxieties and fears lead to a sense of guilt and shame. The Committee on Adolescence of the Group for the Advancement of Psychiatry noted that masturbation is essentially a "normal response in increased sexual development" that is "necessary to the control and integration of new urges and the working out of new relationships through trial acting and fantasy."[3] The committee's report indicates how adolescent masturbation can serve normal development: "The adolescent learns that sexual excitement and engorgement and erection of the penis or the clitoris can be initiated at will, and that orgasmic climax with the ensuing predictable subsidence of tension can be quickly brought about or repeatedly deferred by masturbation. This contributes to a developing sense of mastery over the sexual im-

*We are mindful that the English language does not yet give us a pronoun that adequately recognizes that there are two sexes. We trust the reader will neither be put off nor offended.

pulses and the new sexual capacities and helps the adolescent prepare for heterosexual relationships."[3]

In adulthood a wide variety of sexual behavior and combination patterns exist. These range from total celibacy to a high degree of activity and from exclusive homosexual or heterosexual activity to total indiscretion in partner choice. Those who are sexually active develop a further variety of patterns. Some achieve satisfaction with their sex life, while others are unable to do so. Some struggle with nonorgasmic response or impotence. Others may be obsessive or compulsive in their sexual behavior. Thus we see that sexual activity is not simply a matter of physiologic response, but more importantly it is a psychologic and behavioral response.

The sexual revolution among today's youth is less radical than the one going on among older people according to information Masters and Johnson have published.[4] In spite of this information our society is largely resistant to sexuality and sexual expression in people 50 years of age or older. Obviously, full satisfaction of the sexual needs of older persons cannot take place in a society that ignores or denies the reality of such needs.

Sexual expression has been closely linked to reproductive function for so long that menopause and late middle age are considered to signal the end of sexual life. Compounding this problem is a general prejudice toward older people and the widespread feeling that life, love, and romance belong only to the young. Some older people are made to feel that sex is neither possible nor necessary. If they are active, they are thought of as odd or perverted. Even when it is considered normal, it is thought of as not "nice" for senior citizens to be indulging in sex. Since sexual behavior is a reflection of individual and cultural expectations, this widespread belief about the sexless older years may lead to a self-fulfilling prophecy.

For some older persons continuation of sexual relations is primarily important as a source of psychologic reinforcement, for men at a time when they are facing the loss of prestige and a diminution of self-confidence and for women when they fear the loss of attractiveness and desirability following menopause.[1] "The premature cessation of sexual functioning may accelerate physiological aging, since disuse of any function actually leads to concomitant changes in other capacities."[4]

There are physiologic changes in sexuality that accompany the aging process. The male sexual responsiveness to stimulation decreases with age, and a somewhat longer period is needed to reach orgasm as well as a longer resolution phase. Ejaculation gradually decreases in vigor and becomes scantier. However, the aging male also has some advantage over the younger male. He is able to maintain an erection longer and with greater ejaculatory control; thus more satisfying and imaginative love play is often enjoyed by older couples.[4]

Physical changes that occur in the aging female are less noticeable. Vaginal lubrication (which is the first sign of sexual excitement) occurs more slowly with aging, and less lubricant is produced. However, it has also been found that women who have been sexually active throughout their life keep secreting a normal amount of lubrication. The clitoris may get smaller, but there seems to be no change in its response to sexual stimulation.[4]

There can be little doubt that human beings are capable of enjoying their sexuality from infancy to death. The reason(s) they do not are separate from their physical ability to do so.

■ How is a person's sexuality affected by illness and hospitalization?

From the moment of admission until the time of discharge from a hospital, patients are subjected to many experiences that threaten their self-image. Personal surroundings and belongings of most people reinforce their identities as men or women. When a person is admitted to the hospital, personal effects are removed and usually sent home with the family. The person, who is now called a "patient," is placed in an environment that reflects neither masculine nor feminine tastes (even clothing is essentially asexual). Many people's self-image is linked to personal attractiveness and grooming, and the hospital setting deprives them of many of the devices that enhance their looks and help them express their sexual identity. This is the beginning of the de-

personalization process that continues throughout the hospitalization.

In our culture the male role traditionally has been one of control and dominance. Illness, which places the patient in a submissive role, may be threatening to his sense of masculinity. Although one might very well argue that "masculinity" that is dependent on always being in control is not a particularly realistic (or desirable) model, it must nevertheless be understood in order to deal with it therapeutically. This threat may be further intensified with hospitalization when a man finds himself under the care of and taking directions from staff members, most of whom are women. A woman might also have her sexual identity threatened when she becomes ill. If she views her female role as one of nurturance, it may be uncomfortable for her to become the one to whom care is given.

In a situation where self-image is threatened the patient may feel uncomfortably "on display" to staff and visitors alike. In some areas of the hospital, such as intensive care units, the patient may also be "on display" to patients of the opposite sex. This also might have an impact on a person's sexual self-image.

Another threat to one's self-image may occur because of a change in the partner's conception of the person as a sexual being. Someone who is ill, disabled, or who has just had surgery is sometimes perceived by others as being without sexual identity or interest. The withdrawal of a partner, even when it is motivated by genuine concern, may be experienced as a devastating rejection.

Each person has a certain body space, determined by his culture, that tells him how close to get to another. In our culture this body space is about 2 to 3 feet and is usually entered only by those with whom one is intimate. Throughout hospitalization this space is invaded by many strangers, thus creating uneasy feelings in the patient. Not only is this space entered by many people, but the patient may also be subjected to a number of intrusive events. Some examinations and procedures require that the health care professional's eyes and hands come in contact with areas of the body traditionally reserved for sexual intimacy. Thus the patient may find such things as rectal temperature, complete baths, enemas, and catheterizations to be sexually humiliating.

Lack of privacy and the hospital atmosphere are obvious deterrents to full sexual expression and require changes in the person's sexual behavior patterns. This can be especially difficult for the long-term patient when the hospital stay causes real deprivation. Separation and deprivation are also difficult for the patient's partner, since he/she is well and functioning in a society filled with sexual stimuli. Both the patient and the partner therefore feel a loss of the intimacy they have shared because they have been deprived of their usual means of communicating their bonds of affection.

■ How can a critical care professional be of help?
Self-assessment

The first task for the professional is assessment of self. Basic to this is the recognition that beliefs, values, and attitudes are an important determinant of how one deals with people. Therefore one must begin with the assessment of one's own values and attitudes about human sexuality. Another aspect of self-assessment is the examination of one's professional practice. A question one might ask is "Do I deny, inhibit, or allow for the sexuality of my patients?" Along with this it is important to develop an awareness of how one is perceived by others. Reflect for a moment on the number of patients who have discussed sexual concerns with you. If the answer is none or few, then the next question is "Do the patients I come in contact with have (in fact) no or few sexual concerns, or am I sending nonverbal messages that discourage people from discussing these concerns with me?"

Another aspect of self-assessment is the degree of comfort a person has in discussing sexual concerns with patients. Most patients quickly perceive our comfort or discomfort and react accordingly. Assessment of the extent of one's knowledge of sexual physiology and psychology throughout the life cycle in health and in illness is necessary. Security in doing sexual counseling, as in all other kinds of counseling, is based on knowledge of the subject. It is essential, therefore, that health professionals know what they are

talking about and do not participate in the furtherance of incorrect information, misconceptions, or sexual nonsense.

Before attempting to assist patients, it is essential that health professionals come to terms with their own sexuality. Self-awareness is basic to effective and comfortable interventions with patients. The professional must be able to communicate acceptance without judgment or stereotyping. As expressed by Marianne Zalar, an assistant professor at the University of California School of Nursing, San Francisco: "We must learn not to ignore the disquieting sexual aspects of a patient's humanity; nor should we overtly or covertly stigmatize him or her. We are health care providers, not theologians, law enforcement officers, or moralists. We cannot be committed to total patient care without considering the patient as a sexual being."[5] If the professional feels incompetent, there should be a referral to another professional who is competent. However, all professionals have the responsibility to increase their competencies.

Patient assessment

The second task of the professional is assessment of the patient. One needs to recognize that any alteration in a person's physical or emotional state may affect various aspects of his life pattern —including that of sexual activity. According to Masters, there can be serious medical consequences when health professionals ignore their patient's sexuality. "It depends entirely on the individual care, of course. Sometimes there are no medical consequences at all. In other cases, there may be. Example: many a man has been operated on for a bleeding ulcer without even having been given tests to determine if he is impotent or not. Frequently, the first clinical symptom of impotence is a bleeding ulcer. The field is just beginning to realize that sexual function affects many other aspects of health."[5]

Once it is identified that a patient has a problem or concern, one must distinguish if this is a request for information about normal functioning, a specific sexual problem, a clinical situation that is related to sexual functioning, or a problem requiring temporary or permanent alteration in preferred modes of functioning. Unless the problem is correctly identified, the intervention will not be helpful and could worsen the situation by inhibiting the patient from further exploration.

Skill development

The third task of the professional is the development of interpersonal communication skills. Creating a comfortable atmosphere is essential; the professional who is embarrassed or anxious only augments these reactions in the patient. Managing one's own feelings as well as responding appropriately to those of the patient is essential to good practice.

A natural time to discuss sexuality with a patient is when taking his history. Failure to include sexual information in a person's history reinforces the feeling that sex is a forbidden topic. Likewise the topic may be brought up very naturally during patient education. Many people need to be reassured that it is "OK" to talk about sex, and when it is introduced in this manner, many patients perceive this as permission to discuss their sexual concerns. Sex is still a taboo subject for many people, as well as a source for a good deal of hurt (and pleasure). Thus it is important that the professional be sensitive, gentle, and humane. Perhaps the patient will not respond to questions about his sexuality the first time it is mentioned, but if he knows that it is "OK" to talk about it, and if he feels the professional is competent and caring, that patient may later open up that very private part of his life.

■ In what ways do medications affect sexual functioning?

We do not know much about the complex biochemistry of how medications affect sexual functioning, but the effects are observable. Hence the health practitioner will find that a general knowledge of these effects will be useful in assisting patients.

Antihypertensive drugs

There are a number of the antihypertensive drugs that interfere with sexual function. The central-acting antihypertensive agents such as clonidine (Catapres) infrequently may cause urinary retention and impotence. Rauwolfia alkaloids such as reserpine may delay ejaculation,

and in rare instances there may be a decrease in libido and erectile difficulties. A delay or failure of ejaculation may occur in patients taking adrenergic blocking agents such as guanethidine (Ismelin) as well as ganglionic blocking agents such as mecamylamine (Inversine). Methyldopa (Aldomet) may cause difficulties with libido and potency and difficulty in ejaculation. The aldosterone antagonists such as spironolactone (Aldactone) have been reported to cause impotence.[6] If a patient complains of sexual difficulties, one might try control of the hypertension utilizing diuretics such as hydralazine (Apresoline) or propranolol (Inderal), as these medications do not interfere with sexual functioning.

Central nervous system acting agents

The whole range of CNS drugs have a marked effect on sexuality, sex drive, erectile ability, and ejaculation. They include the opiates (morphine, heroin, and so on); the monoamine oxidase inhibitors such as tranylcypromine (Parnate), phenylethylhydrazine (Nardil), and isocarboxazid (Marplan); the tricyclic antidepressants such as imipramine (Tofranil), desipramine (Norpramin), and amitriptyline (Elavil); the major tranquilizers such as fluphenazine (Prolixin), thioridazine (Mellaril), and chlorpromazine (Thorazine); and finally the cholinergic blocking agents such as atropine, belladonna, and propantheline (Pro-Banthine).[6]

"Recreational" drugs

With one major exception, the effects of the "recreational" drugs on sexuality are not well researched or known. The exception, ethyl alcohol, has a depressive effect on the ability for erection and ejaculation. Chronic alcoholism can lead to persistent impotence.[6]

■ How is sexuality affected by hypertension and stroke?

There is no convincing evidence that hypertensive persons are particularly susceptible to acute cardiovascular catastrophies during sexual intercourse even though many doctors discourage sexual activity. If a person regularly experiences angina during intercourse, he should be advised to use nitroglycerin prophylactically.

In the case of uncontrolled hypertension above 180/110 with target organ disease, maximal sexual activity is contraindicated. For most hypertensive persons, however, it is best to encourage them to lead a normal sexual life. For persons who also have coronary disease it is best to advise positions for passive intercourse to reduce physical stress.

In cases where hypertension is complicated by a cerebrovascular accident a number of things need to be remembered. Stroke is the kind of disorder that touches many of the components of our sexuality. Natural body functions are often affected by stroke (mobility, speech, sensation), and therefore one's body image will also be affected, usually lessened, which in turn often has a negative effect on sexuality. Although actually causing damage by having sexual contact is extremely rare, the *fear* of so doing is a reality to many people. They need reassurance and encouragement to continue their sexual lives. A stroke will not "make" a person impotent, although difficulty in getting and keeping an erection is reported in some instances. The presence of morning erections will tell you that the impotency is psychogenic, and once you know that you can proceed to assist the patient discover the source or make a referral for sex therapy.

The final possibility is that the difficulty with erections is caused by medication. The ganglionic blocking agents and the rauwolfia drugs are almost notorious in their ability to interfere with erection and ejaculation. Again, one might consider changing to medications that do not interfere with functioning.[7,8]

■ How is sexuality affected by a myocardial infarction?

After the initial recovery from an acute myocardial infarction, the cardiac patient oftentimes has doubts and fears about his ability to resume normal physical activities, especially sexual intercourse. The hospitalization itself is a threat to a person's self-image, and superimposed on this are all the accompanying fears of having heart disease. Many men see heart disease as a threat to their masculinity and self-esteem and fear the loss of sexual functioning. Thus it is not uncommon to observe aggressive sexual behavior in the male cardiac patient as a reaction to his fears. This includes seductive comments, frequent references to past sexual abilities, and attempts to touch the nurse or expose the genitals. Nurses who can understand the underlying reasons for this behavior will be able to intervene therapeutically in these problems.

Women, too, suffer from the same threats to their self-image. However, there is less reported aggressive sexual behavior. This may be due to several reasons among them being the cultural image of women being nonaggressive sexually and the scarcity of male nurses with whom to interact.

Cardiac symptoms such as shortness of breath and angina pectoris, as well as the haunting fear of death, may prevent the cardiac patient from experiencing normal and gratifying sexual relationships. If the physician fails to discuss resumption of coital activity, the patient and the partner may falsely assume that the physician believes such activity is beyond his/her cardiovascular limit.

Is sudden death during intercourse a realistic danger for the post myocardial infarction patient? Research has found that sexual activity accounts for less than 1% of sudden deaths and that the few coital deaths caused by coronary disease have usually occurred after extramarital intercourse.[9]

There is an increase in cardiovascular demand during intercourse, but this period of time is short, averaging 4 to 6 minutes. The caloric demand or oxygen consumption is equivalent to climbing one or two flights of stairs, which places sexual intercourse in the light to moderate category of physical activity.[9]

When may the cardiac patient resume sexual activity? The answer to this question depends on the individual situation, the severity of the original myocardial infarction, and whether or not the symptoms are still present. Resumption of sexual activity is usually allowed when the patient can perform exercise at levels of 6 to 8 cal/min without symptoms. For the majority of patients this is usually 8 to 16 weeks after the injury.[9]

Sexual counseling of the cardiac patient and the partner encompasses several areas. The patient must be cautioned to avoid intercourse in situations that are more stressful on the heart. These situations are after a heavy meal, when intoxicated, when fatigued, when in an unfamiliar environment, or when the environment is extremely hot or cold. The patient is also cautioned about extramarital affairs, since these frequently take place after heavy eating and drinking and may be accompanied by guilt feelings and the need to perform exceptionally well.

It is also important to explain to patients that positions requiring prolonged use of the arms and legs for body support should be avoided. This increased isometric muscular activity may increase peripheral vascular resistance, elevate the blood pressure, and set the stage for cardiovascular symptoms.[10]

Another aspect of counseling is teaching the individual to be aware of the signs and symptoms associated with heart problems. They most commonly occur during the resolution phase and may include (1) respiration that does not return to 20/min; 1 minute after orgasm, (2) persistent rapid heart rate beyond 1 minute after orgasm, (3) exhaustion the day after intercourse, and (4) angina during or after intercourse. For the patient who experiences angina, use of prophylactic nitroglycerin before intercourse frequently prevents the occurrence of angina.[10]

In addition, the health professional can counsel the patient to avoid certain forms of activity that do not seem to be as taxing as exercise but represent severe forms of stress on the cardiovascular system. Activities such as fighting heavy traffic or getting into arguments may well be more damaging than climbing two flights of stairs or, indeed, having sexual intercourse.

■ How is sexuality affected by renal disease?

Chronic renal failure, like any life-threatening disorder, does more than physiologic damage to a person and his/her sexuality. When dealing with any chronic disease, you can be sure that the person's body image and self-esteem will be shaken and that added stress will be put on all significant relationships. Once again, it is important to see the total effect chronic illness has on a person.[11]

The physiologic effects of chronic renal failure on sexuality are also serious. We know that sexual desire and activity are inversely proportional to the severity of uremia, with both males and females being affected. In men the testicles become soft and atrophic and spermatogenesis stops. The testicular production of testosterone is also depressed to castrate levels.

Another consequence of the cellular suppression within the testicles is uremic sexual dysfunction, and it is caused by the increase in uremic chemical toxicity. This may be shown by a prolonged metabolic clearance rate of luteinizing hormone that is a result of decreased excretion by the kidney.[12]

There is good evidence that with dialysis there is a resurgence of sexual desire and performance for both men and women.[13] Exact statistics for returning to preuremic levels of functioning have not been done. Preliminary work in this area indicates patients have at least 50% chance of returning to or improving earlier functioning. It has to be remembered that the psychogenic factors far outweigh in importance the physiologic factors once the patient is on dialysis or has had a successful transplantation. At that time if a person is experiencing sexual distress, it is likely to be caused by such things as loss of self-image, an unresponsive partner, a fear of self-injury, a change in basic relationships, or some other such factor. Patients will need to work through issues like these with the health care professional or be referred to someone who does sexual counseling.

It should be remembered also that the physical regimen alone required of a person on hemodialysis can adversely affect sexual desire. If a patient has had a successful transplant, most of the normal functioning can return including sexual functioning.

■ How is sexuality affected by cancer?

Again in the case of working with cancer patients, the health professional will find that most sexual dysfunction and distress is tied to the trauma of having cancer. Threatened or real loss of self-image, physical pain, changes in family structure and significant relationships, strained personal finances, shortened life expectancy, and feelings of great vulnerability and helplessness can all conspire to reduce a person's interest in and desire for sexual contact. Dread of exposing oneself as crippled, damaged, incomplete, or dying may cause sexual inhibition or abstinence.

Sexual functioning and intimacy may also be adversely affected by shame and embarrassment.[14]

Some forms of cancer are especially threatening to a person's sexuality because they involve (1) the genitals, (2) the eliminatory organs, or (3) any part of the body that is closely connected to self-image. It should be remembered also that many people consider cancer such a totally life-threatening disease that the thought of maintaining one's sex life is out of the question. As treatments have and continue to improve, it is increasingly important to give consideration to the quality of life the person will have, not mere survival.

For some people any recognizable loss in the sexual area may be construed as a step closer to death. If there is an avoidance of touching, this tells the person that he/she is repulsive. Thus loneliness may be a great problem for the cancer victim. The need for affection is universal, and at this time of the person's life the need for love and intimacy becomes more intense. Sexual intimacy may be an important primary source of psychologic reinforcement, and self-esteem can be increased by feeling that one is desired by, attractive to, and valued by another.

Cancer of the penis, testicles, vagina, uterus, or ovaries of course will have profound effects on a person's sexuality as well as his or her spouse or significant other. In each case a careful assessment of the amount of tissue and nerve damage will be very important. The chances of a person returning to a satisfactory sex life depends more on the number of neuropathways left unsevered than on the amount of remaining tissue, although tissue damage may call for adjustments in the preferred mode of expression. Vulvectomy or penectomy will no doubt call for such adjustment, but neither case necessarily means that the person is no longer capable of giving or receiving sexual stimulation.

In discussing the effects on sexuality caused by cancer of the bladder and bowel it is important to remember that in our culture eliminatory function is closely linked to sexuality in most people's minds. Therefore when one sees cancer in the colon or bladder or the resulting ostomies, one may be assured that there will be pronounced sexual side-effects. In cases where a total prostatectomy or a cystectomy is performed there is often an interruption in nerve supply. In men this often creates erectile difficulties, although it is impossible to eliminate psychogenic factors in some cases. Women may become secondarily nonorgasmic. In cases where nerve damage has been severe and erection is not possible, some men report that they still can be successfully stimulated to orgasm. The health professional should be ready to suggest that an alternative mode of giving and receiving sexual pleasure might be the treatment of choice. If the patient has a history of untreated sexual dysfunction or great difficulty communicating with his/her partner, a referral for sexual counseling is advised.[15]

With a transurethral prostatectomy, the man needs to be alerted to the likelihood of his experiencing retrograde ejaculation (dry orgasm) because the smooth muscle of the bladder neck has been interfered with during surgery, causing the semen to flow into the bladder. The patient should be counseled that this will neither harm him nor inhibit his performance.[15]

When cancer results in surgery that is radically disfiguring, the critical care professional should be aware that the person's sexual life will surely be affected negatively. The depression and lowered self-image and self-esteem that are normally experienced by such patients will be the cause of most of the sexual distress that they encounter.

One also needs to consider the patient's life functioning before the illness in the areas of work, recreation, family, and community. The professional needs to assess what changes have occurred or will occur that might affect the patient's sexuality. Role changes, financial changes, and recreational changes are a few of the losses that may occur. The more losses in a person's life the greater the potential for sexual problems.

■ What are the effects of spinal cord injury on a person's sexuality?

A spinal cord injury affects a person's sexual function in proportion to the severity of the sensorimotor transection. Since the cognitive and affective components of neurologic processes remain intact, the result may be serious psychosocial problems for the injured person.

Shortly after the injury during the stage of spinal shock, some men experience persistent erection (priapism). This is believed to represent a release of parasympathetic excitation from sympathetic inhibition. This may be a great source of embarrassment for the patient and needs to be handled tactfully by the nurse. Explaining the process matter-of-factly may both reduce his anxiety and give him permission to discuss his sexual concerns.

Some spinal cord–injured men may have reflex erections without emission or ejaculation or some may have difficulty in attaining and maintaining an erection. These disorders are to some extent present in all patients with an injury above T12.

When discussing statistical prognosis, one must make the distinction between complete and incomplete lesions. A complete lesion means that there is total loss of voluntary movement and sensation below a certain body level with preserved anal muscle tone and perineal reflexes. An incomplete lesion means that there is some sensation in the perineal area and/or voluntary control of the anal sphincter or pelvic floor muscles with preserved perineal reflexes. These terms thus describe function and not structure.[16]

Generally altered sexual function of the person with an upper motor neuron type lesion is accompanied by loss of bladder and bowel control. The patient will experience less and less psychogenic erections as the lesion becomes more complete. Men who have upper motor neuron lesions with physiologically complete spinal cord deficits are unable to have psychogenic erection. However, 90% to 95% of these patients are able to have reflex erections, which are usually quite adequate for intercourse.

Of the men who have experienced upper motor neuron incomplete lesions, 25% are able to have psychogenic erections, 95% to 98% are able to have reflex erections, and only 2% experience no erections. Research has shown that men with lower motor neuron complete lesions experience a rate of 25% with psychogenic erections, 25% with reflex erections, and 75% have no erections. In contrast to this, men who have lower motor neuron incomplete lesions are able to have psychogenic erections at an 80% to 85% rate, reflex erections at a 90% rate, and 10% to 15% are unable to have erections.[16]

Gross transecting lesions in women may be accompanied by prolonged periods of amenorrhea, but most women in the appropriate age group resume ovulation and menstruation within a few months. Psychogenic and reflex clitoral erection appear to follow the same rules as in men. Vaginal lubrication may be inadequate, and in that case the woman must be instructed to use a water-soluble lubricant. Fertility accompanies the recovery of the menses and most spinal cord–injured women are able to conceive.[16]

■ **To what extent do spinal cord–injured patients experience sexual pleasure?**

It is of great importance to paraplegics and quadriplegics that they remain sexually active and continue to experience sexual pleasure. The health professional should bear in mind that males who because of their injury experience erectile difficulties nevertheless report that stimulation is still pleasurable and that they may experience orgasm. Women also report a continued enjoyment of stimulation up to and including orgasm. Some men experience reflex erections even when psychogenic erections are dysfunctional. Reflex erections often can be stimulated, so the patient and his partner need to be encouraged to discover ways of evoking the reflex. Often patients report that a warm and wet stroking of the perineum will trigger a reflex erection, many lasting 20 to 30 minutes. Because sexuality is life affirming and because it enhances a relationship, spinal cord–injured patients and their partners need guidance and encouragement from the health professional.

■ **What other types of neurologic pathology affect a person's sexuality?**

It has been reported that lesions in the parietal lobe may produce heightened genital sensation and libido. Frontal lobe lesions, from tumors or strokes, may remove inhibitions, thus causing increased or inappropriate sexual behavior. Altered hormonal production, which reduces libido and potency, may result from tumors or cysts of the hypothalamus. Anterior temporal lobe lesions may produce heightened libido, while posterior or deep temporal lobe lesions usually cause a diminution of libido.[17]

■ **How does respiratory illness affect a person's sexuality?**

Sexual activity puts increased demands on the respiratory system and may be too exhausting to accomplish with even a mild asthmatic episode. It is possible that sexual activity can aggravate or precipitate an attack. Psychogenic factors of anxiety or guilt may also increase the tendency for asthmatic episodes. The patient needs to deal with sexual attitudes that might cause anxiety or guilt.

As in the case of all critical illnesses, patients should be counseled with their partners about the sexual implications of the illness. Try to open the lines of communication between partners and encourage them to state directly what each wants and expects from the other. Each needs to take responsibility for what is satisfying and enjoyable. For a significant number of asthmatics the use of bronchodilator medications before sexual activity may greatly increase the ability to function.[18]

Chronic obstructive lung disease hinders all physical activity including sexual activity, the amount of limitation being related to the extent of the disease. Generally the patient with chronic lung disease will be counseled similarly to the patient with compromised cardiac function. The patient and his or her partner should be taught to give themselves rest periods during prolonged sexual activity and to choose positions for lovemaking that allow the patient to be relatively passive. The patient should avoid any position that requires expenditure of large amounts of energy supporting the body weight. Preferred positions would include side-by-side, the patient on his/her back with the partner straddling, or sitting in an armless chair or at the side of the bed with the partner straddling him or her. Bedside oxygen inhalation can give the patient increased capacity for exertion. The use of nasal prongs connected to the oxygen source allows greater freedom of movement. Psychologic support and encouragement to remain active is very important. Depression in respiratory patients because of reduced life activities and social isolation is very possible. That depression can be a major factor in limiting a person's sex life.[19]

■ What can I teach clients whose sexual functioning has been permanently altered?

It is important to remember in dealing with clients whose sexual functioning has been permanently altered that they will need encourage-ment to communicate frankly with their partners as well as to explore alternative forms of sexual pleasuring.

Couples whose basic relationship has been a good one will be able to make such changes with less difficulty than a couple whose relationship is filled with conflict and anxiety. However, the health professional should bear in mind any condition that significantly alters the way a person functions sexually will require time, attention, and perhaps specific therapy to resolve the problem. Remember that people without disability or disorder may also have serious problems with their sex lives. Any illness would exacerbate that condition, and permanent change in sexual functioning will complicate things further. On the positive side, a person so afflicted may find that the crisis that permanent alteration brings is the deciding factor in making the person seek help for the longer standing sexual problem.

In summary, the critical care health professional needs to be able to do two things: (1) to give specific, accurate, and sensitive information to the patient and partner about how his or her sexuality will be affected by that particular critical illness and (2) in cases where sexuality will be severely affected to refer the patient to a sex therapist.

REFERENCES

1. Berlin, H.: Effect of human sexuality on well-being from birth to aging, Med. Aspects Hum. Sexuality, July, 1976.
2. Kinsey, A. C., Pomeroy, W. B., and Martin, C. E.: Sexual behavior in the human male, Philadelphia, 1948, W. B. Saunders Co.
3. Committee on Adolescence, Group for the Advancement of Psychiatry: Normal adolescence, Report No. 68, New York, 1968.
4. Masters, W. H., and Johnson, V. E.: Human sexual response, Boston, 1966, Little, Brown & Co.
5. Downey, G. W.: Sexuality in a health care setting, Mod. Health Care, May, 1976.
6. Shinn, A. F.: Medications that adversely affect sexual function, Crit. Care Update, February, 1977.
7. Renshaw, D. C.: Sexual problems in stroke patients, Med. Aspects Hum. Sexuality, December, 1975.
8. Muchleray, R. N.: Sex counseling after stroke, Med. Aspects Hum. Sexuality, December, 1977.
9. Heart disease and sex: panel discussion, Med. Aspects Hum. Sexuality, June, 1971.
10. Eliot, R. S., and Miles, R. R.: Advising the cardiac patient about sexual intercourse, Med. Aspects Hum. Sexuality, June, 1975.
11. Moore, G. L.: Psychiatric aspects of chronic renal disease, Postgrad. Med., November, 1976.

12. Hickman, B. W.: All about sex . . . despite dialysis, Am. J. Nurs., April, 1977.
13. Abram, H. S., et al.: Sexual functioning in patients with chronic renal failure, J. Nerv. Ment. Dis., March 1975.
14. Grinker, R. R., Jr.: Sex and cancer, Med. Aspects Hum. Sexuality, February, 1976.
15. Wise, T. N.: Sexual functioning in neoplastic disease, Med. Aspects Hum. Sexuality, March, 1978.
16. Horenstein, S.: Sexual dysfunction in neurological disease, Med. Aspects Hum. Sexuality, April, 1976.
17. Some intracranial pathology which may result in disordered male sexuality, Med. Aspects Hum. Sexuality, September, 1977.
18. Straus, S., and Dudley, D.: Sexual activity for asthmatics— a psychiatric perspective, Med. Aspects Hum. Sexuality, November, 1976.
19. Lyons, H. A.: Sexual relations for male patients with chronic obstructive lung disease, Med. Aspects Hum. Sexuality, April, 1977.

CHAPTER 50

Prognosis for survival in critical care

Bernhard A. Votteri and Mary Jo Tierney

Strong social forces have been at work in the past decade that directly affect decisions about survival. Efforts by physicians to prognosticate survival or death more accurately have been matched by the determination of patients and their families to assume a larger and more responsible role in medical decision making. The debate about survival, which catapulted the Quinlan case into a regular television feature and sparked a broadly shared question in everyone's mind, led to greater awareness on the part of the public of the need for sharing medical decision making with the patient and his family. Social forces have given rise to legislative action that has taken the form of bills, acts, and laws that affect the process of dying.

The high cost of intensive care has become clearly apparent and threatens to consume ever-increasing proportions of the health dollar.[1,2]

With these mounting pressures now evident, a clear need exists to arrive at some perspective about the ethical, moral, medical, and economic considerations of survival.[3]

In this chapter we will review salient questions that are raised often in the discussion of survival. The answers we will provide will possibly reflect current thought only and may be altered by future events. Review of the succeeding questions and answers will, we hope, assist the physician and nurse practitioner in meeting the dilemma presented by the present situation, which offers both the promise for better medical care and the threat of a technically dominated bionic era. The domination of medical practice by technology, primarily because technology is readily at hand, will be emphasized. It will also become apparent that the health practitioner must remain aware of the social and legal forces that are currently molding and transforming the relationship of the patient and physician in their decisions about survival.

■ Can survival of the critically ill patient be predicted?

Although survival or death of individual patients cannot be invariably predicted, a number of workers have been able to identify with reasonable accuracy the critically ill patient who will not survive. Using information obtained within the first 12 to 24 hours of a patient's stay in the intensive care unit, Cullen and associates were able to devise a scoring system that predicted with greater than 90% accuracy patients who would not survive.[4] Nonsurvivors could best be identified by the physical status assessment, disease category, elevated admitting creatinine, rising creatinine, need for renal dialysis, and presence of coma. Although single indicators did not accurately identify patients who would not survive, a combination of indicators that demonstrated the progressive failure of organ systems offered reliable signposts to the health care team about the prognosis for survival.

Accurate prediction of survival for surgical patients also was made possible using a scoring system developed by Goldman and associates.[5] The latter were able to predict a fatal outcome if patients were to undergo emergency intra-abdominal or intrathoracic operation, while manifesting the following abnormalities: cardiac irregularities, frequent premature ventricular contractions, jugular venous distention and third heart sound, significant aortic stenosis, recent myocardial infarction, and poor general medical status.

A scoring system for comatose patients was developed by Caronna and associates, which permitted the identification of patients who would not survive or who would not make a good recovery.[6] Preliminary investigation suggests that death is probable, if not certain, when motor responsiveness and oculovestibular responses are absent in the 24-hour period after onset of coma. Patients without oculovestibular response at 24 hours after injury never survived.[7]

Walker and Molinair reported in a prospective study of over 500 critically ill patients that death could be accurately predicted by the presence of apnea and an unresponsive state, including loss of oculovestibular reflexes and a flat EEG.[8] The reliability of the neurologic examination in predicting death was also confirmed by Powner and Fromm, who noted that the EEG was not a reliable predictor of outcome.[9] Shoemacher and associates[10] could, in a high percentage of patients, discriminate between survivors and nonsurvivors using physiologic parameters for assessment. By measuring cardiorespiratory variables, they were able to predict, more accurately than by clinical assessment alone, the outcome in patients undergoing surgical procedures. Assessment of blood lactate values has also proved useful in predicting the outcome in critically ill patients.[11]

A number of retrospective and prospective studies suggest that prediction of outcome is possible using technical classification systems as just described.[4-12]

■ **Do psychologic factors influence survival?**

Although many people believe that psychologic factors may be related to physical well-being, few authoritative and scientific accounts of these associations have been provided. Engel and associates, after studying the life settings in which patients fell ill, were able to find that illnesses are commonly preceded by a period of psychologic disturbances during which the individual is characterized as unable to cope with stress. The syndrome is characterized as follows: (1) a feeling of giving up, experienced as helplessness or hopelessness; (2) self-depreciation; (3) loss of gratification from relationships or roles in life; (4) disruption of a sense of continuity between past, present, and future; and (5) reactivation of memories of earlier periods of giving up.[13]

The "giving-up" syndrome has also been found in cancer patients who feel that nothing more can be done for them. When these cancer patients discover that another treatment is possible, a remarkable improvement in mental attitude occurs. The mental and subsequent physical improvement noted in patients who came to the Melanoma Clinic at Sydney Hospital was so dramatic that some specialists first attributed it to an organic effect. Subsequent analysis suggested that psychologic factors were responsible for short-term disease remission.[14]

Psychologic events may predispose to life-threatening cardiac arrhythmias in both animals and man.[15] A significant correlation has been demonstrated between failure to survive a myocardial infarction and preexisting dejection, dissatisfaction with achievement, and depression.[16-19] In addition, those patients who had an emotional response to events in a coronary care unit were noted to develop arrhythmias, arrest, or sudden death.[16] In a review of 100 anecdotal accounts of sudden cardiac death, it was noted that prior to their death each subject was in an environment where he felt powerless to avert a real or fancied great personal danger of humiliation or loss of status.[15]

Patients who are in critical care units are frequently in a powerless situation that involves great personal danger. In this setting they are prime candidates for further complications brought about by psychologic stress. To avoid stress-related complications, it is essential to provide patients with a calm environment, an opportunity for choice in their care, and adequate information to allay their fears. Despite the fact that the degree to which stress can modify clinical illness is still not well-defined, the preceding pioneer work should alert clinicians to a need for reducing stress in the critically ill patient.

■ **What interventions should a nurse make when a patient with a good prognosis expresses a desire to die?**

When talking with an individual who expresses a desire to die, the nurse must consider the seriousness of the intent and the underlying meaning of the patient's words. When the patient with a good prognosis says, "I just wish I could die," the nurse has the responsibility to ascertain whether the patient actually has a specific plan and the intent to carry out this plan. If the patient has, the nurse is required to report this to the physician and to initiate precautionary measures.

Many times the expression of a desire to die is not a true indication of a patient's wish. It is, rather, an expression of helplessness, hopelessness, fear, loneliness, exhaustion, or lack of stimulation.[20-22] The patient may be depressed by thoughts of further mutilation, pain, and loss of control over the outcome. He may misinterpret a continued stay in an intensive care unit as an indication that the situation is hopeless. His physical condition and lack of sleep may cause the patient to misperceive reality and to compromise his normal coping mechanism.

What then can a nurse do when a patient expresses a preference to stop living? The nurse must be willing to listen to the patient's expression of feelings, acknowledge turmoil, and search for the patient's inner strengths. If the patient perceives the situation as being more hopeless than it actually is, the nurse can give accurate information. Sleep deprivation can be reduced by providing extended periods of rest and administering sedative-hypnotics when appropriate. Waking and sleeping cycles should be preserved if possible. Personal belongings such as radios and pictures can be brought to the hospital, or the patient's bed can be transported to a place of diversion to increase sensory stimulation. The patient should be allowed to assume more control in those situations in which he feels victimized; thus the patient may choose bath and treatment times and be included in choosing other treatment measures. By giving thorough attention to the patient's psychologic needs, the nurse may provide support during the discouraging parts of a critical illness.

■ Can a patient who attempts suicide be allowed to die?

It appears that in most instances the person who makes a suicide attempt must be resuscitated, although the medical and legal references provide little assistance in answering this question. Even if the patient states a preference for nontreatment, the physician in the emergency room or critical care unit cannot honor such a request, since he does not usually have access to the complete circumstances surrounding the event. Not only is the physician unaware of the patient's mental status at the time of the attempt, but he also has no assurance that the person's impulsive act is truly indicative of his long-term state of mind. Because of the physician's own doubt and the urgency and nature of emergency care, he is compelled to treat the patient, thereby providing the patient a more rational choice at a later time.[23]

The physician is under no obligation to prolong the vital functions of a patient where no real benefit to the person is likely to result. Although this situation may not be common with attempted suicide patients, the physician can withhold procedures when the patient's outcome will be continued vegetative existence.[24]

Medical practitioners should be aware that a distinction has been made between treatment refusal and suicide. An adult person of sound mind has a right to refuse lifesaving treatment when the threat to life is not self-induced. Such refusal of treatment is not defined as suicide. On the other hand, actively setting death in motion is suicide and, although it is no longer considered a crime in most states, it is not a legally protected right.

Can a physician refrain from treating a terminally ill patient who intentionally attempts suicide? An immediate answer is not readily available. The physician must consider such factors as the patient's state of mind and the imminence of natural death. Although there is no legal substantiation for treating the patient, it is probably common practice for a family doctor who has known the patient over a period of time to honor the wishes of the rational, terminally ill patient to hasten death by self-inflicted action. Only in such an exceptional situation might a physician refrain from treatment.

■ May a person make a decision about what he prefers to have done when he develops a severe illness?

Every competent adult is free to choose or reject lifesaving medical treatment.[25-27] The right to refuse treatment is founded on the premise that everyone has the right to determine what shall be done with his body. This right can only be challenged if the patient is incompetent, uninformed, or acting in an irresponsible or negligent manner. The recent Quinlan case focused the attention of the world on the problem that is created when a terminally ill patient is no longer competent to express a preference about medical care.[25,27] The Quinlan case stimulated the public and legal representatives to express concern that decisions about care might come to reside exclusively with others who, without due process, could assume a custodial role over the patient.[28,29] Assemblyman Keene, author of the California Natural Death Act, said "we felt there were peo-

The California Death Act directive that must be completed by the patient and the attending physician is shown below:

Directive made this _____ day of _____(month, year).

I, _____, being of sound mind, willfully, and voluntarily make known my desire that my life shall not be artificially prolonged under the circumstances set forth below, do hereby declare:

1. If at any time I should have an incurable injury, disease, or illness certified to be a terminal condition by two physicians, and where the application of life-sustaining procedures would serve only to artificially prolong the moment of my death, and where my physician determines that my death is imminent whether or not life-sustaining procedures are utilized, I direct that such procedures be withheld or withdrawn, and that I be permitted to die naturally.

2. In the absence of my ability to give directions regarding the use of such life-sustaining procedures, it is my intention that this directive shall be honored by my family and physician(s) as the final expression of my legal right to refuse medical or surgical treatment and accept the consequences from such refusal.

3. If I have been diagnosed as pregnant and that diagnosis is known to my physician, this directive shall have no force or effect during the course of my pregnancy.

4. I have been diagnosed and notified at least 14 days ago as having a terminal condition by _____, M.D., whose address is _____, and whose telephone number is _____. I understand that if I have not filled in the physician's name and address, it shall be presumed that I did not have a terminal condition when I made out this directive.

5. This directive shall have no force or effect five years from the date filled in above.

6. I understand the full import of this directive and I am emotionally and mentally competent to make this directive.

Signed _____

City, County and State of Residence _____

_____

The declarant has been personally known to me and I believe him or her to be of sound mind.

Witness _____

Witness _____

This Directive complies in form with the "Natural Death Act," California Health and Safety Code, Section 7188, Assembly Bill 3060 (Keene).

ple who, in the event of terminal illness, would not want to spend their final days tyrannized by machines when the only purpose of those machines is to postpone the moment of death artificially, when no cure is possible, and where death is in any event imminent."[30]

California signed into law, in January of 1977, The Natural Death Act, which provides a directive prepared by the patient to his attending physician that states that meaningless life-support systems shall be removed if the patient is terminally ill; it provides at the same time freedom from liability for the physician who acts in accordance with the directive.[31]

Although the Natural Death Act would appear to answer some of the problems of patient control over medical destiny, other problems remain. The outstanding problems with the death act are that it is not applicable to persons in good health and patients with chronic illness whose death is not close at hand, and the act leaves the imminence of death undefined. The prediction for survival, which is left to the discretion of the physician may, in many instances, be problematic.[32]

The need for specific legislation such as the California Natural Death Act has been questioned by some workers who indicate that it has always been the patient's privilege to refuse treatment and that this choice has been respected invariably by both physicians and the law. In addition, there has been some concern that the restrictive nature of the law may complicate the dying act for persons who have not signed directives.[29,32]

Although ten states, by 1979, enacted so called "living wills," it is possible that future courts may find that a terminally ill patient has the right to refuse resuscitation before hospitalization without court action if the competent patient's decision is based on information that fully disclosed the diagnosis and available treatment options.[33]

In our experience these legislative actions have had minimal impact on the practice of critical care. Very few patients who are treated in our intensive care units have availed themselves of such directives. Moreover, the patient experiencing catastrophic illness has not usually had warning of his imminent death and, therefore, has not felt compelled to prepare the appropriate direc-

tive. It is of further interest that individuals who have prepared such directives may choose to revoke the directive subsequently and request or demand full and heroic measures when death is imminent.

A recent survey of the experience of physicians with the California Natural Death Act disclosed that 50% of respondents found the act improved relationships with patients. These physicians found that the act clarified the role of the physician and the directive provided a vehicle for discussion that served to bring "out of the closet" the subject of terminal care and dying.[34] An equal number of responders had not utilized the directive and did not believe that such legislation had changed or improved the practice of medicine.

In short, the treatment of patients continues to be based on determinations made between the patient and the physician at the time of the episode. The type of care chosen for the terminally ill patient has probably been more strongly affected by social changes than legislative action. Increasingly, patients and families have come to recognize that only those measures of care that are likely to restore health are necessary. They no longer feel compelled to accept or request heroic measures in the care of every critically ill patient.

■ Should the level of care be related to the patient's prognosis?

It is becoming increasingly clear that the level of care selected by the physician should be based on the expectation that such care will benefit the patient. It is no longer appropriate to persist, in every instance, with unlimited supportive measures until accepted criteria for death supervene.[1,2] Tagge and co-workers proposed that a patient be classified according to prognosis so that the full range of intensive care could be provided only to those patients who reasonably would be expected to recover.[35] They suggested that to provide maximum support to every patient where no reasonable hope for survival existed was illogical, since such a plan demands the full deployment of expensive and time-consuming therapy that would merely prolong the dying process. Moreover, such therapeutic heroism often was followed by frustration, hostility, and guilt affecting both family members and the practitioners.

Tagge's group proposed that the treatment program be based on survival prognosis because such formulation required close communication between patient, primary care physician, consultants, and family members. After classifying the patient's clinical condition, they found that a course of action could then be defined clearly for everyone. When the patient was told that the outcome for survival was very poor, patients and family could better prepare themselves to accept the final outcome. A similar classification system also was formulated by the Clinical Care Committee of the Massachusetts General Hospital.[36]

Guidelines for care according to prognosis also have been used effectively at Presbyterian Hospital in Pittsburg and were described by Loughead.[37] Medical evaluation on admission to the intensive care unit made it possible for Loughead and his associates to assign patients to the following classifications of care according to prognosis:

1. Total support: This group includes patients with acute, potentially reversible illness.
2. All support measures except cardiopulmonary resuscitation: This group includes patients judged to have irreversible cardiopulmonary failure or multiple organ failure.
3. No extraordinary measures: This group includes patients with minimal brain function and no hope for recovery.

Classifications No. 2 and No. 3 are designated after complete disclosure to the patient and family members.

Staff members meet regularly with patients and family members to reassure them that they are not compelled nor morally bound to accept therapy that can provide little promise of benefit for the patient. At the same time, the patient and family are thoroughly informed that heroic measures will not be provided to patients who are classified in groups No. 2 and No. 3 since such measures would only prolong dying.

Using the preceding classification of care, Loughead and co-workers were able to accurately predict outcomes and provide commensurate care in 577 consecutive patients admitted in the ICU. Of the group No. 3 patients 100% died, while only 8% of the group No. 1 patients died. He observed that the ability to provide care commensurate with the prognosis for survival was helpful in avoiding clinical situations where irreversible, critically ill patients are subjected to death-delaying medical therapy.[37]

■ **Should heroic resuscitative measures be given to patients with advanced chronic disorders?**

Resuscitative measures should be applied when medical assessment indicates that such measures may improve the health of the patient.[38] The purpose of heroic measures such as cardiopulmonary resuscitation (CPR) is to prevent sudden, unexpected death. CPR is not conducted in situations where death owing to irreversible illness is expected and resuscitative efforts would be futile.[38] The adverse effect of applying full supportive measures to patients with advanced chronic disease has recently received attention. When heroic supportive measures such as mechanical ventilation were applied to patients with chronic respiratory failure who had not previously benefited from comprehensive supportive care, such heroic measures usually led to prolongation of physical suffering, mental anguish to the patient and family, and did not significantly modify the medical outcome.[39,40] Such findings led Petty and associates to conclude that supportive measures should be applied only when such measures provide hope for recovery. By refusing to apply all technical resources to every critically ill patient, they were able to avoid the dilemma of subjecting patients to a ventilator-bound existence.[39]

Although the legal ramifications of withholding full resuscitative measures will be discussed in greater detail later, it should be mentioned here that a recent court ruling in the Massachusetts Appeals Court by Justice Christopher J. Armstrong found that, where resuscitation will do nothing to cure or relieve terminal illness, physicians may enter "do not resuscitate" orders.[41] The decision in that matter, he observed, was a question peculiarly within the competence of the medical profession to decide what measures are appropriate to ease the imminent passing of an irreversibly, terminally ill, incompetent patient in light of that patient's history and condition and the wishes of his/her family. The Massachusetts court found that withholding treatment that merely prolonged survival, without returning the individual to a normally functioning and integrated existence, did not require judicial review. An order to withhold full resuscitation measures could be initiated by the physician after informed consent was obtained from the competent patient or guardian of an incompetent patient.

Recent publications have reviewed the decision-making process that should be applied when issuing "orders not to resuscitate," and the appropriateness of such orders has been supported by the American Medical Association.[38,42]

■ What is the impact of the Karen Quinlan and Saikewicz cases?

The Karen Quinlan case underscored the difficulty of defining the incompetent patient's rights of self-determination.[25,27-28] The proposed legal solutions raised by the Quinlan case and the subsequent Saikewicz case could add further complexity to the decision-making process involved in providing care for incompetent, critically ill patients.

Karen Quinlan, a 21-year-old woman who incurred irreversible brain damage following ingestion of drugs and alcohol, received continuous mechanical ventilation for 6 months before her stepfather attempted to intervene in the physician's decision to continue treatment. A judicial decision was sought by the stepfather because the physician refused to stop ventilatory support at the family's request. Mr. Quinlan requested that the New Jersey Superior Court appoint him guardian and authorize him to have discontinued "all extraordinary means of sustaining the vital processes of his daughter." On November 10, 1975, Judge Muir of the Superior Court denied Mr. Quinlan's request, stating that the matter was a medical issue not a legal one. He added, "there is no constitutional right to die that can be asserted by a parent for his incompetent adult child."[28]

Mr. Quinlan made an appeal to the New Jersey Supreme Court and, on March 30, 1976, the lower court's ruling was overturned. Joseph Quinlan was named his stepdaughter's guardian. The court stated that if physicians concluded "that there is no reasonable possibility of Karen's ever

emerging from her present comatose condition to a cognitive, sapient state, then the respirator may be withdrawn." The court stipulated that an "ethics committee" of the hospital should assist in making this decision. The court focused attention on Karen's right to privacy in the face of her irreversible status. The ruling held that the court could not "compel Karen to endure the unendurable" and recognized her guardian's right to exercise privacy on her behalf. The court defined less clearly the physician's role when the court implied that it was the responsibility of the doctor and ethics committee to formulate a prognosis, but it was the patient's or guardian's responsibility to accept or refuse treatment.

Considerable consternation in legal circles resulted from the Quinlan court decision, which delegated authority to an ethics committee to make life and death decisions.[25,43,44] This latter provision has been criticized because it would represent an unprecedented delegation of authority by a court to private individuals.[25,43,44] In fact, in a subsequent case in a Massachusetts court, the court in the matter of Saikewicz explicitly rejected the Quinlan solution and stated:

> We take a dim view of any attempt to shift the ultimate decision-making responsibility away from the duly established courts of proper jurisdiction to any committee, panel, or group, *ad hoc* or permanent. ......[45]

The court continued to voice concern that an *ad hoc* committee could adequately represent the rights of incompetent patients when it stated:

> We do not view the judicial resolution of this most difficult and awesome question—whether potentially life-prolonging treatment should be withheld from a person incapable of making his own decision—as constituting a "gratuitous encroachment" on the domain of medical expertise. Rather, such questions of life and death seem to us to require the process of detached but passionate investigation and decision that forms the ideal on which the judicial branch of government was created. Achieving this ideal is our responsibility and that of the lower court, and is not to be entrusted to any group purporting to represent the "morality and conscience of our society," no matter how highly motivated or impressively constituted.[45]

Many physicians perceived this court ruling as a threat to the practice of medicine, since the ruling created the impression that the authority for decision making in issues of life and death would shift from the physician to the courtroom.[46-47] However, it should be recognized that in the case of Saikewicz, a 67-year-old incompetent patient with acute leukemia, the court also ruled that decisions about care would be based on the prognostic determination of physicians and that therapy would not be indicated if it offered no hope of recovery and would only prolong suffering. The court further noted that the interest of the state in saving life was lessened in cases of incurable illness. This ruling was, in fact, more liberal in its scope than the much heralded Quinlan opinion.[43,44]

A recent Massachusetts court ruling may add another important step in clearing the confusion and controversy that surrounded the Karen Quinland and Saikewicz cases.[41,47] The Massachusetts Appeals Court found in the matter of Shirley Dinnerstein that treatment could be withheld without judicial approval if such treatment served only to suspend the act of dying.[41] Although the court did not define clearly the procedure that would be required to withdraw artificial life support from a patient who had irreversible brain damage but who was not in a terminal condition, Schram and associates, who reviewed the recent court findings, believe that judicial review prior to withdrawal of artificial support measures probably is not necessary in terminally ill patients.[47] Baron, however, cautions that such conclusions may be premature and unduly optimistic, since the decision of an appeals court is not a final authority, nor are appeal court findings generally used in defining legal precedents.[48] He further suggests that the body of authority for medical decision making about cases of survival should be developed in the courtroom where he believes that a reaccommodation of the needs of medical practice with the need for protecting the personal integrity of the individual can best be achieved. Many workers really question whether the adversary climate of the courts is the best domain for molding medical practice.[25,46,49] Nevertheless, it is clearly essential that practitioners be prepared to provide the medical input in court decisions to assure that a humane solution is provided, which is based on objective, medical appraisal of the patient's illness. Hopefully, further court rulings will recognize the primary importance of the patient-physician relationship and ensure that most decisions about survival can be provided at the bedside and need not be contested in the courtroom.

■ **Must a nurse initiate resuscitation of a patient who experiences cardiopulmonary arrest when no particular guidelines for intervention have been provided?**

The policy in many hospitals is that a resuscitation effort be made when cardiopulmonary arrest occurs even if guidelines for intervention have not been provided. Confusion about nurse intervention often arises when the primary physician intends to let the patient die peacefully without heroic measures but neglects to write this as a specific order. The attending physician may give a verbal order indicative of his preference to one of the nurses, that is, "resuscitate, but don't try too hard", or "don't be too aggressive in your suctioning." This kind of vague and ambiguous order leaves the nurse in a vulnerable position when a cardiopulmonary arrest occurs. According to Diane Adler, President of the American Association of Critical Care Nurses, a nurse cannot accept a verbal order for "no code."[50]

Such a dilemma could best be avoided if the resuscitation measures to be provided were indicated by the physician in the record of all the critically ill patients. After conferring with the patient, family, and consulting physicians, the primary physician could prepare a summary of the critically ill patient's course that would include the following:

1. Diagnosis
2. Prognosis
3. The competent patient's wishes about resuscitation as elicited by the patient's informed consent
4. Information conveyed to the family
5. Intervention that is appropriate in the light of the above[38,42,47,50,51]

The final decision about the appropriateness of intervention is a matter to be jointly determined by the patient, his guardian, and the attending physician.[49] The decision about the need for resuscitation should be reviewed at least daily and more frequently if appropriate. Since 1974, the American Medical Association has urged that such decisions about resuscitation should be recorded in the patient's hospital record. Rabkin advises that before writing such a directive, the primary physician should verify the irreversible status of the patient's illness with an *ad hoc* committee of the hospital.[42] This opinion was also expressed in the Quinlan proceedings.[28] Although the specific makeup of the *ad hoc* committee was not spelled out by the Quinlan court, Rabkin suggested that the *ad hoc* committee be comprised of physicians who are attending the patient, nurses, and at least one physician who previously has been uninvolved in the patient's care.[42] Although this recommendation is well intentioned, it has not received wide acceptance by physicians and would tend to complicate decision making. In fact, a multidisciplinary committee as envisioned by the Quinlan court would act too slowly to provide useful solutions in critical care decision making. Nor is it clear that such advocates could, more clearly than the primary physician, perceive the needs of the patient or indeed have the legal authority to decide life-and-death issues.[25,51]

A recently proposed revision of the California Hospital Association Consent Manual not only recommended that an order by the primary physician for withholding life-sustaining procedures be accompanied by a concurring statement of the intensive care director, but it even indicated that the primary physician should contact his attorney before writing the order.[52] Such a cumbersome mechanism is contrary to medical practice and is certainly unsuitable in meeting the urgent nature of critical care decisions. Further administrative and legislative solutions should recognize that control in decision making should remain with the patient and the attending physician who are the only individuals who can constantly be responsive to the dynamic changes in health and disease. It is, of course, appropriate in cases when the patient is not competent to provide consent, that the primary physician seek medical consultation with medical peers who have no vested interest in the final treatment decision.[49]

As previously discussed, legal requirements regarding "no code" order writing have not been fully defined. However, some clarification of the physician's role in writing "no code" orders are evolving as is evidenced by the ruling of the Massachusetts Appeals Court.[41] In the Dinnerstein case the court declared that it is within the realm of the medical profession to determine when an incompetent patient is irreversibly, terminally ill. Mandatory judicial review was not determined to be necessary in order to withhold resuscitation measures for every irreversibly, terminally ill, incompetent patient. In that case the court found that the decisions about which measures are appropriate in easing the passing of a terminally ill patient are peculiarly within the competence of the medical profession. Such decision would not require judicial review if the practitioner's action were in keeping with the highest traditions of his profession.

- ### What action should a nurse take when she disagrees with the physician's decision about resuscitation?

The 1965 International Council of Nursing Code of Ethics states, "The nurse is under an obligation to carry out the physician's orders intelligently and loyally . . .".[53] This implies that the nurse must do what the physician says despite her disagreement. However, the 1973 revised code of ethics states, "The nurses' primary responsibility is to those people who require nursing care . . ..".[53] The American Nursing Association Code for Nurses reinforces this statement with, "The nurse acts to safeguard the patient when his care and safety are affected by incompetent, unethical, or illegal conduct of any person."[54] This suggests the nurse must do what she feels is right for the patient and not necessarily what the physician orders. This stance is further supported by existing laws. "Nurses can be held liable for actions they commit even when they are following the orders of physicians."[53] It is clear that ethical behavior is not the exclusive prerogative of the physician when Gaylor points out that "although doctors are licensed to make medical decisions, all men are licensed to make ethical decisions."[55]

Should the nurse then follow her ethical beliefs about what she feels is correct for the patient, despite the physician's preference? Although such action may seem morally justifiable, it is likely to place the nurse in an untenable position vis-á-vis the physician. A more practical approach dictates that the nurse seek consultation not only with the attending physician but also with her peers and with the director of the intensive care unit. Such discussions may objectively define the clinical problems; they also present the opportunity for physicians and nurses to express feelings about providing or not providing resuscitative measures. If, after such discussions, the nurse persists in feeling that her ethical standards are being compromised, her most practical alternative is to ask another nurse to substitute for her. Appealing to the hierarchy of the hospital for resolution is not always practical in the urgent moments required for critical care decisions. Careful consideration and review about the appropriateness of resuscitation prior to the episode is desirable so that the preceding problem can be minimized.

■ **What is the prognosis for survival and recovery after cardiac arrest?**

The prognosis for survival after cardiac arrest is determined by such factors as the underlying clinical disorder, circumstances in which the cardiac arrest occurs, and the skill and speed with which resuscitative measures are undertaken.[56-58] When cardiac status and general health are good and the physiologic derangement can be rapidly reversed as in hypoxemic or drug-induced arrest, recovery and survival occur in the majority of cases. Twenty percent of nonhospitalized patients who are resuscitated after myocardial infarction by well-trained rescuers survive.[59-61] The importance of early intervention in assuring survival has been emphasized by Conley, who noted that a rescuer was immediately present in all patients who survived cardiac arrest.[62] High rates of recovery have also been shown when patients experience cardiac arrests in coronary care units. Up to 30% of such patients who are resuscitated ultimately are discharged from the hospital alive. Connolly noted that even though respiration and cardiac function could be restored in 52% of the patients who were resuscitated in a general hospital, only 12% of those patients ultimately left the hospital alive.[63] Similar findings were demonstrated by LeMire and co-workers, who found that 3% to 7% of all resuscitated inpatients ultimately were discharged from the hospital.[64]

A much poorer prognosis for survival is evident when cardiac arrest occurs in patients with far advanced cardiac disease or life-threatening systemic illnesses. In such patients survival and recovery are rare.[58,65,66] Amey and co-workers found that none of the patients with class four heart disease and congestive heart failure survived for more than 45 days after resuscitation for cardiac arrest.[60] When cardiac arrest occurs in critically ill patients, second resuscitative efforts are rarely followed by survival. These observations led Rogore and associates to the conclusion that second and third resuscitative efforts in poorly responsive patients were futile.[58]

The poor outcome after cardiac arrest in advanced disease should not obscure the fact that patients with transmural myocardial infarction who survive cardiac arrest have a good prognosis, with 76% surviving at the end of 2 years.[62-64,67] It is less well recognized that 47% of those without myocardial infarction who survived cardiac arrest die with a second arrest episode in the subsequent 2 years, probably because of ventricular fibrillation.[67] Efforts to identify patients with electrical instability and to evaluate the impact of antiarrhythmic therapy on the subsequent clinical course are currently under investigation.[62,68,69] It is hoped that such studies may lead to better management with increased survival and recovery following CPR.

A wide spectrum of neurologic syndromes has been described following cardiopulmonary arrest with findings varying from transient confusion to quadriparesis and a vegetative state.[7] Routine neurologic assessment at 1, 12, and 24 hours after arrest has been of predictive value in identifying survivors with intellectual integrity.[7,12,70] Patients who were conscious and/or made purposeful responses to forceful stimuli at 1 to 12 hours after resuscitation usually survived. Although transient neurologic deficit was common, progressive improvement with clearing of neurologic deficit was usually demonstrated by 48 hours.[70]

Patients who were unresponsive to painful stimuli at 1, 12, and 24 hours experienced a 55% mortality. Fifty percent of the unresponsive survivors were severely demented. Decerebrate posturing which persisted 24 hours after arrest implied a poor prognosis, with severe disability, vegetative state, or death resulting.[7] Absence of ocular responses of 3 days' duration was also associated with a grave prognosis. Most patients who had unreactive pupils, absent oculocephalic, oculovestibular, or corneal reflexes sustained severe disability or death.[12] These observations indicate the value of serial neurologic assessment in predicting survival after cardiac arrest.

■ Should a patient be told about his poor prognosis?

Most authorities maintain that a patient should be given his true diagnosis.[71-74] Instead of being plunged into greater despair by the truth, patients rather become quite peaceful and act with purpose in their remaining time. If the patient's prognosis for survival is kept a secret, the patient will discern it by observing the behavior of those around him. Nonverbal communication will usually reveal the truth regardless of the intent to conceal the true prognosis. Wilson states that a patient will "watch a person's face and observe slight changes of expression in the eyes or mouth," will "note the making or evasion of eye contact . . .," and will "see the embarrassed wave of a hand and hear a change in the timbre of the voice."[75] By such gestures, the true prognosis may become painfully apparent. Distrust and anger may result if the patient discovers that the prognosis has been deliberately hidden from him. Regardless of the intent to protect the patient, such subterfuge is rarely successful. Moreover, frankness and honesty are important in preserving the confidence and trust that the patient feels toward the nurse and physician. Preserving such relationships at the time of illness is important. When patients are told their diagnosis, they are able to make religious preparation and arrange their affairs in addition to reconciling relationships in their lives.

The physician who imparts information about a diagnosis also conveys an attitude about that diagnosis.[75] If the physician sees the terminal state as a time for growth, he transmits that perspective to his patient. Affirmation of the patient as an important individual can also be communicated by spending as much time in providing the comforting measures as has been spent in providing active treatment. Open and honest communication about the prognosis promotes an environment of peace rather than creating turmoil during the final stage of life.

■ In what manner can a patient's poor prognosis be conveyed to family members?

Although there are no absolute principles to provide guidance in delivering unpleasant news to family members, several suggestions may be helpful. The physician should be sincere and honest, yet sensitive, in his appraisal of the situation. Family members, on first learning of the critical status of a loved one, may often be so distressed that they are unable to comprehend the full implication of the physician's words.[76] Thorough explanation of all diagnostic and therapeutic options may be inappropriate at such a time, and a physician may only need to provide general information at the first meeting. Two or three sessions may be necessary before full disclosure is possible or can be comprehended.

It may be helpful after the initial meetings to ask family members "Do you have any questions?" In this way the physician can determine what family members are prepared to hear. After giving appropriate information in lay terms, the physician may again inquire, "What does this information mean to you?" Such exchanges permit the physician to reinforce the families' perception of information and offers the physician the opportunity to correct misconceptions.

By acknowledging the emotional turmoil encountered by the family, the physician can often assist the family in adjusting to a poor prognosis.[77] Such acknowledgment may take the following form: "It is natural to feel as you do when someone you love is this ill." In this manner he assures the family that feelings such as guilt, anger, frustration, and so forth are normal and acceptable reactions experienced by grieving family members.

It is helpful for the physician to learn who among the family members will make decisions and who will act as family spokesperson, so that confusion and conflict among family members can be avoided.[77] Medical reports can thus be presented at designated intervals to the spokesperson. Other friends and peripheral family members can then consult with the primary spokesperson for answers to their inquiries.

Hospital staff members also must strive to remain informed of what the physician is telling the family and friends. Information given to staff members must be updated continually as information is given to the family.[78] Staff members can then perform an affirmative role in reinforcing and making clear the physician's reports.

■ **What feelings may be experienced by the patient, family, and health care professionals when the patient is perceived as terminally ill?**

Dr. Elisabeth Kubler-Ross reminds us that feelings of shock, disbelief, anger, bargaining, and depression frequently occur in dying patients.[79] Many patients never progress beyond these stages and die in a state of indignation, bitterness, anguish, and a feeling of futility.[80] Others achieve a stage of acceptance. "These patients are not happy, but they are not terribly sad. They usually have very little physical pain and discomfort, and they slip into a stage which very often reminds us of the beginning of life: when a person has physical needs and needs only one person to give him some tender, loving care and compassion."[81] Such patients show a feeling of equanimity and peace as they ruminate over past events in order to summarize the value and meaning of a lifetime of existence. Whereas in previous stages these patients had a need to inquire about their prognosis and to engage in open communication with their physicians, they now experience detachment and lack of curiosity about worldly affairs.[82] Lorin asserts that even patients who have achieved a certain equanimity about their death still have a need to believe that everything possible for their survival is being done, that they are worthy of maximum efforts, and that there is still a small amount of hope for them.[83]

Family members go through similar phases in their grieving process. However, they may be at a different stage than the critically ill patient. Whereas the patient may be at peace with his terminal status, the family member may still have a need to deny the inevitable. This is particularly true when family members arrive from out of town and have not had time to adjust to the potential loss of a loved one. When the patient's illness occurs without warning, family members feel shock, fright, disbelief, and numbness.[84] They may feel some responsibility for something they failed to do or say. They may be frightened by the foreign sights, sounds, and smells of the ICU. Despair and helplessness may be their response as they sit in the waiting room. This strained situation may conjure up feelings and memories from the past and may force a family member to face his own death for the first time. Family members who are involved in the decision to withdraw active treatment may be overcome by feelings of guilt and doubt over their decision. They may be unprepared for and dismayed by the prolonged period of suffering a loved one goes through before dying.[83] Reassurance, counseling, and emotional support must be available for the dying patient and his family.

Since the training of physicians and nurses is primarily directed at "outwitting" death, the practitioners may be unprepared to provide care, comfort, and counsel to the terminally ill patient. Physicians and nurses may react with frustration, defeat, and feelings of inadequacy to a hopeless clinical situation.[85,86] These feelings may be expressed as withdrawal, intellectualization, cynicism, and preoccupation with tests.[85,87] Resolution of these sentiments requires awareness that continual psychologic replenishment is a necessity for the staff who are caring for hopelessly ill patients. Special seminars incorporating principles of preventive psychiatry have proved helpful in identifying and resolving physicians' anxieties that have arisen during the care of terminally ill patients.[87]

When the physician and nurse can come to accept the premise that care, not cure, must be the goal in care of the terminally ill, they can then begin to regard caring as important and find it emotionally rewarding. Thus the eminence of death that forcefully confronts every practitioner need not be viewed as a threat to his mastery or healing.

■ What care should be provided when there is no hope for survival?

Only comfort giving measures are necessary when there is no hope for survival.[88] Application of lifesaving measures considered mandatory at the onset of illness become optional, and health professionals adjust their interventions according to the wishes of the patient and family. Measures that are often continued include: oxygen that is administered without blood gas monitoring when it makes a dyspneic patient more comfortable, postural drainage and suction to reduce airway obstruction, aspirin to relieve the discomfort of fever, intravenous solutions to prevent excessive dehydration with attendant thirst. In general, optimal management strategy involves treatment that provides comfort with minimum discomfort and maximum psychologic support.

Diagnostic studies that may have guided care and promoted survival during acute, reversible illness become futile and less justifiable in irreversible illness. Routine hematologic and roentgenographic investigations that have no impact on outcome may only contribute to discomfort and increased cost of care. Pain should be alleviated by giving narcotics at regular intervals.[89] Nausea is controlled by using oral, intramuscular, or suppository antiemetics. The patient is repositioned in bed according to his desires and kept warm, clean, and comfortable.

The most important aspect of terminal care is that patients and their families be given greater participation and freedom in making decisions about care. The plan for care should not be dictated solely by the needs of the staff. The patient should choose how he will use his remaining energy.

The hospice movement offers a philosophy of care that may be adapted to a critical care unit.[89] Instead of visiting for short intervals, relatives of dying patients may stay with their loved one for as many hours as is comfortable for the patient. Some family members may choose to sleep in the critical care area; assistance with physical care may be the choice of other relatives. The focus of all efforts by staff and family remains to provide comfort giving measures. The patient and family together choose how to spend the final hours and days.

■ Do the clinical criteria of brain death accurately identify those patients who will not survive in spite of supportive measures?

The Harvard criteria for brain death listed below accurately identify the patient who will develop cardiovascular collapse and somatic death despite supportive measures.[90]

HARVARD CRITERIA FOR BRAIN DEATH[91]

1. Unreceptivity and unresponsivity. "Even the most intensely painful stimuli evoke no vocal or other response. . . ."
2. No movements or breathing. "Observation covering a period of at least one hour by physicians is adequate to satisfy the criteria of no spontaneous muscular movements or spontaneous respiration or response to stimuli . . . the total absence of spontaneous breathing may be established by turning off the respiratory for three minutes and observing whether there is an effort on the part of the subject to breathe. . . ." (This requires that carbon dioxide tension be normal and the patient be breathing room air for 10 minutes before the test.)
3. No reflexes. "The pupil will be fixed and dilated and will not respond to a direct source of bright light. . . . Ocular movement (to head turning and to irrigation of ears with ice water) and blinking are absent. There is no evidence of postural activity" (decerebrate or other). "Swallowing, yawning, vocalizing are in abeyance." "Corneal and pharyngeal reflexes are absent" "As a rule the stretch or tendon reflexes cannot be elicited."
4. Flat electroencephalogram. "Of great confirmatory value is the flat or isoelectric electroencephalogram . . ." (Technical guidelines include 5 V/mm or higher gains, absence of response to a pitch or noise, and 10 minute minimum recording time.) "All of the above tests shall be repeated at least 24 hours later with no change." Hypothermia (temperature below 32.2° C [90° F] and central nervous system depressants such as barbiturates must be excluded. "In situations where . . . electroencephalographic monitoring is not available, the absence of cerebral function has to be determined by purely clinical signs . . . or by the absence of circulation as judged by standstill of blood in the retinal vessels, or by absence of cardiac action. . . ."

These criteria were formulated in 1968 by the *Ad Hoc* Committee of the Harvard Medical School to provide guidelines of care for patients who had lost any hope of a cognitive existence but still had intact cardiovascular function. Such objective criteria of death were necessary to prevent capricious or mischievous medical practices being applied to terminally ill patients that might be motivated by the needs of organ transplantation or the rising cost of caring for the terminally ill.[91] The standards for defining brain death were uniformly accurate in diagnosing a fatal outcome, but many other patients who had equally serious brain damage were excluded by the rigidly defined neurologic criteria that had been chosen.[90,92]

For this reason a reassessment of the criteria for brain death was initiated in 1971-72 by the National Institute of Neurological and Communicative Disorders and Stroke. The nine-hospital cooperative study prepared the modified standards summarized below.

CRITERIA FOR CEREBRAL DEATH (BRAIN DEATH) PROPOSED BY THE COLLABORATIVE STUDY OF CEREBRAL DEATH[92]

PREREQUISITE
1. All appropriate diagnostic and therapeutic procedures have been performed.

CRITERIA (to be present for 30 min at least 6 hr after the onset of coma and apnea)
1. Coma with cerebral unresponsivity (see definition 1)
2. Apnea (see definition 2)
3. Dilated pupils
4. Absent cephalic reflexes (see definition 3)
5. Electrocerebral silence (see definition 4)

CONFIRMATORY TEST
1. Absence of cerebral blood flow

DEFINITIONS
1. Cerebral unresponsivity: a state in which the patient does not respond purposively to externally applied stimuli, obeys no commands, and does not phonate spontaneously or in response to a painful stimulus
2. Apnea: the absence of spontaneous respiration, manifested by the need for controlled ventilation (that is, the patient makes no effort to override the respirator), for at least 15 minutes
3. Cephalic reflexes: pupillary, corneal, oculoauditory, oculovestibular, oculocephalic, ciliospinal, snout, cough, pharyngeal, and swallowing
4. Electrocerebral silence: an electroencephalogram with an absence of electrical potentials of cerebral

origin over 2 V from symmetrically placed electrode pairs over 10 cm apart and with interelectrode resistance between 100 and 10,000 ohms

These latter criteria also accurately identified a fatal outcome in that 100% of patients fulfilling these new criteria died within 3 months of assessment.[1,90,92] Such studies established that the age-old tenet for pronouncing death as the absence of pulse and respiration was clearly inadequate and inappropriate. Moreover, in an era of extraordinary care and cost, somatic life could be maintained by technical means despite the absence of any prospect for restoring a cognitive existence. Thus for moral, legal, and economic reasons, a more appropriate definition of death was required.[93] The redefinition of death based on brain criteria was formulated in 1968 by representatives from medical specialities and the disciplines of ethics, law, and history and was subsequently endorsed by medical societies throughout the world. Simultaneously, and independently, legislation was being proposed in Kansas that would redefine death in order to provide a means to obtain viable organs for transplantation that would ensure protection of the donor and establish a scientific basis for physician's actions. The legislation would be based on the precept that "man dies when the brain dies."[94] Statutory adaption of this new concept of brain death occurred first in Kansas in 1970, and by 1978 more than 15 states, including California, had enacted legislation concerning brain death.[95-97] The wide acceptance of the brain death concept was underscored when the American Bar Association offered the following general model for legal bodies that were considering redefining death: "For all legal purposes, a human body with irreversible cessation of brain function, according to usual and customary standards of medical practice, shall be considered dead."[98] Statutory recognition of brain death would establish consistency under the law and hopefully preclude the need for repeated anguish-producing court cases. Such legislation would also allow physicians to terminate ventilatory support for patients who meet the criteria for death.[99]

The Kansas brain death statute, which incorporated the preceding provisions, has been heralded as particularly noteworthy because it does not specifically define the technical procedures required to assess brain death but sets the criteria as those that are the current standards of medical practice. This approach leaves the door open to changes and advances as the standard of medical care changes.[100-101]

■ When should supportive measures be terminated?

Supportive measures may be terminated when the therapy does not give hope or promise of recovery and serves only to prolong the process of dying.[25,46,49] Although family members of competent, critically ill adults have little legal impact on such decisions, disclosure to them of such contemplated action is strongly recommended. Most family members have no conception of considerations needed to deal with medical issues involved in terminating care and will usually defer such judgments to the physician. Explanation of the considerations should be given to the extent required to enable the lay person to understand the issues. The physician has a moral and social responsibility to objectively present the essential medical facts, alternatives, and expected outcome. This discussion with relatives concerning the patient's hopeless prognosis, the physician's recommendation, and the consent of the family should be noted in the progress record before terminating treatment.[42,47,51]

Family members may, in some instances, insist that treatment of a critically ill incompetent patient be continued even though the prognosis appears hopeless. If the treatment that the family demands will provide no benefit for the patient, it is inappropriate for the physician to persist. The physician is not legally nor morally bound to initiate or continue measures that serve merely to appease distraught relatives. Family members who have major disagreements with the physician can, of course, seek legal recourse.

Surprisingly, few legal claims have been filed regarding the termination of care. Horen, in a legal review, affirmed "there are few, if any, cases when a medical malpractice claim or criminal action has been filed against the physician who ended extraordinary means that were being used to prolong the life of an already terminally ill patient who was in the death process."[102] Thus, although it is clear that the physician has a contractual and moral obligation to his patient to restore health and relieve suffering, he is not legally nor morally obligated to sustain life by means that cannot be expected to have a significant impact on the life process. If inexorable loss of physiologic integrity has occurred, the patient will usually die no matter what the physician does or does not do. In such circumstances therapeutic gestures cannot give life nor can the withholding of elaborate procedures be considered responsible for the advent of death.[25,74]

An important note of caution must be interjected in the patient/physician decision-making process that is used to determine whether to provide or withhold measures. Since the physician, nurse, and health workers may exercise powerful influences over the patient's attitudes toward his continued existence, the patient and family ought to be objectively apprised of the patient's condition so that they may play an active role in expressing their attitudes about the desirability of life or death. The physician's and nurse's preconception about the patient's hopelessness should be recognized as an attitude of the medical care members that may not accurately reflect the attitudes of the patient and family. Where such discordance exists between the patient, patient's family, and medical preconceptions, decision making is often fraught with interpersonal and legal hazards; the ability to support adequately the patient's expectations often are not realized. Thus it must be remembered that the decision to withhold support must be based foremost on the desire and intent to alleviate the suffering of the patient and not the desire to allay the plight of the family or the discomfort of the attending physician or nurse.[25,49]

Physicians and nurses must recognize that medical practice is under great social pressure for change, and medical practitioners could, unthinkingly, yield to the current enthusiasm for premature abandonment of critically ill patients and thereby contribute to premature death.[3]

■ May the physician or nurse intervene actively to terminate the life of a critically ill patient?

Active intervention that is intended to kill and causes the patient to die is considered murder.

Some writers have suggested that active intervention is no different than allowing the patient to die passively.[103] This latter attitude has been firmly rejected by most clinicians and is not accepted by organized American medicine. The AMA House of Delegates in 1973 stated "The intentional termination of the life of one human being by another—mercy killing—is contrary to that for which the medical profession stands, and is contrary to the policy of the American Medical Association."[104] This statement by the American Medical Association would appear to draw a clear distinction between active intervention that causes death and the elective termination of supportive measures in the terminally ill patient that may allow death to supervene. In many instances it may be unclear whether interruption of care represents active intervention or termination of a useless measure. For example, is the act of turning off the respirator to be regarded as active intervention or merely as termination of supportive measures that prolong the dying process? A clear answer cannot be given to this question unless one examines the extenuating circumstances in each clinical situation. For example, if a respirator were discontinued in a patient who had muscular paralysis as a result of d-tubocurarine administration, such intervention clearly would be active intervention and would be unethical, improper, and legally equivalent to killing the patient. If, however, the decision to discontinue the ventilator were based on the medical conclusion that the treatment could not restore health and was serving only to prolong the dying process, then the physician and health care team would be acting appropriately and should not be subjected to the harassment of lawyers or ethicists.[25,49,99] Decisions to terminate supportive measures in patients who are hopelessly ill are commonplace and usually evolve from discussions by the patient, family, and physician without the need of the impersonal intervention of court processes.[49,105-107] In fact, some observers believe that, if adequate consultation between the physician and family members had been pursued in the Quinlan case, it would not have been necessary to create the impersonal carnival that attracted worldwide attention.[25,49] Many physicians and moralists agree that the matter of discontinuing supportive measures in terminally ill patients should only become a matter of court concern when deliberate intent and action to kill has been taken.[25,49]

The recently defined brain death status has clarified the approach to discontinuation of therapy in the patient with irreversible brain damage. Under the brain death statute it is now possible to define the patient as dead even though normal heart rate may still be present. The removal of such a patient from the heart-lung device in a state with a brain death statute is not considered killing because such a patient is legally defined as being dead prior to the intervention. A similar action might have medicolegal implications for persons disconnecting the supportive devices in states that do not incorporate brain death in their statutes.[107] The foregoing legal changes dictate that the nurse and physician become familiar with the statutes of the state in which they practice. Although such legislature clarifies the management of a small number of critically ill patients, the majority of patients who are terminally ill will continue to rely on the judgement and good intention of physicians and nurses who must carefully weigh the benefit and risk of the vast array of technology that stands ready to support the life process. They must then choose that course that will restore health and provide comfort for the patient.

REFERENCES

1. Cullen, D. J., Ferrara, L. C., and Briggs, B. A.: Survival, hospitalization charges and follow-up results in critically ill patients, N. Engl. J. Med. **294:**982, 1976.
2. Turnbull, A. D., et al.: The inverse relationship between cost and survival in the critically ill cancer patient, Crit. Care Med. **7:**20, 1979.
3. Hudson, R. P.: Death, dying and the zealous phase, Ann. Intern. Med. **88:**696, 1978.
4. Cullen, D. J., Ferrara, L. C., Gilbert, J., Briggs, B. A., and Walker, P. F.: Indicators of intensive care in critically ill patients, Crit. Care Med. **5:**173, 1977.
5. Goldman, L., et al.: Multifactorial index of cardiac risk in non-cardiac surgical procedures, N. Engl. J. Med. **297:**845, 1977.
6. Caronna, J. J., et al.: The outcome of medical coma: prediction by bedside assessment of physical signs, Trans. Am. Neurol. Assoc. **100:**25, 1975.
7. Caronna, J. J., and Finkelstein, S.: Neurological syndromes after cardiac arrest. Current concepts of cerebrovascular disease, Stroke **13:**9, 1978.

8. Walker, A. E., and Molinari, G. E.: Criteria of cerebral death, Trans. Am. Neurol. Assoc. **100:**29, 1975.

9. Powner, D. J., and Fromm, G. H.: The electroencephalogram in the determination of brain death, N. Engl. J. Med. **300:**500, 1979.

10. Shoemaker, W. E., Pierchala, C., Chang, P., and State, D.: Prediction of outcome and severity of illness by analysis of the frequency distribution of cardio-respiratory variables, Crit. Care Med. **5:**82, 1977.

11. Cady, L. D., et al.: Quantitation of severity of critical illness with special reference to blood lactate, Crit. Care Med. **1:**75, 1973.

12. Bates, D., et al.: A prospective study of non-traumatic coma: methods and results in 310 patients, Ann. Neurol. **2:**211, 1977.

13. Engel, G. L.: A life setting conducive to illness—the giving up–given up complex, Ann. Intern. Med. **69:**293, 1968.

14. Milton, G. W.: Self-willed death or the bone-pointing syndrome. In Garfield, C. A., editor: Psychosocial care of the dying patient, New York, 1978, McGraw-Hill Book Co., p. 125.

15. Engel, G. L.: Psychologic stress, vasopressor (vasovagal) syncope, and sudden death, Ann. Intern. Med. **89:**403, 1978.

16. Wolf, S.: Psychosocial forces in myocardial infarction and sudden death. In Levi, L., editor: Society, stress and disease, New York, 1971, Oxford University Press, Publishers 1:324-330.

17. Wolf, S.: Central autonomic influences on cardiac rate and rhythm, Mod. Concepts Cardiovasc. Dis. **38:**29, 1969.

18. Bruhn, J. G., Chandler, B., and Wolf, S.: A psychological study of survivors and non-survivors of myocardial infarction, Psychosom. Med. **31:**8, 1969.

19. Bruhn, J. G., Paredes, A., Adsett, A. C., and Wolfe, S.: Psychological predictors of sudden death in myocardial infarction, J. Psychosom. Res. **18:**187, 1974.

20. Platt, M.: Commentary—On asking to die, Hastings Cent. Rep. **5:**9, 1975.

21. Treppasoo, Father: Response to "the patient's right of self-determination," Heart Lung **6**(1):166, 1977.

22. Worrell, J. D.: Nursing implication in the care of the patient experiencing sensory deprivation. In Kintzel, K. C., editor: Advanced concepts in clinical nursing, Philadelphia, 1971, J. B. Lippincott, Publishers, p. 130.

23. Tait, K. M., and Winslow, G.: Beyond consent—the ethics of decision-making in emergency medicine (trauma rounds), West. J. Med. **126:**156, 1977.

24. Bergen, R. P., and Blumberg, E.: Legality of ignoring suicidal patient's request for no resuscitation, J.A.M.A. **218:**1712, 1971.

25. Ramsey, P.: Ethics of the edges of life: medical and legal intersections, New Haven, 1978, Yale University Press.

26. Evans, F. J.: The right to die—a basic constitutional right, J. Leg. Med. **5:**17, 1977.

27. Veatch, R. M.: Death and dying: the legislative options, Hastings Cent. Rep. **7:**5, 1977.

28. In re Quinlan, 70 N.J. 10 (1976).

29. Garland, M.: The right to die in California—politics, legislation and natural death, Hastings Cent. Rep. **6:**5, 1976.

30. California's natural death act (San Francisco: Medical Staff Conference, University of California), West. J. Med. **128:**318, 1978.

31. Keene, B.: The natural death act, Assembly bill **3060:**2, 1977.

32. Jonsen, A. R.: Dying right in California: the natural death act, Clin. Res. **26:**55, 1978.

33. Schram, R. B., Kane, J. C., and Roble, D. T.: No code orders: clarification in the aftermath of Saikewicz, N. Engl. J. Med. **299:**875, 1978.

34. Klutch, M.: Survey results after one year's experience with the natural death act, Sept. 1, 1976-August 31, 1977, West. J. Med. **128:**329, 1978.

35. Tagge, G. F., Adler, D., Bryan-Brown, C. W., and Shoemaker, W. C.: Relationship of therapy in prognosis in critically ill patients, Crit. Care Med. **2:**61, 1974.

36. Optimum care for hopelessly ill patients (Boston, Mass): a report of the clinical care committee of the Massachusetts General Hospital, N. Engl. J. Med. **295:**362, 1976.

37. Hospital Tribune Report: New intensive care unit protocol avoids Quinlan-type dilemma, p. 4, October 4, 1976.

38. Standards for cardiopulmonary resuscitation (CPR) and emergency cardiac care (ECC) v. medicolegal considerations and recommendations, J.A.M.A. **227**(Suppl.):833, 1974.

39. Petty, T. L., Lakshminarayan, S., Sahn, S. A., Zwillich, C. W., and Nett, L. M.: Intensive respiratory care unit: review of ten years' experience, J.A.M.A. **233:**34 1975.

40. Sykes, M. K., McNicol, M. W., and Campbell, E. J.: Respiratory failure, ed. 2, Oxford, 1976, Blackwell Scientific Publications, Ltd., p. 295.

41. Dinnerstein, S., in the matter of: Mass. App. Adv. Sh. 736, 747, n 10, 1978.

42. Rabkin, M., Gillerman, J. D., and Rice, N. R.: Orders not to resuscitate, N. Engl. J. Med. **295:**364, 1976.

43. Annas, G. J.: The incompetent's right to die: the case of Joseph Saikewicz, Hastings Cent. Rep. **8**(1):21, 1978.

44. Glantz, L. H., and Swazey, J. P.: Decision not to treat: the Saikewicz case and its aftermath, Forum Med. **2:**22, 1979.

45. Superintendent of Belchertown State School vs. Saikewicz, 1977, Mass Adv. Sh 1461.

46. Spencer, S. S.: "Code" or "no code": a nonlegal opinion, N. Engl. J. Med. **300:**138, 1979.

47. Schram, R. B., Kane, J. C., and Roble, D. T.: No code orders: clarification in the aftermath of Saikewicz, N. Engl. J. Med. **229:**875, 1978.

48. Baron, C. H.: The "Dinnerstein" decision and "no-code" orders, N. Engl. J. Med. **300:**264, 1979.

49. Relman, A. S.: The Saikewicz decision: a medical viewpoint, Am. J. Law Med. **4:**233, 1978.

50. Adler, D. C.: President's message: "no code"—the unwritten order, Am. Assoc. Crit. Care Nurses **6:**213, 1977.

51. Mills, D. H.: More on brain death, J.A.M.A. **234:**838, 1975.

52. California Hospital Association: Consent manual, ed. 10, 1978, p. 78.

53. Bunzl, M.: A note on nursing ethics in the U.S.A., J. Med. Ethics **1:**184, 1975.

54. Kaserman, I.: A nursing committee and the code for nurses, Am. J. Nurs. **77:**875, 1977.

55. Gaylin, W. M., Sharing the hardest decision, Hosp. Phys. **7:**33, 1972.

56. Lown, B., and Wolf, M.: Approaches to sudden death for coronary artery disease, Circulation **44:**130, 1971.

57. Hofkin, G. A.: Survival after cardiopulmonary resuscitation, J.A.M.A. **202:**652, 1967.

58. Rogore, H. J., Weil, M. H., Thompson, M., and Blair, C.: Cardiopulmonary resuscitation in the hospital, Cardiovasc. Nurs. **13:**7, 1977.

59. Crampton, R. S., Aldrich, R. F., Stillerman, R., and Gascho, J. A.: Prehospital cardiopulmonary resuscitation in acute myocardial infarction, N. Engl. J. Med. **286:**1320, 1972.

60. Amey, B. D., Harrison, E. E., and Straub, E. J.: Sudden cardiac death: a retrospective and prospective study, J. Am. Coll. Emerg. Phys. **5:**429, 1976.

61. Frieden, J., and Cooper, J. A.: The role of the intermediate cardiac care unit, J.A.M.A. **235:**816, 1976.

62. Conley, M. D., McNeer, J. F., Lee, K. L., Wagner, G. S., and Rosati, R. A.: Cardiac arrest complicating acute myocardial infarction, predictability and prognosis, Am. J. Cardiol. **39:**7, 1977.

63. Connolly, T. J., and Wolozen, J. J.: Cardiopulmonary resuscitation, J.A.M.A. **38:**1723, 1977.

64. Lemire, L., and Johnson, A. L.: CPR: is it worthwhile? A decade of experience, N. Engl. J. Med. **286:**970, 1972.

65. Hill, D.: Specialized care for acute myocardiac infarction, Minn. Med. **56:**983, 1973.

66. Camarata, S. J., Weil, M., Hanashiro, P. K., and Shubin, H.: Cardiac arrest in the critically ill, Circulation **44:**688, 1971.

67. Baum, R. S., Alvarez, H., III, and Cobb, L. A.: Survival after resuscitation from out-of-hospital ventricular fibrillation, Circulation **50:**1231, 1974.

68. Green, M. L., Reid, P. R., and Schaefer, A. H.: The repetitive ventricular response in man: a predictor of sudden death, N. Engl. J. Med. **299:**729, 1978.

69. Julian, D. G.: Toward preventing coronary death from ventricular fibrillation, Circulation **54:**360, 1976.

70. Willoughby, J. O., and Leau, B. G.: Relationship of neurological findings after cardiac arrest and outcome, Br. Med. J. **3:**437, 1974.

71. Kubler-Ross, E., Wessler, S., and Avioli, L. V.: Therapeutic grand rounds number 36—on death and dying, J.A.M.A. **221:**174, 1972.

72. Imbus, S. H., and Zawacki, B. E.: Autonomy for burned patients when survival is unprecedented, N. Engl. J. Med. **297:**308, 1977.

73. Blumenfield, M., et al.: Do patients want to be told (letter)? N. Engl. J. Med. **299:**1132, 1978.

74. Veatch, R. M.: Death, dying and the biological revolution, New Haven, 1976, Yale University Press.

75. Wilson, J. M.: Communicating with the dying, J. Med. Ethics **1:**18, 1975.

76. Hogshead, H. P.: The art of delivering bad news, J. Fl. Med. Assoc. **63:**807, 1976.

77. Lipp, M. R.: Respectful treatment: the human side of medical care, Hagerstown, Md., 1977, Harper & Row, Publishers.

78. Gardner, D., and Steward, N.: Staff involvement with families of patients in critical care units, Heart Lung **7:**105, 1978.

79. Kubler-Ross, E.: On death and dying, New York, 1969, MacMillan Inc.

80. Kubler-Ross, E.: Questions and answers to death and dying, New York, 1974, MacMillan Inc.

81. Kubler-Ross, E.: What is it like to be dying? Am. J. Nurs. **71**(1):54, 1971.

82. Abrams, R. D.: The patient with cancer—his changing pattern of communication, N. Engl. J. Med. **274**(6):317, 1966.

83. Lorin, M. I.: The twilight hours. In Patterson, P., et al., editors: Psychosocial aspects of cystic fibrosis, New York, 1973, Columbia University Press.

84. Gardner, D., and Steward, N.: Staff involvement with families of patients in critical care units, Heart Lung **7**(1):105, 1978.

85. White, L. P.: Death and the physician: *mortios vivos docent.* In Feifel, H., editor: New meaning of death, 1977, McGraw-Hill Book Co.

86. Benoliel, J. Q.: Nurses and the human experience of dying. In Feifel, H., editor: New meaning of death, New York, 1977, McGraw-Hill Book Co.

87. Artiss, K. L., and Levine, A. S.: Doctor-patient relation in severe illness: a seminar for oncology fellows, N. Engl. J. Med. **288:**1210, 1973.

88. Schmale, A. H., and Patterson, W. B.: Comfort care only —treatment guidelines for the terminal patient. In Garfield, C. A., editor: First National Training Conference for Physicians on Psychosocial Care of the Dying Patient, University of California, San Francisco, April 29-May 1, 1976.

89. Woodson, R.: Hospice care in terminal illness. In Garfield, C. A., editor: Psychosocial care of the dying patient, San Francisco, 1978, McGraw-Hill Book Co.

90. Black, P. M.: Brain death, N. Engl. J. Med. **299:**338, 393, 1978.

91. A definition of irreversible coma: report of the *Ad Hoc* Committee of the Harvard Medical School to examine the definition of brain death, J.A.M.A. **205:**337, 1968. Copyright 1968, American Medical Association.

92. An appraisal of the criteria of cerebral death: a summary statement—a collaborative study, J.A.M.A. **237:**982, 1976.

93. Beecher, H. K.: Ethical problems created by the hopelessly unconscious patient, N. Engl. J. Med. **278:**1425, 1968.

94. Taylor, L. F.: A statutory definition of death in Kansas, J.A.M.A. **215:**296, 1971.

95. Legislature of the State of Kansas: An act relating to and defining death, KSA:77-202 (suppl.), 1974.

96. Arnett, D., et al.: A legal recognition of death, Assembly Bill **3560:**65, 1974.

97. Curran, W. J.: The brain-death concept: judicial acceptance in Massachusetts, N. Engl. J. Med. **298:**1008, 1978.

98. American Bar Association: Report of the Committee on Medicine and Law, Forum **11:**300, 1975.

99. Veitch, F. J., et al.: Brain death: II, a status report of legal considerations, J.A.M.A. **283:**1744, 1977.

100. Kennedy, M. K.: The Kansas statute on death—an appraisal, N. Engl. J. Med. **285:**946, 1971.

101. The Kansas death statute: bold and innovative, N. Engl. J. Med. **285:**968, 1971.

102. Horan, D. J.: Euthanasia: medical treatment and the mongoloid child: death as a treatment of choice, 27(1) Baylor U.L. Rev. 80, 1975.

103. Rachel, J.: Active and passive euthanasia, N. Engl. J. Med. **292:**78, 1975.

104. Report "B"—The physician and the dying patient, A.M.A. Proceedings of the House of Delegates, 27th Clinical Convention, Anaheim, CA, Dec. 25, 1963, p. 140.

105. Crane, D.: The sanctity of social life: physicians treatment of critically ill patients, New York, 1975, Russell Sage Foundation.

106. Levine, M. D.: Disconnection: the clinicians view, Hastings Cent. Rep. **6:**11, 1976.

107. Thomas, B.: Legal implications, Nurs. Mirror **145:**24, 1977.

Glossary

A-aΔPo$_2$ Difference between alveolar and arterial oxygen tension.

abortion Premature expulsion from the uterus of the products of conception.

abruptio placentae Premature detachment of a normally implanted placenta occurring in the region of maternal transdecidual arterial blood supply and attended by maternal systemic reactions in the form of shock, oliguria, and fibrinopenia.

accelerated conduction Conduction that is faster than expected.

accelerated pathway Portion of the conduction system that transmits impulses more rapidly than normal.

acetylcholine Ester of choline that causes vasodilation and increased flow.

ACH See *Acetylcholine*.

acidosis Chemical state of the blood and body fluids that occurs when there is excess acid or a deficiency of alkali. This may occur in a variety of disease states but is a common concomitant of kidney failure.

ACTH See *Adrenocorticotropic hormone*.

activated charcoal Charcoal treated with steam, air, carbon dioxide, oxygen, zinc chloride, sulfuric acid, phosphoric acid, or a combination of these substances at temperatures ranging from 500° to 900° C to increase its absorptive powers. It has been estimated that 1 ml of charcoal, finely divided, possesses a total surface area of approximately 1000 m²; used as a general purpose antidote.

adenosine triphosphate Enzyme found in all cells. When this substance is split by enzyme action, energy is produced.

ADH See *Antidiuretic hormone*.

Adrenal cortex Outer layer of the adrenal gland; secretes corticosteroids.

adrenal medulla Inner layer of the adrenal gland; secretes catecholamines.

adrenergic receptors Term applied to nerve fibers that, when stimulated, release epinephrine at their endings.

adrenocorticotropic hormone Corticotropin.

aerobic capacity Greatest amount of oxygen that can be transported from the lungs to the working muscles; also known as maximum oxygen uptake (Vo$_{2_{max}}$).

akinesia Complete or partial loss of muscle movement.

albumin Group of simple proteins.

albuminuria Presence of protein (albumin) in the urine. Most commonly this represents an abnormal situation but may not be specific. The test for albumin in the urine serves as a screening test for kidney disease.

aldosterone Hormone secreted by the adrenal cortex that promotes sodium retention and potassium excretion.

Allen's test Test performed by compressing both the ulnar and radial arteries and having the patient repeatedly make a fist, then either the radial or the ulnar artery is released. If the hand fails to blush after release of one artery, this signifies lack of patency to the palmar arch.

allograft Autograft.

α-receptors Sympathetic nerve terminals in certain blood vessels that promote vascular smooth muscle contraction.

alternating current Electric current that reverses its direction at regularly recurring intervals, the frequency being determined by the frequency of the alternator supplying the current and the successive half waves being similar in shape and area.

alveolar ventilation Calculated volume of ventilation that is effective in gas exchange.

alveoli Small hollows or cavities; air cells of the lung.

analgesia Absence of painful sensation in a particular area.

anaphylaxis Hypersensitive state of the body with respect to a foreign protein or drug.

aneurysm Localized abnormal dilation of a blood vessel caused by congenital defect or weakness of the wall of the vessel.

angina pectoris Clinical term for a condition caused by disease of the coronary arteries. The usual symptoms are paroxysmal pain accompanied by a sense of constriction about the chest.

angiocardiography In radiology, the visualization of blood vessels by injection of a nontoxic radiopaque substance.

anoxia Lack of oxygen supply to the tissues.

antibody Protein substance developed by the body usually in response to the presence of an antigen.

anticoagulant Agent that prevents or delays blood clotting.

andiuretic hormone Vasopressin; promotes water retention.

antigen Substance that induces the formation of antibodies.

aortic Pertaining to the large vessel arising from the left ventricle and distributing, by its branches, arterial blood to every part of the body.

aortic stenosis Narrowing of aorta or its orifice because of lesions of the wall with scar formation, infection as in rheumatic fever, or embryonic anomalies.

aortocoronary–saphenous vein bypass Surgical procedure using the saphenous vein segment as a conduit to transport blood from the ascending thoracic aorta to the coronary artery, bypassing obstructions in the coronary artery.

Apgar score Number assigned at birth assessing the condition of the infant; based on color, heart rate, respiratory rate, muscle tone, and responsiveness.

apnea Absence of respiration for a period greater than 10 seconds, producing hypoxia and bradycardia in the neonate; cessation of breathing.

aponeurosis Flat fibrous sheet of connective tissue that serves to attach muscle to bone or other tissues at their origin or insertion.

arborization Interlacing; ramification; applied to nerve processes, terminations, fibers, and arterioles. A structure having the conformation of a tree.

arrhythmia Absence of rhythm; irregularity.

arteriotomy Incision of an artery.

arteriovenous oxygen difference Difference between the oxygen content in the arterial and venous circulations.

arteriovenous shunt (hemodialysis) Direct connection between an artery and a vein surgically created by a conduit that protrudes through the skin.

arteriovenous shunting Passage of blood from the arterial circulation to the venous circulation without transit through the capillaries.

artifacts ECG and EEG waves that arise from sources other than the heart or the brain.

artificial pacemaker Electronic device used to stimulate the heart electrically so that it will depolarize.

assessment Observer's opinion of the patient's mental, physical, or social status or progress or lack of progress from therapeutic and educational assistance based on subjective and objective information.

assisted ventilation Mechanical ventilation in which the initiation of each breath is by the patient's spontaneous inspiratory effort.

asystole Lack of normal cardiac contraction.

atelectasis Collapse or nonexpansion of the alveoli, segment, lobe, or total lung.

ATP See *Adenosine triphosphate.*

atresia Pathologic closure of a normal anatomic opening, or congenital absence of the opening.

atrial fibrillation Rapid irregular atrial depolarization (300 to 700 beats/min).

atrial flutter Rapid regular atrial depolarization with fusing of the "f" and T waves (atrial repolarization) (280 to 340 beats/min).

atrial tachycardia Rapid atrial rhythm (100 to 260 beats/min) from an ectopic focus; may be sustained or paroxysmal.

atrioventricular block Pathologic delay in atrioventricular conduction.

atrioventricular junction Specialized conducting tissue of the AV node, bundle of His, and common AV bundle.

autograft Skin (or tissue) taken from one area of the body for transplant to another area.

autologous grafts Tissue, usually skin, that is moved from one part of the body to another site on the same individual.

autonomic nervous system Part of the nervous system that is concerned with control of involuntary body functions.

A-V See *Arteriovenous.*

AV See *Atrioventricular.*

axon Process of a neuron that conducts impulses away from the cell body.

azotemia Elevation of blood urea concentration.

Babinski reflex (plantar extensor sign, sign of the toe) Pathologic reflex involving extension of the great toe of the foot occurring when a stimulus is applied to the sole of the foot, the calf, or the anterior tibial region. This signifies a lesion in the spinal cord above the lumbar level or in the brain.

baroreceptors Pressure-sensitive nerve terminals in certain blood vessels that send signals to the brain when the systolic blood pressure falls.

basophil Type of white blood cell thought to bring anticoagulant substances to inflamed tissues.

Battle's sign Presence of ecchymosis over a mastoid process, which signifies a petrobasilar fracture.

β-adrenergic blocker Sympathomimetic (adrenergic) drugs stimulate α- and/or β-receptors. Some of the effects of stimulating a β-receptor are (1) stimulation of the heart, (2) dilation of blood vessels, and (3) dilation of the bronchial musculature. A β-adrenergic *blocker* reverses these effects.

bicarbonate precursor Sodium lactate injection, used in

the treatment of metabolic acidosis, that is metabolized in the body to sodium bicarbonate.

bioavailability Amount of drug released from a drug formulation for absorption into the circulation.

bipolar Having or involving the use of two poles.

bougie Slender cylinder for introduction into the cervical canal.

bradycardia Abnormally slow heart rate; in the neonate, less than 90 beats/min.

bronchopulmonary dysplasia Chronic fibrotic lung disease; in the neonate, produced by exposure of the lung to high oxygen concentrations, usually 70% for more than 2 days.

bronchospasm Spasmodic narrowing of the bronchi.

bundle branch block Partial or complete block of one or more of the ventricular bundle branches.

bundle of His Group of fibers; an atrioventricular fasciculus.

calculus Refers to the formation of a stone or "rock"; in the case of the kidney and urinary tract, is called renal or urinary calculus.

calorie (kilocalorie) Heat unit; the amount of heat required to raise the temperature of 1 kg of water from $0°$ to $1°$ C; also known as the large calorie and is used in the study of metabolism. The small calorie is the amount of heat required to raise the temperature of 1 g of water $1°$ C and is one one-thousandth of the large calorie.

calyx Any cuplike division of the kidney pelvis.

capillaries Network of vessels between the arterioles and the veins. Oxygen and nutritive materials diffuse through the walls into the tissues, and carbon dioxide and waste products from the tissues enter the circulatory system.

cardiac arrhythmia Irregular heart action caused by disturbances, either physiologic or pathologic, in the discharge of cardiac impulses from the sinoatrial node or their transmission through conductile tissue of the heart.

cardiac decompensation Inability of the heart to maintain adequate circulation.

cardiac output Blood volume in liters ejected per minute by the left ventricle.

cardiac plexus Cardiac nerves beneath the arch of the aorta.

cardiac tamponade Compression of the heart caused by a collection of fluid in the pericardial sac.

cardiodynamics Study of the forces involved in the heart's action.

cardiogenic Having origin in the heart itself.

cardiogenic shock Condition that interferes with function of the heart as a pump, producing shock.

cardiotonic Substance that stimulates the heart to improve its muscular tension.

cardioversion Procedure of delivering a countershock to the heart that is programmed to occur after the impulse for depolarization has spread across the atrium. The purpose is to interrupt an abnormal rhythm so that the normal rhythm can take over.

carotid sinus (body) Collection of vagal cells near the bifurcation of the carotid artery that is sensitive to pressure and carbon dioxide content of the blood. Massage of these bodies stimulates the vagus and may slow the atrial heart rate.

cartilage Type of dense connective tissue consisting of cells embedded in a ground substance.

cast (in urinary sediment) Cylindric structure that may be seen in the urine when viewed through the microscope. The number and type of casts present are helpful in indicating the type of kidney disease present.

catecholamines Epinephrine, norepinephrine, and similar compounds that have sympathomimetic actions.

causalgia Form of pain, usually severe, in which a usually nonpainful stimulation is perceived as extremely painful. It is spontaneous and usually has a burning quality. This is usually seen in lesions of the CNS and also in proximal portions of damaged nerve roots. In its later stages the involved extremity is pale and cold and may respond favorably to sympathetic blockage.

cell Unit of structure of all animals and plants; the physical basis of all life processes.

cerebrovascular disease Disease of the blood vessels of the brain.

chemoreceptor Sense organ or sensory nerve ending that is stimulated by a chemical substance.

cholinergic Term applied to nerve endings that liberate acetylcholine.

chordae tendineae Tendinous cords that join the papillary muscles of the heart with the valves.

chonotropic Affecting the rate of muscular contraction; term used to describe the cardiac-slowing effect of impulses in certain fibers of the vagus nerve.

chyle Milklike contents of the lacteals and lymphatic vessels in the intestine; consists of the products of digestion.

cicatrix Scar tissue caused by a predominance of white collagen fibers.

cilia Hairlike processes projecting from epithelial cells.

cineangiography Part of the process of cardiac catheterization and angiography that utilizes frames taken at a rapid rate to show movement of the structures and contrast media.

cisternae Reservoirs or cavities.

claudication Weakness of the legs accompanied by cramplike pains in the calves caused by poor circulation of the blood to the legs.

clearance Pertains to measurement of renal function and indicates the volume of blood from which a substance (for example, creatinine or urea) is completely removed in a given unit of time (for example, a minute or day) by the kidneys.

clonus Jerking repetitive movement of a muscle when it is forcibly stretched. Generally performed at the ankles, this indicates a lesion above the lumbar level, either in the spinal cord or brain.

coarctation of the aorta Constriction of the aorta.

cold caloric irrigation Technique of testing integrity of brain stem function carried out by irrigating the external auricular canal of the patient with cold saline solution while the head is flexed at approximately 30 degrees after checking the patency of the ear canal. Stimulation of the labyrinth produces jerky, regular movements of the eyes in the normal patient. Absence may signify damage at the pontine level of the brain stem.

collagen Fibrous insoluble protein found in the connective tissue.

collateral circulation Circulation carried on through secondary channels.

colloid Dissolved proteins of the plasma and interstitial fluids.

conduction Transmission of an impulse from one part of the heart to another.

congestive heart failure (decompensation, cardiac or myocardial insufficiency) Not a disease entitity, but a *syndrome* resulting from many forms of heart disease; a condition that occurs when the heart fails to circulate the optimum amount of blood required by the body. One or both of the ventricles may fail. There is an inadequate emptying of the chambers of the heart.

continuous positive airway pressure Mechanism of gas delivery (under pressure) to the alveoli used to maintain inflation of the alveoli during expiration in the presence of atelectasis.

continuous positive pressure ventilation Positive end-expiratory pressure applied to the airway during mechanical ventilation.

contralateral Opposite side of a point of reference.

controlled ventilation Mechanical ventilation in which the autonomic cycling device in the ventilator initiates inspiration.

convalescence To recover health gradually; the interim between acute illness and recovery.

coronary occlusion Obstruction of the lumen of the coronary artery caused by atheroma, thrombus, or embolus.

coronary thrombosis Formation of a clot in some portion of the coronary arteries, which supply blood to the heart muscle, resulting in obstruction of the artery, which may result in infarction (necrosis) of the area of the heart supplied by the occluded vessel.

corticosteroids Hormones secreted by the adrenal cortex.

corticotropin Hormone secreted by the anterior pituitary that stimulates the adrenal cortex; adrenocorticotropic hormone.

cortisol The principal glucocorticoid secreted by the adrenal cortex; hydrocortisone; 17-hydroxycorticosterone.

cortisone Glucocorticoid that resembles cortisol.

CPAP See *Continuous positive airway pressure.*

CPPV See *Continuous positive pressure ventilation.*

crepitation Crackling feeling or sound commonly used to describe the condition that results when air escapes into the tissue.

crescendo angina Refers to increased frequency, provocation, or change in intensity or character of anginal discomfort and usually associated with ischemic ECG changes.

crystalloid Noncolloid substance able to pass through a semipermeable membrane; forms true solution.

current Movement of positive or negative electric particles (as electrons) accompanied by such observable effects as the production of heat, of a magnetic field, or of chemical transformations.

cyanosis Bluish coloration of the skin and mucous membranes that accompanies inadequate oxygenation of the blood to the tissues.

cytomegalic inclusion disease Transplacentally acquired viral infection. Mothers are asymptomatic. Infants may be asymptomatic but may be affected by deformity or may die.

cytoplasm That portion of the protoplasm other than the nucleus.

data base Information necessary for complete patient care; includes the chief complaint, history of the present illness, patient profile, history, and physical and laboratory tests.

decerebrate posturing Position of the extremities of a patient, generally comatose, in which the arms are extended and internally rotated and the legs are extended with the feet in forced plantar flexion, caused usually by compression of the brain stem at lower levels.

decorticate posturing Position of the extremities in a comatose patient (although not necessarily as deeply unconscious as the decerebrate patient), in which the upper extremities are flexed at the elbows and at the wrists. The legs may be flexed. Decerebrate and decorticate positions are generally produced by the application of painful stimulation to the comatose patient. Decorticate posturing indicates a lesion higher in the brain stem in a mesencephalic region.

default Failure of an impulse to occur or to be transmitted when it would be expected to do so.

defibrillator Machine used to deliver an electric charge to the heart; also termed a depolarizer.

dendrite Branched protoplasmic process of a neuron that conducts impulses to the cell body.

depolarize To prevent, decrease, or remove polarization of (as a dry cell) by adding a substance that prevents the accumulation of reaction products.

dermis Skin.

diabetes insipidus Disorder caused by deficiency of, or renal unresponsiveness to, antidiuretic hormone (vasopressin).

diabetes mellitus Disease characterized by a deficiency of insulin, relative or absolute, and hyperglycemia.

dialysis Diffusion of dissolved particles from one fluid compartment to another across a semipermeable membrane.

dialysis disequilibrium syndrome Syndrome occurring as a result of dialysis; may be manifest by cerebral and other neurologic disturbances, cardiac arrhythmia, and pulmonary edema and is caused by a rapid change in extracellular fluid composition as a result of dialysis.

dialysis fluid Solution flowing on the opposite side of the semipermeable membrane to blood.

diaphoresis Profuse perspiration.

diastole Normal period in the heart's cycle during which the muscle fibers lengthen, the heart dilates, and the cavities fill with blood.

DIC See *Disseminated intravascular coagulation.*

diencephalon Second portion of the brain or that lying between the telencephalon and the mesencephalon.

diffusion Process whereby different gases interpenetrate and become mixed as a result of their constant molecular motion.

direct current Electric current flowing in one direction only and substantially constant in value.

disability Absence or impairment of physical, intellectual, or financial fitness.

disseminated intravascular coagulation Hemorrhagic disease characterized by gross intravascular clotting, consumption of coagulation factors, and excessive bleeding.

diuresis (dried out) Increased excretion of urine.

diuretic Any drug or substance that increases the flow of urine. Such substances are used medically to rid the body of excess salt and water that accumulate in certain kidney diseases, heart failure, and liver disease.

Doppler principle Observation that the pitch of a whistle on a rapidly moving body, like a locomotive, is higher when the body is approaching the listener.

DPT vaccine Diphtheria-pertussis-tetanus vaccine.

dynamic Active, as opposed to static; pertaining to the process of change.

dyskinesia Defect in voluntary movement.

dyspnea Shortness of breath, difficult breathing.

dysrhythmia Disturbance of rhythm, as abnormality of rhythm in speech, or disturbance or irregularity in the rhythm of the brain waves as recorded by electroencephalography.

ecchymosis Extravasation of blood under the skin.

ectopic pregnancy Pregnancy outside of the uterus, usually in the fallopian tube.

effective compliance Ratio of tidal volume to peak airway pressure.

elastin Protein forming the principal substance of yellow elastin tissues.

electrode Contact for introduction or detection of electrical activity.

embolectomy Removal of an embolus through an incision in the blood vessel wall.

embolism Occlusion of an artery by an embolus.

embolized atheroma Embolized fat particle lodged in a vessel.

embolus Bit of matter foreign to the bloodstream that may lodge in some vessel and obstruct the circulation to the area served by the vessel.

emphysema of the lung Condition in which the alveoli become distended and destroyed.

endarterectomy Surgical removal of atheromatous material from the intima of an artery.

endocarditis Inflammation of the lining membrane of the heart or endocardium.

endocardium Inner lining of the heart.

endoneurium Delicate connective tissue sheath that surrounds nerve fibers.

endotoxin Cell wall toxin produced by gram-negative bacteria.

enzymes Catalytic substance formed by living cells and having a specific action in promoting a chemical change.

eosinophil Leukocyte cell that stains readily with acid stain.

epicardium Inner layer of the pericardium.

epimysium Outermost sheath of connective tissue that surrounds a skeletal muscle.

epinephrine Catecholamine secreted by the adrenal medulla; adrenalin. It stimulates β-adrenergic responses.

epineurium General connective tissue sheath of a nerve.

epithelium Layer of cells forming the epidermis of the skin.

erythropoietic factor Substance produced primarily by the kidney that directly or indirectly stimulates the bone marrow to produce red blood cells. This substance may be increased in certain kidney diseases, leading to an excess of red blood cells (erythremia), or decreased in others, leading to a deficiency of red blood cells (anemia).

escape interval Interval between a normal impulse and

an escape focus; usually applies when there is a default.

eschar Slough or scab (layer) of dead skin or tissue.

ethanolism Alcoholic condition or condition involving alcohol.

expressive aphasia Impairment in the formulation and/or expression of language.

extracorporeal circulation (pump perfusion, pump bypass) Circulation that takes place outside the body, as by the use of a mechanical pump and oxygenator.

estrasystole Premature impulse from a focus other than the sinus node.

f waves Either fibrillation or flutter waves.

FIO$_2$ Inspired oxygen; expressed as a fraction.

factor VII Proconvertin, stable factor, or serum prothrombin conversion accelerator; with calcium, is involved in the extrinsic system of prothrombin activation by converting tissue thromboplastin to an active product.

factor XII (Hageman factor) By reacting with foreign products in the circulation and factor XI (plasma thromboplastin antecedent), produces a contact activation product that starts the intrinsic system of prothrombin activation.

fascia Fibrous membrane that unites the skin with underlying tissue.

fasciculus Bundle of nerve or muscle fibers.

fasciotomy Incision of a fascia.

fibril Small filamentous structure that is often the component of a cell.

fibrillation Twitching or quivering of the muscle cells.

fibrin Insoluble protein of a blood clot.

fibrinogen Soluble protein in the blood plasma that, by the action of thrombin, is converted into fibrin.

fibrinogenopenia Condition in which there is a decreased amount of fibrinogen in the blood.

fibrinolytic Agent that has the ability to dissolve a blood clot.

fibroblast Any cell or tissue from which connective tissue is developed.

focal motor signs Refers to the presence of either spastic or flaccid weakness, or clonus in a single area, which implies a lesion at one point in the CNS.

frequency Number of complete alterations per second of an alternating electric current; the number of sound waves per second produced by a sounding body (as a tuning fork); the number of complete oscillations per second of the electric or magnetic component of an electromagnetic wave.

funiculus Division of the white matter of the spinal cord consisting of fasciculi or fiber tracts.

GABA See *γ-Aminobutyric acid*.

gallop rhythm Abnormal heart rhythm having three sounds/cycle, resembling in sound the gallop of a horse.

γ-aminobutyric acid Amino acid found in small amounts in some proteins.

gamma globulin Protein formed in the blood. Ability to resist infection is related to concentration of such proteins.

ganglion Mass of nervous tissue composed principally of nerve cells and lying outside the brain and spinal cord.

gestational age Age of the fetus as calculated from the time of conception: preterm, less than 38 weeks; term, 38 to 42 weeks; postterm, more than 42 weeks.

GFR See *Glomerular filtration rate*.

glia cells Nonnervous or supporting tissue of the brain and/or spinal cord.

globulins Group of simple proteins soluble in neutral solutions of salts of strong acids with strong bases.

glomerular filtration rate Expression of the quantity of glomerular filtrate formed each minute in all nephrons of both kidneys.

glomerulonephritis General name given to diseases that are characterized by inflammatory or other anatomic changes in the renal glomerulus; often the result of an allergic or autoimmune reaction of the glomeruli of the kidney to a streptococcal infection in the body.

glomerulus Tuft of capillaries invaginated into the first part of the kidney tubule where filtration of blood (plasma water) takes place.

glucagon Hormone secreted by the alpha cells of the pancreatic islets that raises the blood glucose level.

glucocorticoids Adrenocortical hormones that promote gluconeogenesis and thus raise the blood sugar.

glycogenolysis Breakdown of glycogen to glucose.

goals Expected outcome as a result of diagnostic, therapeutic, and educational management of the patient's problems: short-term, immediate or day-to-day; long-term, overall or ultimate outcome expected.

Golgi apparatus Network of irregular wavy threads present in the cytoplasm of all nerve cells and many other cells.

graft Skin or other living substance inserted into a similar substance for attachment and growth into an integral part of the original substance.

ground In electricity, to connect (an electrical conductor) with the ground, which becomes part of the circuit, as to *ground* a wire.

growing fracture Fracture, usually linear, of which the x-ray film appearance shows a separation of the fracture edges with the passage of time. This usually indicates a tear of the dura at the time of the injury with gradual pulsatile expansion of the arachnoid through the fracture, forcing the edges apart.

gumma Soft tumor of the tissues characteristic of the tertiary stage of syphilis.

handicap Any disadvantage that makes success more difficult.

hard data Information about the patient that can be observed or measured, as in laboratory data, special tests, or procedures; also referred to as objective data.

health care team Group of professionals and paraprofessionals working together to give and promote health care.

heart block Interruption in the conduction of the electrical impulse through the atrioventricular node.

hematocrit Volume of erythrocytes packed by centrifugation in a given volume of blood.

hematuria Presence of red blood cells in the urine; may be gross or microscopic.

hemianopia, homonymous Defective vision or blindness in half of the visual field.

hemiplegia Paralysis of one side of the body.

hemodialysis Removal of certain elements from the blood by virtue of differences in the rates of their diffusion through a semipermeable membrane while the blood is being circulated outside the body.

hemodynamics Study of the factors affecting the flow and force of the circulating blood.

hemoglobinuria Presence of hemoglobin in the urine.

hemolysis Rupture of erythrocytes with release of hemoglobin into the plasma.

hemopericardium Collection of blood within the fibroserous pericardial sac that surrounds the heart.

hemostasis Arrest of the escape of blood by either natural or artificial means.

hemothorax Accumulation of blood within the thorax, usually in pleural cavity.

Henle's loop U-shaped portion of the renal tubule.

heparin rebound Phenomenon of reactivation of heparin effect (after neutralization with protamine sulfate) occurring from 5 minutes to 5 hours after neutralization.

hepatomegaly Enlargement of the liver.

hepatotoxic Destructive to liver cells.

Hering-Breuer reflex Reflex inhibition of inspiration resulting from stimulation of pressoreceptors by inflation of the lungs.

Hertz Unit of frequency of a periodic process equal to 1 cycle per second.

heterografts Tissue transplanted from one species to another.

hilus Depression or recess at exit or entrance of duct into a gland.

histamine Amine substance found in the body wherever tissues are damaged.

histiocyte Cell present in all loose connective tissues that exhibits marked phagocytic activity.

homeostasis Process of maintaining equilibrium; the maintenance of steady states in the organism by coordinated physiologic processes.

homografts Transfer of tissue from another individual of the same species.

hyaluronidase Enzyme that depolymerizes hyaluronic acid to increase the permeability of connective tissue.

hydrostatic pressure Pertaining to the pressure of liquids in equilibrium and that exerted on liquids.

hypalgesia Refers to a painful stimulus being perceived but not to the same degree as it would be normally.

hyperbilirubinemia Excessive accumulation of bilirubin in blood and tissue; presents the risk of kernicterus in the newborn.

hypercapnia Increase in carbon dioxide content.

hyperemesis gravidarum Severe vomiting during pregnancy, usually during the first trimester, often accompanied by marked and prolonged nausea.

hyperemia Increase in blood flow.

hyperkalemia Elevation of potassium level in blood serum above 5.5 mEq/L.

hypernatremia Elevation of the sodium concentration in the blood serum above 145 mEq/L.

hypertension Elevation of blood pressure above the normal range.

hypertrophy Increase in size of an organ or structure that does not involve tumor formation.

hypervolemia Increase above normal in the volume of circulating blood or blood components.

hypocalcemia Abnormally low level of serum calcium.

hypocapnia Lack of carbon dioxide in the blood.

hypochloremia Decrease in the chloride level in the blood serum below 95 mEq/L.

hypodermis Subcutaneous layer of skin.

hypoglycemia Abnormally low blood sugar concentrations.

hypokalemia Decrease in the level of potassium in the blood serum below 3.5 mEq/L.

hyponatremia Decrease in the level of sodium in the blood serum below 135 mEq/L.

hypotension Blood pressure below the normal range.

hypothalamus Region of the brain adjacent to the pituitary. It secretes hormones or factors that are closely concerned with the regulation of pituitary function.

hypothermia Subnormal temperature of the body.

hypovolemia Decrease below normal in the volume of circulating blood or blood components.

hypoxemia Low oxygen tension of the blood.

hypoxia Lack of adequate amount of oxygen in inspired air such as occurs at high altitudes; reduced oxygen content or tension.

iatrogenic Occurring as a result of medical or surgical treatment.

immunoglobulins Body proteins capable of acting as antibodies.

impedance Apparent opposition in an electric circuit to the flow of an alternating current that is analogous to the actual electrical resistance to a direct current and that is expressed as the ratio of the effective electromotive force to the effective current.

inborn error of metabolism Genetic biochemical disturbance with enzyme deficits that results in metabolic pathology.

infarct Area of tissue death caused by lack of adequate blood supply.

infarct extension Enlargement of an original area of myocardial infarction caused by the death of cells in the marginally ischemic zone.

infarction Interruption of circulation to an area with actual irreversible destruction of cerebral tissue.

inferior vena cava Vein that carries blood from the lower part of the body to the right atrium.

initial plan of care Medical plan of care prepared by the physician.

inotropic Affecting the force of muscular contractions.

inotropic agent Substance that increases myocardial contractility.

inspissation Process of becoming dry or thick by evaporation.

insulin Hormone secreted by the beta cells of the pancreas that promotes the utilization of glucose.

integument Covering, such as the skin.

intermittent positive pressure breathing Principle used in the operation of certain types of respirators.

internal mammary artery bypass Surgical procedure using the internal mammary artery in situ proximal and still attached to the subclavian artery, using the distal end to anastomose to the coronary artery beyond the coronary artery obstruction.

internuncial neuron Connecting neuron in a neural pathway.

interstitial Area between the cells and the intravascular area.

intima Endothelium that lines the blood vessels.

ions Free electron or other charged subatomic particle.

IPPB See *Intermittent positive pressure breathing.*

ipsilateral Same side as point of reference.

ischemia Insufficient blood supply to an area to maintain normal muscle function.

joule From James Prescott Joule, English physicist; metric-kilogram-second unit of work or energy. Adopted in 1948 as the unit of heat.

junctional extrasystole Extrasystole arising from atrioventricular junction.

junctional rhythm Rhythm originating in the atrioventricular junction.

junctional tachycardia Tachycardia (greater than 70 beats/min) originating in the atrioventricular junction, that is, the atrioventricular node, bundle of His, or common bundle.

keloid New growth of skin, that is, scar tissue, caused by a colloidal disorder.

keratinization Process by which the epithelial cells that are exposed to the external environment lose their moisture content and are replaced with a horny substance.

kernicterus Condition with severe neural symptoms associated with high levels of bilirubin in the blood. It is characterized by deep yellow staining of many areas of the brain accompanied by widespread destructive changes.

labile Subject to much variation.

lacteals Lymphatics that originate in the villi of the small intestine.

laminaria Dried seaweed that swells on the absorption of water.

large for gestational age Refers to infant whose weight is above the 90th percentile.

leukocytes White blood corpuscles that are markedly phagocytic.

lidocaine Short-acting antiarrhythmic drug especially effective in ventricular arrhythmias.

ligamentum nuchae Upward continuation of the supraspinous ligament.

long tract signs Includes such signs as clonus, spasticity of muscles, plantar extensor sign, and possible bladder involvement and signifies a lesion generally of the mid- or upper spinal cord or brain.

lumen Passageway inside a blood vessel or other tubular organ.

lung compliance Degree of distensibility of the lung; volume increase per unit of distending pressure increase.

lymph Alkaline body fluid formed in tissue spaces all over the body.

lymphatic Pertaining to the lymph; a vessel conveying lymph.

lymphocyte Lymph cell or white blood corpuscle without cytoplasmic granules.

lysosome Enzyme present in cell fluid that digests substances brought in by phagocytes; an intracellular organelle containing autodigestive enzymes.

malpighian corpuscle Spherical body (renal corpuscle) found in the cortex of the kidney.

mast cells Connective tissue cells that produce histamine and heparin.

master problem list Permanent list of patient problems, current and resolved. List is kept in front of the chart and serves as a "table of contents."

maximum inspiratory force Negative pressure measured in centimeters of water at the airway of a patient who is inspiring maximally against an obstruction.

maximum oxygen uptake Greatest amount of oxygen that can be transported from the lungs to the working muscles; also known as aerobic capacity or $Vo_{2_{max}}$.

mediastinitis Inflammation of the mediastinum.

mesencephalon Midbrain.

mesenchymal cells Diffuse network of cells forming the embryonic mesoderm.

mesoderm Primary germ layer of the embryo lying between the ectoderm and the entoderm.

mesothelium Layer of cells that line the body cavities.

metabolic acidosis Deficiency of base bicarbonate ions that results in a lowered capacity of the blood for buffering and an excessive hydrogen-ion concentration in the body fluids with a decrease in plasma pH below 7.35.

metabolic alkalosis Excessive concentration of base bicarbonate ions with a deficit of hydrogen ions in the body fluids that results in an increase of the plasma pH above 7.45.

metabolic equivalent Heat unit, abbreviated MU or met; the energy expenditure for various activities stated as multiples of the basal metabolic expenditure; commonly accepted as approximately 3.5 cc O_2/kg of body weight/min.

metabolism Sum of the physical and chemical changes that occur within the body.

metaplasia Conversion of one kind of tissue into another.

microampere One millionth of an ampere.

microthermy (diathermy) Heating units used for physiotherapy; heat generated by conversion of radio waves with energy given off as heat.

microwave Very short electromagnetic wave.

milking (stripping) chest tubes Process of compression to the chest tubes beginning at the upper portion of the tubes and working down to the chest bottles to evacuate clots and drainage.

mineralocorticoids Adrenocortical hormones that promote sodium retention and potassium excretion.

minimal occlusive volume Volume of endotracheal cuff inflation that still permits a minimum airway leak during the inspiratory phase of ventilation.

minute ventilation Total ventilation per minute measured by expired gas collection for 1 to 3 minutes.

miosis Excessive contraction of the pupil.

mitochondria Intracellular organelles involved in cellular oxidation.

mitral regurgitation As a result of failure of the valve to close completely, blood is allowed to flow back into the auricle.

MOV See *Minimal occlusive volume.*

mucolytic Tending to dissolve or liquefy mucus.

mural thrombus Blood clot originating from a diseased area of the endocardium.

myelin sheath Fatty semifluid covering of a nerve fiber that serves to insulate the fiber and to speed the rate of impulses.

myocardial infarction Area of necrosis (death of tissue) in the myocardium caused by lack of blood supply resulting from obstruction of the circulation to the heart muscle.

myocarditis Inflammation of the cardiac muscular tissue.

myocardium Muscular wall of the heart that lies between the endocardium on the inside of the heart and the epicardium on the outside of the heart.

myxedema Hypothyroidism; a disease caused by deficiency of thyroid hormones.

nanograms One billionth (10^{-9}) of a gram; abbreviated ng; also called a millimicrogram.

natural pacemaker Any pacing site in the heart.

necrosis Tissue death.

neonate Any infant less than 28 days old.

nephron Functional unit of the human kidney, of which there are more than 1 million in each kidney.

nephrotoxic Quality of being toxic or destructive to kidney cells.

neuron Nerve cell that is the structure and functional unit of the nervous system.

noise Unwanted signal that enters an electronic system.

norepinephrine Catecholamine secreted by the adrenal medulla and sympathetic nerve endings and found also in the brain. It stimulates α-adrenergic responses.

nucleus Vital body in the protoplasm of the cell.

nystagmus Jerky movements of the eyes seen on voluntary or involuntary gaze, particularly with cerebellar and brain stem lesions.

objective data Information about the patient that can be observed or measured as in laboratory data, special tests, or procedures; also referred to as hard data.

obstructive uropathy Any condition that leads to obstruction of the flow of urine. Such obstruction may lead to impairment of kidney function and an increased incidence of urinary infection.

oculocephalic reflex (doll's eye maneuver) Technique of testing integrity of brain stem function in which the patient's head is jerked to one side and then to the other. In a normal individual the eyes will conjugately lag behind the head movement and then slowly assume the midline position. Failure of the eyes to either lag properly or revert back to the midline indicates a lesion on the ipsilateral side at the brain stem level.

ohm Practical meter-kilogram-second system unit of

electrical resistance that is equal to the resistance of a circuit in which a potential difference of 1 V produces a current of 1 amp to the resistance in which 1 watt of power is dissipated when 1 amp flows through it; is taken as standard in the United States.

Ohm's law Law in electricity that holds that the strength or intensity of an unvarying electric current is directly proportional to the electromotive force and inversely proportional to the resistance of the circuit.

oligemia Hypovolemia or reduction in circulating intravascular volume.

oligodendrocytes Neuroglial cells having few and delicate processes.

oliguria Low urine output.

opisthotonus Form of tetanic spasm in which the head and heels are bent backward and the body bowed forward.

organ Collection of tissues organized for the performance of a given function.

organelle Cytoplasmic substance that performs a definite function.

osmolarity Characteristic of a solution determined by the ionic concentration of the dissolved substance per unit of solvent.

osmosis Diffusion of a substance through a semipermeable membrane.

osmotic pressure Pressure generated across a semipermeable membrane separating two solutions of different concentration.

oxidation Originally, the process of combining with oxygen; currently, an increase in the positive valence of an element (or a decrease in negative valence) occurring as a result of the loss of electrons. Each electron so lost is taken on by some other element, thus accomplishing a reduction of that element.

Paco₂ Arterial carbon dioxide tension.

Pao₂ Arterial oxygen tension; expressed in torr.

PIO₂ Partial pressure of inspired oxygen.

Pvo₂ Oxygen tension of a blood sample obtained from the pulmonary artery (mixed venous blood).

pacemaker That area, organ, or instrument that initiates the impulse for heart depolarization.

pancarditis Inflamed condition involving all the structures of the heart.

papillae Small, nipplelike protuberances.

papillary muscles Muscle fibers in the ventricular walls to which the chordae tendineae are attached.

paradoxical pulse Pulse that decreases or disappears during inspiration.

parasympathetic system Craniosacral division of the autonomic nervous system.

parasympatholytic agent Drug that opposes the parasympathetic (cholinergic) nervous system.

paresthesia Abnormal perception of a sensation.

partial bypass Establishment of circulation in which the heart is pumping and maintaining a portion and the remainder of the circulation is performed by mechanical means.

partial pressure Pressure of one gas in a mixture.

passive exercise Movement of a body part of a patient without the voluntary participation of the patient.

patent ductus arteriosus Patency of the duct between the pulmonary artery and the aorta that exists in fetal life but that should close between the third month and the first year of life.

patient's plan of care Plan of care coordinated to include the plans for the patient's care by all members of the health care team.

PEEP See *Positive end-expiratory pressure.*

perception Ability to integrate and interpret messages from the internal and external environment. It is the combined result of activities of end-organs, peripheral nerves, tracts and ganglia, and the integrative sensory cortex.

percutaneous Performed through the skin without an incision.

perforation Hole or break in the containing wall of an organ.

perfusion Passage of a fluid, especially the passage of blood through the vessels of an organ or area.

pericardiocentesis Surgical aspiration of fluid from the pericardial sac.

pericarditis Inflammation of the fibroserous sac that surrounds the heart.

perineurium Connective tissue sheath investing a fasciculus or bundle of nerve fibers.

periodic breathing Prolonged interval between respirations (10 seconds) that is self-resolving and does not result in hypoxia or bradycardia.

peripheral embolic phenomena Clinical signs and symptoms of an embolus in a peripheral vessel.

peripheral resistance Resistance to the flow of blood that is determined by the tone of the vascular musculature and the diameter or caliber of the vasculature.

peripheral vascular disease Disease of any of the blood vessels outside the heart, usually referring to the blood or lymph vessels of the extremities.

peritoneal dialysis Process wherein the patient's peritoneal membrane is used for the same purpose that a hemodialysis apparatus (artificial kidney) is used, that is, for the removal of desired solutes from the body.

phagocytosis Ingestion and digestion of bacteria and particles by phagocytes.

pharmacokinetics Study of the rate of absorption, distribution, metabolism, and excretion of drugs.

phlebitis Inflammation of a vein.

phlebothrombosis Development of venous thrombi in

the absence of antecedent inflammation of the vessel wall.

phlegmasia cerulea dolens Acute fulminating form of deep venous thrombosis with pronounced edema and severe cyanosis of the extremity.

phonocardiogram Mechanical or electronic registration of heart sounds.

physiatrist Physician who tests the patient's physical functioning and supervises the rehabilitation program.

physical fitness Ability to carry out daily tasks with vigor and alertness, without undue fatigue, and with sample energy to enjoy leisure time pursuits and to meet unforeseen emergencies.

pineal gland Structure in the midline of the brain behind the third ventricle that in many individuals may be calcified; serves as a convenient marker on plain x-ray films. A mass lesion on a particular side will often produce a shift of the pineal gland toward the opposite side.

pinocytosis Absorption of liquids of phagocytic cells.

placenta previa Placenta that develops in the lower uterine segment in the zone of dilatation, so that it covers or adjoins the internal cervical os.

plasma Liquid part of lymph and blood.

plasma cell Cell found in bone marrow and loose connective tissue.

pneumothorax Collection of air or gas in the pleural cavity caused by perforation of the chest wall, which may result in collapse of the lung.

polarity Particular either positive or negative state (as of a body) with reference to the two poles or to electrification.

polycystic kidney disease Inherited disease that results in the encroachment of normal kidney tissue by the gradual growth of many cysts in each kidney, leading to kidney failure and high blood pressure.

positive end-expiratory pressure For most patients, positive pressure is only given during the *inspiratory* phase of respiration. For patients such as those with shock lung syndrome, *positive end-expiratory pressure* has been used.

potential difference Difference in electric potential between two points that represent the work involved in the energy released in the transfer of a unit quantity of electricity from one point to another.

P-R interval Period from the onset of the P wave to the onset of the QRS complex.

preeclampsia Disease in which hypertension, edema, and/or proteinuria occur after the twenty-fourth week of pregnancy or in the early puerperium. In severe forms coma or convulsions (eclampsia) may occur.

premature contraction Any contraction of the ventricle or atrium that occurs early with respect to the dominant rhythm.

premature impulse Any impulse that occurs early with respect to the dominant rhythm.

premature rupture of membranes Spontaneous rupture of the amniotic sac prior to the onset of labor.

pressure ventilator Ventilator in which gas delivery is limited by a predetermined pressure.

primary nurse Nurse who has primary responsibility for planning, giving, or supervising the care of the patient and is held accountable for such responsibility.

priming of artificial kidney Preparation of artificial kidney for dialysis.

problem Anything that requires diagnostic, therapeutic, or educational action immediately (active problem) or in the past (inactive problem) as defined subjectively (by the patient) or objectively (by the observer).

problem-oriented medical record Tool of the problem-oriented medical system. It is organized around the patient's problems and is a lasting record of the diagnostic, therapeutic, and educational approaches (relative to each problem) that have been utilized to assist the patient.

proprioceptive Receiving stimuli within the tissues of the body, as within muscles and tendons.

prostaglandins Naturally occurring substances, first found in the semen of man and sheep and subsequently found also in menstrual fluid, that cause strong contraction of smooth muscle and dilation of certain vascular beds.

protoplasm Living substance of the cell that constitutes the physical basis of all living activities.

pulmonary compliance Reflection of the elasticity (expansibility) of the lungs.

pulmonary hypertension Elevation of pulmonary pressures.

pulsatile Characterized by a rhythmic pulsation.

pulse pressure Difference between systolic and diastolic blood pressure.

Purkinje fibers Atypical muscle fibers lying beneath the endocardium of the heart that form the impulse-conducting system of the heart.

pyelogram (urogram) X-ray study whereby the kidneys and urinary tract can be visualized by either injecting an x-ray radiopaque material into a patient's veins (intravenous pyelography) or by introducing the same substance directly into the urinary tract (retrograde pyelography).

pyelonephritis Inflammation of the kidneys and renal pelvis. This implies infection with bacteria and is associated with anatomic abnormalities of the urinary tract.

pyoderma Purulent skin disease.

pyrogenic reaction Syndrome manifested by pyrexia that may be accompanied by rigor and is caused by a reaction to proteins foreign to the patient.

pyuria Presence of pus in the urine.

Queckenstedt's test Technique applied to determine if a complete block exists in the spinal canal; also used to determine if there is obstruction of a lateral sinus. The test is performed by initiating jugular compression while a lumbar puncture needle is present and connected to a manometer. A rise and fall of the spinal fluid column indicates that there is a lack of complete obstruction in the spinal column. When applied unilaterally, its presence indicates patency of the ipsilateral sinus. Its failure to rise when one side is compressed while it does rise when the other side is compressed indicates an obstruction of that lateral or transverse sinus.

Quincke's pulse Capillary pulse caused by a high pulse pressure; seen classically in aortic regurgitation and elicited clinically by applying light pressure to a fingernail.

rale Abnormal sound heart in auscultation of the chest produced by passage of air through the bronchi, which contain secretion or exudate or which are constricted by spasm or a thickening of their walls; may be heard on either inspiration or expiration.

Ranvier's nodes Constrictions in the medullary substance of a nerve fiber at more or less regular intervals.

rate Number of impulses per unit time, usually per minute.

receptive aphasia Sensory aphasia; impairment in the comprehension of language.

receptor Group of cells functioning in the reception of stimuli.

reconstitution Continuous repair of progressive destruction of tissues.

recovery Restoration from illness.

red infarct Pathologic change that occurs in the brain that has first been rendered ischemic by lack of blood and then, with restriction of blood flow, diapedesis of red blood cells occurs into the parenchyma of the brain without actually producing a well-formed hematoma, only infiltration of red blood cells.

rehabilitation Restoration to a disabled individual of maximum independence commensurate with limitations by developing residual capacities. It implies prescribed training and employment of many different methods and professional workers.

renin Hormone produced by the juxtaglomerular cells of the kidneys. It regulates aldosterone secretion by the adrenal cortex and raises blood pressure.

resistance Property of a body whereby it opposes and limits the passage through it of a steady electric current.

resocialization Patient's reintegration into family and community life following critical and/or long-term hospitalization.

resolution Subsidence of problems.

respiratory acidosis Inadequate pulmonary ventilation with retention of carbon dioxide and an increase in carbonic acid.

respiratory alkalosis Decrease in the carbonic acid concentration of the extracellular fluid caused by hyperventilation, which blows off carbon dioxide.

respiratory distress syndrome Lung disease of the preterm infant characterized by atelectasis of the alveoli.

reticular Meshed or in the form of a network.

retrograde To travel in a reverse direction.

revascularization Surgical means of reconstituting vascularization to the heart, organ, or vessel being replaced; usually done by a bypass procedure.

rhythm Relationship of one impulse to its neighbors.

ribosome Submicroscopic ribonucleoprotein particle attached to the endoplasmic reticulum of cells; the site of protein synthesis in cytoplasm.

rouleaux Grouping of red blood corpuscles whose formation resembles a pile of coins.

Sao$_2$ Percent saturation of arterial blood

Svo$_2$ Percent saturation of mixed venous blood.

saltatory conduction Skipping from node to node.

Schwann cells Cells of ectodermal origin that comprise the neurilemma.

sclerosis Thickening or hardening.

semipermeable membrane Barrier to substances above a specific size but allowing passage of substances below that size.

sensory deprivation Decrease in sensory stimulation (sight, sound, touch, and smell) caused either by injury to the brain or lack of dynamic environment.

septicemia Active bacterial infection of the bloodstream.

shock State of inadequate tissue perfusion that results from a decreased effective circulating blood volume.

shock lung Syndrome of pulmonary insufficiency following shock.

shoulder subluxation Separation of humeral head out of the glenoid cavity resulting in pull on the soft tissue of the joint.

shunt Diversion.

Silverman-Anderson score Scoring device for assessing degree of respiratory distress.

sinus bradycardia Sinus rate of less than 60 beats/min in the adult.

sinus pacemaker Primary initiator of a normal cardiac depolarization; located in the right atrium.

sinus tachycardia Sinus rate of 100 or more beats/min in the adult.

small for gestational age Refers to infant whose weight is below the 10th percentile.

soft data Information that only the patient or family can provide, including pain, habits of living, and "feelings"; also referred to as subjective data.

splanchnic Pertaining to the intra-abdominal viscera.

Starling's law of the heart Force of the heart beat is determined primarily by the length of fibers comprising its muscular wall.

status epilepticus Condition in which seizure activity continues for several minutes or hours or consists of interrupted seizures separated by short periods of relative quiet.

stratum corneum Outermost horny layer of the epidermis.

stratum germinativum Innermost layer of epidermis that divides to replace the rest of the epidermis as it wears away.

stratum granulosum Layer of cells found in the epidermis of the skin between the stratum germinativum and stratum lucidum.

stratum lucidum Translucent layer of epidermis lying between the stratum corneum and stratum granulosum.

stenosis Constriction or narrowing of a passage or orifice.

stereotaxis Method of precisely locating areas in the brain.

stroke volume Amount of blood ejected by the left ventricle at each beat.

stroma Foundation supporting tissues of an organ.

subdural hygroma Fluid collection between the dura and the arachnoid resulting from a tear in the arachnoid whereby spinal fluid leaks out into the subdural space.

subjective data Information that only the patient or family can provide, including pain, habits of living, and "feelings"; also referred to as soft data.

superior vena cava Vein that carries blood from the upper part of the body to the right atrium.

supernatant Clear liquid remaining on the top after a precipitate settles.

supine hypotensive syndrome Hypotension characterized by abnormally low blood pressure when the patient is lying down on the back.

surfactant Chemical produced by alveolar cells that is responsible for maintaining intra-alveolar surface tension.

Swan-Ganz catheter Catheter with an inflatable balloon tip that can be manipulated into a peripheral pulmonary artery to measure pressures in the pulmonary artery.

sympathetic nervous system Division of the autonomic nervous system.

sympathomimetic agent Adrenergic agent; a drug whose action mimicks that of the sympathetic (adrenergic) nervous system.

synapse Innervation of one neuron by another.

syndrome Group of symptoms that occur together and are given a name to identify the specific combination of symptoms.

systemic oxygen consumption Amount of oxygen consumed by the body per minute.

system Collection of organs that act together in the performance of a given function.

systole That part of the heart cycle in which the heart is in contraction, that is, when the myocardial fibers are tightening.

T **tube** Apparatus for connecting humidified oxygen to the endotracheal tube to which a spirometer can be attached for the evaluation of tidal volume and the appropriate removal of the endotracheal tube.

tachycardia Rapid heart rate over 100 beats/min; over 180 beats/min in the neonate.

tachyphylaxis Decreasing responses to a drug that follow consecutive injections made at short intervals.

tachypnea Rapid respiratory rate.

telencephalon Embryonic endbrain of the prosencephalon from which the cerebral hemispheres, corpora striata, and rhinencephalon develop.

teratogenic That which produces fetal deformity.

tetralogy of Fallot Combination of four defects: (1) ventricular septal defect, (2) pulmonic stenosis, (3) right ventricular hypertrophy, and (4) overriding of the aorta. (Aorta branches out from just above the ventricular septal defect instead of the left ventricle, so it receives blood from both ventricles.)

thermoneutral environment Environment that keeps body temperature at an optimum point at which the least amount of oxygen is consumed for metabolism.

thoracostomy Incision of the chest wall with maintenance of the opening for the purpose of drainage.

thrombin Enzyme in the blood derived from prothrombin that is responsible for the conversion of fibrinogen into fibrin.

thrombolytic Causing the dissolution of a blood clot.

thrombophlebitis Accumulation of a blood clot within a vein accompanied by inflammation.

thrombus Blood clot inside a blood vessel or chamber of the heart that remains at the place of its formation.

thyrocalcitonin Hormone that lowers the blood calcium level; secreted by the parafollicular cells of the thyroid gland.

thyroxine Hormone secreted by the thyroid gland that increases oxygen consumption and thus increases metabolic rate.

TIA See *Transient ischemic attack.*

tissue Collection of similar cells that act together in the performance of a particular function.

tokodynamometer Instrument for measuring uterine contractions.

torr Abbreviation for torricelli scale; 1 torr is equal to 1 mm Hg and is used in expressing the partial pressure of a gas.

torticollis Contracted state of the cervical muscles producing a twisting of the neck and an unnatural position of the head.

total peripheral resistance (afterload) Degree of constriction of the systemic blood vessels.

toxicity Harmful quality.

transected Cross section; cutting across.

transient ischemic attack Form of minor stroke in which a patient manifests focal neurologic signs caused by temporary interruption of blood flow to an area of the brain that is temporary and reverts within several hours, usually less than 6. Persistence of symptoms indicates infarction of a particular area.

tricuspid atresia Absence of the opening between the right atrium and right ventricle.

triiodothyronine Hormone secreted by the thyroid gland that resembles thyroxine.

trismus Motor disturbance of the trigeminal nerve, especially spasm of the masticatory muscles with difficulty in opening the mouth (lockjaw).

tropocollagen Fundamental units of collagen fibrils obtained by prolonged extraction of insoluble collagen with dilute acid.

tubular necrosis Death of the cells of the small tubes of the kidneys resulting from disease or injury.

tunica Enveloping or covering membrane.

tunica adventitia Outer coat of an artery or any tubular structure.

tunica intima Lining coat of an artery.

tunica media Middle muscular coat of an artery.

ultrafiltration Filtration under pressure through filters with minute pores; results in removal of water by the artificial kidney.

uncal herniation Process whereby the medial portion of the temporal lobe protrudes over the tentorial edge in cases of increased intracranial pressure, particularly from the temporal side. Progression of this process causes pressure directly on the brain stem after first putting pressure on the third cranial nerve. The sign of uncal herniation is a dilated pupil on the side of the herniation.

underwater seal (water trap) Situation where the tube that exits from the patient's chest cavity is placed under water to allow the outflow but no ingress of air, thus establishing a one-way valve.

uremia Clinical state produced when severe functional impairment of the kidneys exists.

V_{DM} Mechanical dead space; the volume of gas contained in inspiratory tubing that does not participate in gas exchange.

V_T Tidal volume; the volume of gas inspired or expired.

Valsalva's maneuver Attempt to forcibly exhale with the glottis, nose, and mouth closed. If the eustachian tubes are not obstructed, the pressure on the tympanic membranes will be increased. Maneuver can also be done with just the glottis closed, but only the intrathoracic pressure will be increased. The maneuver may cause increased intrathoracic pressure, slowing of the pulse, decreased return of blood to the heart, and increased venous pressure.

valvular Pertaining to, affecting, or of the nature of a valve.

valvular insufficiency Inadequate or incomplete closure of a valve that permits a backflow of blood in the wrong direction.

valvulitis Inflammatory process of the heart valves. Valves may be impaired to the extent that they close incompletely or do not open completely.

vasculitis Inflammation of a vessel.

vasoconstrictor Agent that increases the diameter of blood vessels by producing relaxation of the smooth muscles in the walls of the vessels; a drug that decreases total peripheral resistance.

vasopressin Antidiuretic hormone secreted by the hypothalamus and posterior pituitary gland. It promotes the renal reabsorption of water.

vasopressor Drug that increases total peripheral resistance.

ventricular extrasystole Extrasystole arising from the ventricle.

ventricular fibrillation Disorganized rapid and ineffective ventricular depolarization.

ventricular hemiblock Block of only one division of the left bundle branch, that is, either anterior superior or posterior inferior hemiblock.

ventricular septal defect Opening in the ventricular system.

ventricular tachycardia Tachycardia originating from the ventricular Purkinje system.

ventriculotomy Incision of a ventricle of the heart.

ventilation-perfusion defect Occurs when areas of the lung receive inspired air but no blood, or vice versa.

visual verticality Perception of the visual upright.

voltage Electric potential or potential difference; expressed in volts.

voltmeter Instrument (as a galvanometer) for measuring in volts the differences of potential between different points of an electric circuit.

volume ventilator Ventilator that delivers a predetermined volume of gas with each cycle.

wallerian degeneration Degeneration of a nerve fiber that has been severed from its cell body.

watt Unit of electric power, being the work done at the

rate of 1 joule/sec. It is equivalent to a current of 1 ampere under a pressure of 1 V.

wedge pressure Pulmonary or capillary pressure measured at cardiac catheterization by wedging the cardiac catheter in the most distal pulmonary artery branch. It reflects mean left arterial pressure.

Wenckebach block Type of second-degree block characterized by a changing relationship between input, for example, P wave, and output, for example, QRS complex. In atrioventricular Wenckebach block there is a gradual increase in the P-R interval until a nonconducted impulse occurs.

zymogen Inactive precursor that is converted to an active enzyme by the action of acid, another enzyme, or some other means.

Index

Hypoglycemia, 11, 242, 328, 330, 429, 434, 435, 436, 439, 499, 528, 618, 629, 630, 636, 642, 645, 647, 651, 668, 678, 679, 684, 711, 739, 765, 769, 779, 892
  agents, 141, 328
  coma, 128
  insulin-induced, 128
Hypoglycosuria, 678
Hypoinsulinism, 728
Hypokalemia, 128, 148, 208, 210, 267, 327, 328, 330, 342, 364, 373, 384, 387, 388, 434, 435, 502, 519, 528, 540, 678, 679, 689, 708, 892
  ECG manifestations of, 207
Hypomagnesemia, 126, 374, 517, 642, 645, 795
Hyponatremia, 128, 146, 148, 253, 439, 440, 482, 557, 581, 642, 686, 689, 691, 778, 784, 892
  hypochloremic dehydration, 686
Hypoparathyroidism, 432, 581, 647, 701
Hypoperfusion, 716, 727, 733, 743
  persistent, 745
Hypophosphatemia, 145, 483, 484, 503
Hypopituitarism, 146, 431, 439
Hypoproteinemia, 688, 689
Hypotension, 122, 123, 124, 125, 126, 127, 130, 134, 139, 146, 172, 173, 213, 230, 237, 246, 248, 249, 256, 327, 328, 330, 340, 341, 370, 378, 379, 382, 386, 390, 394, 430, 431, 437, 439, 445, 461, 490, 493, 498, 499, 504, 520, 522, 534, 547, 551, 552, 605, 607, 609, 611, 615, 700, 713, 714, 718, 721, 723, 724, 726, 727, 733, 734, 736, 742, 753, 775, 892
  agents, 694
  arterial, 510
  crisis, 141
  episodes, 367
  maternal, 613
  postural, 448, 817
  spinal shock, 11
Hypothalamus, 16, 59, 73, 75, 86, 109, 408, 429, 430, 439, 440, 585, 590, 892
  posterior, 589
  tumor of, 10
Hypothermia, 108, 235, 397, 438, 490, 553, 547, 631, 641, 668, 681, 693, 702, 711, 789, 892
  blanket, 590
  deep, 341
  gastric, 785
  treatment, 347
Hypothyroidism, 11, 155, 438, 439, 535, 894
Hypotonia, 642, 645
Hypotrophic pyloric stenosis, 646
Hypoventilation, 263, 273, 277, 589
  alveolar, 438
Hypovolemia, 131, 146, 148, 172, 178, 250, 252, 301, 312, 319, 336, 343, 350, 351, 384, 387, 394, 559, 569, 615, 633, 704, 719, 745, 746, 747, 750, 769, 775, 790, 892
  systemic, 734
Hypoxemia, 1, 8, 186, 188, 208, 210, 229, 230, 233, 264, 266, 267, 272, 273, 275, 276, 277, 278, 279, 283, 286, 288, 290, 330, 393, 553, 597,

Hypoxemia—cont'd
  605, 642, 680, 685, 689, 712, 731, 735, 745, 747, 750, 769, 850, 852, 853, 892
  arterial, 250
Hypoxia, 8, 15, 128, 150, 170, 171, 173, 175, 184, 186, 246, 248, 251, 257, 311, 382, 390, 393, 553, 557, 568, 569, 574, 588, 597, 617, 630, 631, 633, 637, 638, 642, 643, 644, 650, 679, 680, 682, 686, 687, 688, 689, 702, 709, 711, 716, 719, 721, 722, 724, 725, 726, 727, 730, 733, 736, 737, 739, 743, 892
  acute, 572
  arterial, 250
  carbohydrate metabolism, 184
  cellular, 178
  chronic, 572
  fetal, 624, 625
  myocardial, 220
  tissue, 185
Hysterectomy, abdominal, 230

I

Icterus, 383
  neonatorum, 635
Idiogenic osmoles, 499
Idioventricular rhythm, 216, 234, 241
  hypertrophic subaortic stenosis, 123
  respiratory distress syndrome, 637
IDV; *see* Intermittent demand ventilation
IgA, 46, 48, 49, 632
IgD, 46, 48, 49
IgE, 46, 47, 48, 49
IgG, 45, 46, 48, 49, 632
IgM, 45, 46, 48, 49, 632
Ig's; *see* Immunoglobulins
Ileostomy, 686
Ileus, 502, 519, 521, 526, 535, 556, 557
  conduit, 457
  paralytic, 543
Imipramine, 85, 140, 676, 677, 860
Immune
  deficiency, 51
  system, 45, 48
Immunity
  acquired, 50
    active, 50
    natural, 50
    passive, 50
Immunization, 257
Immunoglobulins, 45, 49, 556, 893
  fetal, 49
Immunosuppression, 401, 402, 459
Immunosuppressive agents, 10, 50, 258, 463, 472, 486, 789
Impotency, 511, 857, 859
Impulse
  ascending, 70
  descending, 70
Imuran, 10, 50; *see also* Azathioprine
Inappropriate secretion of antidiuretic hormone, 146, 439, 440, 581, 707